Operative Gynecology

Operative Gynecology

DAVID M. GERSHENSON, M.D.
Professor and Deputy Chairman,
Department of Gynecologic Oncology,
The University of Texas M.D. Anderson Cancer Center,
Houston, Texas

ALAN H. DeCHERNEY, M.D.
Louis E. Phaneuf Professor and Chairman,
Department of Obstetrics and Gynecology,
Tufts University School of Medicine,
Boston, Massachusetts

STEPHEN L. CURRY, M.D.
Director, Obstetrics and Gynecology,
Hartford Hospital,
Hartford, Connecticut;
Professor of Obstetrics and Gynecology,
University of Connecticut School of Medicine,
Farmington, Connecticut

W.B. SAUNDERS COMPANY
A Division of Harcourt Brace & Company

Philadelphia   London   Toronto   Montreal   Sydney   Tokyo

W.B. SAUNDERS COMPANY
A Division of
Harcourt Brace & Company

The Curtis Center
Independence Square West
Philadelphia, Pennsylvania 19106

Library of Congress Cataloging-in-Publication Data

Gershenson, David M. (David Marc)

Operative gynecology / David M. Gershenson, Alan H. DeCherney, Stephen L. Curry.

   p.   cm.

1. Generative organs, Female—Surgery.   I. DeCherney, Alan H.   II. Curry, Stephen L.   III. Title.   [DNLM: 1. Genital Diseases, Female—surgery.   WP 660 G381o]

RG104.G47   1993

618.1'059—dc20

DNLM/DLC   92–49756

OPERATIVE GYNECOLOGY   ISBN 0–7216–3558–X

Copyright © 1993 by W.B. Saunders Company.

All rights reserved. No part of this publication may be reproduced or transmitted in any form or by any means, electronic or mechanical, including photocopying, recording, or any information storage and retrieval system, without written permission from the publisher.

Printed in the United States of America.

Last digit is the print number: 9 8 7 6 5 4 3 2 1

*This book is dedicated to our wives—
Michelle Gershenson, Dee Dee DeCherney, and Tonja Curry.
Their love, patience, support, and inspiration
have made the completion of this project possible.*

Contributors

Steven R. Bayer, M.D.
Department of Obstetrics and Gynecology, New England Memorial Hospital, Stoneham, Massachusetts
Dilatation and Curettage and Cervical Conization

Matthew Boente, M.D.
Assistant Professor of Obstetrics and Gynecology, Duke University Medical Center, Division of Gynecologic Oncology, Duke University Medical Center, Durham, North Carolina
Preoperative and Postoperative Care

Thomas W. Burke, M.D.
Associate Professor, Department of Gynecologic Oncology, The University of Texas M. D. Anderson Cancer Center, Houston, Texas
Surgery for Malignant Tumors of the Uterine Corpus; Surgery of the Gastrointestinal Tract in Relation to Gynecology; Surgery of the Genitourinary Tract in Relation to Gynecology

Daniel L. Clarke-Pearson, M.D.
Professor of Obstetrics and Gynecology, Duke University Medical Center; Director, Gynecologic Oncology, Duke University Medical Center, Durham, North Carolina
Preoperative and Postoperative Care

Larry J. Copeland, M.D.
Professor of Obstetrics and Gynecology, Director of Gynecologic Oncology, Arthur G. James Cancer Hospital, The Ohio State University, Columbus, Ohio
Reconstructive Surgery in Gynecologic Oncology

Randle S. Corfman, Ph.D., M.D.
Director, The Midwest Center for Reproductive Health; Director, Reproductive Endocrinology and Assisted Reproductive Technologies, Methodist Hospital, St. Louis Park, Minnesota
Gynecologic Endoscopy: Laparoscopy, Falloposcopy, and Hysteroscopy

Stephen L. Curry, M.D.
Director, Obstetrics and Gynecology, Hartford Hospital, Hartford, Connecticut; Professor of Obstetrics and Gynecology, University of Connecticut School of Medicine, Farmington, Connecticut
Embryology and Anatomy of the Female Pelvis

Ann Jeanette Davis, M.D.
Assistant Professor of Obstetrics and Gynecology, Assistant Professor of Pediatrics, Tufts University School of Medicine; Pediatric and Adolescent Gynecologist, New England Medical Center, Boston, Massachusetts
Adnexal Surgery

CONTRIBUTORS

Alan H. DeCherney, M.D.
Louis E. Phaneuf Professor and Chairman, Department of Obstetrics and Gynecology, Tufts University School of Medicine, Boston, Massachusetts
Preoperative and Postoperative Management of Patients Undergoing Reproductive Reconstructive Surgery; Surgery for Endometriosis

Luis Delclos, M.D.
Professor of Radiography, The University of Texas M. D. Anderson Cancer Center, Houston, Texas
Operative Radiotherapeutic Procedures for Gynecologic Cancers

P. D. DePriest, M.D.
Assistant Professor, University of Kentucky Medical Center, Lexington, Kentucky
Surgical Therapy for Cervical Cancer

Michael P. Diamond, M.D.
Associate Professor, Departments of Obstetrics and Gynecology and Surgery; Director, Division of Reproductive Endocrinology and Infertility; Director, Center for Fertility and Reproductive Research, Vanderbilt University Medical Center, Nashville, Tennessee
Prevention of Adhesions

Bruce H. Drukker, M.D.
Professor and Chairperson, Michigan State University College of Human Medicine, East Lansing, Michigan; Active Staff, Sparrow Hospital; Courtesy Staff, St. Lawrence Hospital and Healthcare Services, Lansing, Michigan
Operations for Pelvic Relaxation

David B. Elmer, M.D.
Assistant Clinical Professor of Obstetrics and Gynecology, Tufts University School of Medicine, Boston, Massachusetts; Active Staff, Cape Cod Hospital, Hyannis, Massachusetts; Active Staff, New England Medical Center, Boston, Massachusetts
Benign Procedures for the Vulva and Vagina

Gerald A. Feuer, M.D.
Assistant Professor, Gynecologic Oncology, Brown University; Gynecologic Oncologist, Women and Infants Hospital, Providence, Rhode Island
Instruments for Gynecologic Surgery

Janis H. Fox, M.D.
Instructor, Harvard Medical School; Instructor, Brigham and Women's Hospital, Boston, Massachusetts
Assisted Reproductive Technology (ART): Surgical Aspects

Donald G. Gallup, M.D.
Professor and Director, Gynecologic Oncology, Medical College of Georgia, Augusta, Georgia
Opening and Closing of the Abdomen and Wound Healing

David M. Gershenson, M.D.
Professor and Deputy Chairman, Department of Gynecologic Oncology, The University of Texas M. D. Anderson Cancer Center, Houston, Texas
Surgery for Ovarian Cancer; Operative Radiotherapeutic Procedures for Gynecologic Cancers

David A. Grainger, M.D.
Assistant Professor, Department of Obstetrics and Gynecology, Division of Reproductive Endocrinology, University of Kansas School of Medicine–Wichita, Wichita, Kansas
Preoperative and Postoperative Management of Patients Undergoing Reproductive Reconstructive Surgery

C. O. Granai, M.D.
Associate Professor, Gynecologic Oncology, Brown University; Director of Gynecologic Oncology, Women and Infants Hospital, Providence, Rhode Island
Instruments for Gynecologic Surgery

Lawrence Grunfeld, M.D.
Assistant Professor, Mount Sinai School of Medicine; Assistant Professor, Director of Reproductive Endocrine Fellowship, Mount Sinai Medical Center, New York, New York
Assisted Reproductive Technology (ART): Surgical Aspects

Neville F. Hacker, F.R.C.O.G., F.R.A.C.O.G., F.A.C.O.G., F.A.C.S.
Associate Professor of Obstetrics and Gynaecology, University of New South Wales; Director of Gynaecological Oncology, Royal Hospital for Women, Paddington, Sydney, Australia
Surgery for Malignant Tumors of the Vulva

Lamia Haj-Hassan, M.D.
Assistant Resident, Department of Pediatrics, New England Medical Center, Boston, Massachusetts
Tubal Surgery: Isthmic Tube

R. V. Higgins, M.D.
Associate Director, Gynecologic Oncology, Carolinas Medical Center, Charlotte, North Carolina
Surgical Therapy for Cervical Cancer

Michael P. Hopkins, M.D.
Professor, Department of Obstetrics and Gynecology, Northeastern Ohio Universities College of Medicine, Akron, Ohio
Surgery for Cancer of the Vagina

Ivan Jelen, M.D., F.R.C.S., F.R.C.O.G., F.A.C.S., F.A.C.O.G.
Chief of Gynecology and Associate Professor, The University of Texas Health Science Center at San Antonio; Surgeon, Medical Center Hospital, San Antonio, Texas
Vaginal Fistulas: Operative Management

Gad Lavy, M.D.
Director, New England Fertility Institute; Staff, The Stamford Hospital, Stamford, Connecticut; Staff, Yale–New Haven Hospital, New Haven, Connecticut
Tubal Surgery: Isthmic Tube

Randall A. Loy, M.D.
Active Staff, Florida Hospital; Active Staff, Orlando Regional Health System, Orlando, Florida; Courtesy Staff, Winter Park Memorial Hospital, Winter Park, Florida
Surgery for Endometriosis

Anthony A. Luciano, M.D.
Professor, University of Connecticut Medical School; Attending Faculty, John Dempsey Hospital, Farmington, Connecticut; Attending Faculty, New Britain General Hospital, New Britain, Connecticut
Special Instrumentation

Raymond Lui, M.D.
Assistant Professor, Tufts University School of Medicine; Staff, New England Medical Center, Boston, Massachusetts
Abdominal and Vaginal Hysterectomy

Donald B. Maier, M.D.
Associate Professor, University of Connecticut School of Medicine; Director, Medical Student Education, Department of Obstetrics and Gynecology, University of Connecticut School of Medicine, Farmington, Connecticut; Attending Staff, John Dempsey Hospital, Farmington, Connecticut; Attending Staff, Saint Francis Hospital and Medical Center, Hartford, Connecticut; Attending Staff, New Britain General Hospital, New Britain, Connecticut; Attending Staff, Mt. Sinai Hospital, Hartford, Connecticut
Special Instrumentation

Michele Follen Mitchell, M.D., M.S.
Assistant Professor, Department of Gynecologic Oncology, The University of Texas M. D. Anderson Cancer Center, Houston, Texas
Preinvasive Diseases of the Female Lower Genital Tract

Mitchell Morris, M.D.
Assistant Professor, Department of Gynecologic Oncology, The University of Texas M. D. Anderson Cancer Center, Houston, Texas
Surgery for Malignant Tumors of the Uterine Corpus; Surgery of the Gastrointestinal Tract in Relation to Gynecology; Surgery of the Genitourinary Tract in Relation to Gynecology

Kenneth L. Noller, M.D.
Professor and Chair, Department of Obstetrics and Gynecology, University of Massachusetts Medical School, Worcester, Massachusetts
The History of Gynecologic Surgery

George J. Olt, M.D.
Assistant Professor of Obstetrics and Gynecology, Penn State University School of Medicine; Division of Gynecologic Oncology, Milton S. Hershey Medical Center, Hershey, Pennsylvania
Preoperative and Postoperative Care

Steven J. Ory, M.D.
Associate Professor, Chairman, Division of Reproductive Endocrinology and Infertility, Department of Obstetrics and Gynecology, Mayo Medical School; Consultant, Mayo Clinic, Rochester, Minnesota
Surgery for Ectopic Pregnancy

Jeanne A. Petrek, M.D.
Assistant Professor of Surgery, Cornell University School of Medicine; Attending Surgeon, Breast Service, Department of Surgery, Memorial Hospital of Memorial Sloan-Kettering Cancer Center, New York, New York
Operative Procedures for the Breast

D. E. Powell, M.D.
Professor, University of Kentucky Medical Center; Chairman, Department of Pathology, University of Kentucky Medical Center, Lexington, Kentucky
Surgical Therapy for Cervical Cancer

Raymond J. Reilly, M.B., B.Ch., B.O.A., F.A.C.O.G.
Associate Clinical Professor of Obstetrics and Gynecology and Reproductive Biology, Harvard Medical School; Obstetrician-Gynecologist, Brigham and Women's Hospital, Boston, Massachusetts
Operations for Stress Incontinence and Benign Conditions of the Urethra

Eli Reshef, M.D.
Assistant Professor, Section of Reproductive Endocrinology and Infertility, University of Oklahoma Health Sciences Center; Active Staff, Oklahoma Memorial Hospital and HCA Presbyterian Hospital; Courtesy Staff, Baptist Medical Center of Oklahoma and Mercy Health Center, Oklahoma City, Oklahoma
Tubal Surgery: Distal Fallopian Tube

Gustavo Rodriguez, M.D.
Assistant Professor, Obstetrics and Gynecology, Duke University Medical Center; Division of Gynecologic Oncology, Duke University Medical Center, Durham, North Carolina
Preoperative and Postoperative Care

Jeffrey B. Russell, M.D.
Assistant Professor, Thomas Jefferson School of Medicine, Department of Obstetrics and Gynecology, Philadelphia, Pennsylvania; Director, Division of Reproductive Endocrinology and Infertility, Christiana Hospital, Medical Center of Delaware, Newark, Delaware
Uterine Surgery

Joseph S. Sanfilippo, M.D.
Professor of Obstetrics and Gynecology and Director of Reproductive Biology, University of Louisville School of Medicine; Chairman, Obstetrics and Gynecology, Norton Hospital; Chairman, Gynecology, Kosair/Children's Hospital, Louisville, Kentucky
Tubal Surgery: Distal Fallopian Tube

Vicki Seltzer, M.D.
Professor, Gynecology and Obstetrics, Albert Einstein College of Medicine, New York, New York; Director, Obstetrics and Gynecology, Queens Hospital Center, Jamaica, New York
Operative Procedures for the Breast

José A. Soto-Hunnicutt, M.D.
Instructor, Pediatric and Juvenile Gynecology, Hospital J. M. De Los Rios, San Bernadino, Caracas, Universidad Central de Venezuela, Caracas, Venezuela
Dilatation and Curettage and Cervical Conization

Robert A. Starr, M.D., F.A.C.O.G.
Assistant Professor, Department of Obstetrics, Gynecology and Reproductive Biology, Michigan State University College of Human Medicine, East Lansing, Michigan; Associate, Sparrow Hospital; Courtesy Staff, St. Lawrence Hospital, Lansing, Michigan
Operations for Pelvic Relaxation

J. R. van Nagell, Jr., M.D.
Professor, University of Kentucky Medical Center; Director, Division of Gynecologic Oncology, University of Kentucky Medical Center, Lexington, Kentucky
Surgical Therapy for Cervical Cancer

J. Taylor Wharton, M.D.
Professor and Chairman, Department of Gynecologic Oncology, The University of Texas M. D. Anderson Cancer Center, Houston, Texas
Surgery for Ovarian Cancer; Operative Radiotherapeutic Procedures for Gynecologic Cancers

Preface

When initially approached by senior editors at W.B. Saunders about developing and editing a new textbook on the subject of operative gynecology, we viewed the opportunity with a combination of excitement and trepidation. Our specialty had changed dramatically over the past decade or so, with an information explosion spawned by the emphasis on subspecialization. This transition brought with it several new surgical techniques and sophisticated technologies. Considering this trend, did we really want to propagate another general text in the field? Was there any need for yet another, major textbook of any type within the specialty? After much soul-searching, we arrived at an affirmative answer on both counts, perceived somewhat of a vacuum, and chose to accept the challenge to establish a unique work, *Operative Gynecology*.

As the reader can readily observe, this book is neither a comprehensive textbook of gynecology nor a surgical atlas. It has elements of both, and much more. We designed it to present a systematic approach to the art and science of gynecologic surgery. To accomplish this objective, we believe we have assembled many of the best and brightest men and women within our discipline. Although the list of contributors includes a few "Old Masters" within its ranks, there is a preponderance of "rising young stars" in gynecologic surgery. Such a combination has enabled us to provide the reader with a blend of experience and the most contemporary information.

In addition, contained within these pages are hundreds of new drawings by three world-class medical illustrators—Bill Andrews, Rebekah Dodson, and Richard Fritzler.

Despite the fact that our specialty has expanded to encompass diverse facets of medicine, from chemotherapy administration to critical care medicine to sophisticated outpatient diagnostic and therapeutic techniques, surgery remains the cornerstone of our specialty. Our respect for the historical perspective and the emergence of gynecologic surgery as a distinct entity is evidenced by inclusion of the initial chapter, The History of Gynecologic Surgery. In addition to the usual treatment of indications, techniques, complications, etc., this text attempts to carefully scrutinize the relative merits of various surgical procedures. The latest developments within the fields of infertility and endocrine surgery, benign gynecology, and gynecologic oncology are presented. When appropriate, less radical procedures for gynecologic cancer are discussed.

The book is logically organized according to disease sites. Although it is primarily directed at the practicing obstetrician-gynecologist and the trainee, we believe that subspecialists will also find valuable information herein. During an era when we are vigorously pursuing exciting developments in molecular biology and genetics, there is also mounting concern about the adequacy of surgical training of residents within our discipline and external scrutiny of the level of surgical expertise among practitioners. We hope that *Operative Gynecology* will provide both practitioners and trainees alike the foundation for development of sound surgical judgment and operative technique.

Finally, we would like to acknowledge the constant encouragement of our editor at W.B. Saunders—Avé McCracken—and Martin Wonsiewicz and Joan Meyer, formerly of W.B. Saunders; and of our Developmental Editor—Hazel Hacker. We also acknowledge the assistance of Ms. Ozella Walton at The University of Texas M. D. Anderson Cancer Center, Ms. Betty Albanese at Yale University School of Medicine, and Ms. Carol Kubish and Ms. Marge Serignese at Hartford Hospital.

DAVID M. GERSHENSON
ALAN H. DECHERNEY
STEPHEN L. CURRY

Contents

1
The History of Gynecologic Surgery 1
Kenneth L. Noller

2
Embryology and Anatomy of the Female Pelvis 19
Stephen L. Curry

3
Preoperative and Postoperative Care 29
Daniel L. Clarke-Pearson, George J. Olt, Gustavo Rodriguez, Matthew Boente

4
Preoperative and Postoperative Management of Patients Undergoing Reproductive Reconstructive Surgery 87
David A. Grainger, Alan H. DeCherney

5
Instruments for Gynecologic Surgery 97
C. O. Granai, Gerald A. Feuer

6
Special Instrumentation 107
Donald B. Maier, Anthony A. Luciano

7
Opening and Closing of the Abdomen and Wound Healing 127
Donald G. Gallup

8
Prevention of Adhesions 147
Michael P. Diamond

9
Benign Procedures for the Vulva and Vagina 159
David B. Elmer

10
Surgery for Malignant Tumors of the Vulva 173
Neville F. Hacker

11
Surgery for Cancer of the Vagina 201
Michael P. Hopkins

12
Vaginal Fistulas: Operative Management 213
Ivan Jelen

13
Preinvasive Diseases of the Female Lower Genital Tract 231
Michele Follen Mitchell

14
Dilatation and Curettage and Cervical Conization 257
Steven R. Bayer, José A. Soto-Hunnicutt

15
Surgical Therapy for Cervical Cancer 271
J. R. van Nagell, Jr., P. D. DePriest, R. V. Higgins, D. E. Powell

16
Operations for Stress Incontinence and Benign Conditions of the Urethra 297
Raymond J. Reilly

17
Operations for Pelvic Relaxation 313
Robert A. Starr, Bruce H. Drukker

18
Abdominal and Vaginal Hysterectomy 335
Raymond Lui

19
Uterine Surgery 353
Jeffrey B. Russell

20
Surgery for Malignant Tumors of the Uterine Corpus 371
Thomas W. Burke, Mitchell Morris

21
Surgery of the Gastrointestinal Tract in Relation to Gynecology 395
Mitchell Morris, Thomas W. Burke

22
Surgery of the Genitourinary Tract in Relation to Gynecology 427
Mitchell Morris, Thomas W. Burke

23
Tubal Surgery: Isthmic Tube 453
Lamia Haj-Hassan, Gad Lavy

24
Tubal Surgery: Distal Fallopian Tube 465
Eli Reshef, Joseph S. Sanfilippo

25
Surgery for Ectopic Pregnancy 487
Steven J. Ory

26
Gynecologic Endoscopy: Laparoscopy, Falloposcopy, and Hysteroscopy 501
Randle S. Corfman

27
Adnexal Surgery 513
Ann Jeanette Davis

28
Surgery for Ovarian Cancer 523
David M. Gershenson, J. Taylor Wharton

29
Assisted Reproductive Technology (ART): Surgical Aspects 549
Lawrence Grunfeld, Janis H. Fox

30
Surgery for Endometriosis 569
Randall A. Loy, Alan H. DeCherney

31
Operative Procedures for the Breast 585
Vicki Seltzer, Jeanne A. Petrek

32
Reconstructive Surgery in Gynecologic Oncology 607
Larry J. Copeland

33
Operative Radiotherapeutic Procedures for Gynecologic Cancers 629
Luis Delclos, J. Taylor Wharton, David M. Gershenson

Index 651

The History of Gynecologic Surgery

1

Kenneth L. Noller

In the minds of men and women still alive are memories of a lifestyle so different from the present that reminiscences seem like fiction to today's youth. It is hard to imagine a world in which the internal combustion engine was a novelty, where roads traveled with the terrain rather than through it, and where a journey from New York to California was counted in days or weeks rather than in hours. Very recent inventions make it even harder to recall the past. For example, it is becoming hard to remember how copies of agendas were made for large committees before Xerox machines; carbon paper could make only six. Or, how did one analyze a series of 300 hysterectomies before Hollerith punch cards or personal computers?

The technical advances of the twentieth century leave us in awe. It has been said that more patents, more inventions, more breakthroughs, and more labor-saving devices have been developed in the last 50 years than in the prior 50 centuries. Yet, we must place all things in their proper historical perspective. Although technology may be mind-boggling and useful, it remains but the trade-school application of new ideas. It can be argued (with some success, depending on the occasion) that the invention of the wheel was a far greater feat than the journey to the moon. Certainly, human footsteps never would have appeared in the lunar sand without it.

Modern gynecologic surgery is much like the lunar landing: It is an important and safe experience largely because of radical, new ideas of the past. However, although the advances during the past three decades have been rapid, even a brief trip through the history of gynecologic surgery reveals that very little is truly new in the art. Most of our modern procedures are but modifications of ideas and procedures described long ago. Indeed, one of the widely distributed histories of medicine does not list a single notable advance in gynecologic surgery in the twentieth century!

This brief history of gynecologic surgery is, of course, incomplete. Because we are fortunate that the practitioners of our art have, for centuries, recorded their thoughts and procedures, it would take several volumes to adequately cover the subject, and still many anecdotes would have to be deleted. In the next few pages, we explore the previous 25 centuries of gynecologic surgery in a most superficial manner, discussing only the most important breakthroughs that make modern pelvic surgery safe and effective. This history ends in 1949—the date of the publication of the last truly new gynecologic surgical procedure. Virtually everything since is but a modification of previous work. An additional benefit of the 1949 date allows the author to avoid, with one exception, mention of any surgeon still living. Although there have been tremendously important individuals with equally important techniques practicing since 1950, their stars still shine brightly in our eyes. Their stories will need to be retold in future editions of this book.

ANCIENT MEDICINE (to A.D. 500)
"There Were Giants in the Earth in Those Days"
Genesis 6:4

The fortunes of time have been relatively good to the medical historian. Although it is unfortunate that certain ancient manuscripts, referred to by authorities for centuries, have been lost, it is more positive to marvel over the relatively large body of information still available from these distant times (Fig. 1–1). Three centers of medical learning are paramount in Western civilization: Egypt (Alexandria), Greece, and Rome. The dominance of each center waxed and waned during the early years of recorded history. Interestingly, the influence of an area's physicians was not necessarily related to the dominance of the area's rulers.

Our introduction to ancient medical practice comes from Egypt and its neighbors. Although few original manuscripts remain, the Ebers Papyrus (approximately 1500 B.C., some parts earlier) is extant and some sections discuss gynecology. Physiologic conditions such as pregnancy and lactation are mentioned, as well as pathologic conditions such as sterility and various menstrual disorders. Unfortunately, little more has survived of very ancient Egyptian gynecologic manuscripts.

However, we know that the Egyptians greatly influenced the development of Greek medicine, and much of that body of knowledge survives. From approximately 1250 to 300 B.C. Greek medicine dominated Western healing, and we can begin to recognize the first true foundations of modern practice. Aesculapius (fourteenth century B.C.) is one of the first of the ancients to appear through the mists of time. Although it is often difficult to separate the cult from the man, he is known to have been a real person. His fame came largely from practicing medicine without resorting to magic. Yet by 1250 B.C., in one of the many ironies of history, a temple to Aesculapius had been erected at Titane, and a cult of medicine had arisen from his physician followers. Although little is known about the gynecology practiced by these "priests," the care provided at the temples would seem very familiar to modern practitioners. In effect, the cult of Aesculapius developed the first "hospices." The sick were taken into the temples where soothing music was played, quietly. The patients were bathed and massaged and provided with comfort and dignity as they died from

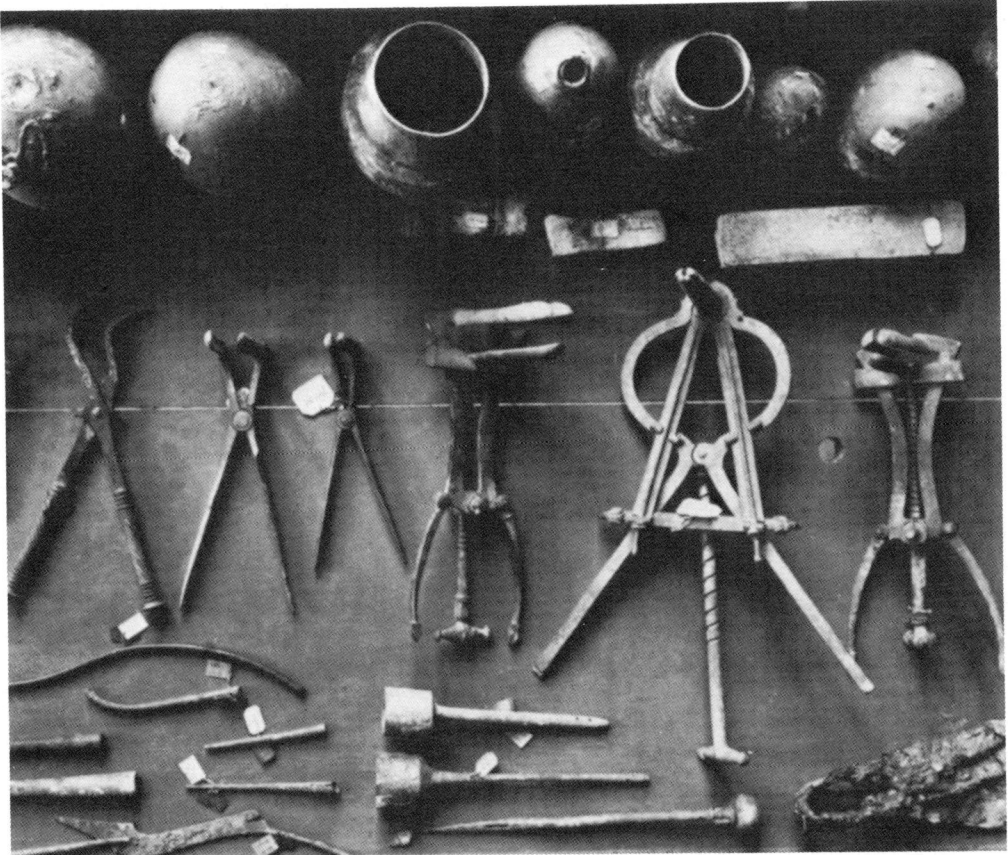

Figure 1–1
Bronze and iron surgical and gynecologic instruments found in the House of the Surgeon (c. A.D. 62–79), Pompeii. Museo Archeologico Nazionale, Naples. (From Lyons AS, Petrucelli RJ: Medicine: An Illustrated History. New York, Harry N Abrams, 1978.)

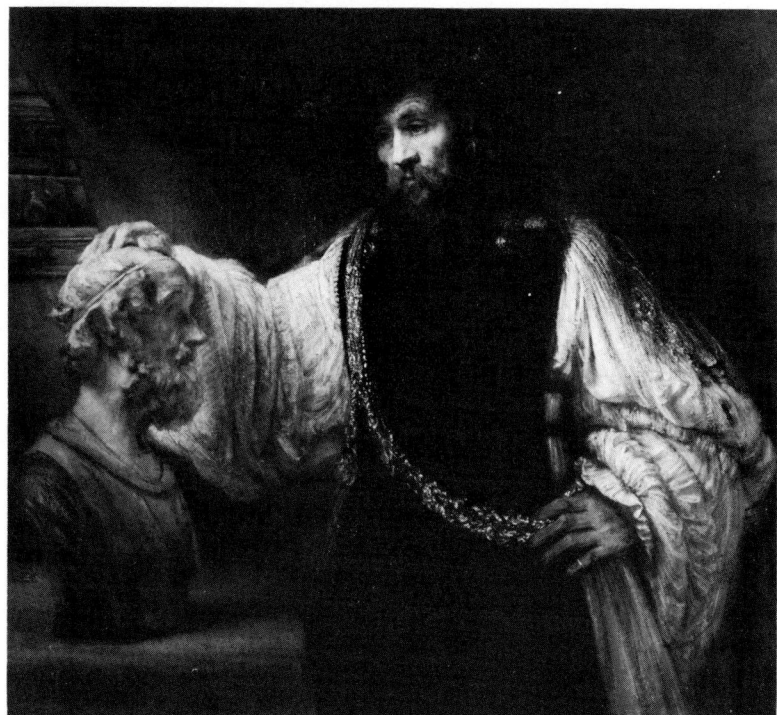

Figure 1–2
Aristotle Contemplating the Bust of Homer (1653), by Rembrandt van Rijn. The importance of Aristotle to Western thought—even some 2000 years after his death—is honored in this painting, in which the great philosopher-scientist also acknowledges a debt to his forebears. (From The Metropolitan Museum of Art, Purchased with special funds and gifts of friends of the Museum, 1961. [61.198] All rights reserved, The Metropolitan Museum of Art.)

slowly progressive illnesses. Interestingly, no patient was allowed to die in the temples, but was carried outside at the last possible moment. The Aesculapian ministers were largely practitioners of medicine who shunned surgery. Thus, it is unusual that Machaon (c. 1250 B.C.) was described as a son of Aesculapius, because he was a practicing surgeon. He is known to have ministered to fallen warriors at the battle of Troy. He is said to have removed arrowheads, stopped bleeding, and likely used tourniquets and possibly even ligatures.

Unfortunately, the study of medicine slowly evolved into a non–hands-on field practiced only by philosophers. No one interested in medicine would dirty his hands by actually touching a patient. After surviving for several hundred years, the philosophic period of Greek medicine ended during the hundred years between 500 and 400 B.C. Once again, great men began the "practice" of medicine, meaning that patients were actually seen and talked to, and on rare occasions, actually examined. In this one brief century lived Euripides, Socrates, Pericles, Aristophanes, Sophocles, and Plato, to name but a few of the most remembered. Although our twentieth-century bias is to describe these men as great "philosophers," in their time they were known for their very practical thinking. Some of these men have left us their thoughts about subjects related to medicine. For example, Aristotle was very interested in anatomy (Fig. 1–2).

Hippocrates (c. 460–377 B.C.) (Fig. 1–3) and his followers lived during the latter part of this remarkable hundred years. Their greatest contribution to medicine was to emphasize the need to observe the individual patient and to make predictions and plan therapy based on each individual's condition. They found it necessary to take medicine out of the temples and to once again remove all vestiges of magic from

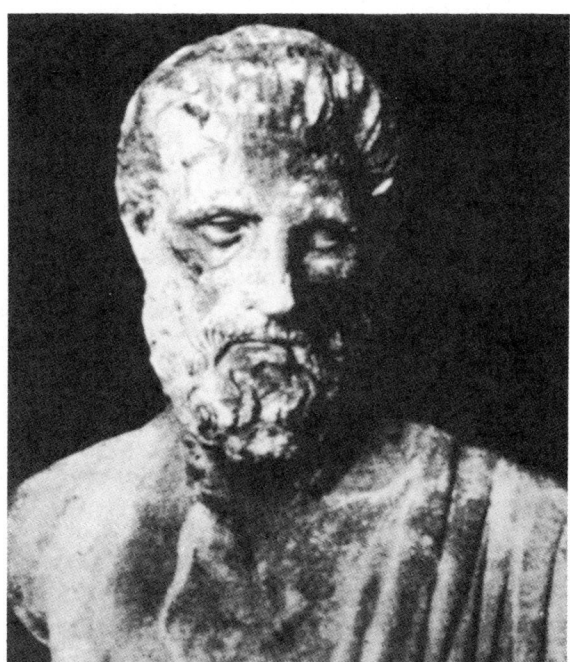

Figure 1–3
Statue, once thought to represent Hippocrates, found on Isle of Cos, where one of the great medical centers of antiquity gained fame late in the fifth century B.C. Cos Museum, Cos, Greece. (From Lyons AS, Petrucelli RJ: Medicine: An Illustrated History. New York, Harry N Abrams, 1978.)

its practice. Although Hippocrates was very interested in the process of disease, he apparently had little interest in anatomy and physiology and was distinctly uninterested in obstetrics and gynecology.

Greek medicine practiced in Greece lost its preeminence after about 300 B.C. The greatest of the Greek physicians moved to Egypt and jointly founded the Alexandrian School of Medicine in 307 B.C. Although this school is not noted for an extensive array of original thought, it did record the writings of Hippocrates and the other Greek physicians, and these thoughts remained the basis for Western medicine for nearly 2000 years. An example of the influence of these writings, *The Nature of the Infant*, said to have been authored by Hippocrates, although this is unlikely, stated that the human maternal pelvic bones separated at birth, allowing for passage of the infant. This error was repeated through the centuries and led to the lack of recognition of cephalopelvic disproportion for centuries. Indeed, it was not until the work of Vesalius, published in 1543, that this error was corrected!

Rome was the next great civilization to emerge in the West. Whereas the Egyptians were the great recorders and builders and the Greeks were the great thinkers, the Romans were the great "users." That is, they drew the very best from all of the known civilizations and applied that information in a practical manner. This is certainly true in the field of medicine. In the late Republic and the glory days of the Empire, Roman-born physicians were not in style and were rarely consulted by the privileged class. Most of the best-known practitioners of the time were actually Greeks who had studied at Alexandria.

As early as 300 B.C. midwifery was a practiced profession in Rome, and Herophilus is known to have written a book of midwifery approximately at this time. Caius Plinius Secundus (c. A.D. 23–79), better known as Pliny the Elder, wrote his famous text, *Historia Naturalis* during the early Empire. This medical text is said to have been the second most commonly read book during the Middle Ages. Unfortunately, the text contains only a little about gynecology, and much of that was incorrect. Pliny, however, did expound on the magical and curative properties of menstrual blood, a falsehood that was believed for centuries because of his stature as one of the greatest Roman physicians. Indeed, in Roman times, cloths soaked with menstrual blood became marketable commodities, with the "first napkin of a healthy virgin" commanding the highest price.

Rufus and Soranus (Fig. 1–4), both of Ephesus, were Greeks who initially studied at the Alexandrian School of Medicine. When they reached Rome, they became the most famous gynecologists of antiquity. Rufus (c. A.D. 99) wrote the first anatomy text that

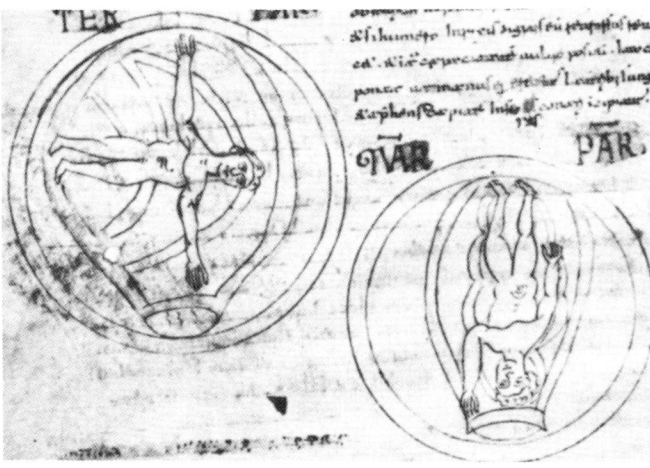

Figure 1–4
Illustration of *fetus in utero*, from a twelfth-century manuscript based on writings of Soranus of Ephesus, a first-century Roman doctor whose writings on obstetrics and the diseases of women were considered authoritative for many centuries. Codex 1653, Royal Library, Copenhagen. (From Lyons AS, Petrucelli RJ: Medicine: An Illustrated History. New York, Harry N Abrams, 1978.)

described the female reproductive system in reasonable detail. His text became the only available anatomy tome for nearly 15 centuries.

Soranus (98–177) was by far the most important gynecologist of ancient times. His *Diseases of Women* became virtually the only text of gynecology until it was supplanted in the Renaissance. Soranus clearly used a speculum to examine women and described uterine prolapse in some detail. Although of course Soranus never performed a vaginal hysterectomy, he is generally credited with conceiving the possibility that such a procedure might be performed. In addition to his gynecologic writings, he recorded considerable information about obstetrics, including a description of puerperal fever and podalic version. It is likely that he actually performed podalic version.

Galen (c. 130–200) was, in his time, the best-known physician in Rome and perhaps the best-known physician who ever lived. Unlike the writings of most of the ancients, his writings were generally available (and read) throughout the Dark Ages. Unfortunately, he had little interest in gynecology. Galen is generally credited with the first description of cancer.

Ancient Rome's last contribution to medicine was the establishment of the first institution that is reminiscent of the modern hospital. At first, these buildings were exclusively for the use of wounded soldiers and closely resembled the cloisters of the later monasteries. Eventually, nonsoldiers were allowed to become inpatients. St. Jerome tells us that in c. A.D. 380, the first hospital in Rome for nonmilitia was established by a female physician, Fabiola.

MEDIEVAL EUROPE (A.D. 500–1500)
Witchcraft, Herbs, and Demons

Every school child knows of the Middle Ages. It was a time of knights and maidens in distress, castles and moats, and sorcerers and magic. Yet the romantic tales that have become a part of our collective memory do little to provide a clear picture of the actual state of affairs during this period of time. Appropriately called the Dark Ages, during the first half of this millennium Western civilization virtually ceased to exist as a recognizable entity, as the extensive central administration of the Roman Empire disintegrated. Life became centered around the local village. Indeed, Western civilization at this time reverted to near tribal status. It is easy to recognize that this type of existence would not support an academy of medicine devoted to philosophic and scientific thought.

Much has been written about the role of the monasteries in the preservation of learning during the Dark Ages. However, it is only recently that we have come to realize that the monasteries did little to maintain the medical works of the ancients and that it was primarily the Alexandrian libraries and schools of thought, and later the important Moslem centers of learning, that preserved for us the medical knowledge of the Egyptian, Greek, and Roman empires. Although the monasteries preserved much ancient learning, they were not particularly interested in medicine. Apparently, for institutions that believed that all misfortune was punishment from God, too many of the illnesses and prescribed remedies resembled witchcraft.

Some few advances were made in Western medicine during this period of history along the fringes of Western civilization, most notably in the Near East and Egypt. Aëtius of Amida (502–575) copied the gynecologic works of Soranus, and these copies became the gynecology texts that were later used at the first medical school at Salerno. Aëtius' contribution to gynecology was to describe the various positions for vaginal examination. Certainly these examinations included the use of a speculum. Paulus Aegina (635–690) is known primarily as the first male midwife in recorded history. Avicenna (980–1037) is credited by some authorities as being one of the greatest physicians of all time, but he was not interested in gynecology.

The establishment of a "medical school" at Salerno in approximately A.D. 650 marked the first major step forward in medicine in several centuries. The founders of this school were wise enough to include scholars from all of the great civilizations. Thus, Christian, Jewish, and Moslem physicians practiced and taught side-by-side. Unfortunately, those of the Moslem faith were later purged; like so many advances, the Salerno school teaches us bittersweet lessons. Medical discussions were once again allowed to be made in the open, the ancient texts were reviewed and updated, and general interest in learning about the nature of diseases laid the groundwork for the rapid advancement that occurred during the Renaissance.

Unfortunately, the school at Salerno also gave credence to the *humoral balance theory*. Although this idea was first conceived in approximately 600 B.C. by the Greek physician Empedocles, it was not generally accepted until it was widely proclaimed by the Salerno scholars. According to this theory, blood (fire), phlegm (earth), black bile (water), and yellow bile (air) were the four physical observations that represented the four basic forces of nature, and harmony of these forces was responsible for good health. It follows from this theory that imbalance of the four "humors" caused all disease, and all cures required restoring them to their native balanced state. Over time, urine and blood became the two signs that were most carefully observed (and remain so to this day). Although this theory led humankind away from the concept of the infectiousness of many diseases, one benefit that is important for this history of surgical gynecology was the need to return the humor blood to its proper balance. This led to the practice of bloodletting, which required that professionals who were willing to stain their hands with blood be employed in the practice of medicine. Thus, after a hiatus of 10 centuries, surgery began to be reintroduced into Western medicine. However, this evolution did not come easily. In 1163, the Council of Tours, predominantly a religious meeting, decreed that surgery should be abandoned by all medical schools and should not be practiced by "decent" physicians.

Europe was nearly ready to lift the veil of the Dark Ages and return to scholarly activities. The rise of nationalism in the thirteenth and fourteenth centuries resulted in the re-emergence of a form of centralized government. Scholars were again able to meet at central points to discuss and advance medicine. Perhaps the best example that times were changing is the work of Mondinus of Bologna (1275–1326). This physician began to perform human dissections for the first time in over 1000 years. His colleagues at the new University of Bologna were stimulated by the remarkable discoveries that were made from this previously sacrilegious activity. Although several human dissections were performed during the next few decades, most of the work was done on animals.

THE RENAISSANCE (A.D. 1450–1600)
Art, Music, and Medicine

The revolution in the fine arts that occurred first in Italy and then in the rest of Western Europe was accompanied by a revival in medicine. Although the Medical Renaissance properly begins in 1315 with Mondinus' first dissection, the start of the Renaissance is usually given as 1453, the date of the fall of the Eastern Roman Empire. This date also marks the end of the Crusades and the gradual decline in the influence of the Church. England, France, Spain, and Portugal were developing as national entities, with central schools and hospitals.

An example of the new attitude toward disease can be recognized by contrasting the approach to the epidemic of syphilis that was rampant in Western Europe in the first years of the sixteenth century with the epidemics of the Dark Ages. During the fourteenth century, the bubonic plague (black death) traveled across Europe in several epidemics, eventually resulting in the death of more than one half of the population. This single disease resulted in the appearance of ghost towns throughout large areas of what are now France and Germany. Despite this devastation, little attempt was made to discover the cause of the disease or its treatment. The monastic centers of learning failed to make any attempt to discover the origin and treatment of this disease. Rather, new religious orders were formed to make the afflicted comfortable in their last days, and to dispose of the bodies.

The syphilis epidemic of the early 1500s resulted in a far different response. Scientists and physicians attempted to learn the origin of the disease and its mode of transmission and to develop forms of therapy. The use of reason, championed by the great philosophers and scientists of the Greco-Roman period, was rediscovered and applied to this disease. Although the humoral disease theory was to persist for another 400 years, almost all of the Renaissance scientists regarded syphilis as a contagious disease linked to sexual activity.

Leonardo da Vinci (1452–1519) extended the work of Mondinus and accurately described his 30 human dissections. Although his books were not studied in any depth for the next 2 centuries, he made unbelievable contributions to anatomy. He was the first to accurately draw the human fetus in the womb and was the first to describe the unilocular nature of the uterus. Because many animals have paired uterine horns that appear to be grossly separate, before Leonardo it was assumed that the human uterus had the same shape.

As great an anatomist as Leonardo was, he was outshone by Andreas Vesalius (1514–1564) (Fig. 1–5). While Leonardo was interested in anatomy, he

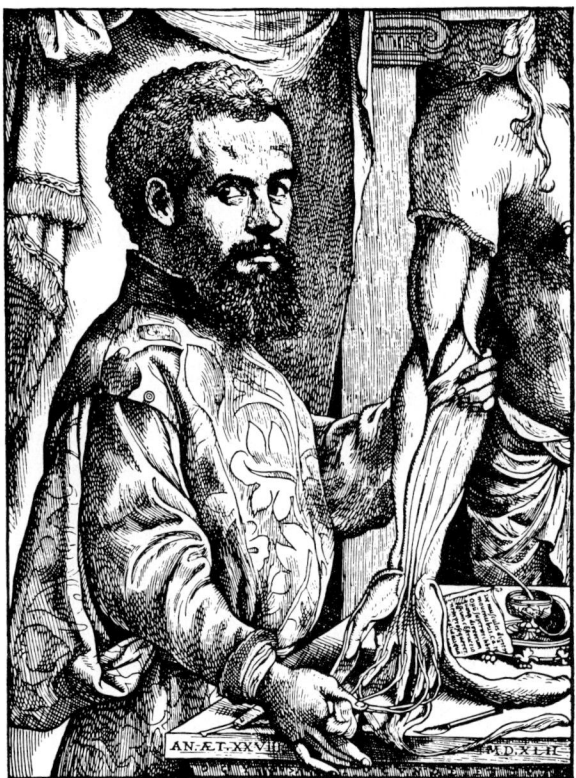

Figure 1–5
Portrait of the great anatomist Andreas Vesalius at the age of 28, from his masterpiece *De humani corporis fabrica* (1543). World Health Organization, Geneva, Switzerland. (From Lyons AS, Petrucelli RJ: Medicine: An Illustrated History. New York, Harry N Abrams, 1978.)

was distracted by so many other interests that he did not concentrate on this field. On the other hand, Vesalius apparently devoted much of his life to accurately describing the human body in anatomical terms. His work *De humani corporis fabrica* is probably the most famous anatomy text ever written. Besides giving accurate illustrations of the correct position of the female genital tract, Vesalius was also the first to demonstrate that the bones of the female pelvis did not separate at the time of delivery; thus he provided the groundwork for the identification of the entity cephalopelvic disproportion. The error of Hippocrates was finally corrected after more than 10 centuries.

Gabriel Fallopius (1523–1562), Vesalius' pupil, apparently subspecialized in female anatomy. His was the first precise description of the clitoris, the ovaries, and the tubes that were later to bear his name.

The field of obstetrics was dominated by midwives, but significant advancements were made by physicians. However, it was a sow gelder, Jacob Nufer (c. 1500), who performed the first successful cesarean section (on his wife). No prior cesarean section had resulted in both a living mother and a living infant. Perhaps as many as 15 additional cesarean sections were successful and were reported during the next century. Scipione Mercurio (Hieronymus) (1550–c. 1595) observed two cesarean sections and described them in detail. He also performed external version—the Braxton Hicks maneuver—250 years before the birth of Braxton Hicks.

However, the most remarkable gynecologist of this era is better remembered as the father of surgery. Quite rightly, he should also be known as the father of gynecologic surgery and the father of obstetrics. Ambroise Paré (1510–1590) (Fig. 1–6), a nonphysician, is the first of several surgeons mentioned in this chapter who combined serendipity (chance) with an acute sense of observation and a keen wit. In 1536, Paré was serving as battlefield surgeon at Tourin. At that time, gunpowder was widely believed to be poisonous and the standard treatment for any gunshot wound was to apply boiling oil to it as soon as possible. Fortunately, Paré ran out of oil during a particularly long battle and was forced to treat the remainder of his patients that day with only cleansing and dressings. His diary reflects his grave concern the next morning when he expected to find ill or dead all of his patients from the previous day who had not been treated with oil. Certainly, he was not the first battlefield surgeon to run out of oil in the heat of battle. However, he was the first to observe and record carefully the fact that the men who had failed to receive the hot oil treatment actually healed more quickly, and with less infection and pain, than those who had been treated with oil. Despite much initial criticism by his colleagues, he never again treated a gunshot wound with oil.

Perhaps Paré would not be well known had his only contribution been to have proved the lack of worth of hot oil. However, Paré extended his interest in wounds and began to experiment with controlling bleeding using ligatures. Although ligatures had probably been used during prehistoric times, certainly were used in India prior to A.D. 400, and were advocated by Celsus in his writings in the 1st century A.D., their use had ceased to be commonplace. Perhaps we will never know why this technique for the control of bleeding was abandoned for so long. However, in the sixteenth century, bleeding was commonly controlled by applying cautery irons to the bleeding vessel. Although this was successful in most cases, it caused considerable pain and slough of tissue. It took Paré to resurrect this simple technique, which is the basis for all modern gynecologic surgery.

It is very clear that Paré frequently used a vaginal speculum to inspect disease in the lower female reproductive tract. He introduced the use of his ligatures to suture the lacerated perineum at the time of delivery and established methods for the induction of labor. He also reintroduced the use of podalic version when rapid delivery was needed. Although surgery was his field (he was not a physician in the usual sense but a barber-surgeon), he did oppose the use of cesarean section for any reason whatsoever.

THE AGE OF SCIENCE AND THE NEW WORLD (1600–1846)
A Time of Thought and Leisure

These 2 centuries represent what is likely the most remarkable outpouring of scientific thought in the history of humankind. Although the twentieth century has rapidly advanced science, the seventeenth and eighteenth provided its basis. The scientific revolution was largely spawned by the development of the "scientific method." Although this system of posing a problem or question, experimenting and observing the results, and forming a hypothesis is largely a result of the work of René Descartes (1596–1650), it must be viewed as a gradually forming concept.

Perhaps the best example of the scientific method as practiced during this era is the description by William Harvey (1578–1657) (Fig. 1–7) of the circulation of the blood (Fig. 1–8). Through careful observation and meticulous documentation, Harvey was able to show that the vascular system was a closed

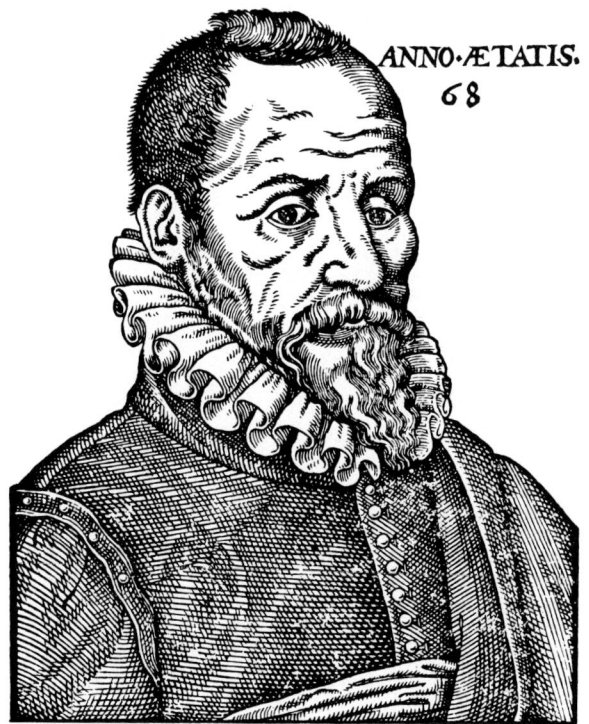

Figure 1–6
Woodcut portrait of Ambroise Paré, at age 68, who, without academic training, revolutionized the treatment of battle wounds and wrote the innovative treatise *A Universal Surgery* (1561). New York Academy of Medicine, New York. (From Lyons AS, Petrucelli RJ: Medicine: An Illustrated History. New York, Harry N Abrams, 1978.)

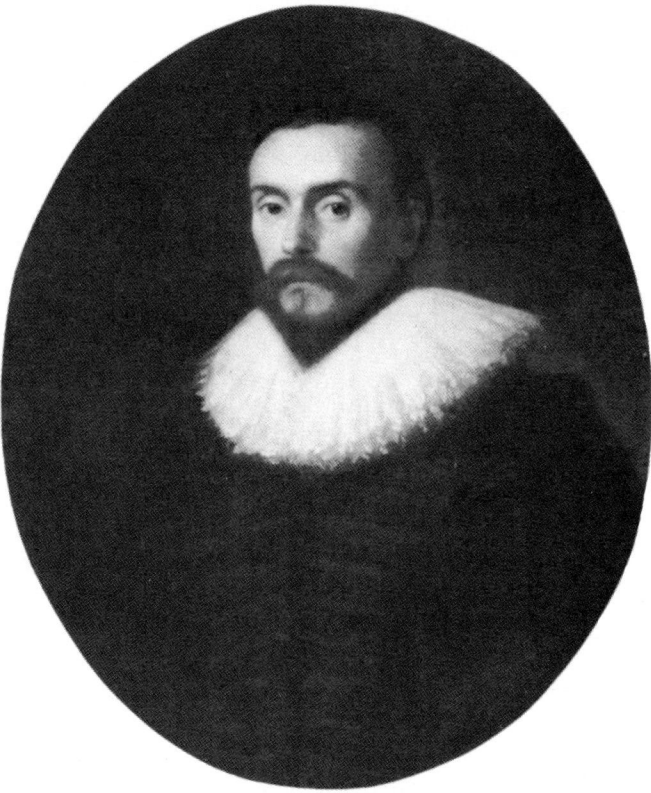

Figure 1–7
William Harvey, whose experiments actually proved for the first time that the blood was pumped around the body in a closed system, is seen here in the Rolls Park portrait of 1627. National Portrait Gallery, London. (From Lyons AS, Petrucelli RJ: Medicine: An Illustrated History. New York, Harry N Abrams, 1978.)

recognizable human fetus. When one reads these, and other, lengthy discourses, repeatedly one asks the question: Why don't you just look? Yet many authors of great repute never touched a patient or completed an experiment. For every active investigator such as Harvey and Leeuwenhoek, there were hundreds of "armchair quarterbacks" ready to speculate upon the true scientists' findings. Not since the Middle Roman Empire had there been so many educated men (and now women) with so little to do.

Many of these men and women of thought and leisure expounded at great length on medical topics, but few of them added anything important to our medical knowledge. It must be remembered that "physicians" were interested almost exclusively in those diseases that affected the inner body and soul. Groups of these physicians would meet and discuss for hours, days, or weeks diseases that would now be known as the endocrinopathies, cirrhosis, diabetes, pneumonia, or mental illness. Although these physicians might, on rare occasion, actually touch a patient or sniff a cup of urine, they practiced "cerebral medicine." Although they wrote voluminously about female disorders, they added little to understanding or cure.

loop. As important as this observation was, it is likely that the recognition that his use of the scientific method led to his discovery was even more important. Scores of "gentlemen scientists" suddenly began to more closely study nature and to arrive at sound conclusions based on their observations.

Although many scientific advances are made by serendipitous observation, Harvey's success was the result of well-planned, meticulous research. It is interesting to note that, after a lengthy education in England, he moved to Padua to be taught by Fallopius, who had been a student of Vesalius, the greatest anatomist of all time.

Despite the work of Harvey and the other gentlemen scientists, a certain frustration comes from reading the works of these centuries. A good example, perhaps, is the research of Anton van Leeuwenhoek (1632–1723). Although Leeuwenhoek used the newly invented microscope to describe spermatozoa for the first time, his simple observations spawned decades of discussion over the nature of the fetus. Literally thousands of pages were written debating whether each sperm (and later each ovary) contained a fully formed miniature human or whether the sperm contained a substance that gradually developed into a

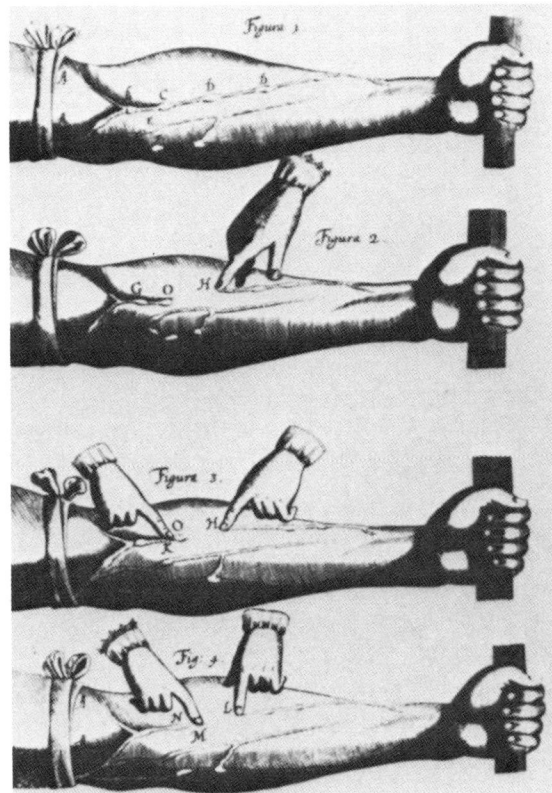

Figure 1–8
Woodcuts used by William Harvey to demonstrate his proof of the circulation of the blood in *De Motu Cordis* . . . (1628), one of the most important books in medicine and biology. World Health Organization, Geneva. (From Lyons AS, Petrucelli RJ: Medicine: An Illustrated History. New York, Harry N Abrams, 1978.)

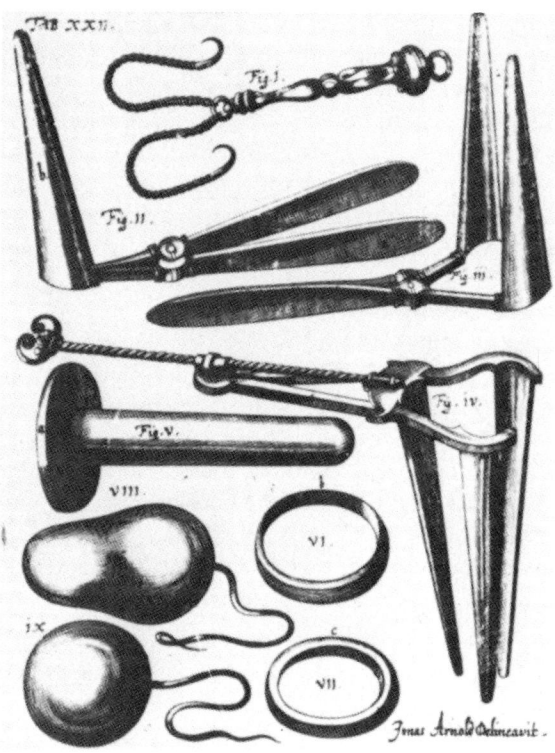

Figure 1–9
Instruments for use in gynecology and obstetrics pictured in J. Scultetus, *Armamentarium Chirurgicum* (1665). By the end of the seventeenth century, male midwifery was the fashion in many cities. National Library of Medicine, Bethesda, Maryland. (From Lyons AS, Petrucelli RJ: Medicine: An Illustrated History. New York, Harry N Abrams, 1978.)

Surgery lagged far behind medicine. Indeed, once the female anatomy had been accurately described by the anatomists, and ligatures, steel knives, and clamps has been invented, there remained but two reasons why thoracic, abdominal, and pelvic surgery could not be performed: pain and infection (Fig. 1–9). The solutions to these problems would not be found until the next century.

In another part of the world, the New World, classically educated physicians were scarce. Rather, the harsh conditions of the frontier required the services of the barber-surgeon. These gutsy, hands-on individuals were rarely trained by any method other than a short apprenticeship to another equally unschooled practitioner. Theirs was not the world of "inner medicine" but the world of trauma and action. They were much more concerned with the extremities than with the trunk, as they understood that they had little to offer the individual who experienced damage to this vital section. Pressure bandages, ligatures, amputations, and immobilization of fractures were commonly practiced. Although these barber-surgeons added little to the practice of gynecology, they did develop a core of nonphysician surgeons who inspired a later generation of trained physicians to inherit their work ethic and their hands-on approach toward patient care.

One of the medical disciplines that is essential for the gynecologic surgeon, the field of pathology, began to be developed during the last part of this period. Although the microscope had been available for some time, two problems prevented it from being applied to the study of human diseases. The first was a problem of philosophy and attitude. Because previously all disease had been diagnosed by actually seeing or feeling the ulceration, tumor, fracture, or other condition, there was reluctance to accept the possibility that disease might be present before it would be perceived by one of the senses. Although it was recognized that tumors grew over time in many cases, apparently no one believed that there was a "microscopic" stage of the disease.

The second problem was of a mechanical nature. Until the development of the microtome, it was virtually impossible to prepare sections of tissue thin enough to be observed by light microscopy. Additionally, tissue stains were not well developed until the early twentieth century.

Perhaps it was the work on the circulation of the blood by Harvey and the recognition that blood contained discrete particles (red and white blood cells) that could be viewed with the microscope that first led to the examination of human tissues using the microscope. Rudolf Virchow (1821–1902) is often called the father of pathology because of his work in this field. He was the first investigator to firmly establish the cellular basis of human disease. Although it may seem to us, in the twentieth century, that such an observation must be accepted immediately as fact, there was much debate concerning this matter. Many "physicians" still clung to the humoral theory of disease. Virchow's work finally ended the plausibility of this ancient mistake. However, it is interesting to note that this man, who singlehandedly put to rest a theory of disease that had existed for more than 2 millennia, later absolutely refused to accept the bacterial theory of disease.

Virchow's work laid the groundwork for the microscopic examination of diseased tissue upon which every gynecologic surgeon relies. The later work of Paul Ehrlich on tissue stains, the remarkable work by George Papanicolaou (Fig. 1–10) on exfoliative cytology, and the description by A. C. Broders of the in situ stage of cancer firmly established the proper place of pathology in a surgical practice.

Thus, the scientific groundwork was laid for the rapid advance in medical treatment that was to occur after 1846: Human anatomy was well known. The scientific method had been described and accepted. The importance of hands-on care and a willingness to try new techniques was ingrained, and most of the tools necessary to perform surgery (clamps, lig-

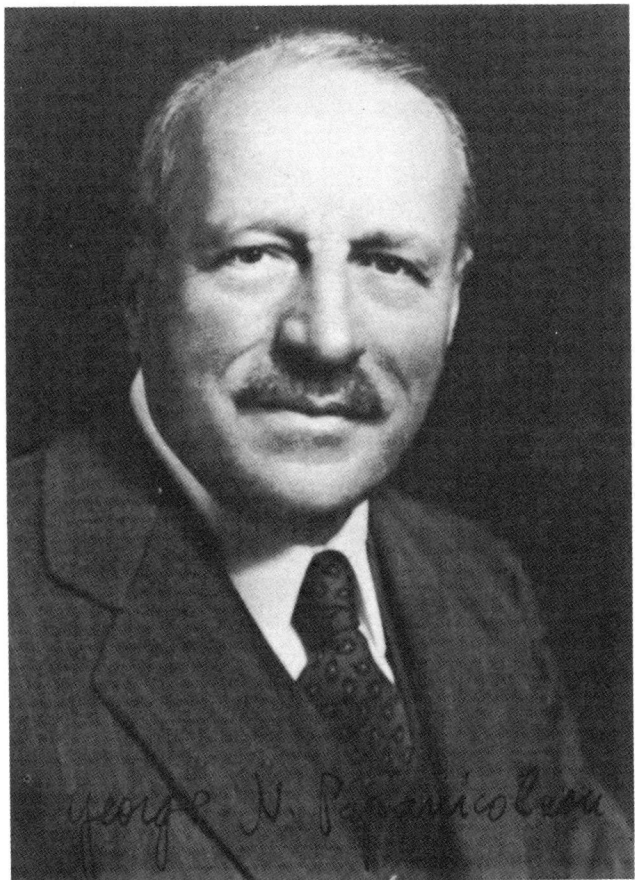

Figure 1-10
George N. Papanicolaou. (From Speert, Harold. Obstetrics and Gynecology in America: A History. The American College of Obstetricians and Gynecologists. Washington, DC, © 1980.)

atures, and so on) were widely available. The world of medicine was ready for the emergence of the surgeon.

MODERN MEDICINE (1846–1950)
"The Century of the Surgeon"
Jurgen Thorwald

Although all other segments of this history have used rounded-off dates, it is very easy to pinpoint the beginning of the modern era of surgery. Indeed, the exact date is October 16, 1846. On that day John Collins Warren, a surgeon of great renown at the Massachusetts General Hospital, allowed William Thomas Green Morton (1819–1868) to administer an unnamed substance to the patient Gilbert Abbott (Fig. 1–11). After the patient fell asleep Warren performed the surgery with his usual great skill. However, unlike other cases, the patient did not move throughout the procedure. Upon awakening, the patient was questioned at length and claimed that he felt nothing during the excision of the tumor of his jaw! Even those of us who practice in the late twentieth century when every patient obtains complete control of pain can appreciate Morton's great breakthrough.

Morton's agent was, of course, ether. In his historical novel, *The Century of the Surgeon*, Jurgen Thorwald portrays all of the characters involved in the early development of general anesthesia. Four individuals claimed "bragging rights" to the development of the technique, eventually resulting in proclamations by the Congress of the United States and the French Academy of Science. However, none of the original four "discoverers" derived fame or fortune from anesthesia. It appears that some innovations are of such magnitude that no one person can claim them. This point is made convincingly by noting that within *1 year* of the demonstration of ether anesthesia in Boston, virtually every surgical procedure throughout the world was performed with the patient under ether anesthesia. A quote from Thorwald's book perhaps summarizes this best:

The history of surgery is the history of the past century. It begins in the year 1846 with the discovery of anesthesia and the possibility of operating painlessly. Everything that went before is but a night of ignorance, of torture, and of fruitless wandering in the dark.

The introduction of anesthesia occurred at exactly the right time for gynecologic surgery. A young physician, James Marion Sims (1813–1883) (Fig. 1–12), of Montgomery, Alabama, was just beginning his pioneering work on vesicovaginal fistula repair. Although his story has been retold many times, it still remains fresh and serves as a model of perseverance.

Sims had been asked to examine and treat three young women who had vesicovaginal fistulas as a result of childbirth. Sims could find no account of there ever being a successful repair of such a condition and had refused to consider the matter further. Later, he admitted that his change of mind occurred entirely because of two accidents. The first accident was that a woman was thrown from a horse and had great pelvic pain. Although examination of the female pelvic organs was distasteful to him, he consented to do a digital examination. His examination revealed a retroverted, incarcerated uterus. In an attempt to correct this condition, he placed the patient in the knee-chest position. At that time, during his vaginal examination, the second accident occurred. Air rushed into the vagina and the weight of the abdominal contents pulled the uterus back into its correct position and allowed Sims to view virtually the entire anterior wall of the vagina easily. Although all events to this point were serendipitous, Sims' single most important contribution to gynecologic surgery was that he recognized that he had found a way to visualize the anterior vaginal wall, the site of the fistulas he had previously refused to treat.

Figure 1–11
Dr. W. T. G. Morton giving ether for Dr. J. C. Warren. (From Thorwald J: The Century of the Surgeon. New York, Pantheon Books, 1957.)

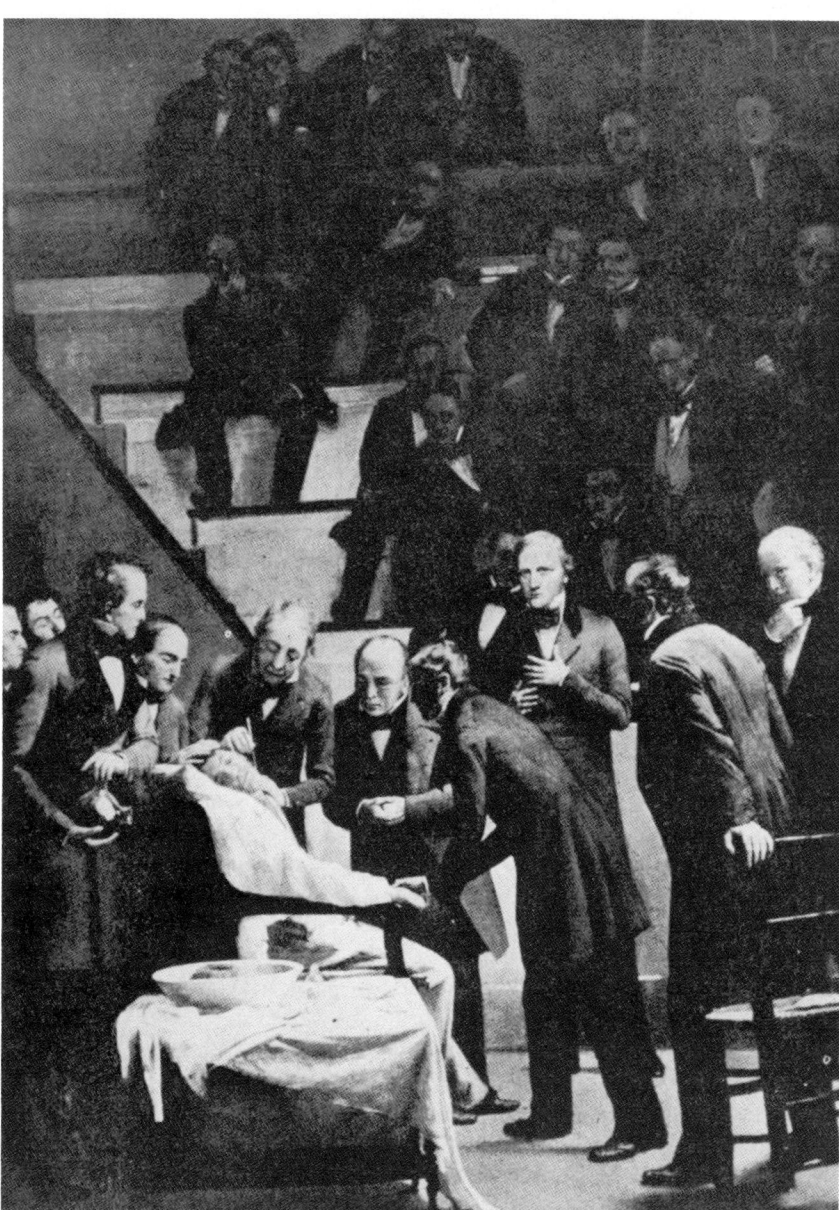

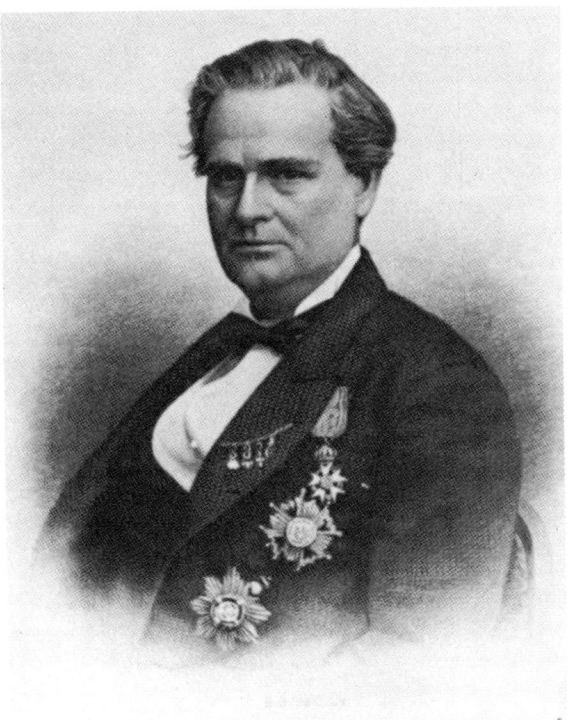

Figure 1–12
James Marion Sims, pioneer investigator of gynecologic and obstetric disorders, laid the groundwork for the specialty of gynecology and founded the Woman's Hospital of the State of New York, the first institution of its kind. National Library of Medicine, Bethesda, Maryland. (From Lyons AS, Petrucelli RJ: Medicine: An Illustrated History. New York, Harry N Abrams, 1978.)

Sims spent the next 3 years attempting to close the fistulas of his first three patients. One of the women was operated on more than 30 times. It is clear that Sims was no better surgeon than his contemporaries and had no better facilities. Rather, he had an unbelievable amount of perseverance. Indeed, most of the breakthroughs in gynecologic surgery during the past hundred years have not been the result of a newly described procedure. Rather, they are the result of a dedicated individual performing the same procedure over and over until it has been perfected.

Sims is a good example of this fact. Although he was unable to find a previous description of repair of vesicovaginal fistula, it had been accomplished at least 200 years before. J. Fatio of Basel identified, treated, and cured vesicovaginal fistulas in the late seventeenth century by denuding the edges of the opening and sewing them together with thread attached to a sharpened goose quill. The lithotomy position was used, and a speculum was placed in the vagina to guide the surgeon. The procedure had even been performed earlier in the United States, by John Peter Mettauer in 1738.

Besides his fistula work, Sims' two other claims to fame were the development of both the vaginal speculum (Fig. 1–13) and the wire suture. It has previously been noted that various vaginal specula had been in use for centuries. Indeed, Ricci has documented 614 varieties between A.D. 97 and 1940. Likewise, wire sutures had been used several times in the past.

Sims eventually left his practice in Alabama and moved to New York City, where he opened the first woman's hospital in the United States in 1855. His fame spread throughout the United States and Europe, and he is correctly regarded as the father of gynecology. He inspired others to join him at the Woman's Hospital, and a cadre of surgeons developed in the United States who were solely interested in women's diseases and, in particular, vaginal surgery.

Although Sims richly deserves to be the first surgeon mentioned in this final chapter in the history of gynecologic surgery, it is appropriate to take a slight step back in time and to recount the work of Ephraim McDowell (1771–1830) (Fig. 1–14) of Danville, Kentucky. Although his contribution to surgery was made before the time of anesthesia, it fits better in this later section. In 1809, McDowell removed a 22-pound ovarian tumor from a 47-year-old patient who had ridden 60 miles on horseback to see him. In many ways it is unclear why this operation should be regarded as the sentinel of abdominal surgery. Although McDowell's operation involved opening the abdominal cavity in a fully awake patient at a time when death from peritonitis usually followed, the abdominal cavity had been opened successfully dozens of times before. Perhaps McDowell's success is yet another example of serendipity: He performed a successful laparotomy, he removed an organ (ovary) that never had been successfully removed before, at a time when it was possible to disseminate the news of his success relatively rapidly. McDowell performed 13 additional oophorectomies with 8 sur-

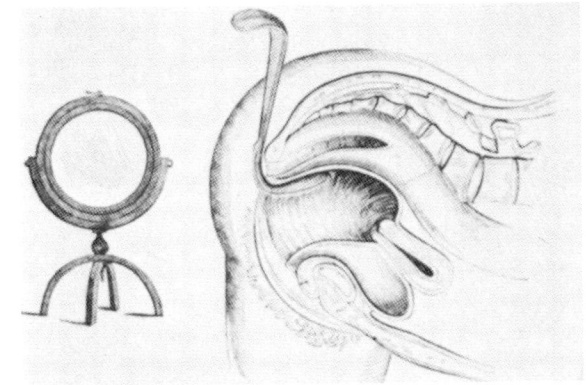

Figure 1–13
Early model of Sims' speculum, with a reflecting glass to direct light. Medical Communications, Inc. (From Lyons AS, Petrucelli RJ: Medicine: An Illustrated History. New York, Harry N Abrams, 1978.)

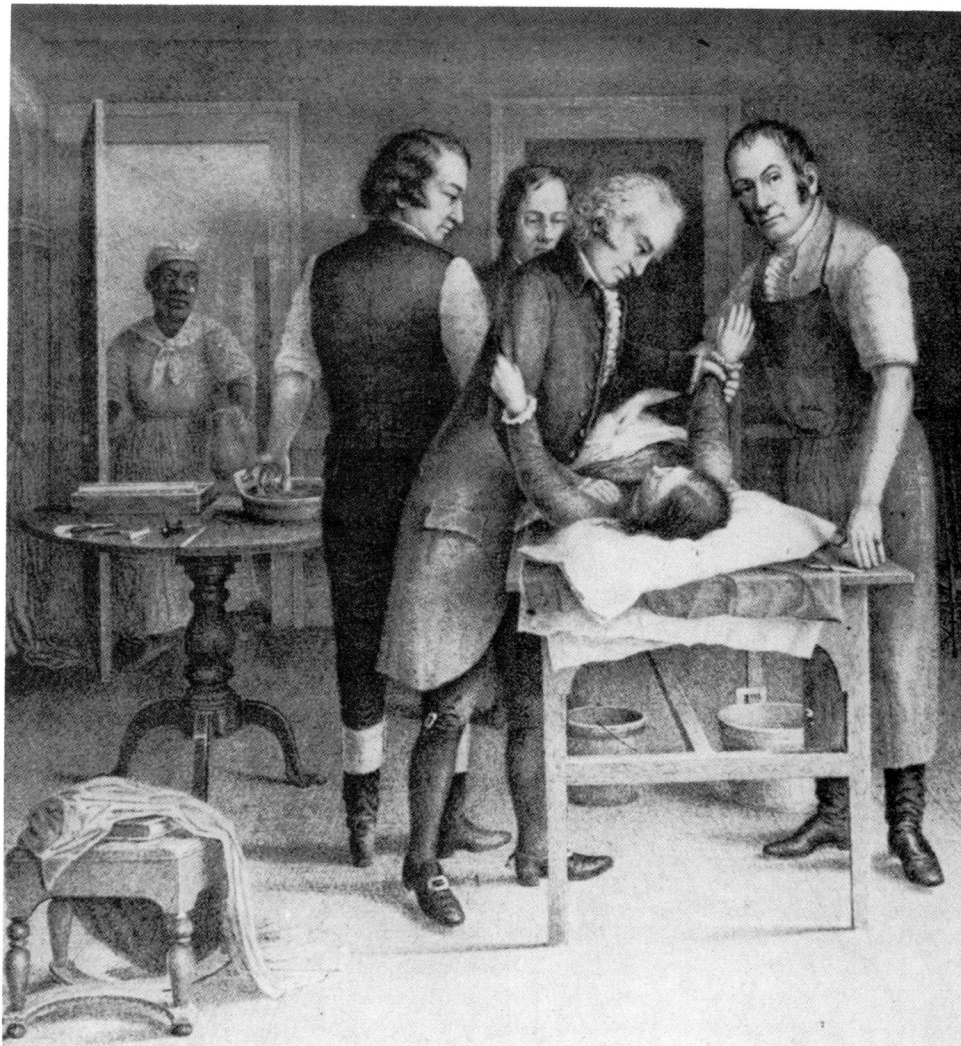

Figure 1–14
Ephraim McDowell. (From Thorwald J: The Century of the Surgeon. New York, Pantheon Books, 1957.)

vivors. Immediately, many other surgeons began to perform unilateral and bilateral ovariotomies, as the procedure was then known.

The work of McDowell and Sims must be considered together in order to understand the development of the specialty of gynecology. Although a few surgeons had been persuaded to devote their careers to vaginal surgery as followers of Sims, it is unlikely that this would have been a successful track for physicians to follow outside of specialized medical centers if transperitoneal pelvic surgery had also not been developed at the same time.

Unfortunately, there were still two major errors of commission to come before gynecologic surgery was to be recognized as an accepted field of practice. The first error has been called by many names, but the "Cervical Erosion Era" perhaps serves well. During this time, physicians interested in female diseases began to inspect the vagina and cervix in detail. The availability of the Sims' speculum and his dynamic personality certainly served as the impetus for this evaluation. For the first time in centuries, physicians began to look into the vagina and to scrutinize what they saw. The uterine cervix was found to be an organ that had many different appearances, and surely because most of the women who were being examined had a gynecologic complaint, these various findings were said to be responsible for the patient's presenting symptoms. Almost immediately after the speculum began to be used, the cervix began to be "treated" by many different methods. "Cervical erosions" were observed for the first time and were treated by hot cautery, silver nitrate, cold compresses, excision, massage, and electricity. Sims and his colleagues at the Woman's Hospital added to this confusion of therapy by writing profusely about many different cervical treatments. Unfortunately, such procedures were never appropriately evaluated.

An alternate line of diagnosis and therapy began in approximately 1860 and lasted for about 20 years. This theory proposed that most gynecologic complaints were due to displacement of the uterus, and the "Manipulation Era" was started. Without any form of objective analysis the uterus was pushed, pulled, turned, twisted, massaged, electrocuted, and operated upon to correct what, in retrospect, was most often a normal condition.

As the nineteenth century was nearing its close, gynecologic surgeons became more adventuresome. Because McDowell and his followers had proved that an ovary could be removed without loss of life, bilateral oophorectomy began to be performed for many gynecologic complaints, including dysmenorrhea, amenorrhea, epilepsy (!), and psychosis (!!). Interestingly, the procedure became known as the *Battery operation* after Dr. Battery of Rome, Georgia, rather than the *McDowell procedure*. Not everyone agreed that the ovaries were responsible for all of these illnesses, and Alexander Skene of periurethral gland fame remarked in 1877 that, ". . . with regard to epilepsy and insanity, I think it would be exceedingly difficult in many cases to decide whether the cause be of uterine or ovarian origin."

Although oophorectomy was accepted as a legitimate procedure, hysterectomy was not. In 1880 Pozzi reported on 119 documented cases of abdominal hysterectomy that had resulted in a 64% mortality rate. C. D. Palmer commented on this paper by saying that, "There are no operations within the domain of surgery more grave. . . ." The problem, of course, was not that the technical part of the procedure could not be done easily, but that infection claimed a large number of patients.

The solution to this problem was now beginning to become well known and represents another example of an allied field of medicine providing the gynecologic surgeon with a tool that is necessary to successfully perform gynecologic procedures. The field is bacteriology, although the first important members of the cast of characters were not bacteriologists. Ignaz Philipp Semmelweis (1818–1865) (Fig. 1–15) is generally regarded as the first important person in this area. Like that of Sims, his story has been retold many times; unlike that of Sims, his story has a tragic ending. As a young, eager, and aggressive member of the medical staff of the First Obstetric Clinic at the Vienna General Hospital, Semmelweis became discouraged about the high rate of postpartum death. Puerperal fever claimed 10–20% of all women who delivered on this obstetric ward. Once again, in retrospect, it seems impossible that someone had not thought previously of the importance of cleanliness to the occurrence of disease. Semmelweis noted that the death rate on the Second Obstetric Service, the midwifery service, was approximately one tenth of that on the physician-run First Service. By a combination of careful observation and chance, Semmelweis eventually determined that the cause of most of the excess deaths was the failure of physicians to wash their hands after leaving the autopsy room before examining patients in labor. By introducing the simple technique of washing with soap and water and a disinfectant before performing examinations, Semmelweis reduced the postpartum death rate to the lowest recorded anywhere in Europe. Unfortunately, his Department Chair was furious with this change in technique, and eventually, Semmelweis was forced to leave. He next went to the St. Rokus Hospital in Pest, Hungary, where he again lowered the postpartum death rate with hand washing. His third success was at the University of Pest.

Despite what appears to us as uncontestable proof, most of his colleagues in Central Europe refused to believe that hand washing was important. Interestingly enough, when his work was finally published and read in the British Isles, it was immediately accepted because they had practiced a minor form of cleanliness for years. The Rotunda Hospital in Dublin, Ireland, had previously had the lowest maternal mortality rate in Europe, largely through similar methods of cleanliness.

Unfortunately, Semmelweis died in a hospital for the mentally insane as a result of septicemia—the same disease from which he had saved so many women. He had truly been a man ahead of his time, proposing a method of salvation for thousands of women too early to be appreciated by his colleagues. Once Louis Pasteur had demonstrated the germ theory of disease, and had proved that many forms of disease were contagious, Semmelweis' great contribution was appreciated, but posthumously.

An interesting marginal note is that Oliver Wendell Holmes, a trained physician but mostly a prolific thinker and writer, had published the article *On the Contagiousness of Puerperal Fever* in 1843, 4 years before Semmelweis' observations and implementation of hand washing (Fig. 1–16). Holmes had developed the cause and cure of the disease purely by sitting in an armchair and thinking.

Although the work of Louis Pasteur (1822–1895) explained why Semmelweis' hand washing was successful and why it is among the most important discoveries of the nineteenth and twentieth centuries, hand washing had little direct application in gynecologic surgery. Perhaps more important was the work of Joseph Lister (1827–1912), who in 1867 began to use antiseptic techniques by spraying carbolic acid across the patient undergoing laparotomy. William Halsted (1852–1922) later introduced the use of rubber gloves, and the gynecologic surgeon now had the appropriate aseptic and antiseptic techniques to result in survival for most patients.

The next important event must be the introduction and widespread use of the technique of vaginal hysterectomy. Although Soranus had originated the idea of vaginal hysterectomy in the second century, Alsaharavius had recommended that it be done in

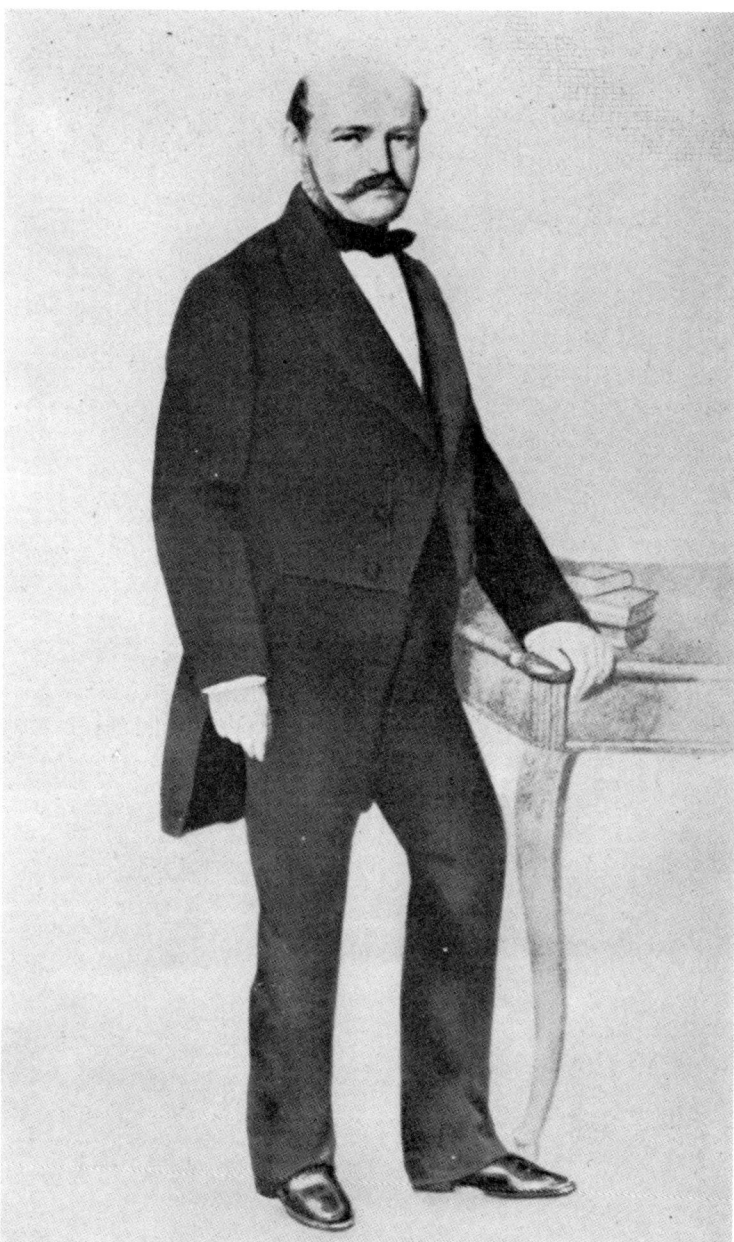

Figure 1–15
Ignaz Philipp Semmelweis (1818–1865). (From Thorwald J: The Century of the Surgeon. New York, Pantheon Books, 1957.)

the eleventh century, and Berengarius of Bologna reported the first authentic description of the procedure in 1507, it was uncommonly performed until the late nineteenth and early twentieth centuries. In 1808, Osiander of Göttingen reported nine successful cases during the previous 7 years. Although it is certain that at least a few of these procedures were complete vaginal hysterectomies, Osiander did state that he had to perform one of the hysterectomies twice on the same patient! The technique rapidly evolved, and perhaps the most important case was that of C. J. M. Langenbeck of Göttingen, which was performed in early 1813 on a patient with severe uterine prolapse. Placing the patient in the lithotomy position, he performed a hysterectomy, suturing all of the bleeders. This patient survived 26 years following the procedure and was examined by a number of distinguished physicians in order to "prove" that a hysterectomy had been performed. The patient was even subjected to autopsy at the time of her death, purely for the purpose of documenting the surgery. The autopsy proved that a hysterectomy had, indeed, been performed. It should be remembered that Langenbeck had no anesthesia, no assistant, and no hemostatic forceps available to him when he performed this procedure.

Vincenz Czerny (1842–1916) is, perhaps, responsible for making this technique an acceptable procedure when, in 1879, he totally extricated a uterus vaginally, applying ligatures to the broad ligaments.

In the United States, a great debate arose regarding whether ligatures or clamps should be used on

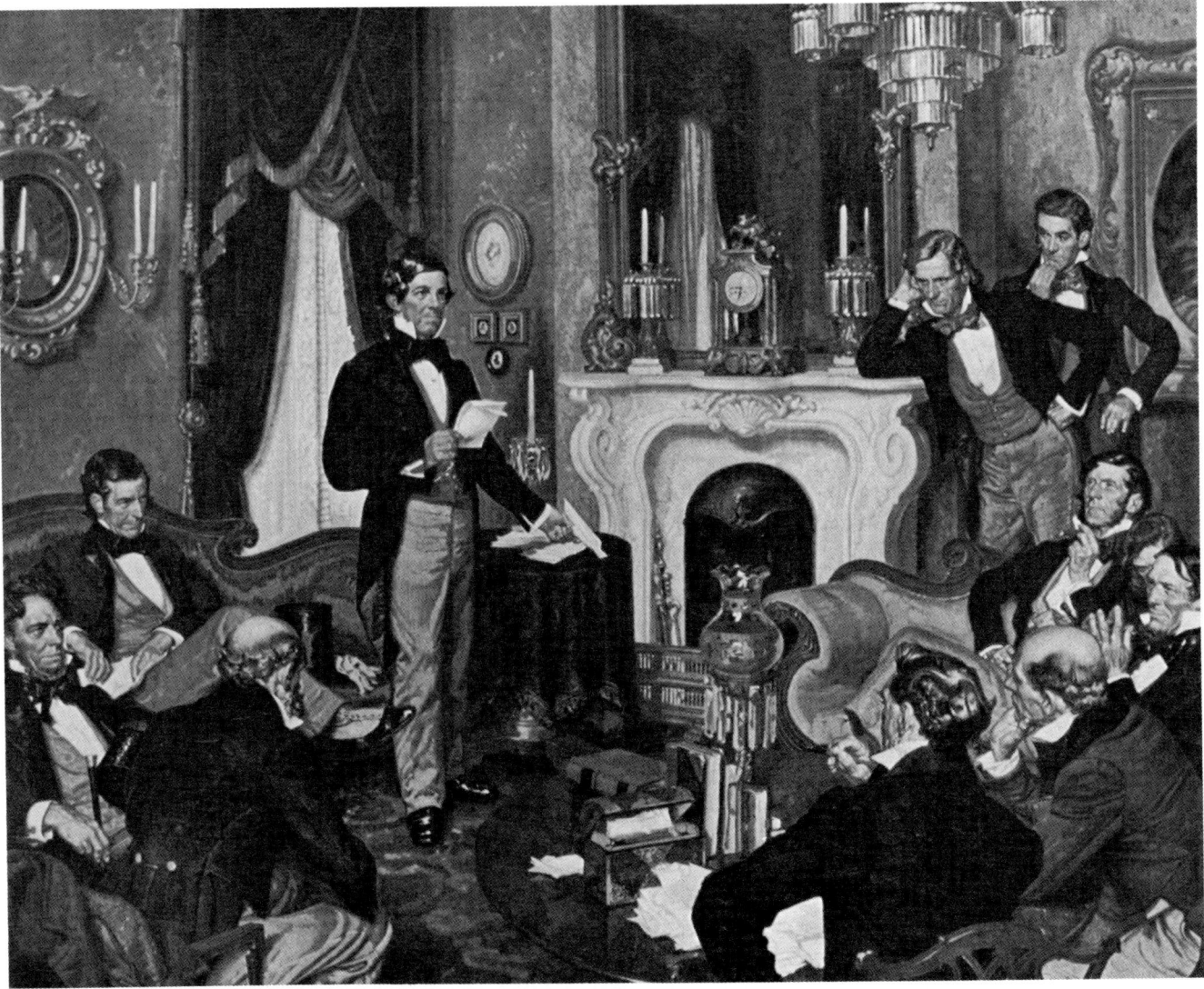

Figure 1–16
Artist's visualization of Oliver Wendell Holmes reading his celebrated essay *On the Contagiousness of Puerperal Fever* before the Boston Society for Medical Improvement in 1843. Wyeth Laboratories, Philadelphia. (From Lyons AS, Petrucelli RJ: Medicine: An Illustrated History. New York, Harry N Abrams, 1978.)

the pedicles following removal of the uterus. Eventually, the suture method won, and it is now, of course, universal practice to ligate the pedicles and to provide support for the vaginal vault by one of several methods. Although names such as Heaney and TeLinde are well recognized and accepted, further specification serves only to hurt those omitted by chance. Likewise, the various procedures for abdominal hysterectomy and radical pelvic surgery for gynecologic malignancy are best mentioned only in passing. Virtually all of these techniques are nearly contemporary, and many of the proponents are still alive.

Once again an important, nongynecologic field of medicine must be mentioned, as it is the final piece in the matrix that allows gynecologic surgery to be safe and successful. That piece is, of course, the development of antibiotics. Although Alexander Fleming (1881–1955) is usually cited as the father of antibiotic therapy, he was not the first to document the antibacterial effects of certain compounds. Various compounds had been used to treat syphilis for centuries. Although these were not very effective, cure appears to have occurred in some cases. Paul Ehrlich (1854–1915) is perhaps the first to describe that certain bacteria "attracted" various chemical compounds. His genius was to theorize that there may be certain of these chemicals that would prove lethal to bacteria. His work is another example of persistence; after trying more than 600 compounds, he discovered that salvarsan was toxic to the syphilis bacteria.

Fleming was not even the first person to identify the *Penicillium* mold. This honor goes to Westling, in

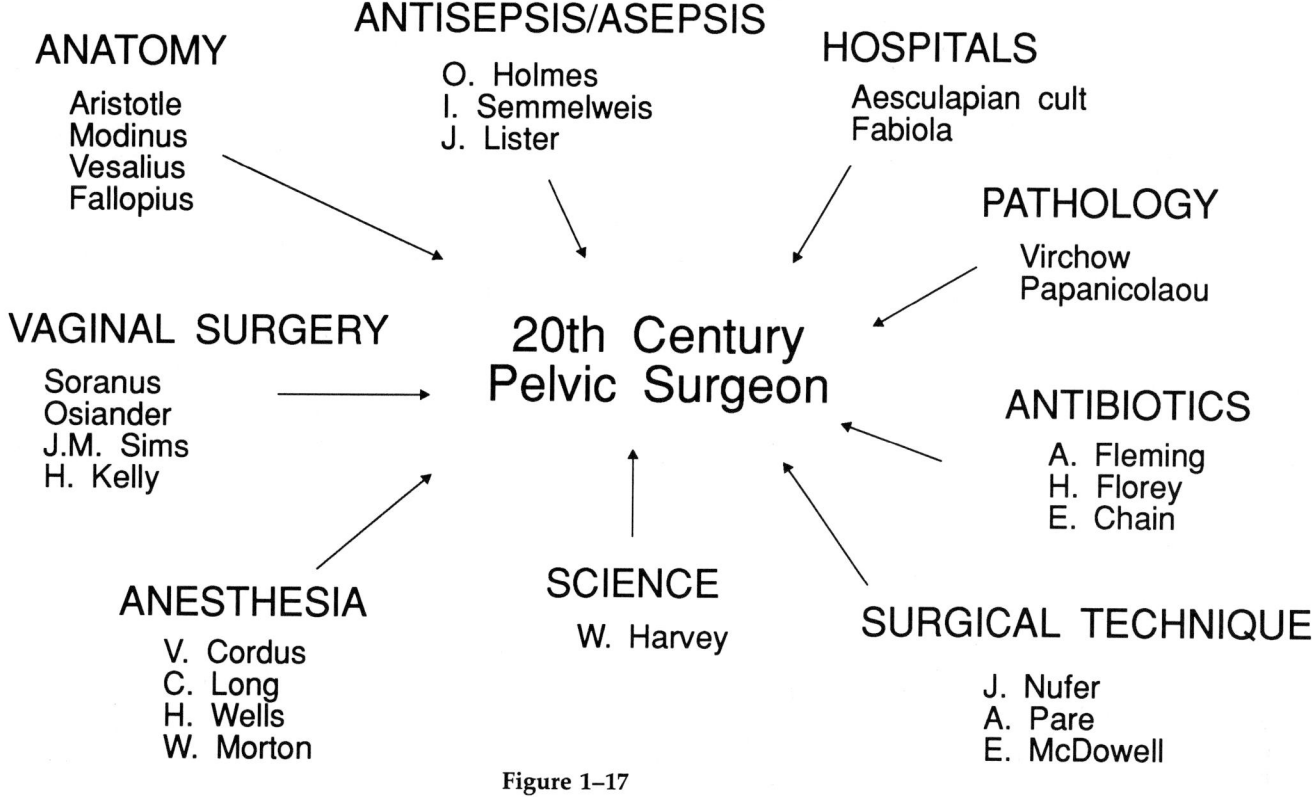

Figure 1–17
The evolution of a pelvic surgeon.

1912. Although there had been many stories told about the observation of the antibacterial activity of *Penicillium* by Fleming, it is not clear that, when he published his studies in 1929, he recognized their tremendous importance. Indeed, little was made of his report until Howard Florey and Ernst Chain began their collaborative work in 1941. A few "sulfur" drugs had previously been found to be effective against specific organisms but their usefulness was limited. When Florey and Chain clearly demonstrated that penicillin could combat heretofore life-threatening septicemia, the importance of this observation became immediately apparent to the United States Government, which was just beginning to be involved in World War II. In an approach similar to that which was to eventually result in the development of the atomic bomb, the United States Government placed vast resources in the hands of both science and industry and rapidly developed methods to synthesize and purify large quantities of penicillin.

The last piece in the armamentarium of the gynecologic surgeon was now in place (Fig. 1–17).

SUMMARY

As we have seen from this brief outline of gynecologic surgery, very little is truly new in surgery. For example, although vaginal hysterectomy only became a safe and frequently practiced technique in the early twentieth century, it had been described 800 years before. The same is true with virtually every standard gynecologic surgery technique. For the most part, "new" techniques are merely refinements of older procedures. Thus, the author has chosen to end this chapter with the year 1949, when the last truly new gynecologic surgical procedure was reported. After years of work, Marshall, Marchetti, and Kranz described the retropubic urethral suspension that bears their names. Their review of the literature convinced them that the technique had not been reported previously. Its simplicity and effectiveness rapidly led to widespread acceptance, although, as expected, modifications have occurred.

It is possible, perhaps even likely, that the MMK will be the last new gynecologic surgery procedure of the classic unmagnified "cut and sew" type. A new era in pelvic surgery has already begun: microsurgery, operative laparoscopy, and hysteroscopy are revolutionizing the field. In addition, medical therapy of women's diseases is improving. In the United States, the rate of hysterectomy has declined dramatically since 1990.

These new techniques *are* our future. The story of their successes and failures awaits a new chapter, in a new book, in the next century.

References

1. Haeger, K: The Illustrated History of Surgery. New York, Bell Publishing, 1988.
2. Kelly, HA: Operative Gynecology. New York, D Appleton, 1898.
3. Kelly HA, Noble CP: Gynecology and Abdominal Surgery. Philadelphia, WB Saunders Co., 1907.
4. Kennedy JW, Campbell AD: Vaginal Hysterectomy. Philadelphia, FA Davis, 1944.
5. Lyons AS, Petrucelli RJ II: Medicine: An Illustrated History. New York, Harry N Abrams, 1978.
6. Ricci JV: The Development of Gynecological Surgery and Instruments. Philadelphia, Blakiston, 1949.
7. Sims JM: Clinical Notes on Uterine Surgery with Special Reference to the Management of the Sterile Condition. New York, William Wood, 1873.
8. Speert H: Obstetrics and Gynecology in America: A History. Washington, American College of Obstetricians and Gynecologists, 1980.
9. Temkin O: Soranus' Gynecology. Baltimore, Johns Hopkins Press, 1956.
10. Thorwald J. The Century of the Surgeon. New York, Pantheon Books, 1957.

Embryology and Anatomy of the Female Pelvis

2

Stephen L. Curry

Because this book is meant to serve as a comprehensive text and atlas of gynecologic surgery, it is critically important for the reader to have a basic understanding of female development from the early embryo through the later years of life. Traditionally, textbooks of embryology have focused on intrauterine development. However, human development is a continuum throughout life. This process impacts directly on the diseases and defects that bring female patients to the physician, occasionally requiring subsequent surgical correction. This chapter highlights the major developmental processes that have a significant impact on gynecologic surgery.

Anatomy is the cornerstone basic science of every surgeon. Rarely is a chapter in a surgical text written in such a way as to allow the reader to develop a mental picture of the structures in relation to a specific procedure or technique. Anatomy is usually written as it is in standard texts or as a small supplement within each description of a specific surgical procedure. The former does not help the surgeon relate to a specific surgical procedure, and the latter may neglect spatial relationships of critical structures not directly involved but closely related.

The anatomic descriptions herein proceed in a functional manner from the prospective of open abdominal procedures and vaginal procedures. Visual locations and the relationships are stressed. The surgeon must understand that variation is common and although basic knowledge is important, it cannot replace careful dissection and reconstruction, always anticipating the unusual. More basic embryology, histology, and anatomy should be reviewed in text devoted to each specific subject. Many other chapters in this text contain anatomic descriptions consistent with the procedures being discussed.

FEMALE GENITAL DEVELOPMENT

Embryology is defined as the science dealing with the formation, early growth, and development of an organism. Unfortunately, most texts of embryology include extensive reviews of the first two areas but completely neglect the third. For the gynecologic surgeon, this last area is equally important and thus must be included. Three basic areas are discussed in this section: the ovary, the genital tract (fallopian tubes, uterus, and vagina), and the mesonephric remnants. Each of these areas has significant clinical import.

Ovarian Development

Around the fifth to sixth week of embryonal development, primordial germ cells migrate from the yolk sac to the genital ridges, thickenings just ventral to the mesonephric ducts. Rarely, germ cells fail to complete migration and thus supernumerary or "third ovaries" occur. Clinically, they are undetectable and unrecognizable; however, they may present as a germ cell tumor of nonovarian origin or as persistent endogenous production of estrogen after bilateral oophorectomy. The latter must include the possibility that there was incomplete resection of one of the two primary ovaries at the original surgery. This is what is commonly referred to as the "ovarian remnant syndrome."

Teratomas of nonovarian origin usually present as a retroperitoneal mass in the pelvis along the midline. Supernumerary ovaries, if visible, present along the medial side of the broad ligament high in the pelvis above the primary ovary. Both of these are examples of possible incomplete germ cell migration.

In the male, the testes migrate into the scrotum and are connected via the ductus deferens. The analogous structure in the female is the utero-ovarian ligament and the round ligament, which are originally a single continuous structure. The surgeon must understand that both of these ligaments have related vascular and lymphatic structures. The round ligament passes out through the canal of Nuck and embeds into subcutaneous tissue medial to the femoral triangle. Thus, there is the possibility of direct extension of uterine malignancy to the inguinal lymph nodes via the round ligament.

In the female, the maximal number of germ cells are available at birth with a constant decrease thereafter. This process impacts directly on fertility and oncology. With increasing age, fewer germ cells are available for fertilization; on the other hand, malignant germ cells are most common in the early years and very rare after age 30.

It is known that the ovarian stroma is functional and yet static in growth. The stroma produces estrogen and androgens and remains the same size throughout its functional life. Ovarian stromal tumors produce hormones and are very slow growing.

Finally, the surface of the ovary, at one time thought to be special germinal epithelium, is now known to be peritoneum continuous with the rest of the peritoneal cavity. The major difference is that this peritoneum through the years may undergo significant injury and repair secondary to ovulation. Thus it is likely that mitosis will occur much more commonly in this small segment of peritoneum, giving it a higher risk of epithelial cancer than other areas or male peritoneum.

In summary, understanding ovarian development allows a basic understanding of ovarian remnant syndrome, extraovarian germ cell tumors, fertility and infertility, and finally ovarian neoplasms. The germ cells migrate to the region and continuously decrease in number until just prior to menopause. The stroma develops the ability to produce hormones and is static in growth pattern throughout menstrual life. Finally, the surface is peritoneum continuous with the rest of the peritoneal cavity and not specific or differentiated germinal epithelium.

The Female Genital Tract

The entire female genital tract, from the hymenal ring to the fimbriated ends of the fallopian tubes, arises from the urogenital sinus (lower one-third of the vagina) and the paramesonephric ducts (the remainder of the vagina, uterus, and tubes). The paramesonephric ducts (müllerian ducts) form during the seventh week of gestation in close proximity to the mesonephric ducts (wolffian ducts). The exact relationship varies, with the most common situation being the paramesonephric duct system being medial to the mesonephric duct system. Without a Y chromosome, no testosterone is present, and thus the wolffian duct of the mesonephric system does not develop. Also, the lack of the Y chromosome results in a lack of müllerian-inhibiting factor (MIF) and thus the paramesonephric or müllerian system continues to develop.

Incomplete unification of the two müllerian ducts results in anomalies of the uterus and vagina (as discussed in Chapter 19). With a complete lack of unification, a horizonal vaginal septum will result. With inappropriate unification of the distal müllerian system and the urogenital sinus, a transversed vaginal septum may result. Usually this occurs at the junction of the lower and middle thirds of the vagina. Because the paramesonephric duct and future müllerian development are so closely linked to the future urinary tract, developmental anomalies in one system mandates a careful search for anomalies in the other.

Early in life, the entire vagina is covered with stratified squamous epithelium. This protects the internal environment from the potentially lethal microbes of the external environment. At the external os of the cervix is the squamocolumnar junction, with the columnar epithelium of the endocervical canal appropriately allowing sperm but not microbes into the peritoneal cavity. At menarche, there is an eversion or turning out of this endocervix, so that now columnar epithelium and its crypts are exposed to the external environment. By a process of reserve cell hyperplasia, new squamous epithelium is developed to recover this area. This is also called squamous metaplasia. Unfortunately, the process does not stop at the external os but continues up into the endocervical canal. Thus, there is a need for endocervical smears as a part of screening for cervical neoplasms (Fig. 2–1).

Finally, exposure of the embryo to diethylstilbestrol (DES) during critical points in the development of the genital tract results in stromal abnormalities that lead to anatomic changes and functional defects throughout the müllerian system. An increased risk of ectopic pregnancy may portend functional defects in the fallopian tubes. Stromal development of the uterus leads to a deformed (T-shaped) endometrial cavity and increased risk of premature delivery. In-

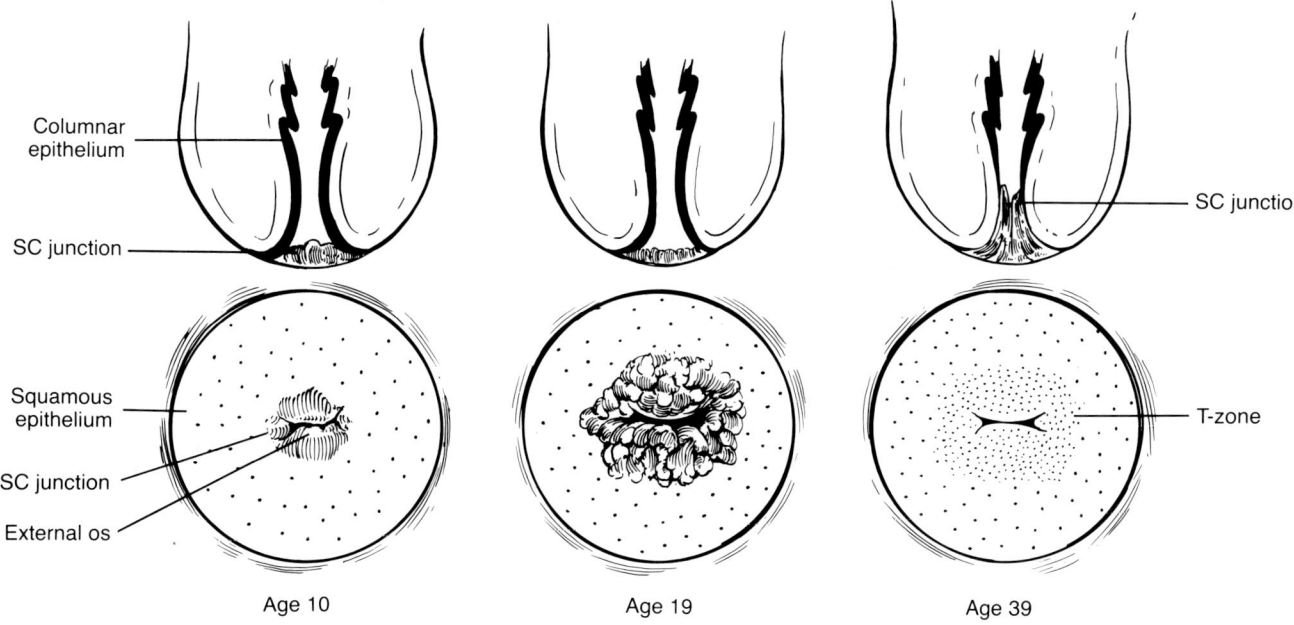

Figure 2–1
Physiologic changes in the cervical epithelium. SC, squamocolumnar.

terrupted migration of squamous epithelium in the upper vagina and cervix results in persistence of columnar epithelium called adenosis. About 1 in 1000 women exposed to DES during their embryonic development may develop a clear cell adenocarcinoma of the cervix or vagina (Fig. 2–2).

Mesonephric Remnants

Mesonephric remnants, persistence of microscopic remnants of the mesonephric system, are not uncommon. As in early development, they are located just lateral to the entire portion of the female genital tract that developed from the paramesonephric (müllerian) system. Near the fimbriated ends of the fallopian tube, teardrop-like ectopic cysts called hydatids of Morgagni develop from mesonephric remnants. Clear-filled cystic structures within the broad ligament are often called parovarian cysts because they are thought to arise from the paroöphoron and epoöphoron, both mesonephric remnants. These cysts can be massive, and the surgeon must understand that the grossly elongated fallopian tube will return to normal size and function after removal of the cysts if appropriately left in place.

Lateral to the upper vaginal wall at three o'clock and nine o'clock, mesonephric remnants may result in cystic structures called Gartner's duct cysts. They are usually asymptomatic and found incidentally on pelvic examination. They may be massive and tense and present as vaginal obstruction resulting in sexual dysfunction (Fig. 2–3).

ANATOMY

Abdominal Approach

The gynecologic surgeon must understand the anatomy of the anterior abdominal wall in order to appropriately plan and carry out entrance to the peritoneal cavity or the retroperitoneal retropubic space. Complete and sufficient closure of an incision also requires a complete understanding of the structures and their function.

As seen in Figure 2–4 the layers include skin, subcutaneous tissue, fascia, muscle, and peritoneum. The blood supply comes from the intercostals, which supply the subcutaneous tissue and skin, and the

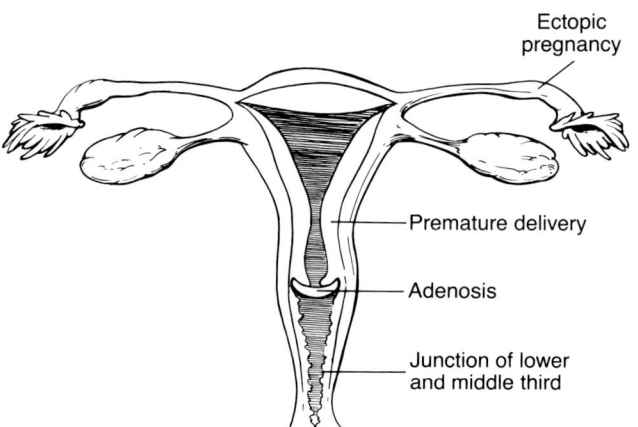

Figure 2–2
The müllerian system and fetal exposure to diethylstilbestrol (DES).

22 EMBRYOLOGY AND ANATOMY OF THE FEMALE PELVIS

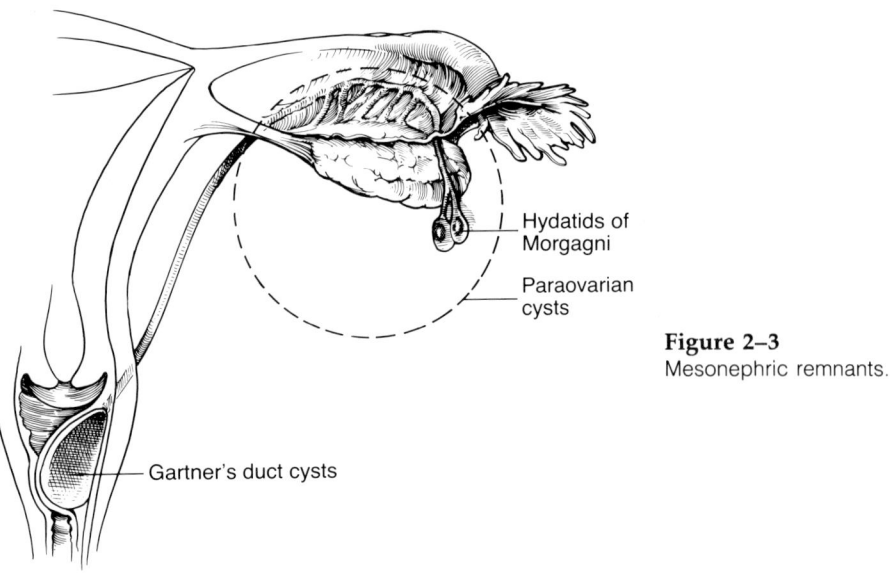

Hydatids of Morgagni
Paraovarian cysts
Gartner's duct cysts

Figure 2–3
Mesonephric remnants.

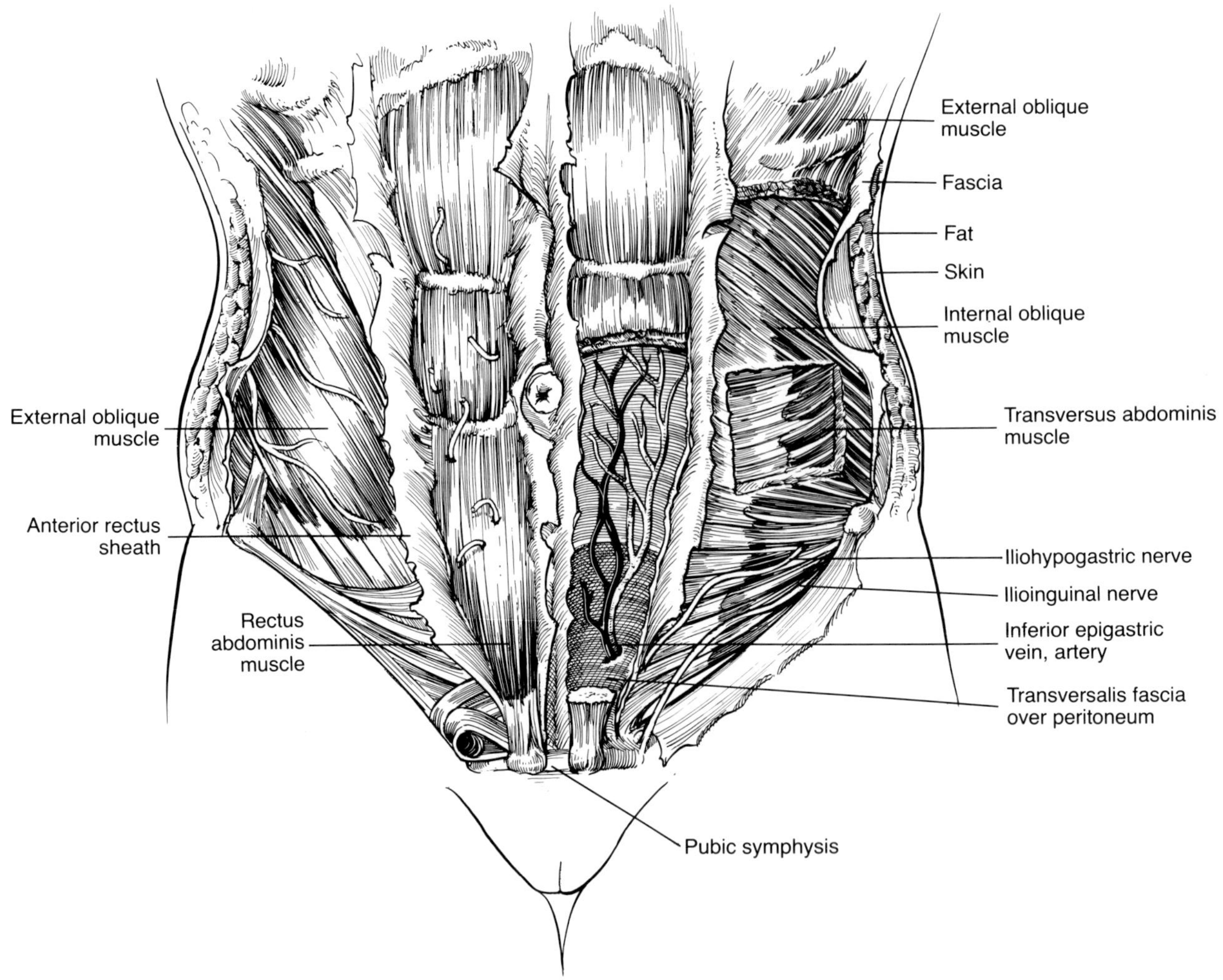

External oblique muscle
Fascia
Fat
Skin
Internal oblique muscle
Transversus abdominis muscle
Iliohypogastric nerve
Ilioinguinal nerve
Inferior epigastric vein, artery
Transversalis fascia over peritoneum

External oblique muscle
Anterior rectus sheath
Rectus abdominis muscle

Pubic symphysis

Figure 2–4
Anatomy of the anterior abdominal wall.

epigastrics (superior and inferior), which supply the muscles and fasciae. Nerves and lymphatics follow the vascular system. Major vessels do not cross the midline, making a midline vertical incision nearly bloodless.

A midline vertical incision from the symphysis pubis to the umbilicus would pass through skin, subcutaneous tissue, the rectus sheath or fascia, and peritoneum. Interiorly, the pyramidal muscle, which is usually small and firmly attached to the midline, must be sharply dissected in order to gain maximum visualization of the pelvis and the retropubic space.

A Pfannenstiel incision is a very low transverse incision approximately 3 cm above the symphysis pubis. The skin and subcutaneous tissue are incised transversely, strict attention being paid to hemostasis because large vessels are commonly encountered. Veins of the anterior abdominal wall below the umbilicus run straight downward and form extensive anastomoses. The fascia of the rectus sheath is open transversely and then the underlining rectus muscles are gently dissected off the fascia superior and inferior to the incision. The strongest attachments are in the midline, and these must be sharply dissected. The peritoneum is then opened vertically. Of critical importance in operative gynecology is the course of the inferior epigastric vessels. In laparoscopic procedures in which multiple puncture sites are involved and in true transverse incisions in which the rectus muscles are divided, these vessels must be identified. The inferior epigastric artery, accompanied by its corresponding vein, arises from the external iliac artery at the level of the inguinal ligament. It pierces the posterior rectus sheath at the lateral border of the rectus muscle and passes superiorly and medially on the posterior surface of the rectus muscle. It is located at the midrectus line about halfway between the symphysis and the umbilicus and then continues in this plane superiorly, being now buried in the substance of the rectus muscle (Fig. 2–5).

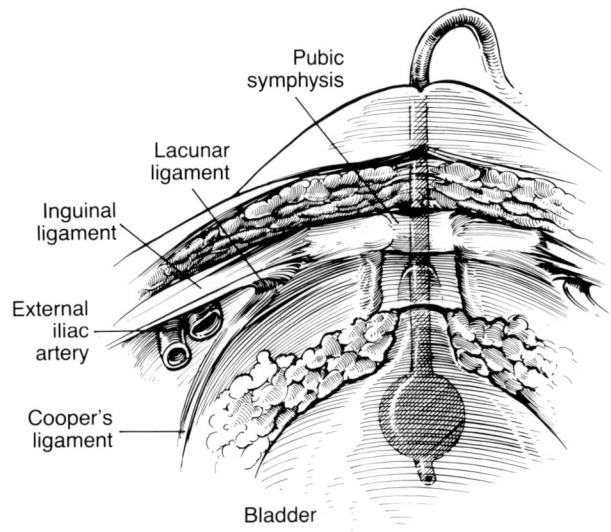

Figure 2–6
Retropubic landmarks.

To enter the rectopubic space, the lower end of the incision must be carried inferiorly to the symphysis and the space is then bluntly dissected from medial to lateral on each side. With a Foley catheter in place, the urethra and neck of the bladder are identified inferiorly. Figure 2–6 depicts the retropubic landmarks that are most commonly used in gynecologic operations.

Pelvic Anatomy

Once an appropriate retractor has been placed and the bowel is packed away, the pelvic contents can be visualized as shown in Figure 2–7. The surgeon should have a clear mental picture of the anterior relationship of the bladder and vagina and the posterior relationship of the vagina, uterosacral ligaments, and rectum in order to avoid an inadvertent injury during vaginal surgery.

Although the opening of the peritoneum of the anterior cul-de-sac is at the level of the junction of the corpus and cervix on the uterine side, it is still high on the posterior surface of the bladder. About 4 cm of posterior bladder wall must be dissected away to reach the level of the vagina. The vaginal fascia is easily identified by its vertical fibers. The lowest portion of the ureter enters the bladder from lateral to medial to form the trigone of the bladder about 5 cm below the cervical vaginal junction. The ureters can be injured here when excessive dissection

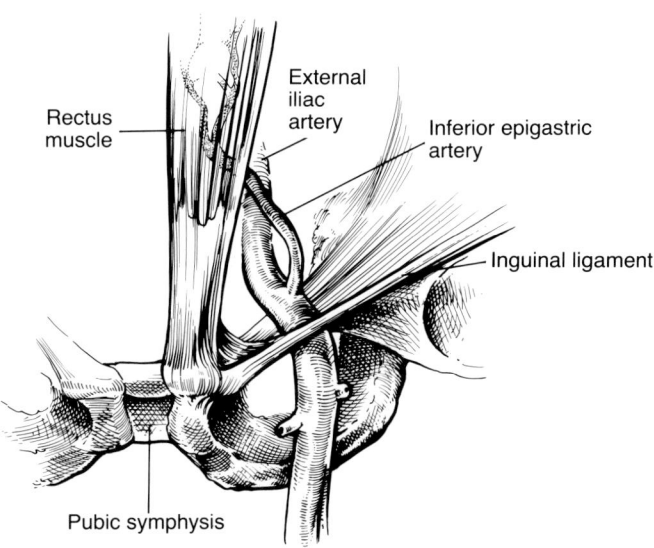

Figure 2–5
Course of the inferior epigastric vessels.

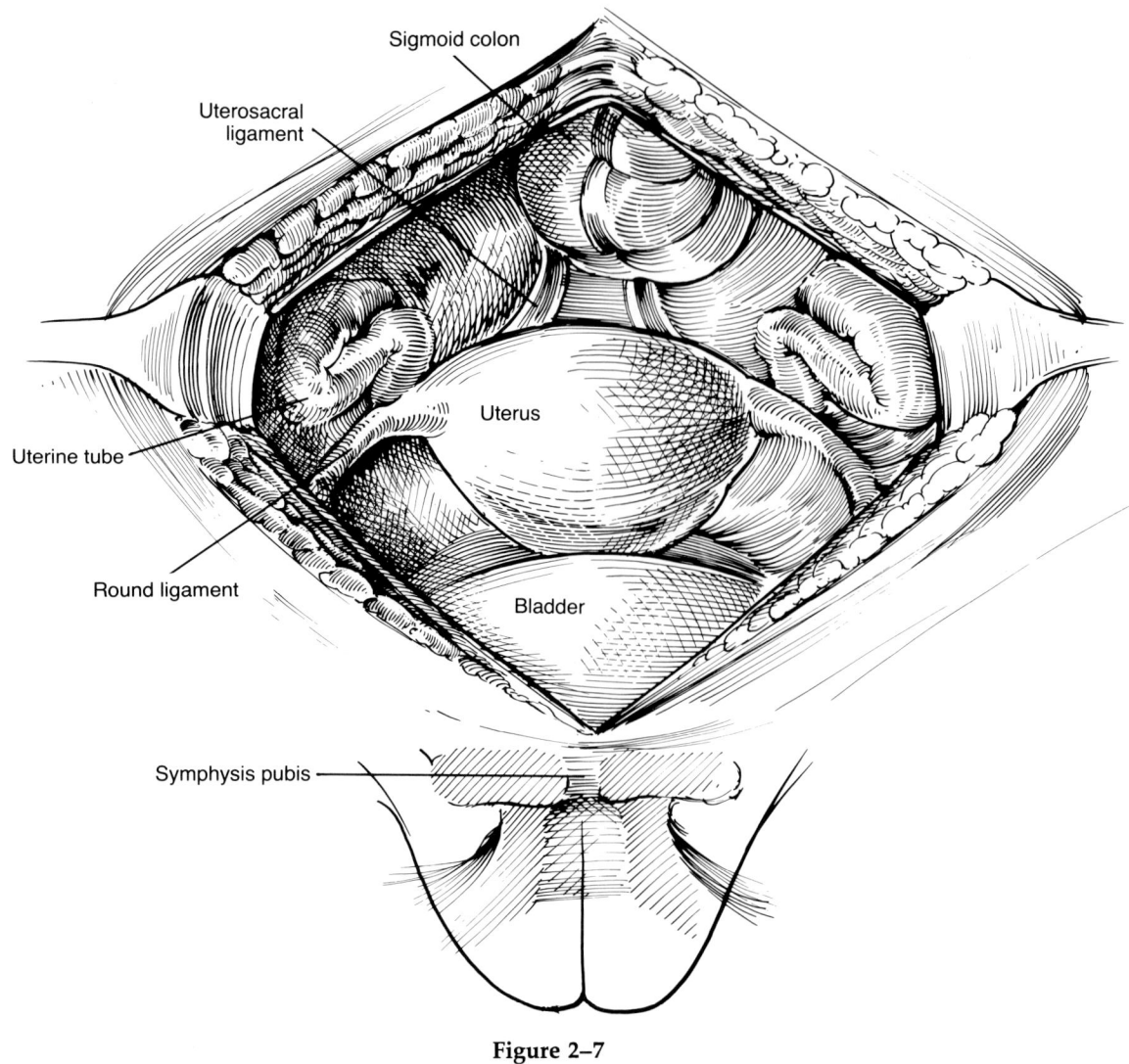

Figure 2–7
Pelvic anatomy.

causes bleeding that is then blindly ligated. The bladder can be damaged if the free space between the two structures is obliterated by previous surgery, making dissection difficult. Also, the bladder must be well dissected away from lower uterine segment and upper vagina. Entering the rectal vaginal space posteriorly requires an incision in the peritoneum deep in the posterior cul-de-sac between the uterosacral ligaments. This area is rarely violated in routine abdominal gynecologic surgery but is critically important for posterior vaginal entrance into the peritoneal cavity (Fig. 2–8).

Most important is a clear understanding of the structures of the lateral retroperitoneal spaces. The round ligament is identified and doubly ligated at the midportion. If one holds the ligament taut, there is a 4–5 cm clear space below and thus bleeding is avoided by appropriate double-ligature placement. It is important to remember that there are vessels and lymphatics that accompany this ligament. The ligament is divided between the ligatures and the peritoneum is incised superiorly over the psoas muscle, the surgeon taking care to stay well lateral to the infundibulopelvic ligament (Fig. 2–9). Using blunt dissection, the space is now opened by moving the medial peritoneal surface towards the midline. This is an avascular space, and the only structures on the retroperitoneal surface of this medial leaf are the ovarian vessels on the superior aspect in the infundibulopelvic ligament and the ureter much deeper. The ureter courses over the pelvic brim at the level of the bifurcation of the common iliac vessel and courses downward on the medial peritoneum to enter the cardinal ligament at the level of the cervical corpus junction approximately 2 cm lateral to the cervix just below the uterine artery. The ureter has very little medial or lateral blood supply from the pelvic brim to the cardinal ligament, and thus blunt dissection for careful identification is without significant complication.

EMBRYOLOGY AND ANATOMY OF THE FEMALE PELVIS 25

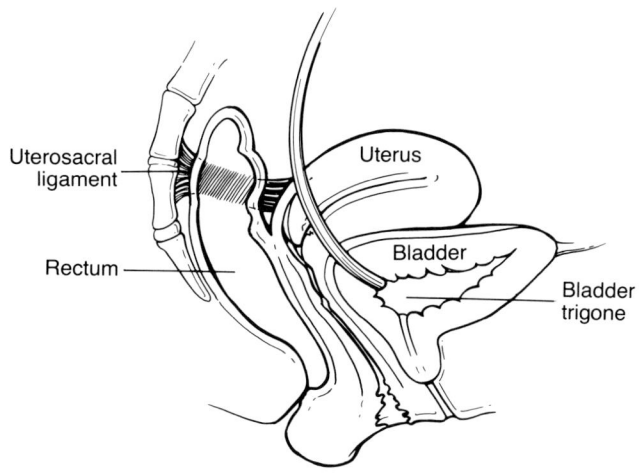

Figure 2–8
Transverse view showing the relationship of the ureter to the uterus and vagina.

The lateral wall of this retroperitoneal space is bordered superiorly by the psoas muscle. Again, at the pelvic brim one can palpate the pulsations of the common iliac artery bifurcating into the external and internal branches. The external iliac, with its larger vein just below, runs along the medial border of the psoas muscle to the inguinal ligament, where it becomes the femoral artery. Its only significant branch is the inferior epigastric, which arises from the anterior surface at the level of the inguinal ligament. There are extensive lymphatics within the adipose tissue surrounding these vessels.

The internal iliac or hypogastric artery is the major blood supply of the pelvis. Again, the corresponding veins run just below. There are four major branches of this artery in order of their origin: the posterior branch, supplying the buttocks; the pudendal, supplying the lower vagina and vulva; the uterine, supplying the uterus and vagina; and the vesicles, supplying the bladder. It is important for the surgeon to understand that ligation of the hypogastric artery for significant pelvic bleeding should be done below the posterior branch. This is approximately 4 cm distal to the common iliac artery. Also, its very large vein lies just below and can be injured during dissection.

The uterine artery transverses the base of the broad ligament to cross over the ureter just lateral to the cervix at the level of the internal os. It then branches into inferior and superior divisions. The inferior division supplies the cervix and the upper vagina. The superior division supplies the corpus and anastomosis with the uterine branch of the ovarian artery at the level of the junction of the broad ligament and the cornu of the uterus just below the insertion of the fallopian tube. Occasionally these vessels are eroded by a cornual ectopic pregnancy, and sudden death is the result (Fig. 2–10).

The ovarian arteries arise from the aorta just below the renal vessels and course downward over the pelvic brim medial to the ureters. They then transverse the apex of the lateral broad ligament to the ovary. This is called the infundibulopelvic ligament. The right ovarian vein empties into the vena cava, but the left ovarian vein empties into the left renal vein.

Finally, the anatomy of the presacral area is important to the gynecologic surgeon. The rectal sigmoid is reflected to the left, and the peritoneum is opened in the midline over the second sacral vertebrasing. This is a very vascular area, with the vessels passing into the retroperitoneal space through the bilateral sacral foramina (Fig. 2–11). The least vascular area is in the immediate midline, and this is where periosteal sutures for sacrovaginal suspension

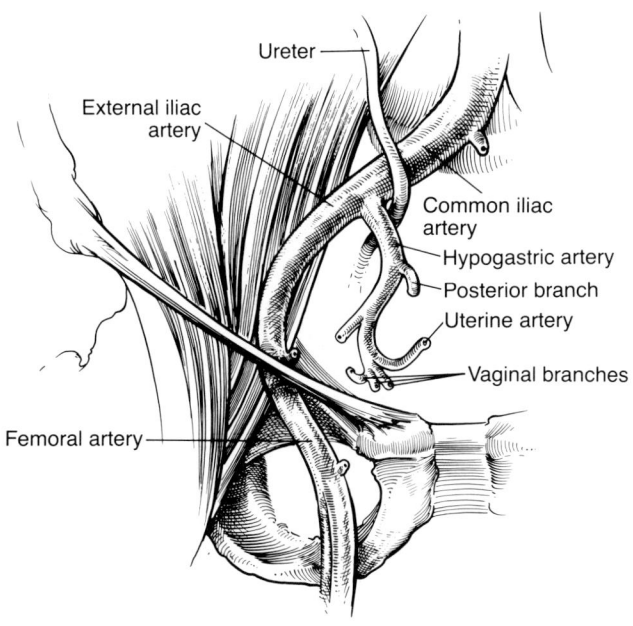

Figure 2–9
Lateral pelvic retroperitoneal space.

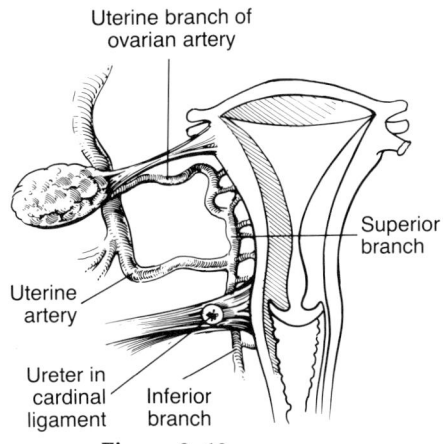

Figure 2–10
Blood supply to the uterus.

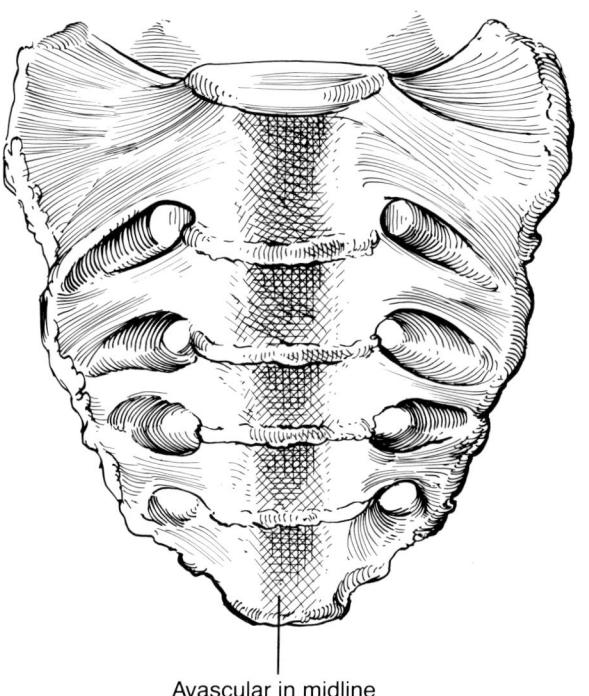

Figure 2–11
Presacral anatomy.

should be placed. This is also where the presacral nerve or sacral plexus is located. Lymphatics from the uterine corpus also traverse the presacral area to go directly to the periaortic nodes.

Vulvovaginal Anatomy

In this text, extensive anatomic descriptions are included in the chapters dealing with specific operative techniques. The pelvis can be likened to a cylinder that in the upright position is vertical and in the supine or lithotomy position is horizontal. The base or bottom is the levator sling, a combination of the levator ani and the coccygeus muscles and their intervening fascia. This sling is perforated by the urethra, vagina, and anus from front to back. External to the sling are the structures of the vulva and vestibule of the vagina.

Internal to the pelvic floor is the majority of the vagina with the urethra and base of the bladder anteriorly and the rectum posteriorly. The major blood supply for the cervix and vagina comes from the inferior branch of the uterine artery, and this is located at three o'clock and nine o'clock, respectively. Dissection anteriorly and posteriorly is relatively avascular. Likewise, the anterior and posterior cul-de-sac of the peritoneal cavity can be entered sharply through the vagina just anterior and posterior to the uterine cervix in the midline without significant bleeding.

The external genital organs are separated from the internal pelvis by the levator sling but more importantly by its external fascial cover. The most important and most dense is Colles' fascia, which continues with the anterior abdominal and lower extremity fasciae. This prevents a hematoma or abscess that is external from entering the pelvis unless it arises in the pararectal or paravaginal spaces. Thus, most hematomas or abscesses of the labia majora will extend up along the anterior abdominal wall but not into the pelvis or retroperitoneal spaces.

The major blood supply to the external genitalia is via the pudendal artery, which is a branch of the hypogastric artery. It follows the same pathway as the pudendal nerve, curving around the sacrospinous ligament. Here these structures can be damaged during sacrospinous suspension.

The gynecologic surgeon must remember that the lower third of the vagina, the vestibule, and the anus arise from the urogenital plate and that the lymphatic drainage for these structures is up along the labial crural folds to the superficial inguinal region (Fig. 2–12).

Nerves and Gynecologic Surgery

Four major areas of concern during gynecologic surgery involve the peripheral nervous system. Foremost is an understanding of where all nerves lie in relationship to other anatomic structures, and the

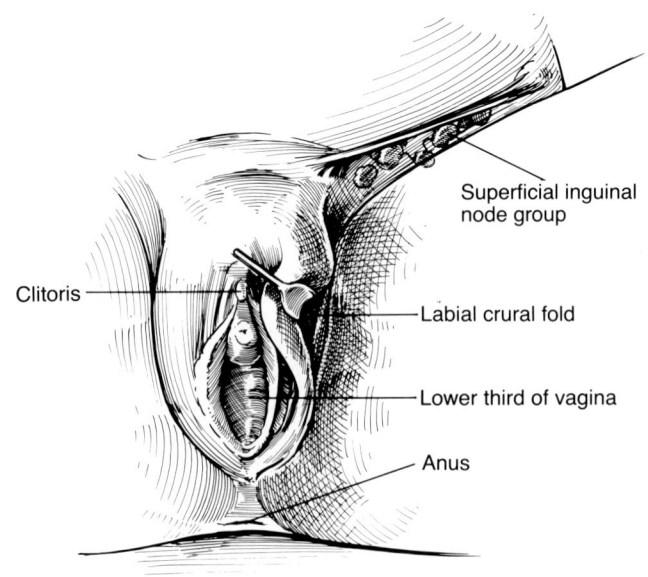

Figure 2–12
Lymphatic drainage of the lower vagina and vulva.

surgeon is referred to standard anatomic texts and other chapters in this text.

The femoral nerve (L2, L3, L4) runs along the medial surface of the psoas muscle and can be injured during surgery by excessive lateral traction, most commonly with a low transverse or Pfannenstiel incision. Prevention involves appropriate padding, using the shortest possible blades on the retractor, and examination to ensure that the blade is not impinging on the psoas muscle. Injury will result in numbness to the anterior surface of the thigh or inability to walk. The former is sensory damage, and the latter is motor damage resulting in inability to flex at the thigh or extend at the knee.

The sciatic nerve (L4, L5, S1, S2, S3) is injured with stretching by inappropriate and/or prolonged positioning for pelvic surgery. Adduction and lateral flexion in the exaggerated dorsal lithotomy position are the most common causes. This nerve can also be injured during sacral spinous suspension because it lies just lateral to the sacral spinous ligament. Injury to the sciatic nerve results in motor and/or sensory loss to the posterior lateral lower leg and the foot. Temporary footdrop is the most common manifestation of this stretch injury.

The pudendal nerve (S2, S3, S4) is injured during lower abdominal incision, resulting in sensory injury usually presenting as some variety of pain in the lower abdominal region, mons, or upper vulva. After ruling out hematoma, abscess, or suture rejection, re-exploration to remove the injured nerve may be required. This should be attempted only if the patient responds to a local nerve block.

Finally, in radical pelvic surgery the innervation of the lower rectum and/or bladder (L1–S4) may be compromised, depending upon the radicality of the uterosacral ligament removal. The obturator nerve (L2, L3, L4) may be inadvertently injured during deep pelvic node dissection. The former would result in inability to void or defecate and the latter in inability to adduct the leg.

SUMMARY

The gynecologic surgeon is encouraged to have a complete understanding of the embryology and anatomy of the female pelvis and all of its related structures in order to provide the most optimal of patient care. The surgeon should understand that even with the most careful dissection and competent surgical technique, injuries may result, and understanding the anatomy of the region will allow for early recognition and appropriate repair.

References

1. Corliss CD: Patten's Human Embryology. New York, McGraw-Hill, 1976, p. 361.
2. Markee JE: The Female Perineum and Pelvis. Durham, NC: Duke University Press, 1963, p. 1.
3. Williams PL, Warwick R, Dyson M, Bannister LH: Gray's Anatomy. Edinburgh, Churchill Livingstone, 1989.
4. Nichols DH: Clinical Problems, Injuries and Complications of Gynecologic Surgery. Baltimore, Williams & Wilkins, 1988.
5. Kuist-Poulson H, Borel J: Iatrogenic femoral neuropathy subsequent to abdominal hysterectomy: Incidence and prevention. Obstet Gynecol 1982; 60:516.

Preoperative and Postoperative Care

3

Daniel L. Clarke-Pearson
George J. Olt
Gustavo Rodriguez
Matthew Boente

The successful outcome of gynecologic surgery is based on thorough evaluation and preoperative preparation of the patient and careful postoperative management. This chapter discusses approaches to the general perioperative management of patients undergoing major gynecologic surgery and discusses specific medical problems that could complicate the surgical outcome.

PREOPERATIVE PREPARATION

Medical History and Physical Examination

The hazards of undertaking surgery without a thorough understanding of a patient's medical history and performing a complete physical examination cannot be overstated. The preoperative medical history should include any significant medical history or medical illnesses that might be aggravated by or complicate anesthesia or surgical recovery. Inquiry should be made as to current medications taken, even those discontinued within the previous months prior to surgery. This should include notation of nonprescription drugs taken, and the use of oral contraceptives, because many patients consider these medications a routine part of their living rather than a medication. Specific instructions must be given to the patient as to the need to discontinue any medications prior to surgery (such as aspirin or oral contraceptives) as well as identifying those medications that should be continued (such as cardiac or antihypertensive medications).

The patient should be questioned as to known allergies to medications (such as sulfonamides and penicillin), as well as other allergies to foods or environmental allergens. A history of sensitivity to shellfish may be the only clue to an iodine sensitivity, which may be significant because iodinated intravenous contrast material is used for intravenous pyelography, enhanced CT scanning, and venography/arteriography. Patients with a history of hypersensitivity to previous intravenously administered iodine-containing compounds or shellfish should be clearly noted, and these patients should not undergo further exposure to iodine-containing compounds unless absolutely mandatory. When intravenous contrast must be used, corticosteroid preparations may prevent life-threatening anaphylactic reactions.

Previous surgical procedures and the patient's course following those surgical procedures should be reviewed in order to identify complications of previous operations that might be avoided. Reaction and response to anesthetic techniques should be evaluated with the anesthesiologist in charge. Inquiries should be made as to specific complications, such as excessive bleeding, wound infection, deep vein thrombosis, peritonitis, or bowel obstruction. A history of prior pelvic surgery should alert the gynecologist to the possibility of distorted surgical anatomy and possible pre-existing injury to adjacent organ systems such as small bowel adhesions in the pelvis or ureteral stenosis from previous periureteral scarring. An intravenous pyelogram may be helpful in such cases to establish ureteral anatomy and patency and to identify any pre-existing abnormality. Many patients may not be entirely certain as to the extent of the previous surgical procedure or the details of intraoperative findings. Therefore, operative notes from previous pelvic operations should be obtained and reviewed to determine the details of the prior surgical procedure and surgical findings. This is particularly important in patients who have had surgery for pelvic inflammatory disease, pelvic abscess, endometriosis, or pelvic malignancy.

Family history may identify familial traits that might complicate planned surgery. A family history of excessive intraoperative or postoperative bleeding, malignant hyperthermia, and other potentially inherited conditions should be sought. General review of systems should also be included in the questioning, searching for any other coexisting medical or surgical conditions. Inquiry as to gastrointestinal and urologic function is particularly important prior to undertaking pelvic surgery, and many gynecologic diseases also involve adjacent nongynecologic viscera.

Although many women undergoing gynecologic surgical procedures are otherwise healthy, with pathology identified only on pelvic examination, other major organ systems must not be neglected in the physical examination. Identification of abnormalities such as a heart murmur or pulmonary compromise should lead the surgeon to obtain additional testing and consultation in order to minimize intraoperative and postoperative complications.

Laboratory Evaluation

The selection of appropriate preoperative laboratory studies depends upon the extent of the anticipated surgical procedure and the patient's medical status. For patients undergoing general anesthesia, a blood count including hematocrit, white cell count, and platelet count should be routinely obtained. Serum chemistries and liver function testing are rarely abnormal in the asymptomatic patient who has no significant medical history and who is not taking medications. Likewise, coagulation studies are of little value unless the patient has a significant medical history.[1] In women under age 40, a chest x-ray and cardiogram are likewise of very low yield in identifying asymptomatic cardiopulmonary disease and may not be necessary.[2,3] On the other hand, women over age 40 and those undergoing major gynecologic surgical procedures should have a chest x-ray, cardiogram, and serum electrolyte study preoperatively. Even if these studies are normal, they will serve as baseline data for comparison with other studies that might be required in the evaluation of a postoperative complication.

Radiographic evaluation of adjacent organ systems should be undertaken in individual cases. For example, an intravenous pyelogram (IVP) is helpful to delineate ureteral patency and course, especially in such cases as a pelvic mass, gynecologic cancer, or congenital müllerian anomaly. However, an IVP is not of significant value in the evaluation of the majority of patients undergoing pelvic surgery.[4] A barium enema or upper GI series with small bowel follow-through may be of significant value in evaluating some patients prior to undergoing pelvic surgery. Because of the proximity of the female genital tract with the lower gastrointestinal tract, the rectum and sigmoid colon may be involved with benign (endometriosis or pelvic inflammatory disease) or malignant gynecologic conditions. Conversely, a pelvic mass could be of gastrointestinal origin such as a diverticular abscess or a mass of inflamed small intestines (Crohn's disease). Clearly, any patient with gastrointestinal symptomatology should be further evaluated with contrast radiographs as well as a proctosigmoidoscopy, or flexible sigmoidoscopy or colonoscopy. Other imaging studies, including ultrasound, CT scan, and MRI, are useful only in selected patients.

Preoperative Discussion and Informed Consent

The verbal and nonverbal rapport and trust that exist between the patient and her gynecologist begins on the initial office visit and should be built upon at each subsequent visit. When surgery is deemed advisable by the gynecologist, initial discussion should explain in sufficient detail to the patient the findings on examination and the results of testing, the natural history of the disease process, and the goals of the surgical procedure. Because most gynecologic surgery is elective, the gynecologist has the opportunity to thoroughly evaluate the patient from a medical point of view, as well as to allow the patient to develop psychologic coping mechanisms and to answer questions that may not have been initially raised. The surgeon should be available to answer these questions in person or by phone prior to actual hospital admission.

This preoperative discussion should serve to allay anxiety and fears that the patient may have and to answer any questions that may have developed in the preoperative period. The discussion should further expand on many issues relative to the surgery, its expected outcome, and risks, and is the basis for obtaining the signed informed consent.[5] This is an educational process for the patient and her family, and explanations need to be made in understandable terms by the physician. The following items should be discussed:

1. The nature and extent of the disease process
2. The extent of the actual operation proposed and potential modifications of this operation, depending upon unexpected intraoperative findings
3. The anticipated benefits of the operation, with a conservative estimate of successful outcome
4. The risks and potential complications of the surgery
5. Alternative methods of therapy and the risks and results of those alternative methods of therapy
6. The results likely if the patient remains untreated

After each item is discussed, the patient and family should be invited to ask questions.

A discussion of the nature and the extent of the disease process should explain in layman's terms the significance of the disease. Is it life-threatening, or will it likely result in significant disability or dysfunction? To what extent does the disease process alter the patient's daily living? If left untreated, could the disease spontaneously resolve, or could it potentially worsen? What is the time course and natural history of the disease?

The goals of the surgery should be discussed in detail. Some gynecologic surgical procedures are performed purely for diagnostic purposes (e.g., dilatation and curettage, cold knife conization, a diagnostic laparoscopy, or staging laparotomy), whereas most are clearly aimed at correcting an anatomic defect or a specific disease process. The extent of the surgery should be outlined, including which organs will be removed. Most patients like to be informed as to the type of surgical incision and the estimated duration of anesthesia.

The expected outcome of the surgical procedure should be explained. If the procedure is being performed for diagnostic purposes, the outcome will depend upon surgical or pathologic findings that are not known prior to surgery. When an anatomic condition is being corrected, the expected success of the operation should be discussed as well as the potential for failure of the operation. This should include a discussion of, for example, the probability of failure of tubal sterilization or the possibility that stress urinary incontinence may not be alleviated. When one is treating cancer, the possibility of finding more advanced disease and the potential need for adjunctive therapy (such as postoperative radiation therapy or chemotherapy) should be mentioned. Other issues of importance to the patient include discussion of loss of fertility or loss of ovarian function. These issues should be raised by the physician to make sure the patient understands adequately the pathophysiology that may result from the surgery, and also to allow her to express her feelings regarding these emotionally charged issues.

The risks and potential complications of the surgical procedure should be discussed with the patient, including the most frequent complications of the particular surgical procedure. For most major gynecologic surgery, the risks include intraoperative and postoperative hemorrhage, postoperative infection, venous thrombosis, and injury to adjacent viscera. If the patient has a pre-existing medical problem, what additional risks might be encountered? Unanticipated findings at the time of surgery should also be mentioned. For example, if the ovaries are found unexpectedly to be diseased, it may be the best surgical judgment that they should be removed.

The usual postoperative course should also be discussed in enough detail so that patient understands what to expect in the days following surgery. The information as to the need for a suprapubic catheter or prolonged central venous monitoring helps the patient accept her postoperative course and avoids surprises to the patient that may be very disconcerting. The expected duration of the recovery period, both in and outside of the hospital, should be noted.

Alternative methods of therapy are also to be mentioned as part of the preoperative discussion. Other medical management or other surgical approaches should be discussed, along with their potential benefits and complications. Finally, the patient should have an understanding as to the outcome of the disease should nothing be done. It should be clear to the patient following this discussion why the proposed surgery is the appropriate next step in her care. Witnesses to the preoperative discussion and signing of the consent form should include a family member and another member of the health care team. The informed consent discussion detailing the information given the patient should be documented in the patient's chart.

The anesthesiologist responsible for the surgical procedure should also have the opportunity to examine the patient, review her laboratory findings, and discuss the proposed anesthetic method with the patient. In many institutions, the consent to the administration of anesthetic is included in the sur-

GENERAL CONSIDERATIONS

Nutrition

Nutritional Assessment

Preoperative preparation that optimizes fluids, electrolytes, and nutritional state results in a more rapid recovery, fewer postoperative infections, and better wound healing.[6,7] The clinician's goal should be to quantify the causes and severity of undernutrition and to provide appropriate preoperative nutritional supplementation.

Carbohydrates, protein, and fat serve as the body's fuel sources that release energy when metabolized. Exogenous protein is needed to satisfy the essential amino acid requirement. In addition to protein, caloric requirements must be sustained to provide energy for the multitude of biologic processes. Glycolytic tissues (e.g., brain, RBCs) use glucose as their metabolic fuel, which, under normal conditions, is derived from carbohydrates, glycogen, or glycogenic amino acids. A second group of organs (e.g., heart, lung) derive energy from free fatty acids, ketone bodies, amino acids, and carbohydrates. The pattern of fuel usage varies greatly with the fasting-feeding cycle and is influenced by the endocrine system and hypermetabolic states such as sepsis, burns, extensive surgery, gastrointestinal disorders, and malignancy. To approximate the caloric needs, the patient's height, weight, sex, age, activity level, type of surgery required, and disease state must be taken into consideration. An example of this estimation can be seen in Table 3–1.[8] In severe hypermetabolic states, the energy requirement for heat loss alone can be up to 4000 kcal/day.[9] Additional problems leading to increased nutritional requirements include drug-nutrient interactions, including those with steroids, anticonvulsants, and antibiotics.[10] Chronic illness such as renal, endocrine, and cardiovascular disease may alter nutritional needs.[11] Gastrointestinal problems, namely short bowel syndrome, obstruction, enteric fistulas, prolonged

Table 3–1

Caloric Needs of Surgical Patients

1. Total daily calorie requirements:
   Basal energy expenditure (E_b) + energy for physical activity (E_{pa}) + energy of injury of surgery (E_{surg})
   a. E_b (kcal/day)
      Men = $66 + (13.7 \times W) + (5.0 \times H) - (6.8 \times A)$
      Women = $655 + (9.6 \times W) + (1.7 \times H) - (4.7 \times A)$
      Simplified: $E_b = 22 \times W$
      where W = weight (kg), H = height (cm), and A = age (yr)
   b. E_{pba} (kcal/kg/hr)

Activity level	Men	Women
Very light	1.5	1.3
Light	2.9	2.6
Moderate	4.3	4.1
Heavy	8.4	8.0

   c. E_{surg}

	(kcal/day)
Minor surgery (e.g., appendectomy)	50–75
Cholecystectomy	100
Partial gastrectomy	150
Severe trauma	200–500
Trauma with sepsis	500–1000
Burns	% burn × 40
Fever	$E_b \times 0.07 \times$ degrees of fever above 98.6° F

2. Net dietary intake = caloric intake (C_I) − caloric loss (C_L)
   a. C_I = (1) enteral
           (2) parenteral
   b. C_L = (1) urinary* = 100 kcal/day
           (2) fecal* = 75 kcal/day
           (3) SDA = 0.6 × total kcal intake/day, where SDA = specific dynamic action

3. Adequacy of energy intake:
   Maintenance: $C_I = C_L$
   Depletion: $C_I < C_L$
   Repletion: $C_I > C_L$

*Values assume normal fecal and urinary losses. Values will be correspondingly higher in uncontrolled diabetes (urinary loss) or malabsorption (fecal loss). When patients are receiving parenteral feedings, stool caloric losses will be reduced.
Adapted from Lubin MF, Walker HK, Smith RB: Medical Management of the Surgical Patient, 2nd ed. Stoneham, MA, Butterworth, 1988, pp. 9–10.

emesis, gastric suctioning, and diarrhea;[12, 13] and cancer-related problems, including side effects of chemotherapy, radiation enteritis, and extensive surgery, also account for increased nutritional requirements.[14-16]

Several measurements can help in the nutritional assessment of the preoperative patient. The most useful and important measurement is body weight. When recorded serially as a percentage of the ideal body weight, it is the single most important reflection of energy and protein reserve. One note of caution is that fluid overload and extracellular fluid deposition may give a false impression that nutritional stores are unaffected. Triceps skin-fold thickness can be used to derive a mid-arm fat area (MAFA), which is the simplest index of adipose stores.[17] The body's total protein reserve is estimated clinically by calculating the approximate muscle mass and visceral protein reserve. Muscle mass can be estimated from a 24-hour urine collection from which a creatinine/height index may be calculated. Visceral protein reserve is estimated by serum albumin and transferrin levels.[17] In general, hypoalbuminemia (≤ 2.5 mg/dl) coupled with weight loss ($\geq 10\%$) is associated with excessive surgical morbidity and mortality.[15, 18]

Preoperative Nutrition

For patients who require additional nutritional support, the route of administration to deliver the nutritional support must be chosen on an individual basis. Enteral nutrition should be considered first because it is the most economical and the easiest to deliver. Relative contraindications include intestinal obstruction, upper gastrointestinal bleeding, and diarrhea. Many different types of enteral feeding solutions exist, each one with varying caloric content, osmolality, fat content, protein content, lactose content, viscosity, and price. Depending on the patient's particular problem, delivery may be through a nasogastric tube, a pharyngotomy, a gastrostomy, or a jejunostomy tube. Adverse symptoms such as vomiting and diarrhea may be alleviated by slowing the rate of the infusion, although for the enteral route to be effective, the patient must be able to tolerate a volume of solution sufficient to deliver an adequate number of calories. Complications of enteral feeding include obstruction, aspiration, pharyngeal and esophageal erosions, vomiting, diarrhea, and electrolyte disturbances.

Peripheral parenteral nutrition can be delivered to supplement enteral feedings or may be given alone as a nutritional supplement. A 900-mOsm solution can be delivered through peripheral veins. Phlebitis, one common side effect, may be overcome by the addition of 5 mg of hydrocortisone to each liter of solution. Additional calories may be provided by peripheral intralipids. Monitoring of both parenteral nutrition and enteral alimentation by measurement of electrolytes, glucose, and transaminase should be performed approximately every 2–3 days for the first week and weekly thereafter, to ensure normality. If the combined route of nutritional support is insufficient or intolerable, central venous nutrition should be initiated.

Parenteral nutrition delivered to a central vein has gained acceptance as a means of providing nutritional support for a wide variety of medical and surgical problems. The gynecologic surgical literature has focused attention on central hyperalimentation in the setting of advanced gynecologic malignancies or in patients receiving chemotherapy. Central venous hyperalimentation (total parenteral nutrition [TPN]) is given when other routes have not or cannot meet the patient's nutritional needs. TPN must be delivered through the subclavian or internal jugular vein. The placement of this catheter must be performed with meticulous sterile technique, and proper daily care must be given to avoid infectious complications. Two to three liters per day of TPN solution usually maintains a eumetabolic patient. Trace metals (Co, I, Mn, Zn) and multivitamins are added to 1 liter each day. Folate and vitamin B_{12} must be added separately, because they are incompatible with the trace metals. Essential fatty acids are supplied weekly, and iron must be given if the hyperalimentation is prolonged or bone marrow stores become depleted. In patients with cardiac, liver, or renal dysfunction, special care must be taken to adjust the sodium, potassium, and amino acid concentration to meet the patient's needs.

Common problems with TPN include fluid overload, metabolic or electrolyte abnormalities, sepsis, pneumothorax/hemothorax, and air/catheter embolism. When TPN is managed by an experienced team, the most frequent serious problem, catheter infection, has been reduced from an incidence of 27% in 1969 to less than 7% in current studies.[19]

The role of preoperative TPN has been reviewed by many authors. Unfortunately, the role of TPN remains controversial because of its inherent risks and the difficulty in selecting patients who will benefit from the treatment. To date, all of the trials performed in a prospective randomized fashion have been done in nongynecologic patient populations. Who, then, should receive preoperative TPN?

A predictive model of nutritional status, designed and validated by Müller, will assist in identifying patients at risk for operative morbidity or mortality.[24] The prognostic nutritional index (PNI) is calculated using the following formula:

$$PNI = 158 - 16.6 [ALB] - 0.78 [TSF] - 0.2 [TFN] - 5.8 [DH]$$

where ALB = serum albumin (mg/ml); TSF = triceps skinfold thickness (cm), TFN = serum transferrin (mg/ml), and DH = delayed skin hypersensitivity (scale, 0–2). Patients with a score of greater than 30% are at high risk for postoperative complications.

There are four prospective, randomized, controlled studies indicating a benefit for administration of preoperative TPN.[20–23] Three studies have shown a decrease in the frequency of early septic events postoperatively.[21, 22, 24] In these studies, the patients received preoperative TPN for 7–20 days. Baseline weight maintenance, increased triceps skinfold thickness, improved immunologic status, and improved PNI were achieved preoperatively.[23] Improvement in survival has also been shown by Müller. However, because of the small number of patients, changing and improving surgical techniques, better antibiotics, and improvements in specific cancer and critical care treatments, all of the improvement in survival may not be due to preoperative TPN. Similarly, it has been impossible to prove or disprove the cost effectiveness of TPN. Other larger, multicenter trials will be necessary to definitively answer these questions.

In general, it is our opinion that because of the expense and potential complications, preoperative TPN should be given only to those patients who would obviously benefit from improving their nutritional status and who would not suffer from a delay in their surgery.

Postoperative Nutritional Support

The routine use of nutritional adjuvants in the postoperative period for gynecologic patients has some appealing theoretical advantages. However, as with the use of these adjuvants preoperatively, the question of whether the improvement in nutritional indices correlates with an improved clinical outcome and whether this therapy is cost effective is a matter of some debate.

If nutritional therapy is delayed until after surgery, the theoretical advantage of correcting the nutritional deficit prior to the stress of surgery is lost. Despite this disadvantage, TPN, if administered early in the postoperative course, has been shown to correct serum albumin and transferrin levels and can reverse a negative nitrogen balance.[25] No prospective, randomized trials in gynecologic patients exist to evaluate the clinical outcome of patients who receive TPN in the postoperative period. However, of several trials from the general surgical literature that have evaluated this issue in depth, one dealing with patients undergoing abdominal-perineal resection contains information that can be useful for gynecologic surgeons. The patients had both benign and malignant diagnoses and were divided into three groups: group I received routine maintenance intravenous fluids postoperatively, group II received 4.25% amino acids only (0.23 ± 0.01 g/kg/day of nitrogen), and group III received a full course of TPN (0.23 ± 0.02 g/kg/day of nitrogen and 25% glucose equivalent to 36.5 ± 3.5 kcal/kg/day). The adjuvant nutrition was started on postoperative day 2 or 3 and continued for 13 days. Group I was slowly advanced to a regular diet as tolerated. Each patient was evaluated postoperatively for transferrin, prealbumin, retinol binding protein, albumin, body composition, and plasma amino acid levels.

Group III (patients receiving full-course TPN) demonstrated significantly shorter healing times for their perineal wounds and shorter hospitalizations. In addition, the TPN therapy spared more body protein and fat and restored plasma amino acids to normal levels as compared with groups I and II. Plasma proteins, which were depleted in all patients in the immediate postoperative period, were restored only in group III. A positive nitrogen balance was observed only in groups II and III. In addition, weight loss was documented in the groups not receiving full TPN. No significant differences could be documented in septic morbidity or mortality between the three groups.

Several additional postoperative problems in gynecologic patients deserve mentioning. Postoperative gastrointestinal fistulas are a well-recognized problem, particularly to the gynecologic oncologist. Furthermore, they are extremely difficult to manage medically or surgically and pose an incredible inconvenience for the patient. Conservative management with TPN, total bowel rest, and appropriate antibiotics occasionally results in complete closure. The use of a somatostatin analogue has been shown to reduce enterocutaneous fistula output and has achieved as high as a 77% spontaneous closure rate. Long half-life somatostatin analogue SMS 201-995 has an inhibitory action on gastrin, pancreatic exocrine function, bile flow, and intestinal secretion, which makes its use more clinically appealing than somatostatin.[26] Its effectiveness in this situation will need to be documented in a large series, but the preliminary results appear encouraging. Even if medical management is not successful, the interval of TPN and the medical management should improve the patient's general status and result in improved surgical outcome when the fistula is ultimately repaired.

Postoperative small bowel obstruction may also be initially managed with nutritional adjuvants. Conservative management with gastrointestinal decompression and TPN should be considered for patients with postoperative small bowel obstruction with the hope that bowel rest and nutritional support will allow resolution of the obstruction. Patients whose medical management requires nothing by mouth for periods of 7 days or longer might also be considered candidates for TPN. In the special case of patients with ovarian carcinoma and intestinal obstruction, tumor burden, serum albumin, and nutritional score have been shown to correlate with postoperative survival and surgical complications.[27] This information may aid the clinician in selecting patients prior to surgery for correction of the bowel obstruction and suggests that preoperative TPN may improve surgical outcome.

A definitive conclusion cannot currently be made as to the efficacy or cost effectiveness of adjuvant nutritional therapy. The variety of TPN formulations as well as the many other clinical variables cannot be directly applied to the gynecologic surgery patient. However, most of the adequately designed studies in the general surgical literature demonstrate trends towards improved outcome in the patients receiving adjuvant nutritional therapy. The use of these agents should be individualized based on age, the magnitude of the proposed surgery, the magnitude of the nutritional deficit, and the particular illness of the patient in question.

Fluid and Electrolytes

In the average woman, total water constitutes approximately 50–55% of body weight. Two-thirds of this water is contained in the intracellular compartment. One-third is contained in the extracellular compartment, of which one-fourth is contained in plasma, and the remaining three-quarters is in the interstitium.

Osmolarity, or tonicity, is a property derived from the number of particles in a solution. Sodium and chloride are the primary electrolytes contributing to the osmolarity in the extracellular fluid compartment. Potassium and, to a lesser extent, magnesium and phosphate are the major intracellular electrolytes. Water flows freely between the intracellular and the extracellular spaces so as to maintain osmotic neutrality throughout the body. Any shifts in osmolarity in any fluid spaces within the body will be accompanied by corresponding shifts in free water from spaces of lower to higher osmolarity, thus maintaining a balance in equilibrium.

The daily fluid maintenance requirement for the average adult is approximately 30 ml/kg/day, or 2000–3000 ml/day.[28] This is offset partially by insensible losses of 1200 ml/day, which includes losses from the lungs (600 ml), skin (400 ml), and gastrointestinal tract (200 ml). Urinary output from the kidney provides the remainder of the fluid loss, and this output will vary, depending on total body intake of water and sodium. Approximately 600–800 mOsm of solute is excreted by the kidney per day. Healthy kidneys can concentrate urine up to approximately 1200 mOsm, and therefore, minimum output can range between 500 and 700 ml/day. The maximal urinary output capability of the kidney can be as high as 20 liters/day, as seen in patients with diabetes insipidus. In the healthy patient, the normal kidney adjusts urine output commensurate with the daily fluid intake.

The major extracellular buffer used in acid-base balance is the bicarbonate–carbonic acid system:[29] $CO_2 + H_2O \rightleftharpoons H_2CO_3 \rightleftharpoons H^+ + HCO_3^-$. Typically, the body will maintain a bicarbonate to carbonic acid ratio of 20:1 in order to maintain an extracellular pH of 7.4. Both the lung and the kidney play integral roles in the maintenance of normal extracellular pH, via retention or excretion of carbon dioxide and bicarbonate. Under conditions of alkalosis, minute ventilation decreases and renal excretion of bicarbonate increases such as to restore the normal bicarbonate to carbonic acid ratio. The opposite occurs with acidosis.

Ultimately, the kidney plays the most important role in fluid and electrolyte balance through excretion and retention of water and solute. Circulating antidiuretic hormone and aldosterone help modulate the process. Hypothalamic release of antidiuretic hormone is sensitive to serum osmolarity, and aldosterone secretion is responsive to renal perfusion. Under states of dehydration or hypovolemia, serum antidiuretic hormone levels increase, leading to increased resorption of water in the distal tubule of the kidney. In addition, increased aldosterone release promotes increased renal sodium and water retention. The opposite occurs in states of fluid excess. As a result, the individual with normal renal function as well as normal circulating antidiuretic hormone and aldosterone levels maintains normal serum osmolarity and electrolyte composition despite daily fluctuation of fluid and electrolyte intake.

Various disease states can alter the normal fluid and electrolyte homeostatic mechanisms, making perioperative fluid and electrolyte management more difficult. In patients with intrinsic renal disease, there is an inability to excrete solute and to maintain acid-base balance. In patients with the stress of chronic starvation or severe illness, there may be an inappropriately high level of circulating antidiuretic hormone and aldosterone, resulting in fluid and sodium retention. With severe cardiac disease, secondary renal hypoperfusion can lead to increased aldosterone synthesis and, therefore, increased sodium and water retention by the kidney. Finally, the patient with severe diabetes can have a significant osmotic diuresis as well as have acid-base dysfunction secondary to circulating ketoacids. Correction and optimization of renal, cardiac, or endocrinologic disorders preoperatively are imperative and will often rectify fluid and electrolyte abnormalities.

Fluid and electrolyte management in the preoperative and perioperative period requires a knowledge of the daily fluid and electrolyte requirements for maintenance, replacement of ongoing fluid and electrolyte losses, and correction of any existing abnormalities. Each of these three factors is considered separately in the following discussion.

Fluid and Electrolyte Maintenance Requirements

The normal daily fluid requirement in the average adult is 2000–3000 ml. The body can and does adjust to higher and lower volumes of intake via changes in plasma tonicity. Alterations in plasma tonicity induce adjustments in circulating antidiuretic hormone, which ultimately regulates the amount of water retained in the distal tubule of the kidney. The daily requirement for various electrolytes is shown in Table 3–2. In the preoperative and the early postoperative patient, it is usually only necessary to replace sodium and potassium. Chloride is automatically replaced concomitant with sodium and potassium because chloride is the usual anion used to balance sodium and potassium in electrolyte solutions. There are various commercially available solutions containing 40 mmol of sodium chloride, with smaller amounts of potassium, calcium, and magnesium, designed to meet the requirements of a patient who is receiving 3 liters of intravenous fluids per day. The daily requirement, however, can be met by any combination of intravenous fluid orders. For example, 2 liters of D5 45 normal saline (NS) (7 mEq sodium chloride each), supplemented with 20 mEq of potassium chloride, followed by 1 liter of D5W with 20 mEq of potassium chloride, would suffice.

Fluid and Electrolyte Replacement

Fluid and electrolyte losses beyond the daily average must be replaced by appropriate solutions. The choice of solutions for replacement depends on the composition of the fluids lost. Often, it is difficult to measure free water loss, particularly in patients who have high "insensible" losses from the lungs or skin, or into the gastrointestinal tract. These insensible losses are difficult to monitor. Procurement of daily weights in these patients can be very useful. Up to 300 g of weight loss daily can be attributable to weight loss from catabolism of protein and fat in the patient who is taking nothing by mouth.[28] Anything beyond this, however, would be due to fluid loss and should be replaced accordingly.

The patient with a high fever can have increased pulmonary and skin loss of free water, sometimes in excess of 2–3 liters/day. These losses should be replaced with free water in the form of D5W. Perspiration typically has one-third the osmolarity of plasma and can be replaced with D5W or, if excessive, with D5 25NS.

The patient with acute blood loss needs replacement with appropriate isotonic fluid and/or blood. There are a wide range of plasma volume expanders, including albumin, dextran, and hetastarch solutions, which contain large molecular weight particles (>50,000 molecular weight). These particles are slow to exit the intravascular space, with about one-half of the particles remaining after 24 hours. These solutions are expensive, however, and for most cases, simple replacement with .9 normal saline or lactated Ringer's solution will suffice. One-third of the volume of lactated Ringer's or normal saline will typically remain in the intravascular space, the remainder going to the interstitium.

Appropriate replacement of gastrointestinal fluid loss is dependent upon the source of fluid loss in the gastrointestinal tract. Gastrointestinal secretions beyond the stomach, and up to the colon, are typically isotonic with plasma (Table 3–3), with similar amounts of sodium; slightly lower amounts of chloride; slightly alkaline pH; and with more potassium, in the range of 10–20 mEq/liter. Under normal conditions, stool is hypotonic. However, under conditions of increased flow (i.e., severe diarrhea), stool contents are isotonic with a composition similar to that of the small bowel. Gastric contents are typically hypotonic, with one-third the sodium of plasma, increased amounts of hydrogen ion, and low pH.

In the patient with gastric outlet obstruction, nausea and vomiting, or nasogastric suction, appropriate replacement of gastric secretions can be provided with a solution such as D5 45 NS with 20 mEq/liter of potassium. Potassium supplementation is particularly important to prevent hypokalemia in these patients, whose kidneys attempt to conserve hydrogen ion in the distal tubule of the kidney, in exchange for potassium ion.

In patients with bowel obstruction, 1–3 liters of fluid can be sequestered daily in the gastrointestinal tract. This fluid should be replaced with isotonic saline or lactated Ringer's solutions. Patients with

Table 3–2

Daily Maintenance Parenteral Requirements

Sodium	100–140 mEq
Potassium	40–60 mEq
Magnesium	30 mEq
Calcium	15 mEq
Carbohydrate	100–150 g
Water	1500 ml/m^2 body surface area

Adapted from Magrina JF: Intravenous fluids and blood component therapy. Clin Obstet Gynecol 1988; 31:686–689.

Table 3–3

Composition of Gastrointestinal Secretions

	Volume (ml/24 h)	Na (mEq/L)	K (mEq/L)	Cl (mEq/L)	HCO_3 (mEq/L)
Salivary	1500 (500–2000)	10 (2–10)	26 (20–30)	10 (8–18)	30
Stomach	1500 (100–4000)	60 (9–116)	10 (0–32)	130 (8–154)	—
Duodenum	(100–2000)	140	5	80	—
Ileum	3000 (100–9000)	140 (80–150)	5 (2–8)	104 (43–137)	30
Colon	—	60	30	40	—
Pancreas	(100–800)	140 (113–185)	5 (3–7)	75 (54–95)	115
Bile	(50–800)	145 (131–164)	5 (3–12)	100 (89–180)	35

From Shires GT, Canizaro P: Fluid and electrolyte management of the surgical patient. In Sabiston DC Jr (ed.): Textbook of Surgery, 14th ed. Philadelphia, WB Saunders Co., 1991, p. 74.

enterocutaneous fistulas or new ileostomies should similarly have isotonic fluid replacement.

Correction of Existing Fluid and Electrolyte Abnormalities

The patient who presents preoperatively with fluid and/or electrolyte abnormalities can pose a diagnostic challenge. The correct diagnosis and therapy are contingent upon a correct assessment of total body fluid and electrolyte status. The management of hyponatremia, for example, may be either fluid restriction or fluid replacement, with the treatment choice dependent upon whether there is an overall extracellular fluid excess and normal body sodium stores or decreased overall total body sodium stores and extracellular fluid. A detailed history is necessary, for documentation of any underlying medical illness as well as for assessment of the amount and duration of any abnormal fluid losses or intake. Initial evaluation should include an assessment of hemodynamic, clinical, and urinary parameters in order to assess the overall level of hydration systemically as well as the fluid status of the extracellular fluid compartment. The patient who has good skin turgor, moist mucosa, stable vital signs, and good urinary output is well hydrated. Nonpitting edema is indicative of extracellular fluid excess, whereas the patient who presents with orthostasis, sunken eyes, parched mouth, and decreased skin turgor clearly has extracellular volume contraction. On a cautionary note, a patient's overall extracellular fluid status does not always reflect the hydration status of the intravascular compartment. A patient can have increased interstitial fluid, yet be intravascularly dry, requiring replacement with isotonic fluid.

Laboratory work-up for patients who may have pre-existing fluid problems should include hematocrit, serum chemistries, glucose, blood urea nitrogen (BUN) and creatinine, urine osmolarity, and urine electrolytes. Serum osmolarity is mainly a function of the concentration of sodium and is given by the following equation:

$$2 \times Na^+ + \frac{glucose\ (mg/dl)}{18} + BUN\ (mg/dl)/2.8$$

Normal serum osmolarity is typically 290–300 mOsm. Blood hematocrit will rise or fall inversely at a rate of 1% for every 500-ml alteration of extracellular fluid volume. The BUN/creatinine ratio is typically 10:1 but will rise to a ratio of greater than 20:1 under conditions of extracellular fluid contraction. Under conditions of extracellular fluid deficit, urine osmolarity will typically be high (>400 mOsm), whereas urine sodium concentration will be low (less than 15 mEq/liter), indicative of an attempt by the kidney to conserve sodium. Under conditions of extracellular fluid excess or in cases of renal disease in which the kidney has impaired ability to retain sodium and water, urine osmolarity will be low with urine sodium high (>30 mEq/liter). Finally, changes in sodium can give insight as to the degree of extracellular fluid excess or deficit. In the average person, the serum sodium concentration rises by 3 mmol/liter for every liter of water deficit and falls by 3 mmol/liter for each liter of water excess. One must, however, be careful in making these estimates, in that the patient with prolonged water and electrolyte loss can present with low serum sodium concentration and marked water deficit.

Specific Electrolyte Disorders

Hyponatremia. Because sodium is the major extracellular cation, shifts in serum sodium are usually inversely correlated with the hydration state of the extracellular fluid compartment. The pathophysiology of hyponatremia, then, is usually expansion of body fluids leading to excess total body water.[29] Symptomatic hyponatremia usually does not occur until the serum sodium concentration is below 120–125 mEq/liter. The severity of the symptoms (nausea, vomiting, lethargy, seizures) is more related to the rate of change of serum sodium than to the actual serum sodium level.

Hyponatremia in the state of extracellular fluid excess can be seen in patients with renal or cardiac failure as well as in conditions such as nephrotic syndrome in which total body salt and water are increased, with a relatively greater increase in the latter. Administration of hypertonic saline to correct the hyponatremia would be inappropriate in this setting. The treatment should include, in addition to correcting the underlying disease process, water restriction with diuretic therapy.

Inappropriate secretion of antidiuretic hormone (ADH) can occur with head trauma, with pulmonary or cerebral tumors, and under states of stress. The abnormally elevated ADH results in excess water retention. Treatment includes water restriction and, if possible, correction of the underlying cause. Demecocycline has been shown to be effective in this disorder via its action in the kidney.

Inappropriate replacement of body salt losses with water alone will result in hyponatremia. This will typically occur in patients who are losing large amounts of electrolytes secondary to vomiting, nasogastric suction, diarrhea, or gastrointestinal fistulas and who are receiving replacement with hypotonic solutions. Simple replacement with isotonic fluids and potassium will usually correct the abnormality. Rarely will rapid correction of the hyponatremia be necessary, in which case hypertonic saline (3%) can be administered. Hypertonic saline should be very cautiously administered in order to avoid a rapid shift in serum sodium, which will induce central nervous system dysfunction.

Hypernatremia. Hypernatremia is an uncommon condition that can be life-threatening if severe (serum sodium level > 160 mEq/liter). The pathophysiology is one of extracellular fluid deficit. The resultant hyperosmolar state results in decreased water volume in cells in the central nervous system, which, if severe, can result in disorientation, seizures, intracranial bleeding, and death. The causes include excessive extrarenal water loss as can be seen in patients with high fever, tracheostomy in a dry environment, or extensive thermal injuries; in patients with diabetes insipidus, either central or nephrogenic; and with iatrogenic salt loading. The treatment involves correction of the underlying cause (correction of fever, humidification of the tracheostomy, vasopressin [Pitressin] for control of central diabetes insipidus) and replacement with free water either by the oral route or intravenously with D5W. As with severe hyponatremia, marked hypernatremia should be corrected slowly.

Hypokalemia. Hypokalemia may be encountered preoperatively in patients with significant gastrointestinal fluid loss (prolonged emesis, diarrhea, nasogastric suction, intestinal fistulas) or marked urinary potassium loss secondary to renal tubular disorders (renal tubular acidosis, acute tubular necrosis, hyperaldosteronism, prolonged diuretic use), or with prolonged administration of potassium-free parenteral fluids in patients who are NPO. The symptoms associated with hypokalemia include neuromuscular disturbances ranging from muscle weakness to flaccid paralysis and cardiovascular abnormalities including hypotension, bradycardia, arrhythmias, and enhancement of digitalis toxicity. These symptoms rarely occur unless the serum potassium level is below 3 mEq/liter. The treatment is potassium replacement. Oral therapy is preferable in patients who are on an oral diet. If necessary, potassium replacement can be given intravenously in doses that should not exceed 10 mEq/hour.

Hyperkalemia. Hyperkalemia is encountered infrequently in preoperative patients. It is usually associated with renal impairment but can also be seen in patients with adrenal insufficiency; with the use of potassium-sparing diuretics; and with marked tissue breakdown as can be seen in patients with crush injuries, massive gastrointestinal bleeding, or hemolysis. The clinical manifestations are mainly cardiovascular. Marked hyperkalemia (potassium level > 7 mEq/liter) can result in bradycardia, ventricular fibrillation, and cardiac arrest. The treatment chosen depends upon the severity of the hyperkalemia and whether or not there are associated cardiac or electrocardiographic abnormalities. Calcium gluconate (10 ml of a 10% solution) given intravenously can offset the toxic effects of hyperkalemia on the heart. One ampule each of sodium bicarbonate and D50 with or without insulin will cause a rapid shift of potassium into cells. Longer term, cation exchange resins such as sodium polystyrene sulfonate (Kayexalate), taken either orally or by enema, will bind and decrease total body potassium. Hemodialysis is reserved for emergent conditions in which other measures are not sufficient or have failed.

Postoperative Fluid and Electrolyte Management

There are several hormonal and physiologic alterations in the postoperative period that may complicate fluid and electrolyte management. The stress of surgery induces an inappropriately high level of circulating ADH. Circulating aldosterone levels are also increased, especially if sustained episodes of hypotension have occurred either intraoperatively or postoperatively. The elevated levels of circulating ADH and aldosterone make the postoperative patient prone to sodium and water retention.

Total body fluid volume may be significantly altered postoperatively. First, 1 ml of free water is released for each gram of fat or tissue that is catabolized and, in the postoperative period, several hundred milliliters of free water is released daily from tissue breakdown, particularly in the patient who has undergone extensive intra-abdominal dissection and who is NPO. This free water is often retained, secondary to the altered levels of ADH and aldosterone. Second, fluid retention is further enhanced by "third spacing," or sequestration of fluid in the surgical field. The development of an ileus may result in an additional 1–3 liters of fluid per day being sequestered in the bowel lumen, bowel wall, and peritoneal cavity.

In contrast to renal sodium homeostasis, the kidney lacks the capacity for retention of potassium. In the postoperative period, the kidney will continue to excrete a minimum of 30–60 mEq/liter daily,[29] irrespective of the serum potassium level and total body potassium stores. If this potassium loss is not replaced, hypokalemia may develop. Tissue damage and catabolism during the first postoperative day usually result in the release of sufficient intracellular potassium to meet the daily requirements. However, beyond the first postoperative day, potassium supplementation is necessary.

Maintenance of fluid and electrolyte balance in the postoperative period starts with the preoperative assessment, with emphasis on establishing normal fluid and electrolyte parameters prior to surgery. Postoperatively, close monitoring of daily weight, urine output, serum hematocrit, serum electrolytes, and hemodynamic parameters will yield the necessary information to make correct adjustments in crystalloid replacement. The normal daily fluid and electrolyte requirements must be met, and any unusual fluid and electrolyte losses, such as from the gastrointestinal tract, lungs, or skin, must be replaced. After the first few postoperative days, third-space fluid begins to mobilize back into the intravascular space and ADH and aldosterone levels revert to normal. The excess fluid retained perioperatively is thus mobilized and excreted through the kidneys, and exogenous fluid requirements decrease. The patient with inadequate cardiovascular or renal reserve is prone to fluid overload during this time of third-space reabsorption, especially if intravenous fluids are not appropriately reduced.

The most common fluid and electrolyte disorder in the postoperative period is fluid overload. The fluid excess can occur concomitant with normal or decreased serum sodium. Large amounts of isotonic fluids are usually infused intraoperatively and postoperatively to maintain blood pressure and urine output. Because the infused fluid is often isotonic with plasma, it will remain in the extravascular space. Under such conditions, serum sodium will remain within normal levels. Fluid excess with hypotonicity (decreased serum sodium) can occur if large amounts of isotonic fluid losses (e.g., blood and gastrointestinal tract) are inappropriately replaced with hypotonic fluids. Again, the predisposition towards retention of free water in the immediate postoperative period compounds the problem. An increase in body weight will occur concomitant with fluid expansion. In the patient who is NPO, catabolism should induce a daily weight loss as great as 300 g/day. Clearly, the patient who is gaining weight in excess of 150 g/day is in a state of fluid expansion. Simple fluid restriction will correct the abnormality. When necessary, diuretics can be employed to increase urinary water excretion.

States of fluid dehydration are uncommon but will occur in the patient who has large daily fluid losses that are not replaced. Gastrointestinal losses should be replaced with the appropriate fluids. Patients with high fevers should be given appropriate free water replacement, in that up to 2 liters/day of free water can be lost through perspiration and hyperventilation. Although these increased insensible losses are difficult to monitor, a reliable estimate can be obtained via the trend in body weight.

Postoperative Acid-Base Disorders

A variety of metabolic, respiratory, and electrolyte abnormalities in the postoperative period can result in an imbalance in normal acid-base homeostasis, leading to alkalosis or acidosis. Changes in the respiratory rate will directly affect the amount of carbon dioxide that is exhaled. A respiratory acidosis will result from carbon dioxide retention in patients who have hypoventilation from central nervous system depression, as seen under conditions of oversedation from narcotics, particularly in the presence of concurrent severe chronic obstructive pulmonary disease. A respiratory alkalosis will result from hyperventilation either due to excitation of the central nervous system from drugs or pain, or iatrogenically from excess ventilator support. Numerous metabolic derangements can result in alkalosis or acidosis, and these are discussed further in this section. Fortunately, proper fluid and electrolyte replacement as well as maintenance of adequate tissue perfusion will help to prevent most acid-base disorders in the postoperative period.

Alkalosis. The most common acid-base disorder encountered in the postoperative period is alkalosis.[29] The alkalosis is usually of no clinical significance and resolves spontaneously. Several etiologic factors may include hyperventilation associated with pain; posttraumatic transient hyperaldosteronism, which results in decreased renal bicarbonate excretion; nasogastric suction, which removes hydrogen ion; infused bicarbonate during blood transfusions in the form of citrate, which is converted to bicarbonate; administration of exogenous alkali; and use of diuretics. Correction of the alkalosis can usually be easily achieved with removal of the inciting cause, as well as with correction of extracellular fluid and potassium deficits (Table 3–4). Full correction can usually be safely achieved over 1–2 days.

Marked alkalosis, with serum pH greater than 7.55, can result in serious cardiac arrhythmias or central nervous system seizures. Myocardial excitability will be particularly pronounced with concurrent hypokalemia. Under such conditions, fluid and electrolyte replacement may not be sufficient to rapidly correct the alkalosis. Acetazolamide (250–500 mg) orally or intravenously can be given two to four times daily to induce renal bicarbonate diuresis. Treatment with an acidifying agent is rarely necessary and should be reserved for acutely symptomatic patients (cardiac or CNS dysfunction) or for patients with advanced renal disease. Under such conditions, HCl (5–10 mEq/hour of a 100-mmol solution) can be given via a central line. Ammonium chloride can also be given orally or intravenously but should not be given in patients with hepatic disease.

Acidosis. Metabolic acidosis is less common than alkalosis in the postoperative period but can be potentially serious as a result of its effect on the cardiovascular system. Under conditions of acidosis, there are decreased myocardial contractility, a propensity for vasodilation of the peripheral vasculature leading to hypotension, and refractoriness of the fibrillating heart to defibrillation.[29] These effects promote decompensation of the cardiovascular system and can hinder attempts at resuscitative efforts.

The primary pathophysiology of metabolic acidosis results from a decrease in serum bicarbonate level as a result of consumption and replacement of bicarbonate by circulating acids, or owing to replacement by other anions such as chloride. The proper work-up includes a measurement of the anion gap:

$$\text{Anion gap} = Na^+ - (Cl^- + HCO_3^-) = 10\text{--}14 \text{ mEq/liter (normal)}$$

The anion gap is composed of circulating protein, sulfate, phosphate, citrate, and lactate.[32]

Patients with metabolic acidosis can be divided into two groups based on the anion gap (increased vs. normal anion gap). An increase in circulating acids will consume and replace bicarbonate ion, thus increasing the anion gap. The causes include an increase in circulating lactic acid secondary to anaerobic glycolysis, such as is seen under conditions of poor tissue perfusion; increased ketoacids, as is seen in cases of severe diabetes or starvation; exogenous toxins; and renal dysfunction, which leads to increased circulating sulfates and phosphates.[33] The diagnosis can be established via a thorough history and measurement of serum lactate (normal < 2 mmol/liter), serum glucose, and renal function parameters. Metabolic acidosis in the face of a normal anion gap is usually the result of an imbalance of the ions chloride and bicarbonate, under conditions leading to excess chloride and decreased bicarbonate. Hyperchloremic acidosis can be seen in patients who have undergone saline loading. Bicarbonate loss will be seen in patients with small bowel fistula, new ileostomies, severe diarrhea, or renal tubular acidosis. Finally, in patients with marked extracellular volume expansion, as is seen commonly postoperatively, the relative decrease in serum sodium and bicarbonate will result in a mild acidosis. A summary of the various causes of metabolic acidosis is shown in Table 3–5.

The treatment of metabolic acidosis depends on the cause. In patients with lactic acidosis, restoration of tissue perfusion is imperative. This can be done through cardiovascular and pulmonary support as needed, oxygen therapy, and aggressive treatment

Table 3–4

Metabolic Alkalosis

Disorder	Source of Alkali	Cause of Renal HCO$_3$ Retention
Gastrric alkalosis		
Nasogastric suction	Gastric mucosa	↓ ECF, ↓ K
Vomiting		
Renal alkalosis		
Diuretics	Renal epithelium	↓ ECF, ↓ K
Respiratory acidosis and diuretics		↓ ECF, ↓ K, ↑ PCO$_2$
Exogenous base	NaHCO$_3$, Na citrate, Na lactate	Coexisting disorder of ECF, K, PaCO$_2$

↓ ECF, extracellular fluid depletion; ↓ K, potassium depletion; ↑ PCO$_2$, carbon dioxide retention.

Table 3–5

Causes of Metabolic Acidosis

	Normal Anion Gap	
High Anion Gap	*Hyperkalemic*	*Hypokalemic*
Uremia	Hyporeninism	Diarrhea
Ketoacidosis	Primary adrenal failure	Renal tubular
Lactic acidosis	NH₄Cl	acidosis
Aspirin	Sulfur poisoning	Ileal and sigmoid
Paraldehyde	Early chronic renal	bladders
Methanol	failure	Hyperalimentation
Ethylene glycol	Obstructive uropathy	
Methylmalonic aciduria		

From Narins RG, Lazarus MJ: Renal system. In Vandam LD (ed.): To Make the Patient Ready for Anesthesia: Medical Care of the Surgical Patient, 2nd ed. Menlo Park, CA, Addison-Wesley Publishing Co., 1984, pp. 67–114.

of systemic infection wherever appropriate. Ketosis from diabetes can be corrected gradually with insulin therapy. Ketosis resulting from chronic starvation or from lack of caloric support postoperatively can be corrected with nutrition. In patients with normal anion gap acidosis, bicarbonate losses from the gastrointestinal tract should be replaced, excess chloride administration can be curtailed, and, where necessary, a loop diuretic can be used to induce renal clearance of chloride. Dilutional acidosis can be corrected with mild fluid restriction.

Bicarbonates should not be given unless serum pH is less than 7.2, or unless there are severe cardiac complications secondary to acidosis. Furthermore, close monitoring of serum potassium is mandatory. Under states of acidosis, potassium will exit the cell and enter the circulation. The patient with a normal potassium concentration and metabolic acidosis is actually intracellularly potassium depleted. Treatment of the acidosis without potassium replacement will result in severe hypokalemia with its associated risks. A summary of the various acid-base abnormalities and associated therapies is shown in Table 3–6.

Pain Management

General Principles

Although satisfactory analgesia is easily achievable with currently available methods, patients continue to suffer unnecessarily from postoperative pain. A number of studies, many reviewed by Edwards,[34] have consistently shown that 30–40% of patients suffer moderate to severe pain in the postoperative period. There are several reasons for the existing inadequacies in pain management. First, patient expectations of pain relief are low. In a study on the perceptions of pain relief after surgery, 86% of pa-

Table 3–6

Acid-Base Disorders and Their Treatment

Primary Disorder	Defect	Common Causes	Compensation	Treatment
Respiratory acidosis	Carbon dioxide retention (hypoventilation)	Central nervous system depression Airway and lung impairment	Renal excretion of acid salts Bicarbonate retention Chloride shift into red cells	Restoration of adequate ventilation Control of excess carbon dioxide production
Respiratory alkalosis	Hyperventilation	Central nervous system excitation Excess ventilator support	Renal excretion of sodium, potassium, bicarbonate Absorption of hydrogen and chloride ions Lactate release from red cells	Correction of hyperventilation
Metabolic acidosis	Excess loss of base Increased nonvolatile acids	Excess chloride versus sodium Increased bicarbonate loss Lactic, ketoacidosis Uremia Dilutional acidosis	Respiratory alkalosis Renal excretion of hydrogen and chloride ions Resorption of potassium and bicarbonate	Increase sodium load Correct underlying process Waste chloride Give bicarbonate for pH <7.2 Restore buffers, protein, hemoglobin
Metabolic alkalosis	Excess loss of chloride and potassium Increased bicarbonate	Gastrointestinal losses of chloride Excess intake of bicarbonate Diuretics Hypokalemia Extracellular fluid volume contraction	Respiratory acidosis May be hypoxia Renal excretion of bicarbonate and potassium Absorption of hydrogen and chloride ions	Increase chloride content Potassium replacement Acetazolamide (Diamox) to waste bicarbonate Vigorous volume replacement Occasional 0.1 N HCl as needed

From Demling RH, Wilson RF (eds.): Fluids, electrolytes, and acid-base balance. In Decision Making in Surgical Critical Care. Philadelphia, BC Decker, 1988, pp. 114–157.

tients had moderate to severe pain after surgery, yet 70% felt that the pain was as severe as they had expected.[35] In a similar study, over 80% of patients were satisfied with their postoperative analgesia, despite the majority of patients reporting significant pain.[36] Patients are not aware of the extent of analgesia that they should expect. Second, there is a lack of formal training in medical school curricula and residency programs. In one review of five well-known surgical textbooks, three of the five textbooks did not discuss postoperative pain management at all, while the other two devoted only several pages to pain management.[37] The end-result of the lack of training in pain management is the commonly written order prescribing a range of narcotic to be given intramuscularly every 3–4 hours prn, leaving pain management decisions up to the nursing staff, and with no attempt to titrate the dose of the prescribed narcotic commensurate with individual patient requirements. Third, nursing attitudes continue to be influenced by the common misconception that the use of narcotics in the postoperative period can result in opioid dependence. In one review, 20% of nurses responding to a staff questionnaire expressed a concern that use of opioid analgesics in the postoperative period could cause addiction.[35] Half the nurses admitted that this misconception influenced their choice of the dose as well as the interval of administration of narcotics when prescribed in a dose range, prn. Studies have confirmed that nurses will administer less than one-quarter of the total dose of narcotic that is prescribed prn.[36, 38] In the final analysis, low patient expectations are fulfilled by their health care providers.

The minimum effective analgesic concentration (MEAC) refers to a serum concentration of a drug below which very little analgesia is achieved.[34] At the MEAC, receptor and plasma concentrations of a drug are in equilibrium.[39] Steady-state drug concentrations above the MEAC are difficult to achieve with intramuscular depot injection. In one pharmacokinetic study, minimal effective drug concentrations were relatively consistent among postoperative patients receiving intramuscular injections with meperidine hydrochloride (Demerol) every 4 hours. However, there were marked intra- and inter-patient variations in narcotic drug peak concentrations as well as the time required to reach these peaks. As a result, serum concentrations of drug were above the MEAC an average of only 35% of each 4-hour dosing interval. The authors concluded that variable pain control following intermittent intramuscular injections was due to inadequate, highly variable, and unpredictable blood concentrations.[40] Adequate analgesia can be achieved through intramuscular or subcutaneous modes of administration, but unpredictable absorption can make titration difficult. Small intravenous boluses can be more easily titrated but may be shorter acting, requiring more frequent injections and thus intensive nursing care, whereas larger intravenous boluses may be associated with a higher incidence of central nervous system and respiratory depression. The patient-controlled analgesia (PCA) technique, which allows patients to self-administer small doses of narcotic on demand, now allows titration of measured boluses of narcotic as needed to relieve pain and can provide a more thorough analgesia with maintenance of steady-state drug concentrations above the MEAC.

Irrespective of the route of administration, analgesics must be front-loaded in order to provide prompt analgesia from the start. Without front-loading, attainment of the MEAC will not occur for at least three elimination half-lives of the narcotic agent that is used. After front-loading, additional small boluses of narcotic can be administered until analgesia is achieved. From the total dose of drug required to achieve analgesia, maintenance drug dosages can then be determined and administered either as a continuous infusion or on a scheduled basis such that the dose of drug administered offsets the amount that is cleared (Table 3–7). Thereafter, prescribed doses of narcotic can be further adjusted as needed.

Patient-Controlled Analgesia (PCA)

In the late 1960s and early 1970s, several investigators reported on the use of patient-controlled analgesia devices.[41–43] The devices were composed of an electronically controlled infusion pump that would deliver a pre-set dose of narcotic into a patient's indwelling intravenous catheter upon patient request. The devices all contained delay intervals or lock-out times during which patient demands for more narcotic would not be met. These devices eliminated the delay between the onset of pain and the administration of analgesic agents, inherent with on-demand prn analgesic orders and a common problem on busy hospital wards.

Not surprisingly, PCA has enjoyed excellent patient acceptance. Compared with conventional intramuscular injections, serum narcotic levels have significantly lower variability in patients on PCA.[44] Patients have been shown to have improved analgesia,[44–46] a lower incidence of postoperative pulmonary complications,[44, 45] and a lower incidence of confusion.[44] Furthermore, the total dose of narcotic used has been lower with PCA than with conventional intramuscular depot injection.[45, 47, 48]

Unfortunately, many of the earlier studies on PCA were poorly controlled and used subjective criteria for determining analgesic effect.[49] More recent studies have shown that carefully supervised regimens

Table 3–7

Guidelines for Front-Loading IV Analgesics*

Drug	Total Front-Load Dose	Increments	Cautions
Morphine	0.08–0.12 mg/kg	0.03 mg/kg q 10 h	Histaminergic effects; nausea; biliary colic; reduce dose for elderly
Meperidine	1.0–1.5 mg/kg	0.30 mg/kg/q 10 h	Reduce dose or change drug for impaired renal function
Codeine	0.5–1.0 mg/kg	⅓ total q 15 h	Nausea
Methadone	0.08–0.12 mg/kg	0.03 mg/kg q 15 h	Do not administer maintenance dose after analgesia
Levorphanol	0.02 mg/kg	50–75 µg/kg q 15 h	Similar to methadone
Hydromorphone	0.02 mg/kg	25–50 µg/kg q 10 h	Similar to morphine sulfate
Pentazocine	0.5–1.0 mg/kg	½ total q 15 h	Psychomimetic effects; may cause withdrawal in narcotic-dependent patients
Nalbuphine	0.08–0.15 mg/kg	0.03 mg/kg q 10 h	Less psychomimetic effect than pentazocine; sedation
Butorphanol	0.02–0.04 mg/kg	0.01 mg/kg q 10 h	Sedation; psychomimetic effects like nalbuphine
Buprenorphine	Up to 0.2 mg/kg	¼ total q 10 h	Long acting like methadone, levorphanol; may precipitate withdrawal in narcotic-dependent patients; safe to give subcutaneous maintenance after analgesia—different from methadone

*A scheme for front-loading the opioids most commonly used in postoperative pain treatment.

using continuous infusions,[48] on-demand intramuscular therapy,[50, 51] or fixed dosage schedules (every-4-hour dosing) with on-demand supplementation[52] can have analgesic efficacy comparable with PCA. PCA does have potential complications (Table 3–8).[53] Nonetheless, the type of close supervision required to achieve adequate on-demand analgesia without PCA is difficult to achieve, particularly in the context of a busy inpatient unit in which nursing is short staffed. Continuous infusion regimens eliminate the delay inherent in on-demand regimens but have been associated with an increased risk of oversedation and apnea.[39] Use of PCA shortens the time delay between the onset of pain and the administration of pain medication, provides more continuous access to analgesics, and allows for an overall steadier state of pain control.

Table 3–8

Problems that Can Occur During Patient-Controlled Analgesia (PCA)

Operator Errors
Misprogramming PCA device
Failure to clamp or unclamp tubing
Improperly loading syringe or cartridge
Inability to respond to safety alarms
Misplacing PCA pump key

Patient Errors
Failure to understand PCA therapy
Misunderstanding PCA pump device
Intentional analgesic abuse

Mechanical Errors
Failure to deliver drug on demand
Defective one-way valve at "Y" connector
Faulty alarm system
Malfunctions (e.g., lock)

From White PF: Mishaps with patient-controlled analgesia (PCA). Anesthesiology 1987; 66:81–83.

Intraspinal Analgesia

Intraspinal anesthetics and/or narcotics administered either in the epidural space or intrathecally are among the most potent analgesic agents available, with efficacy greater than that provided by intravenous PCA techniques.[54] These drugs can be administered in one of several ways, including a single-shot dose given by epidural or intrathecal injection, intermittent injection given either on schedule or on demand, and via continuous infusions.[34]

Intrathecal administration is usually limited to a single dose, owing to the risk of central nervous system infections as well as headaches.[55] Duration of action for a single dose is increased via the intrathecal route as compared with epidural administration as a result of the high concentrations of drug attained in the CSF. However, the risk of CNS and respiratory depression as well as systemic hypotension is also increased. Even low doses of intrathecal morphine have been associated with a high risk of complications. Therefore, some investigators have warned against the use of intrathecal spinal analgesia outside of the intensive care setting.[56]

Epidural administration is the preferred approach and provides for extended (>24 hours) pain control in the postoperative period. Relative contraindications have included the presence of a coagulopathy, sepsis, and hypotension. Both anesthetic and narcotic agents have been used with excellent efficacy. Among the anesthetic agents, bupivacaine has been the most popular, providing excellent analgesia with no motor blockade and minimal toxicity.[55] Epidural analgesia is best suited for pain control in the lower abdomen and extremities. One potential adverse effect is that of sympathetic blockade, precluding the use of this method for attainment of high blocks.

Other adverse effects include urinary retention and hypotension, as well as central nervous system and cardiac depression. In contrast to anesthetic agents, opioids offer excellent analgesia without an accompanying sympathetic blockade. Epidural opioids tend to have a much longer duration of action, and hypotension is a rare complication. Compared with epidural anesthetics, however, there is a higher incidence of nausea and vomiting, respiratory depression, and pruritus.[56] Investigators have been studying the use of anesthetics and narcotic agents in combination in order to take advantage of the potential benefits of each type of agent, while at the same time limiting overall toxicity. In addition, other types of agents are being studied. Initial studies on the use of epidural clonidine have shown encouraging results. In one study comparing epidural sufentanil plus clonidine versus sufentanil, epidural clonidine (1 μg/kg) plus sufentanil (25 μg) afforded greater pain relief than the use of sufentanil (50 μg) alone.[57]

Overall, as compared with analgesics administered intramuscularly or intravenously, epidural analgesia has been shown to be associated with improved pulmonary function postoperatively, a lower incidence of postoperative pulmonary complications, a decrease in postoperative venous thromboembolic complications (most likely secondary to earlier ambulation), fewer adverse gastrointestinal side effects, a lower incidence of central nervous system depression, and faster convalescence. Severe respiratory depression is the most serious potential complication, seen in less than 1% of patients. A lower incidence of respiratory depression is seen with the more lipophilic drugs such as fentanyl which is quickly absorbed within the spinal cord and is therefore less likely to diffuse to the central nervous system respiratory control centers. Pruritus, nausea, and urinary retention[55] are common but can be easily managed and are usually of little clinical significance. Perhaps the main and limiting drawback to epidural analgesia is cost, in that epidural analgesia is much more expensive than more conventional methods.

Close monitoring by nursing staff is required for safe administration of epidural analgesia. However, an intensive care setting is not necessary. Edwards has reviewed his extensive experience with over 3000 patients and has concluded that epidural analgesics can be safely administered in a hospital ward setting, under close nursing supervision.[34] He has recommended close respiratory monitoring with ventilatory checks hourly during the first 8 hours of epidural analgesia.

Antibiotic Prophylaxis

Bacteria that may contaminate the gynecologic surgical field are those that are indigenous to the vaginal tract, including both gram-positive and gram-negative aerobes and anaerobes (Table 3–9). The primary pathogenic bacteria include the coliforms, streptococci, fusobacteria, and bacteroides. Gynecologic operations that carry a significant risk of postoperative infection include vaginal hysterectomy, abdominal hysterectomy, cases involving pelvic abscess or inflammation, select cases of pregnancy termination, and radical surgery for gynecologic cancers. In these cases, organisms indigenous to the vagina may contaminate the pelvic cavity and surgical wound site. Most other gynecologic procedures are considered "clean" and have a low risk (<5%) of postoperative wound infection.[58] Included in these are procedures confined to the abdomen, space of Retzius, perineum, and vagina.

The following are proposed guidelines for antibiotic prophylaxis in gynecologic procedures:[59]

1. The procedure should carry a significant risk of postoperative infection.
2. The surgery should involve considerable bacterial contamination.
3. The antibiotic chosen for prophylaxis should be effective against most contaminating organisms.
4. The antibiotic should be present in the tissues at the time of contamination.
5. The shortest possible course of antibiotic prophylaxis should be given.
6. The prophylactic antibiotic chosen should not be one considered for treatment should postoperative infection occur.
7. The risk of complications from the prophylactic antibiotic should be low.

The existing literature uniformly supports the use of the prophylactic antibiotics for vaginal hysterectomy; however, the use of prophylactic antibiotics for patients who undergo abdominal hysterectomy is controversial. Hirsch reviewed the placebo-controlled trials in the English and non-English literature regarding antibiotic prophylaxis in vaginal and ab-

Table 3–9

Bacteria Indigenous to the Lower Genital Tract

Lactobacillus	Enterobacter agglomerans
Diphtheroids	Klebsiella pneumoniae
Staphylococcus aureus	Proteus mirabilis
Staphylococcus epidermidis	Proteus vulgaris
Streptococcus agalactiae	Morganella morganii
Streptococcus faecalis	Citrobacter diversus
Alpha-hemolytic streptococci	
Group D streptococci	Bacteroides species
Peptostreptococcus	B. bivius
Peptococcus	B. disiens
Clostridium	B. fragilis
Gaffkya ancerobia	B. melaninogenicus
Escherichia coli	
Fusobacterium	
Enterobacter cloacae	

dominal hysterectomy.[60] Included in the review were 48 studies encompassing 5524 patients who underwent vaginal hysterectomy, and 30 studies encompassing 3752 patients who underwent abdominal hysterectomy. In vaginal hysterectomy, prophylactic antibiotics decreased febrile morbidity from 40% in control patients to 15% in treated patients, and lowered the pelvic infection rate from 25% in control patients to 5% in treated patients. The benefits of antibiotic prophylaxis were less pronounced in the abdominal hysterectomy series; febrile morbidity was reduced in 57% of studies, whereas wound infections and pelvic infections were reduced in a minority of the studies. Overall, antibiotic prophylaxis for abdominal hysterectomy reduced febrile morbidity from 28% in control patients to 16% in treated patients, pelvic infections from 10% to 5%, and wound infections from 8% to 3%, respectively. This analysis is further complicated by a lack of series-to-series uniformity regarding criteria for fever or for diagnosis of infection requiring antibiotic therapy. Nonetheless, most investigators would agree that antibiotic prophylaxis should be used in all patients who undergo vaginal hysterectomy, as well as in selected high-risk patients who undergo abdominal hysterectomy. Factors that have been identified as placing patients at high risk for post-hysterectomy infection have included low socioeconomic status, duration of surgery greater than 2 hours, presence of malignancy, and increased number of surgical procedures performed. Obesity, menopausal status, and estimated blood loss have not been shown to be risk factors for postoperative infection when evaluated by multivariate analysis.[61, 62]

The antibiotic chosen for prophylaxis for gynecologic cases should have activity against the broad range of vaginal organisms. The first- and second-generation cephalosporins are well suited, given their activity against gram-positive, gram-negative, and anaerobic organisms. Most classes of antibiotics, including the penicillins, tetracyclines, sulfonamides, broad-spectrum penicillins and cephalosporins, and anaerobic drugs (clindamycin/metronidazole [Flagyl]), have been shown to be effective as prophylactic antibiotics,[63–69] although none has been demonstrated to be consistently more effective than first-generation cephalosporins.

The timing of administration of the prophylactic antibiotic agent is important. Studies dating back to the work by Burke[70] in the 1960s have demonstrated that antibiotics given for prophylaxis against infection are most active if present in tissues prior to contamination with an inoculum of bacteria. For patients who undergo hysterectomy, the antibiotic should be present in the tissues prior to the opening of the vaginal cuff, at which time vaginal organisms gain access to the pelvic cavity. Infusion of an antibiotic, on call to the operating room, within 30 minutes of surgery is ideal for this purpose. For long surgical procedures, particularly where there is a large blood loss or when an antibiotic agent with short half-life is used, a second antibiotic dose should be given intraoperatively.

Many prospective studies have documented that short courses of prophylactic antibiotics (24 hours or less) are as efficacious as longer ones. Several clinical trials have found that one perioperative dose of prophylactic antibiotic is sufficient.[66, 68, 71–73] The use of one dose of prophylactic antibiotic has many advantages, including decreased cost, decreased toxicity, and minimal alteration of host flora (selection of resistant pathogens).

Despite the advantages of using prophylactic antibiotics, the importance of good surgical technique must be emphasized. Antibiotics should not be used in lieu of correct surgical principles such as delicate handling of tissues, good hemostasis, adequate drainage, and avoidance of unnecessarily large pedicles of tissue in ligatures.

Postoperative Surgical Infections

Evaluation of Postoperative Infection

Infections are a major source of morbidity in the postoperative period. Lack of perioperative antibiotic prophylaxis; contamination of the surgical field, either from infected tissues or from spillage of large bowel contents; an immunocompromised host; poor nutrition; chronic and debilitating severe illness; poor surgical technique; and pre-existing focal or systemic infection are all risk factors for infectious morbidity. Sources of postoperative infection can include the lung, urinary tract, surgical site, pelvic side wall, vaginal cuff, abdominal wound, and sites of indwelling intravenous catheters. Early identification and treatment of infections will result in the best outcome from these potentially serious complications.

Although infections are an inevitable complication of surgery, the incidence of infections can be decreased by the appropriate use of simple preventative measures. The use of prophylactic antibiotics has been discussed previously. For patients undergoing hysterectomy, antibiotic prophylaxis decreases colonization of the surgical site from vaginal organisms spilled into the pelvis. In cases that involve transection of the large bowel, spillage of fecal contents also inevitably occurs. A thorough preoperative mechanical and antibiotic bowel preparation in combination with systemic antibiotic prophylaxis will help to decrease the incidence of postoperative pelvic and abdominal infections in these patients. The surgeon can further decrease the risk of postoperative infections by employing meticulous surgical technique. Blood and necrotic tissue are excellent media for the growth of aerobic and anaerobic organisms. In cases in which there is higher than usual potential for serum and blood to collect or spaces that have been contaminated by bacterial spill, closed-suction drainage may reduce the risk of infection. Antibiotic therapy rather than prophylaxis should be initiated at surgery in patients who have frank intra-abdominal infection or pus.

Elective surgical procedures should be postponed in patients who have a preoperative infection. In an epidemiologic study conducted by the Centers for Disease Control, the incidence of nosocomial surgical infections ranged from 4.3% in community hospitals to 7% in municipal hospitals.[74] Urinary tract infections accounted for approximately 40% of these nosocomial infections. Infections of the skin and wound accounted for approximately one-third of the infections, and respiratory tract infections accounted for approximately 16%. These rates of infection were higher with older patients, with increased length of surgery, and with increased length of hospital stay prior to surgery. The relative risk was three times higher in patients with a community-acquired infection prior to surgery. These community-acquired infections included infections of the urinary and respiratory tract. Furthermore, in patients who had any type of infection prior to surgery, the risk of infection at the surgical wound site was increased fourfold.

The standard definition of febrile morbidity for surgical patients has been the presence of a temperature greater than or equal to 100.4° F (38° C) on two occasions at least 4 hours apart in the postoperative period, excluding the first 24 hours. Febrile morbidity is common after gynecologic surgery and has been estimated to occur in as much as one-half of patients.[75] Febrile morbidity often occurs within the first 2 postoperative days[76] and is self-limited, resolving without therapy. Although fever is a sign of infection, the diagnosis of infection is based on the combination of fever and clinical and laboratory evidence of an infected focus.

The work-up of the febrile surgical patient should include a review of the patient's history with regard to risk factors and potential sites for infection, as well as a thorough physical examination with particular emphasis on the potential sites for infection (Table 3–10). This should include inspection of the pharynx, a thorough pulmonary examination, palpation of the kidneys and the costovertebral angles for tenderness, inspection and palpation of the abdominal incision, examination of sites of intravenous catheters, and an examination of the extremities for evidence of deep venous thrombosis or thrombophlebitis. In gynecologic patients, appropriate work-up may also include

Table 3–10

Posthysterectomy Infections

Operative Site	Nonoperative Site
Vaginal cuff	Urinary tract
Pelvic cellulitis	Asymptomatic bacteriuria
Pelvic abscess	Cystitis
Supravaginal, extraperitoneal	Pyelonephritis
Intraperitoneal	Respiratory
Adnexa	Atelectasis
Cellulitis	Pneumonia
Abscess	Vascular
Abdominal incision	Phlebitis
Cellulitis	Septic pelvic
Simple	thrombophlebitis
Progressive bacterial synergistic	
Necrotizing fasciitis	
Myonecrosis	

From Hemsell DL: Infections after gynecologic surgery. Obstet Gynecol Clin North Am 1989, 16:381–400.

inspection and palpation of the vaginal cuff for signs of induration, tenderness, or purulent drainage. A pelvic examination should also be performed in order to identify a mass consistent with a pelvic hematoma or abscess, and to look for signs of pelvic cellulitis.

The laboratory and radiologic evaluation can include a white blood cell count with differential, a catheterized urinalysis and culture, and a chest x-ray for patients with signs and symptoms localizing to the lung. Blood cultures can also be obtained but will most likely be of little yield unless the patient has a high fever (>102° F). In patients with costovertebral angle tenderness, an intravenous pyelogram may be indicated to rule out the presence of ureteral damage or obstruction from surgery, particularly in the absence of laboratory evidence of urinary tract infection. Patients who have persistent fevers without a clear localizing source should have a CT scan of the abdomen and pelvis or scan of the body to rule out the presence of an intra-abdominal abscess. Finally, in patients who have undergone gastrointestinal surgery, a barium enema and/or upper GI series with small bowel follow-through may be indicated late in the course of the first postoperative week if fevers persist, to rule out an anastomotic leak or fistula.

Urinary Tract Infections

The urinary tract has historically been the most common site of infection in surgical patients.[74] However, the incidence reported in the more recent gynecologic literature has been less than 4%.[76, 77] This decrease in urinary tract infections has most likely been due to the increased use of perioperative prophylactic antibiotics. The incidence of postoperative urinary tract infection in gynecologic surgical patients not receiving prophylactic antibiotics has been confirmed to be as high as 40%,[78] and even a single dose of perioperative prophylactic antibiotic has been shown to decrease the incidence of postoperative urinary tract infection from 35% to 4%.[79]

Despite the high incidence of urinary tract infections in the postoperative period, few of these infections are serious. The majority are confined to the lower urinary tract. Pyelonephritis is a rare complication postoperatively.[80] Catheterization of the urinary tract, either intermittently or continuously via the use of an indwelling catheter, has been implicated as a main cause of urinary tract contamination.[81] Therefore, the use of urinary catheters should be avoided when possible.

Symptoms of a urinary tract infection may include urinary frequency, urgency, and dysuria. In patients with pyelonephritis, other symptoms have commonly included headache, malaise, nausea, and vomiting. The diagnosis of urinary tract infection is made microbiologically and has been defined as the growth of greater than 10^5 organisms per ml of urine cultured. The majority of the infections are caused by coliforms, with *Escherichia coli* being the most common pathogen. Other pathogens include *Klebsiella*, *Proteus*, and *Enterobacter* species. *Staphylococcus* organisms are the causative bacteria in fewer than 10% of cases.

The treatment of urinary tract infection includes hydration and antibiotic therapy. Commonly prescribed and effective antibiotics have included penicillins, sulfonamides, cephalosporins, and nitrofurantoin. The choice of antibiotic for treatment should be made with a knowledge of the susceptibility of organisms cultured at each institution. In some institutions, for example, greater than 40% of *E. coli* strains are resistant to ampicillin. For uncomplicated urinary tract infections, an antibiotic should be chosen that has good activity against *E. coli* while awaiting the urine culture and sensitivity data. Patients who have a history of recurrent urinary tract infections, those with chronic indwelling catheters (Foley catheters or ureteral stents), and those who have urinary conduits should be started on antibiotics that will be effective against the less common urinary pathogens such as *Klebsiella*. More resistant organisms, such as *Pseudomonas*, may also be encountered in these patients.

Pulmonary Infections

The respiratory tract is an uncommon site for infectious complications in gynecologic surgical patients. Hemsell noted only six cases of pneumonia in over 4000 women who underwent elective hysterectomy.[76] This low incidence is probably a reflection of the young age and good health status of gynecologic patients in general. In acute care facilities, pneumonia is a frequent hospital-acquired infection, particularly in the elderly.[82] Risk factors include extensive or prolonged atelectasis, pre-existent chronic obstructive pulmonary disease, severe or debilitating illness, central neurologic disease causing an inability to clear oropharyngeal secretions effectively, and nasogastric suction.[82] Early ambulation and aggressive management of atelectasis are the most important preventive measures. The role of prophylactic antibiotics remains unclear.

A significant proportion (40–50%) of hospital-acquired pneumonias are due to gram-negative organisms. These organisms gain access to the respiratory tract from the oral pharynx. Gram-negative colonization of the oral pharynx has been shown to be increased in patients in acute care facilities and has been associated with the presence of nasogastric tubes; pre-existing respiratory disease; mechanical ventilation; tracheal intubation; and with paralytic ileus, which is associated with an increase in the microbial overgrowth in the stomach.[83] Interestingly, the use of antimicrobial drugs seems to significantly increase the frequency of colonization of the oral pharynx with gram-negative bacteria.

A thorough lung examination should be included in the work-up of all febrile surgical patients. In the absence of significant lung findings, a chest x-ray is probably of little benefit in patients at low risk for postoperative pulmonary complications. In patients with pulmonary findings or with risk factors for pulmonary complications, a chest x-ray should be obtained. A sputum sample should also be obtained for Gram's stain and culture. The treatment should include postural drainage, aggressive pulmonary toilet, and antibiotics. The antibiotic chosen should be effective against both gram-positive and gram-negative organisms.

Phlebitis

Intravenous catheter–related infections are common, with a reported incidence from 25% to 35%.[84] The intravenous site should be inspected daily and the catheter removed if there is any associated pain, redness, or induration. Unfortunately, phlebitis can occur even with close surveillance of the intravenous site. In one study, over 50% of the cases of phlebitis developed more than 12 hours after discontinuation of IV catheters.[85] In addition, less than one-third of patients had symptoms related to the intravenous catheter site 24 hours prior to the diagnosis of phlebitis.

Intravenous catheters should be inserted using careful, sterile technique. Furthermore, they should be changed frequently. The incidence of catheter-related phlebitis rises significantly after 72 hours. Therefore, intravenous catheters should be changed at least every 3 days. The institution of intravenous therapy teams has resulted in a decreased incidence of phlebitis by as much as 50%.[84] This decrease was thought to be due not so much to surveillance of the intravenous catheter site by the intravenous therapy teams, but rather to frequent changing of intravenous catheters.

The diagnosis of phlebitis can be made in the presence of fever, pain, redness, induration, and/or a palpable venous cord. Occasionally, suppuration will be present. Phlebitis is usually self-limited and resolves within 3–4 days. The treatment includes application of warm, moist compresses and prompt removal of any catheters from the infected vein. Antibiotic therapy with antistaphylococcal agents should be instituted for catheter-related sepsis. Excision or drainage of an infected vein is rarely necessary.

Wound Infections

A prospective study of over 62,000 wounds revealed a great deal in regard to the epidemiology of wound infections.[86] Clearly, the wound infection rate varies markedly, depending on the extent of contamination in the surgical field. The wound infection rate for clean surgical cases (infection not present in the surgical field, no break in aseptic technique, no hollow viscus entered) is less than 2%, whereas the incidence of wound infections with dirty, infected cases is 40% or greater. Preoperative showers with hexachlorophene slightly lower the infection rate for clean wounds. Preoperative shaving of the wound site with a razor increases the rate of infection. A 5-minute wound preparation immediately preoperatively is as effective as a 10-minute preparation. The wound infection rate increases with increasing length of preoperative hospital stay as well as with longer duration of surgery. In addition, incidental appendectomy may increase the risk of wound infection in patients undergoing clean surgical procedures. The study concluded that the incidence of wound infections could be decreased via the institution of short preoperative hospital stays, hexachlorophene showers prior to surgery, minimizing shaving of the wound site, use of meticulous surgical technique, expediting an operation as much as safely possible, bringing drains out through sites other than the wound, and through dissemination of information to each surgeon of his or her wound infection rate as well as the average infection rate of peers. A program instituting these conclusions led to a fall in the clean wound infection rate from 2.5% to 0.6% over an 8-year period.

In general, the wound infection rate in obstetric and gynecologic services has been less than 5%. The symptoms of wound infection often occur late in the postoperative period, usually after the fourth postoperative day, and may include the presence of fever, erythema, tenderness, induration, and purulent drainage. The management is mostly mechanical and involves opening of the infected portion of the wound above the fascia, with cleansing and débridement of the wound edges as necessary. Wound care, consisting of débridement and dressing changes two to three times daily with mesh gauze, will promote growth of granulation tissue, with gradual filling in of the wound defect by secondary intention. The authors prefer to pack wounds with dry rather than wet gauze because better débridement of the wound edges is achieved upon the removal of dry gauze. Clean, granulating wounds can often be secondarily closed with good success, shortening the time required for complete wound healing.

The technique of delayed primary wound closure can be used in infected surgical cases to lower the incidence of wound infection. Briefly, the technique involves leaving the wound open above the fascia at the time of the initial surgical procedure. Vertical interrupted mattress sutures through the skin and subcutaneous layers are placed 3 cm apart but are not tied. Wound care is instituted immediately after surgery and continued until the wound is noted to be granulating well. Then sutures may be tied and the skin edges further approximated using staples. Using this technique of delayed primary wound closure, the overall wound infection rate has been shown to be decreased from 23% to 2.1% in high-risk patients.[87]

Pelvic Cellulitis

Vaginal cuff cellulitis is present to some extent in most patients who have undergone hysterectomy. It is characterized by erythema, induration, and tenderness at the vaginal cuff. Occasionally, a purulent discharge from the apex of the vagina may also be present. The cellulitis is often self-limited and will not require any treatment. Fever, leukocytosis, and pain localized to the pelvis may accompany a severe cuff cellulitis and most often signifies extension of the cellulitis to adjacent pelvic tissues. In such cases, broad-spectrum antibiotic therapy should be instituted with coverage for gram-negative, gram-positive, and anaerobic organisms. If purulence at the vaginal cuff is excessive or there is a fluctuance or a mass noted at the vaginal cuff, the vaginal cuff should be gently probed and opened with a blunt instrument. The cuff can then be left open for dependent drainage or, alternatively, a drain can be placed into the lower pelvis through the cuff and removed when drainage, fever, and lower pelvic symptoms have resolved.

Intra-abdominal and Pelvic Abscess

The development of an abscess in the surgical field or elsewhere in the abdominal cavity is an uncommon complication after a gynecologic surgery. It is most likely to occur with contaminated cases, particularly if the surgical site is not adequately drained or as a secondary complication in hematomas. The causative pathogens recovered in patients who have intra-abdominal abscess are polymicrobial in nature. The aerobes most commonly identified include *E. coli, Klebsiella, Streptococcus, Proteus,* and *Enterobacter.* Anaerobic isolates are also common, usually from the *Bacteroides* group. These pathogens are mainly from the vaginal tract but also can be derived from the gastrointestinal tract, particularly when the colon has been entered at the time of surgery.

The diagnosis of intra-abdominal abscess is sometimes difficult to make. The evolving clinical picture is often one of persistent febrile episodes with a rising white blood cell count. Findings upon abdominal examination may be equivocal. If an abscess is located deep in the pelvis, it may be palpable by pelvic or rectal examination. For abscesses above the pelvis, diagnosis will depend on radiologic confirmation.

Ultrasound can occasionally delineate fluid collections in the upper abdomen as well as in the pelvis. However, bowel gas interference makes visualization of fluid collections or abscesses in the mid-abdomen difficult. CT scanning is much more sensitive and specific for diagnosing abscesses and is therefore the radiologic procedure of choice. Occasionally, if conventional radiologic methods fail to identify an abscess and the index of suspicion for an abscess remains high, a labeled leukocyte scan may be useful in locating the infected focus.

Standard therapy for intra-abdominal abscess is surgical evacuation and drainage combined with appropriate parenteral antibiotics. Abscesses located low in the pelvis, particularly in the area of the vaginal cuff, can often be reached through a vaginal approach. The ability to drain an abscess by placement of a drain percutaneously under CT guidance has obviated the need for a surgical exploration in many patients. With CT guidance, a pigtail catheter is placed into an abscess cavity and is left in place until drainage decreases. Gram's stain and anaerobic and aerobic cultures should be obtained to guide antibiotic selection. The "gold standard" of initial antibiotic therapy has been the combination of ampicillin, gentamicin, and clindamycin. Adequate treatment can also be achieved with currently available broad-spectrum single agents, including the broad-spectrum penicillins; second- and third-generation cephalosporins; and the sulbactam, clavulanic acid containing preparations.[88-90]

Necrotizing Fasciitis

Necrotizing fasciitis is an uncommon infectious disorder, with approximately 1000 cases occurring annually in the United States.[91] The disorder is characterized by a rapidly progressive bacterial infection involving subcutaneous tissues and fascia, while characteristically sparing underlying muscle. Systemic toxicity is a frequent feature of this disease, as manifested by the presence of dehydration, septic shock, disseminated intravascular coagulation, and multi-organ system failure.

The pathogenesis of necrotizing fasciitis involves a polymicrobial infection of the dermis and subcutaneous tissue. Hemolytic streptococcus was initially thought to be the primary pathogen responsible for the infection in necrotizing fasciitis.[92] However, it is now evident that numerous other organisms are often cultured in addition to streptococcus, including other gram-positive organisms, coliforms, and anaerobes.[93-97] Bacterial enzymes such as hyaluronidase and lipase released in the subcutaneous space destroy the fascia and adipose tissue and induce a liquefactive necrosis. In addition, noninflammatory intravascular coagulation or thrombosis subsequently occurs. Intravascular coagulation results in ischemia and necrosis of the subcutaneous tissues and skin.[93, 94] Late in the course of the infection, destruction of the superficial nerves produces anesthesia in the involved skin. The release of bacteria and bacterial toxins into the systemic circulation can cause septic shock, acid-base disturbances, and multi-organ impairment.

The diagnostic criteria for necrotizing fasciitis have been defined by Fisher.[98] These include extensive necrosis of the superficial fascia with peripheral undermining of the normal skin, a moderate to severe systemic toxic reaction, the absence of muscle involvement, the absence of *Clostridia* in wound and blood culture, the absence of major vascular occlusion despite the presence of microvascular thrombosis, intensive leukocytic infiltration, and necrosis of subcutaneous tissue.

Clinical and laboratory findings commonly seen in patients with necrotizing fasciitis are noted in Table 3–11. The majority of patients suffer pain, which in the early stages of the disease is often disproportionately greater than that expected from the degree of cellulitis present. Late in the course of the infection, the involved skin may actually be anesthetized secondary to necrosis of superficial nerves. Temperature abnormalities, both hyperthermia and hypothermia, are common, concomitant with the release of bacterial toxins as well as with bacterial sepsis, which can be present in up to 40% of patients.[96] The involved skin is initially tender, erythematous, and warm. Edema develops and the

Table 3-11

Clinical and Laboratory Data in 33 Patients with Necrotizing Fasciitis

Clinical Signs and Symptoms	Number of Patients	Laboratory Findings	Number of Patients
Severe pain	31 (94%)	Leukocytosis	29 (88%)
Temperature abnormalities		Anemia	21 (64%)
>101° F	27 (82%)	Hypocalcemia	11 (33%)
<97° F	2 (6%)	Acidosis	9 (27%)
Skin changes	25 (76%)	Gas (x-ray)	8 (24%)
Cellulitis—progressive	24 (73%)		
Crepitus	6 (18%)		

From Sudarsky LA, Laschinger JC, Coppa GF, Spencer FC: Improved results from a standardized approach in treating patients with necrotizing fasciitis. Ann Surg 1987; 206:661–665.

erythema spreads diffusely, fading into normal skin, characteristically without distinct margins or induration. Subcutaneous microvascular thrombosis induces ischemia in the skin, which becomes cyanotic and blistered. Eventually, as necrosis develops, the skin becomes gangrenous and may spontaneously slough. Most patients will have leukocytosis and acid-base abnormalities. Finally, subcutaneous gas may develop, which can be identified by palpation and by x-ray. The finding of subcutaneous gas by x-ray is often indicative of clostridial infection, although it is not a specific finding and may be due to other organisms. These organisms include *Enterobacter*, *Pseudomonas*, anaerobic streptococci, and *Bacteroides*,[99] which, unlike clostridial infections, spare the muscles underlying the affected area. A tissue biopsy specimen for Gram's stain and aerobic and anaerobic culture should be obtained from the necrotic center of the lesion[94] in order to identify the etiologic organisms. Although a diagnosis of necrotizing fasciitis is often made at surgery, a high index of suspicion as well as liberal use of frozen section biopsy[100] can often provide an early life-saving diagnosis and minimize morbidity.

Predisposing risk factors for necrotizing fasciitis include diabetes mellitus, trauma, alcoholism, an immunocompromised state, hypertension, peripheral vascular disease, intravenous drug abuse, and obesity.[91, 93, 96, 97, 99, 101-103] The most frequent site of infection has been in the extremities,[94] but the infection can occur anywhere in the subcutaneous tissues, including the head and neck, trunk, and perineum. Necrotizing fasciitis has been known to occur after trauma, surgery, burns, lacerations; as a secondary complication in perirectal infections or Bartholin's abscesses; and de novo.[91, 93, 94, 97, 103-105] Increased age, delay in diagnosis, inadequate débridement at initial operation, extent of disease upon initial presentation, and the presence of diabetes mellitus are all factors that have been associated with an increased likelihood of mortality from necrotizing fasciitis.[91, 96, 106] Clearly, early diagnosis and aggressive management of this lethal disease have led to improved survival. In an earlier series, mortality was consistently over 30%; in more recent series, the mortality has decreased to less than 10%.[99, 107, 108]

Successful management of necrotizing fasciitis involves early recognition; immediate initiation of resuscitative measures, including correction of fluid, acid-base, electrolyte, and hematologic abnormalities; aggressive surgical débridement and redébridement as necessary; and broad-spectrum antibiotic therapy. Many patients will benefit from central venous monitoring, as well as from high caloric nutritional support.

At surgery, the incision should be made through the infected tissue down to the fascia. An ability to undermine the skin and subcutaneous tissues with digital palpation often will confirm the diagnosis. Multiple incisions can be made sequentially towards the periphery of the affected tissue until well-vascularized, healthy, resistant tissue is reached at all margins. The remaining affected tissue must be excised. The wound can then be packed and sequentially débrided on a daily basis as necessary until it displays healthy tissue at all margins.

Hyperbaric oxygen therapy may be of some benefit, particularly in patients whose cultures are positive for anaerobic organisms. In one retrospective non-randomized study,[91] the addition of hyperbaric oxygen therapy to the standard surgical débridement and antimicrobial therapy appeared to significantly decrease both wound morbidity, as measured by the required number of débridements, and overall mortality in patients with necrotizing fasciitis. The benefit in patients receiving hyperbaric oxygen therapy was particularly impressive because the patients who received hyperbaric oxygen were sicker, with a higher incidence of diabetes, leukocytosis, and shock.

The primary concern after the initial resuscitative efforts and surgical débridement is the management of the open wound. Allograft and xenograft skin can be used to cover open wounds, thus decreasing heat and evaporative water loss. Interestingly, temporary biologic closure of open wounds also seems to decrease wound pain. In addition, allograft skin has an ability to decrease bacterial growth.[109] Amniotic membranes have also been shown to be an effective wound covering in patients with necrotizing fasciitis.[101] Finally, skin flaps can be mobilized to help cover open wounds once the wound infections have resolved and granulation has begun.

Gastrointestinal Preparation and Management

Preoperative Bowel Preparation

Preparation of the lower gastrointestinal tract prior to elective gynecologic surgery has several goals. In most gynecologic surgical procedures, when the gastrointestinal tract is not entered, mechanical preparation of the bowel reduces gastrointestinal contents, thus allowing more room in the abdomen and pelvis and facilitating the surgical procedure. Further, even if there is a rectosigmoid colon enterotomy during surgery, the mechanical bowel preparation eliminates formed stool and reduces the bacterial contamination, thus reducing infectious complications. Mechanical bowel preparation may be accomplished by several methods (Table 3–12). The traditional use of laxatives and enemas requires at least 12–24 hours and generally causes moderate abdominal distention and crampy pain. In addition, nursing supervision of enema administration and the need for intravenous fluid replacement make this regimen relatively expensive. Randomized trials comparing traditional mechanical bowel preparation with oral gut lavage (GoLYTELY) have found that the use of approximately 4 liters of GoLYTELY (administered until the rectal effluent is clear) provides more complete, faster, and more comfortable bowel preparation.[109a] Further, the fluid loss following gut lavage with GoLYTELY appears to be clinically insignificant. Gut lavage can usually be performed at home the day prior to scheduled surgery. Rarely, if the patient cannot drink the 4 liters, the GoLYTELY may be administered through a small-caliber nasogastric tube. The authors recommend mechanical bowel preparation for all patients who will undergo major abdominal, pelvic, or vaginal surgery.

High infection rates after colonic surgery have lead to investigation of methods aimed at reducing these significant complications. Although mechanical bowel preparation is essential and part of all colonic surgery preparation regimens, it does not reduce the infection rate satisfactorily. Reduction of the number of pathogenic flora in the colon is the primary strategy to reducing infection after colonic surgery. The colon has the greatest concentration of bacteria in the body, including both aerobes and anaerobes. Anaerobes outnumber aerobes by 1000:1.

After reducing the bacterial load by mechanical preparation, the addition of antibiotics to the colon can further reduce the bacterial count. Of the many trials reported, the most widely accepted regimen combines erythromycin base and neomycin administered orally (Table 3–13).[110–112] Many surgeons substitute metronidazole for the erythromycin, although there is no significant difference in infection rates. Some patients tolerate metronidazole better than erythromycin. The use of oral antibiotics 24 hours prior to colonic resection has reduced the infection rate from approximately 40% to 5–10% in randomized trials. Because these oral antibiotics are generally poorly absorbed and many do little to reduce infection from vaginal contamination, the authors usually add an intravenous antibiotic (first-generation cephalosporin) to their preoperative regimen. The authors routinely use antibiotic bowel prophylaxis for patients who will likely undergo colorectal surgery (pelvic exenteration, ovarian cancer debulking) and those who are at high risk for rectal injury (such as severe cases of endometriosis or pelvic inflammatory disease).

Postoperative Gastrointestinal Complications

Ileus. Following abdominal or pelvic surgery, most patients will have a component of intestinal ileus. The exact mechanism by which this arrest and disorganization of gastrointestinal motility occurs is

Table 3–12

Mechanical Bowel Preparation Regimens to Begin Day Prior to Surgery

Time	Traditional Mechanical Preparation	GoLYTELY
2400	Clear liquid diet	Clear liquid diet
1200	Magnesium citrate, 240 ml PO	GoLYTELY, 4 L PO over 3 h
2000	Saline enemas to clear IV-D5 ½ NS with 20 mg KCl at 125 ml/h	
2400	NPO	NPO

Table 3–13

Oral Antibiotic Bowel Preparation

1. Mechanical bowel preparation as outlined in Table 3–12 but beginning 48 hours prior to surgery
2. Erythromycin base, 500 mg,* plus neomycin, 1 g PO, at 1:00 P.M., 2:00 P.M., and 11:00 P.M. the day before surgery

*Metronidazole (500 mg) may be substituted.

unknown, but it appears to be associated with the opening of the peritoneal cavity and is aggravated by more extensive manipulation of the intestinal tract and prolonged surgical procedures. Infection, peritonitis, and electrolyte disturbances may also result in an ileus. For most patients undergoing common gynecologic operations, the degree of ileus is minimal and gastrointestinal function returns relatively rapidly, allowing for the resumption of oral intake within a few days of surgery. On the other hand, the patient who has persistently diminished bowel sounds, abdominal distention, and nausea and vomiting requires further evaluation and more aggressive management.

Ileus is usually manifested by abdominal distention and should be initially evaluated by physical examination. Pertinent points of the abdominal examination include assessment of the quality of bowel sounds and palpation searching for tenderness or rebound. The possibility that the patient's signs and symptoms may be associated with a more serious intestinal obstruction or other intestinal complication must also be considered. Pelvic examination should be performed in order to evaluate the possibility of a pelvic abscess or hematoma that may be contributing to the ileus. Further assessment by abdominal x-ray evaluating the abdomen in the flat (supine) position as well as in the upright position usually will aid in the diagnosis of an ileus. The most common radiographic findings include dilated loops of small and large bowel as well as air-fluid levels in the upright position. Sometimes, massive dilation of the colon or stomach may be noted. The remote possibility of distal colonic obstruction suggested by a dilated cecum should be excluded by rectal examination, proctosigmoidoscopy, or barium enema. The flat plate of the abdomen in the postoperative gynecology patient, especially in the upright position, may also show evidence of free air. This is a common finding following surgery, which will last from 7 to 10 days in some instances and is not indicative of a perforated viscus in the great majority of patients.

The initial management of a postoperative ileus is aimed at gastrointestinal tract decompression and maintenance of appropriate intravenous replacement fluids and electrolytes. A well-positioned and properly functioning nasogastric tube should evacuate the stomach of its fluid and gaseous contents. Furthermore, and very importantly, prolonged nasogastric suction continues to remove swallowed air, which is the most common source of air in the small bowel. Some clinicians prefer a longer small intestinal tube (Cantor or Miller-Abbott tube).[113] These tubes, which usually have a mercury-filled bag on their distal tip, may be propelled by peristalsis through the pylorus and into the small bowel, thus allowing a better evacuation of the small bowel. The disadvantage of "long tubes" is that they take a longer time to become positioned and may not enter the small bowel as a result of the decreased intestinal motility associated with ileus. Fluid and electrolyte replacement must be adequate to keep the patient well perfused. Significant amounts of third-space fluid loss occur in the bowel wall, the bowel lumen, and the peritoneal cavity during the acute episode. Further, gastrointestinal fluid losses from the stomach may lead to a metabolic alkalosis and depletion of other electrolytes as well. Careful monitoring of serum chemistries and appropriate replacement are necessary. Most cases of severe ileus will begin to improve over a period of several days. In general, this is recognized by reduction in the abdominal distention, return of normal bowel sounds, and passage of flatus or stool. Follow-up abdominal x-rays should be obtained as necessary for further monitoring. When the gastrointestinal tract function appears to have returned to normal, the nasogastric tube may be discontinued and a liquid diet instituted. On the other hand, if a patient shows no evidence of improvement over the first 48–72 hours of medical management, other causes of ileus should be sought. These may include ureteral injury, peritonitis from pelvic infection, unrecognized gastrointestinal tract injury with peritoneal spill, or fluid and electrolyte abnormalities such as hypokalemia. It has been suggested that in the evaluation of persistent ileus, the use of water-soluble upper gastrointestinal contrast study may assist in the resolution of the ileus. However, prospective randomized data regarding this therapeutic maneuver are lacking.

Small Bowel Obstruction. Obstruction of the small bowel following major gynecologic surgery occurs in approximately 1–2% of patients.[114] The most common cause of small bowel obstruction is adhesions to the operative site. Should the small bowel become adherent in a twisted position, distention and ileus and bowel wall edema may lead to partial or complete obstruction. Less common causes of postoperative small bowel obstruction include herniation of the small bowel into an incisional hernia and an unrecognized defect in the small bowel or large bowel mesentery. Early in its clinical course, a postoperative small bowel obstruction may have signs and symptoms identical to those of an ileus. Initial conservative management as outlined for the treatment of an ileus is appropriate. Because of the potential for mesenteric vascular occlusion and resulting ischemia or perforation, worsening symptoms of abdominal pain, progressive distention, fever, leukocytosis, or acidosis should be evaluated carefully because immediate surgery may be required. In most cases of small bowel obstruction following gynecologic surgery, the obstruction is only partial and the symptoms usually resolve with conservative management. As with an ileus, further evaluation after several days of conservative management may be necessary. Evaluation of the gastrointestinal tract with barium enema and an upper gastrointestinal series with small bowel follow-through is most appropriate. In most cases, complete obstruction is not documented, although a narrowing or tethering of the segment of small bowel may lead to the suspicion as to the site of the gastrointestinal problem. Further conservative management with nasogastric decompression and intravenous fluid replacement may allow time for bowel wall edema or torsion of the mesentery to resolve. If this process becomes prolonged, and the patient's nutritional status is marginal, the use of total parenteral nutrition may be necessary. Conservative medical management of postoperative small bowel obstruction usually results in complete resolution. However, if after full evaluation and an adequate trial of medical management, there remains persistent evidence of small bowel obstruction, an exploratory laparotomy may be necessary in order to surgically evaluate and manage the obstruction. In most cases, lysis of adhesions is all that is required, although a segment of small bowel that is badly damaged or extensively sclerosed from adhesions may require resection and re-anastomosis.

Colonic Obstruction. Postoperative colonic obstruction following surgery for most gynecologic conditions is exceedingly rare. It is almost always associated with a pelvic malignancy, which in most cases will have been known at the time of the initial operation. Advanced ovarian carcinoma is the most common cause of colonic obstruction in postoperative gynecologic surgery patients; it is due to extrinsic impingement of the colon by the pelvic malignancy. Intrinsic colonic lesions may have gone unrecognized, especially in a patient with some other benign gynecologic condition. When colonic obstruction is manifested by abdominal distention and abdominal radiographs reveal a dilated colon and enlarging cecum, further evaluation of the large bowel is required by barium enema and/or coloscopy. Dilation of the cecum on abdominal x-ray to greater than 10–12 cm in diameter requires immediate evaluation and surgical decompression by performing a colostomy. This should be performed at the earliest point at which the obstruction is documented. Conservative management of colonic obstruction is not appropriate because the complication of colonic perforation has an exceedingly high mortality rate.

Diarrhea. Episodes of diarrhea are common following abdominal and pelvic surgery as the gastrointestinal tract returns to its normal function and motility. However, prolonged and multiple episodes may represent a pathologic process such as impending small bowel obstruction, colonic obstruction, or pseudomembranous colitis. Excessive amounts of diarrhea should be evaluated by abdominal x-rays and stool samples submitted for evaluation of the presence of ova and parasites, bacterial culture, and evaluation for *Clostridium difficile* toxin. Proctoscopy and colonoscopy may also be advisable in severe cases. Evidence of intestinal obstruction should be managed as outlined previously. Infectious causes of diarrhea should be managed with the appropriate antibiotics as well as fluid and electrolyte replacement. *Clostridium difficile*–associated pseudomembranous colitis may result from exposure to any antibiotic. Discontinuation of these antibiotics (unless needed for another severe infection) is advisable, along with the institution of appropriate therapy. Because of the expense of vancomycin, the authors usually institute therapy with metronidazole. This therapy should be continued until the diarrhea abates, and several weeks of oral therapy may be required in order to obtain complete resolution of the pseudomembranous colitis.

Fistula. Gastrointestinal fistulas following gynecologic operations are also relatively rare. They are most often associated with malignancy, prior radiation therapy, or surgical injury to the large or small bowel that was improperly repaired or unrecognized. Signs and symptoms of gastrointestinal fistula are often similar to those of small bowel obstruction and/or ileus except that a fever is usually a more prominent component of the patient's symptomatology. When fever is associated with gastrointestinal dysfunction postoperatively, evaluation should include early assessment of the gastrointestinal tract for its continuity. When fistula is suspected, water-soluble gastrointestinal contrast material is advised to avoid the complication of barium peritonitis. Evaluation with abdominal pelvic CT scan may also assist in the identification of a fistula and associated abscess. Recognition of an intraperitoneal gastrointestinal leak or fistula formation usually requires immediate surgery unless the fistula has drained spontaneously through the abdominal wall or vaginal cuff.

Enterocutaneous fistula arising from the small bowel and draining spontaneously through the abdominal incision may on occasion be managed successfully with medical therapy. This should include nasogastric decompression, replacement of intravenous fluids as well as total parenteral nutrition, and appropriate antibiotics to treat an associated mixed bacterial infection. If the infection is under control and there are no other signs of peritonitis, the surgeon may consider allowing potential resolution of the fistula over a period of up to 2 weeks. Some authors have suggested the use of somatostatin in order to decrease intestinal tract secretion and allow for earlier healing of the fistula. In some cases, the fistula will close spontaneously with this mode of management. If, on the other hand, the enterocutaneous fistula does not close with conservative medical management, surgical correction with resection, bypass, and/or re-anastomosis will be necessary in most cases.

A rectovaginal fistula following gynecologic surgery is usually the result of surgical trauma that may have been aggravated by the presence of extensive adhesions in the rectovaginal septum associated with endometriosis, pelvic inflammatory disease, or pelvic malignancy. Management of a small rectovaginal fistula may take a conservative medical approach, hoping that decreasing the fecal stream will allow closure of the fistula. In other patients, a small fistula that allows continence except for an occasional leak of flatus may be managed conservatively for the time being until the inflammatory process in the pelvis resolves. At that point, usually several months later, correction of the fistula is most appropriate. Large rectovaginal fistulas that have no hope of closing spontaneously are best managed by initial diverting colostomy followed by repair of the fistula after inflammation has resolved. Once the fistula closure is healed and established to be successful, take-down of the colostomy should be performed.

Thromboembolism

Risk Factors

Deep venous thrombosis and pulmonary embolism, although largely preventable, are significant complications occurring in postoperative patients. The magnitude of this problem is relevant to the gynecologist, because 40% of all deaths following gynecologic surgery are directly attributed to pulmonary emboli.[115] Pulmonary embolism is also the second leading cause of death in women who undergo a legally induced abortion,[116] and the most frequent cause of postoperative death in patients with uterine[117] or cervical carcinoma.[118]

The causal factors of venous thrombosis were first proposed by Virchow in 1858 and include a hypercoagulable state, venous stasis, and vessel intima injury. When the patient undergoing gynecologic surgery is specifically considered, two prospective studies have evaluated risk factors associated with the postoperative occurrence of deep venous thrombosis. Clayton studied the risk factors of 124 patients undergoing vaginal and abdominal surgery for benign gynecologic disease.[119] Utilizing logistic regression analysis, the five factors identified to be associated with postoperative deep venous thrombosis were age, varicose veins, percentage overweight, euglobulin lysis time, and serum fibrin-related antigen. The risk factors associated with venous thromboembolic complications have also been assessed in 411 patients undergoing major abdominal and pelvic surgery.[120] Of these patients, 84% had gynecologic malignancies. Preoperative risk factors identified in this study included age, nonwhite patients, increasing stage of malignancy, past history of deep venous thrombosis, lower extremity edema or venous stasis changes, varicose veins, weight, and a past history of radiation therapy. Intraoperative factors associated with postoperative deep venous thrombosis included increased anesthesia time, increased blood loss, and transfusion requirements in the operating room. The recognition of these factors, which are associated with postoperative venous thromboembolism, should allow the clinician to stratify patients into low-risk, medium-risk, and high-risk groups.

Prophylactic Methods

Over the past two decades, a number of prophylactic methods have undergone clinical trials showing significant reduction in the incidence of deep venous thrombosis, and a few studies have been completed that have demonstrated a reduction in fatal pulmonary emboli. The ideal prophylactic method would be effective, free of significant side effects, well accepted by the patient and nursing staff, widely applicable to most patient groups, and inexpensive.

The use of small doses of subcutaneously administered heparin for the prevention of deep venous thrombosis and pulmonary embolism is the most widely studied of all prophylactic methods. Over 25 controlled trials have demonstrated that heparin given subcutaneously 2 hours preoperatively and every 8–12 hours postoperatively is effective in reducing the incidence of deep venous thrombosis. The value of low-dose heparin in preventing fatal pulmonary emboli was established by a randomized, controlled, multicenter international trial, which demonstrated a reduction in fatal postoperative pulmonary emboli in general surgery patients receiving low-dose heparin every 8 hours postoperatively.[121]

Trials of low-dose heparin in gynecologic surgery patients are limited, and a clear consensus as to the value of low-dose heparin in all groups of patients has not been established, owing to differences in patient selection and length of follow-up. Three randomized controlled gynecologic surgery studies used the same regimen of low-dose heparin administration: 5000 units subcutaneously 2 hours preoperatively and every 12 hours for 7 days postoperatively. The trials reported by Ballard[122] and by Taberner[123] were conducted in patients with benign gynecologic conditions (98%). All patients were over 40 years of age, and follow-up was discontinued at the time of discharge from hospital. The American study evaluated a larger group of patients on a gynecologic oncology unit.[124] Only 16% had benign gynecologic conditions, and follow-up included the first 6 weeks postoperatively.

The trial by Taberner showed a 23% incidence of deep venous thrombosis in the control group, as compared with a 6% incidence of deep venous thrombosis in the low dose heparin–treated patients.[123] This difference was statistically significant ($P < .05$). Unfortunately, although this was a randomized trial, the control group contained a larger number of patients with malignancy. When the cancer patients were excluded from the trial analysis, there remained no significant value to the use of low-dose heparin in patients with benign conditions. Ballard's study also evaluated a group of patients who had benign gynecologic diseases.[122] The nontreated control group had a 29% incidence of deep venous thrombosis as compared with a 3.6% incidence in the low dose heparin–treated group ($P < .001$). In contrast is a randomized trial of patients undergoing major abdominal and pelvic surgery on a gynecologic oncology service.[124] There was no difference in the incidence of thromboembolic complications between the control group (12.4%) and the low dose heparin–treated group (14.8%). In summary, with regard to gynecologic surgery, only the trial reported by Ballard has found a beneficial effect of low-dose heparin in patients with benign gynecologic conditions.[122] Taberner,[123] in benign gynecology patients, and Clarke-Pearson,[124] in gynecologic oncology patients, did not find low-dose heparin to be of benefit.

In a subsequent trial, two more intense heparin regimens were evaluated in high-risk gynecologic oncology patients.[125] In this study, heparin was given either in a regimen of 5000 units subcutaneously 2 hours preoperatively and every 8 hours postoperatively or in a regimen of 5000 units subcutaneously every 8 hours preoperatively (a minimum of three preoperative doses) and every 8 hours postoperatively. Both of these prophylactic regimens were effective in significantly reducing the incidence of postoperative deep venous thrombosis.

Although low-dose heparin is considered to have no effect on measurable coagulation parameters, most large series have noted an increase in the bleeding complication rate, especially a higher incidence of wound hematoma. Up to 10–15% of otherwise healthy patients develop a prolonged activated partial thromboplastin time (APTT) after 5000 units of heparin is given subcutaneously.[126] These transiently anticoagulated patients have also been noted in one carefully monitored trial of low-dose heparin in gynecology. It was these patients in whom the major bleeding complications were encountered postoperatively. Dockerty also found that estimated blood loss increased from 246 to 401 ml in low dose heparin–treated patients undergoing inguinal or pelvic lymphadenectomy.[127] Retrospective studies have suggested that low-dose heparin contributed to an increased occurrence of lymphocysts,[128, 129] and a prospective study demonstrated a twofold increase in retroperitoneal lymph drainage volume in patients treated with low-dose heparin.[126] Finally, although relatively rare, thrombocytopenia is associated with low-dose heparin use and has been found in 6% of patients after gynecologic surgery.[126] Although many authors feel that no monitoring of coagulation parameters is necessary for effective and safe low-dose heparin use, periodic postoperative assessment of APTT and platelet count seems prudent to maximize the identification of the 22% of patients who had either prolonged APTT or thrombocytopenia and who are most prone to develop major clinical hemorrhagic complications.

Stasis in the veins of the legs has been clearly demonstrated on the operating table, and continues postoperatively for varying lengths of time. Many authors feel that the combination of stasis occurring in the capacitance veins of the calf during surgery and the hypercoagulable state induced by surgery is the prime factor contributing to the development of acute postoperative deep venous thrombosis. Prospective studies of the natural history of postoperative venous thrombosis have shown that the calf veins are the preponderant site of thrombi and that most thrombi develop within 24 hours of surgery.[130] Reduction of venous stasis in the perioperative period by various mechanical methods has been less extensively investigated than pharmacologic methods such as low-dose heparin. However, a growing body of literature supports the important role that these mechanical prophylactic methods may play in the prevention of postoperative deep vein thrombosis.

Although probably of only modest benefit, reduction of stasis by short preoperative hospital stays and early postoperative ambulation should be encouraged for all patients. Elevation of the foot of the bed by 20 degrees, thus raising the calf above heart level, allows gravity to drain the calf veins and should further reduce stasis. More active forms of mechanical prophylaxis include elastic gradient compression stockings and external pneumatic leg compression.

In a survey of general surgeons in the United States, gradient elastic stockings were second only to low-dose heparin as the prophylactic method of choice in high-risk and moderate-high-risk surgical patients.[131] The simplicity of elastic stockings and the absence of significant side effects are probably the two most important reasons that they are included in the routine postoperative orders of many surgeons. Controlled studies of gradient elastic stockings are limited but do suggest modest benefit when carefully fitted.[132] Poorly fitted stockings may be hazardous to some patients, who develop a tourniquet effect at the knee or mid-thigh.[117] Variations in human anatomy do not allow perfect fit of all patients to stocking sizes manufactured.

The largest body of literature discussing the reduction of postoperative venous stasis deals with intermittent external compression of the leg by pneumatically inflated sleeves placed around the calf and/or leg during intraoperative and postoperative periods. Various pneumatic compression devices and leg sleeve designs are available, and the current literature has not demonstrated superiority of one system over another. The single-chambered calf compression device has been studied the most extensively and appears to significantly reduce the incidence of deep venous thrombosis on a par with that of low-dose heparin. In addition to increasing venous flow and pulsatile emptying of the calf veins, external pneumatic compression also appears to augment endogenous fibrinolysis, which may result in lysis of very early thrombi before they become clinically significant.[133]

The duration of postoperative external pneumatic compression has varied in various trials. Because most deep venous thrombosis occurs intraoperatively and in the first 72 hours postoperatively,[134] the authors believe that this time interval should be a minimum length for external pneumatic compression. Several investigators have found external pneumatic compression to be effective when used only in the operating room or in the operating room and for the first 24 hours postoperatively.[135, 136]

External pneumatic compression used in patients undergoing major surgery for gynecologic malignancy has been found to reduce the incidence of postoperative venous thromboembolic complications by nearly threefold.[134] Calf compression was applied intraoperatively and for the first 5 postoperative days. In a subsequent trial of like patients designed to evaluate whether external pneumatic compression might achieve similar benefits when used only intraoperatively and for the first 24 hours postoperatively, there was no reduction of deep venous thrombosis compared with the control group.[130] It appears that patients with gynecologic malignancies remain at risk because of stasis and hypercoagulable states for a longer period of time than the general surgical patients, and if compression is to be effective, it must be used for at least 5 days postoperatively.

External pneumatic leg compression has no significant side effects or risks, although patient tolerance has been cited as a drawback to the use of this equipment. However, the authors have had only two patients of nearly 300 treated with external pneumatic compression request removal because of discomfort. The equipment is easily managed by the nursing staff, and although initial capital outlay for external pneumatic compressors may seem large, Salzman calculated that the cost per patient of this prophylactic method is slightly less than that of low-dose heparin given for 7 days postoperatively.[137]

Management of Postoperative Deep Venous Thrombosis and Pulmonary Embolism

Pulmonary embolism accounts for 40% of deaths following gynecologic surgical procedures.[115] In order to prevent these serious complications, an effective program aimed at the identification of high-risk patients and the use of prophylactic venous thromboembolism regimens has been outlined. In addition, the early recognition of deep vein thrombosis and pulmonary embolism and immediate treatment are critical. Most pulmonary emboli arise from the deep venous system of the leg, although following gynecologic surgery, the pelvic veins are a known source of fatal pulmonary emboli as well. The diagnosis of lower extremity deep venous thrombosis requires a high level of suspicion and the appropriate use of diagnostic tests. The signs and symptoms of deep vein thrombosis of the lower extremity include pain, edema, erythema, and prominent vascular pattern of the superficial veins. These signs and symptoms are relatively nonspecific in that from somewhere between 50 and 80% of patients with these symptoms will not actually have deep vein thrombosis.[138] Conversely, approximately 80% of patients with symptomatic pulmonary emboli have no signs or symptoms of thrombosis in the lower extremities.[139] Because of the lack of specificity when signs and symptoms are recognized by the surgeon, additional diagnostic tests should be performed to establish the diagnosis of deep vein thrombosis. The "gold standard" for diagnosis of deep vein thrombosis has been a contrast venogram. Unfortunately, this study is modestly uncomfortable, requires the injection of a contrast material that may cause allergic reaction or renal injury, and may result in phlebitis in approximately 5% of patients.[140] Fortunately, newer diagnostic tests have been developed that are less invasive yet have a high accuracy rate in most patients. Impedance plethysmography is a noninvasive study that measures the change in electrical impedance of the lower extremity when venous blood flow and volume are altered by an occlusive cuff on the thigh. This study may be performed at the patient's bedside and repeated as often as necessary without any risk to the patient. Correlation with venography in symptomatic patients approaches 95%.[141, 142] The test is very good for the identification of deep venous thrombi in the popliteal, femoral, and external iliac segments. It is less accurate (30%) in identifying calf vein thrombosis and does not identify thrombi occurring in the internal iliac venous system. False-positive results are primarily due to extrinsic venous compression. In gynecology, this might include a large pelvic mass compressing the external iliac or common iliac vein.

Doppler ultrasound has also been used for the noninvasive diagnosis of deep vein thrombosis, although its accuracy is slightly less than that of impedance plethysmography. The reason for this is primarily due to the variable interpretation of audible venous flow patterns, which may be somewhat subjective.[143] B-mode duplex Doppler imaging has been found to be more effective in the diagnosis of symptomatic venous thrombosis, especially when it arises in the proximal lower extremity. With duplex Doppler imaging, the femoral vein can be visualized and clots may be seen directly.[144] Compression of the vein with the ultrasound probe tip allows for assessment of venous collapsibility; the presence of a thrombus diminishes vein wall collapsibility. Color flow studies have also been added to this imaging technique. Doppler imaging is less accurate when evaluating the calf venous system and the pelvic veins. Magnetic resonance imaging (MRI) can also identify thrombi in the deep venous system quite accurately.[145] The primary drawback to MRI is the time involved in examining the lower extremity and pelvis as well as the expense of this technology. All of these diagnostic studies are accurate when performed by a skilled technologist and in most patients may replace the need for routine contrast venography.

The treatment of postoperative deep venous thrombosis requires the immediate institution of anticoagulant therapy. Heparin should be initiated giving a bolus of 5000 units intravenously, followed by a continuous intravenous infusion of 1000 units/hour. Approximately 4 hours after initiation of heparin therapy, an activated partial thromboplastin time (APTT) should be obtained to assess the adequacy of the anticoagulant effect. In general, prolongation of the APTT to 1.5–2.0 times the control level achieves appropriate anticoagulant therapy. The goals of anticoagulant therapy include the prevention of clot propagation or embolization and prevention of re-thrombosis in a high-risk patient; the risks are primarily bleeding complications.[146] Oral maintenance therapy using sodium warfarin (Coumadin) is advised for at least 3 months. Standard treatment regimens called for the use of intravenous heparin for 10 days, followed by continuation of Coumadin for 3 months.[147] However, a randomized trial evaluated a 10-day regimen of heparin compared with a 5-day regimen of heparin and found the 5-day regimen to be equally effective in treating the acute thrombosis and preventing re-thrombosis.[148] Therefore, it is recommended that intravenous heparin be maintained for 5 days and during that time oral Coumadin be initiated. The goals of Coumadin therapy are to achieve an oral dose of medication that will prolong the prothrombin time (PT) to approximately 1.5 times control value. Initially, PT values should be obtained on a daily basis until a stable dose of Coumadin is established. Thereafter, the PT is checked at intervals of every 1–2 weeks for the duration of 3 months' therapy. Anticoagulant therapy may be discontinued in 3 months if the etiology of the deep vein thrombosis episode (such as an acute surgical event or trauma) has been eliminated.

The major hazard of anticoagulant therapy in the postoperative patient is an increased risk of bleeding complications. Therefore, it is important that APTT, PT, platelet count, and hematocrit be followed carefully and that the anticoagulant does not drastically alter the patient to a hypocoagulable state. Heparin-induced thrombocytopenia is a rare complication and has been reported in association with the use of both low-dose prophylactic heparin and standard anticoagulant doses.[149] Therefore, periodic checks of platelet count while the patient is on heparin therapy are advised. Thrombolytic therapy (streptokinase or urokinase) has been advocated by some investigators for the treatment of acute deep vein thrombosis. However, the risk of bleeding complications in a surgical site contraindicate thrombolytic therapy in the postoperative patient.

The diagnosis of pulmonary embolism also requires a high index of suspicion, because many of the signs and symptoms are associated with other, more common pulmonary complications following surgery. The classic findings of pleuritic chest pain, hemoptysis, shortness of breath, tachycardia, and tachypnea should alert the physician to the possibility of a pulmonary embolism. Many times, however, the signs are much more subtle and may only be suggested by a persistent tachycardia or a slight elevation in the respiratory rate. Patients suspected of pulmonary embolism should be evaluated initially by chest x-ray, electrocardiogram, and an arterial blood gas. Any evidence of abnormality should be further evaluated by ventilation-perfusion lung scan, searching for evidence of decreased perfusions in areas of adequate ventilation. Unfortunately, a high percentage of lung scans may be interpreted as "indeterminant." In this setting, careful clinical evaluation and judgment are required to decide whether pulmonary arteriography should be obtained to document or exclude the presence of a pulmonary embolism.

Immediate anticoagulant therapy, identical to that

outlined for the treatment of deep vein thrombosis should be initiated. Respiratory support including oxygen and bronchodilators and an intensive care setting may be necessary. Massive pulmonary emboli are usually quickly fatal, although on rare occasion pulmonary embolectomy has been successfully performed. The use of pulmonary artery catheterization with the administration of thrombolytic agents bears further evaluation and may be important in the patient with massive pulmonary embolism. In situations in which anticoagulant therapy is ineffective in the prevention of rethrombosis and repeated embolization from the lower extremities or pelvis, vena cava interruption may be necessary. This may be accomplished through the percutaneous placement of a vena cava umbrella, filter, or the use of a large clip to obstruct the vena cava above the level of the thrombosis. In most cases, however, anticoagulant therapy is sufficient to prevent repeat thrombosis and embolism and to allow the patient's own endogenous thrombolytic mechanisms to lyse the pulmonary embolus.

MANAGEMENT OF COMMON MEDICAL PROBLEMS

Endocrine Disease

Diabetes Mellitus

In the United States, approximately 200,000 new cases of diabetes mellitus are diagnosed each year, making it the disease of the endocrine system most frequently encountered by gynecologists. Diabetes can lead to significant problems affecting the cardiovascular, renal, nervous, immune, and gastrointestinal systems. If uncontrolled at the time of surgery, there may be up to a twofold increase in morbidity and a threefold increase in postoperative mortality.

In diabetic patients, cardiovascular disease accounts for more than one-half of all deaths.[150] Females with non–insulin-dependent diabetes are four times more likely to suffer from myocardial infarction than similar age-adjusted controls. In addition, diabetic patients can develop cardiomyopathy and congestive heart failure in the absence of coronary artery disease. Therefore, the preoperative evaluation should include a thorough investigation of the diabetic's cardiovascular history, especially for symptoms of early congestive heart failure. The physical examination must evaluate for end-organ (cardiac, renal, ocular) damage secondary to diabetes in order to assess the patient's risk for surgical complications and to prevent sequelae if possible.

After 20 years, 50% of diabetics have some nephropathy and 70% are hypertensive.[150] Relative hyperkalemia secondary to a hyponinemic hypoaldosteronism is also seen in patients with this disease. Therefore, strict attention to fluids and electrolytes is necessary in these patients. In addition, diabetics have an increased risk of acute renal failure after receiving intravenous iodine contrast, especially if their serum creatinine concentration is 2.0 mg/dl or higher, other vascular disease is present, or the onset of diabetes is before 40 years of age.[151]

Neurologic sequelae of diabetes include defects in the autonomic nervous system innervating the esophagus, stomach, and small intestine, which results in a decreased esophageal and intestinal motility and delayed gastric emptying. These physiologic problems increase the risk of aspiration pneumonitis. The autonomic neuropathy also causes labile changes in pulse and blood pressure, and because of this these patients are known to be at increased risk for intraoperative myocardial infarction.[152]

Diabetes mellitus also predisposes patients to infection. There is a known predisposition to gram-negative and staphylococcal pneumonia. There is also an increased incidence of gram-negative and group B streptococcal sepsis.[153] Approximately 7% of all diabetics will have postoperative gram-negative sepsis, compared with a 1% incidence in a nondiabetic population. Sepsis is most often caused by *E. coli* from the urinary tract.[154] On a cellular level, diabetic patients have a defect in the mobilization of inflammatory cells, phagocytosis function, and bactericidal activity in polymorphonuclear neutrophils. It is also interesting that these defects are related to poor glucose control.[155] Decreased amounts of collagen formation, fibroblast growth, and capillary growth also explain the increased incidence of wound dehiscence.[156, 157] In one study, patients with diabetes had a 10.7% rate of wound infection, compared with 1.8% in the nondiabetic population.[158]

Anesthesia and surgically related stress are known to increase serum glucose levels as well as stimulate increases in known insulin antagonists—glucagon, growth hormone, cortisol, norepinephrine, and epinephrine.[160] Interestingly, these adverse effects are not seen when diabetics have a regional anesthetic.

Preoperative management of insulin is a topic of some concern and controversy. Goals include avoiding ketosis, hyperglycemia, and hypoglycemia. Failure to achieve these goals places the diabetic patient at risk for fluid and electrolyte disturbances, decreased immune function, osmotic diuresis, and ketoacidosis. The traditional regimen of giving one-third to one-half of the patient's total daily requirement of insulin as intermediate-acting insulin (e.g., NPH) the morning of surgery is felt by some authors to be inadequate.[161] An alternative is to admit the patient 2 days prior to surgery and begin an insulin drip at 1–3 units/hour. Initially, glucose levels are monitored every 1–2 hours. After stabilization in the 100–200 mg/dl range, glucose monitoring every 4 hours is adequate.[151] For milder forms of diabetes, whether controlled by diet or with oral hypoglycemics, no medication or insulin is given prior to surgery. If the patient is taking long-acting sulfonylureas, they should be discontinued 3 days prior to surgery. Short-acting sulfonylurea agents are discontinued 1 day prior to surgery. Regardless of whether the patient has mild or severe disease, intraoperative glucose control is felt to be important in the overall management of diabetes. Intravenous insulin is given intraoperatively depending on the serum glucose concentration, which is checked every hour.[162] Glucose should be maintained in the 100–200 mg/dl range with 5% dextrose in half-normal or isotonic saline. Compulsive management of diabetes in the perioperative setting will yield better postoperative and long-term results.

Intraoperative and postoperative hypoglycemia and hyperglycemia may also have many adverse effects; therefore, it is imperative that the serum glucose level be controlled. As in the preoperative setting, it is a matter of some debate as to whether the postoperative insulin should be delivered intravenously, as a continuous drip, or as intermittent (every 6 hours) subcutaneous boluses of regular insulin. Although many regimens have been proposed to achieve glycemic control in the postoperative period, very few studies compare the effectiveness of different protocols. Rapid and accurate determinations of blood glucose levels are required for optimal control of blood sugar and adjustment in the dose of insulin administered.

Perioperative hypoglycemia has potential for serious neurologic sequelae and must be avoided. Similarly, hyperglycemia can increase the incidence of perioperative infections, electrolyte abnormalities, hyperosmolar coma, and ketoacidosis. Hyperglycemia also directly impairs wound healing. In addition, experimental data exist that suggest that hyperglycemia can sensitize cerebral tissue to ischemic injury.[163] Finally, it appears that regional anesthesia, may, in fact, lower stress-induced hyperglycemia and may therefore be the preferred route of anesthesia in most gynecologic procedures involving diabetic patients.

There is a well-established association of diabetes, and its thrombotic complications, with the occurrence of disease in the microvasculature.[164] Differences in macroangiopathy and microangiopathy in type 1 and type 2 diabetes suggest important differences in the pathophysiology between the two types of diabetes. Patients with type 1 diabetes have been shown to demonstrate enhanced platelet aggregation and thromboxane A_2 production in response to a variety of stimuli.[165] However, recent data also provide evidence that patients with type 2 diabetes and macroangiopathic disease have enhanced platelet activity in vitro as well as in vivo. This platelet activity is a reflection of an increased production of 11-dehydrothromboxane B_2 from thromboxane A_2 biosynthesis. It is postulated that improved glycemic control and low-dose aspirin may correct these abnormalities in platelet function.[166]

Hyperthyroidism

Diffuse toxic goiter, Graves' disease, is the most common cause of hyperthyroidism and affects women more often than men (10:1). Preoperative recognition and management of this disease are crucial to avoid a catastrophic postoperative course. The typical patient is between 20 and 40 years of age and usually presents with tachycardia, diaphoresis, palpitations, flushing, and weight loss. Physical examination frequently reveals a diffusely enlarged thyroid gland with a smooth or lobular contour. If the patient is severely thyrotoxic, fever, exophthalmos, hyperreflexia, and tremors may be noted. A bruit also may be heard over the lateral lobes of the thyroid gland secondary to increased blood flow. Circulating immunoglobulins and intrathyroidal T-lymphocytes, capable of binding to the thyroid-stimulating hormone (TSH) receptor and mimicking TSH, are responsible for the increased levels of triiodothyronine (T_3) or thyroxine (T_4). Laboratory data, including total T_4, free T_3, free T_4, and TSH, are useful to confirm the clinical diagnosis.

Preoperative management includes treatment with propylthiouracil (PTU), which is well absorbed after oral administration and is given for at least 2 weeks before surgery in doses of 100–200 mg every 6 hours. PTU inhibits thyroglobulin iodination and iodotyrosine coupling. In addition, it reduces extrathyroidal conversion of T_4 to T_3. Iodine blocks hormonal synthesis and release from the thyroid gland by inhibiting iodine uptake and organification by the follicular cell. SSKI (saturated solution of potassium iodide) is given as 6–12 drops twice daily for about 10–14 days prior to surgery. It is useful in hyperthyroidism secondary to Graves' disease but is not appropriate in hyperthyroidism caused by thyroiditis and may exacerbate conditions if toxic nodular goiter exists. In addition, hydrocortisone, 100 mg every 8 hours, decreases extrathyroidal conversion of T_4 to T_3. Sympathomimetic symptoms may be controlled with beta blockers. Propranolol, 10–80 mg every 6–8 hours, is the most commonly used medication for relief of palpitations, tachycardia, diaphoresis, and anxiety. For optimal surgical outcome, these treatments must be implemented at least 2 weeks prior to surgery and be continued postoperatively. Premature improvement of laboratory values prior to 2 weeks of treatment may give the clinician a false sense of security.[167]

Preoperative considerations include a careful examination of the airway by an anesthesiologist to exclude tracheal compression or deviation secondary to goiter. Special care is given to the eye during surgery to avoid injury precipitated by the exophthalmos. In addition, several other anesthetic considerations include avoiding atropine and cyclopropane, because these agents may exacerbate tachycardia and catecholamine release. Avoidance of methoxyflurane, which undergoes toxic biotransformation, is also advised.[168]

The postoperative management of hyperthyroidism is usually uneventful if the proper preoperative care is given. If not recognized preoperatively, however, the most ominous complication postoperatively is that of thyroid storm. Prior to the advent of beta-adrenergic blocking agents, thyroid storm occurred in over 30% of hyperthyroid patients and carried a mortality of up to 70%.[169, 170] Although propranolol does not predictably prevent a thyroid storm, it has dramatically lowered the mortality rate.[171] The key to the management of thyroid storm is the early recognition and treatment of its manifestations. Hyperpyrexia, hypotension, and tachycardia are features that do not diagnose a thyroid storm but that should alert the clinician to the possibility. The differential diagnosis also includes sepsis and malignant hyperthermia, the latter of which can be differentiated from a thyroid storm by elevated creatine phosphokinase (CPK) levels. In a thyroid storm, CPK levels are typically decreased.[172] Critical life-support measures that should be implemented immediately in a thyroid storm include (1) PTU administration, (2) invasive hemodynamic monitoring and crystalloid therapy, (3) oxygen, (4) mechanical cooling devices, and (5) avoidance of aspirin (it displaces T_4 from the binding proteins).[167]

Hypothyroidism

Hypothyroidism is an insidious disease affecting about 0.8% of the population; the diagnosis requires a high index of suspicion. Fifty per cent of all cases are caused by previous thyroid surgery or treatment with radioactive iodine. Symptoms typically consist of lethargy, intolerance to cold, fatigue, weight gain, constipation, dry skin, memory impairment, and apathy. Examination findings include hoarseness, periorbital edema, dry skin, goiter, brittle hair, and increased relaxation phase of deep tendon reflexes. Physical findings or preoperative studies may also reveal cardiomegaly, pleural and pericardial effusions, ascites, and peripheral edema. Severe hypothyroidism may produce a condition known as myxedematous coma, which manifests as decreased consciousness, hypothermia, hypoventilation, and congestive heart failure. Specific laboratory values to diagnose this disease include an elevated TSH and normal or decreased T_4 levels.

Preoperative preparation of the hypothyroid patient requires a slow replacement with levothyroxine. T_3, T_4, and TSH may normalize quickly, but organ-specific abnormalities are slower to resolve. In particular, it should be recognized that T_3, if given too quickly, may cause cardiovascular collapse.[173] A decreased incidence of postoperative CNS depression and improved wound healing are shown to correlate with a preoperative euthyroid state. Hypothyroid patients are exquisitely sensitive to drugs that require metabolic transformation for their elimination. In addition, they are more likely to experience hypoglycemic episodes, anemia, and hypothermia. Furthermore, their ability to excrete free water is impaired and thus they are prone to develop hyponatremia.[174] Evidence shows that hypothyroid patients have an increased incidence of intraoperative hypotension and increased rates of congestive heart failure and ileus after abdominal surgery.[175] However, contrary to previous belief, there is no increased incidence of arrhythmias, blood loss, duration of hospital stay, pulmonary problems, or mortality.[176]

A variety of abnormalities in hypothyroidism have important postoperative consequences. Unfortunately, the symptoms and signs of hypothyroidism are often very subtle. These patients are often overly sensitive to narcotics and other medications that require metabolic transformation for their elimination. Impaired free water clearance with subsequent hyponatremia, hypoglycemia, anemia, hypothermia, adynamic ileus, and delayed gastric emptying have all been associated with the hypothyroid state in postoperative patients.[176] Concomitant adrenal insufficiency has been recognized as one cause for perioperative hypotension in the hypothyroid patient. Therefore, supplemental steroids should be considered if adequate adrenal reserve has not been demonstrated preoperatively. Additionally, the hypothyroid patient has a higher incidence of neuropsychiatric problems.

Mildly to moderately hypothyroid patients represent a group of patients who should have a good postoperative outcome if they receive careful attention. There is, however, very little information regarding the outcome of severely hypothyroid patients after surgery. These patients should be considered at high risk, and the risk-benefit ratio of surgery should be carefully considered preoperatively.

Adrenal Insufficiency/Iatrogenic Steroid Use

Although Addison's disease is uncommon, it should be in the differential diagnosis for perioperative hypotension. On the contrary, patients presenting to their physician for surgery with a history of iatrogenic suppression of their pituitary-adrenal axis with corticosteroids are common. Three important questions regarding steroid use need to be answered. First, what is the duration of steroid use required to produce hypothalamic-pituitary suppression? Second, how long after steroid use does it take for the axis to recover well enough to tolerate the stress of surgery? Third, how does the clinician evaluate the integrity of the axis?

Abnormal cortisol responses to metyrapone or adrenocorticotropic hormone (ACTH) have been observed after only 3 days of steroid administration. Similarly, cortisol response to insulin-induced hypoglycemia is significantly reduced after 2 days of prednisone use (25 mg/day).[171] Studies have also shown that it may take up to 1 year for the axis to recover after supraphysiologic doses of corticosteroids. Therefore, a detailed history regarding any steroid medication should be obtained from all surgical patients. If the patient is unsure, a preoperative ACTH test (250 μg) may be administered and the maximum cortisol response measured. If the cortisol level is normal, it is unlikely that a patient will develop perioperative hypotension secondary to impaired cortisol secretion.[179]

The patient on chronic steroid suppression or with Addison's disease should receive a perioperative steroid "boost." Recommended replacement of glucocorticoids in the perioperative period is as follows: (1) hydrocortisone, 100 mg IM on call to OR; (2) 50 mg IM/IV in recovery room, then every 6 hours for three doses; (3) 25 mg IM/IV every 6 hours for four doses if patient is hemodynamically stable; (4) taper to maintenance dosage over next 3–5 days; and (5) increase cortisol dosage to 200–400 mg over 24 hours if fever, hypotension, or other complications occur[180] that result in stress.

Cardiovascular Disease

In the past, gynecologic surgeons were relatively free of concerns about cardiovascular disease in their patients undergoing surgery. Over the last 20 years, however, there has been a large increase in the postmenopausal population who have a cardiovascular risk similar to their male counterparts. The postmenopausal population also require more surgical intervention as a result of their higher incidence of pelvic malignancies and pelvic relaxation. Despite these factors, the incidence of perioperative cardiovascular complications has decreased markedly.[181] This decrease has resulted from improvements in surgical and anesthetic techniques and especially from preoperative detection of high-risk patients, allowing optimal cardiovascular preparation prior to surgery.

Preoperative Evaluation

The goal of a preoperative cardiac evaluation is to determine the presence of heart disease, its severity, and the potential risk to the patient in the perioperative period. The first step in the evaluation of all patients consists of a thorough history and physical examination. Every patient should be carefully questioned regarding symptoms of cardiac disease such as chest pain, dyspnea on exertion, peripheral edema, wheezing, syncope, claudication, or palpitations. Patients with a prior history of cardiac disease should be closely evaluated for worsening of symptoms, which indicate progressive or poorly controlled disease. Old records are indispensable, and every effort should be made to obtain them, particularly if the patient has received treatment at other institutions. Prescriptions for antihypertensive, anticoagulant, antiarrhythmic, antilipid, or antianginal medications may provide the only hint of prior cardiovascular problems. In patients without known heart disease, the presence of diabetes, hyperlipidemia, hypertension, tobacco use, or a strong family history of heart disease identifies a group of patients at higher risk for heart disease, who should be more carefully evaluated.

Physical examination is important for diagnosis and monitoring of cardiovascular disease. The presence of findings such as hypertension, jugular venous distention, laterally displaced point of maximal impulse, irregular pulse, third heart sound, pulmonary rales, heart murmurs, peripheral edema, or vascular bruits should prompt a more complete evaluation. Laboratory evaluation of patients with known or suspected heart disease should include a blood count and serum chemistries. Anemia is poorly tolerated by patients with heart disease, and serum sodium and potassium levels are particularly important in patients taking diuretics and digitalis. Blood urea nitrogen and creatinine values provide information on renal function and hydration status. Blood glucose levels may detect undiagnosed diabetes mellitus. A chest x-ray and electrocardiogram (ECG) are mandatory as part of the preoperative evaluation and are particularly helpful when compared with previous studies.

Coronary Artery Disease

Coronary artery disease (CAD) is responsible for the major risk to cardiac patients undergoing intra-abdominal surgery. The incidence of myocardial infarction following surgery in an adult population is approximately 0.15%.[182] However, in patients who had a prior myocardial infarction, most studies reported a reinfarction rate of about 5%.[182-184] The risk of reinfarction was inversely proportional to the length of time between infarction and surgery.[183] At 3 months or less, the risk of reinfarction was approximately 30%; from 3 to 6 months, the rate fell to 12%. Six months after myocardial infarction, the risk of death due to a perioperative infarction was similar to that of patients who had no prior history of ischemic heart disease. Fortunately, it has been demonstrated that careful perioperative management could lower the reinfarction rate even in patients with recent infarctions.[185] This is important because the mortality associated with perioperative myocardial infarction approaches 50% in some studies.[184, 186]

Because of the high mortality and morbidity associated with perioperative myocardial infarction, much effort has been made to predict perioperative cardiac risk. Goldman and his colleagues prospectively evaluated cardiac risk factors and using a multivariate analysis identified the independent cardiac risk factors presented in Table 3–14.[187] Using these factors, a cardiac risk index was created that places a patient into one of four risk classes (Table 3–15). Other prospective studies have substantiated the validity of this classification system.[188, 189] Surprisingly, hypertension, diabetes, smoking, stable angina, and hypercholesterolemia were not found to be independent risk factors. Unstable angina, probably because it is relatively uncommon, did not appear as a risk factor. Despite the lack of conclusive data, patients with unstable angina should be considered to be at extremely high risk of perioperative cardiac mortality and should undergo a coronary artery revascularization procedure prior to any gynecologic surgery.

Table 3–14

Goldman Risk Factors for Postoperative Myocardial Infarction

Independent Risk Factors	Points
1. Jugular venous distension or S_3 gallop immediately preoperatively	11
2. Myocardial infarction in preceding 6 months	10
3. Presence of premature atrial contractions on preoperative ECG or any rhythm other than sinus	7
4. More than five premature ventricular contractions per minute preoperatively	7
5. Evidence of significant aortic valvular stenosis	3
6. Age >70 years	5
7. Emergency operation	4
8. Intraperitoneal operation	3
9. Poor general medical condition	3
a. $PO_2 < 60$ or $PCO_2 > 50$ mm Hg	
b. $K < 3.0$ or $HCO_3 < 20$ mEq/L	
c. BUN > 50 or creatinine > 3.0 mg/dl	
d. Liver disease or debilitated patient	

Adapted from information appearing in *The New England Journal of Medicine*, Goldman L, et al.: Multifactorial index of cardiac risk in noncardiac surgical procedures. N Engl J Med 1977; 297:845–850.

Table 3–15

Goldman Risk Classes for Postoperative Myocardial Infarction (MI)

Class	Total Score	Patients	Patients with Life-Threatening Complications or Death*
I	0–5	537	5 (1%)
II	6–12	316	21 (7%)
III	13–25	130	18 (14%)
IV	≥ 26	18	14 (78%)

*Life-threatening complications are documented intraoperative or postoperative MI, pulmonary edema, or ventricular tachycardia without progression to cardiac death.

Adapted from information appearing in *The New England Journal of Medicine*, Goldman L, et al.: Multifactorial index of cardiac risk in noncardiac surgical procedures. N Engl J Med 1977; 297:845–850.

Foster and his colleagues followed patients from the Coronary Artery Surgery Study registry who subsequently underwent major noncardiac surgical procedures.[190] These 1600 patients had coronary artery disease and left ventricular function defined by angiography. Multivariate analysis of potential risk factors found only dyspnea on exertion and left ventricular wall motion score to be independently predictive of perioperative cardiac mortality. Contrary to Goldman's analysis, in this study a history of previous myocardial infarction was not an independent risk factor. The authors felt that this implied that the degree of left ventricular wall dysfunction was more critical than the less objective information provided by a history of infarction. Conversely, preoperative angiography is an invasive procedure that is less clinically feasible than clinical evaluation of risk using the criteria proposed by Goldman.

In an effort to quantitate preoperative cardiac risk, several tests have been utilized to assess cardiovascular function. Exercise stress testing prior to surgery can identify a patient who has ischemic heart disease not manifested when the patient is at rest. These patients have been shown to be at increased risk of developing cardiac complications in the perioperative period.[191] In a study of 130 patients undergoing peripheral vascular surgery, Cutler identified a high-risk group of patients who had ischemic electrocardiographic changes when they exercised to less than 75% of their maximal predicted heart rate.[192] This group had a 25% incidence of perioperative myocardial infarction and an overall 18.5% cardiac mortality rate. Conversely, patients who were able to exercise to greater than 75% of their maximal predicted heart rate and had no electrocardiographic evidence of ischemia had no perioperative myocardial infarctions. The prognostic value of stress testing was not supported in another prospective study by Carliner, who found that only an abnormal preoperative resting ECG was an independent risk factor in a multivariate analysis.[191] The exercise stress test must be selectively applied to a high-risk population, as its predictive value is dependent on the prevalence of the disease. Therefore, it does not appear appropriate to screen all patients preoperatively, but rather it is preferable to rely on a careful history to identify a group with symptoms of cardiac disease for whom the test would be likely to be helpful.

Exercise stress testing is limited in some patients who cannot exercise as a result of musculoskeletal disease, pulmonary disease, or severe cardiac disease. In such patients, the dipyridamole-thallium scan may be used to overcome the limitations of exercise stress testing. This sensitive and specific study relies on the ability of dipyridamole to dilate normal coronary arteries but not stenotic vessels. Normally perfused myocardium readily takes up the thallium given intravenously. On the other hand, hypoperfused myocardium does not demonstrate good uptake of thallium when scanned 5 minutes after injection. Reperfusion and uptake of thallium 3 hours after injection identifies viable but high-risk myocardium. Old infarctions are identified as areas without uptake. Several studies have shown the risk of perioperative myocardial infarction in patients with areas of reperfusion of thallium uptake to range from 20 to 33%.[193–195] The dipyridamole-thallium scan is applicable for patients who are unable to exercise because it uses a medically induced "stress."

The resting gated blood pool (multigated angiogram [MUGA]) study provides another test to evaluate cardiac risk in patients who are unable to exercise. Although this test does not directly evaluate coronary artery disease, it has been shown to correlate with perioperative cardiac risk. Pasternack and colleagues studied 100 patients preoperatively with resting MUGA scans and found that the incidence of postoperative myocardial infarction was 19% if the ejection fraction was greater than 35% but that it increased to 75% with ejection fractions less than 35%.[196]

It is rare for patients who are less than 50 years old and who do not have diabetes, hypertension, hypercholesterolemia, or coronary artery disease to suffer a perioperative myocardial infarction. However, patients with CAD are at increased risk of myocardial infarction in the postoperative period. Prevention, early recognition, and treatment are important because myocardial infarctions that occur in the postoperative period are more highly lethal than those that are not associated with surgery, with mortality rates of approximately 50%.

Nearly two-thirds of postoperative myocardial infarctions occur during the first 3 postoperative days. Although the pathophysiologic factors are complex, the causes of postoperative myocardial ischemia and infarction are related to decreased myocardial oxygen supply coupled with increased myocardial oxygen requirements. Conditions commonly present in postoperative patients that decrease oxygen supply to the myocardium include tachycardia, increased preload, hypotension, anemia, and hypoxia.[197] Those that cause increased myocardial oxygen consumption are tachycardia, increased preload, increased afterload, and increased contractility. Of all these factors, tachycardia and increased preload are the most important causes of ischemia, because both decrease oxygen supply to the myocardium while simultaneously increasing myocardial oxygen demand. Tachycardia decreases the time in diastole, which is when the coronary arteries are perfused, thus decreasing the volume of oxygen available to the myocardium. Increased preload increases the pressure exerted by the myocardial wall on the arterioles within it, thus decreasing myocardial blood flow.

Other factors that have been associated with perioperative cardiac ischemia include physiologic responses to the stress of intubation, intravenous or intra-arterial line placement, emergence from anesthesia, pain, and anxiety. This stress results in catecholamine stimulation of the cardiovascular system, resulting in increased heart rate, blood pressure, and contractility, which may induce or worsen myocardial ischemia. Loss of intravascular volume because of third-spacing of fluids or postoperative hemorrhage can induce ischemia as well.

The diagnosis of postoperative myocardial infarction is often difficult. Chest pain, which is present in 90% of nonsurgical patients with myocardial infarction, may be present in only 50% of patients with postoperative infarction,[185, 198] owing to the masking of myocardial pain by coexisting surgical pain and the use of analgesia. Thus, maintenance of a high level of suspicion for postoperative infarction is extremely important in patients with CAD. The presence of arrhythmia, congestive heart failure, hypotension, dyspnea, or elevations of pulmonary artery pressure may indicate infarction and should prompt a thorough cardiac investigation and electrocardiographic monitoring. Measurement of creatine phosphokinase MB isoenzyme levels is the most sensitive and specific indicator of myocardial infarction and should be obtained on all patients suspected of postoperative infarction.

Despite the high incidence of silent myocardial infarction, routinely obtaining postoperative ECGs on all patients with cardiovascular disease is controversial. Many patients will exhibit P-wave changes that spontaneously resolve and do not represent ischemia or infarction. Conversely, patients with proven myocardial infarctions may show few or no ECG abnormalities. If routine screening of asymptomatic patients is desired, ECGs should be obtained at 24 hours following surgery, as it has been shown that no significant ECG changes will occur immediately postoperatively that do not persist for 24 hours.[199] Although there are no uniform guidelines, it seems prudent to continue with serial ECGs for at least 3 days postoperatively.

Postoperative management of patients with CAD is based on maximizing delivery of oxygen to the myocardium as well as decreasing myocardial oxygen utilization. Most patients benefit from supplemental oxygen in the postoperative period, although special care should be exercised in patients with chronic obstructive pulmonary disease. Oxygenation can be easily monitored by pulse oximetry. Certainly, anemia is detrimental because of loss of oxygen carrying capacity as well as resultant tachycardia and should therefore be carefully corrected in high-risk patients.

Patients with CAD may benefit from pharmacologic control of hyperadrenergic states that result from increased postoperative catecholamine production. Beta blockers decrease heart rate, myocardial contractility, and systemic blood pressure, all of which are increased by adrenergic stimulation. Perioperative beta blockade has been shown to significantly reduce arrhythmias and myocardial infarctions.[200] Certainly, patients receiving beta blockade therapy prior to surgery should continue to receive it in the perioperative period, because abrupt withdrawal results in a rebound hyperadrenergic state.

Labetalol, a mixed alpha- and beta-receptor blocker, may also be useful in patients with CAD who are also hypertensive because reflex tachycardia is limited. Additionally, labetalol has been shown to have antiarrhythmic effects.[20] In patients with asthma, which can be exacerbated by sympathomimetic beta blockers, the use of esmolol is advantageous, because it is a cardioselective beta blocker without intrinsic sympathomimetic activity and thus should not cause bronchoconstriction.

Although prophylactic nitrates have been used in the perioperative period for many years, this practice remains controversial. Nitroglycerin enhances blood flow to ischemic areas, increases collateral flow, increases myocardial oxygenation, and reduces angina.[202] Although studies of nitrate administration during surgery conclusively showed decreased hypertension and increased fluid requirements, results were contradictory about the effect on cardiac ischemia.[203-205] The route of administration, dosage, and duration of therapy are controversial as well; thus, perioperative treatment with nitrates should be initiated in conjunction with consultation with a cardiologist.

Nifedipine, a calcium channel blocker, may be given sublingually in the postoperative period. It lowers blood pressure by selectively dilating arteries and begins to decrease blood pressure in 5 minutes, which plateaus in 30 minutes.[206] The ultimate fall in blood pressure is related to the degree of hypertension initially present because vasodilation is more profound in patients with hypertension.[207] Care must be taken when giving this drug, because ischemia and myocardial infarction have been reported following hypotension associated with nifedipine.[208]

Congestive Heart Failure

Patients with congestive heart failure (CHF) face a substantially increased risk of myocardial infarction during surgery.[187, 209] The postoperative development of pulmonary edema is a grave prognostic sign and results in death in a high percentage of patients.[210] Because patients with heart failure at the time of surgery are significantly more likely to develop pulmonary edema perioperatively, every effort should be made to diagnose and treat CHF prior to surgery.[182] The diagnosis of CHF can often be made by a careful history and physical examination. The signs and symptoms of CHF are listed in Table 3–16. Patients who are able to perform usual daily activities without developing CHF are at limited risk of perioperative heart failure.

To prevent severe postoperative complications, CHF must be corrected preoperatively. Treatment usually relies on aggressive diuretic therapy, although care must be taken to prevent dehydration, which may result in hypotension during the induction of anesthesia. Hypokalemia can result from diuretic therapy and is especially deleterious to patients who are also taking digitalis. In addition to diuretics and digitalis, treatment often includes the use of preload and afterload reducers. Optimal usage of these drugs and correction of CHF may be aided by the consultation of a cardiologist. In general, it is preferable to continue patients on their usual regimen of cardiac medications through the perioperative period. In patients with severe or intractable CHF, the perioperative measurement of left ventricular filling (wedge) pressure with a pulmonary artery catheter (Swan-Ganz) may be extremely helpful to guide perioperative fluid management.

Postoperative CHF results most frequently from excessive administration of intravenous fluids and blood products. Other common postoperative causes

Table 3–16

Signs and Symptoms of Congestive Heart Failure (CHF)

1. Presence of an S_3 gallop
2. Jugular venous distention
3. Lateral shift of the point of maximal impulse
4. Lower extremity edema
5. Basilar rales
6. Increased voltage on ECG
7. Evidence of pulmonary edema or cardiac enlargement on chest x-ray
8. Tachycardia

are myocardial infarction, systemic infection, pulmonary embolism, and cardiac arrhythmias. It is important to determine the cause of postoperative heart failure because successful treatment is based on simultaneous treatment of the underlying cause.

Diagnosis of postoperative CHF is often more difficult, because the signs and symptoms of CHF (listed in Table 3–16) are not specific and may result from other causes. The most reliable method of detecting CHF is by chest radiography, in which the presence of cardiomegaly or evidence of pulmonary edema is a helpful diagnostic feature.

Acute postoperative CHF frequently manifests as pulmonary edema. Treatment of pulmonary edema may include the use of intravenous furosemide, supplemental oxygen, intravenous morphine sulfate, and elevation of the head of the bed. Intravenous aminophylline may be useful if cardiogenic asthma is present. Laboratory evaluation, including an electrocardiogram, arterial blood gases, serum electrolytes, and renal function chemistries, should be expediently obtained. If the patient does not improve rapidly, she should be transferred to an intensive care unit.

Arrhythmias

Nearly all arrhythmias found in otherwise healthy patients are asymptomatic and of limited consequence. However, in patients with underlying cardiac disease, even brief episodes of arrhythmias may result in significant morbidity and mortality. Preoperative evaluation of arrhythmias by a cardiologist and anesthesiologist is important because many anesthetic agents and surgical stress contribute to the development or worsening of arrhythmias. In patients undergoing continuous cardiographic monitoring during surgery, Kuner reported a 60% incidence of arrhythmias excluding sinus tachycardia.[211] Although there has been some disagreement, most authors believe that patients with heart disease have an increased risk of arrhythmias.[212, 213] Commonly these are ventricular arrhythmias. Conversely, patients without cardiac disease are more likely to develop supraventricular arrhythmias during surgery.[209] Those patients taking antiarrhythmic medications prior to surgery should continue on those drugs during the perioperative period. Initiation of antiarrhythmic medications is rarely indicated preoperatively, but patients in whom arrhythmias are detected prior to surgery should receive cardiology consultation.

Patients with first-degree atrioventricular block or asymptomatic Mobitz I (Wenckebach) second-degree AV block require no preoperative therapy. Conversely, those with symptomatic Mobitz II second-degree AV block or third-degree AV block should have a permanent pacemaker implanted before undergoing elective surgery.[214, 215] In emergency situations, a pacing pulmonary artery catheter can be used. Prior to performing surgery on patients with a permanent pacemaker, information as to the type and location of the pacemaker is important because electrocautery units may interfere with demand-type pacemakers.[216] When performing gynecologic surgery on patients with pacemakers, it is preferable to place the electrocautery unit ground plate on the leg to minimize interference. In patients with a demand pacemaker in place, the pacemaker should be converted to the fixed-rate mode by placing a magnet over it.

Surgery is not contraindicated in patients with bundle branch blocks or hemiblocks. Rarely do patients with conduction system disease develop complete heart block during noncardiac surgical procedures.[217–219] However, the presence of left bundle branch block may indicate the presence of aortic stenosis, which can increase surgical mortality if severe.

Valvular Heart Disease

Although there are many forms of valvular heart disease, primarily two types, aortic and mitral stenosis, are associated with significantly increased operative risk.[220] Patients with significant aortic stenosis appear to be at greatest risk; the risk is further increased if atrial fibrillation, CHF, or CAD is also present. In general, patients with significant stenosis of aortic or mitral valves should have them repaired prior to undergoing elective gynecologic surgery.

Severe valvular heart disease is usually evident during physical examination. Common findings in such patients are listed in Table 3–17. The classic history presented by patients with severe aortic stenosis include exercise dyspnea, angina, and syncope;

Table 3–17

Signs and Symptoms of Valvular Heart Disease

Aortic Stenosis
1. Systolic murmur at right sternal border that radiates into carotids
2. Decreased systolic blood pressure
3. Apical heave
4. Chest x-ray with calcified aortic ring, left ventricular enlargement
5. ECG with high R-waves, depressed T-waves in lead I and precordial leads

Mitral Stenosis
1. Precordial heave
2. Diastolic murmur at apex
3. Mitral opening snap
4. Suffused face and lips
5. Chest x-ray with left atrial dilation
6. ECG with large P-waves and right-axis deviation

those with mitral stenosis have paroxysmal and effort dyspnea, hemoptysis, and orthopnea. Most patients have a remote history of rheumatic fever. Stenosis of either valve is considered to be severe if the valvular area is less than 1 cm^2, and this diagnosis can be confirmed by echocardiography or cardiac catheterization.

Patients with any valvular abnormality should receive prophylactic antibiotics immediately preoperatively to prevent bacterial endocarditis. Table 3-18 outlines the American Heart Association recommendations for prophylaxis.

Sinus tachycardias and other tachyarrhythmias are poorly tolerated by patients with aortic and mitral stenosis. In patients with aortic stenosis, it is important to provide sufficient digitalization to correct preoperative tachyarrhythmias, while propranolol may be used to control sinus tachycardia. Patients with mitral valve stenosis often have atrial fibrillation, and, if present, digitalis should be used to reduce rapid ventricular response.

In the postoperative period, patients with mitral stenosis should be carefully monitored for pulmonary edema, as they may not be able to compensate for the amount of intravenous fluid administered during surgery. Patients with mitral stenosis also frequently have pulmonary hypertension and decreased airway compliance. Therefore, they may require more pulmonary support and therapy postoperatively, including prolonged mechanical ventilation.

For patients with significant aortic stenosis, it is imperative that a sinus rhythm be maintained during the postoperative period. Even sinus tachycardia can be deleterious, because it shortens time in diastole. Bradycardia below 45 beats/minute should be treated with atropine. Supraventricular dysrhythmias may be controlled with verapamil or DC cardioversion. Particular attention should be provided to the maintenance of proper fluid status, digoxin levels, electrolyte levels, and blood replacement.

Patients with mechanical heart valves usually tolerate surgery well.[221] Management of these patients requires antibiotic prophylaxis (see Table 3-18) and discontinuation of anticoagulant therapy during the perioperative period. Usually, sodium warfarin (Coumadin) is withheld several days prior to surgery and anticoagulation is obtained by intravenous heparinization.[222] The heparin is discontinued 6-8 hours prior to surgery and resumed several days postoperatively. Ultimately, the patient is returned to oral Coumadin maintenance therapy. Alternatively, some authors recommend stopping the Coumadin 1-3 days preoperatively and restarting it several days postoperatively.[223] Both methods of management had no thromboembolic complications and had similar bleeding complication rates of approximately 15%.

Hypertension

It appears that patients with a history of hypertension alone are at no greater perioperative risk of cardiac morbidity or mortality.[182] However, patients with hypertension and heart disease have a 13% perioperative mortality rate.[220] Therefore, the preoperative evaluation of patients with hypertension should emphasize diagnosis of target organ damage. Laboratory studies should include an ECG, chest x-ray, blood count, urinalysis, serum electrolytes, and creatinine. Patients with evidence of coexistent heart disease should undergo cardiac evaluation.

Patients with diastolic pressures greater than 110 mm Hg or systolic pressures greater than 180 mm Hg should have their hypertension controlled prior to surgery. During surgery, patients with chronic hypertension tend to have increased fluctuations in blood pressure.[224] Chronically hypertensive patients are very susceptible to intraoperative hypotension because of an impaired autoregulation of blood flow to the brain and therefore require a higher mean arterial pressure to maintain adequate perfusion.[225] Additionally, hypertensive patients who also complain of sweating, palpitations, and headaches should be evaluated for a coexisting pheochromocytoma, as this disease is associated with greatly increased perioperative mortality.[226]

The treatment of early postoperative hypertension is usually limited to drugs that can be given parenterally, because absorption via the gastrointestinal mucosa may be diminished and transdermal absorption may be erratic in patients who are cold and are rewarming. Despite these difficulties, it is generally best to maintain antihypertensive medication postoperatively if blood pressures are elevated. Certainly, patients receiving preoperative beta blockade should be maintained on parenteral therapy to prevent rebound tachycardia, hypercontractility, and hypertension. A list of commonly used parenteral antihypertensive drugs is given in Table 3-19.

Table 3-18

Recommendations for Prophylaxis of Bacterial Endocarditis

Standard Regimen
Ampicillin, 2 g IV, and gentamicin, 1.5 mg/kg IM or IV, 30 minutes to 1 hour before

Penicillin-Allergic Patients
Vancomycin, 1 g IV slowly over 1 hour, and gentamicin, 1.5 mg/kg IM or IV 1 hour before; may be repeated once in 12 hours

Oral Regimen for Minor Procedures in Low-Risk Patients
Amoxicillin, 3 g PO, 1 hour before and 1.5 g 6 hours later

From Dajani AS, Bisno AL, Chung KJ, et al.: Prevention of bacterial endocarditis: Recommendations by the American Heart Association. JAMA 1990; 264:2919. Copyright 1990, American Medical Association.

Table 3-19

Common Parenteral Antihypertensives

Drug	Route	Initial Dose	Onset	Duration	Side Effects
Nitroprusside	IV drip	0.5 μg/min	Immediate	2–5 min	Tachycardia, nausea
Labetalol	IV infusion	20 mg	5–10 min	4 h	Bronchospasm, dizziness, nausea
Esmolol	IV infusion	50 μg/min	2 h min	9 min	Headache, somnolence, dizziness, hypotension
Nifedipine	Sublingual	10 mg	5 min	2 min	Hypotension, headache, dizziness, nausea, peripheral edema
Verapamil	IV	5–10 mg	3–5 min	2–5 h	Nausea, headache, hypotension, dizziness, pulmonary edema

Hemodynamic Monitoring

Over the last 20 years, hemodynamic monitoring has become integral to the perioperative management of patients with cardiovascular and pulmonary disease. The major impetus for this advancement resided in the need for the quantitative estimate of cardiac function and resulted in the development of bedside pulmonary artery catheterization. The impact of monitoring of cardiac function is demonstrated by the significant reduction of myocardial infarctions in high-risk patients who are aggressively monitored for 72–96 hours postoperatively.[185]

Prior to the development of the pulmonary artery catheter, central venous pressure (CVP) measurement was used to assess intravascular volume status and cardiac function. In order to measure the CVP, a catheter is placed into the central venous system, most frequently the superior vena cava. A water manometer or a calibrated pressure transducer is connected to the CVP line, and thus an estimation of right atrial pressure may be obtained. Right atrial pressure is determined by the balance between cardiac output and venous return. Cardiac output is determined by heart rate, myocardial contractility, preload, and afterload. Thus, if the pulmonary vascularity and left ventricular function are normal, the CVP accurately reflects the left ventricular end-diastolic pressure (LVEDP). LVEDP reflects cardiac output or systemic perfusion and has been considered the standard estimator of left ventricular pump function. Venous return is determined primarily by the mean systemic pressure, which propels blood towards the heart, balanced against resistance to venous return, which acts in the opposite direction. Thus, if right ventricular function is normal, the CVP accurately reflects intravascular volume.

Unfortunately, left and right ventricular function is frequently abnormal or discordant, and therefore the relationship of CVP to cardiac function or intravascular volume is not maintained. When this occurs, measurement of pulmonary artery occlusion pressures is required to accurately assess volume status and cardiovascular function. The use of a pulmonary artery catheter also allows the detection of changes in cardiovascular function with more sensitivity and rapidity than does clinical observation.

In 1970, Swan, Ganz, and colleagues introduced and popularized the use of a balloon-tipped pulmonary artery flotation catheter (Swan-Ganz catheter) that provided measurement of pulmonary artery and pulmonary artery occlusion pressures.[227] Since then, continued refinements have broadened the capabilities of the catheter to measure cardiac output, obtain intracavitary electrocardiograms, and provide temporary cardiac pacing.

The standard pulmonary artery occlusion catheter is a 7 Fr, radiopaque, flexible polyvinyl chloride, 4-lumen catheter with a 1.5-ml latex balloon at its distal tip. Most often, a right internal jugular cannulation is utilized for placement of the catheter, because this site provides the most direct access into the right atrium. After the catheter is placed into the right atrium, the balloon is inflated and the catheter is "pulled" by blood flow through the right ventricle into the pulmonary artery. The position of the catheter can be identified and followed by the various pressure wave forms generated by the right atrium, right ventricle, and pulmonary artery. As the catheter passes through increasingly smaller branches, the inflated balloon eventually occludes the pulmonary artery. The distal lumen of the catheter, which is beyond the balloon, now measures left atrial pressure (LAP) and in the absence of mitral valvular disease, LAP approximates LVEDP. Thus, pulmonary capillary wedge pressure (PCWP) equals the LAP, which equals LVEDP and is normally 8–12 mm Hg of mercury. Additionally, because the standard pulmonary artery catheter has an incorporated thermistor, thermodilution studies can be performed to determine cardiac output. This thermodilution method is performed by injecting cold 5% dextrose in water through the proximal port of the catheter, which cools the blood entering the right atrium. The change in temperature measured at the more distal thermistor (4 cm from the catheter tip) generates a curve whose area is proportional to cardiac output. Knowledge of the cardiac output is helpful in establishing cardiovascular diagnoses. For example, a patient with hypotension, low to normal wedge pressure, and a cardiac output of 3 liters/minute is most likely hypovolemic. Conversely, the same patient with a cardiac output of 8 liters/minute is probably septic with resultant low systemic vascular resistance.

Despite the great benefit in critically ill patients, the use of pulmonary artery catheters is associated with a small but significant complication rate. The complications can be grouped into those occurring during venous cannulation and those resulting from the catheter or its placement. The most common problems encountered during venous access are cannulation of the carotid or subclavian artery and introduction of a pneumothorax. Problems resulting from the catheter itself include dysrhythmias, sepsis, and disruption of the pulmonary artery. Clearly, pulmonary artery catheters should be placed under the supervision of experienced personnel and in a setting where complications can be rapidly diagnosed and treated.

Hematologic Disorders

Hematologic disorders, although rarely present in preoperative patients, can dramatically increase surgical morbidity and mortality and therefore should be routinely considered preoperatively. All preoperative evaluations should consider the following hematologic problems: (1) anemia and transfusion, (2) disorders of platelets and bleeding, (3) disorders of coagulation, and (4) disorders of white blood cells and immunity.

Anemia

The presence of moderate anemia in itself should not be a contraindication to surgery because it can be readily rectified by transfusion. However, if possible, surgery should be postponed until the cause of the anemia can be identified and the anemia corrected without resorting to potentially hazardous blood transfusions. Current anesthetic and surgical practice usually mandates a hemoglobin of greater than 10 g/dl or a hematocrit greater than 30%. Rather than strictly adhering to these levels, it is important to individualize application of these parameters for several reasons. First, it is the circulating blood volume that provides oxygen carrying capacity and tissue oxygenation. Although in most individuals this is accurately reflected by hemoglobin or hematocrit values, in certain situations it is not. If there has been a recent blood loss, the hematocrit may remain normal although the blood volume is very low until the lost volume is replaced with extracellular fluid, which then results in a drop in hematocrit. Conversely, overly hydrated patients may exhibit low hematocrits or hemoglobins but may have normal red cell mass.

Second, the patient's general physical condition determines her ability to tolerate anemia. The effects of anemia depend on the oxygen requirement of the patient, the rate at which the red cell mass decreases, the magnitude of the anemia, and the ability of compensatory physiologic mechanisms.[228] To maintain the same cardiac output, a patient with a hemoglobin of 10 g/dl requires twice as much coronary blood flow as does a patient with a hemoglobin of 14 g/dl.[229] Clearly, a patient with ischemic heart disease will not tolerate anemia as well as a healthy young patient. Therefore, the presence of cardiac, pulmonary, or other serious illness justifies a more aggressive approach to the management of anemia. Conversely, patients with long-standing anemia may have normal blood volumes and tolerate surgical procedures well. The NIH Consensus Group has pointed out that there is no evidence that mild to moderate anemia increases perioperative morbidity or mortality.[230]

If large perioperative blood losses are anticipated, patients with normal hematocrits are generally able to store at least three units of autologous blood preoperatively.[231] Additionally, the use of recombinant human erythropoietin may increase the amount of blood an autologous donor may store without developing anemia.[232] Planning for intraoperative red cell recovery and reuse can also be useful in eliminating or reducing the need for homologous transfusions in selected patients.

Platelet and Coagulation Disorders

Surgical hemostasis is provided by platelet adhesion to an injured vessel, which plugs the opening as simultaneously the coagulation cascade is activated, forming a stabilizing fibrin clot. Thus, the presence of both functioning platelets and coagulation factors is necessary to prevent excessive surgical bleeding. Platelet disorders are more commonly encountered in the preoperative patient than are coagulation factor abnormalities.

Platelets may be deficient in both number and function. The normal peripheral blood platelet count ranges between 150,000 and 400,000/mm^3, and the normal life span of a platelet is approximately 10 days. Although there is no clear-cut correlation between the degree of thrombocytopenia and the presence or amount of bleeding, several generalizations can be made. If the platelet count is greater than 100,000/mm^3 and the platelets are functioning normally, there is little chance of bleeding during surgical procedures. Patients with a platelet counts greater than 75,000/mm^3 almost always have normal bleeding times, and indeed a platelet count greater than 50,000/mm³ is probably adequate. A platelet count below 20,000/mm³ will often be associated with severe and spontaneous bleeding. Interestingly, platelet counts greater than 1,000,000/mm³ are often paradoxically associated with bleeding.

If the patient's platelet count is less than 100,000 a bleeding time should be obtained. If the bleeding time is abnormal and surgery must be performed, an attempt should be made to raise the platelet count to that level by administering platelet transfusions immediately prior to surgery. In those patients with immune destruction of platelets, human leukocyte antigen (HLA) donor specific platelets may be required to prevent rapid destruction of transfused platelets. If surgery can be postponed, a hematology consultation should be obtained to identify and treat the cause of the platelet abnormality.

Abnormally low platelet counts result from either decreased production or increased consumption of platelets. Although there are numerous causes of thrombocytopenia, most are exceedingly uncommon. Decreased platelet production may be drug induced and has been most often associated with the use of thiazide diuretics or ethanol, although many other drugs have been sporadically implicated. Drugs may also cause immunologic thrombocytopenia by inducing the formation of cross-reacting antibodies that increase platelet destruction. Again, numerous drugs have been occasionally reported in this context, but certainly this mechanism has been convincingly demonstrated with quinine and sulfonamide usage.[233] Frequently, patients receiving cytotoxic chemotherapy or radiation therapy for the treatment of malignancies are thrombocytopenic.

Conditions that are characterized by decreased platelet production include vitamin B_{12} and folate deficiencies, aplastic anemia, myeloproliferative disorders, renal failure, and viral infections. Inherited congenital thrombocytopenia is extremely rare. Much more commonly, thrombocytopenia results from immune destruction of platelets by diseases such as idiopathic thrombocytopenia purpura and collagen vascular disorders. Thrombocytopenia is caused by increased consumption of platelets in patients with disseminated intravascular coagulation (DIC). In a preoperative population, DIC nearly always is associated with the presence of malignancy or sepsis.

Platelet dysfunction may be inherited, but it is much more likely to be acquired. Commonly prescribed drugs such as aspirin, amitriptyline, and nonsteroidal anti-inflammatory agents may cause decreased platelet function as well as numbers. Large doses of penicillin and carbenicillin have been shown to increase bleeding times.[234] Patients who have prolonged bleeding times because of drug therapy should have those drugs withheld for 7–10 days before undergoing surgery. Uremia and liver disease are also common causes of poorly functioning platelets. Von Willebrand's disease is the major inherited congenital disorder of platelet dysfunction. Although it is the second most common inherited coagulation disorder, it is extremely rare in a preoperative population.

Although the diagnosis of an abnormal platelet number is easily made by a blood count, the diagnosis of platelet dysfunction is most often made by a careful history and physical examination.[235] The signs and symptoms of platelet abnormalities are easy bruisability, petechiae, bleeding from mucous membranes, and prolonged bleeding from minor cuts or wounds. A bleeding time will demonstrate clinically important platelet abnormalities. Further laboratory investigation is warranted in patients with abnormal bleeding times and should be done in conjunction with a hematology consultation. The preoperative evaluation must first determine the cause of the platelet abnormality so that corrective treatment can be initiated. Clearly, elective surgery should be postponed until therapy has been effected. Even in those patients in whom surgery must be performed expediently, the evaluation is helpful in predicting the magnitude of perioperative problems that may be encountered.

Disorders of coagulation factors are most often diagnosed by a thorough history and physical examination. Episodes of excessive bleeding following dental procedures, minor surgery, or childbirth; during menses; or a family history of a bleeding diathesis may be indicators of a coagulation disorder. Inherited coagulation disorders are very uncommon, but of these rare disorders Factor VIII deficiency (hemophilia), Factor IX deficiency (Christmas disease), and von Willebrand's syndrome occur most frequently. There are few commonly prescribed drugs that affect coagulation factors, with the exception of Coumadin and heparin. Disease states that may be associated with decreased coagulation factor levels are primarily liver disease, vitamin K deficiency (secondary to obstructive biliary disease, intestinal malabsorption, or antibiotic reduction of bowel flora), and DIC.

The use of preoperative laboratory screening for coagulation deficiencies is controversial. It appears, however, that routine screening in patients without historical evidence of a bleeding problem is not warranted.[1, 236] On the other hand, patients who are seriously ill or who will be undergoing extensive surgical procedures should have a prothrombin time, partial thromboplastin time, fibrinogen level, and platelet count obtained preoperatively.

White Cells and Immune Function

Abnormally high or low white blood cell counts are not an absolute contraindication to surgery. However, they should be considered relative to the need for surgery. Evaluation of an elevated or decreased white blood cell count should be undertaken prior to elective surgery. Clearly, patients with absolute granulocyte counts less than 1000/mm³ are at increased risk of severe infection and perioperative morbidity and mortality and should undergo surgery only for life-threatening indications.[237]

Blood Component Replacement

Nearly all postoperative hematologic problems are related to perioperative bleeding and blood component replacement. The magnitude of the problem is underscored by the fact that two-thirds of all blood transfused in the United States is administered to surgical patients.[238] Although the primary cause of postoperative bleeding, lack of surgical hemostasis, is well known to gynecologic surgeons, other less well-appreciated, nonmechanical factors may compound the problem.

Many patients who are massively transfused (more than 1 blood volume) are noted to develop a coagulopathy. Theories have been postulated that attribute this coagulopathy to dilution of platelets and labile cogulation factors by the use of platelet- and factor poor packed red blood cells (PRBCs), fibrinolysis, or disseminated intravascular coagulation (DIC). Acceptance of these theories has frequently resulted in the use of dogmatic schemes of replacement of fresh-frozen plasma (FFP) and platelets, depending on the number of units of PRBCs given. It is the authors' opinion, however, that it is preferable to use both clinical and laboratory evaluation to individualize blood replacement rather than adhering to a set replacement recipe.

Studies on soldiers receiving massive transfusion reported that those who developed thrombocytopenia following red blood cell replacement manifested bleeding diatheses that responded to infusion of fresh blood but not FFP.[239] The investigators concluded that dilutional thrombocytopenia is a major cause of post-transfusion bleeding. However, more recently in a prospective, randomized, double-blind study, prophylactic platelet administration during massive transfusion was not helpful.[240] Although it seems that these studies are contradictory, they demonstrate the need for obtaining platelet counts during transfusion of large amounts of blood. If clinical evidence of excessive bleeding exists and the platelet count is less than 100,000/mm³, platelets should be transfused because platelets are consumed during surgery and higher levels are required to maintain hemostasis following surgery.

Packed red blood cells, which may have been stored for several weeks, are used for most postoperative transfusions. Most clotting factors are stable for long periods of time with the exception of Factors V and VIII, which decrease to 15 and 50% of normal, respectively. Despite this loss, Factors V and VIII rarely decrease below the levels required for hemostasis. In 1985, the National Institute of Health consensus conference on the use of FFP concluded that there was little or no scientific evidence to support the use of FFP for bleeding diatheses following multiple blood transfusions. FFP should be given, however, if there is clinical bleeding, platelet count greater than 100,000/mm³, and a partial thromboplastin time greater than 1.5 times control.

It appears that the volume of blood transfused does not correlate with the occurrence of a postoperative bleeding diatheses. Rather, it has been shown that the magnitude of abnormalities in coagulation testing correlates with the duration of hypovolemic shock.[241] Also, patients in hypovolemic shock frequently develop DIC, which may compound the bleeding. Thus, most of the problems associated with massive transfusion are the result of inadequate replacement administered too late.

Donor blood is prevented from coagulating by the addition of citrate, which chelates calcium, thus blocking calcium-dependent steps in the coagulation cascade. Therefore, hypocalcemia following transfusion of large amounts of stored blood that contains excess citrate is a theoretical danger. Indeed, it has been shown that at high transfusion rates, ionized calcium levels will transiently fall but return towards baseline levels at the completion of transfusion.[242] Citrate is metabolized at the equivalent rate of 20 units of blood administered per hour, and therefore routine supplemental calcium is not warranted. However, hypothermia, liver disease, and hyperventilation slow the metabolism of citrate, requiring close monitoring of ionized calcium levels when these conditions prevail.

As donor blood is stored, potassium leaches from the red cells and plasma levels may reach as high as 30 mEq/liter. Despite this large potassium load, rarely are serum potassium levels elevated even in patients receiving massive transfusions. Indeed, patients often are hypokalemic as a result of the metabolic alkalosis that follows transfusion, which is caused by the hepatic metabolism of citrate to bicarbonate.

Pulmonary Disease

General Considerations

The incidence of postoperative pulmonary complications in surgical patients ranges from 2 to 5% in healthy individuals to greater than 70% in patients with pre-existing pulmonary disease.[243, 244] Pulmonary physiology changes in the patient who undergoes laparotomy include a decrease in the functional residual capacity (FRC) and vital capacity, an increase in ventilation-perfusion mismatching, and impaired mucociliary clearance of secretions within the tracheobronchial tree. These changes result in transient hypoxemia and atelectasis in the postoperative period.[244-246] They are more pronounced with advanced age, obesity, significant smoking history, surgery that involves the upper abdomen, and pre-existing chronic pulmonary disease.[244]

In a study of over 1000 general surgical patients, postoperative pulmonary complications occurred in 20% of those who had upper abdominal surgery, and in only 2% of those who underwent lower abdominal operations.[247] Most of the complications in the lower abdominal surgery group occurred in patients with pre-existing pulmonary disease or who were smokers. Interestingly, the majority of the patients who developed atelectasis after upper abdominal surgery had no prior history of smoking nor of pulmonary disease, and almost half had normal preoperative spirograms. Most other series have confirmed a lower incidence of postoperative pulmonary complications in patients who undergo lower abdominal surgery and nonthoracic, nonabdominal procedures, although the presence of chronic obstructive pulmonary disease (COPD) markedly increases the risk.[244]

The utility of preoperative pulmonary function testing has been extensively studied in surgical patients.[248,249] Spirometry, although useful in patients undergoing lung resection, is of unproven value in patients who undergo abdominal surgery in whom the risk of postoperative pulmonary complications is low.

Clearly, postoperative pulmonary complications are increased in patients with COPD as well as in patients with a significant smoking history. In addition, patients who present with a history of chronic cough or dyspnea or who have evidence of pulmonary dysfunction by physical examination or chest x-ray should also undergo preoperative spirometric evaluation and arterial blood gas determination. The abnormalities most often associated with postoperative atelectasis and pneumonia are shown in Table 3-20. Spirometry should be performed with and without bronchodilators in order to identify patients who may benefit from preoperative treatment with inhaled beta$_2$ agonists.

The value of preoperative chest x-ray in young, healthy patients has been quite low. In a review of 1000 preoperative chest x-rays, the incidence of significant radiographic findings was only 6.5%.[3] The majority of the patients with chest x-ray abnormalities were over the age of 30 years and were most often found to have cardiomegaly or emphysema, findings that could be either detected or suspected by history or physical examination. Another prospective study reviewed the influence of chest x-ray findings on the decision to operate on 810 patients over the age of 40 who underwent elective noncardiac surgery.[2] In only 5 patients did the preoperative chest x-ray reveal any new relevant information. Furthermore, in only 3 of the 5 patients was the surgical plan changed. In another large series, chest x-ray added new information in only 4% of cases, again mainly in the elderly.[251] A chest x-ray should not be included as a routine preoperative test in all patients undergoing abdominal procedures. Chest x-rays should be limited to patients over the age of 40, patients with a history of smoking, patients with a history of pulmonary disease, and patients who present with cardiac or pulmonary signs or symptoms.

Table 3-20

Predictors of Postoperative Pulmonary Complications*

Parameter	Value
Maximal breathing capacity (MB)	<50% predicted
FEV$_1$	<1 L
FVC	<70% predicted
FEV$_1$/FVC	<65% predicted
PaO$_2$	>45 mm Hg
PaCO$_2$	<60 mm Hg

*Complications defined as atelectasis or pneumonia.
From Blosser SA, Rock P: Asthma and chronic obstructive lung disease. In Breslow MJ, Miller CJ, Rogers MC (eds.): Perioperative Management. St. Louis, CV Mosby, 1990, pp. 259-280.

Asthma

Asthma affects approximately 5% of the U.S. population.[250] The disease is characterized by hyper-responsiveness of the tracheobronchial tree with variable reversible obstruction of the airways. Multiple stimuli have been noted to precipitate or exacerbate asthma, including environmental allergens or pollutants, respiratory tract infections, exercise, cold air, emotional stress, beta-adrenergic blockers, and aspirin.[245] Management of asthma includes removal of the inciting stimuli as well as use of appropriate pharmacologic therapy. Despite advances in pharmacologic management, morbidity and mortality from asthma have been increasing in recent years.[252] This has most likely been due to underdiagnosis and undertreatment.[253]

The preoperative work-up of the asthmatic patient should direct particular attention to the pulmonary examination, chest x-ray, arterial blood gas values, and pulmonary function testing. The pulmonary function testing should be performed with and without inhaled bronchodilators. This work-up is necessary to assess the current state of the airways as well as to reveal the presence of any underlying obstructive pulmonary disease. Asthmatics typically have reduced peak expiratory flow rates that will improve 15% or more with inhaled beta$_2$ agonists. In addition, there is typically a diurnal variation in peak expiratory flow rate, which is worse in the morning or evening but which improves during the daytime hours. Airway hyper-responsiveness may also be documented by the methacholine inhalation test.[254]

There is a significant inflammatory component to asthma, and, in fact, some investigators have referred to asthma as a chronic eosinophilic bronchitis.[253] Various mediators released in the lungs by eosinophils and macrophages induce microvascular leakage, bronchoconstriction, and epithelial damage, which blocks the distal airways. Mast cell degranulation is involved not in this inflammatory component but rather with the bronchoconstriction associated with the early response to allergens. Optimal therapy for asthma involves managing the acute symptoms as well as the inflammatory component.

The beta$_2$-adrenergic agonists are the first-line drugs for bronchodilator therapy of asthma. These drugs, inhaled four to six times daily, relax smooth muscle in the airways very rapidly and are effective for up to 6 hours. They are more effective by inhalation than by the oral route, requiring lower doses and having fewer systemic effects. Beta-adrenergic agonists stabilize mast cells and therefore inhibit release of mediators involved in the early response to allergens. Beta agonists are the agents of choice for treatment of acute exacerbation of asthma as well as of very mild cases of asthma, although they do not have any effect on the inflammatory component of asthma or the late response to allergens or to bronchial hyper-responsiveness.

Methylxanthines, such as theophylline, are weak bronchial dilators, and there is controversy as to whether these drugs add any additional benefit in patients who are already on maximal inhaled bronchodilator therapy. To be effective, adequate serum concentrations are necessary (10–20 µg/ml). Theophylline has mild anti-inflammatory action in asthma, inhibiting the late response to allergens. However, it has no effect on bronchial hyper-responsiveness or on eosinophilic degranulation. In addition, it is important to note that plasma concentrations can be affected by certain drugs, conditions, or factors, and that the theophylline dose should be varied accordingly. Smoking and phenobarbital increase clearance of theophylline by the liver, whereas clearance of theophylline is decreased with hepatic disease, cardiac failure, and the concomitant use of certain drugs, including ciprofloxacin, cimetidine, erythromycin, and troleandomycin.

Anticholinergic agents are weak bronchodilators that work via inhibition of muscarinic receptors in the smooth muscle of the airways, thus decreasing vagal tone. Their use has been limited in the past as a result of undesirable systemic side effects. However, the use of anticholinergic agents has increased secondary to the development of quaternary derivatives such as ipratropium bromide (Atrovent), which are available in an inhaled form that is not absorbed systemically. Anticholinergic drugs may provide additional benefit in conjunction with standard bronchodilator therapy but should not be used as single-agent therapy for asthma because they do not inhibit mast cells or eosinophils, do not have any effect on the late response to allergens, and do not have an anti-inflammatory effect.

Cromolyn sodium is a drug that can be highly effective in some patients for the treatment of asthma. It is one of the first-line drugs for chronic asthma in children, but, in general, it is not as effective in adults. Cromolyn sodium works by an as yet unknown mechanism. The drug comes in an inhaled form and may not be maximally effective until taken regularly for 1 month. It seems to have an anti-inflammatory effect in that it can prevent the late response to allergens as well as decrease bronchial hyper-responsiveness. Cromolyn can provide additional prophylactic benefit to some patients who are on other therapeutic agents, but its role as a single agent is quite limited.

Corticosteroids have become increasingly important in the management of asthma. Because corticosteroids inhibit mediator release from eosinophils and macrophages, inhibit the late response to allergens, and reduce hyper-responsiveness of bronchioles, they have become first-line therapy for chronic asthma.[253] Inhaled steroids (Beclovent) are highly active and have greatly reduced the steroid dose required to achieve optimal results. The steroid effect is dose related, but many asthmatics can be controlled on low-dose inhaled steroid (<500 µg/day). Up to 2 mg/day can be inhaled without adrenal suppression or adverse systemic effects. Onset of action is slow (several hours), and up to 3 months of steroid therapy may be required for optimal improvement of bronchial hyper-responsiveness. Occasionally, a short course of oral steroids may be necessary during acute exacerbations of asthma. However, for adults with chronic asthma, only a minority will require chronic oral steroid therapy. Those patients taking oral steroids should receive a steroid preparation perioperatively.

Elective surgery should be postponed whenever possible until pulmonary function and pharmacotherapeutic treatment are optimized. For the mild asthmatic, this may simply require the use of inhaled beta-adrenergic agonists preoperatively. For the chronic asthmatic, optimization of steroid therapy would greatly decrease alveolar inflammation and bronchiolar hyper-responsiveness. Inhaled beta$_2$ agonists should be added as needed for further control of asthma, and in some patients theophylline may also be required. Each drug prescribed should be used in maximal dosage before adding an additional agent. For patients undergoing nonelective surgery who have significant bronchoconstriction, a multi-modal approach should be instituted. This should include aggressive bronchodilator inhalation therapy and use of methylxanthines, as well as steroid therapy, particularly if the steroid therapy can be instituted 3–6 days preoperatively. In all asthmatics, pharmacotherapeutic response can be monitored with pulmonary function testing as particularly demonstrated by improvement in the peak expiratory flow rate.[254]

Chronic Obstructive Pulmonary Disease

The greatest risk factor for the development of postoperative pulmonary complications is the presence of underlying chronic obstructive pulmonary disease (COPD). The term COPD has been used to encompass both chronic bronchitis and emphysema, disease entities that often occur in tandem. Cigarette smoke is implicated in the pathogenesis of both, and any treatment plan must include cessation of smoking.[255] Chronic bronchitis is defined as the presence of productive cough on most days for at least 3 months per year and for at least 2 successive years.[245] It is characterized by chronic airway inflammation and by excessive mucus production. The histologic changes of emphysema include destruction of alveolar septa and distension of airspaces distal to terminal alveoli. The destruction of alveolar septa is most likely caused by serine elastase, released by neutrophils exposed to cigarette smoke.[255] The destruction of alveoli results in air trapping, loss of pulmonary elastic recoil, collapse of the airways in expiration, increased work of breathing, significant ventilation-perfusion mismatching, and, most importantly, ineffective cough.[250] The impaired ability for effective cough and clearance of secretions predisposes patients with COPD to atelectasis and pneumonia in the postoperative period.

The severity of the obstructive disease can be quantitated via pulmonary function testing.[243, 244, 256] Patients with COPD will typically demonstrate impaired expiratory air flow, manifested by diminished FEV_1, FVC, FEV_1/FVC, and MEFR (maximal expiratory flow rate). Arterial blood gases may show varying degrees of hypoxemia and/or hypercapnia and can be used for prognostic purposes in that a PaO_2 less than 70 mm Hg and $PaCO_2$ greater than 45 mm Hg are associated with a marked increase in the risk of postoperative pulmonary complications and with an increased risk of requirement for postoperative mechanical ventilation.[257]

The risk of postoperative pulmonary complications seems to be particularly increased in patients with COPD who undergo thoracic or abdominal surgery, and the risk is greater with upper than with lower abdominal surgery. Stein and Koota used pulmonary function testing to identify a group of surgical patients at risk for postoperative pulmonary complications.[243] Patients at risk were selected by an abnormal single nitrogen breath test, diminished MEFR (<200 liters/minute), or increased PCO_2 (>45 mm Hg). Patients with abnormal pulmonary function tests had a 70% incidence of postoperative pulmonary complications, as compared with a 3% incidence of complications in patients who had normal spirograms. In patients considered to be at high risk, the incidence of complications was highest in those undergoing abdominal surgery (92%) or thoracic surgery (78%) and lowest in those undergoing surgery outside the abdomen (26%).

In gynecologic surgical patients, the risk of postoperative pulmonary complications is confined mainly to patients with a heavy smoking history and to patients with COPD. In these patients, prophylactic pulmonary measures should be instituted preoperatively and continued postoperatively to minimize the incidence of atelectasis and pneumonia. Several studies have suggested that preoperative pulmonary preparation of patients with pre-existing lung disease can significantly decrease the incidence of postoperative pulmonary complications. In a study including 464 patients with COPD[258] who underwent a variety of surgical procedures, preoperative preparation, including chest physiotherapy, bronchodilators, and antibiotic therapy (for patients with positive sputum cultures), decreased the incidence of pulmonary complications from 43.1% to 23.7%. In another series from the same institution, a 48-hour preoperative preparation in 157 patients with COPD, including inhaled beta-adrenergic agonists, oral theophylline, and chest physiotherapy, resulted in improvement in measured spirometric parameters, improved arterial PO_2 and PCO_2, and a lower postoperative pulmonary complication rate.[259] There was no correlation, however, between the degree of improvement in spirometric parameters and postoperative pulmonary outcome. In one randomized study,[260] poor-risk patients who stopped smoking and received bronchodilator drugs, antibiotics, inhalation of humidified gases, postural drainage, and chest physiotherapy had a significant decrease in the incidence of postoperative pulmonary complications, from 60% to 22%. In addition, the treated group had decreased severity of complications and enjoyed a shorter length of hospital stay. Finally, the timing of administration of perioperative prophylactic pulmonary measures is important in that measures instituted preoperatively and continued postoperatively are more effective in reducing the incidence of postoperative pulmonary complications than measures instituted solely in the postoperative period.[261, 262]

The authors' approach to the preoperative preparation of the patient at high risk for postoperative pulmonary complications includes cessation of smoking for as long as possible preoperatively. Two to three days of smoking abstinence are sufficient for carboxyhemoglobin levels to return to normal.[263] However, 2 months of smoking abstinence is necessary to significantly lower the risk of postoperative pulmonary complications.[264] Inhaler therapy can be started 48–72 hours preoperatively, particularly in patients who have demonstrated either clinical or spirometric improvement on bronchodilators. This can include the use of beta-adrenergic agonists, ipratropium bromide, or both.[265] In addition, up to one-half of patients with COPD may benefit from inhaled steroids. In patients with a suppurative cough and positive sputum culture, a full course of antibiotic therapy may be indicated preoperatively. The antibiotics used should cover the most likely etiologic organisms, *Streptococcus pneumoniae* and *Haemophilus influenzae*. Certainly, in any patient with acute upper respiratory infection, surgery should be delayed if possible. Finally, instruction in deep breathing maneuvers and chest physical therapy are simple to institute and these measures can be started the evening prior to surgery.[246]

Postoperative Pulmonary Management

A number of alterations in respiratory physiology occur postoperatively secondary to surgery and the effects of inhaled anesthetics. First, there is a decrease in the vital capacity, the extent of which is highly dependent on the location of the surgical incision. The vital capacity is impaired most with thoracic and upper abdominal operations. The negative effect on vital capacity is much diminished with surgical procedures in the lower abdomen and is almost negligible with procedures confined to the lower or upper extremities (Fig. 3–1). Second, the functional residual capacity (FRC) decreases as a result of an upper displacement of the diaphragm, which may result from monotonous shallow breathing, increased intra-abdominal pressure due to an ileus, or secondary to maintenance of the patient in a supine position. Third, a decrease in the forced vital capacity as well as an impairment in the mucociliary clearance mechanism of the lung causes a build-up of secretions. Finally, discomfort from the abdominal incision results in a shallow, splinting type of breathing pattern, with diminution of the sighing reflex. Sighing normally occurs several times per hour, inducing release of surfactant from type 2 pneumocytes, which coats the alveoli and is neces-

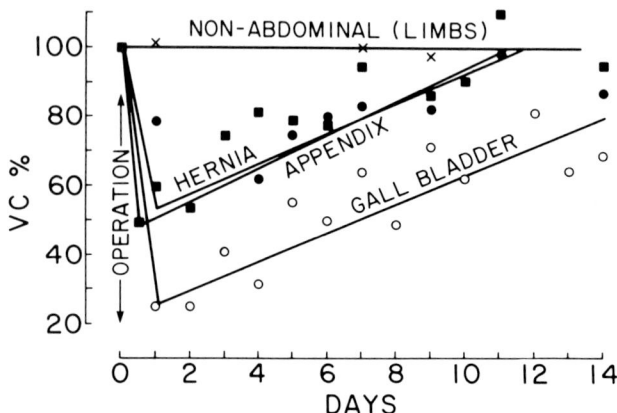

Figure 3–1
Changes in vital capacity (*VC*, in percentage of preoperative value) following operations: gallbladder, ○; hernias, •; appendectomies, ■; and nonabdominal (limbs), x. (Adapted from Churchill ED, McNeil D: The reduction in vital capacity following operation. Surg Gynecol Obstet 1927; 44:483–488. By permission of Surgery, Gynecology & Obstetrics. In Vandam LD (ed.): To Make the Patient Ready for Anesthesia: Medical Care of the Surgical Patient. Menlo Park, CA, Addison-Wesley Publishing Co, 1980, pp. 21–46.)

sary for maintenance of alveolar wall tension. The decrease in FRC, impairment of mucociliary clearance of secretions, and decrease in the alveolar wall tension promote premature closure of the airways upon expiration, resulting in collapse of the alveoli and atelectasis.

Atelectasis. The most common postoperative pulmonary complication is atelectasis, accounting for more than 90% of all postoperative pulmonary complications. The term atelectasis refers to the process of incomplete lung expansion. Irrespective of the cause, the pathophysiology involves a collapse of the alveoli resulting in ventilation-perfusion mismatching, intrapulmonary venous shunting, and a subsequent drop in the PaO_2. Collapsed alveoli are also susceptible to superimposed infection, and if improperly managed, atelectasis will progress to pneumonia. Patients with atelectasis have a decreased FRC as well as decreased lung compliance. This results in an increased work of breathing. In general, despite the decrease in PaO_2, the PCO_2 remains unaffected unless atelectatic changes progress to large volumes of the lung or unless there is pre-existing lung disease.

Atelectasis may be caused by obstruction of the airway, compression or contraction of lung parenchyma, or denaturation of surfactant.[33] Mucus, foreign bodies, or edema may obstruct the smaller airways. Compression of the lung parenchyma can occur from expansion of the pleural space (pneumothorax, hydrothorax) or elevation of the diaphragm. Contraction of the lung parenchyma will occur around foci of infection or fibrosis. Decreased surfactant production will result from lack of alveolar inflation or from direct destruction of the alveoli, as is seen in cases of adult respiratory distress syndrome (ARDS).

Physical findings associated with atelectasis may include a low-grade fever. Auscultation of the chest may reveal decreased breath sounds at the bases or dry rales upon inspiration. Percussion of the posterior thorax may suggest elevation of the diaphragm. Radiologic findings include the presence of horizontal lines or plates noted on posteroanterior chest x-rays, occasionally with adjacent areas containing hyperinflation. These changes are most pronounced during the first 3 postoperative days.

The various treatments for atelectasis are summarized in Table 3–21. Therapy should be aimed at expanding the alveoli and increasing the FRC. The most important maneuvers are those that promote maximal inspiratory pressure, which is maintained for as long as possible. This promotes not only an expansion of the alveoli but also secretion of surfactant. This can be achieved with aggressive supervised use of incentive spirometry, deep breathing exercises, and in some cases the use of positive expiratory pressure with a mask (continuous positive airway pressure [CPAP]). Oversedation should be avoided, and patients should be encouraged to ambulate and change positions frequently. Fiberoptic bronchoscopy should be reserved for patients who fail to improve with the usual measures.

Cardiogenic (High-Pressure) Pulmonary Edema. Cardiogenic pulmonary edema can result from myocardial ischemia, myocardial infarction, or simply from intravascular volume overload, particularly in patients who have low cardiac reserve or renal failure. The process usually begins with an increase in the fluid in the alveolar septa and bronchial vascular cuffs, ultimately seeping into the alveoli. Complete filling of the alveoli impairs secretion and production of surfactant. Concomitant with alveolar flooding, there are a decrease in lung compliance, impairment of the oxygen diffusion capacity, and increase in the arteriolar-alveolar oxygen gradient. Ventilation-perfusion mismatching in the lung results in a decrease in the PaO_2, resulting eventually in decreased oxygenation of the tissues and impairment of cardiac contractility.

Symptoms may include tachypnea, dyspnea, wheezing, and use of the accessory muscles of respiration. Clinical signs may include distention of the jugular veins, peripheral edema, rales upon auscultation of the lungs, and an enlarged heart. Radiographic findings may include the presence of bronchiolar cuffing as well as increased interstitial fluid markings extending to the periphery of the lung. The diagnosis can be further confirmed with the use of central hemodynamic monitoring, which will denote an elevated central venous pressure and, more specifically, an elevation in the pulmonary capillary wedge pressure.

A thorough evaluation of the patient's volume status should be made. In addition, myocardial ischemia or infarction should be ruled out via ECG and cardiac enzymes. The management of cardiogenic pulmonary edema includes oxygen support, aggressive diuresis, and afterload reduction to increase the cardiac output. In the absence of myocardial infarction, an inotropic agent may be used. Mechanical ventilation should be instituted in the case of acute respiratory failure.

Noncardiogenic Pulmonary Edema (Adult Respiratory Distress Syndrome). In contrast to cardiogenic pulmonary edema, in which alveolar flooding is a result of an increase in the hydrostatic pressure of the pulmonary capillaries, alveolar flooding in patients with ARDS is a result of an increase in pulmonary capillary permeability. The primary pathophysiologic process is one of damage to the capillary side of the alveolar-capillary membrane.[33] This results in rapid movement of fluid from the capillaries to the pulmonary interstitial space and thereafter to the alveoli. Lung compliance decreases, and oxygen diffusion capacity is impaired, resulting in hypoxemia. If not managed aggressively, respiratory failure will commonly result.

There are a number of causes of ARDS, and in fact there are several distinct ARDS states. The causes of ARDS include shock, sepsis, massive non-lung

Table 3–21

Treatment of Atelectasis

Obstructive Atelectasis
Remove mucopurulent plugs, foreign bodies
Aggressive pulmonary toilet
Aerosolized bronchodilator
Frequent position changes
Infection and edema control
May need intermittent positive pressure reinflation
Use fiberoptic bronchoscopy if above fail
Adequate control of pain, which can impair cough

Compressive Atelectasis
Chest tube to decompress hemo- or pneumothorax
Nasogastric tube to decrease abdominal distention
Adequate pain control to allow coughing, hyperinflation

Patchy Atelectasis
Requires hyperinflation
Vigorous cough
Frequent need for positive pressure, either CPAP or PEEP to restore FRC
Avoid excess sedation, but maintain adequate control of chest wall pain

CPAP, continuous positive airway pressure; PEEP, positive end-expiratory pressure; FRC, functional residual capacity.
From Demling RH, Wilson RF (eds.): Fluids, electrolytes, and acid-base balance. In Decision Making in Surgical Critical Care. Philadelphia, BC Decker, 1988, pp. 114–157.

trauma as from fractures or burns, multiple red blood cell transfusions, aspiration injury, inhalation injury, pneumonia, pancreatitis, DIC, and fat emboli.[267] Irrespective of the cause, the evolving clinical picture and management are very similar, with the exception that an attempt is made to identify and treat the inciting cause.

The evolving clinical picture of ARDS passes through several stages. Initially, patients develop tachypnea and dyspnea without remarkable findings on clinical evaluation or on chest x-ray. As lung compliance is impaired, functional residual capacity, tidal volume, and vital capacity all decrease. The PaO_2 decreases, and characteristically will increase only marginally with oxygen supplementation. During these early stages, the management plan should include a thorough attempt to identify the inciting cause with treatment initiated as indicated. This can include aggressive hemodynamic and circulatory resuscitation in patients with shock, aggressive broad-spectrum antibiotic therapy in patients who are septic, and aggressive replacement with cyroprecipitate or fresh-frozen plasma in patients who have DIC. An attempt should be made to maintain the arterial oxygen above 90%. This may be achievable initially via oxygen administered by mask. For patients with severe hypoxemia, endotracheal intubation with positive-pressure ventilation should be instituted.

Hemodynamic monitoring is invaluable and should be initiated early in the course of the disease process. Patients with any evidence of fluid overload should be receive aggressive diuresis, whereas others may require fluid resuscitation for maintenance of tissue perfusion, while maintaining the pulmonary-capillary wedge pressure below 15 mm Hg. Other measures for general care should include the placement of a nasogastric tube, gastric acid suppression with H_2 blockers, and steroids in patients with the fat emboli syndrome. Theophylline may be of some benefit, via its inotropic and bronchodilator effects.

With aggressive management, particularly if the inciting cause is identified and treated, ARDS can be reversed during the first 48 hours with few sequelae. Beyond the first 48 hours, progression of the ARDS will cause lung damage that may leave a residual pulmonary fibrosis. With progression beyond 10 days, multi-organ system failure occurs and mortality is greater than 80%.[33] Guidelines for initial ventilatory support can include a respiratory rate greater than 40/minute, arterial PO_2 less than 70 mm Hg, PCO_2 greater than 55 mm Hg, or arterial pH less than 7.30.[267]

Renal Disease

Renal insufficiency (RI) is associated with a high perioperative morbidity and mortality rate.[268] Management of patients with pre-existing renal disease and prevention of iatrogenically induced renal dysfunction in gynecologic surgery patients require an understanding of the underlying causes of renal disease and the metabolic disturbances that develop secondary to renal insufficiency.

The most common etiologic factors leading to end-stage renal disease include glomerulonephritis (28%), pyelonephritis (20%), hereditary factors, diabetes, and hypertensive diseases.[269]

Hematologic and coagulation abnormalities, including a normocytic, normochromic anemia, are common in RI patients. As opposed to normal patients, those with RI tolerate the stress of surgery well at hematocrits around 25%,[270] and routine preoperative transfusion is not usually necessary. Recombinant erythropoietin can be administered to anemic patients to successfully increase their hematocrit if surgery can be delayed several weeks.[271] Patients with chronic renal failure (CRF) are susceptible to incompletely understood bleeding abnormalities that are manifested as increased bleeding times. The increased bleeding time is thought to be due to platelet dysfunction caused by a decreased amount of Factor VIII/von Willebrand antigen in serum of uremic patients. In addition to cryoprecipitate, desmopressin and conjugated estrogens may be given to patients with CRF to shorten the bleeding time.[272, 273] This may be advantageous preoperatively in patients who are expected to have large amounts of blood loss during pelvic surgery. To date, the theoretical risk of potentiating thromboembolic phenomena with these agents has not been carefully studied. Patients with chronic renal insufficiency also are at increased risk for postoperative gastrointestinal bleeding and stress ulcers and should, therefore, receive prophylaxis with antacids, histamine blockers, or sucralfate both pre- and postoperatively. Unless aluminum toxicity is suspected, sucralfate is a desirable choice, owing to its antibacterial effect on enteric flora, which reduces the incidence of nosocomial pneumonia in patients who subsequently aspirate.[274]

Patients with CRF are at high risk for postoperative infections and sepsis. This is accounted for by abnormalities in neutrophil and monocyte function as well as a depressed anergy status.[275, 276] Preoperative nutritional support as well as appropriate antibiotic prophylaxis will reduce these infectious complications.

Chronic renal disease also alters the patient's ability to excrete drugs normally, and metabolic derangements alter the bioavailability of many medications. Because of these factors, and the effect of dialysis on drug availability, the surgeon must be aware of the altered metabolism and availability of many commonly used medications. Narcotics, barbiturates, muscle relaxants, antibiotics, and other drugs that require renal clearance are all significantly affected in patients with renal insufficiency and must be diligently monitored.

Fluid management and cardiovascular hemodynamics are very important in patients with CRF. Although ischemic heart disease is the most common cause of death in patients with RI, it is not a major cause of mortality in surgical patients with impaired renal function.[269] Intravascular fluid volume changes leading to hyper- or hypotension are common and can be difficult to manage because of autonomic dysfunction, acidosis, and other problems inherent to CRF. Physical examination and central venous pressure monitoring correlate poorly with left cardiac filling pressures. Therefore, patients with CRF undergoing major abdominal and pelvic surgery may be optimally managed by invasive intraoperative monitoring using pulmonary capillary wedge pressure measurements to guide fluid replacement and to avoid volume overload. This intensive management should be continued throughout the first postoperative week, because reabsorption of third-space fluid will occur during this time. Prompt dialysis may avoid serious problems associated with fluid overload and hyperkalemia.

Advances in dialysis therapy, including the timing of dialysis, its metabolic consequences, hematologic abnormalities, infectious complications, pharmacology, and cardiovascular and fluid management, may improve the perioperative outcome of dialysis patients. Dialysis-dependent patients should be routinely dialyzed within 24 hours of surgery. A large percentage of perioperative deaths in RI patients are associated with hyperkalemia, which is controlled most efficiently by dialysis.[277] Other methods to manage hyperkalemia include insulin and glucose therapy. Ion-exchange resins given as enemas should be used with caution because they can cause ischemic colitis and death in uremic patients.[278] The management of hypokalemia with bicarbonate is thought to be ineffective.

Cases of perioperative renal failure in previously normal patients may be divided into those caused by decreased renal perfusion, nephrotoxins, or both. Patients with cardiac failure, intravascular volume depletion, sepsis, or hypotension fall into the first category. Nephrotoxic medications such as aminoglycosides, intravenous iodinated contrast agents, some chemotherapeutic drugs, and anesthetic agents fall into the second category.[279–281] If more than one of the risk factors exist at the same time, the risk is cumulative, especially if they occur during a period of intravascular volume depletion.[282, 283]

Several precautions should be taken prior to surgery in all patients with renal insufficiency or chronic renal failure. First, all nephrotoxic drugs should be discontinued. When this is not possible, strict attention should be paid to the pharmacokinetic characteristics of each drug. For example, peak and trough levels are critically important in determining the dose and timing of aminoglycoside administration. If renal impairment develops preoperatively as a result of nephrotoxins, surgery should be delayed until renal function returns to baseline. Patients with diabetes should be given a limited dose of intravenous radiocontrast agents and should be well hydrated, because they are particularly susceptible to renal injury from these materials. Second, adequate intravascular volume assessment should be made and invasive monitoring may be necessary to ensure adequate left ventricular preload. Volume repletion preoperatively have been shown in both animal and clinical studies to lower the incidence of renal impairment postoperatively.[284, 285]

In summary, a review of the patient's history of pre-existing renal disease, including dialysis records, determination of risk factors, and limited exposure to nephrotoxic agents, should be part of the preoperative plan. Physical examination, serum chemistries, and invasive hemodynamic monitoring should provide information regarding the intravascular volume status and estimate renal perfusion. Appropriate steps, including aggressive early dialysis, can control volume overload and electrolyte imbalances and possibly avert intraoperative and postoperative complications. Patients with coagulopathies or prolonged bleeding time should be given cryoprecipitate, desmopressin, or conjugated estrogens in order to circumvent excessive intraoperative bleeding. Invasive central venous monitoring may allow more appropriate fluid management intra- and postoperatively.

Liver Disease

Patients with liver disease may have numerous problems with nutrition, coagulation, electrolytes, encephalopathy, and sepsis following surgery. Therefore, the preoperative assessment should focus particular attention to patients with a history of viral hepatitis, jaundice, intravenous drug use, a personal history of alcohol abuse, previous blood product exposure, or a family history of liver disease. The physical examination should note any jaundice, malnutrition, ascites, or hepatosplenomegaly. In patients with known or suspected hepatic disease,[286] assays of serum transaminases, albumin, prothrombin time, and direct bilirubin are essential. Serum glutamic oxaloacetic transaminase (SGOT) and serum glutamic pyruvic transaminase (SGPT) are nonspecific intracellular proteins in liver, heart, kidney, skeletal muscle, brain, and adipose tissue. However, significant elevation (in the 500–1000 IU/liter range) usually indicates hepatitis and should prompt further investigation. A prolonged prothrombin time also suggests liver dysfunction. Administration of phytonadione

(10 mg, intramuscularly) for 3 days should correct the vitamin K deficiency and thus the prothrombin time.[287] Failure of vitamin K administration to reverse the abnormal prothrombin time indicates severe liver disease.[288] Partial thromboplastin time, thrombin clotting time, and platelet count should also be evaluated in patients with liver disease, although their values may not correlate well with the degree of hepatic dysfunction. Increased splenic sequestration of platelets is seen in liver dysfunction, and patients with less than 60,000 platelets/mm^3 usually require platelet transfusion preoperatively.[289] Careful evaluation of electrolytes, blood urea nitrogen, and creatinine is important because of the well-described relationship between cirrhosis and the hepatorenal syndrome. Serum glucose should be monitored in patients with liver disease because the liver controls glycogenesis, glycogenolysis, gluconeogenesis, and glycolysis.

Acute hepatocellular damage results in increased morbidity and mortality in the surgical patient.[290] Therefore, if after a thorough history, physical examination, and laboratory assessment, the etiology of the liver disease remains unknown, a hepatologist should be consulted. After the specific diagnosis is made, the risk assessment for surgery is made using Child's classification (Classes A, B, and C), which has shown that morbidity and mortality are directly related to the degree of liver dysfunction[291] (Table 3–22). Although originally this classification was used for patients undergoing surgery for bleeding esophageal varices, it has since been shown to be useful in patients undergoing other types of abdominal surgery and is an excellent predictor of surgical morbidity and mortality.[292, 293]

In 100 patients with cirrhosis undergoing abdominal surgery, Garrison reported operative mortalities of 10%, 31%, and 76%, respectively, for each of the three classifications.[293] The Child classification was the best predictor among 53 variables studied and correlates with other postoperative complications such as bleeding, renal failure, wound dehiscence, and sepsis. In these patients, the major cause of perioperative death was sepsis. Experience suggests that patients in Child's Class A may undergo the planned surgery without excessive risk. Patients in Child's Class B or C should not have elective surgery until their hepatic status improves.

Patients with massive ascites due to cirrhosis also frequently have a hydrothorax, a pulmonary ventilation-perfusion mismatch, decreased gastric emptying time, and are at high risk of regurgitation and aspiration. If pulmonary function and arterial blood gases are severely compromised, a therapeutic thoracentesis and paracentesis should be considered preoperatively. Anesthetic considerations include administration of a histamine antagonist, a rapid sequential induction, and an awake intubation because of the high risk of regurgitation and aspiration. The rapid release of hepatic failure–induced ascitic fluid places the patient at high risk for hypovolemic cardiovascular collapse. Intraoperative invasive venous monitoring may greatly assist with fluid replacement decisions.

Because of altered hepatic metabolism, several considerations need to be made with regard to medications. Metabolism of benzodiazepines, narcotics, and muscle relaxants is greatly altered. Diazepam and morphine doses should be lowered and dosing intervals increased because of a prolonged effect of these agents in patients with liver impairment. Muscle relaxants such as D-tubocurarine and pancuronium have increased protein binding, and patients show a relative resistance to their actions. Succinylcholine's duration of action may be lengthened because of a relative decrease in plasma acetylcholinesterase. Hepatic function also is greatly affected by the choice of anesthetic agents because certain drugs alter the flow of blood to the liver and thus change the rate of metabolism. Isoflurane preserves blood flow at clinically effective doses and is the agent of choice in patients with liver dysfunction. Halothane's metabolites possess hepatotoxic potential, and this effect may be genetically influenced. Those at risk of developing halothane hepatitis are patients who have had previous exposure to halothane and patients who are likely to have enzyme induction secondary to barbiturates, smoking, or alcohol ingestion.

Patients with acute viral hepatitis pose a significant surgical problem. First, they should be appropriately diagnosed using serologic markers. Second, because of an increased risk of perioperative morbidity (12%) and mortality (9.5%), only emergency surgery should be performed. After the convalescent phase of the disease has passed and the patient is fully recovered, definitive surgery may then take place. In addition to the increased morbidity and mortality to the patient, there is also increased risk to the health care provider when viral hepatitis is encountered in the surgical patient.

In patients with chronic liver disease (chronic

Table 3–22

Child's Classification of Liver Dysfunction

Parameter	Child Classification		
	A	B	C
Bilirubin	<2.0	2.0–3.0	>3.0
Albumin	>3.5	3.0–3.5	<3.0
Ascites	None	Easily controlled	Poorly controlled
Encephalopathy	None	Mild	Advanced
Nutritional status	Excellent	Good	Poor

From Child CG, Turcotte JG: In Child CG (ed.): The Liver and Portal Hypertension, 3rd ed. Philadelphia, WB Saunders Co., 1964, p. 50.

active hepatitis, chronic persistent hepatitis), steroids may be of some benefit preoperatively. Prednisone 20 mg/day or azathioprine 50 mg and prednisone 10 mg/day have been shown to result in remission in up to 80% of patients. This is still considered experimental, however, and not the standard of care. The regimen is continued only if there is clinical, biochemical, and histologic evidence of remission.[294] A controlled, randomized trial of prednisone and interferon alpha-IIb has documented disappearance of the hepatitis B antigen (HB_eAg) and hepatitis B viral DNA replication in 37% of patients.[295] Although further evaluation of this treatment is needed, it may become part of the preoperative treatment of patients with chronic hepatitis B.

Patients with cirrhosis should be considered for surgery only after evaluation with the Child classification and coagulation studies have been performed. The 30% mortality rate in these patients warrants extensive preoperative preparation. Although limited information is available regarding the gynecologic patient, morbidity and mortality should be considered significant, and infection is a major factor to contend with in these patients.

The precise cause of liver dysfunction following surgery is often difficult to ascertain secondary to the numerous causes and because postoperative patients have often been exposed to numerous hepatic insults (e.g., blood products, hypotension, anesthetics). Postoperative management requires careful assessment of the extent of hepatic involvement and a detailed systematic search for its effects on other organ systems, including the kidneys, central nervous system, gastrointestinal tract (varices), cardiopulmonary system, and the coagulation pathway.

Approximately 70-90% of post-transfusion viral hepatitis falls into the non-A, non-B category.[296] The virus incubation period ranges from 2 weeks to 6 months after exposure and therefore is epidemiologically similar to that of hepatitis B. After this variable incubation period, nausea, vomiting, anorexia, and malaise develop in symptomatic patients. These symptoms usually resolve within 3 months, although a small proportion of cases may progress to chronic liver disease and an even smaller proportion develop into fulminant liver failure. The diagnosis may be secured from serologic methods that exclude other types of hepatitis, including a negative hepatitis B surface antigen and hepatitis A antibody, a negative heterophil test, and the absence of a rising titer to cytomegalovirus. Treatment is entirely supportive in nature.

Intraoperative events such as hypotension, hypoxia, and hypovolemia are known to cause postoperative hepatic dysfunction, though the severity of the incident needed to cause this is not well understood. These insults may cause mild to severe liver damage that may be reversible or irreversible, depending on their severity and on whether preexisting liver disease is present.

The role of anesthetic agents, in particular, halothane, in the development of postoperative liver impairment has, in contrast, been extensively studied. The mechanism of this phenomenon is unknown, although there is some consensus that the pathophysiology involves a halothane metabolite and an autoimmune process. It is of considerable interest that approximately 75-80% of the patients affected have had previous halothane exposure.[297] In addition, if patients who are suspected of having halothane-induced hepatitis are re-exposed to halothane after recovery from the initial episode, they will redevelop hepatitis.[298] Besides prior exposure to halothane, other risk factors for development of this process include obesity and familial susceptibility. These associations, however, have been less extensively studied and are controversial. The clinical features of halothane-induced hepatitis are similar to those described for viral hepatitis except that it occurs between 1 and 2 weeks after the exposure to halothane. Jaundice may develop between 1 and 20 days later and may be associated with palmar erythema, hepatomegaly, ascites, and encephalopathy. Laboratory abnormalities, including elevations in the transaminases, bilirubin, and alkaline phosphatase, are common. Histopathologic criteria for its diagnosis cannot be distinguished from those of viral hepatitis. Halothane-induced hepatitis is fatal in approximately 1 in 35,000 administrations of the drug.

Treatment is supportive in nature, and therefore prevention of this phenomenon should be the gynecologist's goal. General recommendations include avoidance of halothane anesthesia in any patient in whom prodromal symptoms and jaundice followed a prior halothane administration. It is unknown if there exists an interval after which repeated halothane anesthesia would be safe. Therefore, use of an alternate anesthetic agent is preferable.

Treatment of the complications resulting from liver dysfunction involves prompt diagnosis and is mainly supportive in nature. The complexity of liver failure and its effects on numerous organ systems usually require admission to an intensive care unit. Because of the close relationship with the renal system, a thorough evaluation of kidney function is mandatory. Urine output should remain above 30 ml/hour, and close serial monitoring of potassium, bicarbonate, and acid-base balance is usually important. Because of the well-known association with the hepatorenal syndrome, a urine sodium level of less than 10 mEq/liter should alert the clinician to the possibility of this diagnosis. Prompt intervention with a Swan-Ganz catheter to monitor intravascular fluid changes and prompt dialysis when necessary may be life-saving.

Because of massive ascites and other complicated hemodynamic changes, including an excessive protein load, cardiovascular and respiratory compromise is commonly seen in patients with liver failure. Again, a Swan-Ganz catheter may be necessary to identify these labile intravascular changes so that prompt action may be taken. Respiratory failure secondary to volume overload or massive ascites may necessitate mechanical ventilation, thoracentesis, or paracentesis.

As liver function deteriorates, further intervention may be necessary to prevent life-threatening complications secondary to coagulopathies. In mild cases, or early in the course of hepatitis, administration of vitamin K can correct the abnormality. In more severe cases, supportive treatment in the form of FFP and other blood products such as cryoprecipitate or fibrinogen may be necessary.

The postoperative care of patients with cirrhosis is among the most challenging in all of medicine. One of the most serious complications resulting from portal hypertension is bleeding esophageal varices. As this is a life-threatening complication, prompt intervention is necessary. Immediate endoscopy for upper GI bleeding is essential because about 30% of patients with suspected bleeding do not have varices. If bleeding is documented, pharmacologic therapy with vasopressin is indicated. Although controlled trials with vasopressin and nitroglycerin have not shown improved efficacy by the addition of the nitroglycerin, it has lowered the incidence of side effects from the vasopressin.[299] Tamponade of the varices with a four-lumen balloon tube (modified Sengstaken-Blakemore tube) will control acute bleeding in 90% of cases. However, this is only a temporary measure, as more than 60% of these patients will have a recurrence of their bleeding.[300] Therefore, a definitive procedure, preferably within 6–12 hours, is necessary. In two controlled trials, sclerotherapy has been shown to be more effective than balloon tube tamponade alone.[301, 302] It has been recommended as the treatment of choice and may be performed successfully at the time of the first diagnostic endoscopy.[303] Alternatively, staple transection of the esophagus for the emergency control of bleeding has been advocated as a safe and more effective therapy for emergency treatment of bleeding esophageal varices than a single sclerotherapy procedure.[304]

The diagnosis of hepatic encephalopathy is an ominous sign. Daily surveillance for asterixis, inappropriate behavior, and the ability of the patient to write his or her name is useful to detect early signs of encephalopathy. Measurement of serum ammonia levels has also been a routine exercise in the past, although correlation of this parameter with the severity of hepatic encephalopathy is controversial. Administration of lactulose (30 ml four times a day) has been effective in the acidification of the digestive tract, which decreases bacterial production of ammonia.[305] Mannitol infusions, ventilatory support, and other supportive measures for encephalopathy have not been definitively shown to have proven benefit.

The complicated scenario of hepatic failure, in addition to the aforementioned problems, includes an increased risk of infection, serum glucose lability, multiple electrolyte abnormalities, and a host of other problems requiring meticulous and constant surveillance. Although little information in gynecologic patients with these abnormalities exists, analogies to general surgical patients can be made and clear inferences can be drawn. It is obvious that these patients represent a group in whom the advantages and disadvantages of elective surgery must be carefully weighed. In the specific case of cirrhosis, mortality rates approach 30% despite careful patient selection and intensive postoperative care.[293]

References

1. Rohrer MJ, Michelotti MC, Nahrwold DL: A prospective evaluation of the efficacy of preoperative coagulation testing. Ann Surg 1987; 208:554.
2. Lamers RJ, van Engelshoven JM, Pfaff A: Once again, the routine preoperative thorax photo. Nederl Tijdschrift Voor Geneeskunde 1989; 133:2288.
3. Loder RE: Routine preoperative chest radiography. Anesthesiology 1987; 66:195.
4. Piscitelli JT, Simel DL, Addison WA: Who should have intravenous pyelograms before hysterectomy for benign disease? Obstet Gynecol 1987; 69:541.
5. Easley HA, Hammond CB: Informed consent in obstetrics and gynecology. Postgrad Obstet Gynecol 1986; 10:1.
6. Vogel CM, Kingsbury RJ, Baue A: Intravenous hyperalimentation: A review of two and one-half years' experience. Arch Surg 1972; 105:414.
7. Blackburn GL, Bistrian BR: Nutritional care of the injured and/or septic patient. Surg Clin North Am 1976; 56:1195.
8. Lubin MF, Walker HK, Smith RB: Medical Management of the Surgical Patient, 2nd ed. Stoneham, MA, Butterworth, 1988, pp. 9–10.
9. Wilmore DW, Pruitt BA Jr: Parenteral nutrition in burn patients. In Fischer JE (ed.): Total Parenteral Nutrition. Boston, Little, Brown, 1976; pp. 231–252.
10. Theuer RC, Vitale JJ: Drug and nutrient interactions. In Schneider HA, Anderson CE, Coursin DB (eds.): Nutritional Support of Medical Practice. New York, Harper & Row, 1977; pp. 297–305.
11. Abel RM: Nutritional support in the patient with acute renal failure. J Am Coll Nutr 1983; 2:33.
12. Kinney JM, Long CL, Gump FE, Duke JH: Tissue composition of weight loss in surgical patients. I. Elective operation. Ann Surg 1968; 168:459.
13. Aguirre A, Fischer JE, Welch CE: The role of surgery and hyperalimentation in therapy of gastrointestinal-cutaneous fistulae. Ann Surg 1974; 180:393.
14. Copeland EM, MacFadyen BV, Lanzotti VJ, Dudrick SJ: Intravenous hyperalimentation as an adjunct to cancer chemotherapy. Am J Surg 1975; 129:167.

15. Bandy LC, Chin N, Soper JT, et al.: Total parenteral nutrition in poor prognosis gestational trophoblastic disease. Gynecol Oncol 1987; 28:305.
16. Soper JT, Berchuck A, Creasman WT, Clarke-Pearson, DL: Pelvic exenteration: Factors associated with major surgical morbidity. Gynecol Oncol 1989; 35:93.
17. Butterworth CE, Blackburn GL: Hospital malnutrition and how to assess the nutritional status of a patient. Nutr Today 1974; 9:1.
18. Baker JP, Detsky AS, Wesson DE: Nutritional assessment: A comparison of clinical judgement and objective measurements. N Engl J Med 1982; 306:969.
19. Heymsfield SB, Horowitz J, Lawson DH: Enteral hyperalimentation. In Berk JE (ed.): Developments in Digestive Diseases, Vol 3. Philadelphia, Lea & Febiger, 1980; pp. 59–83.
20. Mullen JL, Buzby GP, Waldman TG, et al.: Prediction of operative morbidity and mortality by preoperative nutritional assessment. Surg Forum 1979; 30:80.
21. Heatley RV, Williams RHP, Lewis MH: Preoperative intravenous feeding: A controlled trial. Postgrad Med J 1979; 55:541.
22. Foschi D, Gavagna G, Callioni F, et al.: Hyperalimentation of jaundiced patients on percutaneous transhepatic biliary drainage. Br J Surg 1986; 73:716.
23. Smith RC, Hartemink R: Improvement of nutritional measures during preoperative parenteral nutrition selected by the prognostic nutritional index: A randomized controlled trial. J Parent Ent Nutr 1989; 12(6):587.
24. Müller JM, Keller HW, Brenner U, et al.: Indications and effects of preoperative parenteral nutrition. World J Surg 1986; 10:53.
25. Young GA, Hill GL: A controlled study of protein sparing therapy after excision of the rectum. Ann Surg 1980; 192:183.
26. Nubiola P, Badia JM, Martinez-Rodemas F, et al.: Treatment of 27 postoperative enterocutaneous fistulas with the long half-life somatostatin analogue SMS 201-995. Ann Surg 1989; 210(1):56.
27. Clarke-Pearson DL, DeLong ER, Chin N, et al.: Intestinal obstruction in patients with ovarian cancer. Arch Surg 1988; 123:42.
28. Pestana C: Fluids and Electrolytes in the Surgical Patient. Baltimore, Williams & Wilkins, 1989.
29. Miller TA, Duke JH: Fluid and electrolyte management. In Dudrick SJ, Baue AE, Eiseman B, et al. (eds.): ACS Manual of Preoperative and Postoperative Care. Philadelphia, WB Saunders Co, 1983; pp. 38–67.
30. Magrina JF: Intravenous fluids and blood component therapy. Clin Obstet Gynecol 1988; 31:686.
31. Shires GT, Canizaro P: Fluid and electrolyte management of the surgical patient. In Sabiston DC Jr (ed.): Textbook of Surgery, 14th ed. Philadelphia, WB Saunders Co., 1991, p. 74.
32. Narins RG, Lazarus MJ: Renal systems. In Vandam LD (ed.): To Make the Patient Ready for Anesthesia: Medical Care of the Surgical Patient, 2nd ed. Stoneham, MA, Butterworth, 1984; pp. 67–114.
33. Demling RH, Wilson RF (eds.): Fluids, electrolytes, and acid-base balance. In Decision Making in Surgical Critical Care. Philadelphia, BC Decker, 1988; pp. 114–157.
34. Edwards TW: Optimizing opioid treatment of postoperative pain. J Pain Symptom Manag 1990; 5:S24.
35. Kuhn S, Cook K, Collins M, et al.: Receptions of pain relief after surgery. BMJ 1990; 300:1687.
36. Donovan M, Dillon P, McGuire L: Incidence and characteristics of pain in a sample of medical-surgical patients. Pain 1987; 30:69.
37. Oden V: Acute postoperative pain: Incidence, severity, and the etiology of inadequate treatment. Anesth Clin North Am 1989; 7:1.
38. Marks RM, Sachar EJ: Undertreatment of medical inpatients with narcotic analgesics. Ann Intern Med 1973; 78:172.
39. Smith G: Management of postoperative pain. Can J Anaesth 1989; 36:S1.
40. Austin KL, Stapleton JV, Mather LE: Multiple intramuscular injections: A major source of variability in analgesic response to meperidine. Pain 1980; 8:47.
41. Forest WH Jr, Smethurst PWR, Kienitz ME: Self administration of intravenous analgesics. Anesthesiology 1970; 33:363.
42. Keeri-Szanto M: Apparatus for demand analgesia. Can Anaesth Soc J 1971; 18:581.
43. Sechzer PH: Studies in pain with analgesic demand system. Anesth Analg 1971; 50:1.
44. Egbert AM, Parks LH, Short LM, Burnett ML: Randomized trial of postoperative patient-controlled analgesia vs. intramuscular narcotics in frail elderly men. Arch Intern Med 1990; 150:1897.
45. Lange MP, Dahn MS, Jacobs LA: Patient-controlled analgesia versus intermittent analgesia dosing. Heart Lung 1988; 17:495.
46. De Conno F, Ripamonti C, Gamba A, et al.: Treatment of postoperative pain: Comparison between administration at fixed hours and "on demand" with intramuscular analgesics. Eur J Surg Oncol 1989; 15:242.
47. Rose PG, Piver MS, Batista E, Lau T: Patient-controlled analgesia in gynecologic oncology: A comparative analysis. J Reprod Med 1989; 34:651.
48. Zachiarias M, Pfeifer MV, Herbison P: Comparison of two methods of intravenous administration of morphine for postoperative pain relief. Anaesth Intens Care 1990; 18:205.
49. White PF: Patient-controlled analgesia: An update on its use in the treatment of postoperative pain. Anesth Clin North Am 1989; 7:63.
50. Ellis R, Hames D, Shah R, et al.: Pain relief after abdominal surgery: Comparison of IM morphine, sublingual buprenorphine, and self-administered IV pethidine. Br J Anaesth 1982; 54:421.
51. Welchew FA: On-demand analgesia: A double-blind comparison of on-demand intravenous fentanyl with regular intramuscular morphine. Anaesthesia 1983; 38:19.
52. Dahl JB, Daugaard JJ, Larsen HV, et al.: Patient-controlled analgesia: A controlled trial. Acta Anaesthesiol Scand 1987; 31:744.
53. White PF: Mishaps with patient-controlled analgesia (PCA). Anesthesiology 1987; 66:81.
54. Rapp SE, Ready LB, Greer BE: Postoperative pain management in gynecologic oncology patients utilizing epidural opiate analgesia and patient-controlled analgesia. Gynecol Oncol 1989; 35:341.
55. Lutz LJ, Lamer TJ: Management of postoperative pain: Review of current techniques and methods. Mayo Clin Proc 1990; 65:584.
56. Dodson ME: Post-operative pain relief. In Nunn JF, Utting JE, Brown BR Jr (eds.): General Anesthesia, 5th ed. Stoneham, MA, Butterworth, 1989, Chap. 94.
57. Vercauteren M, Lauwers E, Meert T, et al.: Comparison of epidural sufentanil plus clonidine with sufentanil alone for postoperative pain relief. Anaesthesiology 1990; 45:531.
58. Flynn NM: Reducing the risk of infection in surgical patients. In Bolt RJ (ed.): Medical Evaluation of the Surgical Patient. Mt Kisco, NY, Futura, 1987, pp. 195–240.
59. Ledger WJ, Gee C, Lewis WP: Guidelines for antibiotic prophylaxis in gynecology. Am J Obstet Gynecol 1975; 121:1038.
60. Hirsch HA: Prophylactic antibiotics in obstetrics and gynecology. Am J Med 1985; 78:170.
61. Shapiro M, Munoz A, Tager IB, et al.: Risk factors for infection at the operative site after abdominal or vaginal hysterectomy. N Engl J Med 1982; 307:1661.
62. Haley RW, Culver DH, Morgan WM, et al.: Identifying patients at high risk of surgical wound infection. A simple multivariate index of patient susceptibility and wound contamination. Am J Epidemiol 1985; 121:206.
63. Roy S, Wilkins J, Galaif E, Azen C: Comparative efficacy and safety of cefmetazole or cefoxitin in the prevention of postoperative infection following vaginal and abdominal hysterectomy. J Antimicro Chemo 1989; 23:109.
64. Trimbos JB, van Lindert ACM, Heintz APM, et al.: Piperacillin for prophylaxis in gynecological surgery. Eur J Obstet Gynecol Reprod Biol 1989; 30:141.
65. Davey PG, Duncan ID, Edward D, Scott AC: Cost-benefit analysis of cephradine and mezlocillin prophylaxis for ab-

dominal and vaginal hysterectomy. Br J Obstet Gynaecol 1988; 95:1170.
66. Munck JM, Jensen HK: Preoperative clindamycin treatment and vaginal drainage in hysterectomy. Acta Obstet Gynecol Scand 1989; 68:241.
67. Gerber B, Retzke F, Wilken H: Effectiveness of perioperative preventive use of antibiotics with ampicillin/gentamicin or cefoxitin in abdominal cesarean section. Zentralbl Gynakol 1989; 111:658.
68. Friese S, Pricker GJ, Willems FT, et al.: Single-dose prophylaxis in gynecological surgery: Amoxicillin/clavulanic acid versus the combination of cefuroxim and metronidazole in a randomized prospective comparison. Eur J Obstet Gynecol Reprod Biol 1988; 27:313.
69. Chodak GW: Use of systemic antibiotics for prophylaxis in surgery. Arch Surg 1977; 112:326.
70. Burke JF: The effective period of preventive antibiotic action in experimental incisions and dermal lesions. Surgery 1961; 50:161.
71. Hemsell DL, Martin JN Jr, Pastorek JG II, et al.: Single-dose antimicrobial prophylaxis at abdominal hysterectomy. Cefamandole vs. cefotaxime. J Reprod Med 1988; 33:939.
72. Hemsell DL, Johnson ER, Heard MC, et al.: Single-dose piperacillin versus triple-dose cefoxitin prophylaxis at vaginal and abdominal hysterectomy. South Med J 1989; 82:438.
73. Orr JW Jr, Sisson PF, Patsner B, et al.: Single-dose antibiotic prophylaxis for patients undergoing extended pelvic surgery for gynecologic malignancy. Am J Obstet Gynecol 1990; 162:718.
74. Brachman PS, Dan BB, Haley RW, et al.: Nosocomial surgical infections: Incidence and cost. Surg Clin North Am 1980; 60:15.
75. Garibaldi RA, Brodine S, Matsumiya S, et al.: Evidence for the noninfectious etiology of early postoperative fever. Infect Control 1985; 6:273.
76. Hemsell DL: Infections after gynecologic surgery. Obstet Gynecol Clin North Am 1989; 16:381.
77. Bartzen PJ, Hafferty FW: Pelvic laparotomy without an indwelling catheter. A retrospective review of 949 cases. Am J Obstet Gynecol 1987; 156:1426.
78. Kingdom JCP, Kitchener HC, MacLean AB: Postoperative urinary tract infection in gynecology: Implications for an antibiotic prophylaxis policy. Obstet Gynecol 1990; 76:636.
79. Ireland D, Tacchi D, Bint AJ: Effect of single-dose prophylactic co-trimoxazole on the incidence of gynaecological postoperative urinary tract infection. Br J Obstet and Gynaecol 1982; 89:578.
80. Boyd ME: Postoperative gynecologic infections. Can J Surg 1987; 30:7
81. Kunin CM: Urinary tract infections. Surg Clin North Am 1980; 60:223.
82. Harkness GA, Bentley DW, Roghmann KJ: Risk factors for nosocomial pneumonia in the elderly. Am J Med 1990; 89:457.
83. Eikhoff TC: Pulmonary infections in surgical patients. Surg Clin North Am 1980; 60:175.
84. Tomford JW, Hershey CO, McLaren CE, et al.: Intravenous therapy team and peripheral venous catheter–associated complications. Arch Intern Med 1984; 144:1191.
85. Hershey CO, Tomford JW, McLaren CE, et al.: The natural history of intravenous catheter–associated phlebitis. Arch Intern Med 1984; 144:1373.
86. Cruse PJE, Ford R: The epidemiology of wound infection: A 10-year prospective study of 62,939 wounds. Surg Clin North Am 1980; 60:27.
87. Brown SE, Allen HH, Robins RN: The use of delayed primary wound closure in preventing wound infections. Am J Obstet Gynecol 1977; 127:713.
88. Crombleholme WR, Schachter J, Ohm-Smith M, et al.: Efficacy of single-agent therapy for the treatment of acute pelvic inflammatory disease with ciprofloxacin. Am J Med 1989; 87:142.
88a. Crombleholme WR, Ohm-Smith M, Robbie MO, et al: Ampicillin/sulbactam versus metronidazole/gentamicin in the treatment of soft tissue infections. Am J Obstet Gynecol 1987; 156(2):507.
89. Cunningham FG: Treatment and prevention of female pelvic infection: The quest for single agent therapy. Am J Obstet Gynecol 1987; 157:485.
90. Hemsell DL, Heard MC, Hemsell PG: Single agent therapy for women with acute polymicrobial pelvic infections. Am J Obstet Gynecol 1987; 157:488.
91. Riseman JA, Zamboni WA, Curtis A, et al.: Hyperbaric oxygen therapy for necrotizing fasciitis reduces mortality and the need for debridements. Surgery 1990; 108:847.
92. Meleney RL: Hemolytic streptococcus gangrene. Arch Surg 1925; 9:317.
93. Umbert IJ, Winkelmann MD, Oliver GF, Peters MS: Necrotizing fasciitis: A clinical, microbiologic, and histopathologic study of 14 patients. J Am Acad Dermatol 1989; 20:774.
94. Wikerson R, Pauli W, Coville FV: Necrotizing fasciitis: Review of the literature and case report. Clin Orthop 1987:187.
95. Marrie TJ, Costerton JW: In vivo ultrastructural study of microbes in necrotizing fasciitis. Eur J Clin Microbiol Infect Dis 1988; 7:51.
96. Clayton MD, Fowler JE, Sharifi R, Pearl RK: Causes, presentation and survival of fifty-seven patients with necrotizing fasciitis of the male genitalia. Surg Gynecol Obstet 1990; 170:49.
97. Sudarsky LA, Laschinger JC, Coppa GF, Spencer FC: Improved results from a standardized approach in treating patients with necrotizing fasciitis. Ann Surg 1987; 206:661.
98. Fisher JR, Conway MJ, Takeshita RT, Sandoual MR: Necrotizing fasciitis: Importance of roentgenographic studies for soft tissue gas. JAMA 1979; 241:803.
99. Hirn M, Niinikoski J: Management of perineal necrotizing fasciitis (Fournier's gangrene). Ann Chir Gynaecol 1989; 78:277.
100. Stamenkovic I, Lew PD: Early recognition of potentially fatal necrotizing fasciitis. The use of frozen-section biopsy. N Engl J Med 1984; 310:1689.
101. Rothman PA, Wiskind AK, Dudley AG: Amniotic membranes in the treatment of necrotizing fasciitis complicating vulvar herpes virus infection. Obstet Gynecol 1990; 76:534.
102. Hoffman MS, Turhquist DT: Necrotizing fasciitis of the vulva during chemotherapy. Obstet Gynecol 1989; 74:483.
103. Cruikshank SH, McLauchlan L: A de novo case of vulvar synergistic necrotizing fasciitis. Obstet Gynecol 1987; 69:516.
104. Frolich EP, Schein M: Necrotizing fasciitis arising from Bartholin's abscess: Case report and review of literature. Isr J Med Sci 1989; 25:644.
105. Cederna JP, Davies BW, Farkas SA, et al.: Necrotizing fasciitis of the total abdominal wall after sterilization by partial salpingectomy. Am J Obstet Gynecol 1990; 162:138.
106. Ahrenholz DH: Surgical spectrum. Clinical skin and soft tissue infection. Physicians World Communications (monograph). West Point, PA: Merck, Sharpe, and Dohme, 1988, pp. 16–24.
107. Eltora IM, Hart GB, Strauss MB, et al.: The role of hyperbaric oxygen in the management of Fournier's gangrene. Int Surg 1986; 71:53.
108. Kaiser PE, Cerra FB: Progressive necrotizing surgical infections: A unified approach. J Trauma 1981; 21:349.
109. Robson MC, Krizek TJ, Koss N, Samburg JC: Amniotic membranes as a temporary wound dressing. Surg Gynecol Obstet 1973; 136:904.
109a. Bech DE, Harford FJ, DiPalma JA: Comparison of cleansing method in preparation for colonic surgery. Dis Colon Rectum 1985; 28:491.
110. Clarke JS, Condon RE, Bartlett JG, et al.: Preoperative oral antibiotics reduce septic complications of colon operations. Ann Surg 1977; 1986:251.
111. Fry DE: Antibiotics in surgery: An overview. Ann J Surg 1988; 155(5A):11.
112. Menaker GJ: The use of antibiotics in surgical treatment of the colon. Surg Gynecol Obstet 1987; 164:581.
113. Wolfson PJ, Bauer JJ, Gelerut IM, et al.: Use of the long tube in the management of patients with small intestinal obstruction due to adhesions. Arch Surg 1985; 120:1001.
114. Ratcliff JB, Kapernick P, Brooks GG, et al.: Small bowel obstruction and previous gynecologic surgery. South Med J 1983; 75:1349.
115. Jeffcoate TNA, Tindall VR: Venous thrombosis and embolism

in obstetrics and gynecology. Aust N Z J Obstet Gynaecol 1965; 5:119.
116. Kimball AM, Hallum AV, Cates W: Deaths caused by pulmonary thromboembolism after legally induced abortion. Am J Obstet Gynecol 1978; 132:169.
117. Clarke-Pearson DL, Jelovsek FR, Creasman WT: Thromboembolism complicating surgery for cervical and uterine malignancy: Incidence, risk factors, and prophylaxis. Obstet Gynecol 1983; 61:87.
118. Creasman WT, Weed JC Jr: Radical hysterectomy. In Schaefer G, Graber EA (eds.): Complications in Obstetrics and Gynecologic Surgery. Hagerstown, MD, Harper & Row, 1981, pp. 389–398.
119. Clayton JK, Anderson JA, McNicol GP: Preoperative prediction of postoperative deep vein thrombosis. Br Med J 1976; 2:910.
120. Clarke-Pearson DL, DeLong E, Synan IS, et al.: A prospective study of risk factors associated with postoperative venous thromboembolism in gynecology. Obstet Gynecol 1987; 69(2):146.
121. Kakkar VV: Prevention of fatal postoperative pulmonary embolism by low dose heparin. An international multicenter trial. Lancet 1975; 2:145.
122. Ballard M, Bradley-Watson PJ, Johnstone ED, et al.: Low doses of subcutaneous heparin in the prevention of deep venous thrombosis after gynecologic surgery. J Obstet Gynaecol Br Commonw 1973; 80:469.
123. Taberner DA, Poller L, Burnstein RW, et al.: Oral anticoagulants controlled by British comparative thromboplastin versus low dose heparin prophylaxis of deep venous thrombosis. Br Med J 1978; 1:272.
124. Clarke-Pearson DL, Coleman RE, Synan IS, et al.: Venous thromboembolism prophylaxis in gynecologic oncology: A prospective controlled trial of low-dose heparin. Am J Obstet Gynecol 1983; 145:606.
125. Clarke-Pearson DL, DeLong E, Synan IS, et al.: A controlled trial of two low-dose heparin regimens for the prevention of postoperative deep vein thrombosis. Obstet Gynecol 1990; 75:684.
126. Clarke-Pearson DL, DeLong E, Synan IS, et al.: Complications of low-dose heparin prophylaxis in gynecologic oncology surgery. Obstet Gynecol 1984; 64:689.
127. Dockerty PW, Goodman JDS, Hill JG, et al: The effect of low-dose heparin on blood loss at abdominal hysterectomy. Br J Obstet Gynecol 1983; 90:759.
128. Catalona WJ, Kadmon D, Crane DB: Effect of mini-dose heparin on lymphocele formation following extraperitoneal pelvic lymphadenectomy. J Urol 1979; 123:890.
129. Piver MS, Malfetano JH, Lele SB, et al.: Prophylactic anticoagulation as a possible cause of inguinal lymphocyst after radical vulvectomy and inguinal lymphadenectomy. Obstet Gynecol 1983; 62:17.
130. Clarke-Pearson DL, Creasman WT, Coleman RE, et al.: Perioperative external pneumatic calf compression as thromboembolism prophylaxis in gynecologic oncology: Report of a randomized controlled trial. Gynecol Oncol 1984; 18:226.
131. Conti S, Daschbach M: Venous thromboembolism prophylaxis: A survey of its use in the United States. Arch Surg 1982; 117:1036.
132. Scurr JH, Ibrahim SZ, Faber RG, et al.: The efficacy of graduated compression stocking in the prevention of deep vein thrombosis. Br J Surg 1977; 64:371.
133. Allenby F, Boardman L, Pflug JJ, et al.: Effects of external pneumatic intermittent compression on fibrinolysis in man. Lancet 1976; 2:1412.
134. Clarke-Pearson DL, Synan IS, Hinshaw W, et al.: Prevention of postoperative venous thromboembolism by external pneumatic calf compression in patients with gynecologic malignancy. Obstet Gynecol 1984; 63:92.
135. Salzman EW, Ploet J, Bettlemann M, et al.: Intraoperative external pneumatic calf compression to afford long-term prophylaxis against deep vein thrombosis in urological patients. Surgery 1980; 87:239.
136. Nicolaides AN, Fernandes e Fernandes J, Pollock AV: Intermittent sequential pneumatic compression of the legs in the prevention of venous stasis and postoperative deep venous thrombosis. Surgery 1980; 87:69.
137. Salzman EW, Davies GC: Prophylaxis of venous thromboembolism: Analysis of cost effectiveness. Ann Surg 1980; 191:207.
138. Haegger K: Problems of acute deep vein thrombosis. Angiology 1969; 20:219.
139. Palko PA, Namson EM, Fedonik SO: The early detection of deep venous thrombosis using ^{131}I-tagged fibrinogen. Can J Surg 1964; 7:215.
140. Athanasoulis CA: Phlebography for the diagnosis of deep leg vein thrombosis, prophylactic therapy of deep venous thrombosis and pulmonary embolism. DHEW Publication No. (NIH) 76–866, 1975.
141. Wheeler HB, O'Donnell JA, Anderson FA: Occlusive cuff impedance phlebography: A diagnostic procedure for venous thrombosis and pulmonary embolism. Prog Cardiovasc Dis 1974; 17:199.
142. Clarke-Pearson DL, Creasman WT: Diagnosis of deep vein thrombosis in obstetrics and gynecology by impedance phlebography. Obstet Gynecol 1981; 58:52.
143. Yao JST, Gourmos C, Hobbs JT: Detection of proximal vein thrombosis by Doppler ultrasound flow-detection method. Lancet 1972; 1:1.
144. Anthonie WA, Lensing MD, Paolo P, et al.: Detection of deep-vein thrombosis by real-time B-mode ultrasonography. N Engl J Med 1989; 320:342.
145. Mintz MC, Levy DW, Axel L, et al.: Puerperal ovarian vein thrombosis: MR diagnosis. AJR 1987; 149:1273.
146. Clarke-Pearson DL, Synan IS, Creasman WT: Anticoagulation therapy for venous thromboembolism in patients with gynecologic malignancy. Am J Obstet Gynecol 147:369, 1983.
147. Moser KM, Fedullo PR: Venous thromboembolism: Three simple decisions. Chest 1983; 83:256.
148. Hull RD, Raskob GE, Rosenbloom D, et al.: Heparin for 5 days as compared with 10 days in the initial treatment of proximal venous thrombosis. N Engl J Med 1990; 322:1260.
149. Bell WR, Royal RM: Heparin induced thrombocytopenia: A comparison of three heparin regimens. N Engl J Med 1980; 303:902.
150. Unger RH, Foster DW: Diabetes mellitus. In Wilson JD, Foster DW (eds.): Williams Textbook of Endocrinology, 8th ed. Philadelphia, WB Saunders Co., 1992, pp. 1255–1333.
151. Droegemueller W, et al.: Preoperative management. In Droegemueller W, et al. (eds.): Comprehensive Gynecology. St. Louis, CV Mosby, 1987, p. 643.
152. Page MM, Watkins PJ: Cardiorespiratory arrest and diabetic autonomic neuropathy. Lancet 1978; 1(Part 1):14.
153. Wheat LJ: Infection and diabetes mellitus. Diabetes Care 1980; 3:187.
154. Abbott TR: Anesthesia in untreated myxedema: Report of 2 cases. Br J Anaesth 1967; 39:510.
155. Rayfield EJ, et al.: Infection and diabetes: The case for glucose control. Am J Med 1982; 72:439.
156. McMurry JF Jr: Wound healing with diabetes mellitus. Surg Clin North Am 1985; 64:35.
157. Weringer EJ, et al.: Effects of insulin on wound healing in diabetic mice. Acta Endocrinol 1982; 99:101.
158. Cruse PJE, et al.: A five-year prospective study of 23,649 surgical wounds. Arch Surg 1973; 107:206.
159. Nesto RW, et al.: Angina and exertional myocardial ischemia in diabetic and non-diabetic patients: Assessment by exercise thallium scintigraphy. Ann Intern Med 1988; 108:170.
160. Goldberg NJ, et al.: Insulin therapy in the diabetic surgical patient: Metabolic and hormone response to low dose insulin infusion. Diabetes Care 1981; 4:279.
161. Walts LF, et al.: Perioperative management of diabetes mellitus. Anesthesiology 1981; 55:104.
162. Meyers EF, et al.: Perioperative control of blood glucose in diabetic patients: A two-step protocol. Diabetes Care 1986; 9:40.
163. Sieber FE, et al.: Glucose: A reevaluation of its intraoperative use. Anesthesiology 1987; 67:72.
164. Mustard JF, Bierman EL: Arteriosclerosis: Progress and evolution. Arteriosclerosis 1984; 4(1):1.

165. Halushka PV, Mayfield R, Wohltmann HJ: Increased platelet arachidonic acid metabolism in diabetes mellitus. Diabetes 1981; 30(Suppl. 2):44.
166. Davi G, Catalano I, Averna M: Thromboxane biosynthesis and platelet function in type II diabetes mellitus. N Engl J Med 1990; 322:1769.
167. Goldman DR: Surgery in patients with endocrine dysfunction: Preoperative consultation. Med Clin North Am 1987; 71:499.
168. Roizen MF: Endocrine abnormalities and anesthesia: Implications for the anesthesiologist. Refresher Course in Anesthesiology 1984; 13:161.
169. Ingbar SH: Thyrotoxic storm. N Engl J Med 1966; 274:1242.
170. Waldstein SS, et al.: A clinical study of thyroid storm. Ann Intern Med 1960; 52:626.
171. Stehling LC: Anesthetic management of the patient with hyperthyroidism. Anesthesiology 1974; 41:585.
172. Nevins MA, et al.: Pitfalls in interpreting serum creatine phosphokinase activity. JAMA 1973; 224:1382.
173. Murkin JM: Anesthesia and hypothyroidism: A review of thyroxine physiology, pharmacology, and anesthetic implications. Anesth Analg 1982; 61:371.
174. Anderson A, Hausmann W: Triiodothyronine in myxedema coma (letter). Lancet 1956; 2:999.
175. Siddiq YK, Gebhart SS: Disorder of the thyroid gland. In Lubin MF (ed.): Medical Management of the Surgical Patient, 2nd ed. Stoneham, MA, Butterworth, 1988, p. 297.
176. Ladenson PW: Complications of surgery in hypothyroid patients. Am J Med 1984; 77:261.
177. See ref. 176.
178. See ref. 178.
179. Kehlet H, Binder C: Value of an ACTH test in assessing hypothalamic-pituitary-adrenocortical function in glucocorticoid-treated patients. Br Med J 1973; 2:147.
180. Baxter JD, Tyrell JB: The adrenal cortex. In Felig P (ed.): Endocrinology and Metabolism. New York, McGraw-Hill, 1981, p. 462.
181. Becker RC, Underwood DA: Myocardial infarction in patients undergoing noncardiac surgery. Cleve Clin J Med 1987; 54:25.
182. Goldman L, et al.: Cardiac risk factors and complications in non-cardiac surgery. Medicine 1978; 57:357.
183. Steen PA, Tinker JH, Tarhan S: Myocardial reinfarction after anesthesia and surgery. JAMA 1978; 239:2566.
184. Von Knorring J: Postoperative myocardial infarction: A prospective study in a risk group of surgical patients. Surgery 1981; 90:55.
185. Rao TLK, Jacobs KH, El-Etr AN: Reinfarction following anesthesia in patients with myocardial infarction. Anesthesiology 1983; 59:499.
186. Tarhan S, Moffitt EA, Taylor WF, Giuliani ER: Myocardial infarction after general anesthesia. JAMA 1972; 220:1451.
187. Goldman L, et al.: Multifactorial index of cardiac risk in noncardiac surgical procedures. N Engl J Med 1977; 297:845.
188. Zeldin RA: Assessing cardiac risk in patients who undergo noncardiac surgical procedures. Can J Surg 1984; 27:402.
189. Detsky AS, et al.: Predicting cardiac complications in patients undergoing non-cardiac surgery. J Gen Intern Med 1986; 1:211.
190. Foster ED, et al.: Risk of noncardiac operation in patients with defined coronary disease: The Coronary Artery Surgery Study (CASS) registry experience. Ann Thoracic Surg 1986; 41:42.
191. Carliner NH, Fisher ML, Plotnich GD, et al.: Routine preoperative exercise testing in patients undergoing major noncardiac surgery. Am J Cardiol 1985; 56:51.
192. Cutler BS, Wheeler HB, Paraskos JA, Cardullo PA: Applicability and interpretation of electrocardiographic stress testing in patients with peripheral vascular disease. Am J Surg 1981; 141:501.
193. Boucher CA, et al.: Determination of cardiac risk by dipyridamole-thallium imaging before peripheral vascular surgery. N Engl J Med 1985; 312:389.
194. Eagle KA, et al.: Dipyridamole-thallium scanning in patients undergoing vascular surgery: Optimizing preoperative evaluation of cardiac risk. JAMA 1987; 257:2185.
195. Leppo J, et al.: Noninvasive evaluation of cardiac risk before elective vascular surgery. J Am Coll Cardiol 1987; 9:269.
196. Pasternack PF, et al.: The value of the radionuclide angiogram in the prediction of postoperative myocardial infarction in patients undergoing lower extremity revascularization procedures. Circulation 1985; 72(Suppl. II):13.
197. Kaplan J: Hemodynamic monitoring. In Kaplan J (ed.): Cardiac Anesthesia. New York, Grune & Stratton, 1987, pp. 179–226.
198. Goldman L: Cardiac risks and complications of non-cardiac surgery. Ann Intern Med 1983, 98:504.
199. Driscoll AC, Hobika JH, Etsten BE, Proger S: Clinically unrecognized myocardial infarction following surgery. N Engl J Med 1961; 264:633.
200. Pasternack PR, et al.: The hemodynamics of beta blockade in patients undergoing abdominal aortic aneurysm repair. Circulation 1987; 76(Suppl. III):1.
201. Poquized SM, Sharma AD, Corr PB: Influence of labetalol, a combined alpha and beta adrenengic blocking agent, on the dysrhythmias induced by coronary occlusion and reperfusion. Cardiovasc Res 1982; 16:398.
202. McGregor M: The nitrates and myocardial ischemia. Circulation 1982; 66:689.
203. Coriat P, et al.: Prevention of intraoperative myocardial ischemia during noncardiac surgery with intravenous nitroglycerin. Anesthesiology 1984; 61:193.
204. Gallagher J, et al.: Prophylactic nitroglycerin infusions during coronary artery bypass surgery. Anesthesiology 1986; 64:785.
205. Thomson I, Mutch W, Culligan J: Failure of intravenous nitroglycerin to prevent intraoperative myocardial ischemia during fentanyl-pancuronium anesthesia. Anesthesiology 1984; 61:385.
206. Lacche A, Basaglia P: Hypertensive emergencies: Effects of therapy by nifedipine administered sublingually. Curr Ther Res 1983; 34:879.
207. Pedersen O, Christensen N, Ramsch K: Comparison of acute effects of nifedipine in normotensive and hypertensive man. J Cardiovasc Pharmacol 1980; 2:357.
208. O'Mailia J, Saunder G, Giles T: Nifedipine associated myocardial ischemia or infarction in the treatment of hypertensive urgencies. Ann Intern Med 1987; 107:185.
209. Howat DDC: Cardiac disease, anesthesia and operation for noncardiac conditions. Br J Anaesth 1971; 43:288.
210. Cooperman LH, Price HL: Pulmonary edema in the operative and postoperative period: A review of 40 cases. Ann Surg 1970; 172:883.
211. Kuner J, et al.: Cardiac arrhythmias during anesthesia. Dis Chest 1967; 52:580.
212. Vanik PE, Davis HS: Cardiac arrhythmias during halothane anesthesia. Anesth Analg 1968; 47:299.
213. Bertrand CA, et al.: Disturbances of cardiac rhythm during anesthesia and surgery. JAMA 1971; 216:1615.
214. Vandam LK, McLemore GA Jr: Circulatory arrest in patients with complete heart block during anesthesia and surgery. Am J Med 1957; 47:518.
215. Frye RL, et al.: Guidelines for permanent cardiac pacemaker implantation, May 1984: A report of the joint American College of Cardiology/American Heart Association task force on assessment of cardiovascular procedures (subcommittee on pacemaker implantation). Circulation 1984; 70:331A.
216. Lerner SM: Suppression of a demand pacemaker by transurethral electrocautery. Anesth Analg 1973; 52:703.
217. Rooney SM, Goldner PL, Muss E: Relationship of right bundle branch block and marked left axis deviation to complete heart block during general anesthesia. Anesthesiology 1976; 44:64.
218. Bellocci F, Santarelli P, DiGennaro M, et al.: The risk of cardiac complications in surgical patients with bivasicular block. A clinical and electrophysiologic study in 98 patients. Chest 1980; 77:343.
219. Berg GR, Kofler MN: The significance of bilateral bundle branch block in the preoperative patient. A retrospective electrocardiographic and clinical study in 30 patients. Chest 1971; 59:62.
220. Skinner JF, Pearce ML: Surgical risk in the cardiac patient. J Chron Dis 1964; 17:57.

221. Maille JG, et al.: Patients with cardiac valve prostheses: Subsequent anesthetic management for noncardiac surgical procedures. Can Anaesth Soc J 1973; 20:207.
222. Katholi RE, Nolan SP, McGuire LB: The management of anticoagulation during noncardiac operations in patients with prosthetic heart valves: A prospective study. Am Heart J 1978; 96:163.
223. Tinker JH, Tarhan S: Discontinuing anticoagulant therapy in surgical patients with cardiac valve prostheses: Observations in 180 operations. JAMA 1978; 239:738.
224. Ryhanen P, Saarela E, Hollmen A, et al.: Blood pressure changes during and after anesthesia in treated and untreated hypertensive patients. Ann Chir Gynaecol 1978; 67:180.
225. Strandgaard S, Olesen J, Skinhoj E, Lassen NA: Autoregulation of brain circulation in severe arterial hypertension. Br Med J 1973; 1:507.
226. Samaan HA: Risk of operation in a patient with unsuspected pheochromocytoma. Br J Surg 1970; 57:462.
227. Swan HJC, Ganz W, Forrester J, et al.: Catheterization of the heart in man with the use of a flow-directed balloon-tipped catheter. N Engl J Med 1970; 283:447.
228. Linman JW: Physiologic and pathophysiologic effects of anemia. N Engl J Med 1968; 279:812.
229. Lundsgaard-Hansen P: Blood transfusion and capillary function. In Ikkala E, Nyhanen A (eds.): Transfusion and Immunology. Helsinki, International Society of Blood Transfusions, 1975.
230. National Institutes of Health: Summary of NIH consensus development conference on perioperative red cell transfusion. Am J Hematol 1989; 31:144.
231. Goodnough LT: Autologous blood donation. JAMA 1988; 260:65.
232. Goodnough LT, et al.: Increased preoperative collection of autologous blood with recombinant human erythropoietin therapy. N Engl J Med 1989; 321:1163.
233. Kelton JG, et al.: Drug-induced thrombocytopenia is associated with increased binding of IgG to platelets both in vivo and in vitro. Blood 1981; 58:524.
234. Brown CH, et al.: Defective platelet function following the administration of penicillin compounds. Blood 1976; 47:949.
235. Marengo-Rowe AJ, Leveson JE: Evaluation of the bleeding patient. Postgrad Med 1977; 62:171.
236. Olt GJ, et al.: Preoperative assessment of fragment D-dimer as a predictor of postoperative venous thrombosis. Am J Obstet Gynecol 1990; 162:772.
237. Bodey GP, et al.: Quantitative relationships between circulating leukocytes and infection in patients with acute leukemia. Ann Intern Med 1966; 64:328.
238. Stehling L: Preoperative blood ordering. Int Anesth Clin 1982; 20:45.
239. Miller R, et al.: Coagulation defects associated with massive blood transfusions. Ann Surg 1971; 174:794.
240. Reed RL, et al.: Prophylactic platelet administration during massive transfusion. Ann Surg 1986; 203:40.
241. Harke H, Rahman S: Hemostatic disorders in massive transfusion. Bibl Haemat 1980; 46:179.
242. Kahn R, et al.: Massive blood replacement: Correlation of ionized calcium, citrate, and hydrogen ion concentration. Anesth Analg 1979; 58:275.
243. Stein M, Koota GM, Simon M, Frank HA: Pulmonary evaluation of surgical patients. JAMA 1962; 181:765.
244. Mohr DN, Jett JR: Clinical reviews. Preoperative evaluation of pulmonary risk factors. J Gen Intern Med 1988; 3:277.
245. Hensley MJ, Fencl V: Lungs and respiration. In Vandam LD (ed.): To Make the Patient Ready for Anesthesia: Medical Care of the Surgical Patient. Menlo Park, CA, Addison-Wesley, 1984, pp. 18–41.
246. Hotchkiss RS: Perioperative management of patient with chronic obstructive pulmonary disease. Int Anesth Clin 1988; 26:134.
247. Forthman HJ, Shepard A: Postoperative pulmonary complications. South Med J 1969; 62:1198.
248. Lawrence VA, Page CP, Harris GD: Preoperative spirometry before abdominal operations. A critical appraisal of its predictive value. Arch Intern Med 1989; 149:280.
249. Zibrak JD, O'Donnell CR, Marton K: Indications for pulmonary function testing. Ann Intern Med 1990; 112:763.
250. Blosser SA, Rock P: Asthma and chronic obstructive lung disease. In Breslow MJ, Miller CJ, Rogers MC (eds.): Perioperative Management. St. Louis, CV Mosby, 1990, pp. 259–280.
251. Sagel SS, Evens RG, Forrest JV, Branson RT: Efficacy of routine screening and lateral chest radiographs in a hospital based population. N Engl J Med 1974; 291:1001.
252. Galant SP: Treatment of asthma. New and time-tested strategies. Postgrad Med 1990; 87:229.
253. Barnes PJ: A new approach to the treatment of asthma. New Engl J Med 1989; 321:1517.
254. Hargreave FE, Dolovich J, Newhouse MT: The assessment and treatment of asthma: A conference report. J Allergy Clin Immunol 1990; 85:1098.
255. Flenley DC: Chronic obstructive pulmonary disease. Dis Mon 1988; 34:543.
256. Schwaber JR: Evaluation of respiratory status in surgical patients. Surg Clin North Am 1970; 50:637.
257. Milledge JS, Nunn JF: Criteria of fitness for anaesthesia in patients with chronic obstructive lung disease. Br Med J 1975; 3:670.
258. Tarhan S, Moffitt EA, Sessler AD, et al.: Risk of anesthesia and surgery in patients with chronic bronchitis and chronic obstructive pulmonary disease. Surgery 1973; 74:720.
259. Gracey DR, Divertie MB, Didier EP: Preoperative pulmonary preparation of patients with chronic obstructive pulmonary disease. Chest 1979; 76:123.
260. Stein M, Cassara EL: Preoperative pulmonary evaluation and therapy for surgery patients. JAMA 1970; 211:787.
261. Thoren L: Post-operative pulmonary complications. Observations on their prevention by means of physiotherapy. Acta Chir Scand 1953; 107:193.
262. Castillo R, Haas A: Chest physical therapy: Comparative efficacy of preoperative and postoperative in the elderly. Arch Phys Med Rehabil 1985; 66:376.
263. Anderson ME, Belani KG: Short-term preoperative smoking abstinence. AFP 1990; 41:1191.
264. Warner MA, Offord KP, Warner ME, et al.: Role of preoperative cessation of smoking and other factors in postoperative pulmonary complications: A blinded prospective study of coronary artery bypass patients. Mayo Clin Proc 1989; 64:609.
265. Easton PA, Jadue C, Dhingra S, Anthonisen NR: A comparison of the bronchodilating effects of a beta-2 adrenergic agent (albuterol) and an anticholinergic agent (ipratropium bromide), given by aerosol alone or in sequence. New Engl J Med 1986; 315:735.
266. Hensley MJ, Fencl V: Lungs and respiration. In Vandam LD (ed.): To Make the Patient Ready for Anesthesia: Medical Care of the Surgical Patient. Menlo Park, CA, Addison-Wesley, 1984, pp. 18–41.
267. Wellman JJ, Smith BA: Respiratory complications of surgery. In Lubin MF (ed.): Medical Management of the Surgical Patient. Boston, Butterworth, 1988, pp. 9–10.
268. Pinson CW, et al.: Surgery in long-term dialysis patients: Experience with more than 300 cases. Am J Surg 1986; 151:567.
269. Broyer M, et al.: Demography of dialysis and transplantation in Europe, 1984. Nephrol Dial Transplant 1986; 1:1.
270. Lundin AP, et al.: Fatigue, acid-base and electrolyte changes in exhaustive treadmill exercise in hemodialysis patients. Nephron 1987; 46:57.
271. Eschbach JW, et al.: Correction of the anemia of end-stage renal disease with recombinant erythropoietin: Results of a combined phase I and II clinical trial. N Engl J Med 1987; 316:73.
272. Mannucci PM, et al.: Desamino-8-D-arginine vasopressin shortens bleeding time in uremia. N Engl J Med 1983; 308:8.
273. Livio M, et al.: Conjugated estrogens for the management of bleeding associated with renal failure. N Engl J Med 1986; 315:731.
274. Driks MR, et al.: Nosocomial pneumonia in intubated patients given sucralfate as compared with antacids or hista-

mine type 2 blockers: The role of gastric colonization. N Engl J Med 1987; 317:1376.
275. Lewis SL, Van Epps DE: Neutrophil and monocyte alterations in chronic dialysis patients. Am J Kidney Dis 1987; 9:381.
276. Mullen JL, et al.: Reduction of operative morbidity and mortality by combined preoperative and postoperative nutritional support. Ann Surg 1980; 192:604.
277. Blumberg A, et al.: Effect of various therapeutic approaches on plasma potassium and major regulating factors in terminal renal failure. Am J Med 1988; 85:507.
278. Lillemoe KD, et al.: Intestinal necrosis due to sodium polystyrene (Kayexalate) in sorbitol enemas: Clinical and experimental support for the hypothesis. Surgery 1987; 101:267.
279. Bullock ML, et al.: The assessment of risk factors in 462 patients with acute renal failure. Am J Kidney Dis 1985; 5:97.
280. Hou SH, et al.: Hospital-acquired renal insufficiency: A prospective study. Am J Med 1983; 74:243.
281. Wilkes M, Mailloux LU: Acute renal failure: Pathogenesis and prevention. Am J Med 1986; 80:1129.
282. Meyer RD: Risk factors and comparison of clinical nephrotoxicity of aminoglycosides. Am J Med 1986; 80 (S6B):119.
283. Shusterman N, et al.: Risk factors and outcome of hospital-acquired acute renal failure: Clinical epidemiologic study. Am J Med 1987; 83:65.
284. Barry KG, Mazze RI, Schwartz FD: Prevention of surgical oliguria and renal-hemodynamic suppression by sustained hydration. N Engl J Med 1964; 270:1371.
285. Bush HL, et al.: Prevention of renal insufficiency after abdominal aortic aneurysm resection by optimal volume loading. Arch Surg 1981; 116:1517.
286. Friedman LS, Maddrey WC: Surgery in the patient with liver disease. Med Clin North Am 1987; 71(3):453.
287. Roberts HR, Cederbaum AI: The liver and blood coagulation: Physiology and pathology. Gastroenterology 1972; 63:297.
288. Maze M: Hepatic physiology. In Miller RD (ed.): Anesthesia 2nd ed., Vol. 1. New York, Churchill Livingstone, 1986, p. 585.
289. Isaacs JH, Byrne MP: Pelvic Surgery: A Multidisciplinary Approach. Mount Kisco, NY, Futura, 1987, p. 14.
290. Harvill DD, Summerskill WH: Surgery in acute hepatitis: Causes and effects. JAMA 1963; 184:257.
291. Child CG, Turcotte JG: Surgery and portal hypertension. In Child CG (ed.): The Liver and Portal Hypertension, 3rd ed. Philadelphia, WB Saunders Co., 1964, p. 50.
292. Bloch RS, Allaben RD, Walt AJ: Cholecystectomy in patients with cirrhosis: A surgical challenge. Arch Surg 1985; 120:669.
293. Garrison RN, et al.: Clarification of risk factors for abdominal operations in patients with hepatic cirrhosis. Ann Surg 1984; 199:648.
294. Czaja AJ, Summerskill WH: Chronic hepatitis. To treat or not to treat? Med Clin North Am 1978; 62:71.
295. Perrillo RP, et al.: A randomized controlled trial of interferon alpha-IIB alone and after prednisone withdrawal for the treatment of chronic hepatitis B. N Engl J Med 1990; 323:295.
296. Hernandez JM: Post-transfusion hepatitis in Spain: A prospective study. Vox Sang 1983; 44:231.
297. McPeek B, Gilbert JP: Onset of postoperative jaundice related to anesthetic history. Br Med J 1974; 3:615.
298. Tzakis AG: Clinical considerations in orthopedic liver transplantation. Radiol Clin North Am 1987; 25:289.
299. Gimson AE, Westaby D, Hegarty J: A randomized trial of vasopressin and vasopressin plus nitroglycerin in the control of acute variceal hemorrhage. Hepatology 1986; 6:410.
300. Panes J, Teres J, Bosch J, et al.: Efficacy of balloon tamponade in the treatment of bleeding gastric and esophageal varices. Dig Dis Sci 1988; 33:454.
301. Barsoum MS, Bolous FI, El-Roohy AA, et al.: Tamponade and injection sclerotherapy in the management of bleeding oesophageal varices. Br J Surg 1982; 69:76.
302. Paquet KJ, Feussner H: Euroscopic sclerosis and esophageal balloon tamponade in acute hemorrhage from esophageal varices: A prospective controlled randomized trial. Hepatology 1985; 5:580.
303. Shubert T, Smith O, Kirkpatrick S, et al.: Improved survival in variceal hemorrhage with emergent sclerotherapy. Am J Gastroenterol 1987; 82:1134.
304. Burroughs AK, Hamilton G, Phillips A, et al.: Comparison of sclerotherapy with staple transection of the esophagus for emergency control of bleeding from esophageal varices. N Engl J Med 1989; 321:857.
305. Siefkin AD, Bolt RJ: Preoperative evaluation of the patient with gastrointestinal or liver disease. Med Clin North Am 1979; 63:1309.

Preoperative and Postoperative Management of Patients Undergoing Reproductive Reconstructive Surgery

4

David A. Grainger
Alan H. DeCherney

By definition, patients undergoing "reproductive reconstructive surgery" are doing so to promote fertility. The first and most important question to address when contemplating a reconstructive procedure is: Should we operate? Have alternatives to surgery been adequately explored? Have confounding variables in the pursuit of conception been evaluated? The obligation of reproductive surgeons to their patients is to answer these questions adequately prior to surgery. If pregnancy—the desired goal—is best achieved nonsurgically, it is disadvantageous to subject the patient to the risks and expense of reconstructive surgery. This mandates a thorough knowledge of disease processes affecting fertility and pregnancy rates achieved by different modalities of therapy—to be touched on briefly in this chapter and covered in greater detail in the ensuing chapters.

SHOULD WE OPERATE?

In a life-threatening surgical crisis, options for both the patient and the physician are limited, and the decision to operate is a life-preserving one. However, this is not so for most reproductive surgical procedures. Indeed, insurance companies and attorneys—in contrast to the patient and her husband—view these procedures as quite elective. What does this mean in practical terms for the pelvic reconstructive surgeon?

First, the procedure under consideration must offer the patient a reasonable chance of success when compared with other modalities of therapy, including medical therapy or in vitro fertilization. These alternatives of therapy must be discussed with the patient, and this discussion must be documented in the chart.

Second, the more elective a procedure is, the more detailed the informed consent should be regarding potential risks of the surgery.[1] This is not to imply that every reported complication from the surgery or anesthesia need be discussed; however, the patient should be aware of the more common complications that could occur. Fortunately, in reproductive surgery, even the common complications are rare. Although much of reproductive surgery is endoscopic and outpatient in nature, it should not be implied that these are "minor" procedures. The patient should consent to a laparotomy that may be needed to repair damage to bowel, bladder, blood vessels, and ureters.[2-4] Consents are preferably obtained with both the husband and wife present, so that all questions regarding the proposed surgery can be answered; this visit needs clear and complete documentation in the patient's chart.

SURGICAL ALTERNATIVES

In Vitro Fertilization

It may be in the best interest of the patient to select in vitro fertilization (IVF) as an alternative to reconstructive surgery. Each patient is different, and there are few "rules" governing the next step. However, a knowledge of the current literature regarding pregnancy rates for both IVF and the surgical procedure under consideration should guide the clinician in the right direction.

The use of IVF in the treatment of infertility is increasing rapidly. In 1988, 13,000 retrievals were performed in the United States alone; this number jumped to 25,000 in 1989. Unfortunately, there was not a commensurate increase in clinical pregnancy rates per embryo transfer (ET) (Fig. 4–1). Although there are IVF programs with pregnancy rates of 30–40% per ET, the overall rate remains below 20%.[5-7] Gamete intrafallopian transfer (GIFT) appears to offer increased pregnancy rates for patients in whom the fallopian tubes are open (Fig. 4–2). The most encouraging results have been demonstrated with tubal embryo (or zygote) transfer.[8-10] Fertilization occurs in vitro, and the embryo is then transferred to the fallopian tube. Increased pregnancy rates (34–50% per ET) are presumably due to the advantageous environment of the fallopian tube, and improved endometrial-embryonic synchrony. This technique has also been successful in the treatment of women with premature ovarian failure,[11] and the procedure has been performed transcervically.[12]

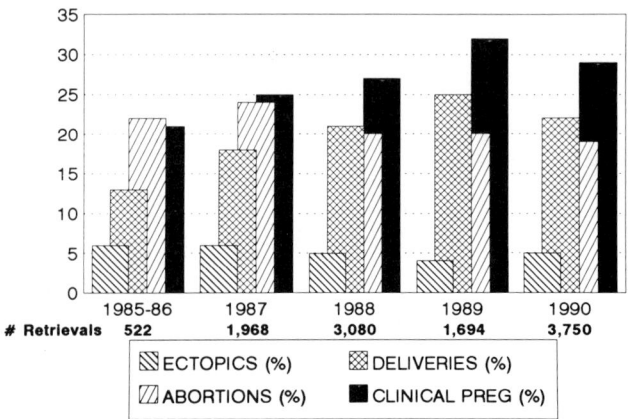

Figure 4–2
Gamete intrafallopian transfer (GIFT). (Data from IVF Registry.)

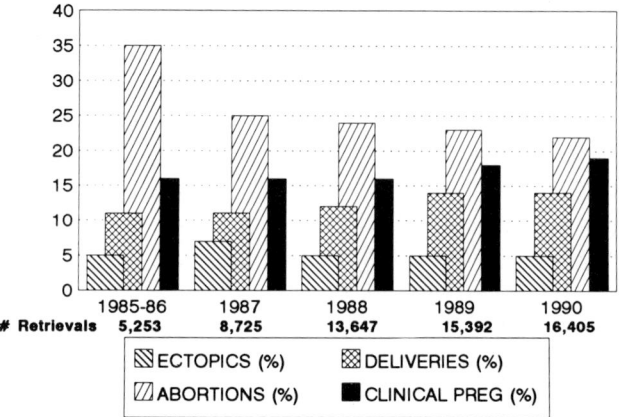

Figure 4–1
In vitro fertilization. (Data from IVF Registry.)

The preceding statistics regarding the success of IVF or other assisted reproductive techniques reflect the state of the art in 1990. The reader must compare contemporary results of these alternatives to surgery when deciding whether to perform a reconstructive surgical procedure.

Medical Treatment

Pelvic diseases that may be amenable to medical therapy include endometriosis, leiomyoma, and tubal pregnancy. (The medical therapy of ectopic pregnancies is discussed in Chapter 25.) Medical therapy for endometriosis and leiomyoma consists of danazol, progestins, or gonadotropin-releasing hormone (GnRH) analogues.[13-17] These treatments appear to exert their efficacy by antagonizing the tropic effects of estrogens. It is doubtful, for the following reasons, that medical therapy in and of itself will exclude surgical procedures.

First, endometriosis is generally diagnosed laparoscopically, and most, if not all, reproductive surgeons would treat the disease in that initial setting. Exceptions may include severe disease, in which laparoscopic resection of tissue is impossible. However, severe disease almost always involves extensive pelvic adhesions, for which medical therapy will exert a negligible effect. At the other end of the disease spectrum, one must bear in mind that there is no clear evidence that fertility is improved following laparoscopic treatment or medical therapy of minimal to mild endometriosis.[18]

Second, although most leiomyomas will shrink 50% or more during the first 3 months of treatment with GnRH analogues, nearly all will show immediate and rapid regrowth after the medication is discontinued.[15-17] This makes medical therapy adjunctive, rather than therapeutic, for this disorder.

Medical therapy may offer some advantages when used preoperatively. Benefits of preoperatively treating endometriosis patients with GnRH analogues may include a decrease in inflammation and vascularity, facilitating the surgical procedure.[19] There are also instances in which the preoperative treatment of patients with uterine fibroids may be useful. In patients with large submucous fibroids (>4–6 cm), hysteroscopic resection may be possible following therapy with GnRH analogues.[20] Also, patients not wishing to preserve fertility, and undergoing hysterectomy for large symptomatic leiomyomas, may be candidates for vaginal versus abdominal procedures following shrinkage with 3 months of GnRH analogues. There is some evidence that blood loss with abdominal myomectomy may be less following treatment with GnRH analogues; conversely, small fibroids may shrink and be undetected at the time of laparotomy. Certainly, the choice of surgical incisions and intraoperative exposure may be beneficially altered following 3 months of treatment. In addition, this treatment period usually induces amenorrhea and allows time for correcting anemia, if present, and/or banking autologous blood preoperatively.

In summary, most medical therapy will be adjunctive. There is no clear evidence that fertility rates are improved with preoperative or postoperative medical therapy for endometriosis.[18] Medical therapy may convert a procedure that could have only been accomplished at laparotomy to one that can be performed endoscopically, for either endometriosis or submucous myomas, thereby decreasing the morbidity of the procedure.

PREOPERATIVE COUNSELING

The infertile couple are vulnerable to the suggestions and recommendations of health care professionals. It is the responsibility of reproductive surgeons to provide accurate information regarding not only the current literature but also their individual/clinic pregnancy rates with surgery and IVF. Exploitation—providing substandard or unnecessary medical care—should not occur.[21]

Patients should be counseled preoperatively regarding not only the benefits (pregnancy rates) of the procedure but also the cost of the procedure. It should be clearly established what financial responsibility the patient will incur for the proposed treatment. These costs should be weighed against the cost/benefits of IVF.

In summary, the surgeon must honestly ask, "Is this operation really in the patient's best interest?" and proceed only when the answer is affirmative.[21]

PREOPERATIVE EVALUATION

The patient undergoing reproductive reconstructive surgery is generally healthy and a low surgical risk. Exceptions exist; these surgical risk factors must be elucidated from the history and physical examination. Of paramount importance is the exclusion of other significant fertility factors that may coexist with the patient's surgical problem. The following discussion outlines an infertility evaluation that should be completed prior to surgery, identify pertinent historical and physical findings, and address laboratory and radiologic examinations that may be useful preoperatively.

Evaluation of the Infertile Couple

In order for pregnancy to occur, viable sperm must gain access to the fallopian tubes and fertilize a recently released oocyte, forming a zygote, which must then traverse the tube and implant in a properly prepared endometrium. Therefore, the basic tenets of the infertility work-up are a semen analysis, postcoital test to evaluate cervical mucus-sperm interaction, hysterosalpingography to demonstrate tubal patency, basal body temperature charts to give evidence of ovulation, and an endometrial biopsy to demonstrate both ovulation and an adequate luteal phase. Each of these tests is to be briefly discussed.

Semen Analysis

The semen analysis is performed after 2 days of sexual abstinence, and the specimen is preferably collected by masturbation. Time to liquefaction is noted, as is the viscosity. The count is performed either manually, with a Makler chamber, or by a computer-assisted semen analysis. Sperm concentration is expressed as number (million)/ml; counts greater than 60 million/ml were initially thought to reflect fertility, until closer evaluation of fertile men was performed.[22] The current definition of "normal" includes a concentration of greater than 20 million/ml, with greater than 60% of the sperm being motile and greater than 60% showing normal morphology.[23] It must be realized that there is great individual day-to-day variability in semen analyses; multiple counts must be performed to document a persistent problem. Azoospermia is the only condition in which the male can definitely be presumed to be sterile. Significant male factor infertility may influence the decision to perform pelvic reproductive surgery. In these circumstances, a cycle of IVF may provide needed information regarding the fertilizing potential of the husband's sperm, and also offer a chance of pregnancy.

Postcoital Test

There is no clear consensus on what constitutes a normal postcoital test. The test should be performed around the time of ovulation, preferably using a urinary luteinizing hormone (LH) surge predictor kit. The mucus is assessed for clarity and elasticity, and is examined microscopically for the presence of spermatozoa. A normal postcoital test should have greater than 5 progressively motile sperm per high-power field; most will have greater than 20 motile sperm per high-power field.[24] If immotile sperm are identified or signs of infection are present, the couple should be treated with a broad-spectrum antibiotic and the test repeated the following cycle. Persistent abnormalities may indicate the presence of antisperm antibodies (ASA). Significant ASA should be identified prior to surgery, because the best treatment for certain classes of antibodies is IVF.

Hysterosalpingogram (HSG)

The HSG provides indirect visualization of the endometrial cavity, and ideally should predict the likelihood of tubal patency and peritubal adhesions identified at subsequent laparoscopy. Applying the criteria of convolution of the fallopian tube, loculation of contrast, a tube with a double contour, a vertical fallopian tube, and ampullary dilatation will correctly predict pelvic adhesions 75% of the time.[25] The HSG should be performed after menses has ceased and prior to ovulation. It is the authors' practice to screen these patients with a white blood count and an erythrocyte sedimentation rate (ESR) prior to the procedure; if either are elevated, the procedure is cancelled, the patient treated with a broad-spectrum antibiotic, and the procedure rescheduled for the next cycle. In patients at risk for infectious morbidity, or those in whom hydrosalpinx is identified, broad-spectrum antibiotic coverage is recommended.[26] The HSG provides useful preoperative information regarding the presence of intrauterine lesions and tubal obstruction, either proximal or distal. The surgical procedure may need to be tailored to evaluate these abnormalities; indeed, factors such as very large hydrosalpinges may influence either the decision to operate or the modality used (laparoscopy or laparotomy).[27]

Ovulation

A history of regular menses accompanied by moliminal symptoms is a fairly reliable indicator of ovulation.[28] Basal body temperature charting that demonstrates a luteal elevation, combined with positive urinary LH testing, adds to the evidence that ovulation is occurring.[29, 30] Secretory changes on the endometrial biopsy and luteal progesterone greater than 4 ng/ml are also indicative of ovulation and luteal function. If the patient is anovulatory, an evaluation regarding the etiology should be undertaken and should include a serum prolactin concentration and thyroid function studies. Restoration of ovulatory cycles with appropriate medical therapy should precede surgical intervention.

Endometrial Biopsy

The endometrial biopsy is routinely included in the evaluation of the infertile patient. The biopsy, obtained in the late luteal phase, is an attempt to quantify luteal function through the use of a bioassay—that is, the end-organ response to progesterone. However, several limitations should be noted. First, there is great variability in interpretation or dating of the biopsy between pathologists.[31, 32] Second, out-of-phase biopsies (defined as either 2 or 3 days out of phase, depending on the study) appear to be as common in fertile populations as in infertile ones.[33] This test is painful and expensive, and if out of phase, the recommendation is to repeat the biopsy in the next cycle. Although subtle changes in luteal function may be quite common, the endometrial biopsy is a relatively insensitive test. Other endometrial pathology such as polyps, hyperplasia, or fibroids may rarely be diagnosed on the routine endometrial biopsy.[34] Overall, in an ovulatory patient contemplating reconstructive reproductive surgery, the endometrial biopsy may be unnecessary.

History and Physical Examination

In the initial evaluation of the couple seeking help for infertility, it is important to establish rapport in addition to obtaining a complete medical and surgical history. Patients are often uncomfortable discussing intimate and personal issues. The understanding clinician will create an environment of trust and cooperation.

The man should be questioned regarding a history of undescended testicle; testicular injuries; or a history of any genital infections, including mumps orchitis. Any genital surgeries should be noted, including varicocele repair. A medical history of systemic diseases, including diabetes mellitus and other endocrine disorders, should be elicited. In addition, any medications that affect sexual functioning should be noted. He should be questioned regarding current sexual functioning; the ability to maintain an erection, and ejaculatory disturbances; such as retrograde or premature ejaculation. Although the World Health Organization (WHO) recommends physical examination of the male partner of the infertile couple, one study demonstrated that when the male partner does not have an abnormal semen analysis and there is no psychosexual or ejaculatory dysfunction, there is no independent relationship between male physical characteristics and fertility outcome.[35] If the male is examined, attention should be paid to hair distribution, stature, obesity, and stigmata of thyroid or adrenal disease. Examination of the genitalia should note the presence of varicoceles, prostatic tenderness, urethral discharge, testicular volume, and appropriate Tanner stage development.

The woman's history should begin with age, gravidity, and parity. Details of menarche and subsequent menstrual patterns including, molimina and dysmenorrhea, should be noted. Sexual functioning, including dyspareunia, frequency, and the use of artificial vaginal lubricants, should be recorded. Prior use of contraceptives, particularly intrauterine devices, or a history of any previous tubal infections are documented. Questions should address any changes in bowel or bladder functioning, including dysuria, dyschezia, or hematochezia. Changes in weight or level of stress that might affect hypothalamic-pituitary-ovarian function are ascertained. Any other medications or systemic illnesses are recorded. Importantly, all previous surgical procedures, including copies of the operative reports, should be reviewed and recorded. If the patient presents for reversal of sterilization, the records become extremely important. Success rates are dependent on the type of sterilization procedure the patient had, with reversal of Falope's ring or clips yielding the highest pregnancy rates.[36, 37]

The physical examination includes palpation of the thyroid; a breast examination for masses or galactorrhea; cardiovascular and pulmonary examinations; abdominal examination for masses or tenderness; and a pelvic examination, including a Papanicolaou smear if not current. The pelvic examination, including a rectal examination, should identify uterine or adnexal tenderness or fixation of the uterus. If any adnexal or uterine enlargement is noted, ultrasonography may be of benefit prior to surgery. Dermatologic manifestations of diseases such as Addison's or Cushing's disease or acanthosis nigracans should be noted and investigated prior to taking the patient to the operating room.

Preoperative Laboratory Evaluation

There are only two requisite laboratory tests for the young, healthy patient undergoing reconstructive reproductive surgery. First, the anesthesiologist will not anesthetize the patient without knowing the hematocrit. Second, when operating on female patients of reproductive age, a recent negative pregnancy test should be on the chart prior to surgery. Other laboratory testing should be dictated by the patient's medical condition and the proposed procedure. For example, in patients taking aspirin or nonsteroidal anti-inflammatory agents, or in patients with a history of blood clotting disorders, a bleeding time, prothrombin time, and partial thromboplastin time may be indicated. In patients taking diuretics, serum electrolyte values should be obtained. If excessive blood loss from the procedure is a concern (e.g., with a myomectomy), a type and screen may be advisable. However, these tests obtained routinely are probably not cost effective.[38]

Serum CA-125 levels, which are commonly elevated in patients with ovarian malignancies, are also elevated in patients with endometriosis.[39, 40] This marker may be useful in the patient with pelvic pain, although most of these patients will go to laparoscopy regardless of the CA-125 concentration. The marker may also be useful postoperatively to predict recurrence of endometriosis.

Preoperative Radiologic Evaluation

Chest Roentgenogram

Surgeons have been ingrained to "avoid surprises." This mentality may explain the overuse of preoperative radiologic studies, preponderantly the chest roentgenogram. There is no evidence that routine preoperative chest roentgenograms are appropriate for any group of patients. Patients who have cardiopulmonary disease, or those who are suspected of having such a disorder after the history and physical examination may benefit from a chest roentgenogram.[41] Even in high-risk groups of patients, routine chest roentgenograms to detect lung cancer have not been demonstrated to improve survival.[42] Therefore, routine chest roentgenograms should not be obtained in young, healthy women undergoing reproductive surgery, unless there is a suspicion of cardiopulmonary disease elicited from the history or physical examination.

Ultrasound

The evaluation of the pelvic mass using ultrasound may provide useful information preoperatively. Vaginal ultrasound can identify simple, unilocular ovarian cysts, which are almost always benign regardless of the size of the cyst or age of the patient. Endometriomas have a characteristic high intensity, homogeneous internal echo pattern (Fig. 4–3). Multicystic, complex masses are more likely to be neoplasms, either benign or malignant.

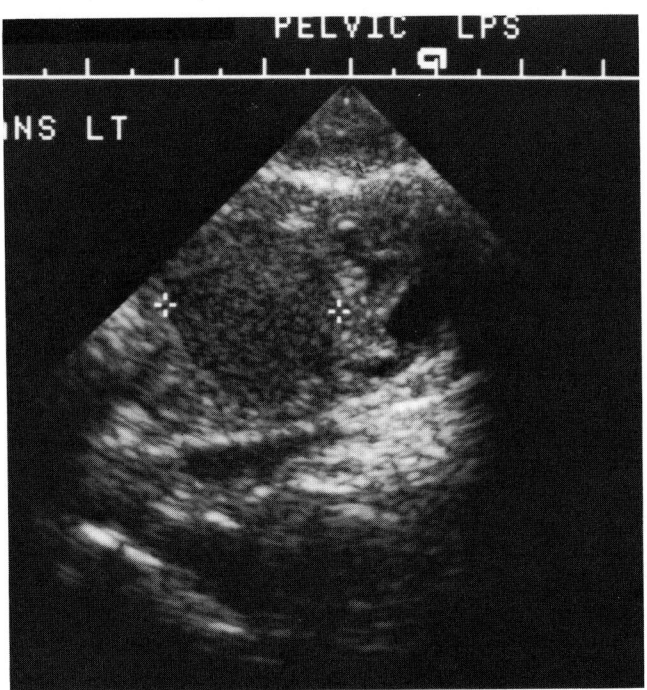

Figure 4–3
Vaginal ultrasonogram demonstrating characteristic pattern seen with ovarian endometriomas.

Hysterosalpingography

Hysterosalpingography is useful preoperatively in assessing the uterine cavity, as well as in documenting tubal patency or obstruction, as demonstrated in Figure 4–4. In patients with distal tubal obstruction, it is often difficult to judge the severity of tubal epithelial damage. Falloposcopy, a means of transcervical assessment of the tubal lumen, may prove to be useful in determining which patients with distal obstruction would be best served by IVF.[43]

Proximal tubal obstruction, as demonstrated in Figure 4–5, may be a result of tubal spasm or occlusion by a mucous plug. The HSG should be repeated, preferably using selective tubal catheterization, prior to cornual resection and anastomosis. Newer techniques utilizing transcervical canalization and balloon tuboplasty may obviate the need for an abdominal procedure.

If filling defects are noted on the HSG, hysteroscopy should be performed to identify polyps, synechiae, or submucous myomas. Uterine septae can also be visualized, as shown in Figure 4–6A, with a postoperative film shown in Figure 4–6B. The HSG appearance of a septum is also consistent with a bicornuate uterus; laparoscopy should be performed prior to transcervical resection.

HSGs have characteristically been performed prior to reversal of tubal ligation to estimate the length of the proximal tube. This practice does not influence the decision to perform the anastomosis, which is made at the time of laparoscopy using chromopertubation.[44] If there are questions regarding the endometrial cavity in these patients, hysteroscopy can be performed with the diagnostic laparoscopy.

Magnetic Resonance Imaging (MRI)

Many pelvic diseases can be imaged using MRI, including endometriosis and uterine fibroids. Endometriosis has a characteristic brightness on T1-weighted images. MRI may also be used preoperatively to determine structural relationships in the patient with congenital anomalies of the müllerian system.[45] These patients should also have a preoperative intravenous pyelogram, as 10–20% will have either congenital absence of a kidney or other malformations of the collecting system.

Electrocardiography

In the healthy young female, with a normal history and physical examination, there is no indication for

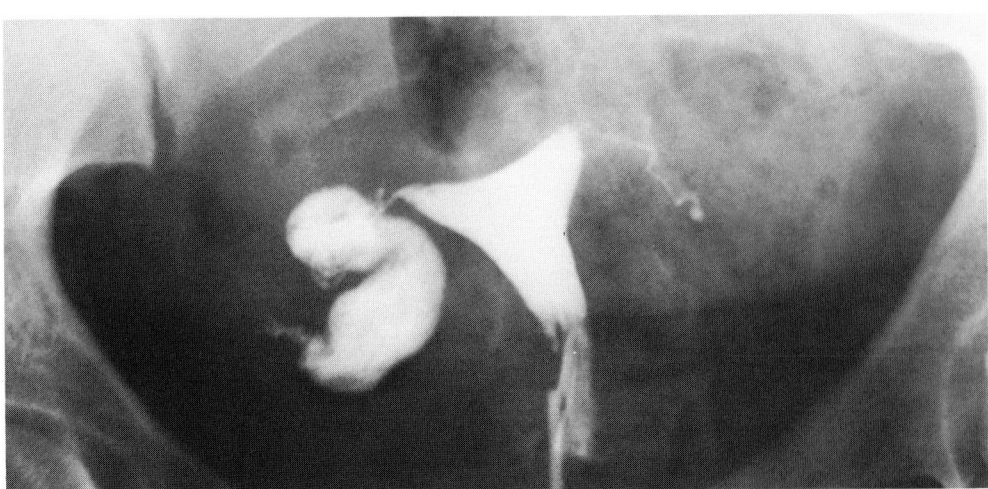

Figure 4–4
Hysterosalpingogram demonstrating a right hydrosalpinx.

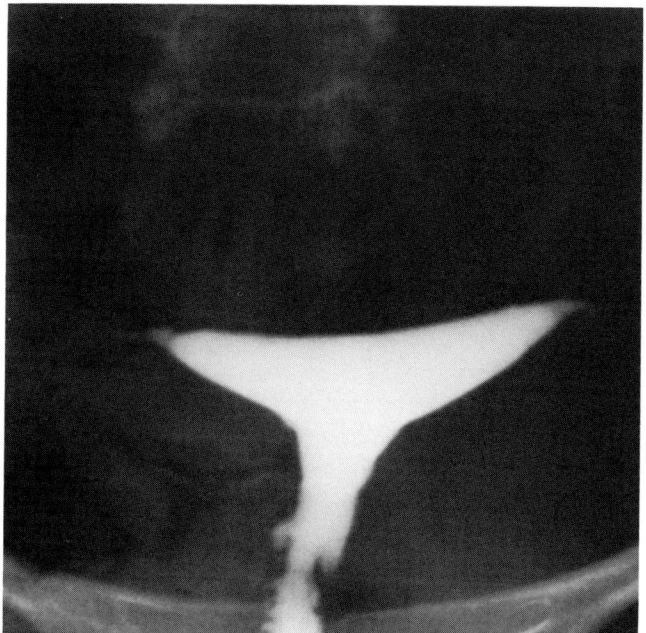

Figure 4–5
Hysterosalpingogram demonstrating bilateral proximal tubal obstruction.

Contraindications to Surgery

Absolute contraindications to surgery include an active pelvic infection and a medical illness that makes surgery a risk to life. In addition, if the intent of the surgery is to promote fertility, any medical condition that would be severely compromised as a result of pregnancy would constitute a contraindication to surgery. End-stage tubal disease, in which the chance of a successful outcome is very low, should also be considered a contraindication to surgery.

The age of the female deserves special mention. It is clear that fecundity decreases with increasing age, most notably after the age of forty.[47, 48] This decrease in fecundity appears to be related to aging eggs; donor oocytes have been utilized with great success in patients over the age of forty. It should be considered a relative contraindication to perform extensive reconstructive surgery on patients over the age of forty.

Summary: Preoperative Evaluation

Prior to reconstructive reproductive surgery, other factors affecting fertility need to be examined and corrected if abnormal. A careful history and physical examination will guide the clinician in preoperative laboratory and radiologic testing. The work-up must be thorough and complete but should also be cost effective. Most importantly, it must be in the patient's best interest to perform the procedure; all alternatives

a routine ECG. Patients with a mid-systolic click, particularly when accompanied by a holosystolic murmur, should be evaluated for mitral valve prolapse prior to surgery. Patients with mitral valve prolapse, and particularly those with mitral regurgitation, should receive antibiotic prophylaxis prior to surgery.[46]

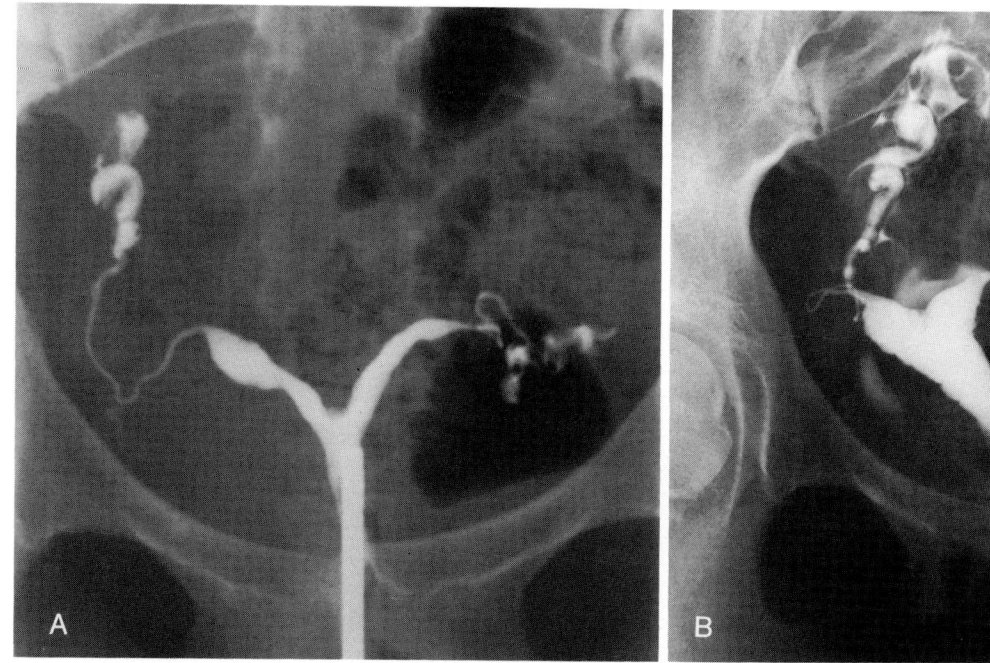

Figure 4–6
Hysterosalpingogram showing uterine septum, preoperatively (A) and 3 months after hysteroscopic resection (B).

should have been explored and discussed with the patient and her husband.

POSTOPERATIVE CARE

The first responsibility of the surgeon is to inform the patient and/or her husband of the operative findings, the procedure that was performed, and a realistic prognosis for pregnancy. It is often helpful to see the patient back in the office within 2–4 weeks after surgery to explain the findings and, most importantly, to generate a plan for the ensuing months. The plan will vary, depending on the disease process, but might include observation for a specified length of time, ovulation induction with or without inseminations, or medical suppression of residual endometriosis.

Immediate Care

Most of reproductive surgery is accomplished endoscopically, including extensive lysis of adhesions, tuboplasties, excision of endometriosis, and adnexectomy.[49,50] These patients are generally dismissed 4–6 hours postoperatively. The operative morbidity is less from a laparoscopic procedure than from a similar procedure performed at laparotomy. However, the recuperation time from operative laparoscopy is greater than that from diagnostic laparoscopy and appears to be related to the extent of intraabdominal surgery performed.[51]

Complications can occur from these procedures. The patient who presents with abdominal pain, fever, peritonitis, and leukocytosis must be evaluated for a hollow viscus injury. In addition, ureteral injury occurring at the time of laparoscopy can present with a similar picture. An intravenous pyelogram should be performed, such that if ureteral injury has occurred, early intervention with stents can be accomplished.[4]

Hysteroscopic procedures utilize distention media in order to visualize the uterine cavity. The use of these solutions can present some unique postoperative complications, particularly when the procedure is operative as opposed to diagnostic in nature. Large volumes of 5% dextrose in water, when intravasated, can induce hyponatremia and hyperglycemia.[52] Crystalloids, when intravasated, can cause respiratory compromise secondary to pulmonary edema. These patients should be carefully observed in the recovery room. One other distention medium 32% dextran-70, has been rarely associated with an anaphylactic reaction and disseminated intravascular coagulation.[53] Large volumes of dextran-70 can also induce fluid overload; central monitoring is generally recommended when greater than 500 ml of this distention medium is used.

Surgery Through First Month

Activity

With extensive laparoscopic procedures, most patients will be dismissed on the same day as the surgery and will be fully recovered within 7–9 days. When a laparotomy is performed, diet is advanced as tolerated, and the patients are released on the second or third postoperative day. Early ambulation to reduce the risk of deep venous thrombosis is encouraged. Four weeks generally provides time for adequate wound healing to occur; patients are then allowed to return to normal activity.

Hydrotubation

There are no well-controlled studies demonstrating any efficacy of postoperative hydrotubation, and studies advocating this procedure are flawed.[54] In a prospective, randomized, controlled study, there was no demonstrable efficacy of hydrotubation.[55] Given the potential infectious risks of the procedure and the lack of benefit, hydrotubation should have no place in the postoperative management of patients undergoing tubal surgery.

Adhesions: Second-Look Laparoscopy

The formation and pathogenesis of adhesions are discussed in detail in Chapter 8; however, a word seems appropriate when considering postoperative care. Postoperative adhesions form nearly 100% of the time, regardless of whether the procedure is performed laparoscopically or at laparotomy.[56] It is attractive to speculate that early second-look laparoscopy would improve the success of the initial procedure. However, although adhesion reformation and de novo adhesion formation are present and are easily lysed at early second-look laparoscopy, no study to date has clearly demonstrated a significant improvement in pregnancy rates.[57] Until studies demonstrate improved pregnancy rates, it would appear that the best course of action is a meticulous first surgery, with possibly a repeat laparoscopy in 12–18 months if conception has not occurred. Newer adjuvants that have been demonstrated to reduce postoperative adhesion reformation include INTERCEED (Johnson and Johnson Patient Care, New Brunswick, NJ), a barrier that can be applied either at laparoscopy or laparotomy.[58] Despite these advances, adhesion reformation remains the bane of the reproductive surgeon. Many adhesion prevention regimens are widely practiced, including postoperative steroids and antibiotics. However, none of these have been demonstrated to be effective in reducing adhesion formation.

Delayed Care

A typical patient goes to the operating room because she believes that she will conceive following the procedure. This may or may not occur. It is the surgeon's responsibility to understand the disease process, to represent the chances of conception fairly to the patient and her husband, and to know when to intervene with alternative therapies. Disease processes that will be described in detail in the following chapters are characterized by cumulative pregnancy rates, or pregnancy rates as analyzed by life table analysis. In general, with reconstructive reproductive surgery, most patients who are going to conceive as a result of the surgery do so by 12–18 months postoperatively. At this juncture, regardless of the etiology of the infertility, in vitro fertilization becomes a viable option. It is important to realize that many options may theoretically exist, but for the patient, they may not be practical. The authors provide their patients with accurate information, and they decide when enough is enough.

References

1. Shane JA: Putting res ipsa loquitor and informed consent in perspective. In Roberts DK, Shane JA, Roberts ML (eds.): Confronting the Malpractice Crisis: Guidelines for the Obstetrician-Gynecologist. Kansas City, KS, Eagle Press, 1985, p. 97.
2. Schwimmer WB: Electrosurgical burn injuries during laparoscopy sterilization: Treatment and prevention. Obstet Gynecol 1974; 44:526.
3. Soderstrom RM: Hazards of laparoscopic sterilization. In Sciarra JW (ed.): Gynecology and Obstetrics. Philadelphia, Harper & Row, 1982, p. 1.
4. Grainger DA, Soderstrom RM, Schiff SF, et al.: Ureteral injuries at laparoscopy: Insights into diagnosis, management, and prevention. Obstet Gynecol 1990; 75:839.
5. Medical Research International: In vitro fertilization/embryo transfer in the United States: 1985 and 1986 results from the National IVF-ET Registry. Fertil Steril 1988; 49:212.
6. Medical Research International: In vitro fertilization/embryo transfer in the United States: 1987 results from the National IVF-ET Registry. Fertil Steril 1989; 51:13.
7. Medical Research International: In vitro fertilization/embryo transfer in the United States: 1988 results from the IVF-ET Registry. Fertil Steril 1990; 53:13.
8. Hamori M, Stuckensen JA, Rumpf D, et al.: Zygote intrafallopian transfer (ZIFT): Evaluation of 42 cases. Fertil Steril 1988; 50:519.
9. Balmaceda JP, Gastaldi C, Remohi J, et al.: Tubal embryo transfer as a treatment for infertility due to male factor. Fertil Steril 1988; 50:476.
10. Pool TB, Ellsworth LR, Garza JR, et al.: Zygote intrafallopian transfer as a treatment for nontubal infertility: A 2-year study. Fertil Steril 1990; 54:482.
11. Rotsztejn DA, Remohi J, Weckstein, et al.: Results of tubal embryo transfer in premature ovarian failure. Fertil Steril 1990; 54:348.
12. Scholtes MCW, Roozenburg BJ, Alberda AT, Zeilmaker GH: Transcervical intrafallopian transfer of zygotes. Fertil Steril 1990; 54:283.
13. Dmowski WP, Radwanska E, Binor Z, et al.: Ovarian suppression induced with buserelin or danazol in the management of endometriosis: A randomized, comparative study. Fertil Steril 1989; 51:395.
14. Henzl MR, Corson SL, Moghissi K, et al.: Administration of nasal nafarelin as compared with oral danazol for endometriosis: A multicenter double-blind comparative clinical trial. N Engl J Med 1988; 318:485.
15. Friedman AJ, Harrison-Atlas D, Barbieri RL, et al.: A randomized, placebo-controlled, double-blind study evaluating the efficacy of leuprolide acetate depot in the treatment of uterine leiomyomata. Fertil Steril 1989; 51:251.
16. Friedman A: Treatment of leiomyomata uteri with short-term leuprolide followed by leuprolide plus estrogen-progestin hormone replacement therapy for 2 years: A pilot study. Fertil Steril 1989; 51:526.
17. Letterie GS, Coddington CC, Winkel CA, et al.: Efficacy of a gonadotropin-releasing hormone agonist in the treatment of uterine leiomyomata: Long-term follow-up. Fertil Steril 1989; 51:951.
18. Olive D, Haney AF: Endometriosis-associated infertility: A critical review of therapeutic approaches. Obstet Gynecol Surv 1986; 41:538.
19. Donnez J, Lemaire-Rubbers M, Karaman Y, et al.: Combined (hormonal and microsurgical) therapy in infertile women with endometriosis. Fertil Steril 1987; 48:239.
20. Donnez J, Schrurs B, Gillerot S, et al.: Treatment of uterine fibroids with implants of gonadotropin-releasing hormone agonist: Assessment by hysterography. Fertil Steril 1989; 51:947.
21. Blackwell RE, Carr BR, Chang RJ, et al.: Are we exploiting the infertile couple? Fertil Steril 1987; 48:735.
22. MacLeod J, Gold RE: The male factor in fertility and infertility: II. Spermatozoon counts in 1000 men of known fertility and 1000 cases of infertile marriage. J Urol 1951; 66:436.
23. Rehan NE, Sobrero AJ, Fertig JW: The semen of fertile men: Statistical analysis of 1300 men. Fertil Steril 1975; 26:492.
24. Collins JA: The postcoital test as a predictive of pregnancy among 355 infertile couples. Fertil Steril 1984; 41:703.
25. Karasick S, Goldfarb AF: Peritubal adhesions in infertile women: Diagnosis with hysterosalpingography. AJR 1989; 152:777.
26. Stumpf PG, March MM: Febrile morbidity following hysterosalpingography: Identification of risk factors and recommendations for prophylaxis. Fertil Steril 1980; 33:487.
27. Rock JA, Katayama KP, Martin EF: Factors influencing the success of salpingostomy techniques for distal fimbrial obstruction. Obstet Gynecol 1978; 52:591.
28. Grinsted J, Jacobsen JD, Ginsted L, et al.: Prediction of ovulation. Fertil Steril 1989; 52:388.
29. Corsan GH, Ghazi D, Kemmann E: Home urinary luteinizing hormone immunoassays: Clinical applications. Fertil Steril 1990; 53:591.
30. Bieglmayer C, Fischl F, Janisch H: Evaluation of a simple and fast self-test for urine luteinizing hormone. Fertil Steril 1990; 53:842.
31. Scott RT, Snyder RR, Strickland DM, et al.: The effect of interobserver variation in dating endometrial histology on the diagnosis of luteal phase defects. Fertil Steril 1988; 50:888.
32. Li TC, Dockery P, Rogers AW, Cooke ED: How precise is histologic dating of endometrium using the standard dating criteria? Fertil Steril 1989; 51:759.
33. Davis OD, Berkeley AS, Naus GJ, et al.: The incidence of luteal phase defect in normal, fertile women, determined by serial endometrial biopsies. Fertil Steril 1989; 51:582.
34. McNeely MJ, Soules MR: The diagnosis of luteal phase deficiency: A critical review. Fertil Steril 1988; 50:1.
35. Dunphy BC, Kay R, Barratt CLR, Cooke ID: Is routine examination of the male partner of any prognostic value in the routine assessment of couples who complain of involuntary infertility? Fertil Steril 1989; 52:454.

36. Gillett WR, Herbison GP: Tubocornual anastomosis: Surgical considerations and coexistent infertility factors in determining the prognosis. Fertil Steril 1989; 51:241.
37. Rock JA, Guzick DS, Katz E, et al.: Tubal anastomosis: Pregnancy success following reversal of Falope ring or monopolar cautery sterilization. Fertil Steril 1987; 48:13.
38. Kaplan EB, Sheiner LB, Boekman AJ, et al.: The usefulness of preoperative laboratory screening. JAMA 1985; 253:3576.
39. Moretuzzo R, DiLauro S, Jenison E, et al.: Serum and peritoneal lavage fluid CA-125 levels in endometriosis. Fertil Steril 1988; 50:430.
40. Pittaway DE, Douglas JW: Serum CA-125 in women with endometriosis and chronic pelvic pain. Fertil Steril 1989; 51:68.
41. Gagner A, Chiasson A: Preoperative chest x-ray films in elective surgery: A valid screening tool. CJS 1990; 33:271.
42. Epstein DM: The role of radiologic screening in lung cancer. Radiol Clin North Am 1990; 28:489.
43. Kerin J, Daykhovsky L, Segalowitz J, et al.: Falloposcopy: Microendoscopic technique for visual exploration of the human fallopian tube from the uterotubal ostium to the fimbria using a transvaginal approach. Fertil Steril 1990; 54:390.
44. Groff TR, Edelstein JA, Schenken RS: Hysterosalpingography in the preoperative evaluation of tubal anastomosis candidates. Fertil Steril 1990; 53:417.
45. Letterie GS, Wilson J, Miyazawa K: Magnetic resonance imaging of Müellerian tract abnormalities. Fertil Steril 1988; 50:365.
46. Devereux RB, Kramer-Fox R, Kligfield P: Mitral valve prolapse: Causes, clinical manifestations, and management. Ann Intern Med 1989; 111:305.
47. Schwartz D, Mayaux MJ: Female fecundity as a function of age. Results of artificial insemination in 2193 nulliparous women with azoospermic husbands. Federation CECOS. N Engl J Med 1982; 306:404.
48. Stovall DW, Toma SK, Hammond MG, Talbert LM: The effect of age on female fecundity. Obstet Gynecol 1991; 77:33.
49. Gomel V: Operative laparoscopy: Time for acceptance. Fertil Steril 1989; 52:1.
50. Murphy AA: Operative laparoscopy. Fertil Steril 1987; 47:1.
51. Azziz R, Steinkampf MP, Murphy A: Postoperative recuperation: Relation to the extent of endoscopic surgery. Fertil Steril 1989; 51:1061.
52. Carson SA, Hubert GD, Schriock ED, Buster JE: Hyperglycemia and hyponatremia during operative hysteroscopy with 5% dextrose in water distention. Fertil Steril 1989; 51:341.
53. Trimbos-Kemper TC, Veering BT: Anaphylactic shock from intracavitary 32% dextran-70 during hysteroscopy. Fertil Steril 1989; 51:1053.
54. Tulandi T, Cherry N: Clinical trials in reproductive surgery: Randomization and life-table analysis. Fertil Steril 1989; 52:12.
55. Rock JA, et al.: The efficacy of postoperative hydrotubation: A randomized prospective multicenter clinical trial. Fertil Steril 1984; 42:373.
56. Jansen RP: Early laparoscopy after pelvic operations to prevent adhesion: Safety and efficacy. Fertil Steril 1988; 49:26.
57. DeCherney AH, Mezer HC: Timing of postoperative laparoscopic evaluation of tubal surgery patients. Fertil Steril 1983; 39:402.
58. INTERCEED (TC7) Adhesion Barrier Study Group: Prevention of postsurgical adhesion by INTERCEED (TC7), an absorbable adhesion barrier: A prospective, randomized multicenter clinical study. Fertil Steril 1989; 51:933.

Instruments for Gynecologic Surgery

5

C. O. Granai
Gerald A. Feuer

After a century-long struggle, gynecology is now well established as a medical specialty, but expertise in pelvic surgery must continue to progress if gynecology is to maintain its validity in the surgical arena. What will make this possible is an eye toward creativity, improved training in anatomy and operative technique, and better use of current surgical instrumentation.

Every surgeon, in preparing for an unusual operation, has found it difficult to decide what instruments and materials should be selected. The surgeon, harassed with the care of many patients, will not infrequently find that in his selection, some things will be omitted which would have greatly expedited the work.[1]

So begins *Care of Patients Undergoing Gynecologic and Abdominal Procedures Before, During and After Operation*, by E.E. Montgomery, published in 1916. The admonition is still relevant today. Montgomery's textbook is also illustrative of gynecology as having evolved from general surgery, and as such, inheriting instrumentation not always ideal for the particular needs of the female pelvis (Fig. 5-1). Fortunately, today's gynecologic surgeons, respectful of the timelessness of classic surgical instrumentation, can also avail themselves of the advances in surgical tools that, taken in conjunction with improvements in anesthesia, antibiotics, and medical management, have led to better care of patients requiring gynecologic surgery.

When classified according to fundamental functions, surgical instruments are asked to meet surprisingly few needs: to cut, expose, hold, arrest (hemostasis), and secure. Historically, these functions have been well met by the limited categories of basic surgical tools—knives, scissors, retractors, clamps, and sutures—which have nevertheless afforded a great diversity of operative procedures. It would, however, be close minded to think that surgery has reached a point at which further improvements cannot be made through evolution in these basic tools or through new ideas in instrumentation. Indeed, surgical tools have been and are being greatly improved by better design, better materials, better engineering, and new insights into human physiology.

Why, then, do some surgeons continue to use a "Kelly" or "Kocher" for everything? The answer is that as with all patterns of human behavior, changing one's selection in surgical tools is emotionally difficult. The reluctance of human nature aside, stalwart general purpose clamps used in gynecology should in many instances give way to more refined, specialized effective instruments such as Adson's and Rogers' clamps (Fig. 5-2). Classic suture materials, such as cotton, silk, and even catgut, are being superseded by nonreactive, stronger, absorbable synthetic counterparts. Surgical retractors, once available in only simplistic designs, are now present in a startling array, permitting access to the most difficult anatomic

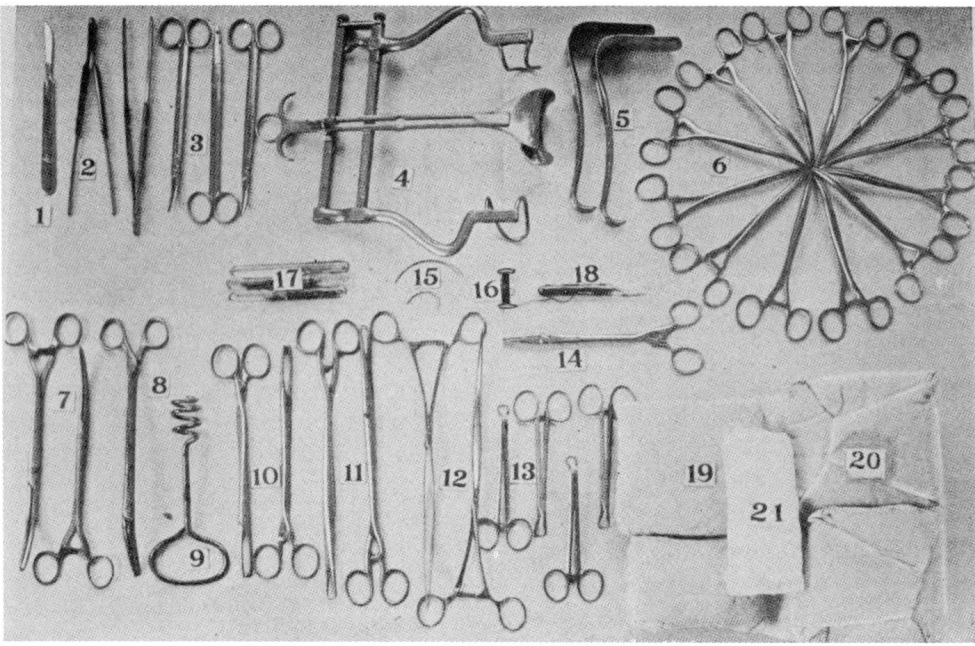

Figure 5–1
Instruments and preparations for abdominal hysterectomy, in E.E. Montgomery's 1916 *Care of Patients Undergoing Gynecologic and Abdominal Procedures Before, During and After Operation*, published by WB Saunders Company. *1*, Scalpel, *2*, Tissue forceps, *3*, Scissors, *4*, Combined retractor (self-retaining), *5*, Long retractors, *6*, Hemostatic forceps, *7*, Pedicle forceps, *8*, Right-angled clamp forceps, *9*, Myoma screw, *10*, Fixation forceps, *11*, Double tenacula, *12*, Intestinal clamp, *13*, Towel clips, *14*, Needle holder, *15*, Curved needles, *16*, Sterile silk, *17*, Catgut, chromic, *18*, Catgut, plain, *19*, Sterile gauze packs and sponges, *20*, Sterile gowns, sheets, and towels, *21*, Iodoform gauze.

locations. Other technologies, such as surgical drains, surgical stapling instruments, laser, ultrasound guided imaging,[2] and intraoperative video, all improve surgeons' ability to perform gynecologic surgery.

In short, today's gynecologic surgeons, unlike their forefathers, have access to instrumentation specific to the patients' surgical needs. However, to avail oneself of this potential requires not only education and imagination but also personal introspection on the part of the surgeon to be sure that superstition, ego, pride, ignorance, or even fear do not create a barrier to change. The paraphrased cliché, "You can't teach an old surgeon new tricks," is, of course, wrong.

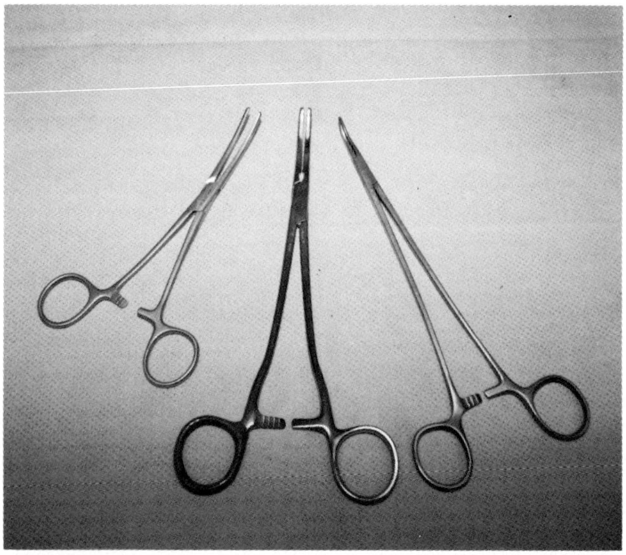

POSITIONING THE PATIENT

Proper positioning of the patient under anesthesia facilitates optimal surgical exposure and patient safety. It is often useful, in difficult gynecologic cases, to employ a modified lithotomy position, which is maintained by multipositional stirrups, where the weight of the leg is borne by the sole of the patient's foot (e.g., Allen stirrups)[3] (Fig. 5–3). This positioning permits a second surgical assistant to participate more directly in the operation and affords simultaneous access via the abdomen and the vagina to pelvic pathology. The importance to the final surgical outcome of optimal patient positioning, made possible by unheralded modern stirrups, is often overlooked by even the most experienced pelvic surgeons.

OPENING THE ABDOMEN

Outside the development of superior materials, little genuine improvement has been made over the classic scalpel as a mechanism for incising the skin and opening the abdomen. Complementary techniques such as the Bovie do offer some degree of hemostasis but cause more necrosis to the adjacent tissues than the knife.[4, 5] The laser, particularly the neodymium-yttrium-aluminum garnet laser, has been proposed as a futuristic sterilizing alternative to the scalpel;[6, 7] however, at present it is hard to recommend use of the laser because it is a slower, more costly option.

Figure 5–2
Left to right, The general purpose Kelly clamp in comparison with more refined and specific alternatives—the Rogers and the Adson.

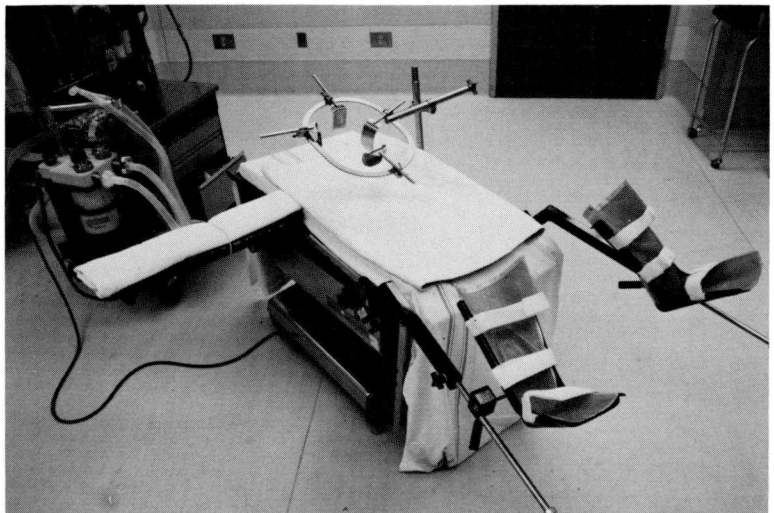

Figure 5–3
Allen stirrups in conjunction with the Bookwalter attached to operating room table.

EXPOSURE OF THE ABDOMEN AND PELVIS

Retractors

To facilitate safe and effective surgery, there is no substitute for an adequate incision and maximal exposure of the surgical field. In the latter role, the value of self-retaining retractors is unsung yet often critical to the success of the operation. The classic two-way or three-way Balfour retractor has long been a standard part of the armamentarium of the gynecologic surgeon. Less well known is the simple but creative modification to the standard three-way Balfour retractor, the "fourth arm," which with a quick turn of a screw easily attaches to the parent device and inexpensively converts the old classic Balfour into a far more effective four-way retractor (Fig. 5–4). The potential utility and cost effectiveness of the "fourth arm" is one of the most unimplemented mechanical upgrades available to today's operating suites.

A number of specifically designed four-way retractors are in fact commercially available. The most common version employed in gynecology is the O'Connell-O'Sullivan retractor. This device provides good exposure to a small, central-pelvic field but is not engineered to retract tissues in a deep pelvis or where a large field of view is necessary. In the latter instance, the creative Bookwalter retractor (see Fig. 5–3), or various competitors (Fig. 5–5), can provide remarkable exposure in even obese patients or when complex surgical fields are encountered. Bookwalter's innovations of attaching the retractor directly to the surgical table, rather than to the patient, and his

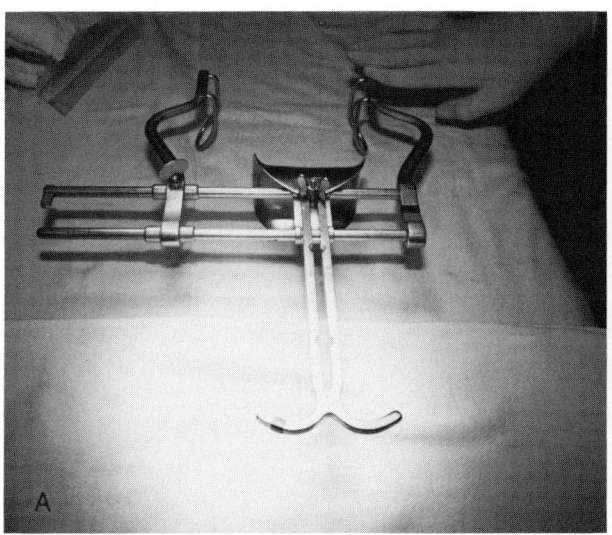
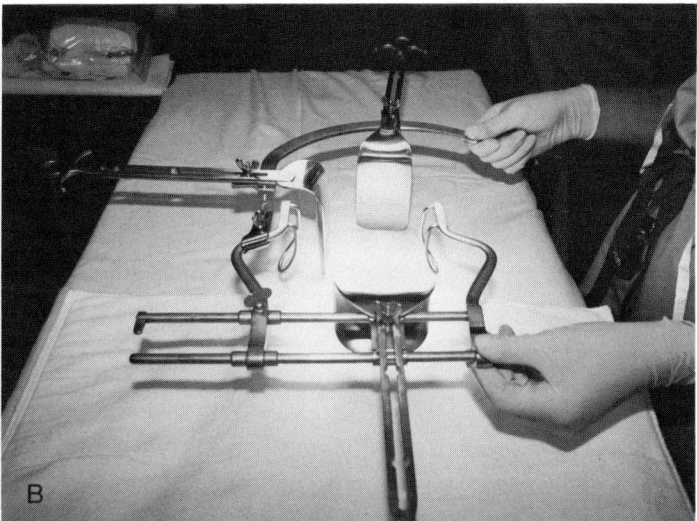

Figure 5–4
A, The Balfour three-way retractor. *B*, The Balfour three-way retractor with the fourth arm attached.

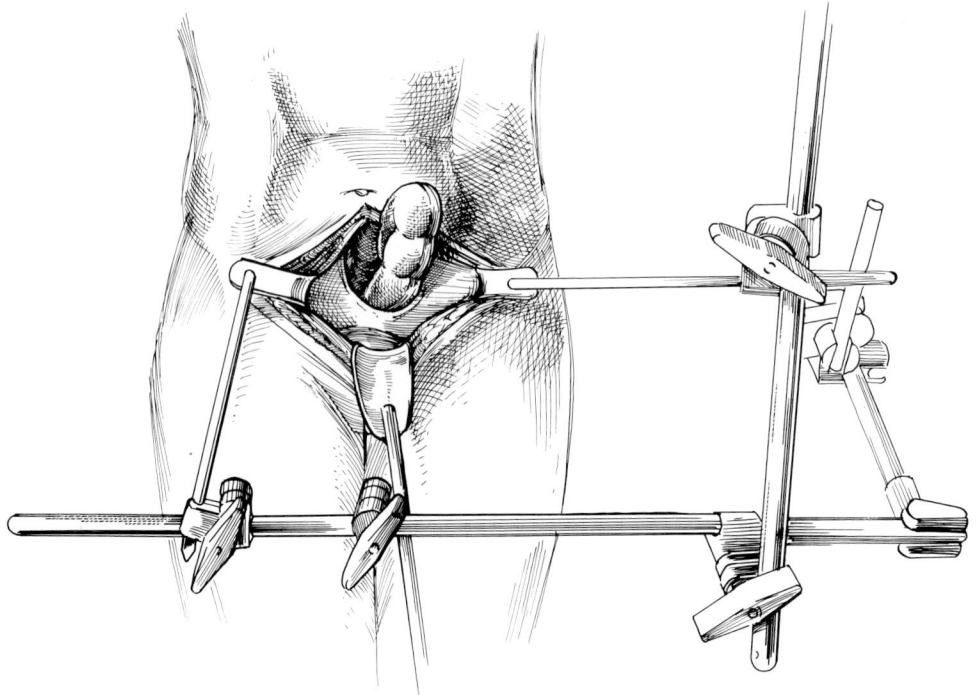

Figure 5–5
The Thompson retractor.

design of specific blades for retracting afford a wide variety of mechanical options yielding good exposure, even with large incisions. Similar, attached-to-the-table retractors are available to facilitate exposure during vaginal surgery.

Whereas the value of sophisticated modern retractors in specific patients is unquestionable, few hospitals can afford the luxury of having one, let alone two, such devices dedicated to each surgical suite. Fortunately, for most pelvic surgery, including complex radical surgery, simple modification of the classic three-way Balfour retractor by the attachment of the fourth arm and its blades produces superb operative exposure while being highly cost effective.

Packing

Visualization of the surgical field, even when employing the best of retractors, can be influenced significantly by the "packing" selected by the surgeon. Toward that end, various devices have been introduced that form walls/barriers around the pelvis in hopes of preventing the upper abdominal contents from falling into and obscuring the pelvic field. In the final analysis, however, none of these more "scientific" devices are superior to, or cheaper than, moist towels used to pack the intestines superiorly and held in that barrier position by the upward blade of a four-way retractor. If necessary, lysis of adhesions should precede any packing effort if maximal success is to be attained.

Lighting

As with retracting and packing, the importance of the illumination of the surgical field is often underestimated, particularly in times of emergency, when there is truly no substitute for good vision/lighting. Unfortunately, all too often the overhead lighting in the assigned gynecologic operating room is inadequate to meet the surgical needs of the female pelvis. At least two and preferably three mobile, adjustable light banks are necessary if overhead lighting is to be used alone. To augment room lighting, many pelvic surgeons have realized the utility of wearing headlamps (Fig. 5–6), which permit the accustomed surgeon a great adjunct to the illumination of the pelvis, especially at revealing difficult angles. In a similar vein, "flashlights" for intra-abdominal/pelvic use are commercially available. Particularly clever, though expensive, is a device that combines a light source attached to a hand-held suction and irrigating spout. Occasionally, the illuminated tip of this device can become quite hot and may theoretically cause minor thermal injury. Nevertheless, this tool can be useful in those difficult situations deep in the pelvis where vision is obscured by darkness and bleeding.

EXPLORING THE ABDOMEN-PELVIS

Proper exploration of the abdomen and pelvis requires a keen understanding of human anatomy and

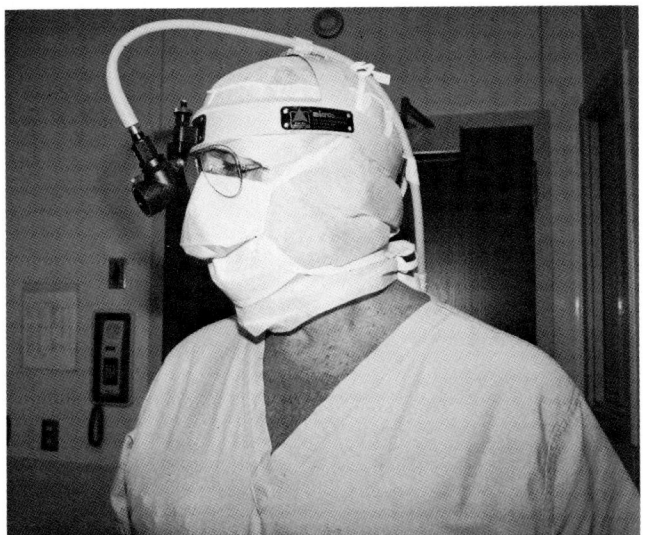

Figure 5-6
Headlamp.

RESECTION

Surgical resection requires a knowledge about the anatomy and physiology of the structure being removed, and an expertise with the appropriate operative procedure. Here, too, a delicate dissection and precise atraumatic technique using refined instruments will result in the ultimate surgical outcome. Long, sensitive, exacting tools properly utilized will often obviate the need for cruder, historic surgical tools. Good examples of the former category are the various graceful clamps capable of artful holding, dissecting, and tying (Fig. 5-8). Refined clamps such as the Adson, employed as part of a precise dissection, eliminate the need for the nondescript Kelly clamp applied grossly across large bulks of tissue. Similarly, long, slender needle holders permit a surgical delicacy, sense of touch, and improved vision of the tissues to be sutured. Contrary to their less substantial, even frail, appearance when properly used, these refined instruments can usually drive the needle through the thickest tissues.

Another important surgical tool used for resections and elsewhere in the operation is the right-angle clamp. Similar to its less curved counterpart, the Adson clamp, the right-angle clamp can be em-

surgical techniques, including those that give access to the retroperitoneum. Confronted with complicated pelvic pathology, it is often critical to enter the retroperitoneum to define disease and to identify vascular pedicles and the ureter. In so doing, more precise, delicate, and effective surgery can be performed. Refined surgical instrumentation enhances these difficult and other, less complex procedures (Fig. 5-7). For example, scissors as a basic tool are available in many styles, but long, sleek, sharp instruments such as the Metzenbaum series permit a graceful precision and a feel for the tissues not possible using bulkier, cruder counterparts. Occasionally, large, heavy scissors are needed to cut thick, dense tissues, but properly used, more refined prototypes are usually capable and superior. By analogy, many excellent, long, delicate, precise, non-toothed forceps (e.g., DeBakey) are available and have supplanted the need to use bulky, wide, tooth forceps with their inherent tissue trauma. In light of the newer atraumatic alternatives, the indication for traumatic forceps is increasingly rare.

Finally, the supreme tools of surgical exploration, but not often conceptualized as such, are the surgeon's own fingers. Fingers with dexterous expertise implement the knowledge of anatomy and facilitate dissection in ways unequaled by synthetic, mechanical counterparts. The "hands-on" yet delicate surgeon employs to the patient's advantage all possible human senses, including touch. Curiously, some schools of surgical thought dogmatically forbid "vulgar fingers" in the abdomen, preaching instead a stylistic approach that is at times guilty of the accusation "form without substance."

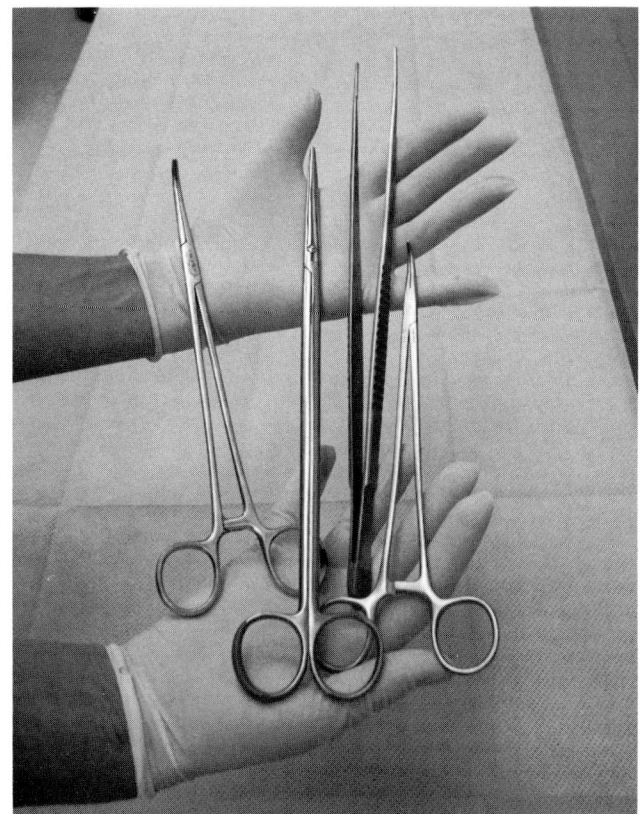

Figure 5-7
An array of delicate tools.

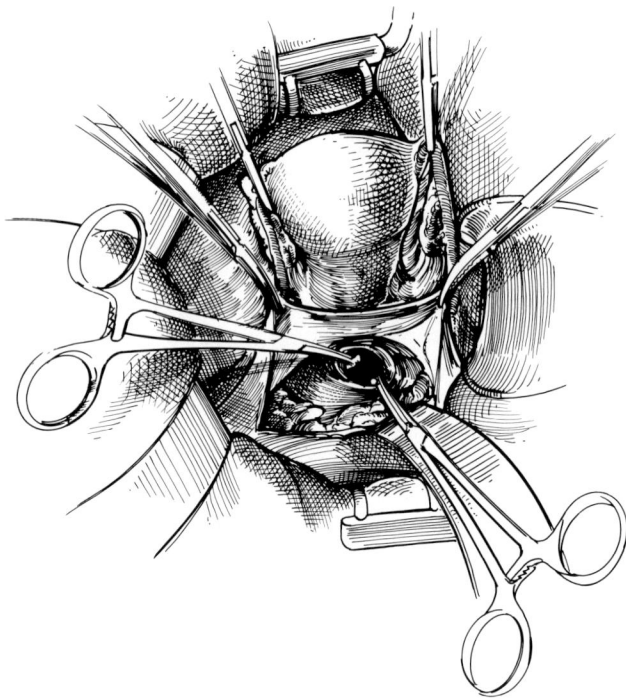

Figure 5–8
A retroperitoneal dissection facilitated by exacting instrumentation.

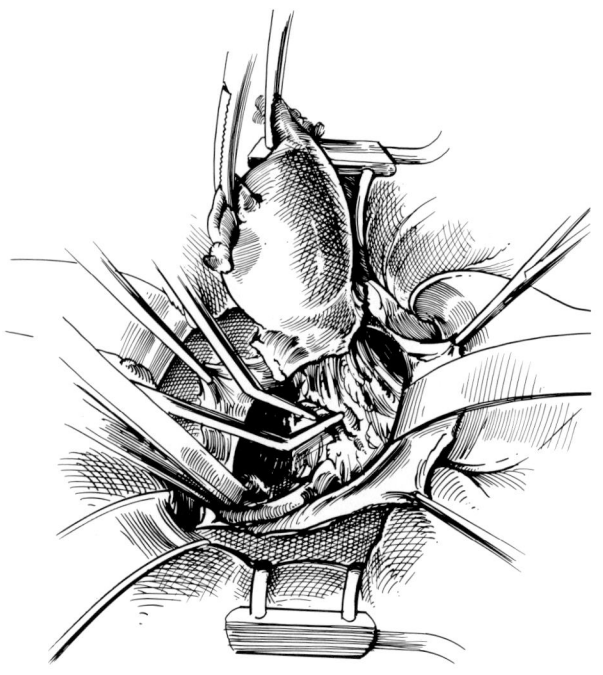

Figure 5–9
Untunneling the ureter in a radical hysterectomy.

ployed to meticulously dissect and clamp tissues in those instances where more acute angulation is needed. Examples of good applications of the right-angle clamp working in awkward anatomic locations are untunneling the ureter in a radical hysterectomy and clamping and tying blood vessels deep in the pelvis (Fig. 5–9).

For the occasional circumstance when stronger or heavier clamps than those mentioned thus far are needed, modern revisions of classic bulky clamps incorporate newer materials and better engineering (Fig. 5–10). The use of historic all-purpose clamps such as Kochers and Heaneys should be reconsidered in deference to the more precise, secure, and less tissue-damaging equivalent instruments such as the curved or straight Rogers clamp.

SURGICAL STAPLING

Although conceived near the turn of the century, surgical stapling is only now overcoming physician skepticism and beginning to demonstrate its potential surgical roles. Despite such obstacles, intra-abdominal stapling has already revolutionized surgical resections in certain areas of the body.[8, 9] Effective instruments such as the GIA,* TA,* and EEA* devices (Fig. 5–11) have significantly reduced the time for bowel resections and reanastomoses because of their capacity to quickly apply staggered rows of B-shaped staples while simultaneously transecting the tissues. In the same philosophy, the LDS* instrument makes it possible to perform an omentectomy (Fig. 5–12) or resection of the bowel mesentery in only minutes. Additionally, biochemical advances in the materials used to make absorbable staples have allowed for their application across the vaginal cuff, expediting

---

*Trademark of the United States Surgical Corporation.

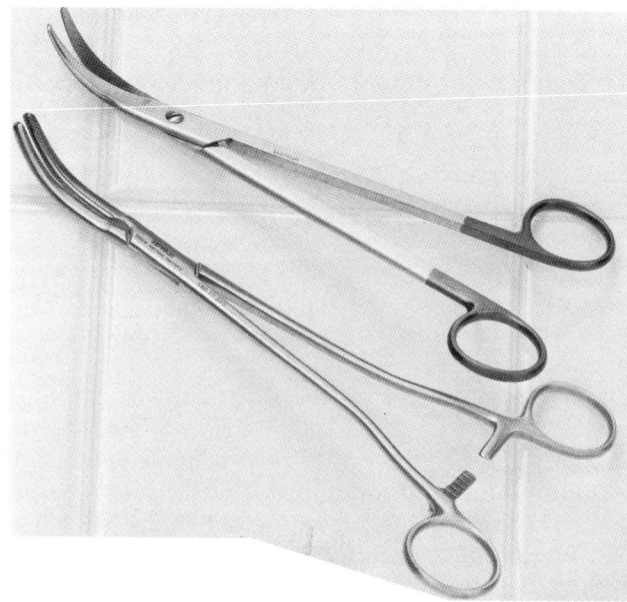

Figure 5–10
Modern revisions of classic bulky clamps and scissors.

---

*Trademark of the United States Surgical Corporation.

INSTRUMENTS FOR GYNECOLOGIC SURGERY 103

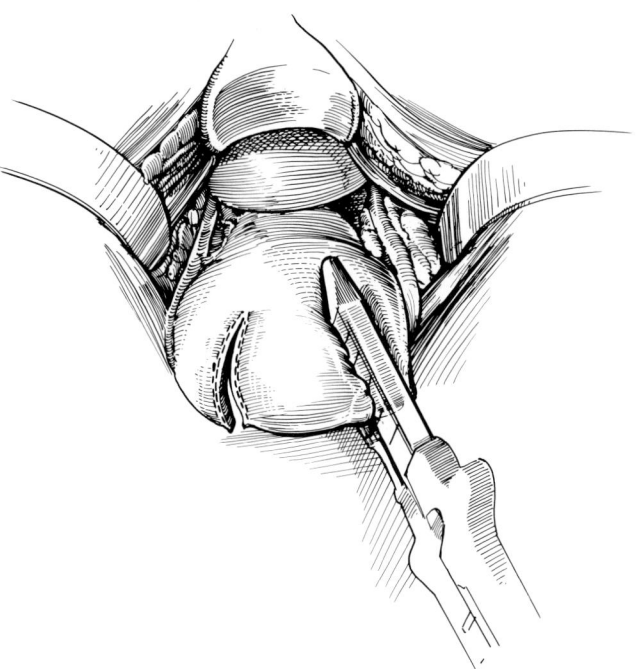

Figure 5–11
Surgical stapling using the GIA stapler to transect the adnexa.

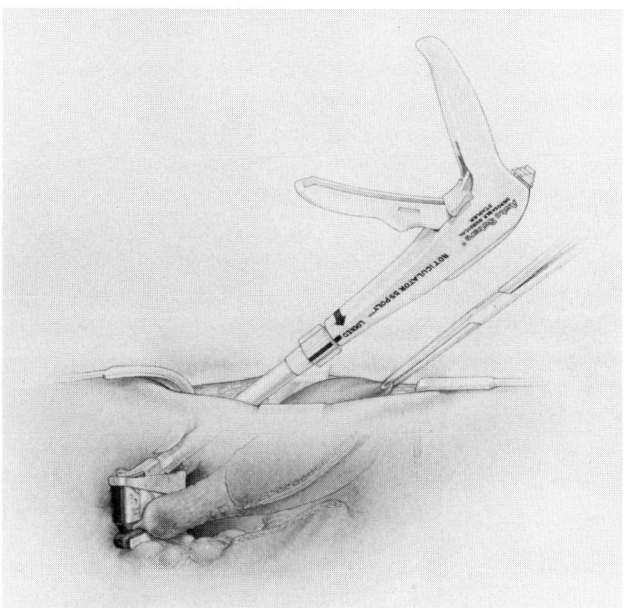

Figure 5–13
Stapling across the vaginal cuff, using the Roticulator 55 Poly.

the resection of the uterus and closure of the vagina (Fig. 5–13) in comparison with standard suturing techniques.[10] By virtue of being highly effective and significantly faster, stapling has found many applications in gynecologic oncology, on both irradiated and nonirradiated patients.[11–13] Applications of surgical stapling on patients undergoing non-oncologic procedures, although in some ways less dramatic, can also have real advantages for these patients.[14]

Overall, although not a panacea, surgical stapling is a major technologic advancement that, when mastered and employed, has significant benefits to selected patients. Unfortunately, for reasons that may have more to do with egos than with science, surgeons not familiar with this technology tend to impede its application. Despite this reluctance, new ideas for stapling in pelvic surgery, as in all other anatomic areas, are evolving, and they deserve to be objectively evaluated.

HEMOSTASIS

Maintaining control of bleeding is an undisputed principle of any surgery. Although generally not portrayed as a tool, sutures have always been an essential part of obtaining hemostasis. Despite their long history, dramatic progress has been made recently in sutures themselves, progress that enhances the surgical value of this basic tool. Biochemical technology has brought an array of polyglycolic acid sutures that are absorbed through simple, nonreactive hydrolysis at a predictable rate of degradation.[15] In marked contradistinction to the original absorbable sutures (e.g., catgut), polyglycolic acid sutures retain significant tensile strength throughout the critical phases of healing without engendering much inflammatory response.[16, 17] As such, sutures like Vicryl (Ethicon, Inc.) and Dexon (Davis & Geck) have re-

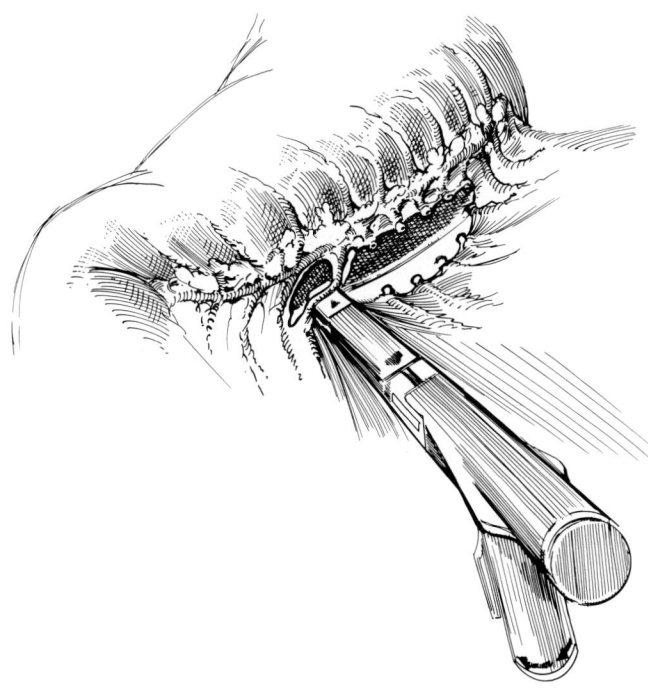

Figure 5–12
An omentectomy being performed with the LDS stapling instrument.

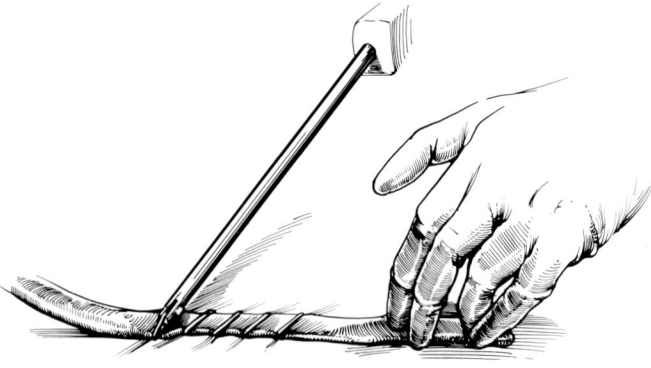

Figure 5–14
Surgical clips as mini-tools.

placed, or should replace, their predecessors in almost all aspects of pelvic surgery. More recently, suture technology has improved the monofilament suture, hence the introduction of synthetic monofilament sutures with a prolonged tensile strength and slow absorption.[18, 19] With these sutures, it is possible to perform closures requiring maximal strength without leaving bulkier, braided suture at the site or leaving a monofilament material, such as nylon, that will not absorb.

Today, the hemostatic value of electrocautery is accepted by surgeons of all types. Devices such as the Bovie have proved to be great time savers in preventing and controlling small bleeders encountered in all phases of a major operation. Various improvements in electrocautery devices, including bipolar cautery, are advocated under some circumstances because they conduct less current to the adjacent tissues, thus reducing the total amount of tissue trauma and necrosis.

Surgical clips, actually an extended form of surgical stapling, are a meaningful addition to the hemostatic armamentarium of the pelvic surgeon. With improvements in the clips themselves and in their applicator, much operating time can be saved by using clips to ligate even sizable vessels. Surgical clips as mini-tools can be expeditiously and accurately placed without adjacent tissue trauma (Fig. 5–14). For instance, surgical clips are useful in radical hysterectomies for efficiently ligating the uterine artery and, in conjunction with electrocautery, expediting lymph node dissection. Given the great potential of surgical clips, it is unfortunate that their advantages go underutilized by many gynecologic surgeons.

CYTOREDUCTIVE SURGERY

The rationale for maximal surgical debulking as a cornerstone in the management of ovarian cancer is now widely accepted.[20–22] Attaining optimal cytoreduction often demands a supreme effort on the part of the surgical team. Creativity by the surgeons employing virtually all types of instrumentation makes it possible to achieve optimal debulking in a surprising 80% of cases.[23] Even a higher success rate may be possible as new instruments are introduced that theoretically can play a complementary role to standard surgical tools. For example, the dynamic technology of the laser may be part of the surgical management of ovarian cancer as it will be a part of many aspects of future medical care. Already, the cytoreductive capabilities of intra-abdominal laser enhanced by photoabsorptive dyes are being tested in hopes of obtaining near-complete vaporization of the ovarian cancer implants.[24]

Through remarkable advances in a different technology, ultrasound is also finding increasing numbers of medical applications.[25, 26] Aside from its well-known imaging functions, ultrasound can also be used as a means of destroying tissues. As an example, the Cavitron device (Cavitron Surgical Systems) (Fig. 5–15) has made it possible for neurosurgeons to ultrasonically disrupt brain tissues and simultaneously aspirate them from the surgical field.[27] This same technology has been reported to be of value in attaining maximal cytoreductive surgery for ovarian carcinoma.[28] At the moment, it remains to be seen what the ultimate role of laser and ultrasound will be, but undoubtedly these representatives of super technology[29] will be an integral part of surgery.

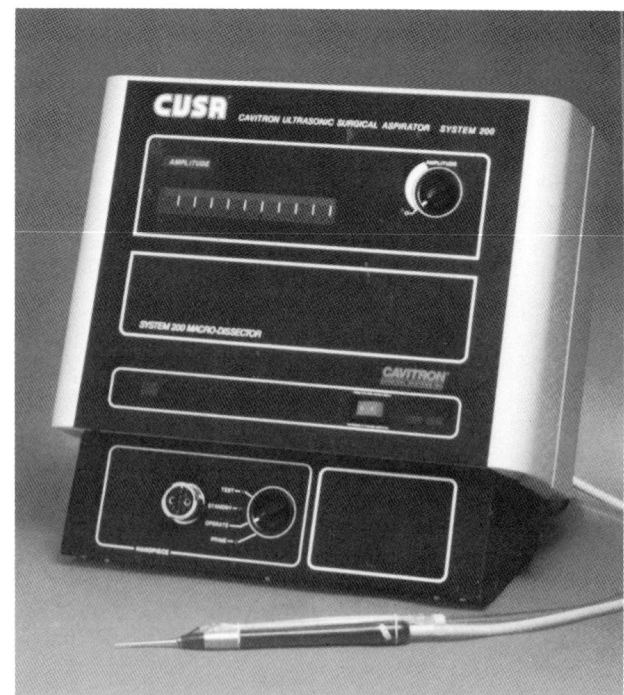

Figure 5–15
Cavitron Ultrasonic Surgical Aspirator.

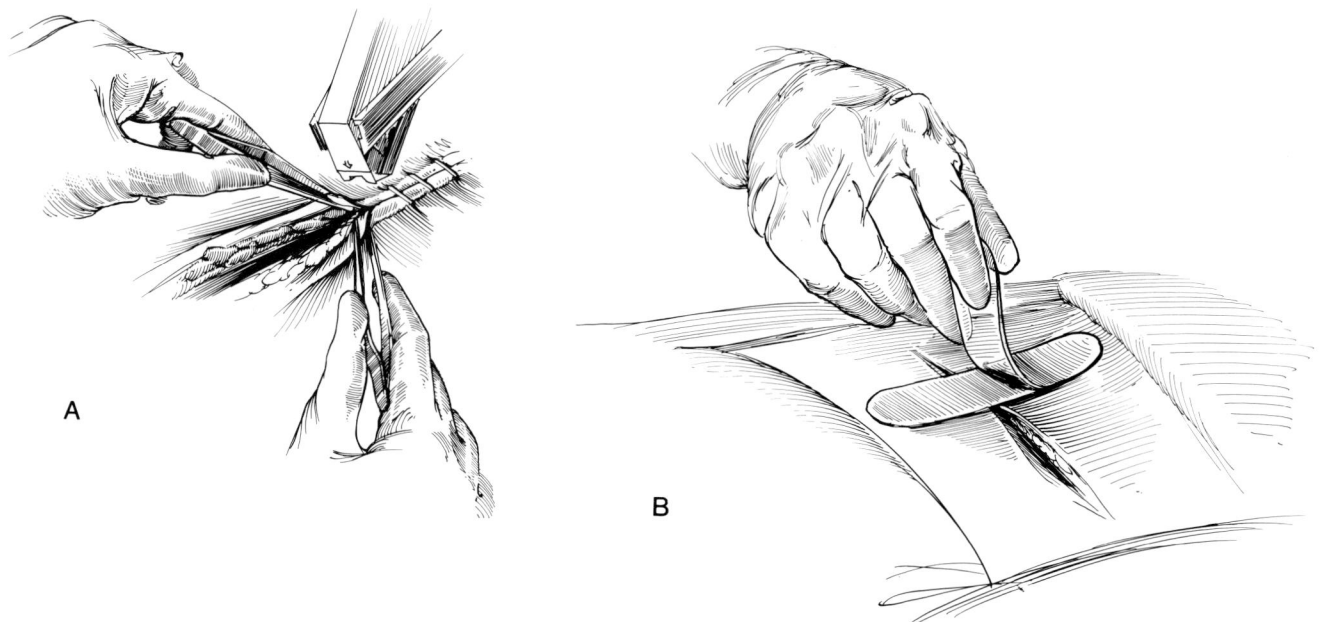

Figure 5–16
Stapling *(A)* and taping *(B)* as closure methods.

CLOSING THE ABDOMEN

Ironically, the actual success of a complex operation is, in the end, held hostage to the mundane—that is, the closing of the laparotomy incision. Fortunately, progress in suture materials and a better understanding of wound healing have lead to improvements in the closure of the abdomen.[30–32] Large, curved needles with heavy monofilament sutures can now be employed in continuous bulk closures of the abdomen. This type of continuous abdominal closure yields surgical results at least equivalent to those of older, slower, more suture burdening techniques, including the Smead-Jones method.[33–37] Mass closure techniques, made possible by remarkably strong yet entirely absorbable suture such as PDS No. 2 (Ethicon, Inc.), allow the surgeon to capitalize on the physiology of wound healing and reduce operative time. For closure of the skin, surgical clips further decrease procedure time, but at a minor financial cost. Surprisingly, closure of abdominal skin incisions with modern tapes may prove to be the best all-around option[38] (Fig. 5–16).

SPECIAL INSTRUMENTS

Creatively applying often obscure but current surgical instrumentation, or designing a new instrument to meet a specific need, is a hallmark of the resourceful surgeon. "Borrowing" select tools from the existing menu of allied surgical specialties, such as vascular surgery and urology, can be very helpful to the gynecologic surgeon. In addition, enterprising companies engaged in research and development offer an ever-expanding array of new and sometimes clever instruments to meet the special requirements of abdominal, vaginal, and laparoscopic operations (Fig. 5–17). Most of these "new" devices are in some way modifications of the basic knife, scissors, for-

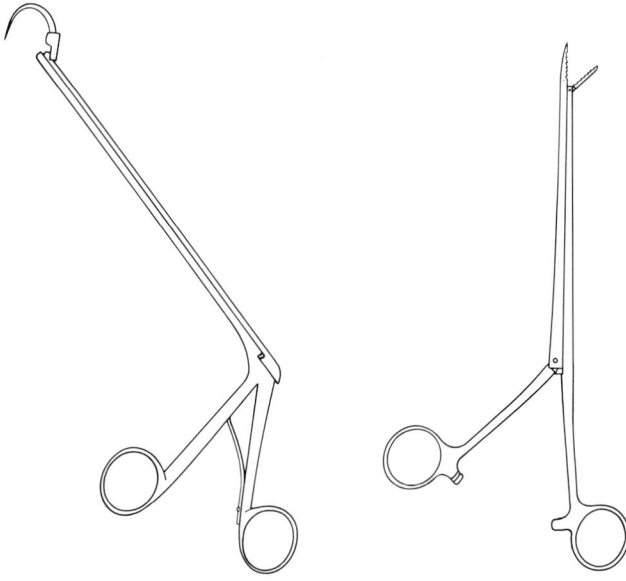

Figure 5–17
Examples of an ever-expanding array of specialty instruments.

ceps, etc. Nevertheless, it behooves pelvic surgeons to be aware of what instruments exist and use the best options. The timeless "caveat emptor" will always apply, as long as it is possible to fall trap to technical gimmickry over the basic, proven performance of standard techniques and classic tools.

Postscript

If this book, as it passes from his hands, by lessening the anxiety of the surgeon, promotes better work, facilitates the labor of nurses and interns, but, above all, adds to the comfort and satisfaction of the patients, the author will feel well repaid for his efforts.

E.E. MONTGOMERY, 1916

References

1. Montgomery EE: Care of Patients Undergoing Gynecologic and Abdominal Procedures Before, During and After Operation. Philadelphia, WB Saunders Co., 1916.
2. Granai CO, Doherty F, Allee P, et al.: Ultrasound for diagnosing and preventing malplacement of intrauterine tandems. Obstet Gynecol 1990; 75:110.
3. Adler LM, Loughlin JS, Morin CJ, Haning RV: Bilateral compartment syndrome after a long gynecologic operation in the lithotomy position. Am J Obstet Gynecol 1990; 162:1271.
4. Rossi EC: Comments on the early history of hemostasis. Med Clin North Am 1972; 56:9.
5. Glover J, Bendick P, Link W: Use of thermal knives in surgery. Curr Probl Surg 1978; 15:1.
6. Dolsky RL: Argon laser skin surgery. Surg Clin North Am 1984; 64:861.
7. Maker VK, Kaplan RL: Contact neodymium-yttrium-aluminum garnet laser acts as a sterilizing scalpel. Surg Gynecol Obstet 1990; 170:17.
8. Steichen FM, Ravitch MM: Stapling in Surgery. Chicago, Year Book Medical Publishers, 1984, p. 33.
9. Wheeless CR: Stapling techniques in operations for malignant disease of the female genital tract. Surg Clin North Am 1984; 64(3):591.
10. Buka NJ: Absorbable staples in abdominal hysterectomy. Surg Gynecol Obstet 1988; 166:174.
11. Delgado G: Use of the automatic stapler in urinary conduit diversions and pelvic exenterations. Gynecol Oncol 1980; 10(1):93.
12. Rubin SC, Benjamin I, Hoskins WJ, et al.: Intestinal surgery in gynecologic oncology. Gynecol Oncol 1989; 34:30.
13. Chalas E, Mann WJ, Westermann CP, Patsner B: Morbidity and mortality of stapled anastomoses on a gynecologic oncology service: A retrospective review. Gynecol Oncol 1990; 37:82.
14. Beresford JM: Automatic stapling techniques in abdominal hysterectomy. Surg Clin North Am 1984; 64(3):609.
15. Sanz LE: Sutures: A primer on structure and function. Contemp OB/GYN 1990; 35(2):99.
16. Pavan A, Bosio M, Longo T: A comparative study of poly (glycolic acid) and catgut as suture materials. Histomorphology and mechanical properties. J Biomed Mater Res 1979; 13:477.
17. Sanz LE, Patterson JA, Kamath R, et al.: Comparison of Maxon suture with Vicryl, chromic catgut and PDS sutures in fascial closure in rats. Obstet Gynecol 1988; 71:418.
18. Ray JA, Doddi N, Regula D, et al.: Polydioxanone (PDS): A novel monofilament absorbable suture. Surg Gynecol Obstet 1981: 153.
19. Katz AR, Mukherjee DP, Kagonov AL, Gordon S: A new synthetic monofilament absorbable suture made from polytrimethylene carbonate. Surg Gynecol Obstet 1985; 161(3):213.
20. Griffiths CT: Surgical resection of tumor bulk in the primary treatment of ovarian carcinoma. Natl Cancer Inst Monogr 1975; 42:101.
21. Hacker NF, Berek JS, Lagasse LD, et al.: Primary cytoreductive surgery for epithelial ovarian cancer. Obstet Gynecol 1983; 61:413.
22. Richardson GS, Scully RE, Nikrui N, et al.: Common epithelial cancer of the ovary. N Engl J Med 1985; 312:415.
23. Eisenkop S, Spirtos N, Montag T: The impact of subspecialty training in the management of advanced ovarian cancer. Women's Cancer Center, San Jose/Burlingame, CA. Abstract presented at 21st Annual Meeting, Society of Gynecologic Oncologists, February 1990.
24. Brand E, Choi H-S, Braunstein GD, et al.: Photodynamic therapy of human choriocarcinoma transplanted to the hamster cheek pouch. II. Intralesional photosensitization. Gynecol Oncol 1989; 34:289.
25. Kelman CD: Phaco-emulsification and aspiration: A report of 500 consecutive cases. Am J Ophthalmol 1973; 75:764.
26. Andrus CH, Kaminski DL: Segmental hepatic resection utilizing the ultrasonic dissector. Arch Surg 1986; 121:515.
27. Fasano VA, Zeme S, Frego L, et al.: Ultrasonic aspiration in the surgical treatment of intracranial tumors. J Neurosurg Sci 1981; 25:35.
28. Adelson MD, Baggish MS, Seifer DB, et al.: Cytoreduction of ovarian cancer with the Cavitron ultrasonic surgical aspirator. Obstet Gynecol 1988; 72(1):140.
29. Brand E: Electrosurgical cytoreduction of ovarian adenocarcinoma using the argon beam coagulator. University of Colorado Health Sciences Center, Denver, CO. Abstract presented at 21st Annual Meeting of Society of Gynecologic Oncologists, February 1990.
30. Raftery AJ: Regeneration of parietal and visceral peritoneum. An electron microscopical study. J Anat 1973; 115:375.
31. Elkins TE, Stovall TG, Warren J: A histological evaluation of peritoneal injury and repair: Implications for adhesion formation. Obstet Gynecol 1987; 70:225.
32. Metz SA, Chegini N, Masterson BJ: In vivo tissue reactivity and degradation of suture materials: A comparison of Maxon and PDS. J Gynecol Surg 1989; 5(1):37.
33. Van Rijssel EJ, Brand R, Admiraal C, et al.: Tissue reaction and surgical knots: The effect of suture size, knot configuration and knot volume. Obstet Gynecol 1989; 74(1):64.
34. Kenady DE: Management of abdominal wounds. Surg Clin North Am 1984; 64:803.
35. Archie JP Jr, Feldman RW: Primary wound closure with permanent continuous running monofilament sutures. Surg Gynecol Obstet 1981; 153:721.
36. Fagniez P, Hay JM, Lacaine F, Thomsen C: Abdominal midline incisions closure. A randomized prospective trial of 3,135 patients, comparing continuous vs. interrupted polyglycolic acid sutures. Arch Surg 1985; 120:1251.
37. Gallup DG, Talledo OE, King LA: Primary mass closure of midline incisions with a continuous running monofilament suture in gynecologic patients. Obstet Gynecol 1989; 73(4):675.
38. Pepicello J, Yavorek H: Five year experience with tape closure of abdominal wounds. Surg Gynecol 1989; 169:310.

Special Instrumentation

6

Donald B. Maier
Anthony A. Luciano

Reproductive surgery differs from other types of gynecologic and obstetric surgery. The primary goal is restoration of normal anatomy and function, as opposed to excision or destruction. The condition of the tissue that remains in the pelvis after surgery is more important than the tissue that has been sent to Pathology. Specialized training and instrumentation are required for the reproductive surgeon to be able to meet this goal. This chapter focuses on the instrumentation essential for reproductive surgery.

There are several guiding principles of reproductive surgery. These include magnification; prevention of tissue ischemia, drying, and abrasion; delicate handling of tissue; absence or minimization of foreign bodies; and the use of no suture or fine, nonreactive suture without placing tissue on tension. The goal of these principles is the prevention of postoperative adhesions, a topic that is discussed at length in Chapter 8. These principles apply whether surgery is performed either via laparotomy or via laparoscopy, and proper use of the correct instruments will help the surgeon in reaching that goal.

It is essential that the reproductive surgeon have adequate training. A well-trained surgeon using inadequate instruments may have better results than an inexperienced surgeon using the correct instruments. Adequate training is a prerequisite for use of the instruments discussed in this chapter. The purpose of this chapter is to provide an overview of the types of instrumentation available to the reproductive surgeon. Because the types and varieties of instrumentation available change frequently, this chapter is not a directory to specific manufacturers' instruments.

When the surgeon chooses his or her particular instruments, several factors will need to be kept in mind. These include cost and the comfort that the instrument affords the specific surgeon. It is important that the surgeon be able to distinguish essential instruments from unnecessary gadgets. Too many instruments will clutter the operative field and increase the time for surgery. Not all surgeons need all the instruments discussed in this chapter.

INSTRUMENTATION FOR LAPAROTOMY

Magnification

The use of magnification has greatly improved the outcome of delicate reproductive surgery. Magnification may be obtained with loupes, microscopes, and video equipment.

Loupes are the simplest and least expensive form of magnification. They are used at laparotomy, and several types of optical systems are available (Fig. 6–1). In order of increasing cost, complexity, and usefulness, these include a simple lens system, Galilean lens systems, and Kepler prisms. Loupes are mounted on eyeglasses or are available as headbands. For surgeons who already require eyeglasses, loupes that attach to the surgeon's own lenses are available. Loupes give a fixed magnification at a fixed

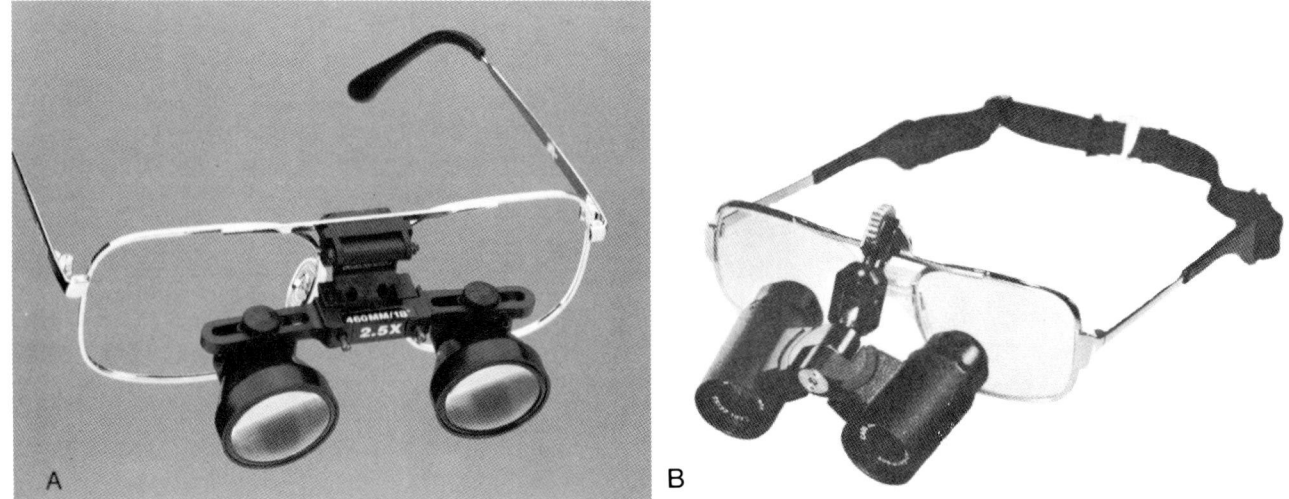

Figure 6–1
Two types of loupes. A, Galilean lens system. B, Kepler prism.

distance. The magnification range available is 1.8× to 8×, with most loupes providing 2.5× to 3.5×. The two major disadvantages of loupes are the limited range of magnification and the neck fatigue brought about by the need to limit head motion. Loupes are especially useful when magnification is required for a short period of time, but they may not provide sufficient magnification for the finer types of surgery, such as an intramural tubal re-anastomosis. Nevertheless, for the surgeon who performs few reproductive surgery cases or who is at a hospital where an operating microscope is not available, loupes may be useful for adhesiolysis and distal tubal surgery.

The operating microscope has become a standard tool for most reproductive surgeons (Fig. 6–2). A microscope is expensive but can be shared with other surgical services such as Neurosurgery and ENT. Magnification is adjustable from 2× to 40×. The microscope is usually mounted on a floor stand, which must be heavy enough to prevent vibrations and tipping but also be mobile enough to be easily moved during the procedure. Angled eyepieces are essential, and a two-headed microscope that provides the assistant with the same view as the surgeon is preferable. Optimally, the second head should be positioned directly opposite from the surgeon and should provide binocular vision. Some operating microscopes have a motorized head through which the height, zoom, focus, and lateral movement can be controlled by a foot pedal. This is a helpful but expensive addition.

The reproductive surgeon needs to be thoroughly familiar with the microscope that he or she will be using. Before each procedure, the correct functioning of the microscope, light source, and video system must be checked and the focus, height of the microscope, and interpupillary distance of the eyepieces should be adjusted by both surgeons. Attempting to do so during the procedure is both cumbersome and time consuming.

Operating microscopes can have video cameras attached to them, allowing the surgeon's view to be seen by the entire operating room staff. This decreases boredom among nurses and second assistants and also allows for recording cases for teaching or patient education. Alternatively, still photography may be performed for documentation.

Magnification may also be obtained using a video system. This is especially helpful during laparoscopy, where the video system not only provides magnification but also lessens back strain for the operating

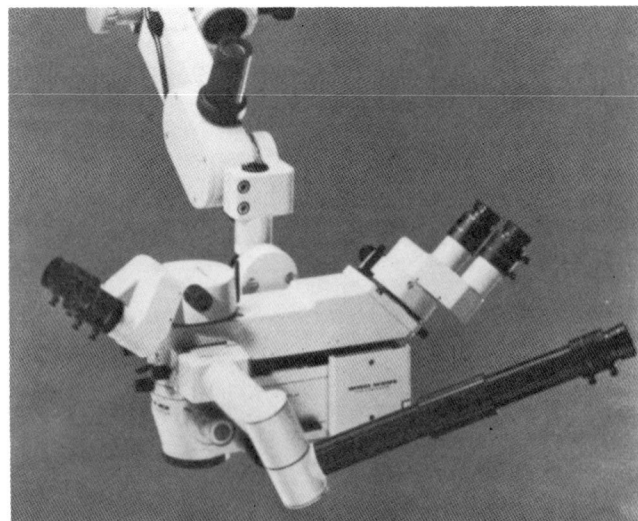

Figure 6–2
An operating microscope with two opposite heads. (From Bermant MA, Shively RE: In Hunt RB (ed.): Atlas of Female Infertility Surgery. Chicago, Year Book Medical Publishers, 1986, p. 92.)

surgeon and provides a view for the assistants. Magnification with the laparoscope alone can be up to fourfold, whereas the additional magnification from the video system depends on the size of the television screen. Video laparoscopy is discussed further in the chapter on laparoscopy (Chapter 26).

Instruments for Tissue Handling

Delicate handling of tissue is one of the primary rules of reproductive surgery. Proper instruments are essential and should only be used for the specific task for which they were designed. Instruments are usually available in both stainless steel and titanium. The latter is more lightweight but also more expensive. Instruments are usually 12–14 cm in length but are available in various lengths for operating in different depths of the pelvis. The instruments must be easy to use, fit the surgeon's hand well, be well balanced, and not be fatiguing with long use. It is also important that instruments that may come in contact with needles be nonmagnetic or be frequently demagnetized.

Delicate instruments require special care and are best cared for by a designated nurse who inspects them routinely for sharpness and any damage. They must not be used for purposes other than those for which they are designed and should not be borrowed by other services.

Tissue forceps are used for a variety of purposes (Fig. 6–3). Forceps that are used to elevate or grasp normal tissue should be lightweight, gentle, and have smooth tips; tissue damage must be avoided. To put tissue on stretch, instruments that hold more firmly should be used, and toothed forceps may be required. However, it is best to avoid the use of toothed forceps on tissue that is not being excised. Forceps may also be used to hold sutures or needles. These forceps should have a flat surface. Platform forceps used for tying suture may also be appropriate for tissue handling. Use of incorrect types of forceps will result either in a slippage of tissue or suture or, conversely, in excessive tissue trauma.

Special types of forceps are available for handling specific tissues. Tubal forceps that gently grasp the tube at the tubal mesentery are preferable to Babcock forceps, which are heavy, lock, and are less flexible. Also available are ovarian forceps, which gently cradle the ovary over a broad surface rather than grasp it tightly over a small surface. Ring forceps, which have a small opening at the tip, are useful in picking up tissue because they distribute pressure over a broader surface and therefore decrease trauma. They can also be used as platform forceps for tying suture; additionally, the ring can be used to help grasp the needle by passing it through the ring and closing the forceps.

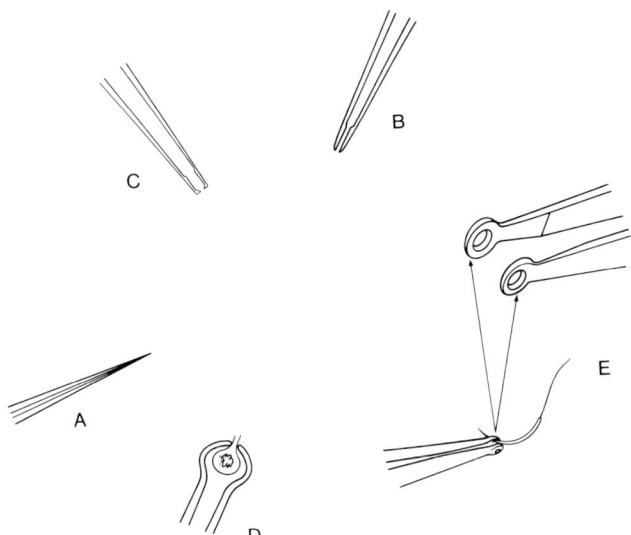

Figure 6–3
Tissue forceps. *A*, Delicate forceps for tissue handling. *B*, Platform forceps for suture tying or tissue handling. *C*, Toothed forceps for handling tissue to be excised. *D*, Tubal forceps for tubal elevation. *E*, Micro-ring forceps for tissue grasping or needle holding.

Scissors

Several types of scissors are required in reproductive surgery (Fig. 6–4). During tubal re-anastomosis, the blunt ends of the tubes must be transsected in order to reach the patent portions. This is best done using relatively large, sharp scissors for a single clean cut. Iris scissors are excellent for this purpose. Scissors are also used to cut through scar tissue and adhesions; in these instances, fine microscissors with slightly rounded tips are best, because the rounded

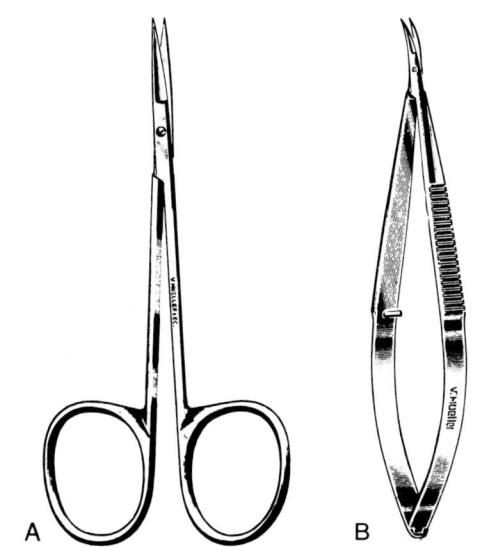

Figure 6–4
Scissors for microsurgery. *A*, Iris scissors for resecting tubal segments prior to tubal re-anastomosis. *B*, Fine scissors for cutting tissue or adhesions.

tips will decrease the chance for inadvertent tissue trauma. Scissors are also necessary for cutting suture; to avoid dulling them, the use of microscissors for cutting large suture must be avoided.

Tissue may also be cut with laser or electrosurgery. There is no evidence that these modalities provide a practical advantage over scissors in terms of tissue healing and ultimate outcome. Laser and electrosurgery are discussed later in this chapter.

Needle Holders

The needle holders used in reproductive surgery must be especially adapted for use with fine needles (Fig. 6–5). Micro needle holders allow the needle to be grasped firmly over a small surface to avoid bending or damaging it. A bent or misshapen needle will cause tissue trauma as it is passed through the tissue. Suture that is greater than 8–0 should be handled with small, traditional needle holders because the larger needles used with this type of suture will damage the jaws of micro needle holders. The needle holder must also allow proper needle handling so that the needle can be passed smoothly through tissue with minimal force.

Different types of micro needle holders are available. The handles of the needle holder may be either flat or round; round ones are preferable because they allow the surgeon to pass the needle smoothly with a simple finger rotation. The tips of most needle holders are flat. Those that have concave and convex surfaces on opposite sides allow for a firmer grasp of the needle, but only if the needle is being held at a right angle. The tips may also be either straight or curved, with the curved tips being more appropriate for suturing at angles. Needle holders are also available in either locking or nonlocking varieties. The advantage of a lock is that the needle can be mounted by the nurse and then passed to the surgeon without fear of the needle falling from the holder and being lost. There is also decreased finger fatigue if the surgeon is not required to grasp the needle holder firmly at all times. However, the unlocking of the needle holder after suture placement produces vibrations that can damage delicate tissue. It is therefore advised that if the surgeon prefers a locking needle holder, the needle holder should be unlocked just before the needle is passed through the tissue. Most reproductive surgeons prefer to use nonlocking needle holders.

Sutures and Needles

Postoperative adhesion formation is promoted when large, reactive suture is used, and the use of fine, nonreactive suture has greatly improved the success of reproductive surgery. However, tissue reaction is least when no suture is used, and data are now accumulating that indicate that the surgeon should think twice before using any suture, especially in the ovary.[1] After ovarian cystectomy, it is possible to leave the ovarian capsule open, rather than placing sutures to approximate the tissue, as long as hemostasis has been obtained. Use of sutures for hemostasis should be limited to large vessels that are not controllable by either defocused laser or bipolar electrocautery. Suturing can cause adhesions by inciting a local reaction, by causing necrosis of the tissue compressed by the knot, and by the tissue trauma from the passage of the needle. If suture is to be used, the surgeon must choose between absorbable or nonabsorbable types. If absorbable suture is used, nonreactive types are essential. These include polyglycolic acid, polyglactin, and polydioxanone, which are absorbed by hydrolysis instead of by macrophage activity. There appear to be minimal differences between these nonreactive sutures, and the individual surgeon's preference may be based on other factors such as the different handling characteristics of the suture. If nonabsorbable suture is used, a nonreactive type such as polypropylene or nylon is needed.

Use of suture for tissue approximation and alignment is obviously important for tubal re-anastomosis. In the future, however, tissue glue may replace sutures in this procedure.

Instruments for Establishing Tubal Patency

During reproductive surgery, the surgeon often needs to establish that the tubes are patent. Tubal

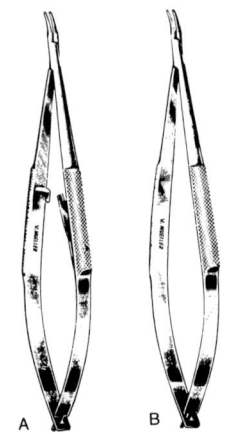

Figure 6–5
Micro needle holders. *A*, Locking. *B*, Nonlocking.

patency is established with minimal trauma using fluids instilled either antegrade or retrograde. This is essential with tubal re-anastomosis, but it is also very helpful with repair of distal tubal occlusion because distention of the distal tube with fluid will reveal the thinnest area of the hydrosalpinx and guide the surgeon to the best areas for incising the tube. Tubal trauma and infection must be minimized, and the perfusion system should not get in the way of the surgeon. At laparotomy, two approaches are possible: transcervical or transfundal. The transcervical apparatus needs to be set up before surgery begins. This may involve either a pediatric Foley catheter placed in the uterus or a specialized device such as the Harris uterine manipulator (HUMI) (Fig. 6–6A). Tubing may be brought up onto the operative field for the surgeon to use during the procedure. If a Foley is used, care must be taken not to overinflate the balloon, because this may fill the uterine cavity and occlude the tubal ostia or kink the tip of the Foley. This error will lead the surgeon to believe that cornual occlusion exists and may result in unnecessary tissue removal. It is also important to ensure that the tubing is not kinked as it is brought up into the operative field.

The transfundal approach usually involves placing a Buxton clamp around the cervix (Fig. 6–6B) and passing an Intracath through the fundus into the uterine cavity. The surgeon needs to be able to enter the uterine cavity at the first attempt; otherwise, the instillation of fluid into the myometrium may compress the cavity and make it impossible to enter on subsequent attempts. The Buxton clamp itself is cumbersome, especially when an operating microscope is also in the field. At times, after the needle is removed from the fundus, troublesome bleeding may occur from the needle track. However, when a transcervical perfusion system has not been placed before laparotomy, or if the system fails, it may be necessary to resort to the transfundal approach.

Although tubal patency is usually established with chromotubation, tubal probing is occasionally needed. A variety of tubal probes are available but should be used only when necessary. Probing increases the potential for intratubal bleeding, which may be difficult to stop and may result in adhesions. Any probe that is used needs to have a blunted tip. Lacrimal duct probes are frequently used and are available in several sizes. Use of an intravenous catheter or pediatric feeding tube is another method for tubal cannulation that provides a flexible probe. At tubal re-anastomosis, it is sometimes helpful to pass a suture through the distal portion of the tube from the fimbriated end into the proximal portion and then into the uterus to act as a temporary stent while sutures are being placed in the tube. To cannulate the distal segment, a special probe with a blunted obturator is passed through the distal tubal segment, the obturator is removed, and the suture is then passed through the hollow probe (Fig. 6–7).

Other Instrumentation

Malleable Teflon rods are available for use as backstops for electrosurgery (Fig. 6–8). These blunt rods are available in numerous sizes and lengths and are useful for elevating adhesions during adhesiolysis. They cannot be used at laser surgery, when titanium rods must be used.

During delicate microsurgical procedures, the sur-

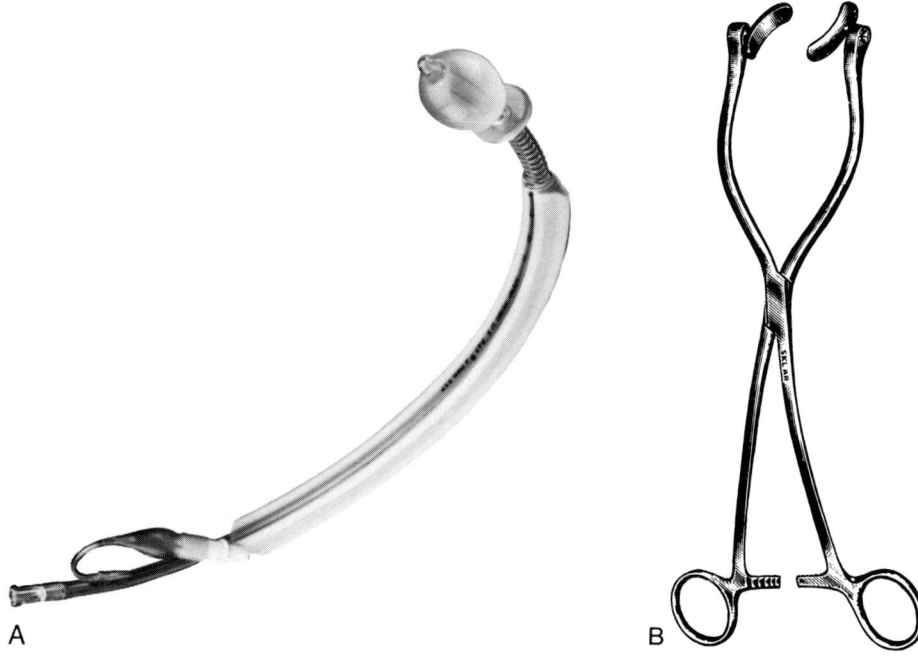

Figure 6–6
Special instrumentation for documenting tubal patency. A, Harris uterine manipulator. This device is inserted into the cervix and held in place by inflating the balloon at the distal end. The rigid nature of the device allows it to be used to manipulate the uterus, and chromopertubation is accomplished through the hollow channel. (HUMI® [Harris Kronner Uterine Manipulation/Injector] available from: UNIMAR,® Inc., Wilton, Connecticut.) B, Buxton clamp. This instrument occludes the cervix at abdominal procedures. Transfundal tubal perfusion can then be accomplished without dye flowing out through the cervix.

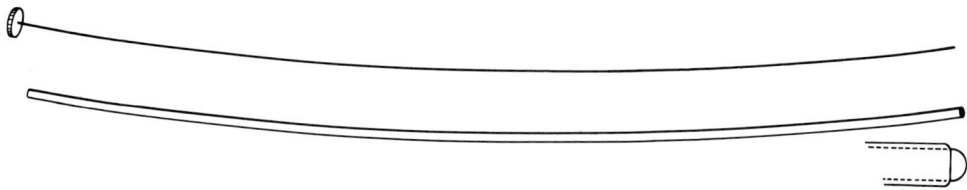

Figure 6–7
A hollow guide that can be used for tubal cannulation and placement of an intratubal stent. The tip of the obturator is rounded to decrease tissue trauma. At tubal re-anastomosis, the assembled device is passed through the fimbriated end of the tube to the proximal end of the distal tube. The obturator is removed, and a 0 suture is passed though the hollow guide from the fimbriated end and then into the distal end of the proximal segment, forming a stent for aligning the tubal segment during re-anastomosis. The guide is removed after the suture has been passed.

geon's hands must rest on the patient's abdomen in order to reduce tremor. Bulky retractors, such as the O'Connor-O'Sullivan, can interfere with this. Some reproductive surgeons prefer the Kirchner, which has a low profile and no screws or bolts and therefore interferes less with hand movement (Fig. 6–9). The Kirchner retractor also allows for more flexible placement of blades and has shallow blades that decrease the chance for lateral pelvic wall compression and nerve damage.

An irrigation system is essential in reproductive surgery. It allows the surgeon to wash away blood in order to pinpoint bleeders, and helps to keep tissues moist to prevent drying and reduce postoperative adhesions. The irrigation source needs to be able to deliver a precise stream of irrigating fluid. The simplest system is a syringe with an intravenous catheter attached to it. Specific irrigators or irrigators-aspirators are available for use at laparotomy, and some surgeons prefer to use them. As will be discussed, the use of an irrigator-aspirator is essential at laparoscopy.

LAPAROSCOPIC INSTRUMENTATION

Laparoscopic procedures are discussed in Chapter 26. In this section, the focus is on laparoscopic instrumentation. As noted previously, the same microsurgical principles apply in all types of reproductive surgery, regardless of whether those procedures are being performed at laparoscopy or laparotomy. Laparoscopy facilitates the utilization of some of those principles: tissue handling is decreased, tissue trauma with sponges and sutures is eliminated or reduced, and the closed abdomen decreases the potential for tissue drying. However, utilization of other microsurgical principles is sometimes more difficult at laparoscopy, at least for the less experienced surgeon. These include the use of fine suture and provisions for precise hemostasis.

Laparoscopy also imposes limits on instrument design, because the instrument must fit through a trocar that is 3 mm, 5 mm, 10 mm, 12 mm, or 20 mm in diameter. Nevertheless, the same types of

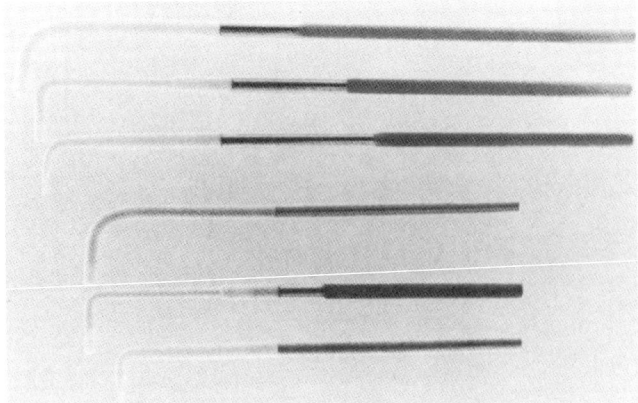

Figure 6–8
Teflon rods. These may be used as backstops for adhesiolysis with electrosurgery or to elevate pelvic structures. The Teflon tips may be bent and are either pointed or blunt. (From Hunt RB: In Hunt RB (ed.): Atlas of Female Infertility Surgery. Chicago, Year Book Medical Publishers, 1986, p. 159.)

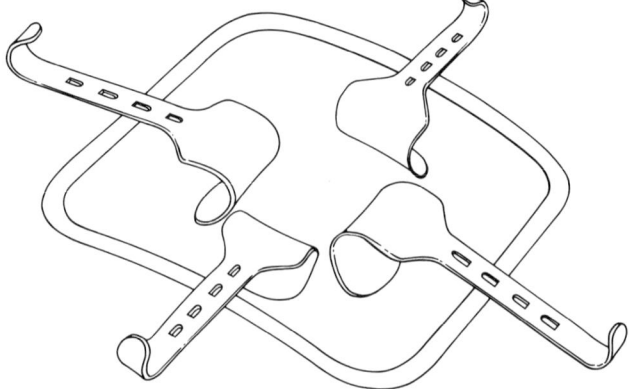

Figure 6–9
Kirchner retractor. The blades may be placed at different sites along the square frame. The low profile allows the surgeon to rest his or her hands on the abdomen and thereby decreases tremor.

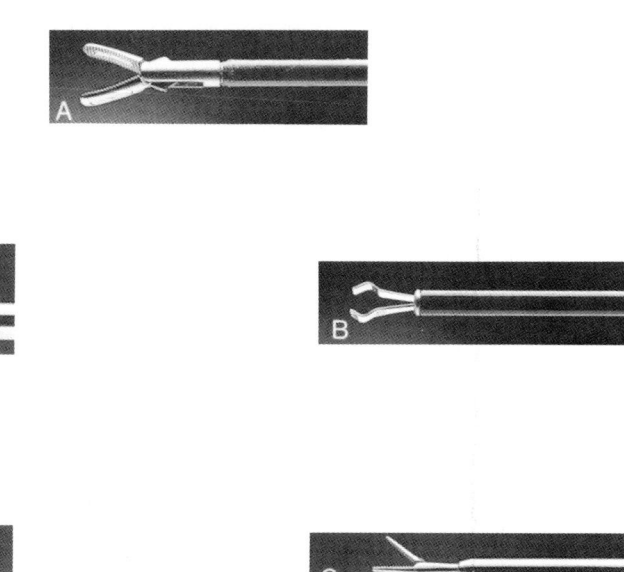

Figure 6–10
Laparoscopic instruments. *A*, Standard forceps. *B*, Atraumatic forceps. *C*, Fine forceps. *D*, Small toothed forceps. *E*, Needleholder. *F*, Myoma claw forceps.

instruments are available for laparoscopy as for laparotomy (Fig. 6–10). Forceps must be able to grasp tissue firmly but not damage it. The laparoscopic forceps initially used were too broad for precise tissue pickup, and finer and less traumatic forceps are now available. As at laparotomy, the surgeon should use forceps appropriate for the task at hand: pointed, fine forceps for fimbrioplasty; heavier toothed graspers for traction on fibroids or cyst walls; and rounded, wide forceps for removing ectopic pregnancies.

Standard laparoscopic scissors have blades that are too large for fine dissections, and microscissors should be used for delicate tasks (Fig. 6–11). However, many laparoscopists prefer the use of the laser or electrosurgery for tissue cutting. The laser is well suited to use through the laparoscope because the CO_2 beam or the laser fibers can be easily introduced through the primary or secondary laparoscopic sites. Electrosurgical instruments designed specifically for use in laparoscopic reproductive surgery are being introduced (Fig. 6–12). These include microbipolar cautery for coagulation and fine unipolar electrodes for cutting. Instruments initially designed for tubal cautery and destruction are not well designed for control of small bleeding points or cauterization of thin adhesions prior to division with the scissors. Microelectrosurgical systems are much less expensive than laser systems and are becoming increasingly popular with laparoscopists. Laser and electrosurgical principles are discussed later in this chapter.

Laparoscopic suturing is still difficult. The need

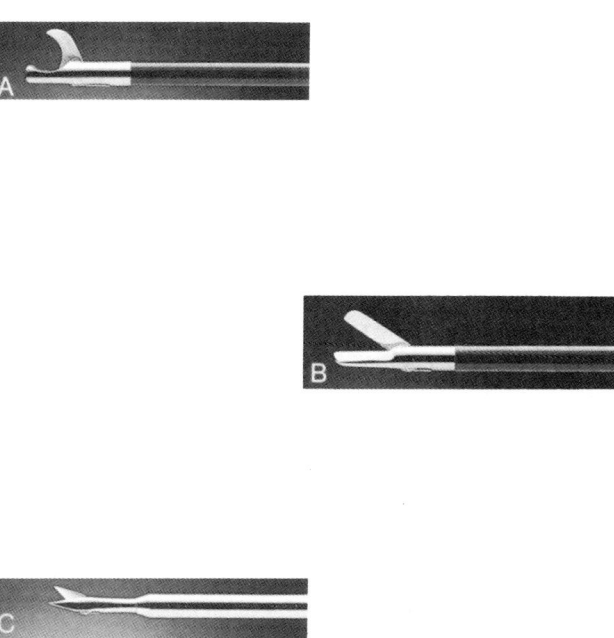

Figure 6–11
Laparoscopic scissors. *A*, Large hook scissors. *B*, Large scissors with teeth. *C*, Microscissors.

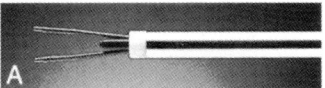

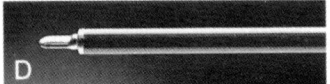
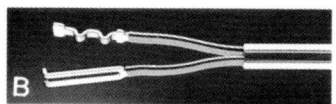

Figure 6–12
Laparoscopic electrosurgical instrumentation. A, Microbipolarforceps. B, Large bipolar forceps. C, Unipolar microelectrode. D, Large unipolar electrode.

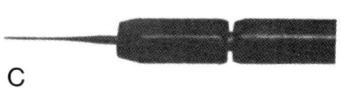

for suturing in most laparoscopic surgery cases has been questioned, but the difficulty in obtaining needles or suture especially adapted for laparoscopic use has also been an important factor in limiting laparoscopic suturing. Learning the technique for suture placement through the laparoscope requires considerable practice. Suture tying with intra-abdominal instrument ties or extra-abdominal knotting is difficult for the novice. Needle holders are generally not well adapted for small, atraumatic needles, and only a limited range of suture sizes and types are available. One useful suturing option is the Roeder loop, which can be used to ligate bulky tissue such as the infundibulopelvic ligament, tubal mesentery, or omentum (Fig. 6–13).

Irrigation and suction are very important in laparoscopic surgery. Irrigation is used for washing away char from laser procedures and for better visualization of small bleeding vessels prior to cautery. Irrigation can also be used, at high pressure, for tissue dissection and for creating planes during surgery. Because of the large quantities of fluid used during laparoscopic procedures, an adequate mechanism for suctioning the pelvis is required. Instruments that are combination aspirators-irrigators and that can also be employed as laser backstops are some of the most useful instruments for laparoscopic procedures (Fig. 6–14).

Other specialized instruments for laparoscopic surgery are available. These include tissue morcellators, which reduce large masses of tissue to smaller fragments that can be removed through the small laparoscopic trocar, and ampullary dilators for breaking up fine adhesions at the fimbriated end of the tube (Fig. 6–14). As laparoscopic surgery becomes more commonplace, the range of instruments will expand, so that almost all types of reproductive surgical procedures may be performed through the laparoscope; whether or not a specific procedure should be performed that way will depend primarily on the skill and training of the reproductive surgeon.

Magnification can be easily obtained with the laparoscope by use of a video system, and the use of video laparoscopy has added to both the ability to magnify and the use of surgery. The television monitor is as important a laparoscopic instrument as any other. By allowing the surgeon to perform these sometimes long and complicated laparoscopic pro-

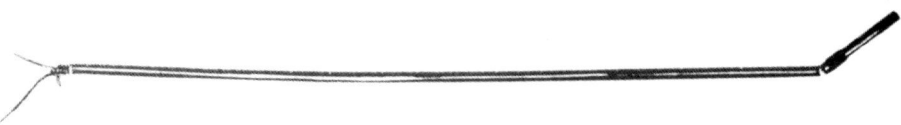

#6663-1 Ethibinder Looped Suture

Figure 6–13
Roeder loop for tissue ligation.

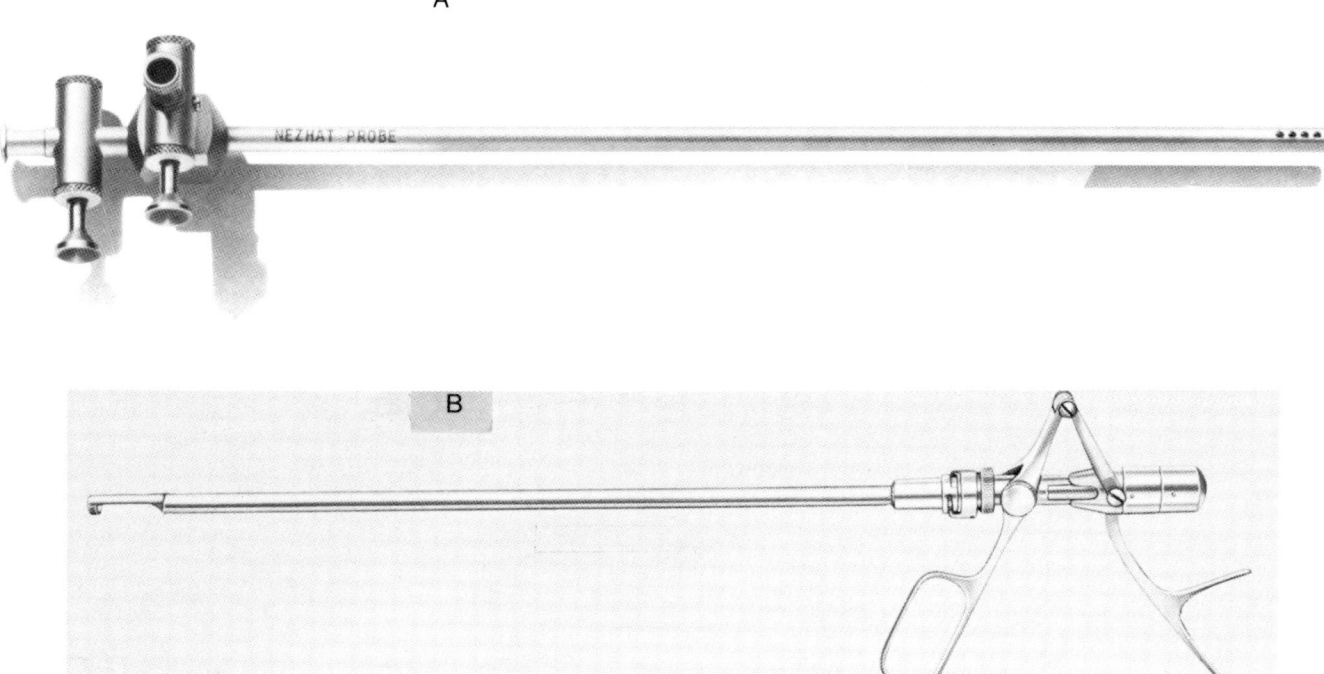

Figure 6–14
Other laparoscopic instruments. A, Aspirator-irrigator that can also be used as a backstop for laser surgery. B, Morcellator used to reduce large, bulky tissue, such as fibroids, to smaller pieces for removal from the abdomen.

cedures in the much more comfortable upright position, the use of a video monitor helps reduce back strain and fatigue for the surgeon and allows the assistants and nurses to actively participate in the surgical procedure as it unfolds on the video monitor screen. With practice, the reproductive surgeon can become as proficient or more proficient operating while viewing the video monitor as operating while looking through the laparoscope.

The impact of operative laparoscopy on the current and future practice of gynecologic surgery in the United States is not difficult to imagine. The question is not whether or not operative laparoscopy is going to have a place in our surgical armamentarium, but how extensive it is going to be. Because of high patient acceptance and decreased morbidity, discomfort, and cost associated with laparoscopic surgery,[2] in the future the ability to perform laparoscopic surgery will be a skill demanded of all reproductive surgeons. The techniques of operative laparoscopy do not differ from other delicate surgical techniques that require a combination of knowledge, proper training, practice, and caution. If the results from endoscopic surgery continue to compare favorably with those obtained with the more invasive laparotomy, endoscopic surgery will profoundly change our specialty and future reproductive surgeons may be more accurately referred to as microsurgical endoscopists.

HYSTEROSCOPIC INSTRUMENTATION

Hysteroscopic surgery in general is discussed in Chapter 26. In this chapter, the discussion is limited to the different types of hysteroscopic instruments available.

The type of hysteroscope determines the types of instruments that are usable. This differs from the situation with laparoscopy, in which the optics and the instrumentation are usually separate. Flexible hysteroscopes allow passage of only thin, flexible catheters, and are therefore not useful for operative hysteroscopy. Most traditional hysteroscopes allow for passage of flexible instruments, with rigid instruments being limited to hysteroscopes with offset optics or to hysteroscopes with the instrument permanently mounted at the distal end of the sheath (Fig. 6–15). This latter arrangement decreases the flexibility of the instrument, because the scissors or forceps are fixed and cannot be retracted within the hysteroscope. Larger rigid instruments require a larger diameter hysteroscope, which requires more cervical dilatation and may be more traumatic. Laser fibers, however, may be used through smaller hysteroscopes.

The same types of instrumentation are available in both flexible and rigid varieties (Fig. 6–16). Instruments are available either for tissue cutting or for

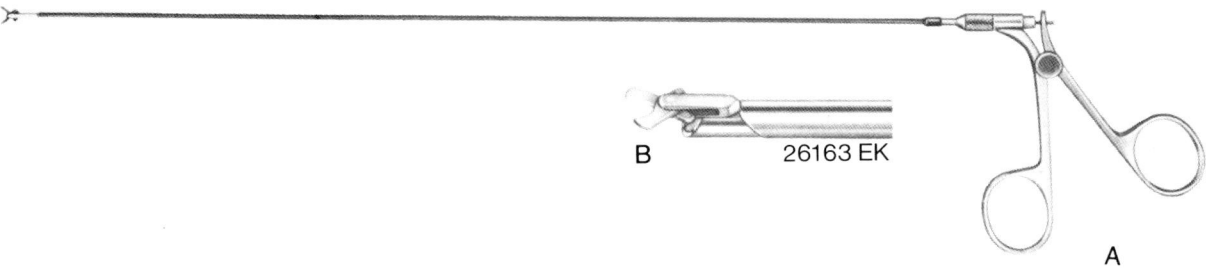

Figure 6–15
Types of hysteroscope instrumentation. A, Flexible scissors. B, Rigid scissors fixed to end of hysteroscope sheath.

cautery. Cutting is used for uterine septa, adhesions, or fibroids. Scissors are commonly used, but some hysteroscopes allow for passage of a small knife that may be used either as a cold knife or with cautery. Cutting may also be performed with a laser (Argon, KTP, or Nd:YAG) or with a thin electrocautery loop. Cauterization may be required for hemostasis, as in the case of bleeding after resection of a septum; for excision, as in the removal of a fibroid; or for tissue ablation, as in endometrial ablation. Coagulation or ablation is best obtained when a large electrode, such as a roller ball, is used. The resectoscope allows more flexibility because the electrical element can move separately from the body of the scope, and electrical loops are available in a variety of shapes and sizes (Fig. 6–17). The basic electrosurgical principles discussed in the next section apply for use with the hysteroscope. It is also important to keep in mind that uterine perforation during electrosurgery may result in electrical damage to bowel.

The variety of types of different hysteroscopic media is also discussed in Chapter 26 and is not discussed in detail here. However, the choice of media does have some impact on instrumentation. If Hyskon is used, it is essential that instrumentation be cleaned promptly after the procedure to avoid drying of Hyskon and freezing of moving parts, especially with small scissors. If low-viscosity fluids are used, it is important to remember that some fluids, such as saline, will conduct electricity and cannot be used during electrosurgery.

ELECTROSURGERY AND LASERS

This section describes the two available energy forms that can be used in reproductive surgery—electrical and laser. Each form is considered separately, including a discussion of necessary basic physics. Finally, the different modalities are compared. The reproductive surgeon must understand the underlying principles of both modalities in order to use the instrumentation safely and effectively; whereas the instrumentation will continue to evolve and change, the physical principles will not.

Electrosurgery

Electrosurgery is underutilized and misunderstood by many surgeons. Electrosurgery was initially used for procedures such as tubal cautery and became associated with destructive, not reconstructive, surgery; it also became associated with unexpected and unpredictable complications such as bowel burns. However, these complications are more often the result of faulty or incorrectly used instrumentation rather than a flaw in the surgical theory itself. Because they do not understand basic electrosurgical principles, many surgeons consider electrosurgery to be mysterious and untrustworthy. However, with correct use of electrosurgical instruments, the reproductive surgeon can use this modality as a major tool in tissue cutting and hemostasis. This section reviews the necessary electrosurgical terms and concepts and then discusses the available electrosurgical instruments.

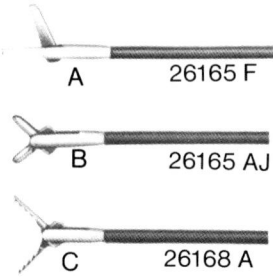

Figure 6–16
Hysteroscopic instrumentation. A, Scissors. B, Biopsy forceps. C, Grasper.

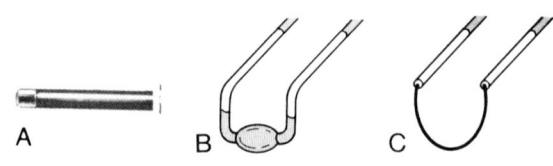

Figure 6–17
Hysteroscopic electrosurgical instrumentation. A, Ball cautery. B, Roller ball. C, Loop electrode. Instruments shown in B and C are used with the resectoscope.

Electrosurgical Principles

Electrical energy comes from the flow of electrons. This current is described by several important, interrelated terms. The ampere is the *rate of current flow*, the volt is the *unit of force* driving the flow, the ohm is the *resistance* of the tissue to the flow, and the watt is the *amount of work* produced by the flow. A current of one ampere is produced by one volt applied across a resistance of one ohm. Wattage is equal to volts multiplied by amperes. In the clinical situation, the voltage is determined by the generator and the resistance is determined by the tissue involved. Tissue resistance ranges from 100 to 1000 ohms, but changes during electrosurgery. With tissue coagulation, evaporation of water leads to increased resistance, which eventually becomes so high that current will no longer flow. At this point, if high voltage is being applied, the energy will seek other outlets and sparking will occur. If low voltage is used, flow will simply and safely stop. It is therefore very important that the surgeon be aware of the characteristics of the generator being used, especially with delicate reproductive surgery. Generators providing more than 100 watts are unnecessarily powerful for gynecologic surgery.

Electron flow is not unidirectional; with alternating current, the flow is constantly changing direction. These changes, resulting in the voltage increasing to maximum in one direction, dropping to zero, and then increasing to maximum in the other direction, result in a wave form (Fig. 6–18). The frequency with which the current changes direction is measured in hertz (Hz). Normal household current is 60 Hz. Nerves and muscles respond to frequencies below 10,000 Hz, and therefore for electrosurgery the normal alternating current must be converted into a much higher frequency to avoid unwanted tissue effects. Normal generators provide frequencies between 300,000 and 4,000,000 Hz.

Different wave patterns produce different tissue effects (Fig. 6–19). A continuous high-frequency flow of electrons will provide intense heat and cut through the tissue by exploding the cells (cutting current). The energy is actually transferred by a spark jumping from the electrode to the tissue. On the other hand, bursts of rapidly increasing current interrupted by intervals without current result in cell heating and dehydration with hemostasis and charring but no cutting (coagulating current). With coagulating current, there is less tissue heating because the pause between bursts of current allows the heat to dissipate. Many generators provide a blended current combining these two types. In this situation, there is a continuous but altering wave form that will simultaneously cut and provide coagulation. Blended current is preferable to pure cutting current in almost all situations.

Electrons will flow only when there is a completed circuit. Unipolar and bipolar systems differ with respect to how much of the patient's tissue is in the circuit (Fig. 6–20). In a unipolar system, current flow proceeds from the electrode to the tissue being cut or cauterized. Flow then spreads out through the rest of the body and leaves through a return plate attached over a broad surface such as the buttocks or a leg. As the electrical energy spreads out, the electron density is diffused and the tissue is not heated. Situations that inadvertently concentrate electron flow may result in tissue damage; examples include a small loop of bowel adherent to the tube or an incompletely applied return plate. Therefore, with a unipolar system, potential damage to adjacent organs is a constant concern. This concern decreases when a bipolar system is used. A bipolar system does not involve use of a return plate, and only a

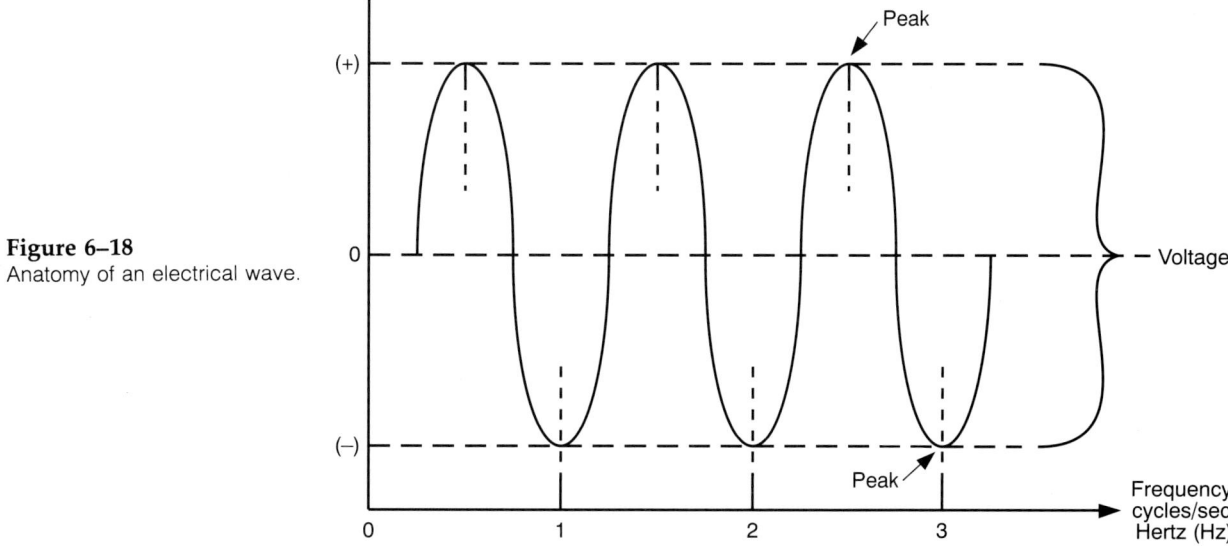

Figure 6–18 Anatomy of an electrical wave.

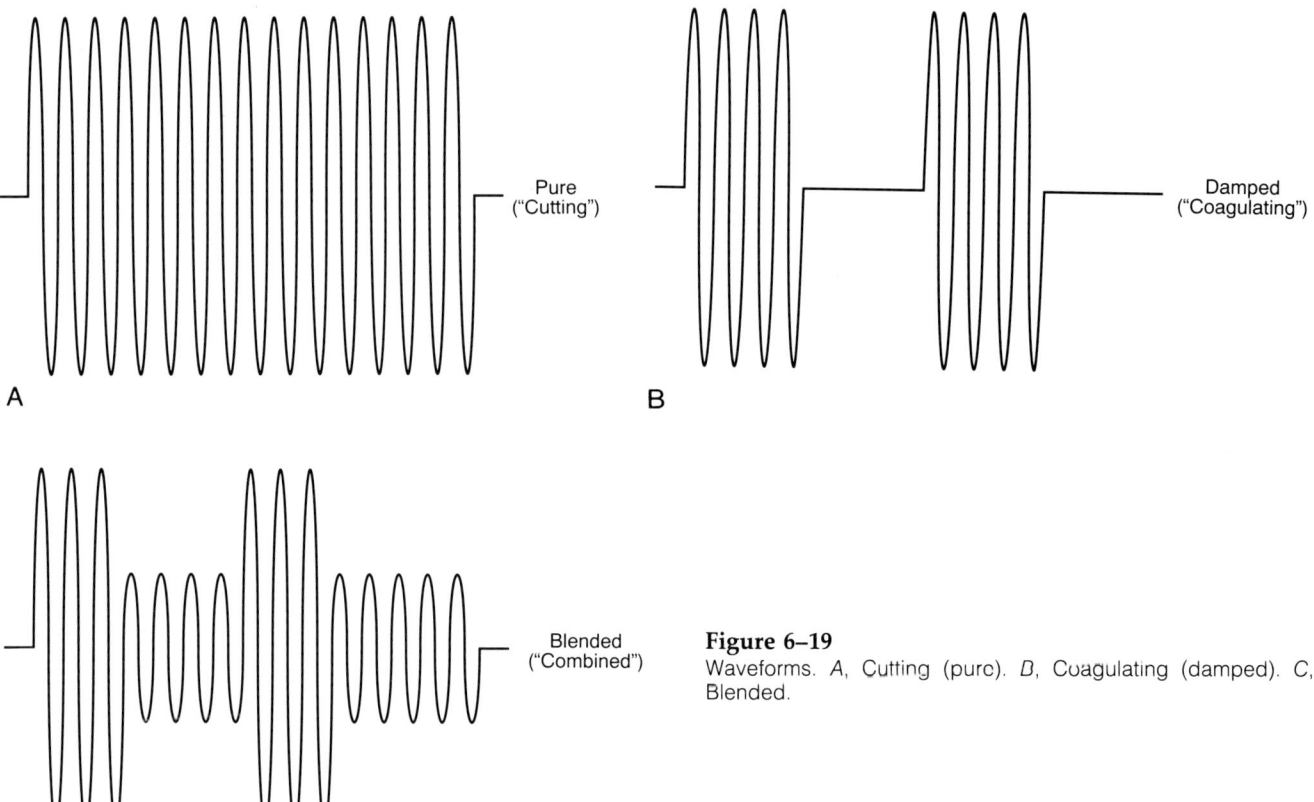

Figure 6–19
Waveforms. A, Cutting (pure). B, Coagulating (damped). C, Blended.

small amount of tissue is included in the circuit. With bipolar systems, the return electrode is adjacent to the active electrode and current flows only between them. An example is the Kleppinger tubal forceps, in which one prong of the forceps is the active electrode and the other is the return (Fig. 6–21). The tube that is grasped between the prongs is the only tissue that current flows through, and adjacent organs are not part of the circuit. There will, however, be transmission of some heat to surrounding tissue. Although it increases the margin of safety, bipolar cauterization requires that the tissue being coagulated be surrounded by the forceps and is therefore more difficult to use with retracted vessels. This grasping of tissue can coapt the walls of vessels before the current is passed, which further helps to seal the vessels. Bipolar current can only provide coagulation and cannot be used to cut tissue.

The distinction between unipolar and bipolar cautery is especially important at laparoscopy, where most unipolar electrodes are large and the potential for complications is therefore increased. The development of unipolar microelectrodes for laparoscopy has increased the safety of laparoscopic unipolar electrosurgery, but the surgeon still needs to be aware of the basic differences between unipolar and bipolar systems. At laparotomy, for adhesiolysis or pinpoint coagulation, the handheld unipolar electrode is extremely small and precise. As to be discussed, a comparison of state of the art unipolar electrosurgery and laser surgery reveals them to be similar in terms of adjacent tissue damage.

Electrosurgical Instrumentation

There are two principal parts of electrosurgical instrumentation: the generator and the electrode. The generator supplies the current flow and is adjustable to enable the surgeon to deliver the correct energy levels for the situation at hand. As discussed previously, use of a generator at excessively high settings may result in tissue damage. It is also important that the electrosurgical generator be matched with the proper electrode. A large electrode will produce coagulation effects even with cutting current. For tissue cutting, fine electrodes that deliver a more concentrated flow of electrons will result in cutting with minimal charring. When using microelectrodes, a low current is necessary. Use of a high current will result in sparking, adjacent tissue damage, and burning of the electrode wire. An electrosurgical generator designed for microsurgery is required when a microelectrode is being used; attempting to adapt macrosurgical equipment to microsurgical cases will result in unsatisfactory results. A variety of types of microelectrodes are available. Some are insulated, with

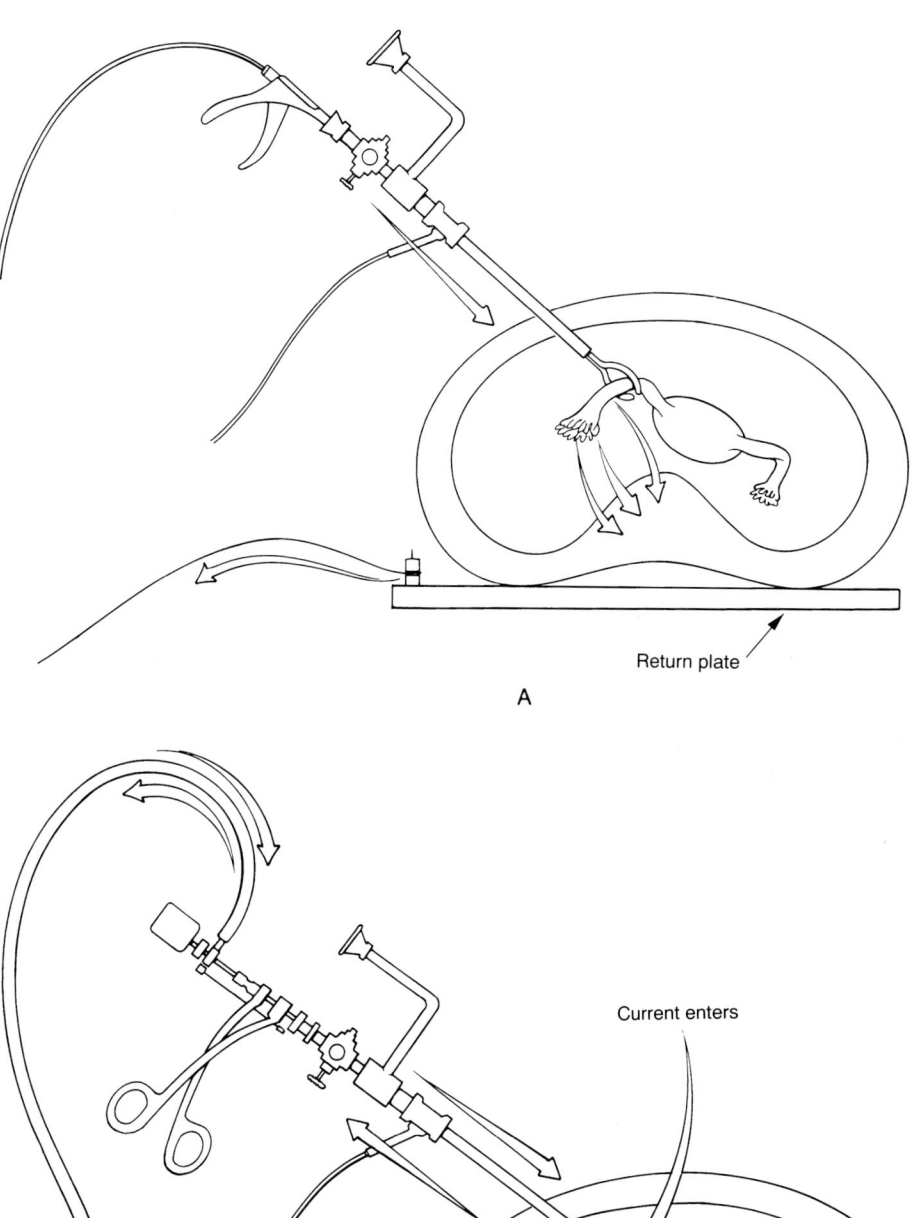

Figure 6–20
Unipolar and bipolar circuitry compared. *A*, Unipolar current enters through the electrode, is concentrated at the point of contact with the tissue, and then spreads out to exit through the large return plate. The circuit is large. *B*, Bipolar current enters through one electrode, passes through a small amount of tissue, and leaves through the other electrode. The circuit is small.

120 SPECIAL INSTRUMENTATION

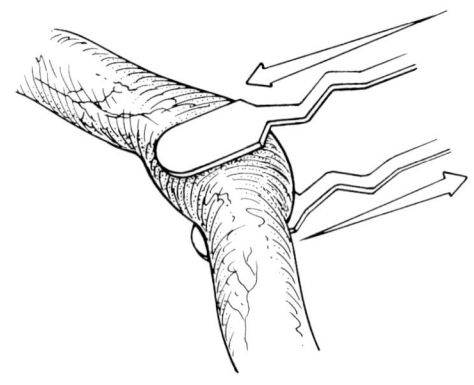

Figure 6–21
Detail of Kleppinger bipolar forceps for tissue cautery. Electrons pass from one electrode, through the tissue, and then exit through the opposite electrode.

only the tip being exposed. This will decrease the chance of inadvertent damage to lateral tissue during adhesiolysis.

With reproductive surgery, the principles of microsurgery must be followed when using electrosurgery. Therefore, tissue damage and spread of thermal and electrical damage to surrounding tissue must be kept to a minimum. Electrosurgery provides the surgeon with a wide range of options: type of current, power level, unipolar or bipolar systems, and type of electrode. Given the proper equipment and an understanding of the electrosurgical principles, the reproductive surgeon can use electrosurgery in many useful ways. Faulty or improper equipment, or lack of understanding by the surgeon, will result in poor surgical outcome and a higher possibility of unnecessary complications.

Lasers

Often referred to as "the light that heals," the surgical laser was first introduced by Fox in 1969.[3] In 1979, Bruhat and colleagues introduced the use of the CO_2 laser via laparoscopy, which further expanded its role and potential usefulness in gynecologic surgery.[4] Like all innovations, the laser has had both strong advocates who have made glowing and sometimes unrealistic claims regarding its usefulness and its share of skeptics who have too quickly dismissed it as just another gimmick. Although not a panacea, the usefulness of lasers in our specialty is no longer in question and, as more versatile lasers are developed and introduced, its role in reproductive surgery will continue to expand.

Laser Principles

Laser is an acronym for "light amplification by stimulated emission of radiation." The laser is a device that produces and amplifies light energy to create intense, coherent electromagnetic radiation. However, unlike the ionizing radiation of x-rays and gamma rays, which result from nuclear destruction, the radiation emitted by a laser results from the release of photons that occurs when stimulated electrons circling their nuclei return from their "excited" (E2) to their "resting" (E1) states (E2 − E1 = photon) (Fig. 6–22). These intermediate-energy photons induce molecular vibration and create heat.

The electromagnetic energy of lasers is both a propagated wave and a discrete photon with energy and momentum. The energy, wavelength, and frequency of a photon depend upon the quantum of energy released by the electron. Because each lasing substance has a unique atomic and/or molecular structure, with its characteristic electron orbits and energy levels, the wavelength, amplitude, and frequency of photons emitted by each substance (CO_2, KTP, etc.) will be unique and uniform. Although powerful and penetrating, laser light is neither mutagenic nor carcinogenic.

Unlike incandescent light, laser light is totally uniform, being monochromatic, coherent, and collimated (Fig. 6–23). Monochromatic light consists of a single wavelength that cannot be separated into any other components; regular light, in contrast, can be separated into all colors of the spectrum by passing it through a prism. When all the light waves are exactly in phase with one another and all waves are parallel, the light is said to be coherent and collimated, respectively. Because the laser light waves have exactly the same length, are in phase with one another, and always run parallel, the laser light can be precisely focused by lenses into a very small spot, which can develop an extremely high power density.

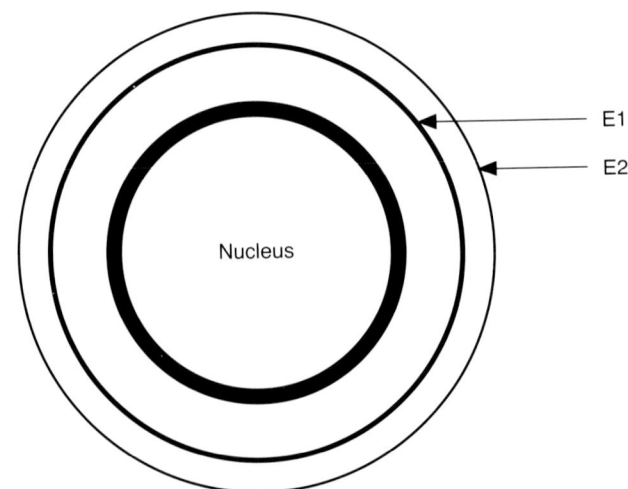

Figure 6–22
Excited (E2) and resting (E1) states of electrons. Laser radiation is released when the electron drops from the E2 state to the E1 state.

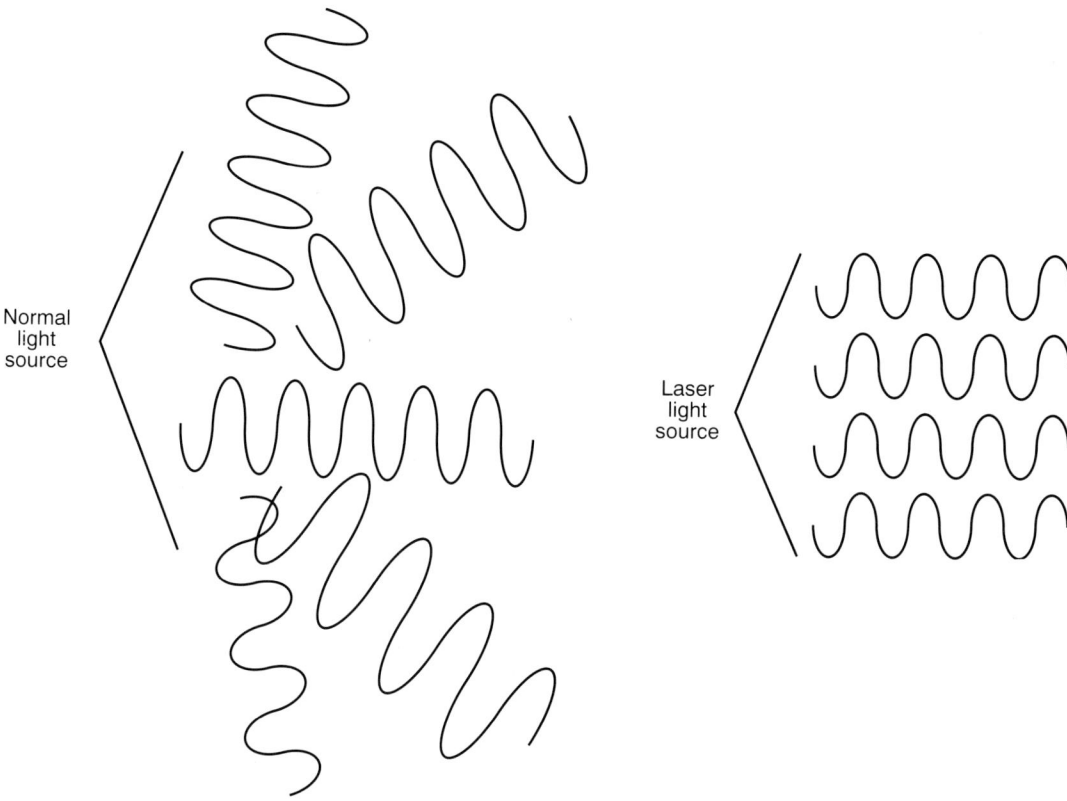

Figure 6–23
Laser light waves compared with regular light waves. With regular light, different wavelengths emerge at many angles; with laser, the waves are of uniform length (monochromatic), in phase with each other (coherent), and parallel (collimated).

The amount of power delivered by lasers is measured in watts. However, the penetrating power of the laser depends largely on the diameter of the laser spot. Thus, the power density is a much better indicator of the penetrating force of the laser energy than the wattage setting on the laser machine. The power density is directly related to the wattage and inversely related to the spot size, as illustrated by the following formula:

$$\text{Power density (watts/cm}^2) = \frac{\text{watts} \times 100}{\text{spot diam}^2 \text{ (cm}^2)}$$

As the laser beam strikes the tissue, the cells at the site of impact are rapidly heated and then vaporized, ablated, or coagulated, depending on the power density employed. Tissue effects of different power densities are as follows:

10–100 watts/cm^2: surface heating and coagulation
400–1200 watts/cm^2: vaporization and some hemostasis
4000–25000 watts/cm^2: rapid vaporization and less hemostasis
>25000 watts/cm^2: very rapid vaporization with minimal hemostasis

Although these general guidelines for power densities and tissue effects were developed for the CO_2 laser, they can be applied to other types of lasers and to electrosurgery as well.[5]

Besides the power density, other determinants of the tissue effects of laser include the degree to which a specific laser is absorbed, refracted, or reflected by the impacted tissue. For example, the CO_2 laser is fully absorbed by water; therefore, tissue, being made up mostly of water, will absorb all of the laser energy, boil, and vaporize immediately. Argon, KTP, and Nd:YAG lasers are not absorbed by water or clear tissues but are fully absorbed by pigmented tissues containing hemoglobin. Consequently, they have been successfully employed to coagulate bleeding on the retina of the eye without affecting the clear structures in front of it. Similarly, they have been successfully used to coagulate bleeding esophageal varices and to ablate endometrium and vascular tumors. Table 6–1 describes the commonly used lasers in gynecologic surgery and their properties.

The major types of lasers currently used in surgery are the CO_2, argon, KTP-532, and Nd:YAG. Developmental work involves the use of the krypton, excimer, free electron, and tunable lasers, which may have surgical applications in the future. The carbon dioxide laser was the first laser to be used in our specialty. The CO_2 laser emits photons with a wavelength of 10.6 micra, which is within the infrared of

Table 6–1
Properties of Lasers Commonly Used in Gynecologic Surgery

	CO_2	Nd:YAG	Argon	KTP-532
Wavelength (μm)	10.6	1.064	0.458–0.515	0.532
Visible light	No	No	Yes	Yes
Flexible fibers	No	Yes	Yes	Yes
Color dependent	No	Yes	Yes	Yes
Effects of fluid on beam	Strongly absorbed	Slightly absorbed	Not absorbed	Not absorbed
Degree of scatter	Minimal	Significant	Moderate	Moderate
Approximate depth of tissue destruction (mm)	0.1	4.0	0.5	0.4
Cutting capabilities	Very good	Fair with sapphire tips	Fair	Fair
Coagulation capabilities	Poor	Very good	Good	Good

the electromagnetic spectrum and therefore cannot be seen. Therefore, the CO_2 laser is delivered together with the helium-neon (He-Ne) laser, which is visible and serves as the aiming beam. The CO_2 laser offers high power density and high efficiency and is ideally suited for cutting and vaporizing. It is highly absorbed by nonreflective solids and liquids, is not dependent upon the color of tissue for absorption, and is not significantly scattered from the target point. Thus, the thermal damage to tissue is limited to the target tissue and deeper or adjacent layers are spared. The CO_2 laser cannot be delivered through fluids, is a poor coagulator, and, as of this writing, cannot be delivered by fibers. A large range of power densities are available with the CO_2 laser by varying the output wattage or the diameter of the laser spot. Low power densities, being more hemostatic, are used for the cervix and myomas, where hemostasis is important and thermal damage is not a major concern. Higher power densities are preferred for reconstructive adnexal surgery, where thermal damage must be minimized.

KTP-532 and argon lasers are very similar in their characteristics and clinical applications, because they have similar wavelengths of 0.532 and 0.458–0.515 micra, respectively. Both release a visible green light that travels through clear fluids and is absorbed by dark-pigmented tissue, and both can be delivered through flexible fibers, making them well suited for endoscopic use. Because they are not absorbed by clear fluids or unpigmented tissue, these lasers are ideal for coagulation of retinal bleeding or for ablation of peritoneal endometriosis, where tissue coagulation can be effected without disrupting the clear overlying tissue. The argon laser is available in two models—5 and 16 watts—for abdominal and pelvic surgery. The 16-watt model is more useful for reproductive surgery and ablation of endometriosis. This model requires high electrical current energy, triple phase, in excess of 200 volts at 60 amps. The laser fibers range in size from 300 to 600 micra in diameter and can be introduced through the small channels of the operating laparoscope or ancillary trocars, and may be steered toward the target with special bridges. The laser beam is at maximal focus at the tip of the fiber; as the distance from the tissue increases, the spot size increases (the beam diffuses) and the power density diminishes.

Because of back-scatter and the potential for retinal damage, protective goggles or eyewear is absolutely necessary when operating the argon laser. When using the laser through the laparoscope, the operator may choose to cover the eyepiece of the laparoscope with the "monoshutter"—an electronically triggered eyepiece that attaches to the laparoscope and interposes a protective filter between the operator's eye and the laparoscope when the laser is fired. The monoshutter may be used equally well with the video cameras for video surgery and documentation.

The Nd:YAG laser is a crystal laser with a wavelength of 1.064 micra, in the near-infrared part of the spectrum. The YAG laser is invisible, highly color dependent, and passes through fibers and clear fluids. The YAG laser penetrates deeply into tissue, which is advantageous in coagulating tumors, in hemorrhaging ulcers, and in endometrial ablation. Although it is an excellent coagulator, the YAG laser is a poor cutter unless used with sapphire tips to increase the power density and produce the ability to vaporize as well as ablate. The YAG laser is not a good choice for reconstructive adnexal disease because of the large amount of scatter and excessive thermal damage to tissue.

Laser Components

The laser consists of a pumping system, lasing medium, optical cavity, and controls (operating system). The pumping system is the power source that energizes the atoms of the lasing medium to higher energy states. The lasing medium may be a solid such as a ruby crystal or Nd:YAG, a gas such as CO_2 or He-Ne, or a liquid such as gallium arsenide diode. The optical cavity, also referred to as a resonator cavity, consists of a tube with parallel mirrors on either side, which allow continuous reflection of photons back and forth in all directions as they strike other excited atoms to effect "stimulated emission of radiation." At one end of the optical cavity, the mirror is only partially reflective, thus allowing escape of only those photons that are exactly in phase (coherent) and are traveling in the same parallel direction (collimated). As the photon is repeatedly reflected back and forth between the parallel mirrors of the optical cavity, it progressively accelerates, building in intensity until it finally flashes out of the partially reflective mirror. This amplification is similar to the amplification in the resonator chamber of a musical instrument.

The operating system controls the delivery of the laser to the tissue. It determines the power in watts and the mode at which the laser is delivered from the unit. The power is adjusted by the power control knob. The mode of delivery of the laser energy may be continuous, pulsed, or superpulsed (Fig. 6–24). In the continuous mode, the laser energy is delivered to the tissue without interruption as long as the control pedal remains depressed. The pulsed mode may be in single or repeated pulses. With single pulses, the operating system releases one burst of energy for a specified interval (range 0.05–0.5 seconds) with every depression of the pedal. To discharge a second laser pulse, the pedal must be released and depressed again. The repeat pulse mode delivers intermittent bursts of laser of predetermined width and intervals (number of pulses per second), for as long as the pedal remains depressed. Finally, the superpulse mode of the CO_2 laser releases very rapid pulses at short intervals, delivering extremely high peak power (10 times continuous peak), alternating with refractory very short periods when the laser energy is not delivered. By releasing "bursts" of peak powers, the power density can be increased by fourfold or more over the average obtained with continuous power output. The refractory periods between laser output allow heat to dissipate into the atmosphere rather than being conducted to adjacent tissue, thus minimizing thermal injury.[5] The use of the superpulse mode results in very precise and rapid vaporization with decreased tissue desiccation, carbonization, thermal injury, and smoke plume.

Baggish and ElBakry determined from animal studies that pulse intervals between 0.6 and 0.2 milliseconds, at rates below 700 pulses per second, permit effective ablation with minimal thermal injury.[6] Thus we recommend that for the superpulse mode the pulse duration be set at 0.3 milliseconds at a frequency of 300 pulses per second. These high power densities are desirable when ablating or vaporizing avascular adhesions involving the ovaries and/or fallopian tubes, where thermal tissue injury should be minimized and coagulation effects of the laser are not important. However, when incising vascular tissue, it may be desirable to use lower power densities to take advantage of the coagulation effects obtained.

Delivery Systems

The CO_2 laser beam leaves the optical resonator and is delivered to the end of an articulated arm by

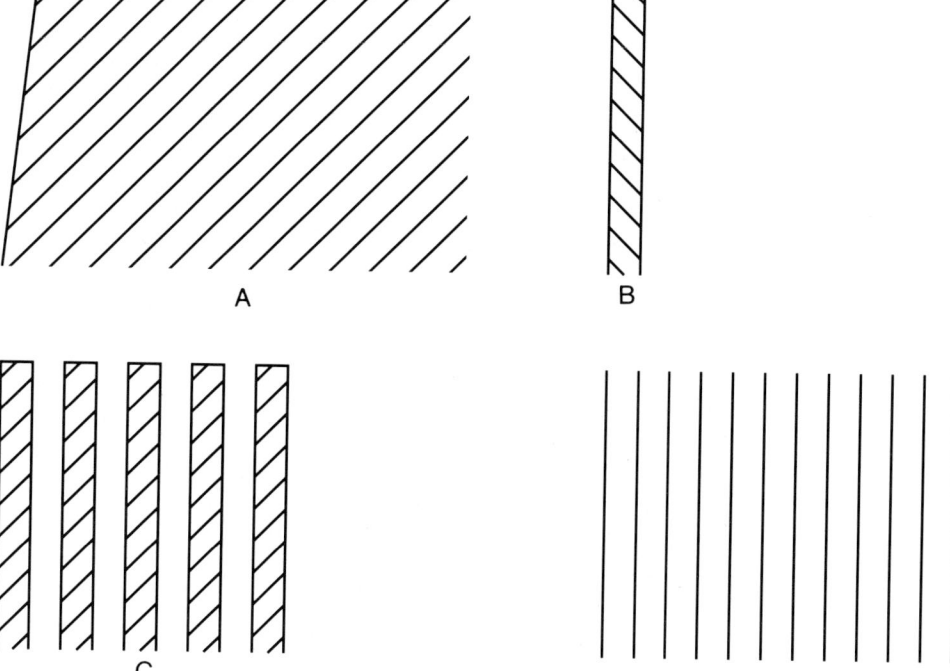

Figure 6–24
Comparison of different modes of laser delivery. A, Continuous. B, Single pulse lasting 0.05–0.5 seconds. C, Repeat pulses. D, Superpulse; each pulse lasts milliseconds.

several metallic mirrors, which are precisely aligned to preserve the configuration and power of the beam as it leaves the generator. When it leaves the arm, the CO_2 laser beam and the He-Ne beam are composed of parallel waves, which need to be focused to increase the power density of the laser. Coupling lenses of various focal lengths are used to focus the beams at the end of the hand-held probe or laparoscope. One type of coupling lens is a fixed lens that is easily assembled between the arm of the laser and the laparoscope. Its focal length may be set at 28 cm if the laser is delivered through the operating channel of the laparoscope or at 18 cm if the laser is delivered through a second puncture site to focus at the end of the shorter accessory trocar. In laparoscopic procedures, the focal point is usually 2.0 cm from the tip of the laparoscope. Instead of a fixed lens, the laser couplers can have a Galilean system with variable focal lengths that allows the surgeon to focus and defocus the laser beam and change the spot size by simply turning a knob on the coupler. This system allows for the focal length to be adjusted between 100 and 315 mm and the spot size to be varied between 0.5 and 2.0 mm in diameter.

It is obvious from the foregoing that the quality of the CO_2 laser output depends largely on the proper alignment of the directing mirrors in the articulated arm of the laser, on the quality and performance of the coupling lens, and on the integrity of the operative channel of the laparoscope. A disturbance of any part of these three systems will result in poor beam alignment and loss of laser power. To avoid this problem, rigid wave guides have been developed that guide the focused laser beam from the articulated arm through the operative channel of the laparoscope to its end, where it is always in perfect focus and in close proximity to the tissue to be lasered. The impact site of the beam lies immediately beyond the tip of the wave guide, which protrudes a few millimeters from the end of the laparoscope. Rigid wave guides are usually composed of ceramics with a high index of refraction so that high power densities may be transmitted with less than a 10% power loss. A purge of continuous carbon dioxide of up to 1000 cc per minute flows down the wave guide channel to keep it cool and clear of smoke. This carbon dioxide serves as an additional source of insufflation to replace the gas evacuated with suctioning of the smoke.

The availability of fiber delivery systems is a major advantage of the argon, KTP and Nd:YAG lasers. These quartz fibers are flexible, light, and thin. They can also be delivered at a greater distance from the laser generator than the CO_2 laser, which needs to be close to the operative field because of its relatively short articulated arm. The laser beam is at maximal focus at the tip of the fiber, which may deliver the laser with or without contact with the tissue (Fig. 6–25). By varying the diameter of the fiber, or the distance between the fiber and the impacted tissue, the power density of the argon or KTP lasers may be adjusted to vaporize, ablate or coagulate. The Nd:YAG laser may be modified with sapphire tips to effect coagulation or vaporization.

In addition to providing a delivery system for the laser beam, fiberoptics may also be used in the future to monitor laser surgery. Sensor data can be returned to console computers for an analysis of tissue effects through the same fiberoptic bundles used to deliver the beam. This type of back-and-forth transmission of light is commonplace in the communication industry today, and may in the future make laser application in surgery much safer and more useful.

Clinical Considerations

Lasers have several unique characteristics that differentiate them from other medical tools. The primary difference is that the tissue is not touched by surgical instruments but only by the laser beam. Thus, the depth of the incision is not controlled by the pressure exerted on the tissue but by the amount of time that the laser is focused on any one spot. This "action at a distance" allows for greater accessibility to the target tissue and perhaps less tissue trauma.

When used at open laparotomy, the CO_2 laser may be delivered with a hand-held probe or it may be attached to the operating microscope. The former has the advantage of a shorter focal distance and therefore a smaller spot size, which results in greater power density. The greater power density, as discussed earlier, yields much higher penetrating power and significantly less thermal damage to the contig-

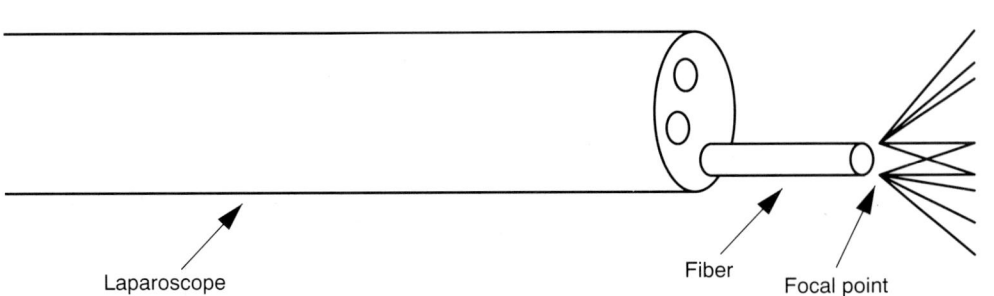

Figure 6–25
Laser fiber used through the operating channel of the laparoscope. The focal point is at the tip of the fiber, and the beam becomes less focused as it diverges from the tip.

uous normal tissue. The hand-held probe, however, is subject to hand tremor and less accurate beam delivery. Attaching the laser to the microscope increases precision as a result of both the magnification and the absence of hand tremor; however, because of the longer focal length, the spot size is larger. Nevertheless, with more sophisticated lasers, very high power density may also be achieved through the microscope or the laparoscope by the use of higher wattage (50–100 watts) or with superpulse mode.

Electrosurgery Versus Laser

Electrosurgery and laser are currently being used at laparotomy, laparoscopy, and hysteroscopy. At laparotomy, whether or not the laser has any advantages over microelectrosurgery is uncertain. Laser proponents claim shorter operative time; better hemostasis; and, because of the "no-touch" technique, less tissue trauma, less risk of infection, reduced postoperative adhesion formation, and improved pregnancy rates. To date, none of these claims has been documented or supported by either clinical[6,7] or experimental animal studies.[8,9] Tulandi prospectively randomized patients to either microlaser or microdiathermy for salpingo-oophorolysis at laparotomy and found similar postoperative adhesion reduction and pregnancy rates with both techniques.[8] Initial animal studies reported variable results when comparing tissue damage and postoperative adhesion formation following electromicrosurgery versus laser surgery. However, when power densities were made comparable between the two techniques, Luciano and associates found no difference in the depth of thermal damage, extent of collagen deposition, or postoperative adhesion formation following CO_2 and electromicrosurgery at laparotomy in rabbits.[8] Therefore, for intra-abdominal surgical procedures at laparotomy, laser may not be superior to the more traditional approach of microelectrosurgery. Laser may be preferable to electrosurgery in some cases of endometriosis involving the bowel, bladder, or pelvic sidewalls because the CO_2 laser beam is completely absorbed by the impacted tissue to a depth of only 0.1 mm, thus preserving the integrity of the adjacent tissue and vital organs.

Perhaps the major advantage offered by the laser is its application via the laparoscope that allows the gynecologist to perform major pelvic operative procedures through puncture wounds without the need for abdominal incision and the concomitant morbidity, potential disability, and expenses of hospital admission. Laser laparoscopy is being successfully employed for pelvic adhesiolysis, neosalpingostomy, ovarian cystectomy, ablation and excision of endometriosis, removal of benign tumors, treatment of ectopic pregnancy, and essentially all reproductive surgical procedures except for tubal anastomosis.[10–13] Data from animal studies indicate that following laser surgery by laparoscopy, postoperative adhesion formation is significantly lower and adhesion reduction significantly greater than following laser surgery at laparotomy.[14] In addition, whereas de novo adhesion formation is a common occurrence in reconstructive surgery performed by laparotomy,[15] this does not appear to occur following operative laparoscopy in both animal[14] and clinical[16] studies. Studies have reported that successful pregnancy rates following operative laser laparoscopy for mild to severe endometriosis or ectopic pregnancy are comparable with and in many cases significantly better than those obtained following laparotomy.[11–13]

CONCLUSION

Reproductive surgery is a rapidly changing field, and many advances have been made over the last decade. New instrumentation, especially for the laparoscope, can be anticipated in the future. It is important for the gynecologic surgeon to keep aware of changes in instrumentation, because the correct use of current and future instrumentation is crucial to the surgeon's ability to maintain or restore fertility.

References

1. Brumsted JR, Deaton J, Lavigne E, Riddick DH: Postoperative adhesion formation after ovarian wedge resection with and without ovarian reconstruction in the rabbit. Fertil Steril 1990; 53(4):723.
2. Luciano AA, Lowney J, Jacob SL: Endoscopic treatment of endometriosis-associated infertility: Therapeutic, economic, and social benefits. J Reprod Med 1992; 37:573.
3. Fox JA: The use of laser as a surgical knife. J Surg Res 1989; 9:199.
4. Bruhat M, Mage G, Manhes M: Use of CO_2 laser via laparoscopy, laser surgery III. In Kaplan I (ed.): Proceedings of the Third International Society for Laser Surgery, Tel Aviv, OT-PAZ, 1979, pp. 175–179.
5. McKenzie AL: How far does thermal damage extend beneath the surface of CO_2 laser incision? Phys Med Biol 1983; 28:905.
6. Baggish MS, ElBakry MM: Comparison of electronically superpulsed and continuous-wave CO_2 laser on the rat uterine horn. Fertil Steril 1986; 45:120.
7. Daniell JF, Diamond MP, McLaughlin DS, et al.: Clinical results of terminal salpingostomy with the use of CO_2 laser: Report of the Intraabdominal Laser Study Group. Fertil Steril 1986; 45:175.
8. Tulandi T: Salpingo-ovariolysis: A comparison between laser surgery and electrosurgery. Fertil Steril 1986; 45:489.
9. Luciano AA, Whitman G, Maier DB, et al.: A comparison of thermal injury, healing patterns and postoperative adhesion formation following CO_2 laser and electromicrosurgery. Fertil Steril 1987; 48:1025, 1029.
10. Filmar S, Gomel V, McComb PF: The effectiveness of CO_2 laser and electromicrosurgery in adhesiolysis: A comparative study. Fertil Steril 1986; 45:407.

11. Olive DL, Martin DC: Treatment of endometriosis-associated infertility with CO_2 laser laparoscopy: The use of one and two parameter exponential models. Fertil Steril 1987; 48:18.
12. Nezhat C, Crowgey S, Nezhat F: Videolaseroscopy for the treatment of endometriosis-associated infertility. Fertil Steril 1989; 51:237.
13. DeCherney AH, Diamond MP: Laparoscopic salpingostomy for ectopic pregnancy. Obstet Gynecol 1987; 70:948.
14. Gomel V: Salpingo-ovariolysis by laparoscopy in infertility. Fertil Steril 1983; 60:607.
15. Luciano AA, Maier DB, Nulsen JC, et al.: A comparative study of postoperative adhesion formation following laser surgery by laparoscopy versus laparotomy in the rabbit model. Obstet Gynecol 1989; 74:220.
16. Diamond MP, Daniell SF, Feste S, et al.: Adhesion re-formation and de novo adhesion formation after reproductive pelvic surgery. Fertil Steril 1987; 47:874.
17. Nezhat C, Nezhat F, Metzger DA, Luciano AA: Adhesion re-formation following reproductive surgery by videolaseroscopy. Fertil Steril 1990; 53:1008.

Opening and Closing of the Abdomen and Wound Healing

7

Donald G. Gallup

Abdominal incisions and their closure vary with the urgency for operative intervention; the indications for the operation; and associated preoperative conditions, such as the presence of ascites or bowel obstruction, suspicion of upper abdominal pathology, and a previous abdominal scar. Incisions for gynecology surgery should be highly individualized. Incisions should meet certain basic criteria, including reasonably rapid entry, minimal nerve damage, adequate exposure, and a closure that will leave minimal chance of infection or fascial dehiscence. Additionally, for gynecologic oncology patients, the need for colostomies, urinary diversions, and extraperitoneal approaches to node-bearing areas must be considered. This chapter is designed to allow the surgeon to compare classic techniques with recently reported modifications.

ANATOMY OF THE ANTERIOR ABDOMINAL WALL

To avoid injury to nerves and vessels and to close any incision with minimal chance of dehiscence, abdominal wall anatomy should be thoroughly understood. Cephalad, the anterior abdominal wall is bounded by the costal margins and the xiphoid process of the sternum. The costal cartilages of the seventh, eighth, ninth, and tenth ribs form part of the cephalad boundary. Lateral boundaries include the iliac crests. The caudad boundaries include the inguinal ligaments, the pubic crests, and the upper border of the symphysis pubis. The lines of tension (Langer's lines) of the skin of the abdomen are almost transverse. Vertical scars have a tendency to stretch, whereas the scars associated with transverse incisions tend to be more cosmetic as time passes. In addition to the skin, the other components of the anterior abdominal wall include muscles, fascia, subcutaneous tissue, and the nerve and vascular supply to these structures.

Muscles and Fascia

Two groups of muscles form the musculature of the anterior abdominal wall. The "flat muscles" include the external oblique, the internal oblique, and the transverse. Their fibers run transversely. The second group, composed of the rectus muscles and pyramidal muscles, have vertically running fibers. The rectus muscle with its thin investing fascia is a muscle of locomotion and posture. The integrity of the anterior abdominal wall is not greatly associated with this muscle.[1]

The external oblique muscle and its aponeurosis form the most anterior layer of the flat muscles. It originates from the lower eight ribs. Superiorly, the fibers of this muscle run transversely; inferiorly, they assume an oblique downward course. A portion of the muscle gives rise to a broad fibrous aponeurosis, which courses medially, anterior to the rectus muscle. The next posterior fan-like muscle is the internal oblique, which originates primarily from the iliac crest, the thoracolumbar fascia, and the inguinal ligament. The midportion of the muscle runs an upward oblique course and gives rise to the aponeurosis of the internal oblique. At the lateral border of the rectus, the aponeurosis splits and forms a sheath around the rectus muscle, rejoining medial to the rectus to help form the linea alba (Fig. 7–1). The third "flat" muscle, the transverse abdominis, arises from the lower six costal cartilages, thoracolumbar fascia, and the internal lip of the iliac crest. It has a truly transverse course. Above the midway point between the umbilicus and pubis, the aponeurosis of this muscle passes behind the rectus muscle and contributes to the posterior rectus sheath. Below this point, the aponeurosis passes anterior to the rectus muscle, contributing to the anterior rectus sheath (Fig. 7–1). Medial to the rectus muscle, the fascia of all three flat muscles insert to form the linea alba.

The lower limit of the upper portion of the transverse aponeurosis, which is situated posterior to the rectus muscle, forms a crescentic border, the arcuate or semilunar line. Below the arcuate line, near the level of the anterior superior iliac spines, the posterior rectus sheath is absent. Thus, if proper closure methods are not utilized, hernias or fascial dehiscence is more likely to occur in this area. In the lower abdomen, the force required to approximate the edges of a vertical incision is 30 times greater than the force required to approximate the edges of a transverse incision.[2]

The rectus abdominis muscle arises from the pubic crest. It courses superiorly and inserts into the fifth, sixth, and seventh ribs (costal cartilages) and the xiphoid process. Its upper attachment is three times as broad as its pubic insertion. It has three to four fibrous insertions, the linea transversae. One is at the level of the umbilicus; and two, usually one-half way between the umbilicus and the insertions. Importantly, the fibrous insertions are tightly adherent to the anterior rectus sheath. These limit the muscle's retraction when it is cut.[3] As mentioned, the rectus abdominis is also enclosed in an aponeurotic sheath (rectus sheath), which is made up of the aponeuroses of the three flat muscles. The pyramidalis, a triangular muscle, usually lies anterior to the rectus. It arises from the anterior portion of the symphysis and inserts into the inferior portion of the linea alba. The midportion of this muscle usually has an avascular raphe, which can easily be incised for adequate exposure of the space of Retzius.

Blood Supply

The anterior abdominal wall has an abundant blood supply; it is supplied by the superior epigastric, musculophrenic, deep circumflex iliac, and inferior epigastric arteries. The medial abdominal wall receives blood from the epigastric arteries, while the lateral wall is supplied by the musculophrenic and deep circumflex iliac arteries. The lumbar and intercostal arteries also contribute to the blood supply. Because of the rich anastomosis, vascular deficiency is usually not a complication of abdominal wall surgery (Fig. 7–2). The linea is relatively bloodless. Therefore, wound healing is felt to be relatively impaired when midline incisions are used.

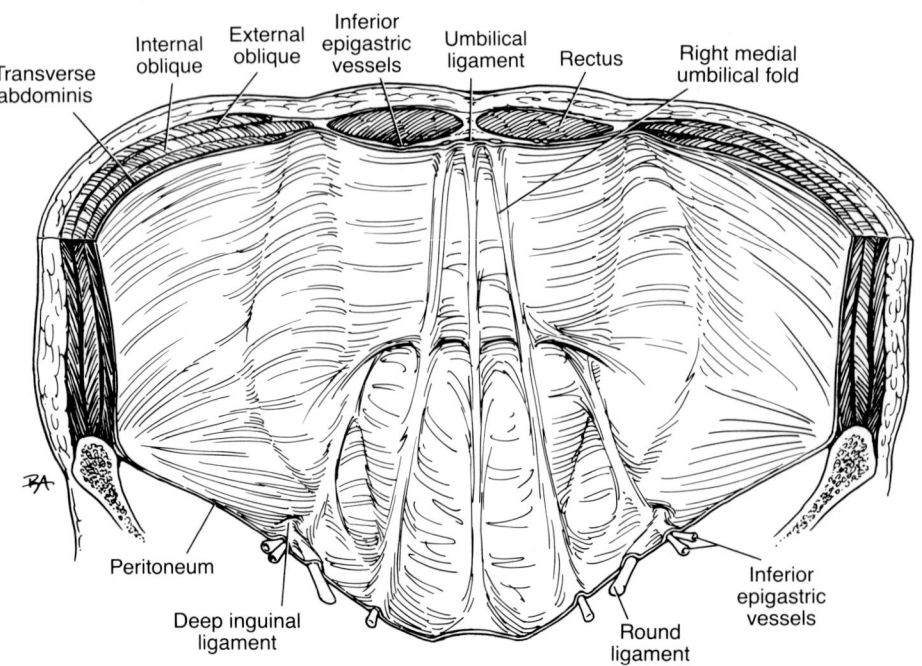

Figure 7–1
Cross-section of the lower abdominal wall. In this section, cephalad to the arcuate line, the posterior sheath, formed by the fascial aponeuroses of the flat muscles, is intact. The inferior epigastric vessels are approaching the medial portion of the undersurface of the rectus muscle.

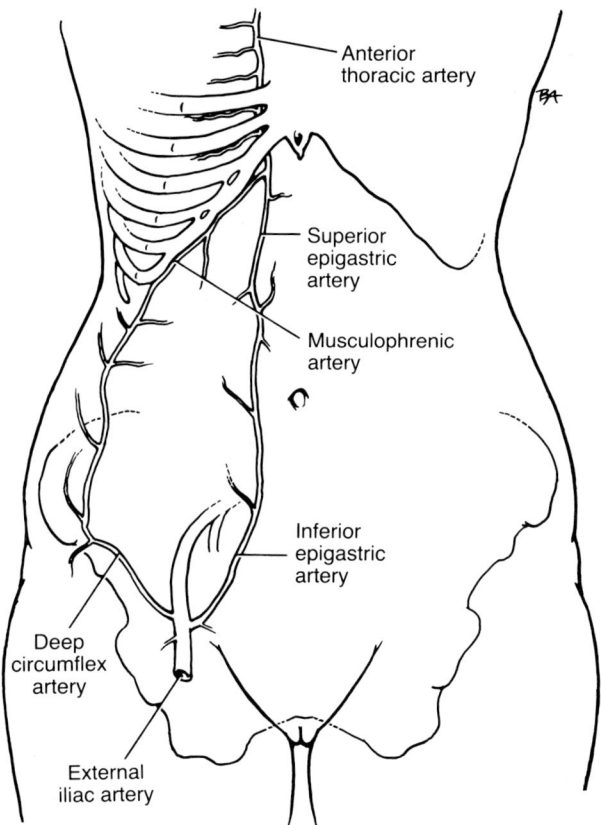

Figure 7–2
The major arterial blood supply of the anterior abdominal wall. The four major vessels, two medial and two lateral, contribute to the rich anastomosis.

Conversely, the epigastric vessels are subject to injury, particularly when a muscle splitting incision is used. Also, the deep circumflex or musculophrenic vessels can be injured when an extraperitoneal approach is chosen.

The superior epigastric artery is a continuation of the internal thoracic (mammary) artery. It enters the sheath of the rectus from behind the seventh costal cartilage and descends posterior to the rectus. It has multiple branches in the substance of the rectus muscle and anastomosis to the inferior epigastric artery. In the upper abdomen, cephalad to the umbilicus, the main branch of the artery tends to lie posterior to the *midportion* of the rectus muscle (Fig. 7–3). The inferior epigastric artery arises from the external iliac artery near the midinguinal point. It continues in a cephalad course along the posterior *lateral* portion of the rectus muscle and has an anastomosis with the superior epigastric arteries. The lower a transverse incision is made, the more lateral the inferior epigastric arteries will be encountered. The veins lie in close approximation to the main trunks of these arteries.

The musculophrenic artery, arising from the internal thoracic, courses along the costal margin behind the cartilages. It has an anastomosis with the deep circumflex artery, which originates from the external iliac at about the same level as the inferior epigastric. The deep circumflex courses behind the inguinal ligament and along the iliac crest, eventually piercing the transversus muscle and digitating between that muscle and the internal oblique. Prior to its anastomosis with the musculophrenic, it can be relatively large. Care must be taken when these muscles are incised laterally.

Innervation

The anterior abdominal wall is supplied by thoracoabdominal nerves, the iliohypogastric nerves, and the ilioinguinal nerves. The thoracoabdominal nerves, which are the seventh to eleventh intercostal nerves, leave the intercostal spaces and travel caudad and anterior between the transversus and internal oblique. They supply these muscles and the external oblique. They enter the sheath of the rectus, and their branches supply the rectus and the overlying skin. The majority of the nerves are supplied by several trunks. Any one nerve in the anterior abdominal wall contains fibers from the last two to three intercostal nerves.[2] When an incision is made lateral to the midline, a transverse type is least likely to cause injury to nerves. In the upper abdomen, an obliquely caudad and out incision is least likely to cause significant nerve injury. In the lower part of the abdomen, an obliquely directed cephalad and out incision is relatively nerve sparing.

A vertical incision that passes lateral to the rectus muscle or through the muscle will denervate medial lying tissue, depending on the length of the incision. Atony or atrophy of the muscle may sometimes occur. The iliohypogastric and ilioinguinal nerves are sensory in function (Fig. 7–4). Injury to the former, when wide transverse incisions are used, may result in sensation changes in the skin over the mons, whereas injury to the latter may result in sensation changes to the labia majora. Both are chiefly derived from the first lumbar nerve root. Although they lie for a distance between the internal oblique and the transversus, they do not enter the rectus sheath. They do not supply the external oblique or the rectus muscle.[4] Both nerves supply the lower fibers of the internal oblique and transversus. If damage occurs to these nerves at the level of the anterior superior iliac spine, these muscle fibers are denervated. A weakening of the normal canal controlling mechanism may occur, predisposing the patient to an inguinal hernia.

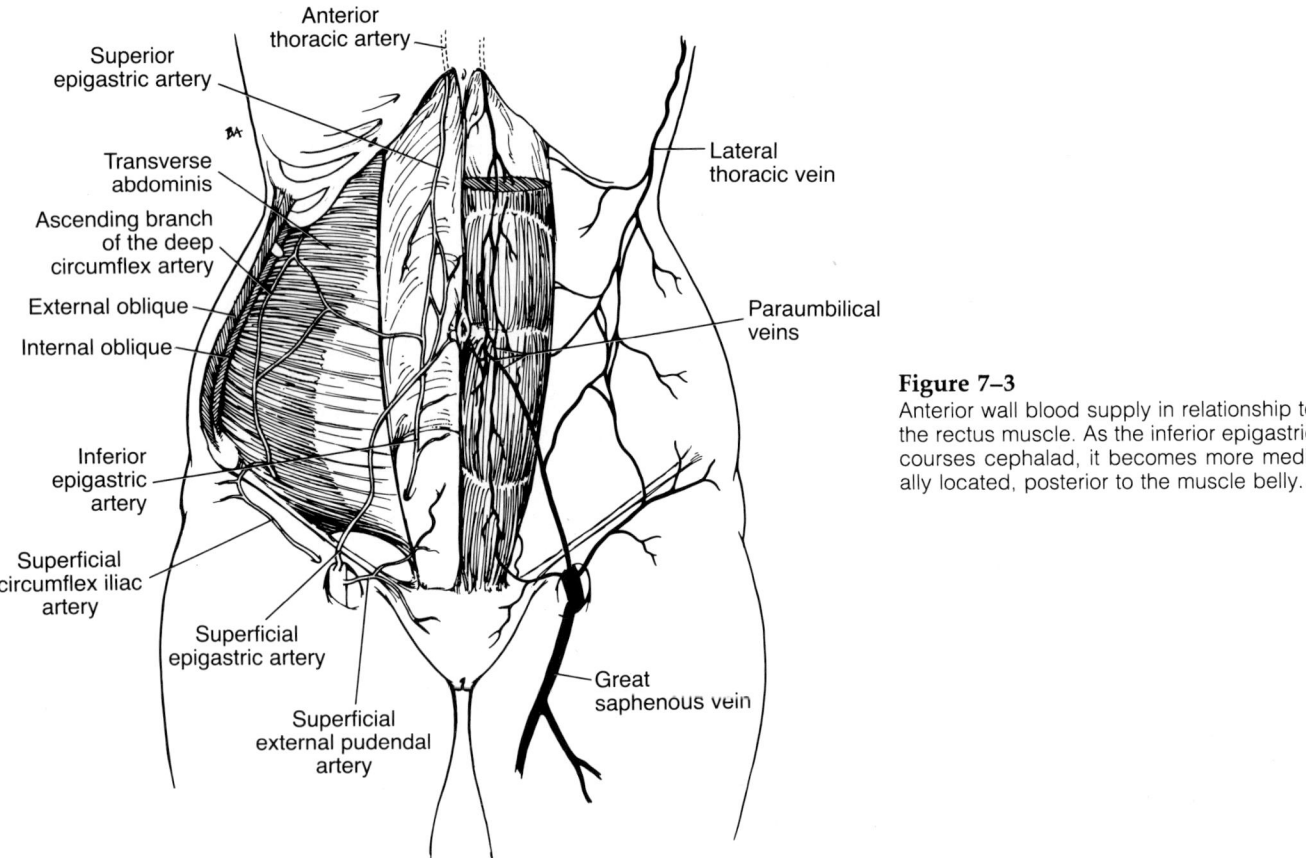

Figure 7–3
Anterior wall blood supply in relationship to the rectus muscle. As the inferior epigastric courses cephalad, it becomes more medially located, posterior to the muscle belly.

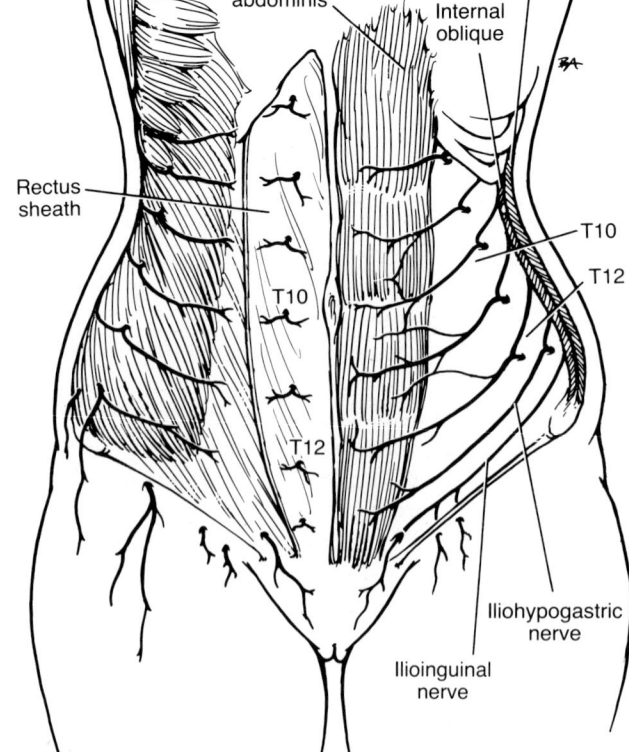

Figure 7–4
Major innervation of the anterior abdominal wall. The iliohypogastric nerves and ilioinguinal nerves supply the sensory innervation of the lower abdominal wall.

PHYSIOLOGY OF WOUND HEALING

Wound complications are a psychologic and economic problem for the patient and basically include infections, dehiscence, and evisceration, and late occurring problems, such as incisional hernias and wound sinus formation. Factors negatively affecting proper wound healing include diabetes, malnutrition, prior irradiation or chemotherapy, older patient age, alcoholism, preoperative shaving the evening before on the ward, the duration of preoperative hospitalization, the duration of the operation, the use of Penrose type drains brought out through the incision, ascites, malignancy, immunosuppression (including long-term corticosteroid therapy), and obesity.[5-8] Additionally, factors affecting wound disruption that usually occur in the absence of infection include choice of suture material, closure technique, occurrence of excessive coughing due to pulmonary disease, retching and vomiting, and intestinal obstruction.

The four phases of wound healing include inflammation, migration, proliferation, and maturation. Breaks in the normal cycle of wound healing can occur anywhere, depending on pre-existing conditions. Importantly, the fibroblastic-proliferation phase lasting from about day 5 through day 20, provides the most strength to the wound. By day 21, most wounds will have regained almost 30% of their original tensile strength. Any wound contamination or foreign bodies can cause chronic inflammation, sinuses, delayed incisional hernias, or the early postoperative problems of infection and dehiscence.

The risks of wound infections are directly related to the classification of wounds (Table 7–1).[9, 10] Obviously, few surgeons would primarily close a dirty wound. Most of the abdominal procedures performed by gynecologists include a hysterectomy. The vagina is entered, and this procedure is classified as being associated with a clean-contaminated wound with the attendant risk.

SUTURES

Suture choice is basically a surgeon's prerogative, but the characteristics of suture material intended for fascial closure should be well known to the surgeon. Additionally, suture choice should be based on the patient's condition, the type of incision, and the strength and reaction of the suture (Table 7–2). In general, the ideal suture material should have the following characteristics: knot security, inertness, adequate tensile strength, flexibility, ease in handling, nonallergenic, resistant to infection, and absorbability at a predictable rate. Neither plain catgut nor chromic catgut maintains tensile strength during the critical time of wound healing. They should not be used for fascial closure of the abdominal wall, no matter what type of incision is used. Estimation of tensile strength of chromic suture after 14 days is 34% whereas plain gut has none.[11]

In general, sutures are classified as nonabsorbable if they maintain tensile strength for over 60 days. In the permanent suture group, monofilament sutures yield less inflammation than polyfilament sutures. Wire has been the traditional suture used by surgeons for decades in high-risk patients, particularly when infection was an associated operative finding. Wire has several disadvantages. It is difficult to tie and breaks easily if bent sharply. It may cut through

Table 7–1

Wound Classification

Class	Category	Definition	Wound Infection Rate (%)
I	Clean	Wounds are made under ideal operating room conditions. The procedures are usually elective, and no entry is made into the oropharyngeal cavity or the lumen of the respiratory, alimentary, or genitourinary tract. Inflammation is not encountered, and no break in technique occurs. The wounds are always primarily closed and seldom drained. Almost 75% of all operations are included in this group.	<5
II	Clean-contaminated	Wounds occur from entry into the oropharyngeal cavity, respiratory, alimentary, or genitourinary tract without significant spillage. Clean wounds are included in this category when there is a minor break in surgical technique. These procedures include approximately 16% of all operations.	5–10
III	Contaminated	This category includes open, fresh, traumatic wounds; operations with a major break in sterile technique; and incisions encountering acute, nonpurulent inflammation, such as in cholecystitis or cystitis.	15–20
IV	Dirty	Old traumatic wounds (older than 4 hours), perforated viscera, or operations involving clinically evident infections are included in this category. Wounds containing foreign bodies or devitalized tissue are also considered dirty.	>30

Table 7-2

Commonly Used Sutures for General Closure

Suture Type	Tissue Reaction (1–4)	Relative Strength (1–4)
Absorbable		
Plain gut	4	1
Chromic gut	3	2
Polyglycolic acid (Dexon, Dexon 2)	2	3
Polyglactin 910 (Vicryl)	2	3
Polydioxanone, polyglyconate (Maxon)	1	4
Nonabsorbable		
Natural (silk, cotton)	4	2
Polypropylene monofilament (Surgilene, Novofil, Prolene)	1	4
Braided synthetics (Dacron, Mersilene, Ti-Cron, Ethibond, Tevdek)	2	4
Stainless-steel wire (Flexon)	1	4
Nylon (Dermalon, Ethilon, Surgilon)	2	4

tissues if placed too close to incisional edges. It may cause prickling sensations in some patients. It may penetrate the surgeon's gloves, a particular problem with some infectious diseases prevalent in the 1990s. Furthermore, in animal models, both monofilament nylon and monofilament polypropylene sutures have elicited less infection in contaminated tissue than has wire.[12] The durability of these sutures may be even greater. Both cotton and silk are highly tissue reactive sutures. Silk, usually considered a nonabsorbable suture, loses all of its tensile strength after 1 year, and cotton loses 50%, after a year.[13,14] If a permanent suture is chosen for closure, one of the monofilament polypropylene sutures or monofilament nylon should be used.

Over the last two decades, synthetic absorbable sutures have been added to the surgeon's armamentarium. Two early developed sutures, polyglycolic acid and polyglactin, have been extensively studied. They maintain an estimated 55% of their original tensile strength at 14 days. A newer polyglycolic acid suture, Dexon 2, appears to have better knot security. Many surgeons use one of these for various types of transverse incision closures. In 1985, Fagniez and colleagues reported few fascial dehiscences in a large series of patients who had midline incisions closed with polyglycolic acid sutures.[15]

Polyglyconate (Maxon) and polydioxanone (PDS) represent a new class of monofilament absorbable sutures. In animal studies, both of these sutures have been noted to have a much less inflammatory response than polyglactin.[16] These investigators have also estimated that Maxon and PDS retain about 95% of their tensile strength by postoperative day 10 and retain 50% by postoperative day 28. In one study of degradation patterns of Maxon and PDS in rabbit fascia, PDS was noted to be superior.[17] Rodeheaver and associates found no significant difference in knot breaking strength in these two sutures.[18] Maxon appeared to have less stiffness in handling. Another study in rabbits also noted the tensile strength superiority of Maxon and PDS to polyglycolic acid and polyglactin. Maxon was felt to have the best knot security.[19] These investigators also noted that the most consistent knot security was achieved when six square knots were used. The author's own clinical impression is that there is little difference in suture handling and knot security when Maxon and PDS II are compared. When wound healing is anticipated to take longer than 2 weeks, particularly for fascial closure in midline incisions, one of these two delayed absorbable sutures should be highly considered. Finally, knot security also depends on suture size and the tissue needing approximation. Although sliding knots may be safely used for pelvic viscera, sutures used to close abdominal wall fascia should be tied with square knots. van Rissel and colleagues have noted poor knot performance when a surgeon's knot plus a square knot was made with monofilament sutures.[20] Nonabsorbable synthetic monofilament sutures, such as Prolene or Surgilene, should be used for closing the fascia in the presence of infection.

DRAINS

The use of prophylactic drains in the subcutaneous space or "wet" subfascial space remains controversial. Some investigators suggest that the lowest clean wound infection rate will be found in patients who have no drains.[7,21] Little controversy should exist about the use of drains in a few conditions. Most surgeons would use some type of closed drainage system when an unavoidable large potential space remains, for example, in dissection of a large incisional hernia or when mesh or a fascial graft is used. Most gynecologic oncologists use a closed drainage system when performing inguinal-femoral lymphadenectomies or in the space created by mobilizing myocutaneous flaps. Drainage may be necessary for persisting defects in blood coagulation to prevent a subsequent hematoma. As will later be discussed, two published series on pelvic-abdominal surgery in obese patients seem to indicate an advantage in the use of subcutaneous drains.[22,23] On the other hand, Scott and coworkers operated on 56 consecutive patients whose panniculi measured 6–11 cm in thickness.[24] They used systemic and oral antibiotics, transverse incisions, copious lavage, and tape to close the skin. No drains were used, and only one patient had a wound infection.

Few randomized prospective studies with a significant number of patients exist. In some series, perhaps only patients at high risk for wound infection were drained subcutaneously or subfascially.

Farnell and associates,[25] in a prospective study, analyzed 3282 incisions of the wound varieties listed in Table 7-1. They noted that subcutaneous closed drainage systems, alone or with antibiotics or saline irrigation, were not superior to primary closure in clean-contaminated wounds or contaminated wounds. However, a trend favoring subcutaneous catheter and antibiotic irrigation was noted in patients with dirty wounds. Irrigating wounds may affect wound healing. In one study, irrigating solutions in vitro and in laboratory animals, such as 1% povidone-iodine, 0.25% acetic acid, or 0.5% sodium hypochlorite, were noted to have cytotoxic effects when applied to human fibroblasts.[26] The one cytotoxic agent in that study that did not retard wound healing was hydrogen peroxide, but it also had minimal bactericidal potency. Irrigation of drains in subcutaneous, or even subfascial, spaces may be harmful. Drains, if used, should be utilized for evacuation of suspected relatively increased fluid output from tissues.

Drains may be classified into two basic categories—passive or active. The former function primarily by overflow and are sometimes assisted by gravity. The latter are connected to some type of suction.[27] The use of passive drains in wounds may be one reason why wound drainage has been associated with increased infection rates. The two types used, a Penrose or cigarette (a Penrose drain with gauze placed inside it to enhance capillary activity) should never be brought out through the incision itself. The author and colleagues prefer a closed drainage system such as a Jackson-Pratt or a Blake. Both have small reservoir systems (100 ml), which are relatively easy for paramedical personnel to manage on the ward. In the author's experience, the Blake drain, with its longitudinal ridges, seems to offer less chance of obstruction from small tissue fragments than the Jackson-Pratt (Fig. 7-5). However, no large prospective trials comparing these systems are currently available. To avoid clot formation causing obstruction, early suction should be used.[28] The author connects the drain to wall suction while completing closure of the incision. Active drains in the subfascial or subcutaneous space should be removed, not advanced, when the drainage is less than 50 ml/24 hours, usually by postoperative day 2 or 3. Again, drains should never be brought out through the incisions.[9]

PREVENTION OF WOUND COMPLICATIONS

In two large studies, Cruse and Foord added to our knowledge about wound infections and their causes.[7, 9] Preoperative showering with hexachlorophene lowered the infection rate in clean wounds

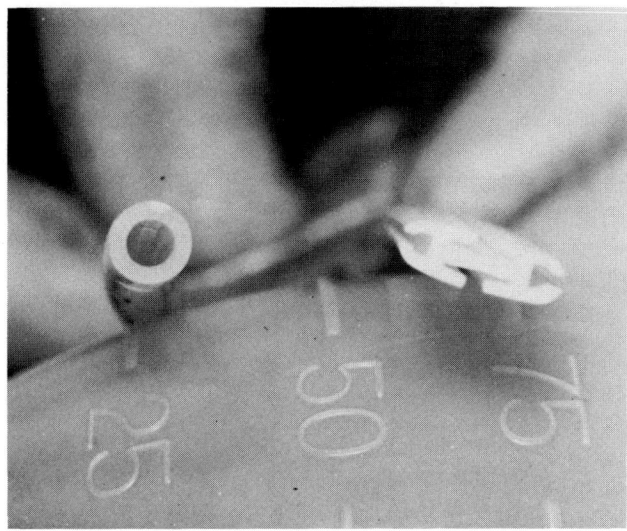

Figure 7-5
Cross-section of a Jackson-Pratt drain on the left and a Blake drain on the right. These lie over the 75-ml reservoir, which can be used for either drain. Note the longitudinal ridges of the Blake, as opposed to the perforations of the Jackson-Pratt.

(1.3%) versus no shower (2.3%). They also noted, as have others, that a clip preparation of abdominal pubic hair versus a shave preparation the evening prior to surgery resulted in fewer wound infections. Smaller series also support this concept.[29] Probably the only reason to remove hair is that its presence may interfere with wound approximation in some incisions. Depilatories have been advocated by some surgeons, but they are relatively expensive.[30, 31] In the series reported by Seropian and Reynolds,[31] the wound infection rate for depilatory preparations versus no shaving was equal (0.6%). The author and his colleagues prefer to use an electric razor in the operating room, whenever feasible.

Skin preparations and draping do not need to be complex or lengthy. Using a povidone-iodine skin preparation for 3 minutes is adequate. An alternative solution is chlorhexidine.[9] Plastic adhesive drapes have no advantage in preventing wound infections. In fact, they may prove to be harmful if they lift from the skin.[32] Furthermore, the time-honored 10-minute scrub of the surgeon's hands is unnecessary. Galle and coworkers noted no difference in infection rates between a 5-minute versus a 10-minute scrub time. A lesser time obviously decreases total operative time and water usage.

Incisions of the skin or fascia should not be made with cautery. The wound infection rate was reportedly doubled when a Bovie device was used compared with a knife.[7, 9] In a randomized prospective study, the rate of postoperative wound infections was not significantly different following the use of one or two scalpels for the incision.[34] The same scalpel can be safely used for superficial and deep incisions. The incision should be made in a bold strike in order to minimize dead space. Subcutaneous sutures should be avoided in obese patients. In general, the subcutaneous tissue does not provide support. An alternate method is the use of a fine (4.0) running polyglycolic acid type suture to remove tension from the approximated skin edges. Chromic catgut should never be used to close the fascia and should not be used in subcutaneous closure. In general, delayed closure should be used for contaminated or dirty wounds.

TYPES OF ABDOMINAL INCISIONS

Transverse Incisions

Transverse incisions offer several advantages over vertical incisions. They are the best cosmetic incisions for pelvic surgery. Proponents of transverse incisions have suggested that they are as much as 30 times stronger than midline incisions. Additionally, they are less painful and result in less interference in postoperative respirations when placed in the lower abdomen. Wound dehiscence is allegedly more common with vertical incisions.[35] The older literature suggests that wound evisceration was three to five times more common and hernia occurrence was two to three times more common when vertical incisions were used, as compared with transverse incisions.[36-38] Many earlier studies of reported increased incidence of eviscerations with midline incisions could be associated with inappropriate closures. Some studies actually show an advantage of midline incisions could be associated with inappropriate closures. Some studies actually show an advantage of midline incisions over transverse incisions in avoiding dehiscence or show no difference.[25, 39] Transverse incisions do have certain associated disadvantages: inability to explore the upper abdomen, relatively more bleeding, division of multiple layers of fascia and muscle with formation of potential spaces; more time consuming, and occasionally nerves are divided.[36]

Pfannenstiel's Incision

When the Pfannenstiel incision is employed, the cosmetic results are superb but exposure is limited. Thus, it should not be used for patients with known gynecologic malignancies. It should not be used when pelvic exposure is needed in operating on patients with nonmalignant conditions—that is, severe endometriosis or large leiomyomas with distortion of the lower uterine segment, or when reoperating on a patient for hemorrhage. The Pfannenstiel incision should not be used when speed in entering the abdomen is essential.

The incision may be "wet" and require subfascial drainage. Regarding fascial closure, a running technique can be used in patients with clean wounds or clean-contaminated wounds. Polyglycolic acid, polyglactin 910, or one of the delayed absorbable sutures can be used. In assessing the use of running versus interrupted polyglycolic acid sutures in midline incisions, Fagniez and colleagues noted no difference in fascial dehiscence in a randomized prospective trial of 3135 patients.[15] Subcutaneous sutures are unnecessary. The skin can be closed with staples or a subcuticular suture.

Cherney's Incision

The Cherney incision is about 25% longer than a midline incision from the umbilicus to the symphysis.[40] It provides excellent access to the space of Retzius for stress urinary incontinence procedures. It provides excellent exposure of the pelvic sidewall when needed—that is, in patients who require hypogastric artery ligation. Occasionally, the surgeon who uses a Pfannenstiel incision will find the incision inadequate for exposure for hemostasis or not large enough to adequately expose areas of associated abnormal conditions. Under these circumstances, the safe approach is not to "half-transect" the rectus muscles; the safe approach is to perform a Cherney incision.

Even if the peritoneum is opened, the space of Retzius can be bluntly dissected (Fig. 7–6). The inferior epigastric vessels, which course more laterally in the caudad portion of the abdominal wall, are identified. The pyramidal muscles are sharply dis-

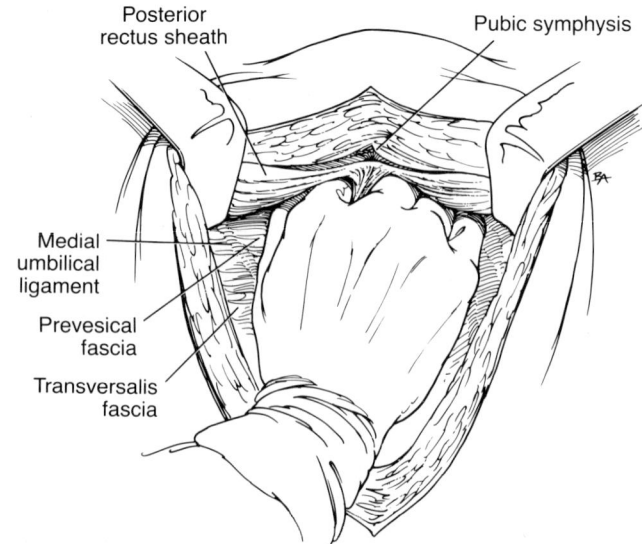

Figure 7–6
Developing the space of Retzius. The weight of the hand of the operator easily separates the bladder from the overlying symphysis in the relatively bloodless midline.

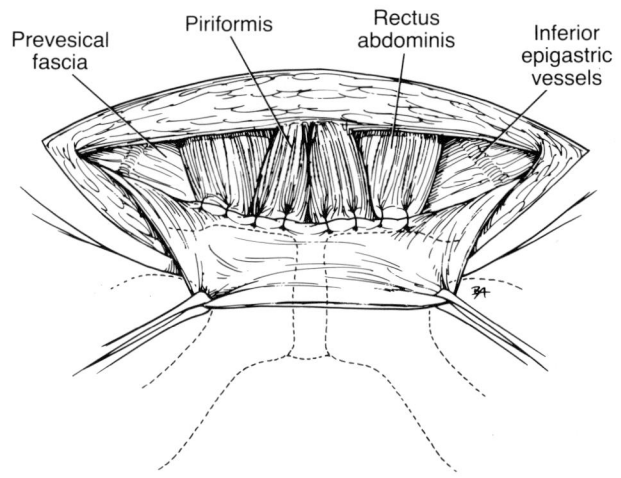

Figure 7–7
Reuniting the rectus tendons to the inferior portion of the lower flap of the rectus muscle after a Cherney transverse incision.

sected. The fibrous tendinous rectus muscles are then dissected sharply from their insertion into the symphysis pubis. Bleeding is negligible in this area, and the inferior epigastric vessels do not need to be ligated. The peritoneal incision can be extended laterally about 2 cm cephalad to the bladder while visualizing the vessels. The peritoneum is closed separately with a running polyglycolic acid suture. Drainage of the subfascial space may be necessary. The ends of the rectus tendons are united to the inferior portion of the lower flap of the rectus sheath. Five to six permanent sutures, interrupted or horizontal mattress, should be used (Fig. 7–7). The rectus muscles should not be sutured to the symphysis pubis, in order to avoid osteomyelitis. Fascial closure can be accomplished with a running continuous suture of No. 1 or No. 2 delayed absorbable suture, as in the Pfannenstiel. Although the lines of tension favor transverse incisions as opposed to vertical, running sutures should be placed at least 1.5 cm from the fascial edge. The remainder of the closure can be similar to the Pfannenstiel closure, depending on the surgeon's preference.

Maylard's Incision

In 1907, Ernest Maylard, a British surgeon, advocated a muscle cutting incision.[41] This incision provides excellent pelvic exposure and is used by many surgeons for radical pelvic surgery, including radical hysterectomy with pelvic lymph node dissection and pelvic exenteration. Although the author prefers midline incisions for patients with suspicious adnexal masses, young patients with adnexal masses that are questionable for malignancy by radiographic studies may be candidates for this cosmetic incision. Patients must be informed that if malignancy is found, the transverse incision will be "hockey sticked" in a J-shaped fashion (see Incisions for Extra-peritoneal Approaches) or a separate upper abdominal incision will be used to adequately evaluate the upper abdominal cavity and retroperitoneal para-aortic nodes.

The original Maylard-Bardenheuer incision has been modified in several aspects since its original description. The transverse skin incision is made about 3–8 cm above the symphysis, depending on patient age and weight and indications for surgery. Following a transverse fascial incision, well lateral to the borders of the rectus muscles, the inferior epigastric vessels, lying on the posterior lateral border of each muscle, are identified. (Some surgeons suggest preservation of these vessels even when the rectus muscles are transected.[42]) Using gentle finger dissection, the vessels are teased away from their attachments. The vessels are ligated with permanent suture *prior* to incising the rectus muscles, in order to avoid tearing of the vessels, vessel retraction, and hematoma formation (Fig. 7–8). The fingers of the surgeon tease the overlying rectus muscle from the peritoneum, and the muscles are sectioned using the knife or a Bovie. For better approximation of the muscles during closure, the author prefers to suture the underlying muscle to the overlying fascia prior to entering the peritoneum. A 2–0 delayed absorbable

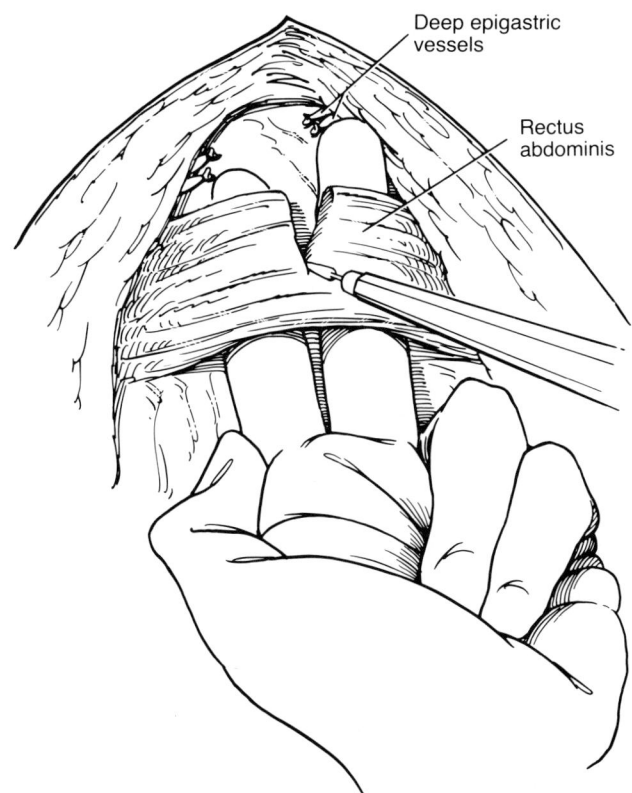

Figure 7–8
The Maylard incision. The rectus muscle is transected using a knife or a Bovie device. Note that the inferior epigastric vessels have been previously isolated, sectioned, and ligated.

"U-suture" is used, and the knots are placed anterior to the fascia. The peritoneum is incised transversely. Closure of the fascia is similar to the running technique for other transverse incisions. The muscles do not need to be reapproximated with individual sutures. A subfascial drain is indicated if hemostasis is not absolute.

Vertical Incisions

In general, vertical incisions afford excellent exposure, can be easily extended, and provide for rapid entry. Whether midline or paramedian, the resulting scar may be wide.

Paramedian Incisions

Paramedian incisions have been advocated over midline incisions because of alleged greater strength. In a prospective study, Guillou and coworkers found no significant difference in respiratory complications, wound infections, and dehiscence when comparing midline, medial paramedian, and lateral paramedian incisions.[43] None of the patients with lateral paramedian incisions developed incisional hernias. The incidence of hernia in midline and medial paramedian incisions was the same. Increased infection rates, increased intraoperative bleeding, increased operating time, and the possibility of nerve damage atrophy to the rectus muscle are relative disadvantages of the paramedian incision. Long paramedian incisions may increase pain with respirations.

Midline Incisions

As noted in the section on anatomy, the midline incision is the least hemorrhagic incision. Rapid entry is feasible. Exposure is excellent, and minimal nerve damage occurs. Dehiscence and hernias are said to be more common, particularly in the area caudad to the arcuate line. Abdominal wound disruption is one of the most serious postoperative problems associated with gynecologic surgery. The "burst abdomen" or evisceration, seen more frequently in general surgery patients, occurs with a frequency of 0.3–0.7% in gynecologic patients. It is associated with a mortality of 10–35%.[44-46] The choice of incision is not the only factor associated with evisceration. Wound infection is present in up to 50% of associated cases. Use of chromic catgut for fascial closure is associated with a higher incidence of dehiscence than with use of other sutures. Mechanical factors, such as wound hematomas, paroxysmal coughing associated with chronic lung disease, or gastrointestinal problems (retching, vomiting, ileus), may lead to evisceration. Newer closure techniques can help avoid the problems with hernia and dehiscence, but the cosmetic result is relatively poor.

The midline incision is the most easily mastered gynecologic incision, because the fascial area is relatively bloodless and because the rectus muscles are usually separated in parous women. If the patient has had a prior midline incision, one should incise the peritoneum more cephalad to the prior incision, in order to avoid injury to possibly adherent bowel. In patients undergoing radical pelvic surgery, or surgery for deeply seated, adherent pelvic masses, the author and colleagues prefer to develop the space of Retzius. This maneuver allows for incision extension between the pyramidal muscles and gives better exposure in the deep pelvis. Because it can easily be extended, the midline incision is the most versatile of all incisions used by gynecologists.

In closing midline incisions, many surgeons prefer a layered closure (Fig. 7–9). This type of closure is probably unnecessary for the vast majority of patients operated on for any gynecologic disorder. If used, sutures should always be loosely tied. The major cause of wound evisceration is too many sutures placed too close together, too close to the

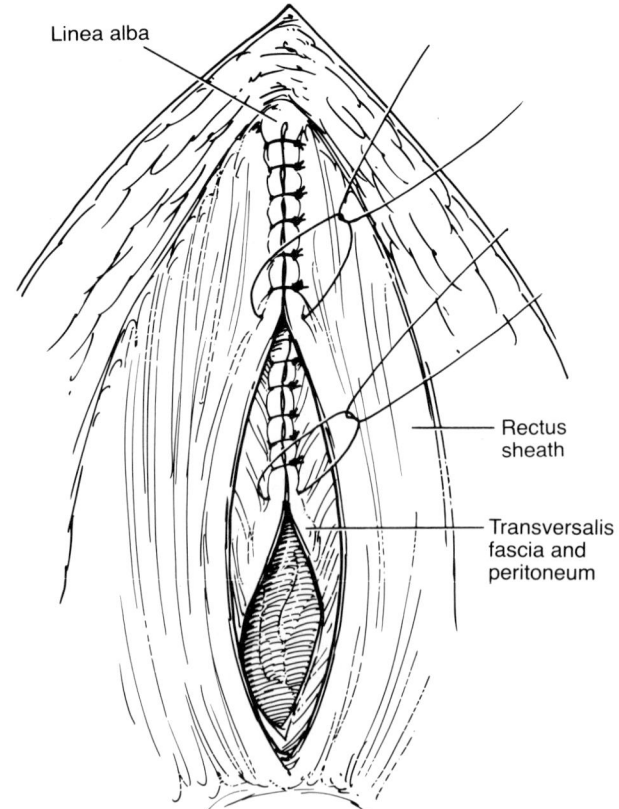

Figure 7–9
Layered closure of the anterior abdominal wall after a midline incision. The peritoneum has been closed with a continuous fine 2-0 absorbable suture. The posterior fascia may be closed with interrupted or figure-of-eight sutures, followed by closure of the anterior fascia.

Table 7–3

Closure with Running Sutures in Midline Incisions

Authors	No. of Patients	Material	No. of Patients with Fascial Dehiscence
Archie and Feldman (1981)[50]	120	MFPP (No. 1)	1
Murray and Blaisdell (1978)[51]	255	PGA (No. 1)	1
Shepherd et al. (1983)[52]	200	MFPP (No. 2)	0
Knight and Griffen (1983)[53]	419	MFPP (No. 1)	4
Gallup et al. (1989)[54]	210	MFPP (No. 2)	0
Total	1204		6 (0.5%)

MFPP, monofilament polypropylene; PGA, polyglycolic acid.

fascial edge and tied too tightly.[47] Often at reoperation for evisceration, the sutures and knots are intact, but the suture has simply torn through the fascia. To avoid wound disruptions in high-risk patients, several investigators have advocated a Smead-Jones closure technique.[22, 23, 48] This is a far-far, near-near suturing technique, and only the anterior fascia is included in the near-near bite. A No. 1 nylon or No. 1 polypropylene suture is used. The key to the success of this closure is using wide far-far bites, 1.5–2.0 cm. The Smead-Jones closure is time consuming.

In 1976, Jenkins proposed that bursting of abdominal wounds could be prevented by using wide bites of nonabsorbable continuous suture through fascia, muscle, and peritoneum.[49] Some investigators, particularly those who perform general surgery, have advocated a single-layer running mass closure technique as expedient yet safe.[50–53] The author and his colleagues began using this technique in high-risk patients in 1984 and noted no fascial dehiscences in 210 patients. One patient later developed an incisional hernia.[54] When the author added this series to four studies of patients who had running mass closures, the incidence of fascial dehiscence was only 0.5% (Table 7–3). Fagniez and associates noted that polyglycolic acid could be safely used in a running manner when midline incisions were employed.[15] Many of the more recent studies are from trauma centers, and Stone and colleagues in a randomized, prospective trial, also noted no difference in dehiscence rates between interrupted and running mass closures.[55]

In the author's study, the midline incisions were closed with a continuous No. 2 polypropylene suture.[54] Closely spaced bites were taken and placed 1.5–2.0 cm from the fascial edge. Bites should include the peritoneum, if easily located, the fascial layers, and the intervening muscle (Fig. 7–10). One suture should be started from each end of the incision, and the single ends should be tied in the middle. Six throws should be used for each knot. In the original series, a small hemoclip was placed above each knot to prevent unraveling. A double strand should never be tied to a single strand. The sutures should not be pulled too tightly, because the major advantage of this closure is that tension is equally distributed over a continuous line.

One problem with the use of large-bore permanent suture for mass closure is occasional late occurring wound sinus formations.[52, 53] This occurred in two of our previously reported patients.[54] With research leading to the development of monofilament (delayed) absorbable sutures (Maxon and PDS), the

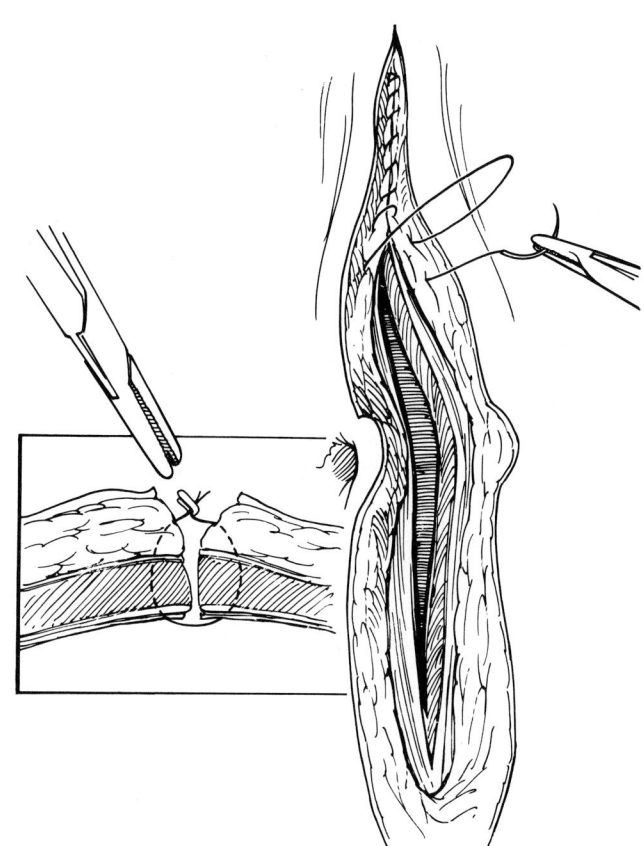

Figure 7–10
Closure of a midline incision using a No. 2 polypropylene, running mass closure. As noted in the insert, the anterior fascia, muscle, posterior fascia, and peritoneum are included in the bites, which are taken 1.5–2.0 cm from the fascial edge. These bites should be taken approximately 1 cm apart. With permanent polypropylene suture, a hemoclip may be used on the short end to avoid suture unraveling.

author and colleagues changed their running closure technique to avoid the problem with large knots causing sinus formation. They used No. 1 Maxon suture because of its relatively easier handling and knot security. The running mass closure was similar to the closure with polypropylene, except seven throws were used for each knot. Also, the knots were buried. Most of the 285 patients with midline incisions closed with this suture were at high risk for wound disruption. Of these, seven developed superficial wound infections, one developed a ventral hernia, and one had an evisceration on the fourth postoperative day.[56] At re-exploration of this last patient, the central knot of the intact suture had untied, and later questioning of the surgeons involved revealed that only four throws had been used per knot. A delayed absorbable suture can also be safely used in running midline closures for high-risk patients.

Incisions for Obese Patients

Obesity is a recognized high-risk factor for wound infections. Pitkin noted a 4% wound complication rate in nonobese women undergoing abdominal hysterectomy, compared with a 29% rate in obese patients.[57] Krebs and Helmkamp reported a wound infection rate of 24% in massively obese patients when a periumbilical transverse incision was used.[58] Because muscle cutting may be needed for this transverse incision, entry time can be lengthy and the resulting incision relatively bloody. If any transverse incision is chosen for obese patients, it should be far removed from the anaerobic moist environment of the subpannicular fold.

In 1977, Morrow and colleagues suggested modifications of preoperative care, intraoperative techniques, and postoperative care in obese gynecologic patients and noted only a 13% wound infection rate.[22] The author subsequently modified Morrow's techniques and operated on a group of 97 mostly high-risk obese patients and retrospectively compared them with obese patients not operated on by the author's protocol. The wound infection rate in obese patients not operated on by protocol was 42%, as compared with a 3% rate in protocol-operated obese patients.[23]

The author's original protocol, which is still used for obese patients, has only been modified by fascial closure techniques. All patients have careful cleansing of the umbilicus and undergo preoperative showering. Mini-dose subcutaneous heparin (5000 to 8000 U) is used 2 hours prior to surgery, and every 12 hours after surgery, until patients are fully ambulating. Prophylactic antibiotics are not routinely given. Clip preparation of abdominal hair is used. The midline incision is made by first retracting the panniculus caudad, below the inferior margins of the symphysis, in order to avoid an incision in the anaerobic subpannicular fold (Fig. 7–11). The skin incision is a periumbilical incision, as it is usually extended around the umbilicus. A wound protector is used to improve exposure in the pelvis and to protect the skin edges. The fascial incision is always extended to the symphysis. Once the uterus and/or other organs are removed, the pelvic peritoneum is not closed. The cuff is closed. Most patients require a closed drain, placed posterior to the redundant sigmoid. Fascia may be closed with a Smead-Jones or running mass closure. The author and colleagues prefer the latter. Subcutaneous sutures are not used, but a Jackson-Pratt or Blake drain is placed anterior to the fascia, after irrigating the tissues with normal saline. This drain is removed in 72 hours, or when the output is less than 50 ml in 24 hours. The skin is closed with a suture stapler, and these staples are left in place for 2 weeks. A nasogastric tube is inserted during surgery and is left in place for 24 hours, in order to avoid abdominal distention. The author's relatively low wound infection rate in obese patients supports this type of operative management.[54, 56]

Nevertheless, no randomized prospective studies exist regarding prophylactic antibiotics or the use of subcutaneous sutures versus subcutaneous drains. A time-honored surgical principle is to eliminate dead space. Subcutaneous areas rarely contain adequate supportive tissues to approximate subcutaneous tissues. If one wishes to use sutures, a running technique using fine, polyglycolic acid suture should be performed. Of the patients who had wound infections in the series reported by Morrow and colleagues, none had subcutaneous drains.[22]

Incisions for Extraperitoneal Approaches

The value of a staging laparotomy to assess para-aortic nodes in patients with advanced stage (IIB–IV) cervical cancer has been established in the past two decades.[59, 60] The incidence of positive para-aortic nodes is progressively higher as the stage of disease increases, prompting such organizations as the Gynecologic Oncology Group to require para-aortic node sampling prior to placing patients with advanced cervical cancer on phase 3 studies. Serious bowel complications have been noted in cervical cancer patients who have had operative evaluation through a transperitoneal approach, followed by radiation therapy.[61] When extraperitoneal approaches to para-aortic nodes are compared with transperitoneal approaches in later irradiated patients, more

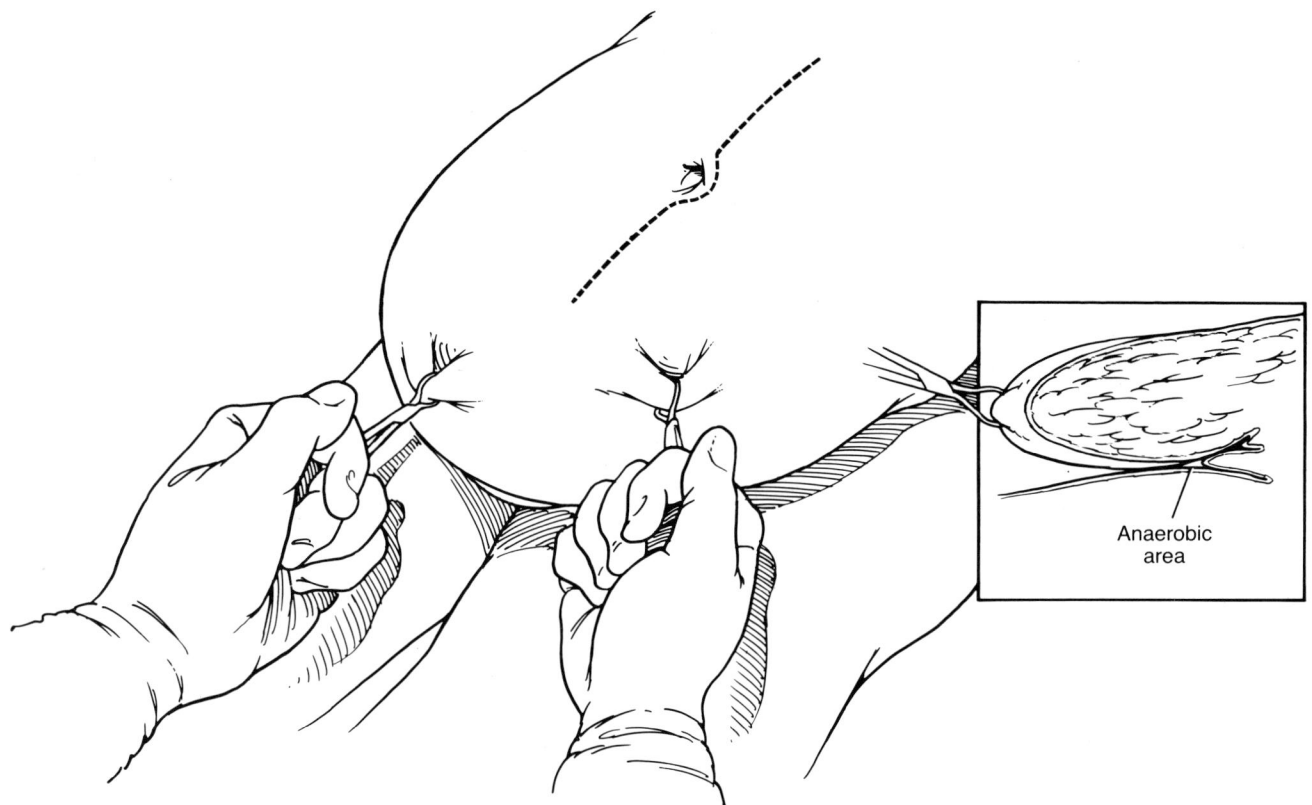

Figure 7–11
Retraction of the panniculus caudad with towel clips. The incision is made cephalad to the anaerobic subpannicular fold.

serious, later occurring small bowel problems are associated with the latter approach.[62, 63] To avoid these complications, an extraperitoneal approach has been advocated by means of bilateral superior groin incisions, a unilateral J-shaped incision, or an upper abdominal incision.

Bilateral Groin Incisions

In 1950, Nathanson suggested this extraperitoneal approach to eradicate regional node metastases in cervical cancer patients.[64] His study led to a later study of Stage IB cervical cancer patients, who initially had a staging procedure, in order to modify their later treatment.[65] The survival in the latter study was equivalent to Stage IB cancer patients managed by more traditional methods.

The procedure begins with an incision made 2.5 cm cephalad and parallel to the inguinal ligament. In obese patients, the incision is extended upward and outward, 2–4 cm beyond the anterior superior iliac spine. The external oblique fascia is divided medially to the internal ring. Laterally, the fibers of the internal oblique and transversalis muscles are divided in line of the skin incision. The round ligament is identified and usually divided, as are the deep inferior epigastric vessels. Beginning with the inferior portion of the incision, the peritoneum can gently be manipulated from the underlying tissues and retracted cephalad and medially (Fig. 7–12). Once the vessels are exposed, nodal dissection can be carried out as described later for midline incisions.

The disadvantages to this approach are obvious: no access to the para-aortic nodes and the need for two incisions. Nevertheless, this extraperitoneal approach may be indicated in the previously heavily irradiated patient who requires hypogastric artery ligation, when the artery is not easily obliterated by radiographic methods, or in the patient who needs exploration of the retroperitoneal pelvic space to rule out recurrence.

J-Shaped Incision

A modification of the extraperitoneal inguinal incision was described in the gynecologic literature by Berman and associates.[62] This is actually a modified Gibson incision (Fig. 7–13). The group from UCLA prefers to make the skin incision on the left, because the left para-aortic lymphatic channels are lateral and posterior to the aorta. They believe it is easier to dissect the precaval nodes from a left-sided incision, if a single incision is to be used for extraperitoneal para-aortic node sampling.

Access is gained by a vertical skin incision, starting just cephalad to the umbilicus and 3 cm medial

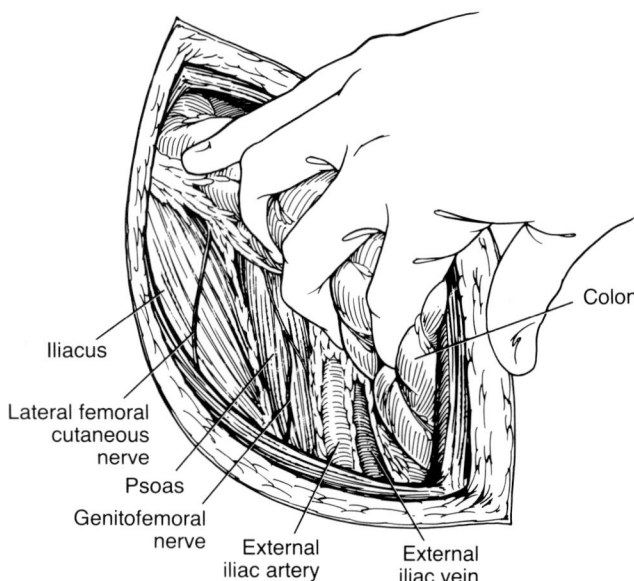

Figure 7–12
Gentle mobilization of the peritoneum off the lateral pelvic wall. This mobilization should begin caudad and the tissue swept medially and cephalad.

complications.[67–69] In the author's initial report of 30 patients who had pelvic node dissections by this approach, no significant complications were noted.[70] Two patients developed lymphocysts, and one had a superficial wound infection. The mean operating time to complete the bilateral pelvic node dissection was 48.7 minutes.

Following a vertical midline incision from umbilicus to pubis, the underlying fascia is sharply incised. (The incision can easily be extended around the umbilicus to the left for an extraperitoneal approach to para-aortic nodes.) The space of Retzius is bluntly dissected (see Fig. 7–6) in the midline, using the weight of the operator's hand. Any bleeding along Cooper's ligament can be controlled with cautery. The patient can be tilted 15 degrees laterally away from the side of surgery to aid dissection. The loose areolar tissue is further mobilized with a sponge stick to the pelvic floor. One hand of the operator assists in pulling the bladder and peritoneum from the opposite sidewall (see Fig. 7–12). The obturator nerve should be clearly seen. The fibroareolar and lym-

to the left iliac crest. Just caudad to the crest, the incision is carried medially about 3 cm cephalad and parallel to the left inguinal ligament. The fascial layers are incised separately. Exposure of the extraperitoneal space is developed by rolling the peritoneum medially, as shown from the right side in Figure 7–12. The round ligament and inferior epigastric vessels are ligated and sectioned to improve exposure. Following identification of the left ureter, a left para-aortic node dissection is performed. The left common iliac, external and internal iliac, and obturator nodes are subsequently removed. The peritoneum overlying the vena cava and right pelvic vessels is then elevated off the underlying vessels. After identification of the right ureter, all right-sided node chains are removed. The table should be tilted toward the patient's right to facilitate dissection.

Berman and associates caution that gentle traction must be used on the peritoneum when dissecting the right para-aortic (precaval) nodes, to avoid injury to the inferior mesenteric vessels. In an updated report from the same institution, Ballon and coworkers noted that 2 of 95 patients had avulsion of the inferior mesenteric artery, repaired without sequela.[66] In addition to the relative difficulty in sampling right-sided nodes, the lower portion of the incision may be in future radiation fields in some patients.

Midline Incisions

A single midline incision for extraperitoneal pelvic node lymphadenectomy has been used extensively in patients with prostatic and penile cancer with few

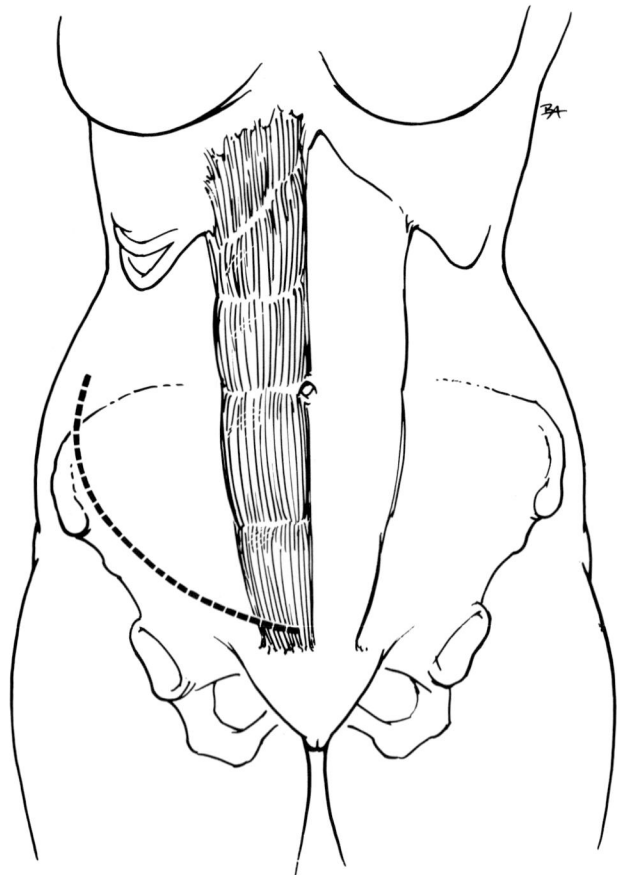

Figure 7–13
A modified Gibson incision. The incision is shown on the right. It may be started cephalad to the umbilicus or just 2–3 cm above and parallel to the inguinal ligament. The incision may also be initiated on the left side, depending on the preference of the operator.

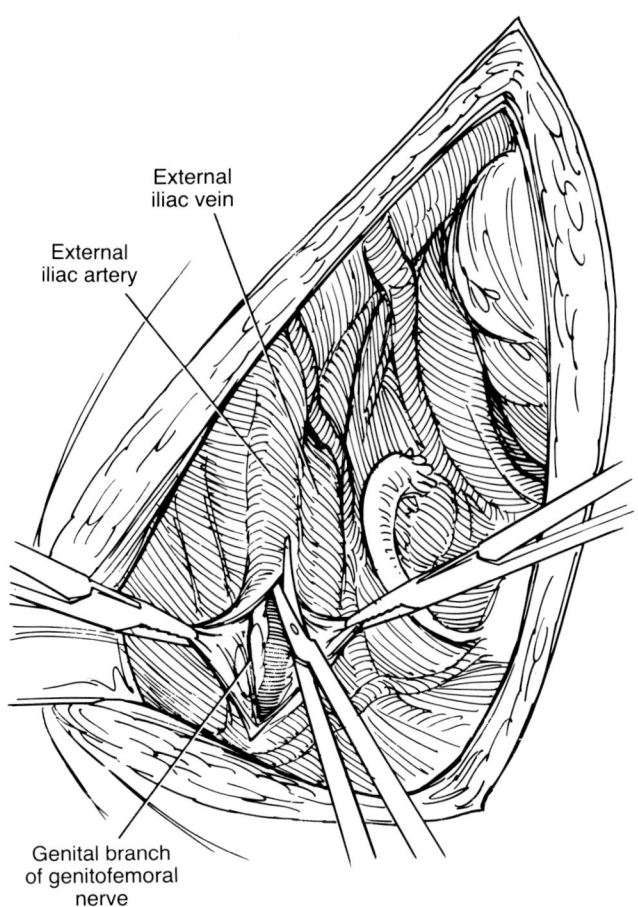

Figure 7–14
A midline incision has been made, and the peritoneum retracted medially. The areolar tissue over the external iliac artery is incised, and the genitofemoral nerve is clearly identified prior to removing any lymphatic tissue over the external iliac artery.

phatic tissue over the external iliac vein and artery is mobilized from cephalad to caudad, beginning at the bifurcation of the iliacs and ending at the caudad limits of dissection—the circumflex iliac artery and vein. The genitofemoral nerve should be clearly identified and cleaned prior to sectioning the proximal tissue bundle (Fig. 7–14). The finger of the surgeon is then passed lateral to the vessels down to the obturator space in order to ensure an avascular plane. The Singley forceps are used to mobilize all lymphatic tissue beneath the artery and vein to clear lymphatic tissue from the underlying muscles to the distal limits of dissection (Fig. 7–15). At this point, a Kitner dissector is used to strip the remaining areolar tissue overlying Cooper's ligament. All lymphatic tissue, now in one bundle, can be mobilized medially with the use of a right-angle clamp. A large clamp, such as a Carmalt, is rocked off of Cooper's ligament, and the lymphatic bundle is clamped, sectioned, and tied with a permanent suture.

By using the Singley forceps, the lymphatic bundle is bluntly dissected from the obturator nerve and mobilized cephalad. Often, the obturator vein and artery must be sacrificed to obtain access to tissue posteriorly and lateral to the nerve. Small vessels in the obturator space are individually clipped and sectioned. The bundle is mobilized superiorly to the bifurcation of the common iliacs. The ureter is identified. A Carmalt clamp is used to clamp the bundle at this level, and the tissue bundle is sectioned and removed en bloc. A large-bore closed drainage system is inserted into each obturator space and left in place for 5–10 days, depending on the amount of drainage.

The major disadvantage of this approach is that the incision must be healed if pelvic irradiation is needed. The access to nodes on both pelvic sidewalls is feasible, and easier access to the obturator space is obtained. The peritoneum can be used as a pack when performing the node dissection, of particular value in obese patients. This approach or the OIPE incision is used for all patients undergoing radical hysterectomy at the author's institution. If matted, large, bilateral nodes are found, they can be removed without entering the peritoneum, and the patient can be irradiated at the operator's discretion. Downey and colleagues have noted an advantage to debulking

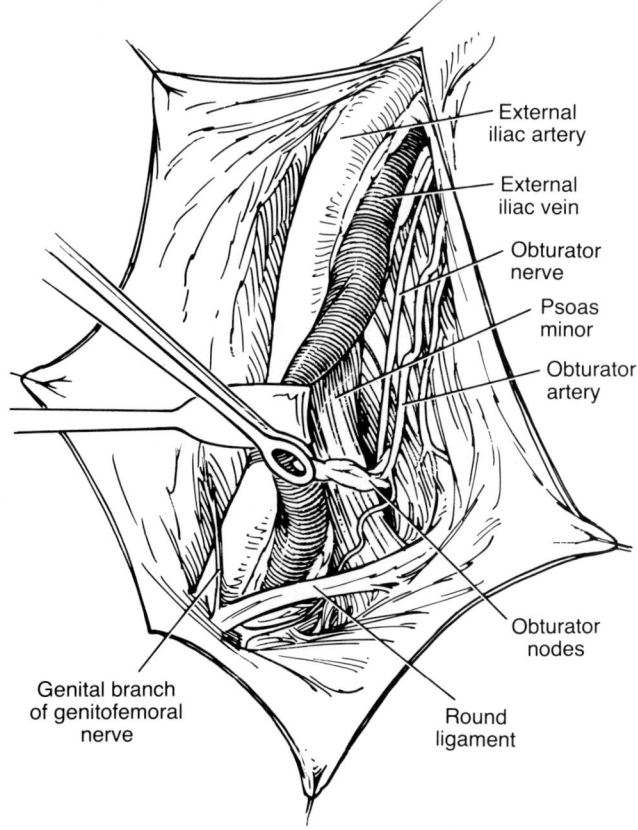

Figure 7–15
A vein retractor elevates the external iliac vein. The lymphatic bundles surrounding the obturator nerve may be mobilized cephalad or caudad and removed in one bundle.

pelvic nodal disease in later irradiated cervical cancer patients.[71] When a radical hysterectomy is to follow the node dissection, the uterine artery can be easily identified and sectioned at its insertion.

OIPE Approach

Kelâmi described a transverse approach that offers excellent exposure to the pelvic nodes.[72] This one-incision, pararectal, extraperitoneal (OIPE) approach is an extended (toward the anterior superior iliac spine) lower abdominal incision (Fig. 7–16). Once the fascia is incised, it is dissected cranially and caudally by blunt and sharp dissection. The peritoneum is then mobilized medially and cephalad to gain excellent exposure to the nodes. Because of the extensive fascial mobilization, a subfascial drain is usually needed.

This incision will allow excellent exposure to the common iliacs. However, its disadvantage is the inability to adequately sample the para-aortic nodes.

Upper Abdominal Incision

Schellhas described a right mid-rectus upper abdominal incision.[73] The incision described is short (7–8 cm) and made longitudinally from the level of the umbilicus toward the right costal margin. However, the incision usually has to be extended in the obese patient. Following the skin incision, the anterior rectus sheath is incised and freed laterally from the rectus muscle. Branching vessels from the epigastrics are ligated, and the rectus muscle is retracted medially. The posterior rectus sheath is opened in the mid-rectus line and is dissected from the underlying peritoneum by a hemostat. It is then retracted laterally, and peritoneum is freed from its muscular attachments to the lateral abdominal wall with sharp scissor dissection. The posterior peritoneum is bluntly dissected and mobilized medially. The space is more easily exposed if the manual dissection begins caudad, near the psoas. The right ureter and ovarian vessels are identified and may be left attached to the peritoneum or dissected off and retracted laterally. The vessels may be transected.

The disadvantages of this approach are difficulty in dissecting the left para-aortic nodes and inability to remove bulky low common iliac or pelvic nodes. Moreover, in obese patients, when the incision needs to be extended, the likelihood of nerve damage to the intercostal nerves increases. A significant transection of these nerves could result in partial rectus muscle paralysis and hernia formation. The incision is usually well removed from pelvic radiation fields.

"Sunrise" Incision

The author has used an upper abdominal transverse incision for extraperitoneal nodal staging in cervical cancer patients, which allows early postoperative irradiation (Fig. 7–17). The skin incision is made in a curved transverse manner, lying about 2 cm cephalad to the umbilicus in the center. The rectus muscle on the right is transected. The peritoneum is mobilized medially, after being separated from its lateral attachments with sharp dissection. The blunt dissection begins caudad, at the level of the common iliacs. With transection of the right rectus, exposure to both precaval and left para-aortic nodes is usually readily obtained. However, in obese patients, the left rectus muscle occasionally needs to be transected and peritoneum mobilized from the left side for adequate left para-aortic node dissections. After the nodes are removed, the peritoneum can be incised, cell washings obtained, and manual evaluation of the abdominal cavity performed, including pelvic nodes. (Figure 7–18 illustrates the Steri-Stripped incision far removed from the outlined proposed irradiation fields.)

The advantages of this incision are a relatively low chance of intercostal nerve injury and the ability to easily extend the incision laterally below the iliac crest to remove any discovered bulky pelvic nodes by an extraperitoneal approach.

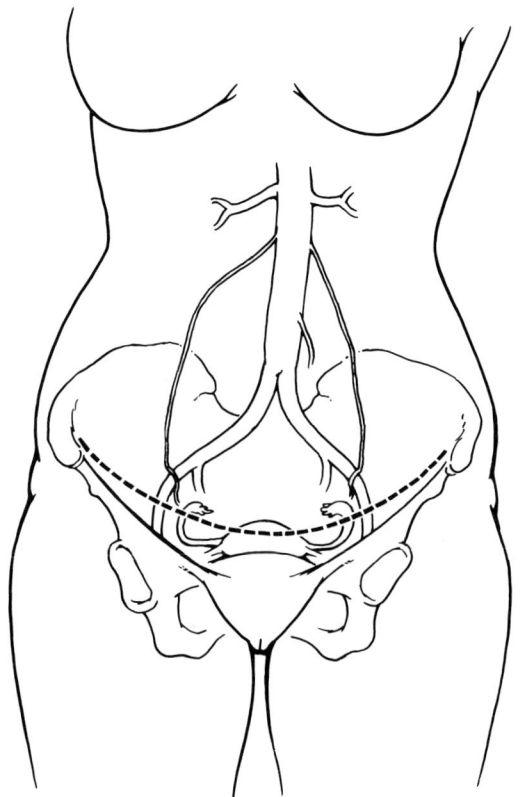

Figure 7–16
The one-incision, pararectal, extraperitoneal (OIPE) incision. This is an extended transverse incision. Once the fascia is incised, it is dissected cranially and caudally by blunt and sharp dissection. Peritoneum may be mobilized medially for an extraperitoneal approach to the pelvic nodes.

Transperitoneal Approaches to Para-aortic Nodes

Para-aortic node sampling is indicated in some patients with ovarian carcinoma or malignant corpus tumors. Patients have usually been explored through a midline incision. Three approaches are used by most gynecologists. An incision can be made over the right common iliac artery in the posterior parietal peritoneum. This approach may not give adequate exposure in some ovarian carcinomas, in which the entry point for metastatic spread may be at the level of the renal vessels on the left and approximately 1–2 cm below the renal vessels on the right.

An alternative approach, particularly in high-risk ovarian cancer patients, is to use an entry popularized for testicular cancer and described in the gynecologic literature.[74] The incision is initiated in the parietal peritoneum 2–3 cm caudal and lateral to the cecum. It is extended cephalad, along the line of Toldt, parallel to the right colon and extended all the way to the hepatic flexure. For better exposure, the lower portion of the incision can be extended medially just anterior to the right common iliac artery.

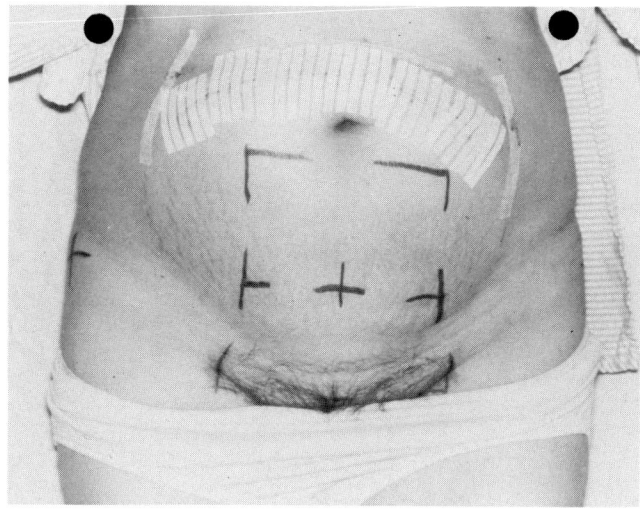

Figure 7–18
The "sunrise" incision made 3 days prior to this illustration shows Steri-Strips approximating the skin. The radiation field in this postoperative patient has been outlined for early irradiation following a staging procedure for carcinoma of the cervix.

Care must be taken at this point to avoid injury to the underlying ureter (Fig. 7–19). The colon and small bowel with their respective mesentery are gently mobilized by sharp and blunt dissection medially and cephalad. Care must be taken not to avulse the inferior mesenteric vessels. For maximum exposure, these can be sacrificed. The ureters should be freed from their attachment to the peritoneum. In those patients undergoing oophorectomy, the ovarian vessels may be isolated and divided as close as possible to their junction with the aorta or vena cava. This approach will afford excellent exposure to the cephalad portion of the great vessels. The incision can also be initiated in the left lateral peritoneal gutter, and the sigmoid and descending colon mobilized medially.

DELAYED SECONDARY CLOSURE

The value of delayed primary wound closure in managing possible contaminated wounds has been recognized by military surgeons for many years. Grosfeld and Solit noted that patients with perforating appendicitis had a reduction in wound infection rates from 34.1 to 2.3% when delayed closure was used.[75] In a high-risk group of patients, which included patients with obesity, cancer, possible contamination from "above and below" procedures, infection, and bowel content contamination, Brown and colleagues found a marked reduction in wound infection rates when delayed primary closure was used as compared with immediate closure in matched patients.[76] The infection rate for the former group was 2.1%; for the latter, 23.3%. Possible candidates

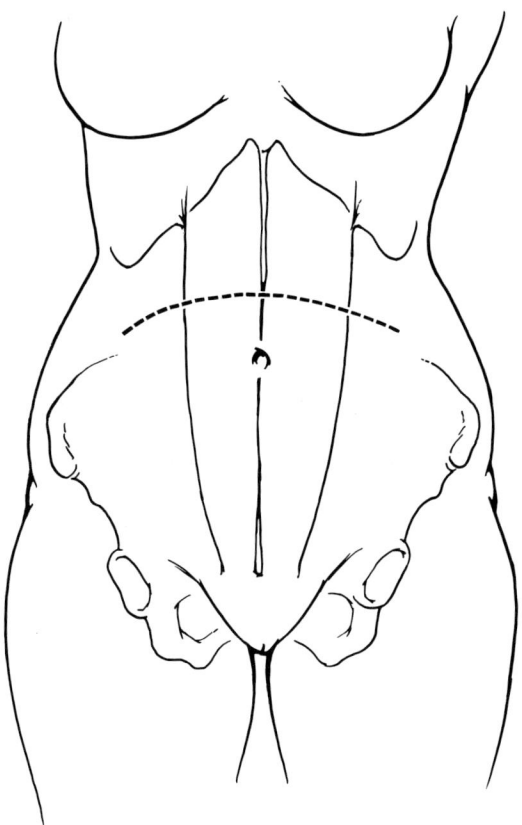

Figure 7–17
An upper abdominal transverse incision is made approximately 2–3 cm cephalad to the umbilicus. This is a "sunrise" incision and may be extended caudally to remove enlarged pelvic nodes. The incision is designed for an extraperitoneal para-aortic lymph node sampling for cervical cancer.

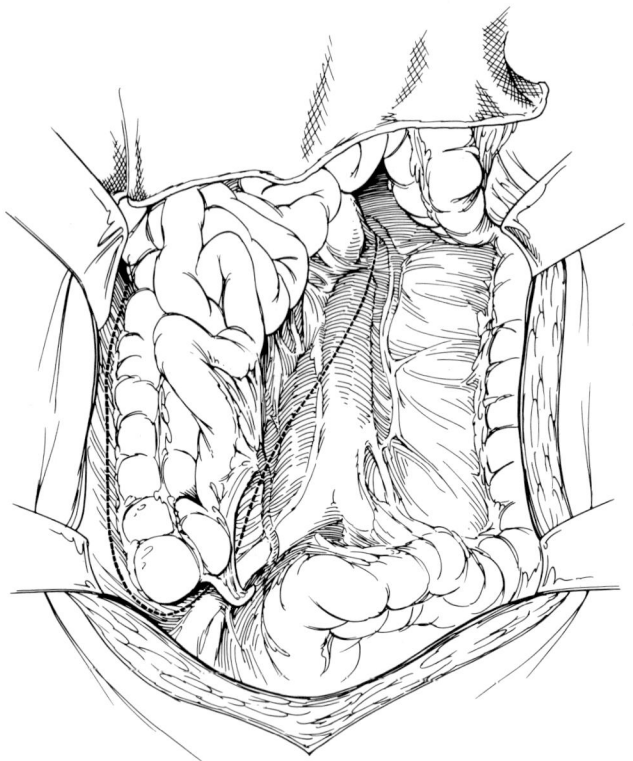

Figure 7–19
An incision for mobilization of the right colon to adequately expose the high para-aortic nodes in patients in whom they are palpable or when nodes in the area of the renal vessels should be removed, as in some patients with ovarian carcinoma. This is also a useful incision in the obese patient, in whom exposure is limited. The incision may be utilized on the left to expose the left para-aortic nodes, depending on the operator's preference.

for such a closure include patients with suppurative appendicitis, ruptured tubo-ovarian abscess, extensive bowel injury in the "unprepared" bowel, or diverticulitis with contamination. Delayed closure may also be of value in select patients who have had groin incisions associated with radical vulvectomy procedures.

Following closure of the fascia, the wound is irrigated with copious amounts of saline. Some investigators prefer to then spray the solution with a combined broad-spectrum antibiotic spray.[76, 77] Vertical interrupted mattress sutures of 3-0 nylon or 3.0 monofilament polypropylene are placed 2–3 cm apart. They are loosely tied over dilute povidone-iodine dressing gauze. The 4 × 8 dressing sponges are changed three times a day with a "wet-to-dry" technique, using sterile saline. Some surgeons use bridges, consisting of rolled gauze on the lateral borders of the incision, to support these sutures.[78] In 4–5 days, depending on the appearance of the subcutaneous tissues, the previously placed sutures are tied to approximate the skin edges. In obese patients, a closed drainage system is placed anterior to the fascia and removed in 1–3 days. Tincture of benzoin is placed at the lateral edges of the closed incision, and Steri-Strips are used to approximate uneven skin edges.

COMPLETE WOUND DEHISCENCE AND EVISCERATION

Technically, wound dehiscence means separation of layers of the abdominal incision. Incomplete or partial dehiscence means separation of the layers posteriorly, sometimes including the fascia. If the peritoneum is included in the disruption, the dehiscence is considered complete. If the intestine protrudes through the wound, the term evisceration is used.

Evisceration is one of the most feared and dangerous postoperative complications. The mortality associated with evisceration is reported from 10 to 35%,[44–46, 79] and this mortality is usually associated with other complications such as sepsis. Evisceration is less likely to occur in gynecology patients, as compared with general surgery patients.

Many of the predisposing factors for complete wound disruption or evisceration are metabolic and include malnutrition, poorly controlled diabetes, corticosteroid use, and older age.[80] Mechanical factors include obesity, intra-abdominal distention, infection, retching, and coughing, often associated with chronic lung disease. Rapid postoperative reaccumulation of ascites has been associated, and radiation therapy may lead to poor wound healing. As noted, complete wound dehiscence and evisceration are usually problems associated with tissue failure, not suture failure.[80] In one series, 88% of eviscerated wounds had tearing of suture through the fascia with knots and suture intact.

Eviscerations usually occur from day 5 to 14 following operations, with a mean of around 8 days. One of the early signs of complete dehiscence and impending evisceration is the seepage of serosanguineous pink discharge from an apparently intact wound. It may be present for several days before evisceration occurs. Although occult hematomas are usually the cause of such discharge, these patients' wounds should be carefully examined at frequent intervals (every 6–8 hours).

With very few exceptions, complete dehiscence or eviscerations should be closed as soon as they are recognized. In case of evisceration, when a delay of several hours is anticipated because of a recent meal, the bowel can be replaced using sterile gloves and gently packed in place with lap pads soaked in povidone-iodine.[81] An abdominal binder should be placed over the lap pads. Broad-spectrum antibiotics should be initiated, and baseline blood counts and serum electrolyte studies should be obtained.

When the patient is in the operating room (never on the floor), the wound should be meticulously explored to determine the extent of dehiscence. Necrotic tissue, clots, and suture material should be removed. The bowel and omentum should be inspected and thoroughly cleansed with several liters of warm normal saline. If the fascial margins can be located and are not ragged, a Smead-Jones closure with large-bore polypropylene or nylon can be used. The subcutaneous tissue and skin are packed open for later delayed closure.

If the wound edges are ragged and/or the patient's condition is poor, a through-and-through suture of No. 2 nylon or polypropylene is used. The sutures are placed at least 2.5–3.0 cm from the skin edges and are passed through all layers. To allow for edema, they are placed 2 cm apart. To prevent inclusion of the underlying intestine in a suture, all sutures are held up before the first one is tied. Skin edges unopposed between the through-and-through sutures can be approximated with interrupted 3-0 polypropylene. The through-and-through sutures should be left in for 3 weeks.[44, 82] A nasogastric tube should be used in the immediate postoperative period to avoid abdominal distention.

References

1. Daversa B, Landers D: Physiologic advantages of the transverse incision in gynecology. Obstet Gynecol 1961; 17:305.
2. Rees VL, Coller FA: Anatomic and clinical study of the transverse abdominal incision. Arch Surg 1943; 47:136.
3. Thorek P: Anatomy in Surgery, 3rd ed. New York, Springer-Verlag, 1985, p. 368.
4. McMinn RMH, Hutchings RJ, Logan BM: Color Atlas of Applied Anatomy. Chicago, Year Book Medical Publishers, 1984, p. 110.
5. Cruse PJE: Infection surveillance: Identifying the problem and the high-risk patient. South Med J 1977; 70(Suppl. 1):40.
6. Mead PB: Managing infected abdominal wounds. Contemp OB/Gyn 1979; 14:69.
7. Cruse PJE, Foord R: A five year prospective study of 23,649 surgical wounds. Arch Surg 1973; 107:206.
8. Dineen P: A critical study of 100 conservative wound infections. Surg Gynecol Obstet 1961; 113:91.
9. Cruse PJE, Foord R: The epidemiology of wound infection: A 10 year prospective study of 62,939 wounds. Surg Clin North Am 1980; 60:27.
10. Olson M, O'Connor MO, Schwartz ML: A 5-year prospective study of 20,193 wounds at Minneapolis VA Medical Center. Ann Surg 1984; 199:253.
11. Sanz LE, Smith S: Mechanism of wound healing, suture material, and wound closure. In Buchsbaum HJ, Walton LA (eds.): Strategies in Gynecologic Surgery. New York, Springer-Verlag, 1986, p. 53.
12. Edlich RF, Panek RH, Rodeheaver GT, et al.: Physical and chemical configuration of suture in the development of surgical infection. Ann Surg 1973; 177:679.
13. Postlethwait RW: Long-term comparative study of nonabsorbable sutures. Ann Surg 1970; 171:892.
14. Macht SD, Krizek TJ: Sutures and suturing—current concepts. J Oral Surg 1978; 36:240.
15. Fagniez P, Hay JM, Lacaine F, Thomsen C: Abdominal midline incisions closure. A randomized prospective trial of 3,135 patients, comparing continuous vs. interrupted polyglycolic acid sutures. Arch Surg 1984; 120:1351.
16. Sanz LE, Patterson JA, Kamath R, et al.: Comparison of Maxon suture with Vicryl, chromic catgut, and PDS sutures in fascial closure in rats. Obstet Gynecol 1988; 71:918.
17. Metz SA, Chegini N, Masterson BJ: In vivo tissue reactivity and degradation of suture materials: A comparison of Maxon and PDS. J Gynecol Surg 1989; 5:37.
18. Rodeheaver GT, Powell TA, Thacker JG, Edlich RF: Mechanical performance of monofilament synthetic absorbable sutures. Am J Surg 1987; 154:544.
19. Bourne RB, Bitar H, Andrese PR, et al.: In-vivo comparison of four absorbable sutures: Vicryl, Dexon Plus, Maxon and PDS. Can J Surg 1988; 31:43.
20. van Rissel EJC, Baptisttrimbos J, Booster MH: Mechanical performance of square knots and sliding knots in surgery: A comparative study. Am J Obstet Gynecol 1990; 162:93.
21. Higson RH, Kettlewell MGW: Parietal wound drainage in abdominal surgery. Br J Surg 1978; 65:326.
22. Morrow CP, Hernandez WL, Townsend DE, DiSaia PJ: Pelvic celiotomy in the obese patient. Am J Obstet Gynecol 1977; 127:335.
23. Gallup DG: Modification of celiotomy techniques to decrease morbidity in obese gynecologic patients. Am J Obstet Gynecol 1984; 150:171.
24. Scott HW, Law HD, Sandstead HH, et al.: Jejunoileal shunt in surgical treatment of morbid obesity. Ann Surg 1970; 171:770.
25. Farnell MB, Worthington-Self S, Mucha P Jr, et al.: Closure of abdominal incisions with subcutaneous catheters. Arch Surg 1986; 126:641.
26. Lineweaver W, Howard R, Soucy D, et al.: Topical antimicrobial toxicity. Arch Surg 1985; 120:1985.
27. Helmkamp BF, Krebs HB, Amstey MS: Correct use of surgical drains. Contemp OB/Gyn 1984; 23:123.
28. Moss JP: Historical and current perspective on surgical drainage. Surg Gynecol Obstet 1981; 152:517.
29. Balthazar ER, Colt JD, Nicols RL: Preoperative hair removal: A random prospective study of shaving versus clipping. South Med J 1982; 75:799.
30. Hamilton HW, Hamilton KR, Lone FJ: Preoperative hair removal. Can J Surg 1977; 20:269.
31. Seropian R, Reynolds BM: Wound infections after preoperative depilatory versus razor preparation. Am J Surg 1971; 121:251.
32. Alexander JW, Aerni S, Plettner JP: Development of a safe and effective one-minute preoperative skin preparation. Arch Surg 1985; 120:1367.
33. Galle PC, Homesley HD, Rhyne AL: Reassessment of the surgical scrub. Surg Gynecol Obstet 1978; 147:214.
34. Hasselgren AO, Harbery E, Malmer H, et al.: One instead of two knifes for surgical incision. Arch Surg 1984; 118:917.
35. Mowat J, Bonnar J: Abdominal wound dehiscence after cesarean section. Br Med J 1971; 2:256.
36. Tollefson DG, Russell KP: The transverse incision in pelvic surgery. Am J Obstet Gynecol 1954; 68:410.
37. Thompson JB, Maclean KF, Collier FA: Role of the transverse abdominal incision and early ambulation in the reduction of postoperative complications. Arch Surg 1949; 59:1267.
38. Helmkamp BF: Abdominal wound dehiscence. Am J Obstet Gynecol 1977; 128:803.
39. Greenburg G, Salk RP, Peskin GW: Wound dehiscence. Pathophysiology and prevention. Arch Surg 1979; 114:143.
40. Cherney LS: A modified transverse incision for low abdominal operations. Surg Gynecol Obstet 1941; 72:92.
41. Maylard AE: Direction of abdominal incision. Br Med J 1907; 2:895.
42. Parsons L, Ulfelder H: Atlas of Pelvic Surgery, 2nd ed. Philadelphia, WB Saunders Co., 1968, p. 156.
43. Guillou PJ, Hall TJ, Donaldson DR, et al.: Vertical abdominal incisions—a choice? Br J Surg 1980; 67:359.
44. Pratt JH: Wound healing—evisceration. Clin Obstet Gynecol 1973; 16:126.
45. Alexander HC, Prudden JF: The causes of abdominal wound disruption. Surg Gynecol Obstet 1966; 122:1223.
46. Richards PC, Balch CM, Aldrete JS: Abdominal wound closure. Ann Surg 1983; 197:238.
47. Jurkiewicz MJ, Morales L: Wound healing, operative incisions, and skin grafts. In Hardy JD (ed.): Hardy's Textbook of Surgery. Philadelphia, JB Lippincott, 1983, p. 108.

48. Wallace D, Hernandez W, Schlaerth JB, et al.: Prevention of abdominal wound disruption utilizing the Smead-Jones closure technique. Obstet Gynecol 1980; 56:226.
49. Jenkins TPN: The burst abdominal wound: A mechanical approach. Br J Surg 1976; 63:873.
50. Archie JP, Feldman RW: Primary wound closure with permanent continuous running monofilament sutures. Surg Gynecol Obstet 1981; 153:721.
51. Murray DH, Blaisdell FW: Use of synthetic absorbable sutures for abdominal and chest wound closures. Arch Surg 1978; 113:477.
52. Shepherd JH, Cavanagh D, Riggs D, et al.: Abdominal wound closure using a nonabsorbable single-layer technique. Obstet Gynecol 1983; 61:248.
53. Knight CD, Griffen FD: Abdominal wound closure with a continuous monofilament polypropylene suture. Arch Surg 1983: 118:1305.
54. Gallup DG, Talledo OE, King LA: Primary mass closure of midline incisions with a continuous running monofilament suture in gynecologic patients. Obstet Gynecol 1989; 73:67.
55. Stone HH, Holfling SJ, Strom PR, et al.: Abdominal incisions, transverse vs. vertical placement and continuous vs. interrupted closure. South Med J 1983; 76:1106.
56. Gallup DG, Nolan TE, Smith RP: Primary mass closure of midline incisions with a continuous polyglyconate monofilament absorbable suture. Obstet Gynecol 1990; 76:872.
57. Pitkin RM: Abdominal hysterectomy in obese women. Surg Gynecol Obstet 1976; 142:532.
58. Krebs HB, Helmkamp F: Transverse periumbilical incision in the massively obese patient. Obstet Gynecol 1984; 63:241.
59. Averette HE, Dudan RC, Ford JH: Exploratory celiotomy for surgical staging of cervical cancer. Am J Obstet Gynecol 1972; 133:1090.
60. Nelson JH, Boyce J, Macasaet M, et al.: Incidence, significance, and follow-up of para-aortic lymph node metastases in late invasive carcinoma of the cervix. Am J Obstet Gynecol 1977; 128:336.
61. Wharton JT, Jones HW, Day TG, et al.: Preirradiation celiotomy for invasive carcinoma of the cervix. Obstet Gynecol 1977; 49:333.
62. Berman ML, Lagasse LD, Watring WG, et al.: The operative evaluation of patients with cervical carcinoma by an extraperitoneal approach. Obstet Gynecol 1977; 50:658.
63. Weiser EB, Bundy B, Hoskins WJ, et al.: Extraperitoneal versus transperitoneal selective paraaortic lymphadenectomy in the pre-treatment surgical staging of advanced cervical carcinoma (a Gynecologic Oncology Group study). Gynecol Oncol 1989; 33:283.
64. Nathanson IT: Extraperitoneal iliac lymphadenectomy in the treatment of carcinoma of the cervix. Prog Gynecol 1950; 2:565.
65. Quigley MM, Knab DR, McMahon EB: Carcinoma of the cervix: A third treatment. Obstet Gynecol 1975; 45:650.
66. Ballon SL, Berman ML, Lagasse LD, et al.: Survival after extraperitoneal pelvic and paraaortic lymphadenectomy and radiation therapy in cervical carcinoma. Obstet Gynecol 1981; 57:90.
67. Skinner DG: Pelvic lymphadenectomy. In Glen JF (ed.): Urologic Surgery, 2nd ed. New York, Harper & Row, 1983, pp. 589–594.
68. Brendler CB, Cleeve LK, Anderson EE, et al.: Staging pelvic lymphadenectomy of the prostate: Risk versus benefit. J Urol 1980; 124:849.
69. Lieskovsky G, Skinner DSA, Weisenburg T: Pelvic lymphadenectomy in the management of carcinoma of the prostate. J Urol 1980; 124:635.
70. Gallup DG, Jordan GH, Talledo OE: Extraperitoneal lymph node dissections with use of a midline incision in patients with female genital cancer. Am J Obstet Gynecol 1986; 155:559.
71. Downey GO, Potish RA, Adcock LL, et al.: Pre-treatment surgical staging in cervical carcinoma: Therapeutic efficacy of pelvic lymph node dissection. Am J Obstet Gynecol 1989; 160:1055.
72. Kelâmi A: One-incision, pararectal, extraperitoneal (OIPE) approach for bilateral procedures on lower two thirds of ureters. Urology 1980; 15:296.
73. Schellhas HF: Extraperitoneal para-aortic node dissection through an upper abdominal incision. Obstet Gynecol 1975; 46:444.
74. Lubicz S: Approach to abdominal retroperitoneum in patients with gynecologic malignancies. Gynecol Oncol 1985; 22:32.
75. Grosfeld JL, Solit RW: Prevention of wound infection in perforated appendicitis. Experience with delayed primary wound closure. Ann Surg 1968; 168:891.
76. Brown SE, Allen HH, Robins RN: The use of delayed primary wound closure in preventing wound infections. Am J Obstet Gynecol 1977; 127:213.
77. Stone HH, Hester TR: Topical antibiotic and delayed primary closure in the management of contaminated surgical incisions. J Surg Res 1972; 12:70.
78. Mendenez MA: The contaminated wound. In O'Leary JP, Waltering EA (eds.): Techniques for Surgeons. New York, John Wiley & Sons, 1985, pp. 36–37.
79. Keill RH, Keitzer WF, Henzel J, DeWeese MS: Abdominal wound dehiscence. Arch Surg 1973; 106:573.
80. Kenady DE: Management of abdominal wounds. Surg Clin North Am 1984; 64:803.
81. Morris DM: Preoperative management of patients with evisceration. Dis Colon Rectum 1982; 25:249.
82. Helmkamp BF: Abdominal wound dehiscence. Am J Obstet Gynecol 1977; 128:803.

Prevention of Adhesions

8

Michael P. Diamond

Teleologically, adhesions can probably be thought of as representing an attempt by the body to provide vascular supply to a traumatized, relatively ischemic area of tissue. As such, adhesions constitute a part of the normal healing process. However, when adhesions so formed interfere with normal function (e.g., tubal ovum pickup, propagation of food through bowel, etc.) or result in pain, they constitute a normal process gone awry.

Probably the greatest impediment to attempts at reducing adhesion development is lack of physician recognition of their clinical significance, and of the frequency with which adhesions occur postoperatively. All too often, comments are made by individual surgeons that "adhesions are not a problem for (my) patients" or that they "don't get any adhesions after surgery," and thus they don't have to be concerned with trying to prevent postsurgical adhesions. Unfortunately, as will be illustrated, this is not usually the case.

Although most clinical studies directly assessing postsurgical adhesion development have been performed by infertility surgeons, this issue really should be of interest to the broader category of all gynecologic surgeons, and actually, all intra-abdominal surgeons in general. Postoperative adhesion development is not only a concern in the immediate future after infertility surgery when functional maximization of the tubal ovum pickup mechanism is desired. It is also an issue for fertility years later, after treatment of pelvic inflammatory disease, ovarian cysts, ectopic pregnancies, and appendectomies, as well as for minimization of future intra-abdominal pain, bowel obstruction, and bowel fixation (which can result in bowel damage following abdominal radiation therapy).

Nevertheless, most clinical studies assessing acute postoperative adhesion development have been described in the infertility literature. The explanation is the clinical significance of the occurrence of postoperative adhesions, as well as the clinical practice on the part of many reproductive pelvic surgeons to recommend early second-look laparoscopy to their infertility patients.[1] At the time of these early second-look surgeries, the surgeon is able to directly assess where, and to what extent, adhesions have developed after the initial surgical procedure. Thus, the efficacy of surgical techniques and adjuvants can be evaluated, and adhesions that have developed since the initial procedure can be treated.

Evaluations performed at the time of early second-look laparoscopy have clearly demonstrated the high frequency with which adhesions re-form after adhesiolysis.[2-7] As shown in Table 8–1, adhesion re-formation occurred in 55–100% of infertility patients initially treated at laparotomy. This high frequency of postoperative adhesion development occurs despite application of the tenets of gynecologic microsurgery, the widespread use of surgical adjuvants, and use of laser technology in many of these series.

More specifically, despite adherence to the use of these state of the art techniques, in the reports of the Intraabdominal Laser Study Group, adhesiolysis at laparotomy in 121 women was followed by reduction of the pelvic adhesion score in 91 women; however, in 14 women the adhesion scores remained the same, whereas adhesion scores actually increased in 16 women.[8] Further analysis of these data dem-

Table 8–1

Pelvic Adhesions Noted at Second-Look Laparoscopy

	Time from Initial Procedure	Total No. of Patients	Total No. with Adhesions	Percentage with Adhesions
Diamond et al.[2]	1–12 wk	106	91	86
DeCherney and Mezer[3]	4–16 wk	20	15	75
	1–3 yr	41	31	76
Surrey and Friedman[4]	6–8 wk	31	22	71
	≥6 mon	6	5	83
Pittaway et al.[5]	4–6 wk	23	23	100
Trimbos-Kemper et al.[6]	8 days	188	104	55
Daniell and Pittaway[7]	4–6 wk	25	24	96

From Sciarra J (ed.): Gynecology and Obstetrics. Philadelphia, Harper & Row, 1988.

onstrates the rate of adhesion re-formation at individual sites within the pelvis (as a function of whether the initial adhesions were fine and filmy, or dense and vascular): the ovary (Fig. 8–1A), the fimbria (Fig. 8–1B), and other locations in the pelvis (the omentum, large bowel, small bowel, pelvic sidewall, and cul-de-sac [Fig. 8–1C]). In this series, the frequency with which adhesions were observed at second-look laparoscopy was independent of the type of adhesion (fine and filmy or dense and vascular) present at the time of the initial procedure. Similarly, the type of adhesion observed at second-look laparoscopy was independent of the initial type of adhesion. These data therefore suggest that concern for postoperative adhesion development is not limited to those more complex in nature, but extends to those adhesions with "Saran Wrap" characteristics as well.

Thus, when appropriate evaluations are conducted to assess postoperative adhesion development, the presence of peritoneal scarring is an all too frequent occurrence.

Furthermore, the same group illustrated that postoperative adhesion development is not limited to adhesion re-formation, but also includes de novo adhesion formation.[8] De novo adhesion formation is defined as the presence of adhesions at a second-look procedure at sites that did not undergo adhesiolysis at the time of the initial operative procedure. As such, de novo adhesions represent adhesions that form at sites undergoing primary procedures (e.g., neosalpingostomy, fimbrioplasty, ovarian wedge resection) as well as sites with no primary surgery. As shown in Table 8–2, following the performance of reproductive pelvic surgery at laparotomy, de novo adhesion formation occurred with a relatively high frequency throughout the pelvis, and in fact was present at nearly one-third of available sites at early second-look laparoscopy. Furthermore, the frequency with which de novo adhesions formed following operative procedures was approximately 50%. Consequently, the frequency of de novo adhesion formation at nonoperated sites is nearly the same.

PATHOGENESIS OF ADHESIONS

In order to consider prevention of postoperative adhesion development, it is important to understand normal peritoneal healing, and how this process is altered by prior damage to the peritoneum. Unfortunately, we are as yet still in our infancy in under-

Table 8–2

De Novo Adhesion Formation*

	Total No. of Sites	Adhesions at Initial Procedure	Structures Excised	Sites Available for De Novo Adhesion Formation	Sites with Occurrence of De Novo Adhesions	Percentage of Available Sites with De Novo Adhesions
Ovaries	164	84	8	72	42	58
Tubes	164	50	10	104	26	25
Omentum	82	4	—	78	13	17
Small Bowel	82	8	—	74	19	26
Colon	82	11	—	71	13	18
Cul-De-Sac	82	26	—	56	16	29
Sidewall	82	27	—	55	30	55
Total	738	210	18	510	159	31

*Frequency of de novo adhesion formation identified at early second-look laparoscopy at sites throughout the pelvis after reproductive pelvic surgical procedures performed at laparotomy.
From unpublished data of Diamond MP, Daniell JF, Feste J, Surrey MW, McLaughlin DS, Friedman S, Vaughn WK, and Martin DC.

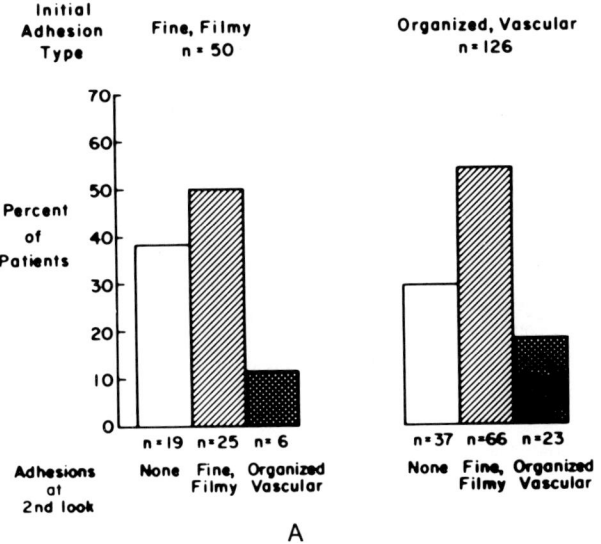
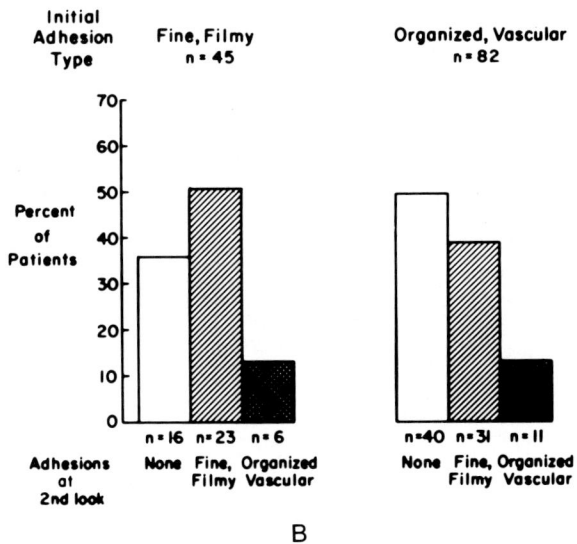
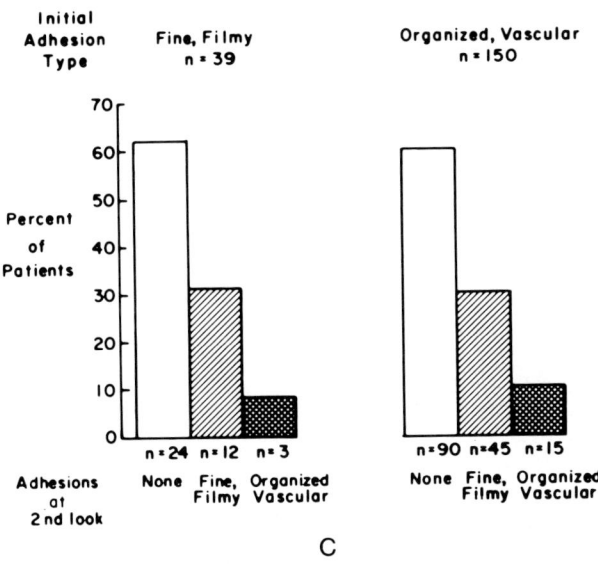

Figure 8–1
Frequency of postoperative adhesion re-formation following adhesiolysis at laparotomy at (A) ovaries, (B) fimbria, and (C) other pelvic locations (omentum, large bowel, small bowel, pelvic sidewall, and cul-de-sac). (Modified from Diamond MP, et al.: Adhesion reformation and de novo adhesion formation following reproductive pelvic surgery. Fertil Steril 1987; 47:864.)

standing the physiologic process of healing, and know even less regarding how this process is altered during healing of previously damaged peritoneum. The following sequence represents a combination of postulated theories and established observations of peritoneal repair.

It appears that healing of peritoneum differs from healing of skin. Repair of a skin defect occurs by proliferation of normal epithelial cells surrounding the wound, with resultant healing from the edges into the center. In contrast, peritoneal healing following surgical trauma is thought not to generally occur by this mechanism, but rather by differentiation of primordial cells at the base of the entire defect into fibroblasts that repair the wound.[9] Another alternative mechanism—seeding of the defect by free-floating peritoneal macrophages—is also not thought to be likely. At the present time, there appears to be no reason to suspect that peritoneal defects from causes other than surgical trauma (e.g., infection, ruptured viscus, endometriosis, etc.) heal by alternative mechanisms; however, this question has not as yet been appropriately addressed.

The question thus becomes what initiates and

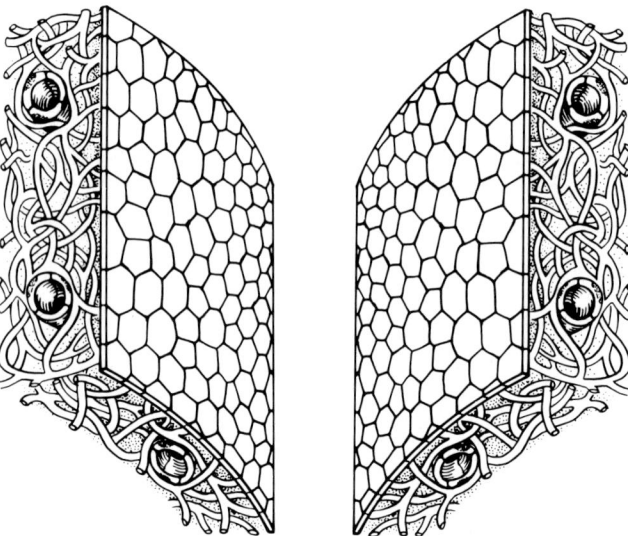

Figure 8–2
Diagrammatic representation of neighboring peritoneal surfaces.

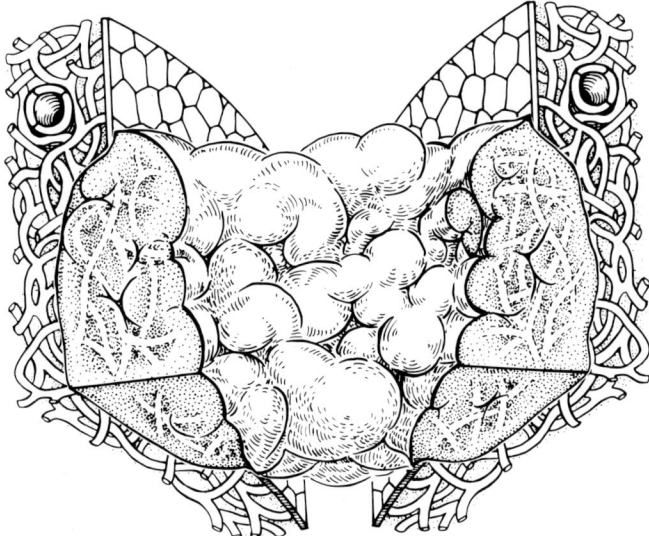

Figure 8–4
Proteinaceous exudate forming over the injured peritoneal surfaces as a consequence of vascular damage and increased vascular permeability, resulting in connection of adjoining peritoneal surfaces by the proteinaceous exudate.

regulates the fibroblast proliferation, and over what time course does this process occur. In normal peritoneum (Fig. 8–2) in response to peritoneal trauma, there is establishment of a defect that can involve underlying connective tissue and vascular structures (Fig. 8–3). As a result, there is immediate elaboration of a proteinaceous exudate that is rich in fibrin and other proteins in the clotting cascade, as well as in a variety of white blood cells, including macrophages, plasma cells, and polymorphonucleocytes (Fig. 8–4).[9, 10] The exudation of the proteinaceous products is thought to be due to increased vascular permeability, which is propagated by release of histamine from mast cells at the wound site. Monokines, particularly interleukin-one (IL-1), are also thought to be involved in this process and to result in subsequent adhesion development.[11] The exudation of these products results in deposition of a fibrinous mass at the traumatized site (Fig. 8–5). Whether an adhesion subsequently develops is based on whether this mass connects adjoining structures, and whether it is dissipated (as occurs with normal healing of serosal surfaces, with no resultant adhesions) or whether it persists during the time of fibroblast proliferation with resultant collagen deposition into

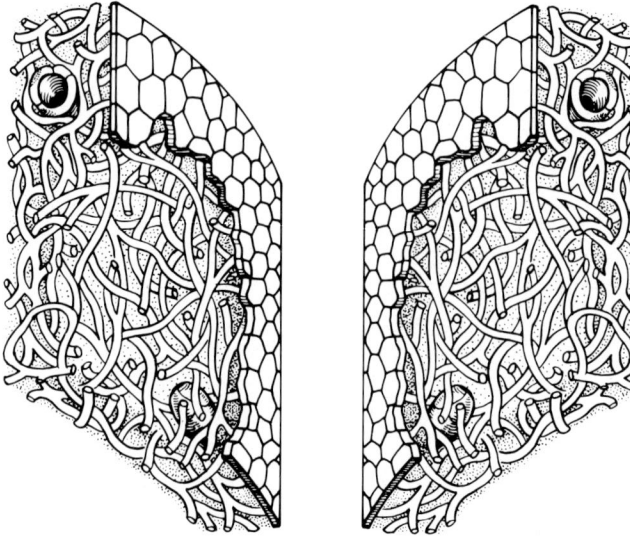

Figure 8–3
Peritoneal defect extending into subperitoneal tissues with resultant damage to peritoneum, underlying connective tissue, and vessels.

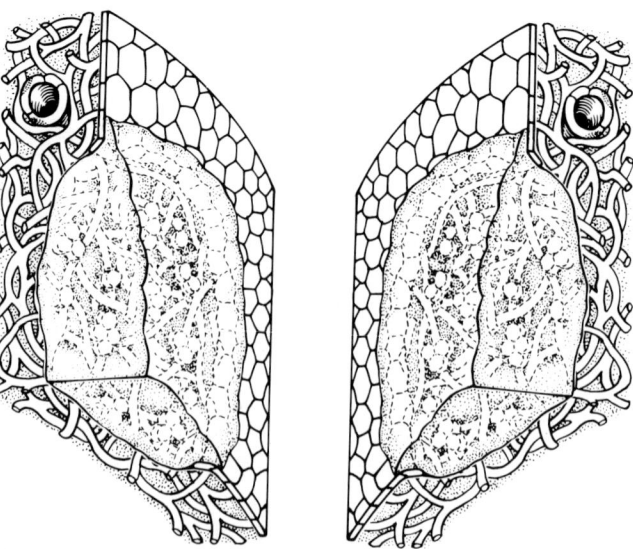

Figure 8–5
As a result of endogenous fibrinolytic activity residing in the peritoneum, the proteinaceous mass has been partially degraded. Note that the mass no longer connects adjoining peritoneal surfaces. Also note initial generation of new peritoneal cells at base of defect.

the fibrin mass connecting two adjacent surfaces, thus creating an adhesion.

Resolution of the fibrinous mass is the result of plasminogen activator activity that resides primarily in peritoneal cells (Fig. 8–6). Plasminogen activator is responsible for conversion of plasminogen into the active form, plasmin, which cleaves fibrin to form fibrin split products.[9, 10] If plasminogen activator activity is normal (e.g., as occurs in normal peritoneum), the fibrin mass can be completely degraded. However, if there is diminished plasminogen activator activity, there may be impairment in resolution of the fibrin mass with resultant subsequent adhesion development. Situations associated with diminished plasminogen activator activity include tissue ischemia, such as occurs with peritoneal grafts. Ellis has demonstrated that plasminogen activator activity increases after peritoneal trauma and reaches a maximum approximately 48–72 hours after lesioning. However, in the presence of an autologous peritoneal graft, plasminogen activator activity is significantly suppressed. However, pathophysiology of this process is more involved, because plasminogen activator inhibitors have now been identified, their regulation remaining poorly understood.

Regardless of whether the fibrinous mass persists, the final stage in the healing process involves proliferation of fibroblasts with collagen deposition.[9, 10] If no fibrin mass persists, proliferation will occur solely along the parietal and visceral surfaces, with re-epithelialization without adhesions (Fig. 8–7). In contrast, if the fibrinous mass does persist, fibroblast proliferation extends into the mass, collagen is deposited, and an adhesion develops. The entire time course over which the events described so far occur

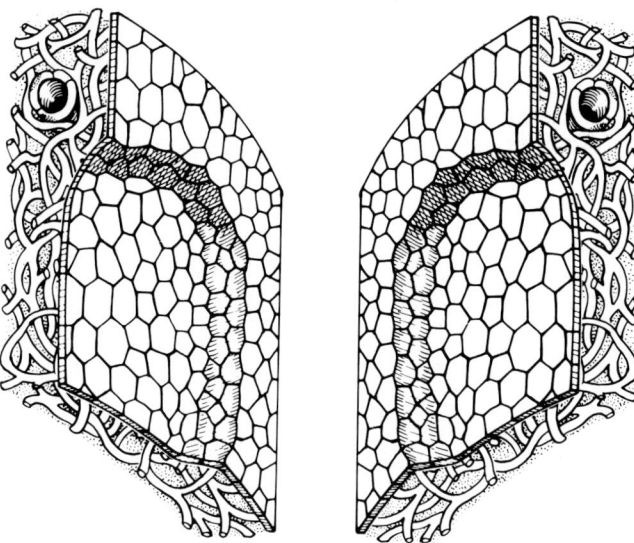

Figure 8–7
Completed healing of peritoneal surface without adhesion development.

is the initial 2–4 days after peritoneal trauma. Concomitantly, vascular ingrowth occurs and subsequently continues beyond this time, particularly in relatively ischemic areas of tissue healing in which oxygen supply is reduced. The stimulus for the vascular ingrowth is not well defined but is likely to involve growth factors, particularly fibroblast growth factor (FGF).

Having now illustrated the extent of the problem that adhesions present, and described the likely mechanism by which they develop, one can ask, "What can be done to prevent or reduce postoperative adhesion development?" The potential answers are shown in Table 8–3, which lists five ways to impact on postoperative adhesions.

REDUCTION IN PERITONEAL TRAUMA

Several approaches have been advocated for the purpose of reducing intraoperative peritoneal trauma. These proposals include the use of "microsurgical" as compared with macrosurgical techniques, use of lasers as opposed to non-laser techniques, and per-

Table 8–3

Approaches to Reduction of Postoperative Adhesion Development

Reduction in peritoneal trauma
Anti-inflammatory agents
Anticoagulants
Thrombolytic agents
A barrier

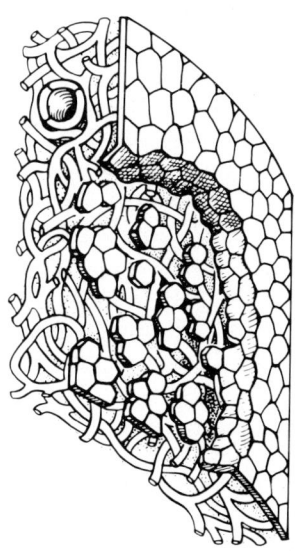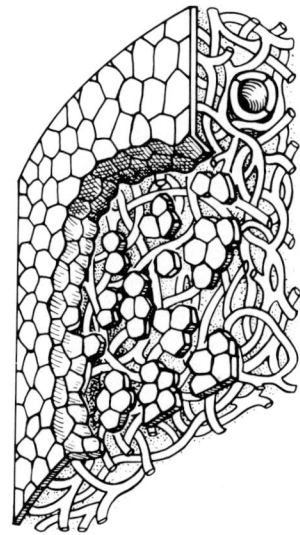

Figure 8–6
Continued fibrinolytic activity has resulted in total resolution of the proteinaceous mass. Peritoneal cells continue to proliferate.

formance of procedures at laparoscopy rather than at laparotomy.

Macrosurgery Versus Microsurgery

The tenets of gynecologic microsurgery include minimization of tissue handling; prevention of tissue desiccation; achievement of meticulous hemostasis; avoidance of introduction of foreign bodies; use of fine, nonreactive sutures; application of magnification where needed; and precise approximation of tissue planes.[1] Among these issues, the hazard of use of larger, more reactive suture and the combination of tissue drying and the presence of blood have been well established. Probably of greatest controversy among these dictums is the benefit of precise approximation of tissue planes. One study has shown that leaving the anterior abdominal wall peritoneum open after laparotomy results in less postoperative adhesion formation than closure of the anterior incision.[12] (However, that study utilized chromic suture for closure; if a less reactive suture had been utilized, a difference may have been noted.) Additionally, several studies have now suggested that ovarian bisection in animals results in fewer adhesions when the ovary is left open rather than closed.[13, 14] Whether this observation can be extended to ovarian cystectomies or to treatment of ovarian endometriomas remains to be established.

Lastly, it has been proposed that surgical adjuvants can be utilized to "lubricate" peritoneal surfaces beginning as soon as the abdomen is opened.[15] The adjuvant is repeatedly applied throughout the surgical procedure, thus reducing peritoneal trauma and subsequent de novo adhesion formation.

Role of Lasers

It was initially hoped that the application of lasers to the performance of reproductive pelvic surgical procedures would reduce or prevent postoperative adhesion development. Unfortunately, after reflecting on a decade of experience, one must conclude that this goal has not been achieved. In fact, there is little evidence to suggest differences in postoperative adhesion development or pregnancy outcome as a result of the use of a laser for performance of an operative procedure.[16]

Although early animal studies suggested reduction in adhesions when lesions were created with the carbon dioxide (CO_2) laser, the studies were critically flawed by lack of use of equivalent power densities for the laser and non-laser techniques.[17, 18] More recently, Luciano and colleagues have directly examined lesions created with equivalent power densities from the carbon dioxide (CO_2) laser and microelectrocautery.[19] Regardless of whether examining tissue destruction, postoperative fibrosis, or postoperative adhesions, no significant differences between these two modalities were identified either on uterine peritoneum or on the ovarian cortex. Similarly, in comparison of postoperative adhesion formation and re-formation in women following surgery utilizing the CO_2 laser with non-laser techniques, no consistent trend was identifiable.[20] These observations are consistent with reports describing equivalent pregnancy outcomes following the use of laser or non-laser techniques for the performance of adhesiolysis or neosalpingostomies.[21, 22]

Thus at this time, there does not appear to be an advantage in terms of adhesion development or pregnancy outcome with the use of the laser per se. However, this will be a question that will be repeatedly posed as newer lasers are introduced into clinical use.

Laparotomy Versus Laparoscopy

Performance of surgery at laparotomy is increasingly being replaced by laparoscopy. Therapeutic laparoscopic procedures are no longer limited to adhesiolysis and treatment of mild to moderate tuboperitoneal disease, but have extended to virtually all intra-abdominal reproductive pelvic surgical procedures.[23] Moreover, laparoscopy is also utilized by gynecologists for nonreproductive procedures such as salpingectomy, oophorectomy, and even hysterectomy, and by the general surgeons for cholecystectomies, appendectomies, and lymphadenectomies. This transition has been fueled by technologic innovations that allow improved visualization of the operative procedure and introduction of a wide variety of methods for incision, excision, and coagulation, as well as for control of vascular and nonvascular pedicles, organs, ducts, and other structures. The advantage of endoscopic therapy is claimed to be reductions in patient morbidity, hospital stay, and expense. However, appropriate comparative assessment of efficacy of procedures performed at laparoscopy and laparotomy remain scarce.

One of the claims of many proponents of laparoscopic surgery is a subsequent reduction in postoperative adhesion development. Such a conclusion is supported intuitively by the concepts of lack of use of retractors and packs at laparoscopy, maintenance of a closed abdomen with presumed reduction in peritoneal drying, less likelihood of introduction of foreign bodies, a reduced likelihood of blind manual dissection of adhesions during abdominal exploration, and less tissue damage (as assessed by length of laparotomy and laparoscopy incisions). Support for this hypothesis of reduced adhesions after endoscopic surgery can be extracted from several clinical trials, although none of these were specifically designed to examine this question and are potentially biased by the assignment of procedures to performance at laparoscopy or laparotomy.[24, 25] However, Luciano and coworkers have directly assessed this issue in rabbit studies in which lesions of the uterine horn were made at laparoscopy or laparotomy at wattages calculated to yield equivalent power densities.[26] This study demonstrated no intra-abdominal adhesions in those animals with the lesions created laparoscopically, whereas those lesions created at laparotomy were consistently followed by adhesion formation. Furthermore, the investigators then assigned the latter animals (those with adhesions) to adhesiolysis at laparotomy or laparoscopy and demonstrated greater reduction in adhesion re-formation following laparoscopic adhesiolysis.

However, questions regarding laparoscopic surgery remain, including whether dissections are as complete as when performed at laparotomy, whether the dissections are as meticulous, and whether equivalent degrees of hemostasis are achieved at the conclusion of the procedure. Additionally, fine suturing is less amenable endoscopically.

One report describes postoperative adhesion development at early second-look procedures following laparoscopic adhesiolysis.[27] This multicenter report described a high (97%) incidence of adhesion re-formation in women following laparoscopic adhesiolysis. Moreover, adhesion re-formation was a frequent occurrence regardless of the vascularity or consistency of the initial adhesion. This incidence is consistent with that previously reported following adhesiolysis at laparotomy, and thus suggests that adhesion re-formation will not be able to be eliminated by utilization of endoscopic techniques. Of note, however, was the reduced incidence of de novo adhesion formation following laparoscopic surgery, as compared with the previous report.

ANTI-INFLAMMATORY AGENTS

Several varieties of anti-inflammatory agents have been employed in attempts at reducing postoperative adhesion development, including glucocorticoids, nonsteroidal anti-inflammatory agents, and antihistamines.[28] These agents would be anticipated to reduce vascular permeability, thereby minimizing exudation of the proteinaceous mass during peritoneal repair (see Fig. 8–2), or to limit white blood cell elaboration.

The challenge with the use of these classes of adjuvants, as well as those that follow in subsequent sections, is to reduce intra-abdominal scarring (the undesired process) without interfering with the necessary healing process of the abdominal wall.

Several authors have reviewed animal studies demonstrating the ability of each of these adjuvant classes in reducing postoperative adhesions.[28-31] However, the human literature is relatively limited and does not establish a clear advantage of these agents. Horne and associates described a regimen of pre- and postoperative use of glucocorticoids and promethazine hydrochloride (Phenergan), and reported improved pregnancy outcome after infertility surgery.[32] However, their report did not include a control group, but rather used historical controls. Subsequently, neither Jansen[33] nor Harris and Daniell[34] have been able to demonstrate a benefit of glucocorticoids in women.

ANTICOAGULANTS

The theory behind the use of anticoagulants for reduction of postoperative adhesion development is the reduction of congealing of the proteinaceous exudate as a result of peritoneal injury. The agent most commonly utilized for this purpose has been heparin. For this purpose, heparin has been added to peritoneal irrigants with concentrations of approximately 5 U/ml. Again, although this is frequently utilized, clinical data establishing its efficacy are minimal. In animal studies, beneficial actions of heparin have been described.[35, 36] The mechanisms by which it may act are severalfold. First, heparin may interact in the clouding cascade by a combination with antithrombin III.[37] This results in activation of the serine estrace activity with subsequent inhibition of the clotting cascade. As a consequence, deposition of fibrin is reduced. Second, heparin directly stimulates the activity of plasminogen activator, thereby promoting breakdown of fibrin clots once they form.[38] An additional action of heparin may be through its binding to fibroblast growth factor (FGF), which results in marked improvement in healing of cutaneous wounds.[39] Whether the same activity will be able to be demonstrated in peritoneal injuries remains to be established. Heparin has also been applied to material barriers and placed on peritoneal surfaces with resultant improvement of the efficacy of the barrier.[40, 41] This may in part relate to delivery of heparin to the traumatized surface. Alternatively, it may result from reduction of deposition of fibrin within the interstices of the barrier material.

In a human trial, a comparison was made of postoperative adhesions in patients in whom heparinized irrigation solution was used during the performance of laparotomy.[42] In these patients, no reduction in adhesion development postoperatively as a result of heparin use in the irrigation fluid was able to be established.

THROMBOLYTIC AGENTS

The use of thrombolytic agents for reduction of postoperative adhesions is based upon the principle of degradation of previously established fibrin clots. Agents initially used for this purpose included streptokinase and urokinase. Difficulties with many of the earlier studies using these agents included postoperative hemorrhagic complications in the animals. More recently, the advent of techniques to manufacture plasminogen activator has allowed examination of the role of this enzyme in directly reducing postoperative adhesions. In animal studies conducted by Doody and colleagues, this agent has repeatedly been shown to offer efficacy.[43] Its use has not been associated with hemorrhagic complications. This agent thus by both the available animal trials and by theory would appear to have great promise. However, its utility will need to be established by the performance of appropriate human clinical trials.

USE OF BARRIERS

The philosophy behind use of a barrier for the reduction of postoperative adhesions is that it will allow separation of peritoneal surfaces during the early days of the healing process in the immediate postoperative period. Use of a barrier is different from the other adjuvants described earlier in as much as it does not affect the healing process per se but separates potentially opposing surfaces during the time of healing.

Barriers fall into three classes—one is of endogenous tissue such as a peritoneal graft, the second is exogenous nonresorbable material, and the last is exogenous resorbable material.[44] The advantage of the first is that it does not involve introduction of foreign bodies into the abdominal cavity. However, the use of peritoneal grafts or omental patches results in placement of devascularized tissue that in and of itself may be adhesiogenic. These agents require suturing in place with the resultant suture material and tissue ischemia caused by suturing being potential initiating factors of adhesions. Generally, such techniques have fallen in disfavor at this time.

The second class of barriers is exogenous nonresorbable material. A wide variety of agents have been utilized for this purpose, as previously described. For most of these, efficacy has failed to be established. Animal studies have been conducted using Gore-Tex Surgical Membrane,[45, 46] composed of expanded polyfluoroethylene. The pore size of this material is very small, such that individual cells cannot grow into the material. This is thus distinct from other prostheses made of the same material in which the intent is for fibroblast ingrowth, such as vascular grafts. Two animal studies have been conducted utilizing Gore-Tex Surgical Membrane. The first was designed so that the control side developed only a few adhesions and no correction was made for the fact that the material had to be sutured in place.[45] This study failed to show efficacy of this material, and in fact showed worse adhesions on the side on which the membrane was placed. The second report, by Boyers and coworkers, compared deperitonealized, devitalized abdominal wall surfaces that were randomized to placement of the Gore-Tex Surgical Membrane.[46] Stay sutures were placed on both surfaces with material being applied in random fashion on one side in each animal. This study was able to clearly demonstrate reduction of adhesions using the Gore-Tex Surgical Membrane. This material is currently available for use as a peritoneal substitute and has been used by cardiothoracic surgeons for years as a pericardial substitute without adverse effects. Use of this material necessitates either a second operative procedure to remove it, or a decision to allow it to remain in place permanently.

The third class of barrier is resorbable agents. These can consist of either fluids (which may have other properties to reduce adhesions as well) or materials. Although administration of large volumes of instillates has also been suggested to reduce postoperative adhesion development, this claim remains to be established. One purported advantage of instillation of large volumes of irrigation solution at the completion of a laparoscopic procedure is the elimination of gas from the abdominal cavity, thereby reducing postoperative shoulder pain referred from diaphragmatic irritation. However, crystalloid left in the abdominal cavity is relatively rapidly absorbed and may not be present during the entire period of the initial several days when adhesion development occurs.

In an attempt to prolong the benefits of hydroflotation, several viscous solutions have been used in both animal and human studies. The agent that has probably seen the greatest use in this regard is 32% dextran-70 (Hyskon). The animal literature regarding efficacy of Hyskon is mixed, but many studies do suggest benefit of this compound (see review, ref. 47). In addition to its action by hydroflotation effect, its activity has also been postulated to be related to a "siliconizing" effect, and stimulation of plasminogen activator activity.

There have been four large clinical trials evaluating the efficacy of Hyskon for reduction of postoperative adhesions.[48-51] Each of these involve randomization of patients to use or non-use of Hyskon at the completion of laparotomy for infertility purposes. Subsequently, adhesions were graded again at the time of an early second-look laparoscopy. In the initial two reports published by the Adhesion Society

Group[48] and by Rosenberg and Board,[49] a benefit of Hyskon in reducing postoperative adhesions was able to be demonstrated. However, the two subsequent studies by Jansen[50] and Larsson[51] failed to establish a benefit of Hyskon. Although each of these studies has potential criticisms, they nevertheless represent very reasonable clinical trials. Thus, the clinician is left with a mixed data base when trying to make the decision as to whether or not to use Hyskon at the conclusion of the operative procedure.

Use of Hyskon appears to be reduced over the last several years. This may in part be related to anecdotal reports of anaphylactic-like reactions associated with the use of Hyskon, but these are primarily associated with the use of large volumes of 32% dextran-70 at the time of hysteroscopy. There does not appear to be a detrimental effect of 32% dextran-70 on electrolyte balance.[52] The ability of this material to promote bacterial growth has been debated in the literature,[53, 54] but has not been a common clinical problem.

Other viscous solutions have also been utilized for reduction of postoperative adhesion development. Carboxymethylcellulose (CMC) has been utilized by many investigators,[55–58] each of whom has been able to demonstrate efficacy of this material in reducing postoperative adhesion development. To date, however, no clinical trials using this material have been performed.

Several proteoglycans have been utilized in an attempt to reduce postoperative adhesions, including chondroitin sulfate, dermatan sulfate, and hyaluronic acid.[59–61] Although several of these agents have been shown to be efficacious, this effect has not been universal, thus implying that the benefit appears to be specific to the individual agents rather than to this class of agents as a whole.

Resorbable barriers in the form of oxidized regenerated cellulose have also been utilized to reduce postoperative adhesion development.[62] In the early animal trials that utilized Surgicel, a variety of results have been obtained. More recently, oxidized regenerated cellulose has been developed in the form of a knitted fabric with small pore sizes called INTERCEED (TC7). This material has now been examined in several animal models and has been shown to reduce adhesion formation in most of these trials.[63–65] Based on these initial animal studies, a human clinical trial was conducted. This study utilized each subject as her own control and examined adhesion re-formation on the pelvic sidewall after adhesiolysis at laparotomy. This multicenter study was able to demonstrate in 74 subjects that use of this material significantly reduced the incidence and area of postoperative adhesion re-formation.[66] Additionally, the material was able to remain in place without requiring suturing and in all but three patients was resorbed by the time of the early second-look laparoscopy. Animal studies have shown that in fact this material commonly is resorbed within 4 days in most situations, exceptions being when the material is placed in multiple layers or when it bunches up.[67] Of utmost importance in use of INTERCEED (TC7) is that meticulous hemostasis be achieved prior to application of the barrier.

The efficacy of INTERCEED (TC7) has been able to be further improved in animal studies by moistening the material with heparin after it is in place on peritoneal surfaces, rather than with saline as originally described. Using INTERCEED (TC7) plus heparin, significant reduction of adhesion formation has been observed in animal models,[40, 41] and adhesion re-formation has also been able to be significantly reduced.[68] The improved efficacy of the combination of INTERCEED (TC7) plus heparin remains to be established in human clinical trials.

Another "barrier" undergoing evaluation is poloxamer 407, a compound that is a liquid below body temperature but that gels at body temperature. Using this compound, Leach and colleagues have demonstrated a reduction in postoperative adhesions in the rat.[69] Future evaluation of this family of compound appears warranted.

Lastly, Steinleitner and associates have described two classes of compounds that have potential effects on many of the steps in the adhesion development cascade. Use of calcium channel blockers (which alter prostaglandin production, mast cell activation, platelet activation, and vascular permeability) has significantly reduced adhesion formation and re-formation in several animal species.[70–72] Also, pentoxifylline (which reduces leukocyte activities, decreases phagocytic tissue injury, and stimulates plasminogen activator activity) significantly reduced adhesion formation in hamsters.[73]

PREGNANCY OUTCOME AFTER ADHESIOLYSIS

Implicit in performance of adhesiolysis for infertility patients is the assumption that adhesiolysis will improve pregnancy outcome. Although this concept is held by many physicians, strong support for this idea in the literature is not definitively established. Several investigators have demonstrated establishment of pregnancy after adhesiolysis in previously infertile women. Tulandi and coworkers extended these observations by identifying patients with pelvic adhesions at laparoscopy.[74] A subgroup of these patients subsequently underwent adhesiolysis at laparotomy while a second subgroup did not. Comparing subsequent pregnancy outcome among these two patient populations, pregnancy rates were significantly higher among those women undergoing adhesiolysis. In both subgroups, those patients with the more severe adhesions had reduced pregnancy rates.

An extension of this concept and the realization that postoperative adhesion development follows frequently after reproductive pelvic surgery both at laparotomy and at laparoscopy are the need for second-look laparoscopy. At the time of second-look laparoscopy, the adhesions can be identified and treated with the hope of further improving the likelihood of conception. Additionally, second-look laparoscopy allows the surgeon to assess relative efficacy of the surgical techniques and/or adjuvant utilization. Finally, in this day of widespread availability of in vitro fertilization, those patients who fail to have a good outcome from their initial operative procedure can be so informed, and referred either for adoption or for in vitro fertilization. The frequency with which this poor surgical outcome (worse adhesions than at the time of the initial operative procedure) occurs is approximately 10% by several reports.[75, 76]

Despite these potential advantages of early second-look laparoscopy, it needs to be realized that there has yet to be a clinical trial that shows that performance of early second-look laparoscopy improves subsequent pregnancy rate. Trimbos-Kemper and colleagues have demonstrated that performance of early second-look laparoscopy does reduce adhesions observed at the time of a third-look procedure, but this did not correlate with any improvement in pregnancy outcome.[77] There was, however, one subgroup of patients undergoing neosalpingostomy who had a reduced incidence of ectopic pregnancies after early second-look laparoscopy.

An additional issue is whether the presence of pelvic adhesions affects ovarian function. When in vitro fertilization was initially introduced, many patients underwent preparative pelvic surgery to allow improved ovarian access for oocyte aspiration at laparoscopy.[78] However, with the increasingly frequent utilization of ultrasound-guided aspiration of follicles transvaginally, the need to be able to visualize the ovaries at the time of laparoscopy has been

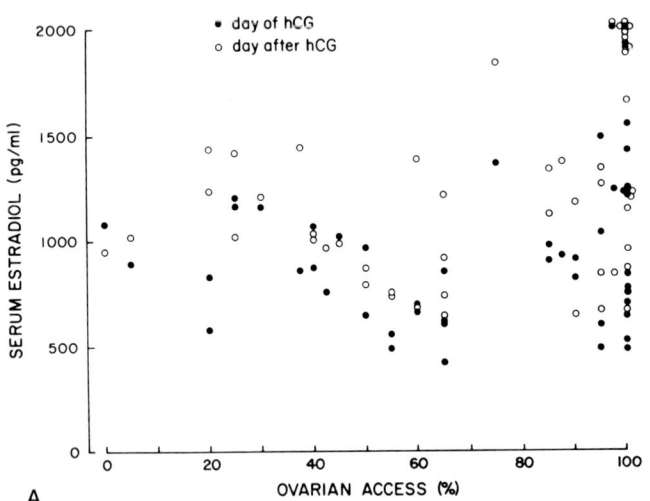
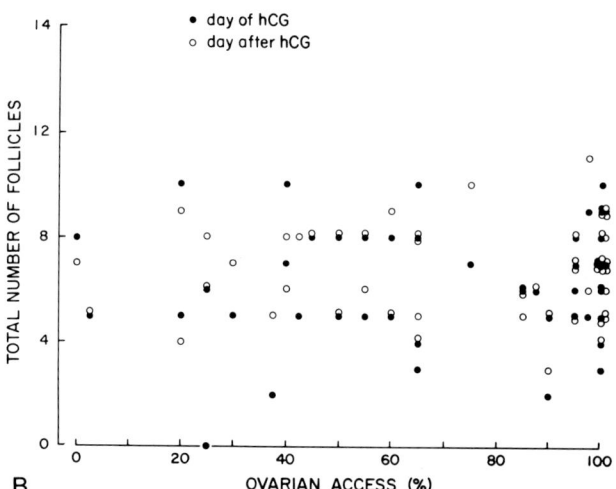
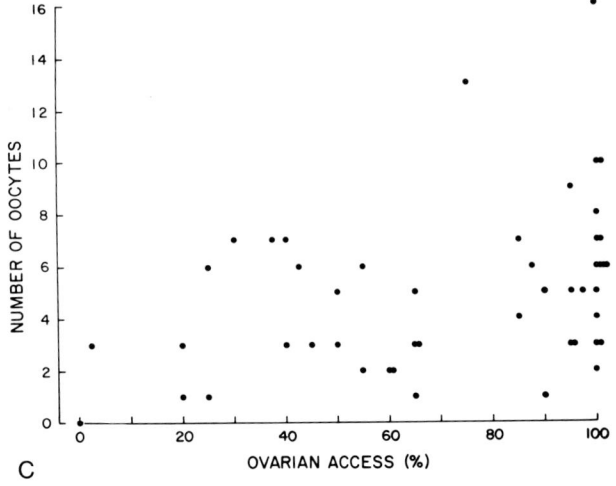

Figure 8–8
Relationship between periovarian adhesions and ovarian function as assessed by (A) serum estradiol levels, (B) follicular development, and (C) oocyte recovery in women undergoing laparoscopic follicular aspiration for in vitro fertilization. hCG, human chorionic gonadotropin. (From Diamond MP, et al.: The effect of periovarian adhesions on follicular development in patients undergoing ovarian stimulation for in vitro fertilization–embryo transfer. Fertil Steril 1988; 49:100.)

reduced. Two groups have suggested that ovarian function is reduced by the presence of extensive pelvic adhesions.[79,80] However, as shown in Figure 8–8, this has not been the experience of the author.[81] In these patients, the presence of adhesions was assessed at the time of laparoscopy for oocyte recovery. Whether looking at estradiol levels or follicular development, no significant correlation was identified between the extent of ovarian adhesion and ovarian response to gonadotropin stimulation. Subsequently, in animal studies, the author has examined the number of corpora lutea and the nidation index as a function of adhesion development after ovarian bisection.[13] These studies also failed to identify detrimental effects of adhesions on ovarian function.

References

1. Diamond MP: Surgical aspects of infertility. In Sciarra J (ed.): Gynecology and Obstetrics, Vol. 5. Philadelphia, Harper & Row, 1988, pp. 1–23.
2. Diamond MP, Daniell JF, Feste J, et al.: Pelvic adhesions at early second look laparoscopy following carbon dioxide laser surgery procedures. Infertility 1984; 7:39.
3. DeCherney AH, Mezer HC: The nature of post-tuboplasty pelvic adhesions as determined by early and late laparoscopy. Fertil Steril 1984; 41:643.
4. Surrey MW, Friedman S: Second-look laparoscopy after reconstructive pelvic surgery for infertility. J Reprod Med 1982; 27:658.
5. Pittaway DE, Daniell JF, Maxson WL: Ovarian surgery in an infertility patient as an indication for a short-interval second-look laparoscopy: A preliminary study. Fertil Steril 1985; 43:395.
6. Trimbos-Kemper TCM, Trimbos JB, van Hall EV: Adhesion formation after tubal surgery: Results of the eighth-day laparoscopy in 188 patients. Fertil Steril 1985; 43:395.
7. Daniell JF, Pittaway DE: Short-interval second-look laparoscopy after infertility surgery: A preliminary report. J Reprod Med 1983; 28:281.
8. Diamond MP, Daniell JF, Feste J, et al.: Adhesion reformation and de novo adhesion formation following reproductive pelvic surgery. Fertil Steril 1987; 47:864.
9. diZerega GS: The Cause and Prevention of Postsurgical Adhesions. Bethesda, Pregnancy Research Branch, National Institutes of Health, 1980.
10. diZerega GS: The peritoneum and its response to surgical injury. In diZerega GS, Malinak LR, Diamond MP, Linsky CB (eds.): Treatment of Post-Surgical Adhesions. New York, Wiley-Liss, 1990, pp. 1–12.
11. Hershlag A, Otterness IG, Bliven ML, et al.: Interleukin-1 (IL-1) potentiates adhesion formation in the rat. Thirty-seventh Annual Meeting of the Society for Gynecologic Investigation, St. Louis, March 1990.
12. Tulandi T, Collins JA, Burrows E, et al.: Treatment-dependent and treatment-independent pregnancy among women with periadnexal adhesions. Am J Obstet Gynecol 1990; 162:354.
13. Meyer WR, Grainger DA, DeCherney AH, et al.: Ovarian surgery: The effect of closure on adhesion formation and ovarian function in the rabbit. Sixteenth Annual Meeting of the Society of Gynecologic Surgeons, Inc., New Orleans, March 1990.
14. Brumsted JR, Deaton J, Lavigne L, Riddick DH: Postoperative adhesion formation after ovarian wedge resection with and without ovarian reconstruction in the rabbit. Fertil Steril 1990; 53:723.
15. Yaacob Y, Goldberg EP, Kaelin D, et al.: Hyaluronic acid and other hydrophilic high polymer solutions: Tissue-protective devices to prevent surgical adhesions (abstract). International Symposium for the Treatment of Post-Surgical Adhesions, Phoenix, September 1989.
16. Diamond MP: Assessment of results of laser surgery. In Sutton CJG (ed.): Bailliere's Clinical Obstetrics and Gynaecology: Laparoscopic Surgery, Vol. 3. London, Bailliere Tindall, 1989, p. 649.
17. Klink F, Grosspietzsch R, von Klitzing L, et al.: Animal in vivo studies and in vitro experiments with human tubes for end-to-end anastomotic operation by a CO_2 laser technique. Fertil Steril 1978; 30:100.
18. Baggish MS, Chong AP: Carbon dioxide laser microsurgery of the uterine tube. Obstet Gynecol 1981; 58:111.
19. Luciano AA, Whitman G, Maier DB, et al.: A comparison of thermal injury, healing patterns, and postoperative adhesion formation following CO_2 laser and electromicrosurgery. Fertil Steril 1987; 48:1025.
20. Diamond MP, Wentz AC, Herbert CM, et al.: One ovary or two: Difference in ovulation induction, estradiol level, and follicular development in a program for in vitro fertilization. Fertil Steril 1984; 41:519.
21. Mage G, Bruhat M-A: Pregnancy following salpingostomy: Comparison between CO_2 laser and electrosurgery procedures. Fertil Steril 1983; 40:472.
22. Tulandi T, Vilos GA: A comparison between laser surgery and electrosurgery for bilateral hydrosalpinx: A 2-year follow-up. Fertil Steril 1985; 44:846.
23. Martin DC, Diamond MP, Yussman MA: Laser laparoscopy for infertility surgery. In Sanfilippo Jr, Levine R (eds.): Operative Gynecologic Endoscopy. New York, Springer-Verlag, 1989, pp. 211–235.
24. Fayez JA, Schneider PJ: Prevention of pelvic adhesion formation by different modalities of treatment. Am J Obstet Gynecol 1987; 157:1184.
25. Luciano AA: Laparotomy versus laparoscopy. In diZerega GS, Malinak LR, Diamond MP, Linsky CB (eds.): Treatment of Post-Surgical Adhesions. New York, Wiley-Liss, 1990, pp. 35–44.
26. Luciano AA, Maier DB, Koch EL, et al.: A comparative study of postoperative adhesions following laser surgery by laparoscopy versus laparotomy in the rabbit model. Obstet Gynecol 1989; 74:220.
27. Diamond MP, Daniell JF, Johns DA, et al.: Adhesion formation and reformation after operative laparoscopy: Assessment at early second-look procedures (abstract). Forty-sixth Annual Meeting of the American Fertility Society, Washington, October 1990.
28. Diamond MP, DeCherney AH: Pathogenesis of adhesion formation/reformation: Application to reproductive pelvic surgery. Microsurgery 1987; 8:103.
29. Pfeffer WH: Adjuvants in pelvic surgery. Fertil Steril 1980; 33:245.
30. DeCherney AH: Preventing postoperative pelvic adhesions with intraperitoneal treatment. J Reprod Med 1984; 29:157.
31. Holtz G: Prevention and management of peritoneal adhesions. Fertil Steril 1984; 41:497.
32. Horne HW, Clyman M, Debrovren C, et al.: The prevention of postoperative pelvic adhesions following conservative operative treatment for human infertility. Int J Fertil 1973; 18:109.
33. Jansen RPS: Failure of intraperitoneal adjuncts to improve the outcome of pelvic operations in young women. Am J Obstet Gynecol 1985; 153:363.
34. Harris WJ, Daniell JF: Use of corticosteroids as adjuvant in terminal salpingostomy. Fertil Steril 1983; 40:785.
35. El-Chalabi HA, Otubo JAM: Value of a single intraperitoneal dose of heparin in prevention of adhesion formation: An experimental evaluation in rats. Int J Fertil 1987; 32:332.
36. Fukysawa M, Girgis W, diZerega GS: Inhibition of post-surgical adhesions in a standardized rabbit model: Intraperitoneal treatment with heparin. Int J Fertil, in press.
37. Rosenberg RD: Heparin antithrombin and abnormal clotting. Ann Rev Med 1978; 29:267.
38. Andrade-Gordon P, Strickland S: Interaction of heparin with plasminogen activators and plasminogen: Effects on the activation of plasminogen. Biochemistry 1986; 25:4033.

39. Gospodarowicz D, Ferrara N, Schweigerer L, Neufeld G: Structural characterization and biological functions of fibroblast growth factor. Endocr Rev 1987; 8:95.
40. Diamond MP, Linsky CB, Cunningham T, et al.: Synergistic effects of INTERCEED (TC7) and heparin in reducing adhesion formation in the rabbit uterine horn model. Fertil Steril 1991; 55(2): 389.
41. Diamond MP, Linsky CB, Cunningham T, et al.: Adhesion reduction in the rabbit sidewall/uterine horn model with INTERCEED (TC7)/heparin. Sixteenth Annual Meeting, American Association of Gynecologic Laparoscopists, San Francisco, November 1987.
42. Rock JA, Cohen SM, Franklin RR, et al.: Clinical evaluation of INTERCEED (TC7) Absorbable Adhesion Barrier: Role of adhesiolysis techniques and heparin irrigation on adhesion formation (abstract). American Fertility Society, November 1989, p. 525.
43. Doody KG, Dunn RC, Buttram VC: Recombinant tissue plasminogen activator reduces adhesion formation in a rabbit uterine horn model. Fertil Steril 1989; 51:509.
44. Schwartz LB, Diamond MP: Formation, reduction, and treatment of adhesive disease. Semin Reprod Endocrinol, in press.
45. Golberg JM, Toledo AA, Michell DE: An evaluation of the Gore-Tex surgical membrane for the prevention of postoperative peritoneal adhesions. Obstet Gynecol 1987; 70:846.
46. Boyers SP, Diamond MP, DeCherney AH: Reduction of postoperative pelvic adhesions in the rabbit with Gore-Tex Surgical Membrane. Fertil Steril 1966; 49:1066.
47. diZerega GS, Hodgen GD: Prevention of postoperative tubal adhesions: Comparative study of commonly used agents. Am J Obstet Gynecol 1980; 135:173.
48. Adhesion Study Group. Reduction of postoperative pelvic adhesions with intraperitoneal 32% dextran 70: A prospective, randomized clinical trial. Fertil Steril 1983; 40:612.
49. Rosenberg SM, Board JA: High-molecular-weight dextran in human infertility surgery. Am J Obstet Gynecol 1984; 148:380.
50. Jansen RPS: Failure of intraperitoneal adjuncts to improve the outcome of pelvic operations in young women. Am J Obstet Gynecol 1985; 153:363.
51. Larsson B, Lalos O, Marsk L, et al.: Effect of intraperitoneal instillation of 32% dextran 70 on postoperative adhesion formation after tubal surgery. Acta Obstet Gynecol Scand 1985; 64:437.
52. Tulandi T, Hilton J: Effect of intraperitoneal 32% dextran 70 on blood coagulation and serum electrolytes. J Reprod Med 1985; 30:431.
53. Bernstein J, Mattox JH, Ulrich JA et al.: The potential for bacterial growth with dextran. J Reprod Med 1982; 22:77.
54. Elkins TE, Trenthem L, McNeeley SG, et al.: Potential for in vitro growth of common bacteria in solutions of 32% dextran 70 and 1.0% sodium carboxymethylcellulose. Fertil Steril 1985; 43:477.
55. Elkins TE, Bury RJ, Ritter JL, et al.: Adhesion prevention by solutions of sodium carboxymethylcellulose in the rat. Fertil Steril 1984; 41:926.
56. Kotry I, Frederick CM, Holtz G, et al.: Adhesion prevention in the rabbit with sodium carboxymethylcellulose solutions. Am J Obstet Gynecol 1986; 155:667.
57. Diamond MP, DeCherney AH, Linsky CB, et al.: Assessment of carboxymethylcellulose and 32% dextran 70 for prevention of adhesions in a rabbit uterine horn model. Int J Fertil 1988; 33:278.
58. Diamond MP, DeCherney AH, Linsky CB, et al.: Adhesion reformation in the rabbit uterine horn model. I. Reduction with carboxymethylcellulose. Int J Fertil 1988; 33:372.
59. Diamond MP, Linsky CB, Cunningham T, et al.: Effect of the combination of glycosaminoglycans with TC7 (INTERCEED) in the reduction of adhesions. Forty-fourth Annual Meeting, American Fertility Society, Atlanta, October 1988.
60. Oelsner G, Graebe R, Pan S, et al.: Chondroitin sulphate: A new intraperitoneal treatment for postoperative adhesion formation in the rabbit. J Reprod Med 1987; 32:812.
61. Grainger DA, Meyer WR, Diamond MP: Evaluation of a proteoglycan, hyaluronic acid, in the prevention of ovarian adhesions. Forty-fifth Annual Meeting, American Fertility Society, San Francisco, November 1989.
62. Soules MR, Dennis L, Bosarge H, Moore DE: The prevention of postoperative pelvic adhesions: An animal study comparing barrier methods with dextran 70. Am J Obstet Gynecol 1982; 143:829.
63. Linsky CB, Diamond MP, Cunningham T, et al.: Adhesion reduction in a rabbit uterine horn model using TC7. J Reprod Med 1987; 32:17.
64. Diamond MP, Linsky CB, Cunningham T, et al.: A model for sidewall adhesions in the rabbit: Reduction by an absorbable barrier. Microsurgery 1987; 8:197.
65. Maxson WS, Herbert CM, Oldfield EL, Hill G: Efficacy of a modified oxidized cellulose fabric in the prevention of adhesion formation. Gynecol Obstet Invest 1988; 26:160.
66. INTERCEED(TC7) barrier adhesion study group: prevention of postsurgical adhesions by INTERCEED (TC7), an absorbable adhesion barrier: A prospective randomized multicenter clinical study. Fertil Steril 1989; 51:933.
67. Diamond MP, Cunningham T, Linsky CB, et al.: INTERCEED(TC7) as an adjuvant for adhesion reduction: Animal studies. In diZerega GS, Malinak LR, Diamond MP, Linsky CB (eds.): Treatment of Post-Surgical Adhesions. New York, Wiley-Liss, 1990.
68. Diamond MP, Linsky CB, Cunningham T, et al.: Synergistic effects of INTERCEED (TC7) and heparin in reducing adhesion formation in the rabbit uterine horn model. Fertil Steril 1991; 55(2):389.
69. Leach RE, Henry RL: Reduction of postoperative adhesions in the rat uterine horn model with poloxamer 407. Am J Obstet Gynecol 1990; 162:1317.
70. Steinleitner A, Lambert II, Montoro L, et al.: The use of calcium channel blockade for the prevention of postoperative adhesion formation. Fertil Steril 1988; 50:818.
71. Steinleitner A, Lambert H, Montoro L, et al.: Use of diltiazem for preventing postoperative adhesions. J Reprod Med 1988; 33:891.
72. Steinleitner A, Kazensky C, Lambert H: Calcium channel blockade prevents postsurgical reformation of adnexal adhesions in rabbits. Obstet Gynecol 1989; 74:797.
73. Steinleitner A, Lambert H, Kazensky C, et al.: Use of pentoxifylline as an adjuvant to reduce primary postsurgical adhesion formation: Preliminary investigations in a rodent model. J Gynecol Surg 1989; 5:367.
74. Tulandi T, Collins JA, Burrows E, et al.: Treatment-dependent and treatment-independent pregnancy among women with periadnexal adhesions. Am J Obstet Gynecol 1990; 162:354.
75. Garcia JE, Jones HW Jr, Acosta AA, Andrews MC: Reconstructive pelvic operations for in vitro fertilization. Am J Obstet Gynecol 1985; 153:172.
76. Diamond MP, Feste J, McLaughlin DS, et al.: Pelvic adhesions at early second-look laparoscopy following carbon dioxide laser surgery. Infertility 1984; 7:39.
77. Trimbos-Kemper TCM, Trimbos JB, van Hall EV: Adhesion formation after tubal surgery: Results of the eighth-day laparoscopy in 188 patients. Fertil Steril 1985; 43:395.
78. DeCherney AH, Tarlatzis BC, Laufer N: A simple technique for ovarian suspension in preparation for in vitro fertilization. Fertil Steril 1985; 43:659.
79. Mahadevan MM, Wiseman D, Leader A, et al.: The effects of ovarian adhesive disease upon follicular development in cycles of controlled stimulation for in vitro fertilization. Fertil Steril 1985; 44:489.
80. Molloy D, Martin M, Speirs A, et al.: Performance of patients with a "frozen pelvis" in an *in vitro* fertilization program. Fertil Steril 1987; 47:450.
81. Diamond MP, Pellicer A, Boyers SP, DeCherney AH: The effect of periovarian adhesions on follicular development in patients undergoing ovarian stimulation for in vitro fertilization–embryo transfer. Fertil Steril 1988; 49:100.

Benign Procedures for the Vulva and Vagina

9

David B. Elmer

Surgical conditions of the vulva and vagina are commonly encountered by the practicing obstetrician-gynecologist. Many, however, go undetected because they are not looked for. Careful attention during the most "normal" of examinations may lead to early diagnosis and treatment of many vulvar and vaginal disorders. With the rising occurrence of lesions related to the human papillomavirus, one wonders how often subtle lesions are overlooked during a hurried examination.

Examination of the vulva and the vagina is best performed with the patient in the dorsal lithotomy position. Appropriate draping of the patient will place her more at ease and maintain professionalism. An adequate light source is necessary, but care must be taken to protect the patient from high temperatures generated by many lights. Inspection of the vulva should include the mons pubis, where lesions from parasitic infestation may be apparent. All surfaces of the labia majora and minora should be examined for pigmented or depigmented lesions. Dermatoses and evidence of venereal warts should be noted. Abnormalities of Bartholin's duct and the ducts of the minor vestibular glands should be sought. The introitus should be inspected for evidence of cyst formation or other changes. An appropriate vaginal speculum will allow evaluation of all vaginal surfaces. If the lateral vaginal walls obscure the examiner's vision, the speculum may be placed through a single finger of a latex examination glove, from which the end has been cut. This should retract the vaginal sidewalls and allow complete vaginal visualization. Bimanual examination allows further assessment of vaginal as well as pelvic lesions. Finally, rectovaginal examination is critical to the complete evaluation of the lower genital tract.

VULVAR LESIONS

Multiple lesions occur on the vulva, representing variants of normal, benign neoplasms, malignancies, or systemic manifestations of non-gynecologic disease. Historically, many vulvar lesions were termed leukoplakia, a term used for any lesion with white discoloration. Because this term may be applied to benign and malignant lesions alike, it should be abandoned for more specific pathologic classification. The following is the currently recommended classification of non-neoplastic epithelial disorders of vulvar skin and mucosa (previously termed vulvar dystrophies):[1]

1. Lichen sclerosis (lichen sclerosis et atrophicus)
2. Squamous cell hyperplasia (formerly hyperplastic dystrophy)
3. Other dermatoses

Few vulvar lesions have a gross appearance so characteristic as to allow diagnosis without biopsy. It is also important to remember that there are no normal pigmented lesions of the vulva. Three to five per cent of all melanomas of the skin occur on the vulva.[2] Therefore, vulvar biopsy of any pigmented or suspicious lesion is a critically important procedure for accurate diagnosis and proper treatment.

Many lesions are associated with pruritus as the presenting symptom. Accurate diagnosis and treatment are necessary because of the irresistible attraction of these lesions for the fingernail, a structure that over time is related to the degeneration of benign lesions to malignancies. *Candida albicans*; *Trichomonas*; and various soaps, detergents, perfumes, and fabric softeners are well-known, nonpathologic causes of pruritus. After infectious agents, allergens, and vaginitides have been ruled out, biopsy must be used to arrive at a specific pathologic diagnosis. Only then should local antipruritic agents such as fluorinated steroids be used to control pruritus or other symptoms.

Vulvar Biopsy

Biopsy of a vulvar skin lesion is best accomplished using a Keyes punch. The 4–7 mm size provides adequate tissue for pathologic evaluation. With larger lesions, a leading edge of the abnormal area should be selected as the biopsy site. This will produce a specimen including the lesion as well as a margin of normal squamous epithelium. After using a local anesthetic to infiltrate the biopsy site, the punch should be rotated back and forth using light to moderate downward pressure. Rotation of the skin itself should be minimized by applying stretch to the surrounding area. Downward pressure should be continued until a full thickness of the skin is obtained. Elevating the biopsy specimen will then allow the deep attachment to be cut with a scissors or scalpel. The specimen may then be placed in formalin or other appropriate fixative.

Easy and successful hemostasis at the biopsy site may be achieved by using the same biopsy punch to cut a corresponding piece of absorbable gelatin sponge (Gelfoam). The sponge is then placed in the defect at the biopsy site and held in place with moderate pressure for 1 minute. Use of electrocautery or silver nitrate to coagulate the base of the biopsy area is a reasonable alternative. Rarely should a hemostatic suture be required.

Once a histologic diagnosis is made, appropriate therapy may be initiated. Most of the depigmented lesions can be treated medically, whereas vulvar intraepithelial neoplasia, carcinoma in situ (Bowen's disease), Paget's disease, and frank malignancies require more extensive excision.

Lichen sclerosis is the most common white lesion of the vulva.[3] It is characterized by loss of the rete pegs and development of a hypocellular, homogeneous layer beneath the epidermis. It is most commonly found in postmenopausal, light-skinned women, although it has been described among all age groups and races. Treatment with 2% testosterone compounded in lanolin or petrolatum base and applied topically is usually effective in relieving pruritus and limiting extension.

Squamous cell hyperplasia is believed to represent the reaction of vulvar skin to a local irritant. Various microorganisms, synthetic fabrics, perfumes, fragrances, and laundry products have been implicated in initiating a local dermatitis and its attendant pruritus. Long-term abrasions from scratching result in the characteristic excoriations seen in these lesions. Histologically, there is thickening of the epithelium, and the rete pegs are elongated and blunted (acanthosis). A chronic inflammatory infiltrate is present throughout the dermis. Treatment with topical corticosteroids should follow the elimination of possible irritants.

Wide Local Excision

Wide local excision should be considered for lesions not clearly defined by biopsy results, or when complete excision is otherwise indicated. Because vulvar skin is very pliable, it is recommended that the margins of the desired incision be defined with a surgical marker prior to the excision. After appropriate preparation of the skin, infiltration of local anesthesia should be accomplished with care. Because of the obvious sensitivity of the area along with the patient's anxiety, adequate anesthesia should be ensured prior to use of a scalpel. Infiltration of the anesthetic itself often represents the most painful part of this otherwise straightforward procedure. By using a 30-gauge needle when available and injecting the anesthetic agent very slowly, pain can be minimized, thus ensuring that the patient is better able to tolerate the excision.

The skin incision should follow the marked area, with care being taken to see that the initial incision passes entirely through the dermis. When the incision is performed in several passes, irregular edges are likely to result. Once the entire circumference of the lesion has been incised, the lesion should be undermined sharply, ensuring that no unnecessary subcutaneous tissue is included in the specimen. Closing the defect occasionally places the skin edges under unusual tension. This can be avoided by undermining beneath the dermis for several centimeters. It is strongly recommended that 5-0 absorbable suture be used for closure.

Vulvar Condylomata

Genital warts represent one of the most common lesions of the vulva.[4] Caused by the human papillomavirus (HPV), vulvar condylomata are usually found in clusters around the introitus and may involve the vagina, cervix, anus, and urethra as well.[5] The typical raised lesions appear with a wide verrucous surface arising from a narrower stalk. Corresponding lesions on opposite sides of the labia minora are common. Extension may occur until the warts are nearly confluent. The lesions are believed to be spread by sexual contact with an affected person. Infection appears more commonly in association with pregnancy; with diabetes mellitus; and in immunosuppressed individuals such as those with an underlying malignancy, those undergoing chemotherapy, and transplant patients.

Occasionally, lesions occur on the vulva or within the vagina that take on a papillary form similar to a condyloma. Papillary remnants of the hymenal ring are often confused by patients and practitioners as representing condylomata because their appearance and location may be common for warts. Distinction can often be made by use of a 5% acetic acid solution (household vinegar). Applied to the suspicious lesion, the acetic acid solution will turn HPV-infected lesions white. The distinction is clearer still when viewed through a colposcope.

There is no treatment available for condylomata that ensures eradication of the HPV infection. Therefore, recurrences are common with all current modalities of treatment, and the patient should be so warned. Smaller lesions, even when multiple, often respond to topically applied trichloroacetic acid, podophyllin, or liquid nitrogen. Care should be taken to protect uninvolved skin from run-down of these caustic chemicals. Treatment should be repeated at 1–2 week intervals. Condylomata that persist after three treatments will require some alternate form of therapy, such as cryotherapy, laser ablation, loop excision, or electrodesiccation with cautery. Intralesional injection of interferon has shown some promise in treating resistant lesions. Use of the carbon dioxide laser is gaining increasing popularity, with success rates at least equivalent with other modalities. Specific treatment guidelines are beyond the scope of this text but are well reported in the literature.[6,7]

Large lesions or those that fail to respond to other therapies require surgical excision. This also has the added benefit of providing tissue for histopathologic evaluation. Local excision should be accomplished in the manner described previously. The patient should again be warned that excision does not eradicate the virus and that recurrence is common.

VULVAR CYSTS

Cyst or abscess formation of the female external genitalia represents a commonly encountered problem in ambulatory gynecology. Understanding the function of the vestibular glands and their duct system leads to an intelligent approach to the management of cystic or inflammatory changes. Remnants of the wolffian duct system can also result in cystic structures of the vulva and vagina. Cysts of the canal of Nuck arise from peritoneal inclusions along the distal course of the round ligament. Other dermatologic cysts, such as mucinous cysts of the vaginal mucosa and keratinous cysts of the vulva, are commonly encountered.

Vestibular Gland of Bartholin

The greater vestibular glands of Bartholin are paired glands that produce clear mucous secretions and deliver that secretion through a duct system that terminates at the posterolateral aspect of the introitus, just external to the hymenal ring. Blockage of the duct results in accumulation of the gland products and subsequent cystic dilation of the duct. Infection, classically with *Neisseria gonorrhoeae*, results in abscess formation. Bartholin's duct abscesses can range from less than 1 cm to a size replacing much of the labia majora.

The uninfected cyst of Bartholin's duct presents as a cystic enlargement at the introitus. There should be little if any surrounding erythema and minimal tenderness to light palpation. Needle aspiration of the cyst provides accurate diagnosis when only mucous products are seen and cultures demonstrate no growth of microorganisms. However, with the duct orifice still obstructed, recurrence is predictable, often complicated by infection introduced during needle aspiration. It is therefore necessary to either excise the gland or ensure patent egress for the gland secretions. Bartholin's gland lies just inferior to the venous sinusoids of the vestibular bulb. Dissection in this area during attempted excision of Bartholin's gland risks significant bleeding and hematoma formation. It is for this reason that most gynecologic surgeons will opt to provide a patent tract for drainage of the cyst.

Excision of the gland should not be attempted during acute infection of the gland or duct. Most initial occurrences of cyst or abscess formation can be managed with incision and drainage, leaving a wick or catheter to prevent closing of the incision and subsequent reaccumulation of fluid or pus.

Incision and Drainage

An area of fluctuance of the cyst or abscess should be present prior to attempted incision and drainage (Fig. 9–1A). Ideally, the incision should be just exterior to the hymenal ring, into the area of fluctuance. The incision should be approximately 1–2 cm in

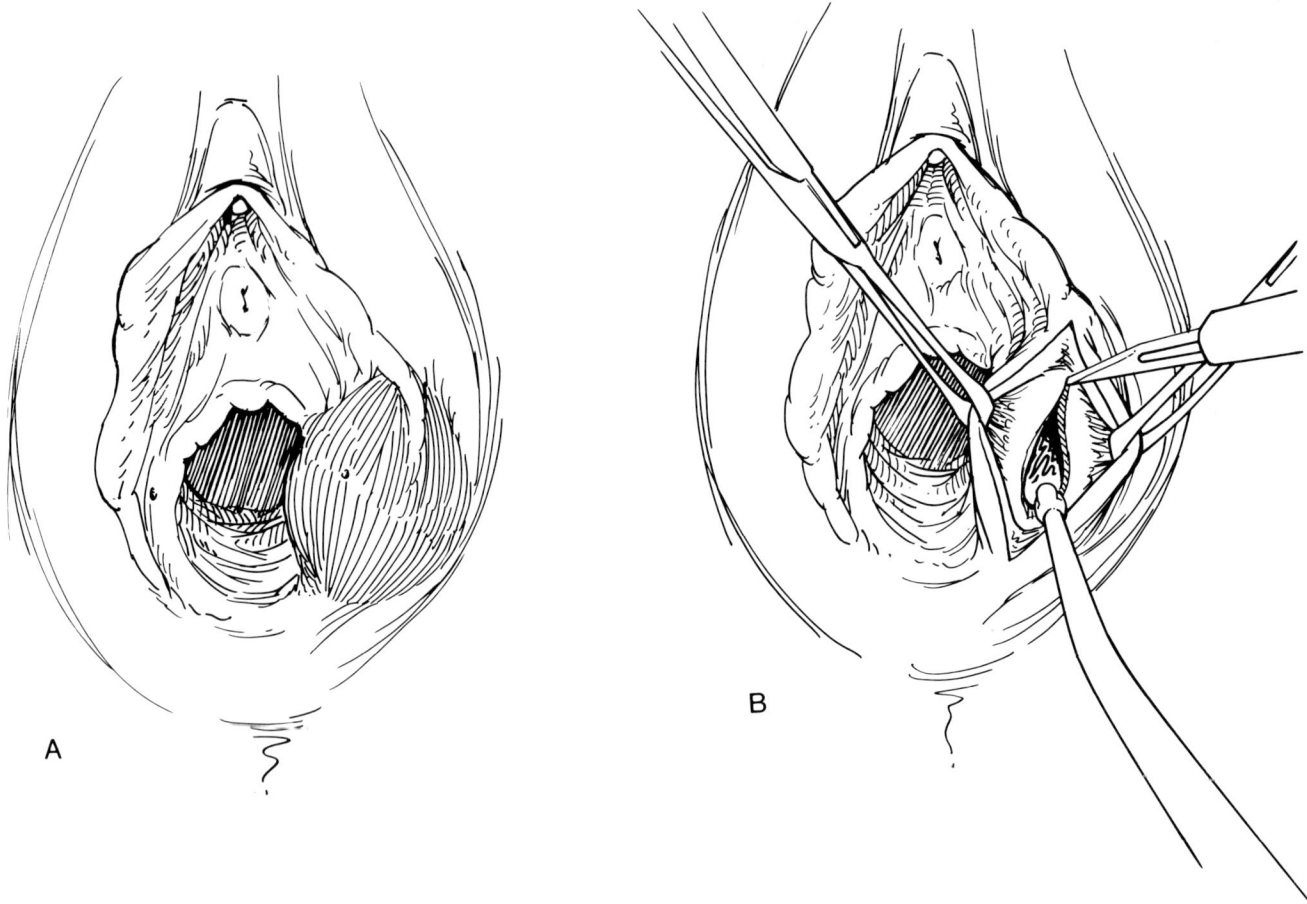

Figure 9-1
A, Bartholin duct cyst—typical appearance and location. B, 1-2 cm incision is made just external to the hymenal ring remnant, entering the cyst or abscess cavity.

length and run parallel with the hymenal ring (Fig. 9-1B). A larger incision will not allow the retention of a Word catheter.[8] Because the contents of Bartholin's abscesses are often under considerable pressure, protective eyewear should be worn to minimize the risk of gonococcal conjunctivitis to the operator. The abscess or cyst cavity may contain multiple loculations; therefore, these partitions must be broken by blunt dissection using an operating finger or a Kelly clamp. Only by doing this will recurrence be minimized.

Once the pus or cyst fluid has been completely drained, the drainage access must be maintained by placement of a wick or Word catheter. Seeing their efforts fail because of wick dislodgment has convinced many surgeons of the superior results obtained by a Word catheter. The bulb end of the catheter should be placed into the cyst cavity and inflated with 2 ml of saline. The free end will be less vulnerable if placed within the vagina. The catheter should be left in place for approximately 3 weeks. This will allow epithelialization of the incision tract, which will then maintain patency following the removal of the catheter.

Marsupialization of Bartholin's Cyst

A large cyst may not resolve using a Word catheter. It is then advisable to marsupialize the cyst wall, thereby creating a permanent fistulous tract. This procedure avoids the bleeding complications often encountered in cyst excision. An elliptical incision should be made through the vestibular skin as though a skin excision were to be performed. The incision should, however, be carried deeper in order to incorporate the underlying cyst wall. This "window" is then completely excised. Adhesions and loculations should then be broken down using blunt technique. The base of the cyst must be palpated. If it feels thickened or a solid "nubbin" is palpated, that area should be biopsied to exclude adenocarcinoma of Bartholin's gland or transitional or squamous cell carcinoma of Bartholin's duct. Malignancy is more likely in patients over 40 years of age;

therefore, these patients should be evaluated with a higher level of suspicion.[9]

Marsupialization is completed with the suturing of the cyst wall to the skin of the vestibule (Fig. 9–2). Interrupted sutures of a synthetic, delayed-absorbable material provide an excellent result.

Removal of a "window" of vestibular skin and cyst capsule has been advocated as an alternative to marsupialization.[10] In this variation, a 2 × 3 cm ellipse of vulvar skin is incised. The incision is then carried deeper to include the cyst or abscess capsule. The ellipse is finally excised and is available for pathologic examination.

Excision of Bartholin's Gland

For a "minor" procedure, excision of Bartholin's gland is associated with major potential complications. Bleeding from venous sinuses as well as branches of the pudendal and hemorrhoidal vessels can obscure the operative field. Hematomas in this area can extend and dissect from the anterior perineal compartment into a more superficial, potential space beneath Colles' fascia. From there, it may continue over the mons pubis and further under Scarpa's fascia. "Blind" hemostatic sutures are often ineffective and may compromise the vulvar blood supply such that fenestrations of the labium minus occur.

When it is necessary to perform Bartholin's gland excision, the initial incision should be made on the vaginal mucosal side of the hymen. Leaving a small strip of vaginal mucosa attached to the cyst wall affords a stronger surface for traction than using the cyst wall alone. Blunt dissection should be used whenever possible to free the cyst wall. Often, past inflammation has caused more dense adherence of the cyst wall. Blunt-tipped dissecting scissors will often allow further progress without leaving cyst wall behind. Once the cyst is excised, the dead space must be closed using multiple layers of fine, synthetic, delayed-absorbable suture material. Bed rest, pressure dressing, and ice packs are useful adjuncts in minimizing hematoma formation.

Minor Vestibular Glands

The minor vestibular glands form a ring adjacent to the hymen. Cysts occurring associated with these glands may become quite large. They generally enlarge along the longitudinal axis of the vaginal tube. When drainage using a Word catheter is unlikely, marsupialization as described previously is often effective. Large cysts, once marsupialized, can leave a large defect in the vaginal wall, but one that is usually asymptomatic.

Cyst of the Canal of Nuck

A cyst of the canal of Nuck in the female is the equivalent of a hydrocele in the male. It represents a sac lined with peritoneum that accompanies the round ligament along its course through the inguinal canal to its insertion in the labium majus. Fluid may accumulate in this peritoneal sac, giving rise to a cystic structure appearing in the labia majora.

It is important to distinguish the uncommon cyst of the canal of Nuck from the commonly encountered Bartholin's cyst. A cyst of the canal of Nuck will remain external to the hymenal ring, whereas a Bartholin's cyst often extends within the hymenal ring. Attempts to treat a hydrocele as a Bartholin's cyst will result in recurrence of the cyst.

Surgical management of a cyst of the canal of Nuck is indicated when the cyst becomes large or symptomatic. The cyst should be entered from an incision through the labium majus. The round ligament should be palpated along its course to the external inguinal ring. The cyst wall should then be excised and the inguinal ring closed with interrupted, delayed-absorbable sutures. The dead space created by the cyst should be closed in a similar fashion. On rare occasion, an inguinal hernia will coexist with a cyst of the canal of Nuck, as a loop of intestine herniates through the inguinal ring and enters the peritoneal lined cyst.[11] In this situation, an inguinal herniorrhaphy must be performed in conjunction with excision of the cyst.

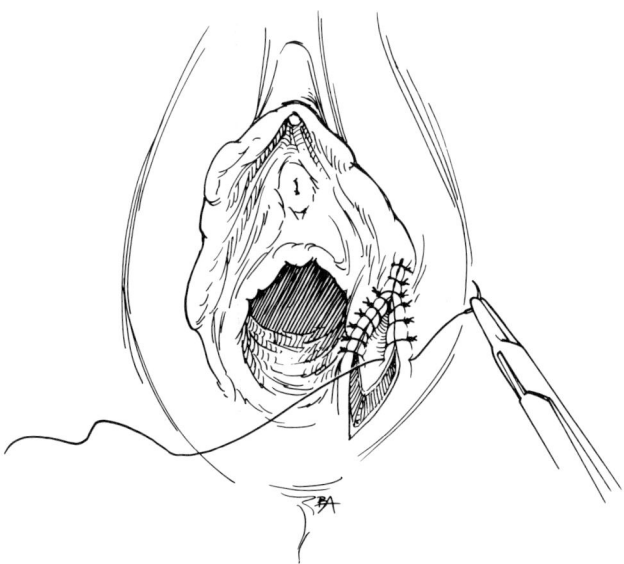

Figure 9–2
Marsupialization of a Bartholin duct. After the cyst cavity is entered, the cyst wall is sutured to the skin of the vestibule, allowing continued drainage.

EPISIOTOMY

Perhaps the most commonly performed operation in obstetrics and gynecology is the episiotomy, so much so that many texts make no mention of it as an operative procedure. The proper performance and repair of an episiotomy or perineal laceration may, therefore, represent the single greatest impact a practitioner has on his or her patient population. Despite multiple studies, obstetric practitioners remain sharply polarized as either harsh critics or enthusiastic proponents of this 2–4 cm incision. Patients, similarly, either refuse it months prior to the birth of their infant or demand it just moments before. Beyond the controversy lies a common goal of practitioners and patients from both persuasions. All parties seek childbirth with a minimum of pain and morbidity to the mother and the infant. In pursuit of this common goal, performance and repair of an episiotomy should be undertaken when failure to perform an episiotomy is likely to result in more extensive repair, an assessment that can be properly made only by the delivering practitioner in the moments just prior to delivery. Factors to consider include size of the perineal body, distensibility of old scarring from past repairs, size of the fetal presenting part, and fetal well-being. Attention should also be given to proper anesthesia during the operation and during repair. Failure to attend to this point can erase a positive "birth experience," leaving only nightmarish memories of the episiotomy.

As though there were not enough controversy surrounding this procedure already, midline versus mediolateral episiotomy arguments create their own heated discussions. Again, common intent can be found if each practitioner performs the operation which he or she feels best attains the goal of maximum benefit with minimal risk. Traditionally, midline episiotomy is criticized for frequent extension to third- or fourth-degree lacerations of the perineum. Hematoma formation, difficulty of repair, and pain limit widespread use of mediolateral episiotomy.

Midline Episiotomy

Midline episiotomy is not a procedure whose utility is limited to obstetrics. It can be a simple remedy to prevent aborting an otherwise difficult vaginal procedure that is hampered by a restricted vaginal orifice. The vaginal surgeon should retain this procedure as a useful adjunct in such cases.

Most frequently, however, the midline episiotomy is used as an obstetric procedure to limit perineal laceration, avoid future pelvic relaxation, and expedite delivery in cases of fetal distress. As the presenting part of the fetus distends the perineum during the second stage of labor, the entire introitus undergoes significant stretch. This is often more apparent in primigravid patients. When these distending forces appear so great that a significant perineal laceration seems imminent, many practitioners choose to perform a midline episiotomy. Many texts describe a relative anesthesia of the perineum when so distended and therefore advise performance of the episiotomy without use of a local anesthetic. The occasional patient in whom this does not prove to be true will never forget the experience. It is therefore recommended that the perineum be infiltrated with a lidocaine solution. Attention to avoiding intravascular injection is crucial. Local anesthesia often lessens the discomfort experienced by the patient, because she is then able to push in labor without the pain and burning of perineal stretching. In addition, the use of local anesthesia does not commit the practitioner to the performance of an episiotomy.

An adequate incision should be made vertically in the midline, through the perineal body, using blunt-tipped tissue or bandage scissors. It is imperative for the operator to ensure that no fetal parts lie between the blades of the scissors before performing the episiotomy. The incision should also not extend through the puborectalis muscle under routine circumstances. If pressure from the crowning vertex does not cause a tamponade of the vessels encountered, digital pressure can be maintained until delivery of the neonate.

Following delivery, the vagina and vulva should be carefully examined to assess the extent and severity of vaginal and perineal laceration. Oxytocic medications should be used to limit uterine bleeding and selective hemostatic sutures employed to control vaginal and perineal bleeding so that the practitioner may have a clear view of the operative field. Rectal examination may be useful if a fourth-degree perineal extension cannot be excluded. Third-degree extension is apparent when a cylindrical muscle bundle is present at the site of the anal sphincter, or bilateral hollows are present at the same site, representing the area of sphincter retraction.

Attempts to repair an extensive perineal laceration without adequate anesthesia are both counterproductive for the surgeon and torturous for the patient. If adequate anesthesia or exposure cannot be obtained with local infiltration, regional anesthesia should be employed without hesitation. Repair should be in a stepwise fashion, initially repairing fourth-degree extension by reducing the laceration to a third degree. Attention to technique at this point will avoid the devastating development of a rectovaginal fistula. Similarly, proper repair of a third-degree extension avoids fecal incontinence.

With vaginal and submucosal tissues adequately

retracted, the apex of the rectal tear should be identified. A running suture of a fine, absorbable material on an atraumatic needle should be selected. A suture of 3-0 chromic gut provides a reasonable balance of strength and fairly rapid absorption. Longer lasting synthetic materials may promote fistula formation. Care should be taken to see that the suture does not pierce the rectal mucosa. Once the first layer is completed to the mucosal junction of the anus, it should be oversewn by a second layer of synthetic delayed-absorbable suture such as 2-0 polyglycolic acid in interrupted fashion. This layer should include submucosal and muscularis tissue, thereby providing strength to the closure. Rectal examination at this point should confirm the absence of a persistent defect in the rectal mucosa or penetrating suture material.

Successful repair of a third-degree perineal laceration requires identification of the muscle fibers and capsule of the rectal sphincter. Often one or both free ends of the sphincter will retract into the perirectal connective tissue. They may be retrieved using an Allis clamp advanced into the recess produced by the retracted muscle. Approximating the Allis clamps in the midline, encircling an examiner's rectal finger will confirm retrieval of both halves by creating the feel of an intact sphincteric ring. At this time, gloves should be changed and further rectal examinations avoided for 6 weeks.

The intent of third-degree laceration repair is to approximate the *capsule* or fascia of the rectal sphincter. The muscle fibers themselves will not reliably hold a suture. Three figure-of-eight sutures should be placed evenly around the circumference of the muscle capsule (Fig. 9–3A). A strong, synthetic, delayed-absorbable suture material should be employed. By not tying any suture until all three are placed, the operator will allow easier placement of the sutures behind the sphincter. Successfully completing this step should reconstruct a substantial perineal body.

Uncomplicated healing of a third- or fourth-degree perineal laceration will be enhanced by keeping the patient on stool softeners for 1 month postoperatively. The serious complications of rectovaginal fistula and fecal incontinence will usually occur within 3 weeks of repair, but patients may not present for treatment until years afterward. Therefore, careful questioning of patients recovering from a third- or fourth-degree laceration is important.

Repair of the uncomplicated midline episiotomy should be accomplished with care but not obsession. Excessive attention to cosmetic closure of the perineal skin can result in excessive pain for the patient without any improvement in final results. The apex of the vaginal incision should be identified and a suture placed above the apex. This will afford hemostatic control of vessels at the apex. Continuing in a running, locking fashion, the vaginal incision should be reapproximated until the hymenal ring is reached (Fig. 9–3B). By bringing the suture through the vaginal suture line out to the midline of the perineal defect, no knot will remain in the vagina, avoiding future dyspareunia.

The so-called crown stitch will restore shape and strength to the introitus. This is achieved by entering the perineal connective tissue deep in the midline and exiting superficially at the apex of the perineal incision where the exposed connective tissue meets the skin. On the contralateral side, the needle should enter at the superficial junction of connective tissue and skin and exit deep in the midline. This stitch should then be tied securely.

The perineal defect can be closed by either continuing with the same suture or using interrupted sutures to approximate the bulbospongiosus muscles in the midline (Fig. 9–3C). Once this is completed, the proximity of the skin edges should be evaluated. If there is minimal distance between skin edges in the lithotomy position, the skin edges should spontaneously oppose once the patient is at rest. The patient will experience less episiotomy discomfort and the final result will be excellent if no further suturing is done. Few if any postpartum patients will voluntarily assume a lithotomy position during the 7–10 days required for episiotomy healing. If the operator feels that the skin defect remains too great to ensure a satisfactory result, an absorbable, subcuticular suture beginning at the anal margin of the defect up to the introital margin may be used (Fig. 9–3D). This suture is, however, often responsible for the majority of episiotomy discomfort. Those who have not eliminated this final closure from their routine should try omitting it on several patients with close approximation of skin edges following bulbospongiosus closure. Later questioning has shown many practitioners that those patients experience minimal discomfort with no compromise in final outcome. The results may be surprising.

Mediolateral Episiotomy (Schuchardt's Incision)

Use of a mediolateral episiotomy is felt to minimize obstetric lacerations of the rectal sphincter and rectal mucosa. Laterality of the incision is at the discretion of the operator, although most right-handed surgeons perform a right-sided mediolateral episiotomy with greater facility. Left-handed operators prefer the left-sided procedure. Adequate repair and final outcome critically depend on achievement of excellent hemostasis. Enormous hematoma formation threatens the less-than-compulsive surgeon.

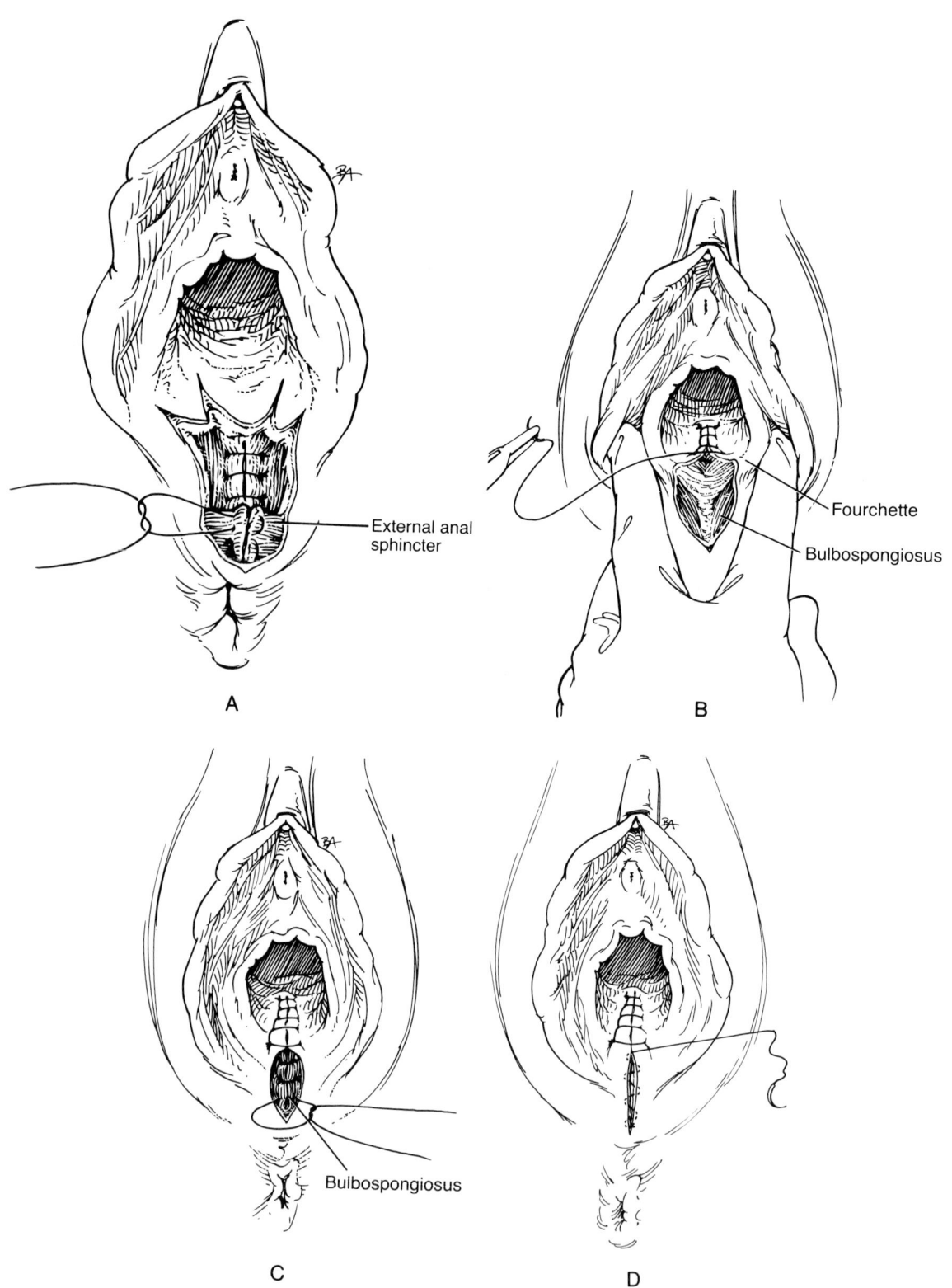

Figure 9-3
A, Third-degree perineal laceration. The capsule of the anal sphincter is reapproximated using three figure-of-eight sutures. B, Repair of a second-degree perineal laceration begins with a running, locking suture initiated at the apex of the vaginal defect. C, The bulbospongiosus muscles are reapproximated in the midline, restoring the perineal body. D, A subcuticular suture may be used to complete perineal repair.

Repair of a mediolateral episiotomy is begun in a fashion similar to that described for a midline repair, with the closure of the vaginal mucosa. Beyond the hymenal ring, the repair differs. Attention should then be directed to placing interrupted absorbable sutures such that the opposing halves of the perineal defect are returned to their proper anatomic relationship. This can be facilitated by using a surgical marker to draw horizontal lines on the perineum prior to performing a mediolateral episiotomy. Because patients generally complain of greater pain following a mediolateral episiotomy, consideration should again be given to avoiding too tight approximation of the perineal skin. Ice packs and judicious pressure applied to a perineal pad further reduce the likelihood of hematoma formation.

THE IMPERFORATE HYMEN

An imperforate hymen is rarely encountered in the clinical practice of gynecology. Even in tertiary referral centers, few groups report large series of patients. However, it is incumbent upon all gynecologists to be familiar with the presentation and management of the unusual developmental aberration, because prompt treatment avoids potential lifelong complications.[12]

The incidence of imperforate hymen is unknown. The hymen is felt to represent the embryologic septum separating the urogenital sinus externally and the sinovaginal bulbs internally.[12] As such, it is not of müllerian origin. Therefore, other anomalies of the müllerian or mesonephric duct system are not to be expected in association with an imperforate hymen.

An imperforate hymen is usually asymptomatic prior to menarche, although occasionally it will be recognized prepubertally by an astute mother. At the time of menarche, the adolescent with an imperforate hymen will have no visible menstrual flow. Instead, the menstrual blood will collect in and distend the vaginal vault (hematocolpos), causing few if any symptoms. With the second or third menstruation, the menstrual fluid will exceed the capacity of the vagina, backing up into the uterine cavity (hematometra). Low abdominal pain, suprapubic cramps, and difficulty or pain with urination or defecation are common presenting symptoms of the young woman with an imperforate hymen. Amenorrhea despite other appropriate pubertal milestones further supports the diagnosis. Prompt evaluation and treatment limit retrograde menstruation, hemoperitoneum, and development of endometriosis.

Physical examination occasionally demonstrates a tender, low midline abdominal mass—the hematometra. Inspection of the vulva may reveal a bluish apparent mass bulging between the labia. Palpation of the mass confirms the imperforate nature of the hymen.

Prompt surgical management is necessary. In prepubertal girls, the hymen may be incised at the 2, 4, 8, and 10 o'clock positions (Fig. 9–4A). Mucus rather than blood would be expected because only the glandular secretions will have accumulated. The four hymenal tabs may then be sharply excised and the mucosal defects approximated (Fig. 9–4B). Once hematocolpos or hematometra has developed, significant blood loss and hypotension may accompany incision of the hymen. Incision should be accomplished as described previously, but the hymenal tabs should not be excised during primary drainage. Gentle cervical dilation to a maximum of a No. 10 dilator may improve resolution of a hematometra. Under no circumstances should the uterine cavity be curetted or explored, because the distended uterine wall is prone to perforation. Four to six weeks following drainage, excess hymenal tissue may be excised when the vagina and related structures have returned to their normal anatomic relation. At this time, patency of the endocervical canal and contour of the endometrial cavity can be carefully assessed.

VAGINAL SEPTAE

The vagina is derived embryologically from the fused müllerian ducts, which form the upper two-thirds; and the vaginal plate of the urogenital sinus, which forms the lower third. At the point of fusion, incomplete canalization of the tube or incomplete fusion of the two structures can result in a transverse vaginal septum (Fig. 9–5). A longitudinal vaginal septum indicates incomplete fusion of the paired müllerian ducts. In cases of longitudinal vaginal septae, associated anomalies of the müllerian and mesonephric systems should be sought, particularly uterus didelphys.

Transverse Vaginal Septum

When complete, a transverse vaginal septum causes symptoms similar to those seen with an imperforate hymen. Because the septum usually occurs at the junction of the upper third of the vagina with the lower two-thirds,[13] less vaginal distention is possible and symptomatic hematometra occurs earlier than with an imperforate hymen. A partial transverse septum may cause dyspareunia because of the functional shortening of the vagina but is often an incidental finding during a routine pelvic examination.

A complete septum should be incised to allow drainage of a hematometra 6 weeks or more before excision is attempted. When excision is undertaken, traction should be applied to the center of the sep-

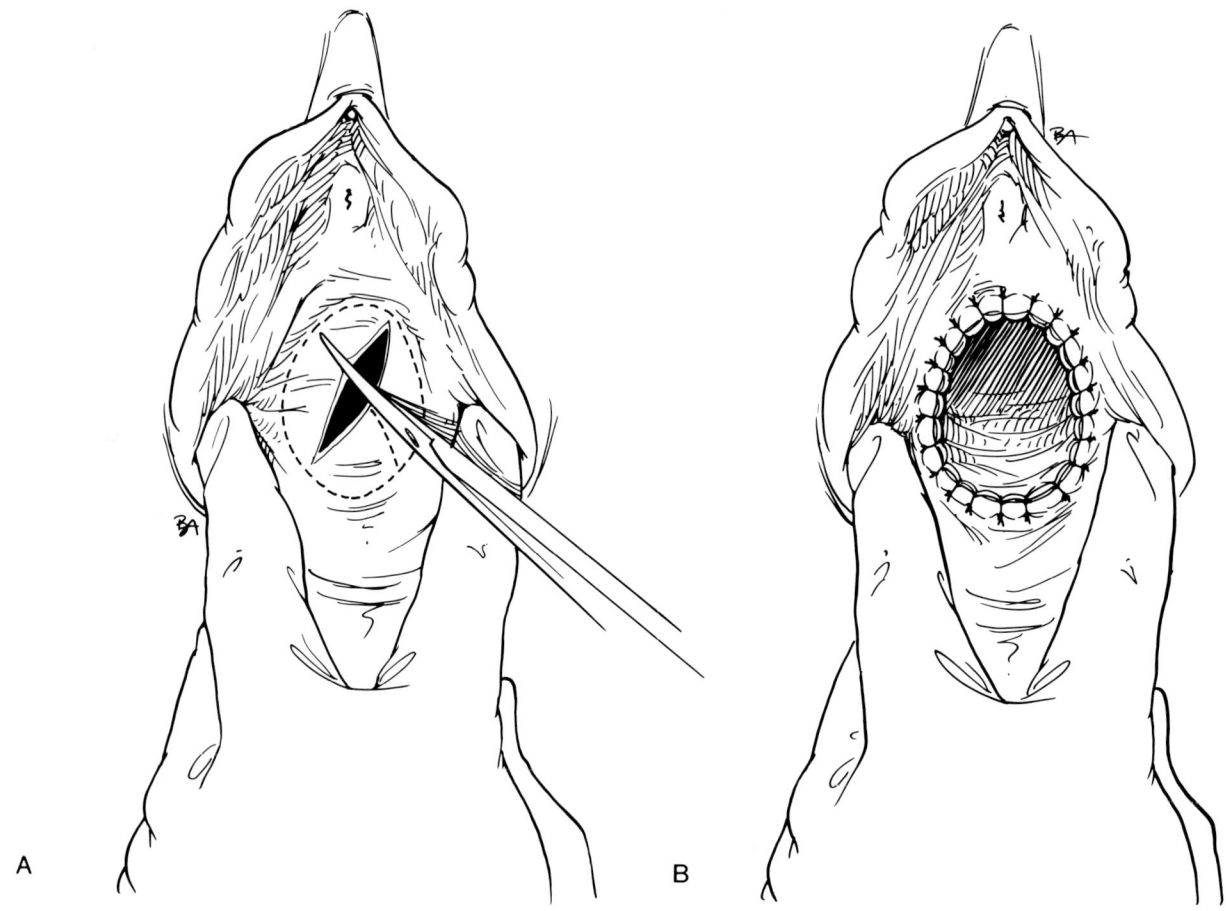

Figure 9–4
A, The imperforate hymen, with incision at the 2, 4, 8, and 10 o' clock positions. B, Final result following repair of imperforate hymen.

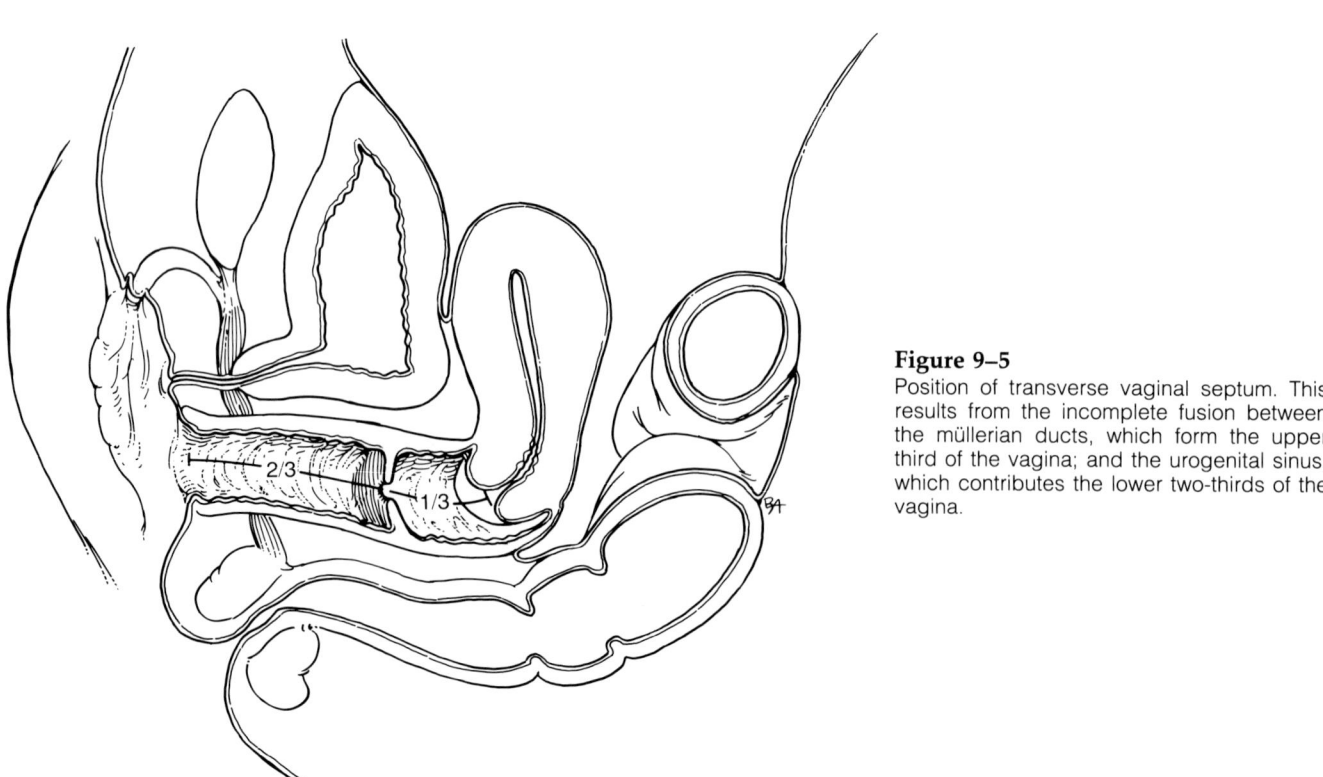

Figure 9–5
Position of transverse vaginal septum. This results from the incomplete fusion between the müllerian ducts, which form the upper third of the vagina; and the urogenital sinus, which contributes the lower two-thirds of the vagina.

tum. A vertical incision is carried through the septum, dividing it into halves (Fig. 9–6A). Each half is sharply excised from the vaginal mucosa (Fig. 9–6B). Finally, the residual mucosal defect is closed using interrupted, delayed-absorbable suture (Fig. 9–6C and D). Complete excision of a thick septum may produce an unacceptably foreshortened vagina. In those cases, the septum should be widely fenestrated without final excision from the vaginal mucosa.

Longitudinal Vaginal Septum

As mentioned previously, when a longitudinal septum is encountered (Fig. 9–7A), the patient should be evaluated for other müllerian malformations. An intravenous pyelogram must also be performed to identify mesonephric anomalies.[14] Once this preliminary evaluation is complete, excision of the longitudinal septum may be undertaken. Patients who are free of dyspareunia may still benefit from excision of the septum, which can cause obstruction at the time of vaginal delivery.

Prior to excision of the septum, the bladder must be emptied. A clamp should be placed along the septum, applying gentle traction (Fig. 9–7B). (Excessive pressure on the clamp could draw the urethra or bladder tissue into the area of excision from above, or rectal tissue from below.) The septum is then sharply separated from the vaginal mucosa above

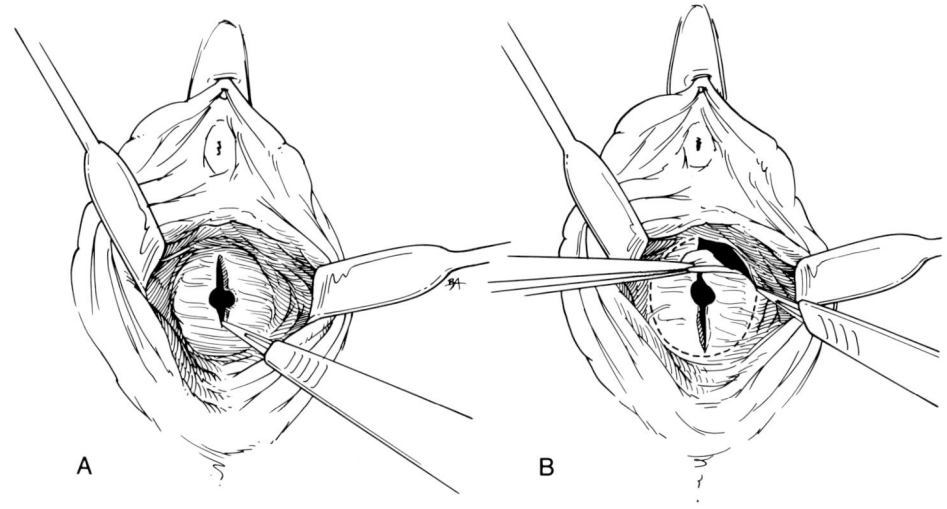

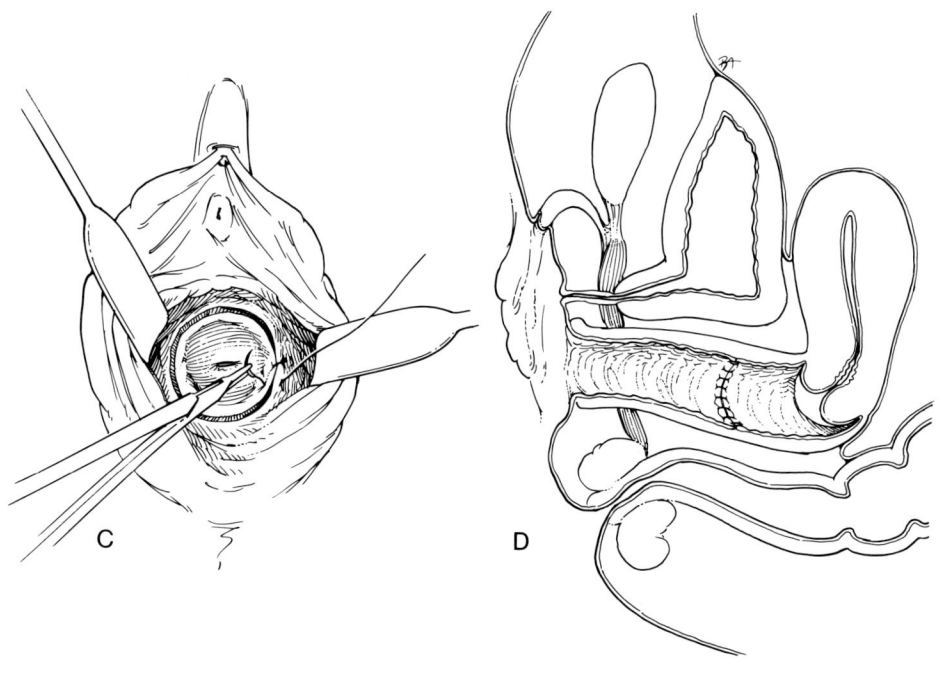

Figure 9–6
A, The initial vertical incision is made in the transverse vaginal septum. B, The septum is then sharply excised from the vaginal mucosa. C and D, The defect in the vaginal mucosa is finally repaired with interrupted sutures.

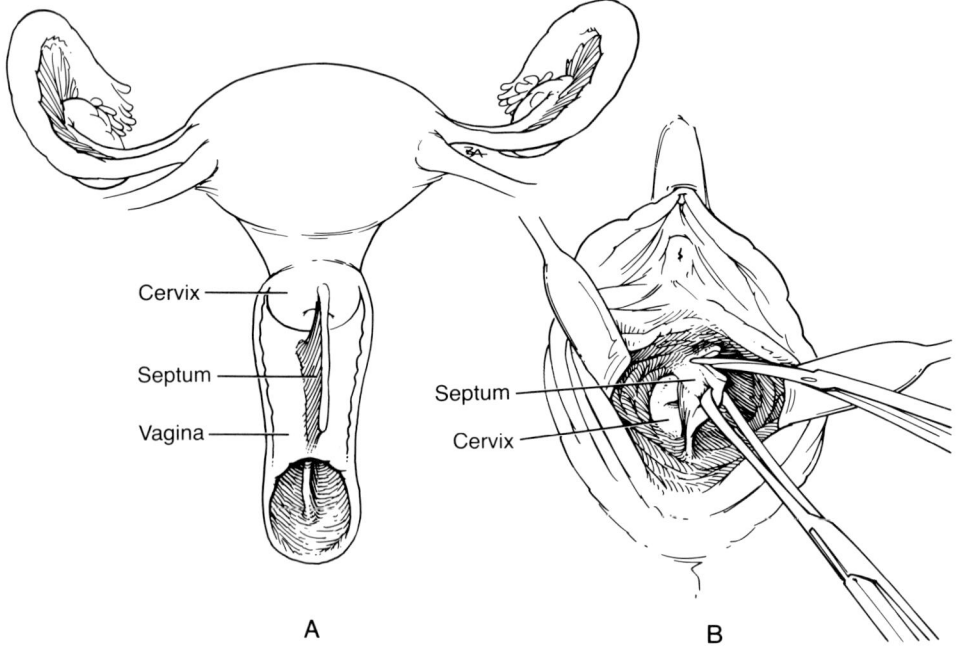

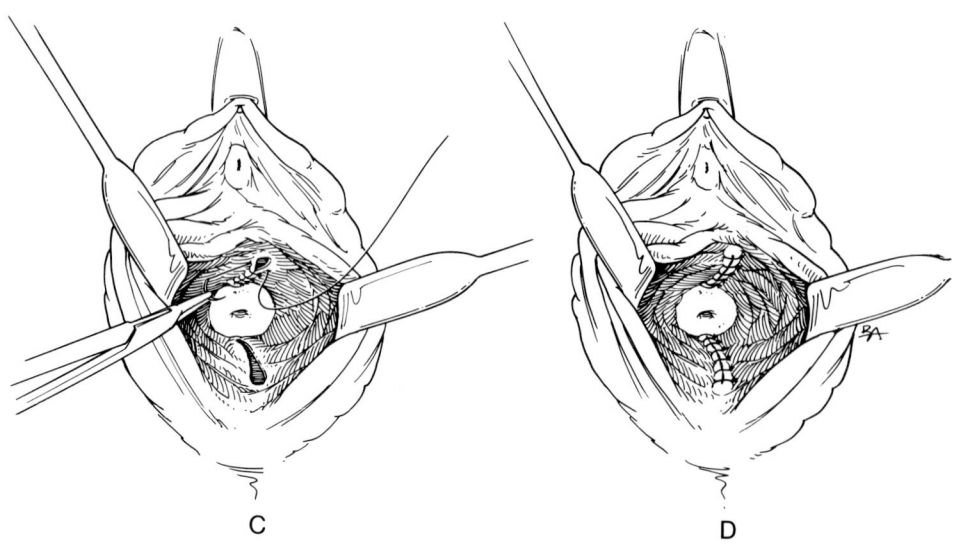

Figure 9–7
A, Longitudinal vaginal septum results from the incomplete fusion of the paired müllerian ducts. Other anomalies of the müllerian and mesonephric ducts should be sought. *B*, Gentle traction is applied as the septum is sharply excised. *C* and *D*, Finally, the mucosal defect is closed.

and below, using tissue scissors. The mucosal defect can then be closed using delayed-absorbable suture (Fig. 9–7C and D).

References

1. Report of the ISSVD Terminology Committee, Proceedings of the Seventh World Congress, Stockholm. J Reprod Med 1987; 31:973.
2. Lundwall F: Cancer of the vulva. Acta Radiol (Stockh) 1961; 208 (suppl.).
3. Hewitt J: Lichen sclerosis. J Reprod Med 1986; 31:781.
4. Lynch PJ: Condylomata acuminata (anogenital warts). Clin Obstet Gynecol 1985; 28:142.
5. Oriel JD, Almeida JD: Demonstration of virus particles in human genital warts. Br J Vener Dis 1970; 46:37.
6. Baggish MS: Carbon dioxide laser for condylomata acuminata venereal infections. Obstet Gynecol 1980; 55:711.
7. Calkins JW, Materson BJ, Magina JF, et al.: Management of condylomata acuminata with the carbon dioxide laser. Obstet Gynecol 1982; 59:105.
8. Word B: Office treatment of cyst and abscess of Bartholin's gland duct. South Med J 1968; 61:514.
9. Chamlian DL, Taylor HB: Primary carcinoma of Bartholin's gland: A report of 24 patients. J Obstet Gynecol 1972; 39:489.
10. Cho JY, Ahn MO, Cha KS: Window operation: An alternative treatment method for Bartholin gland cyst and abscess. Obstet Gynecol 1990; 76:886.
11. Kucera PR, Glazer J: Hydrocele of the canal of Nuck: A report of four cases. J Reprod Med 1985; 30:439.
12. Huffman JW: Gynecology of Childhood and Adolescence, 2nd ed. Philadelphia, WB Saunders Co., 1981.
13. Bowman JA, Scott RA: Transverse vaginal septum. Obstet Gynecol 1954; 3:144.
14. Thompson DP, Lynn HB: Genital anomalies associated with solitary kidney. Mayo Clin Proc 1966; 41:538.

Surgery for Malignant Tumors of the Vulva

10

Neville F. Hacker

Vulvar cancer is uncommon, representing about 4% of all female genital tract malignancies. Even busy gynecologic cancer units seldom see more than one vulvar cancer each month, therefore, worthwhile reported series have usually been accumulated over at least a 20-year period.

Surgery is the mainstay of treatment for vulvar cancer, and during the past 60 years, surgical opinion has come full circle. In the early part of the century, conservative operations such as simple vulvectomy were often performed, but a 5-year survival of only about 20–25% was achieved.[1, 2] These poor results encouraged the Frenchman Antoine Basset to advocate a more radical en bloc dissection of the vulva and regional lymph nodes.[3] Using the Basset approach, Frederick Taussig in the United States[4] and Stanley Way in Britain[5] reported 5-year survival rates of 60–70%. Both physical and psychologic morbidity was high with this radical approach, and in recent years a more conservative surgical approach has again been advocated, particularly for the primary tumor. With careful patient selection, survival does not seem to be compromised.

In addition to a less radical surgical approach, the appropriate integration of radiation therapy into the management of vulvar cancer is receiving increasing attention, and guidelines for preoperative or postoperative radiation therapy are slowly evolving.

SURGICAL ANATOMY

As with any surgical procedure, a full appreciation of the relevant anatomy is necessary if the best results are to be obtained.

The vulva includes the mons veneris; the labia majora and minora; the clitoris; and the vulvar vestibule, which contains the urethral meatus and vaginal orifice (Fig. 10–1).

The mons veneris, a fatty prominence anterior to the pubic symphysis, becomes covered with hair at the time of puberty. The labia majora are pigmented and covered with hair on their lateral surface, whereas medially they contain sebaceous glands. The labia minora lie between the labia majora and meet posteriorly in a skin fold called the fourchette. Anteriorly, they split to enclose the clitoris, forming the prepuce anteriorly and the frenulum posteriorly. The internal surfaces of the labia minora contain numerous sebaceous glands.

The clitoris is an erectile structure consisting of a glans, a body, and two crura. Only the glans is visible externally. The vestibular bulbs (equivalent to the corpora spongiosa of the penis) extend posteriorly from the glans on either side of the lower vagina. Each bulb is covered by the bulbocavernosus muscle and is attached to the inferior surface of the perineal membrane or inferior fascia of the urogenital

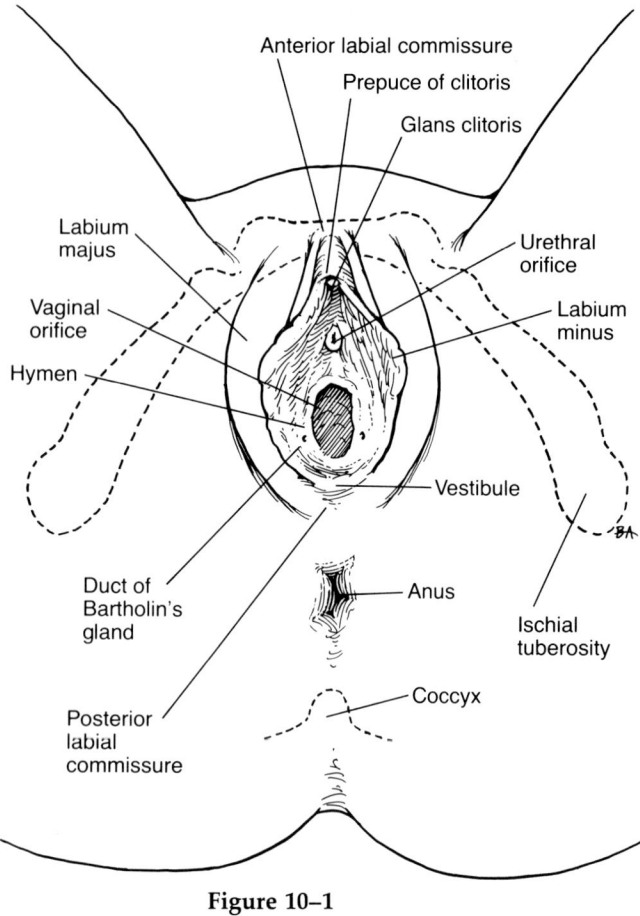

Figure 10-1
Female external genitalia.

the sciatic artery.) The artery emerges from the pelvis around the ischial spine, then travels forward along the outer wall of the ischiorectal fossa on the obturator internus muscle. During this part of its course, it is contained in a sheath of the obturator fascia (Alcock's canal) and accompanied by the internal pudendal nerve and vein. On the vulva, each artery has the following branches: the superficial perineal artery, which supplies the labia; the artery of the bulb, which supplies the vestibular bulb and the erectile tissue of the vagina; the artery of the corpus cavernosum, which supplies the corresponding organ; and the dorsal artery of the clitoris, which supplies the dorsum of that organ and terminates in the glans.

The main nerve supply is from the internal pudendal nerve, which is the direct continuation of the lower cord of the sacral plexus. It derives its fibers mainly from the third and fourth sacral nerves. The nerve follows the corresponding artery throughout its course and has similar branches on the vulva.

The pathways of lymph flow from the vulva have been well described by Plentl and Friedman.[6] More recently, Iversen and Aas confirmed and quantified previous observations with a scintigraphic study.[7]

Lymphatics from the vulva course anteriorly towards the mons veneris, turning laterally at the mons to terminate mainly in the inguinal lymph nodes.

diaphragm (Fig. 10-2). The body of the clitoris is composed of a pair of corpora cavernosa and extends superiorly beneath the labia for some distance before dividing into two crura, which are attached to the undersurface of either pubic ramus. Each crus is covered by the corresponding ischiocavernosus muscle.

The vaginal orifice is guarded in the virgin by a thin mucosal fold, the hymen, which tears at first coitus. After childbirth, nothing is left of the hymen but a few rounded tags known as carunculae myrtiformes.

Bartholin's glands (the greater vestibular glands) are a pair of pea-sized mucus-secreting glands lying deep to the posterior parts of the labia majora. Each gland drains via a simple duct, which opens into the vulvar vestibule in the angle between the hymen and the corresponding labium minus. The glands are impalpable when healthy but become readily palpable if malignant transformation of the gland or its duct occurs.

The main arterial supply is from the internal pudendal artery, the smaller of the two terminal branches of the anterior trunk of the internal iliac (hypogastric) artery. (The larger terminal branch is

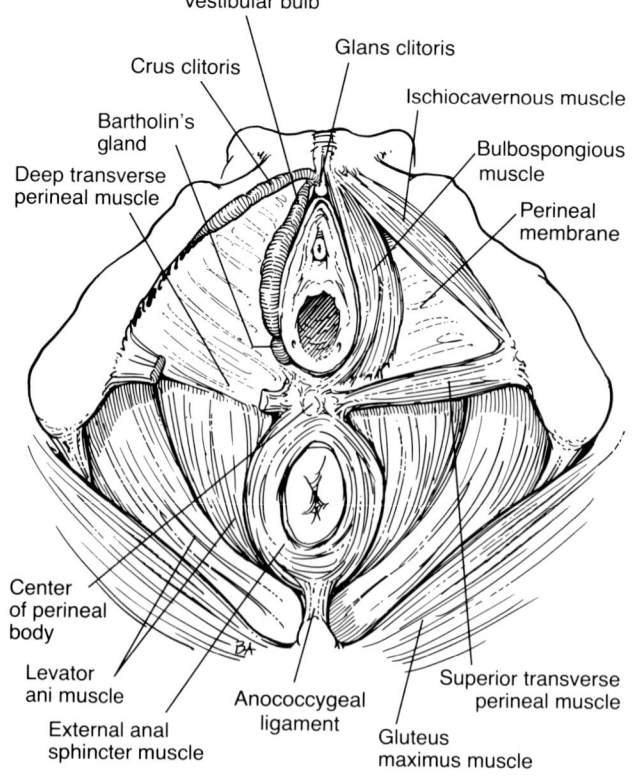

Figure 10-2
The perineum.

The latter are situated along the line of the inguinal ligament, slightly below it, and along the saphenous vein. They lie above the fascia lata and cribriform fascia, and below Camper's (superficial) fascia (Fig. 10–3). Lymphatic channels from both sides anastomose, and some contralateral spread is theoretically possible. There are usually about 10–12 inguinal nodes present on each side.

Beneath the cribriform fascia are the femoral lymph nodes. These lie along the femoral vein, and there are usually only two or three nodes present. The most cephalad node of the group is known as the lymph node of Cloquet or Rosenmüller, and it is situated under the inguinal ligament in the femoral canal. The femoral nodes receive efferents from the inguinal nodes, but may also receive some direct channels through the cribriform fascia, particularly from the clitoris and anterior vulva. From the femoral nodes, efferents pass to the external iliac nodes, particularly the medial group.

Iversen and Aas injected different areas of the vulva with 99m-Tc colloid in 54 patients prior to Wertheim hysterectomy and pelvic lymphadenectomy for Stage Ib carcinoma of the cervix.[7] The radioactivity in the groin and pelvis was measured with a scintillation camera and in the removed pelvic nodes with a well counter. These investigators confirmed that there was bilateral lymph flow from the perineum and clitoris. The vast majority of radioactivity from the remainder of the vulva was to the ipsilateral groin nodes, but 67% of patients did have a low, but detectable, contralateral lymph flow. All patients injected in the anterior labium minus showed contralateral flow. Of the removed pelvic nodes, 73% of the total radioactivity was in the medial external iliac group with Cloquet's node containing 47% of the activity. However, in 13% of cases, the activity in the lateral external iliac nodes was higher than in the medial group, suggesting that not all lymph travels to the pelvis via Cloquet's node.

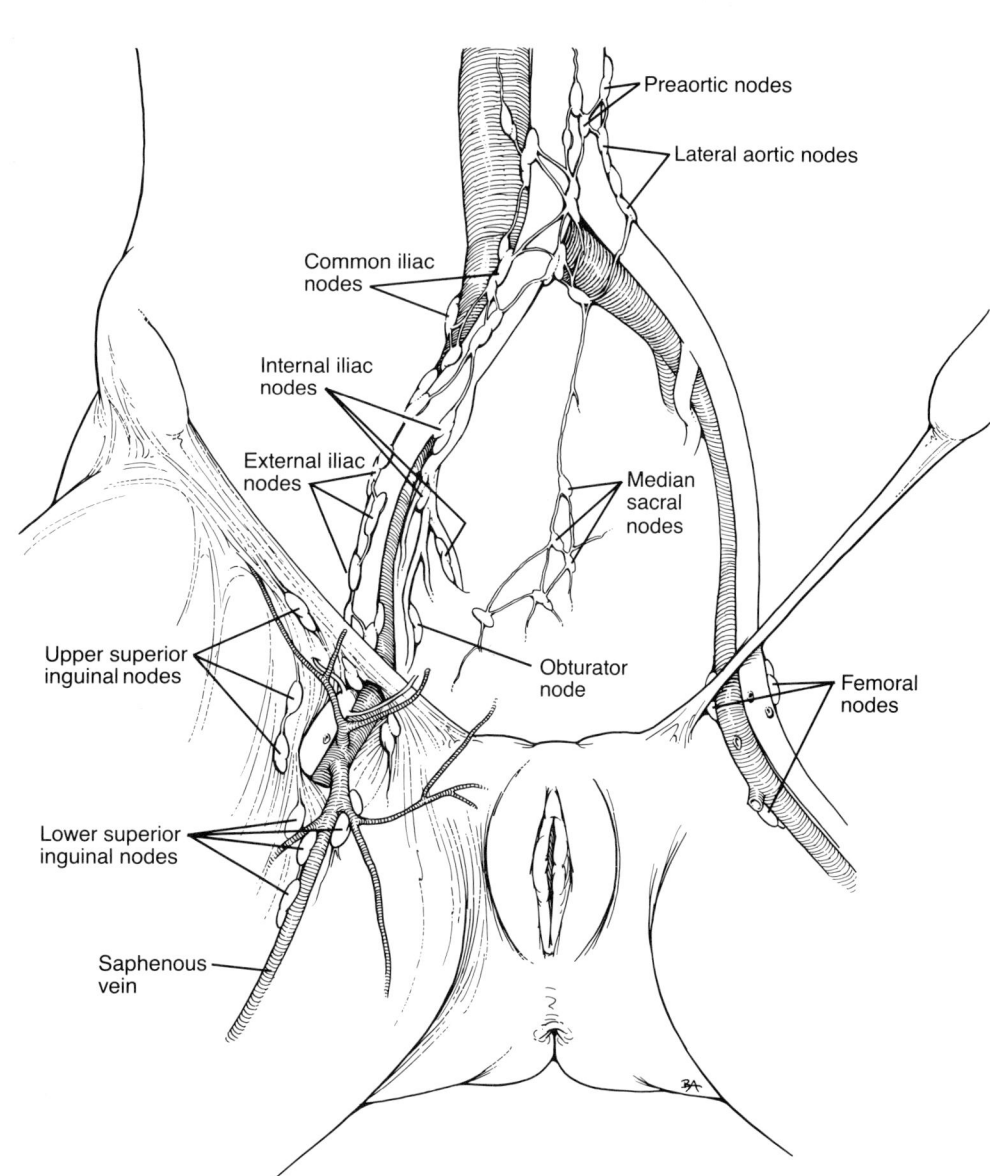

Figure 10–3
Inguinal-femoral lymph nodes.

No direct pathway from the clitoris to the pelvic nodes could be demonstrated.

HISTOLOGIC CLASSIFICATION OF TUMORS

About 90% of primary vulvar malignancies are squamous cell carcinomas. Less common tumors are melanomas, adenocarcinomas (often underlying Paget's disease), basal cell carcinomas, Bartholin's gland carcinomas, sarcomas, verrucous carcinomas, and lymphomas. The relative proportion of vulvar malignancies is seldom stated in papers, but the cumulative statistics from three reports published in the last decade are shown in Table 10–1.

STAGING

Until 1989, vulvar cancer was staged clinically by the Federation Internationale de Gynecologie et d'Obstetrique (FIGO). At their meeting in Rio de Janiero in 1989, the Cancer Committee of FIGO approved a surgical staging for vulvar cancer (Table 10–2). Surgical staging recognizes the prognostic significance of the status of the lymph nodes and acknowledges the inability of palpation of groin nodes to adequately determine the presence or absence of metastatic disease.

Because of the change in FIGO staging, all reports in the current literature are based on the old FIGO staging, which was adopted in 1969. Hence, this staging is also reproduced (Table 10–3).

SQUAMOUS CELL CARCINOMA

Squamous cell carcinoma is preponderantly a disease of postmenopausal women, the mean age at diagnosis being about 65 years.

The etiology of vulvar cancer is uncertain and is most likely multifactorial. Like cervical cancer, vulvar carcinomas may be preceded by intraepithelial neoplasia (VIN), but the natural history of the latter is unclear. Women with vulvar cancer are generally of lower socioeconomic status and may be obese, hypertensive, and diabetic.[11] Smoking has been implicated,[12] and many patients have a previous history of other lower genital tract malignancies, particularly cervical cancer.[13] In some countries, chronic granulomatous venereal diseases are associated with an earlier age at onset of vulvar cancer. Such diseases include lymphogranuloma venereum, granuloma inguinale, and syphilis.[14]

Viral agents have been implicated in a number of studies. Kaufman and colleagues have demonstrated

Table 10–1

Primary Malignancies of the Vulva

Histologic Type	Number	Percentage
Squamous cell carcinoma	689	87.9
Melanoma	50	6.4
Adenocarcinoma	15	1.9
Basal cell carcinoma	14	1.8
Bartholin's gland carcinoma	8	1.0
Verrucous carcinoma	5	0.6
Sarcoma	2	0.3
Lymphoma	1	0.1
Totals	**784**	**100.0**

Data from refs. 8–10.

Table 10–2

FIGO (1989) Staging of Vulvar Carcinoma

Stage	Clinical Findings
0	Carcinoma in situ, intraepithelial carcinoma
I	Tumor confined to the vulva and/or perineum, 2 cm or less in greatest dimension. No nodal metastasis
II	Tumor confined to the vulva and/or perineum, more than 2 cm in greatest dimension. No nodal metastasis
III	Tumor of any size with: 1. Adjacent spread to the urethra and/or the vagina, or the anus, and/or 2. Unilateral regional lymph node metastasis
IVA	Tumor invades any of the following: upper urethra, bladder mucosa, rectal mucosa, pelvic bone, and/or bilateral regional node metastasis
IVB	Any distant metastasis, including pelvic lymph nodes

Table 10–3

Old FIGO Staging for Vulvar Cancer (1969)

FIGO Stage	Clinical Findings
0	Carcinoma in situ—e.g., vulvar intraepithelial neoplasia type 3, noninvasive Paget's disease
I	Tumor confined to the vulva, up to 2 cm in diameter, and no suspicious groin nodes
II	Tumor confined to the vulva, more than 2 cm in diameter, and no suspicious groin nodes
III	Tumor of any size with: 1. Adjacent spread to the urethra and/or the vagina, the perineum, and the anus, and/or 2. Clinically suspicious lymph nodes in either groin
IV	Tumor of any size: 1. Infiltrating the bladder mucosa, or the rectal mucosa, or both, including the upper part of the urethral mucosa, and/or 2. Fixed to the bone, and/or 3. Other distant metastases

herpes simplex virus type 2 (HSV-2)–induced cytoplasmic antigens in 9 of 10 in situ squamous vulvar carcinomas,[15] while human papillomavirus particles and capsid antigens have also been located adjacent to in situ or invasive squamous carcinoma.[16] Type 16 seems to be the most frequently implicated wart virus.[17]

Chemical carcinogens such as shale oil and arsenic may be involved in specific cases,[18] while the immune status of the patient is always an important factor to consider. Immunosuppressed women such as those on high doses of corticosteroids or those on immunosuppressant drugs following organ transplantation are at increased risk of developing vulvar neoplasms.[19]

Clinical Features

Most patients present with a lump or a mass, although a long history of vulvar itching is common. Less common presenting symptoms include bleeding, discharge, and dysuria. In affluent societies, about half the patients have early lesions at presentation; in poorer areas, advanced cases are still common, and such patients may present with a large mass in the groin.

On physical examination, the lesion is usually raised and may be fleshy, ulcerated, leukoplakic, or warty in appearance. Warty tumors have been reported to account for 20% of vulvar squamous tumors.[20] They may be misdiagnosed as condylomata acuminata.

Most squamous carcinomas occur on the labia majora, but the labia minora, clitoris, and perineum may also be primary sites. Only about 5% of cases are multifocal.

Diagnosis

There are no pathognomonic features of vulvar diseases, and a wedge biopsy (or excisional biopsy for smaller lesions) should be performed on any vulvar abnormality. Physician delay is still distressingly common with vulvar cancer, particularly if the lesion has a warty appearance or has a large component of vulvar intraepithelial neoplasia (VIN). Any confluent mass of "warts" should be biopsied to exclude an underlying squamous cell carcinoma before treatment.

Patterns of Spread

Vulvar cancer spreads by the following routes:

1. Direct extension to adjacent organs, including the vagina, urethra, and anus
2. Lymphatic embolization to regional lymph nodes
3. Hematogenous spread to distant organs such as the liver, lungs, and bone

Although lymphatic spread is usually initially to the inguinal lymph nodes, patients with metastases to the femoral nodes without involvement of the inguinal nodes have been reported.[21-23] The author has now personally seen three such cases. One of these women had an inguinal-femoral lymphadenectomy as primary treatment by the author. She had negative inguinal nodes but one positive femoral node, and remains alive and well at 24 months. The other two patients were treated by other surgeons with inguinal lymphadenectomy only, and in spite of negative inguinal nodes, experienced recurrence within 12 months in a femoral node. Both died of disseminated disease over the groin, thigh, and lower abdomen.

From the inguinal-femoral nodes, spread occurs to the pelvic nodes, particularly the external iliac group. Although direct lymphatic pathways have been described from the clitoris and Bartholin's gland to the pelvic nodes, these channels seem to be of minimal clinical significance.[24-26]

The overall incidence of lymph node metastases in vulvar cancer is about 30% (Table 10–4). The

Table 10–4

Incidence of Lymph Node Metastases in Operable Vulvar Cancer

Author	No. of Cases	Positive Nodes	Percentage
Rutledge et al., 1970[27]	110	40	36.4
Green et al., 1978[28]	142	54	38.0
Krupp and Bohm, 1978[29]	195	40	20.5
Benedet et al., 1979[30]	120	34	28.3
Curry et al., 1980[24]	191	57	29.8
Iversen et al., 1980[31]	268	86	32.1
Hacker et al., 1983[32]	113	31	27.4
Podratz et al., 1983[33]	175	59	33.7
Monaghan and Hammond, 1984[34]	134	37	27.6
Totals	**1448**	**438**	**30.2**

From Hacker NF: Vulvar cancer. In Berek JS, Hacker NF (eds.): Practical Gynecologic Oncology. © 1989, the Williams & Wilkins Co., Baltimore.

incidence correlates well with the old FIGO stage, being approximately 10% for Stage I lesions, 26% for Stage II, 65% for Stage III, and 90% for Stage IV.[35] For Stage I lesions, the incidence also correlates well with depth of stromal invasion, as shown in Table 10–5. Pelvic node metastases occur in about 5% of patients,[41] and virtually never occur in the absence of clinically suspicious (N2) groin nodes and three or more positive groin nodes.[24, 32, 33]

Treatment

Early attempts at the surgical management of invasive vulvar cancer yielded 5-year survivals of about 20–25% because of inadequate dissection of both the primary tumor and the regional lymph nodes.[1, 2] However, the excellent results achieved with an en bloc dissection by Taussig[4] and by Way[5] established en bloc radical vulvectomy, bilateral groin dissection, and bilateral pelvic node dissection as the treatment of choice for all patients with operable vulvar cancer.

Although the survival improved markedly with a more aggressive surgical approach, postoperative morbidity was high, with most patients experiencing breakdown of the groin and vulvar dissections, difficulty with approximation of tissue over the pubic symphysis, infection of the wounds and surrounding soft tissues, and prolonged hospitalization. In addition, the psychologic sequelae of radical vulvectomy were often devastating for the patient.[42]

Over the past decade, a number of significant advances have occurred in the management of squamous cell vulvar cancer. These include the following:

1. Vulvar conservation for patients with unifocal lesions and an otherwise normal vulva[40, 43–45]
2. Elimination of routine pelvic lymphadenectomy[24, 32, 46]
3. Omission of groin dissection for patients with T1 tumors and less than 1 mm of stromal invasion[40, 43]
4. Omission of the contralateral groin dissection in patients with lateral lesions and negative ipsilateral nodes[40, 47, 69]
5. The use of separate incisions for the groin dissections[48, 49]
6. Use of preoperative radiation therapy to obviate the need for exenteration in patients with advanced disease[50, 51]
7. Use of postoperative radiation to decrease the incidence of groin recurrence in patients with multiple positive groin nodes[52]

Hence, modern treatment for vulvar cancer must be individualized. There is no longer a standard operation appropriate for all cases. Optimal management requires careful consideration of the most appropriate surgical procedure for both the vulva and the groin, and the appropriate integration of surgery and radiation therapy. With careful patient selection, a more conservative surgical approach can be offered without compromising survival.

Management of Early Vulvar Cancer (T1, N0–1)

There is no "standard" operation applicable to every patient with early vulvar cancer. Treatment must be individualized, and it is necessary to determine independently the most appropriate operation for the following:

1. The primary lesion
2. The groin lymph nodes

Prior to any treatment, all patients should have colposcopy of the cervix, vagina, and the vulva, because preinvasive (and occasionally invasive) lesions may be present at other sites in the lower genital tract and will need appropriate management.

Management of the Primary Lesion

The trend is towards a more conservative resection of the primary lesion,[40, 43, 44, 53] sparing as much of the vulva as possible. The depth of invasion is of no clinical significance in determining the management of the primary tumor, because all resections should be to the level of the inferior fascia of the urogenital diaphragm. The two factors that must be taken in account are as follows:

1. The condition of the remainder of the vulva
2. The age of the patient

If the remainder of the vulva is healthy, radical local excision is the appropriate treatment regardless of the patient's age. Whether a radical vulvectomy or a radical local excision is performed, both the lateral and deep margins adjacent to the tumor will be the same. There has been some uncertainty regarding the radicality required to prevent local recurrence,

Table 10–5

Incidence of Lymph Node Metastases in Relation to Depth of Invasion in Stage I Vulvar Cancer

Depth of Invasion	Number	Positive Nodes	Percentage
≤1 mm	120	0	0.0
1.1–2.0 mm	121	8	6.6
2.1–3.0 mm	97	8	8.2
3.1–4.0 mm	50	11	22.0
4.1–5.0 mm	40	10	25.0
>5.0 mm	32	12	37.5
Totals	**460**	**49**	**10.7**

From Hacker NF: Vulvar cancer. In Berek JS, Hacker NF (eds.): Practical Gynecologic Oncology. © 1989, the Williams & Wilkins Co., Baltimore.

Table 10-6

Treatment of the Primary Tumor vs. Local Invasive Recurrence for T1 Vulvar Cancer

	Number	Recurrence	Percentage
Radical local excision	74	5	6.7
Radical vulvectomy	223	18	8.1

Data from refs. 22, 40, 43–45, 55.

but a recent clinicopathologic review of the UCLA data by Heaps, Fu, and colleagues has indicated that lateral and deep margins should clear the tumor by at least 1 cm.[54]

An analysis of the available literature indicates that for patients with T1 tumors, the incidence of local invasive recurrence following radical local excision is not higher than that following radical vulvectomy (Table 10–6). In addition, local vulvar recurrence can usually be successfully treated by further resection, with or without the addition of radiation therapy.

If the vulvar cancer arises in the presence of widespread VIN or dystrophy, treatment will be influenced by the patient's age. In elderly women, radical vulvectomy will usually be the best approach, although this will need adequate discussion with the patient. Most elderly women have had many years of chronic vulvar itching; the vulva is quite sore and excoriated, and they are only too pleased to have it removed. In a younger woman, it will usually be desirable to treat the primary tumor with radical local excision, and then treat the remainder of the vulva in the most appropriate manner. For example, vulvar dystrophy will require topical steroid therapy, whereas VIN may require superficial local excision with primary closure, or laser therapy. It is unwise to perform laser therapy on VIN III lesions, because some of these will have areas of occult invasion.

Clitoral lesions in younger patients present a unique problem. Resection of the clitoris will have major psychosexual sequelae, and wide dissection of this area will interrupt the lymphatic channels passing forward in the labia. This will often cause marked edema of the posterior vulva, which may ultimately require completion vulvectomy for relief.

The only cosmetically acceptable option for treating clitoral lesions in young patients is to use radiation therapy. Small vulvar lesions will respond well to about 5000 cGy of external radiation, and biopsy can be performed following therapy to confirm the absence of residual disease. The treatment may be combined with the radiation sensitizer 5-fluorouracil (1000 mg/m^2 by continuous intravenous infusion for 4 days at the beginning and end of treatment). In either case, the treatment will induce quite a brisk desquamative vulvitis, and it may need to be interrupted for a week or two. The reaction will settle within a few weeks of stopping therapy.

Technique for Radical Local Excision

A number of terms have been used to describe this procedure, including wide local excision,[44] modified radical vulvectomy,[56] and radical wide excision.[45] The term *radical local excision* is preferred, because the adjective "radical" implies both a wide and a deep dissection of the local (primary) lesion.

For lateral lesions, an ellipse of skin is removed to allow closure of the defect. In general, the lateral incision will be in the labiocrural fold, whereas the medial incision will be at the introitus, provided that clearance of at least 1 cm is obtained on all sides of the tumor. If margins are closer than this, the incisions should be extended up the vagina or out onto the thigh. The deep plane of dissection is at the level of the inferior fascia of the urogenital diaphragm, which is coplanar with the fascia over the pubic symphysis, and the fascia lata.

For perineal lesions, proximity to the anus may compromise the posterior margin. If the tumor is within 5 mm of the anal resection margin, it will be preferable to use preoperative or postoperative radiation. Conservative surgery for a small posterior vulvar carcinoma is shown in Figures 10–4 and 10–5.

If there is a large defect in the perineum following the resection, rhomboid flaps may be mobilized to close the defect. These are described later.

Management of the Groin Lymph Nodes

Groin dissection is associated with postoperative wound infection and breakdown, and chronic leg edema.[27] The use of separate groin incisions has significantly reduced the risk of wound breakdown,

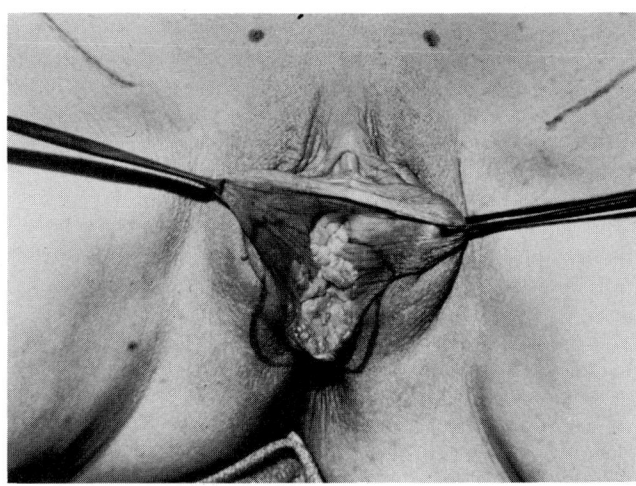

Figure 10–4
Small (T1) posterior vulvar carcinoma.

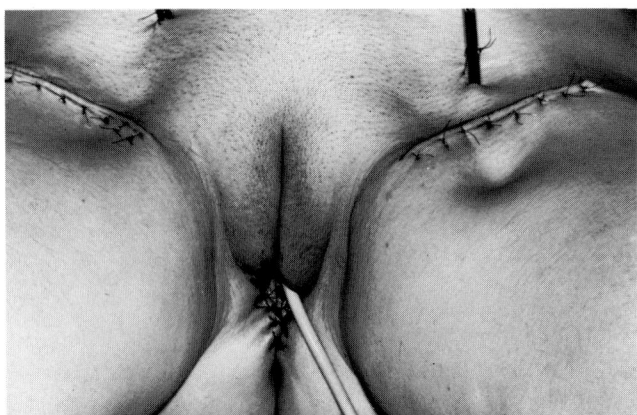

Figure 10–5
Resection of lesion shown in Figure 10–4.

because closure is no longer under tension.[49] However, chronic leg edema remains a major problem.

The initial reports on early vulvar cancer suggested that it was reasonable to omit the groin dissection in most patients with Stage I disease, provided that the depth of stromal invasion was less than 5 mm.[22, 57] However, as an increasing number of reports appeared in the literature, two points became clear:

1. The only patients without risk of lymph node metastases were those whose tumors invaded the stroma to less than 1 mm (see Table 10–5).
2. Patients who developed recurrent disease in an undissected groin had a very high mortality (Table 10–7).

Hence, it became clear that appropriate groin dissection was the single most important factor in decreasing mortality from early vulvar cancer.

In 1984, the International Society for the Study of Vulvar Disease (ISSVD) made the following statements:[58]

1. The current definition of microinvasion is misleading and dangerous, and should be dropped.
2. The term *Stage Ia carcinoma of the vulva* should be adopted for a single lesion, which is
   a. 2 cm or less in diameter, with
   b. 1 mm or less of stromal invasion

Patients with more than one site of invasion are not included in this definition. Although an occasional patient with less than 1 mm of stromal invasion has had documented groin metastases,[59] the incidence is so low that it is of no practical significance.

Measurement of Depth of Invasion

A commonly used method for determining depth of invasion is that originally proposed by Wilkinson, which measures the distance from the most superficial dermal papilla adjacent to the tumor, to the deepest focus of invasion.[38] This method of measurement is also the recommendation of the Nomenclature Committee of the International Society of Gynecological Pathologists. Other investigators have measured from the surface of the epithelium (tumor thickness),[36, 60–62] the deepest rete pegs,[55] or the base of the epithelium.[22, 63] Fu and Reagan estimate that the average difference between tumor thickness and depth of invasion as determined by the Wilkinson method is only 0.3 mm.[64]

Evaluation of the Risk of Lymph Node Metastases

A wedge biopsy specimen should be taken from the primary tumor under local anesthesia, and depth of invasion determined. If depth is less than 1 mm, the entire lesion should be locally excised and analyzed histologically to allow a more accurate determination of the depth of invasion. If there is still no invasive focus greater than 1 mm, groin dissection may be omitted. In frail, elderly patients, it may be reasonable to omit groin dissection in patients with up to 3 mm invasion, provided that the tumor is not poorly differentiated, the tumor does not have a "spray" pattern of infiltration, and there is no vascular space invasion.[21, 65]

From the accumulated experience now available in the literature, it is clear that for T1 tumors, it is not necessary to perform bilateral groin dissection if the lesion is unilateral and involves the labium majus, because the risk of positive contralateral nodes in the absence of positive ipsilateral nodes is less than 1% in such cases.[35] Midline lesions require bilateral dissections.

Primary Groin Irradiation

Groin irradiation has been considered a possible alternative to groin dissection for patients with N0 or N1 lymph nodes.[66] However, the Gynecologic Oncology Group (GOG) has concluded a study in which patients with N0 and N1 groin nodes were

Table 10–7

Death from Recurrence in an Undissected Groin

Author	Recurrence	Death from Disease
Rutledge et al., 1970[27]	4	3
Magrina et al., 1979[36]	4	3
Hoffman et al., 1983[39]	4	4
Hacker et al., 1984[40]	3	3
Monaghan and Hammond, 1984[34]	4	4
Totals	**19**	**17 (89%)**

From Hacker NF: Vulvar cancer. In Berek JS, Hacker NF (eds.): Practical Gynecologic Oncology. © 1989, the Williams & Wilkins Co., Baltimore.

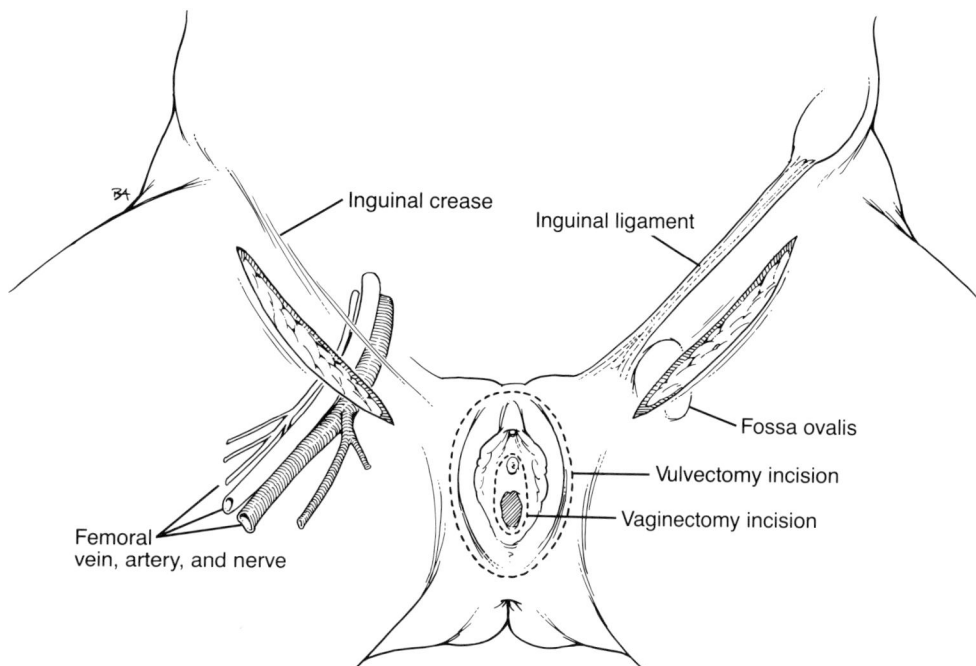

Figure 10–6
Skin incision for groin dissection through separate incisions. A line is drawn 1 cm below and parallel to the groin crease, and a narrow elipse of skin is removed.

randomized between groin dissection and groin irradiation. Patients in the surgical arm of the study with positive nodes were given postoperative irradiation. The study was closed prematurely because of the high incidence of groin recurrence in the group receiving irradiation.[66a]

Technique for Groin Dissection

The inguinal lymph nodes lie between the superficial fascia and the fascia lata over the femoral triangle and inguinal ligament. To remove them, an ellipse of skin is removed 1 cm below and parallel to the groin crease (Fig. 10–6). The incision should extend from the lateral border of the adductor longus muscle medially to the medial border of the sartorius muscle laterally. After removing the skin, the incision is carried down through the subcutaneous tissue to the superficial (Camper's) fascia. The latter is incised, then grasped with artery forceps to place it on traction (Fig. 10–7). Skin flaps are developed superiorly and inferiorly, care being taken to preserve all subcutaneous tissue above the superficial fascia. This is the most important step in avoiding skin necrosis.

This dissection removes all the fatty tissue over the femoral triangle, and is carried 2 cm above the inguinal ligament to ensure removal of all inguinal lymph nodes. The saphenous vein is tied off at the apex of the femoral triangle and at its point of entry into the femoral vein. The fascia lata over the lateral half of the femoral triangle is not removed, because there are no lymph nodes beneath it, and retention of the fascia lata helps decrease femoral nerve injury (Fig. 10–8).

The fascia lata over the femoral vessels is split longitudinally, and the fatty tissue containing the femoral lymph nodes is removed from around these vessels. All lymph node bearing tissue is medial to the femoral vein, and there are usually only two or three femoral nodes present. Transposition of the sartorius muscle, by detaching it from the anterior-superior iliac spine and suturing it to the medial border of the inguinal ligament and adductor longus fascia to protect the femoral vessels, was popularized by Way.[5] However, with prophylactic antibiotics and less radical removal of groin skin, wound breakdown is much less common, and many surgeons no longer perform this procedure.

A suction drain is placed in the groin, and the

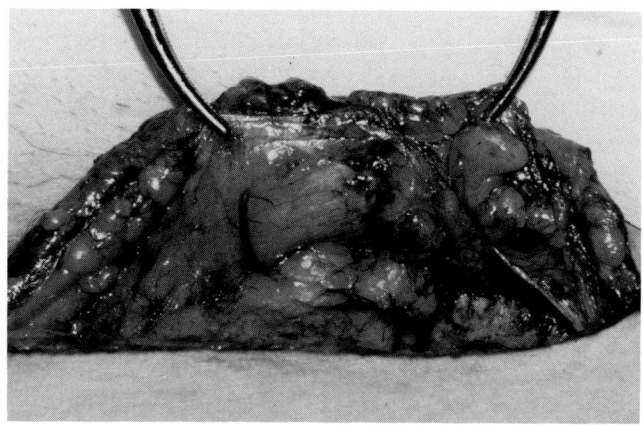

Figure 10–7
Elevation of superior groin skin flap. Traction is placed on the superficial (Camper's) fascia, and all subcutaneous fat above the fascia is preserved.

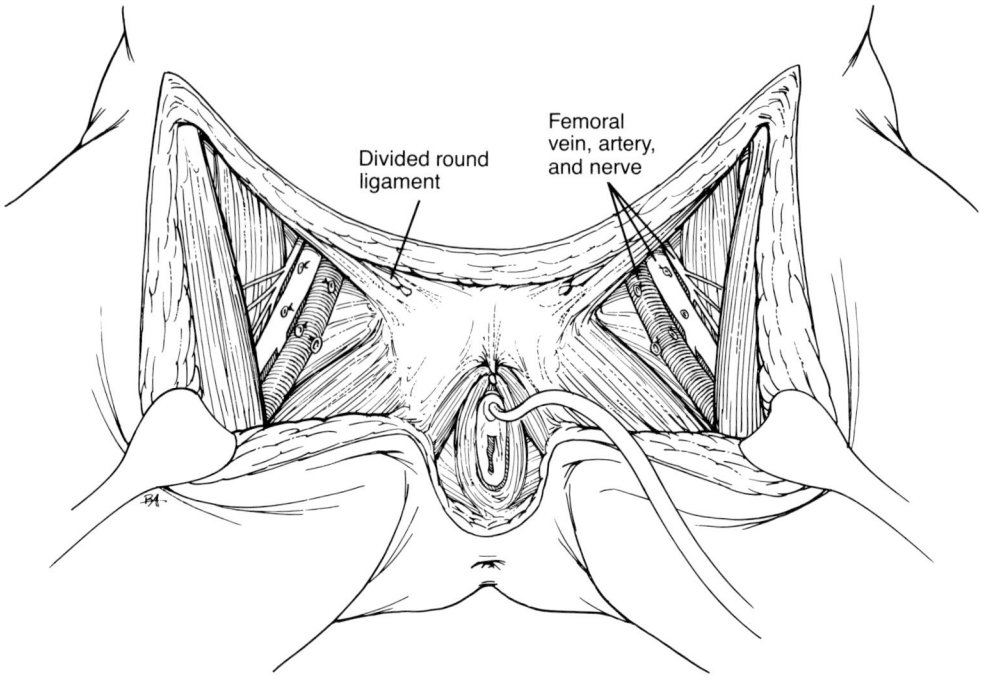

Figure 10–8
Femoral triangle after dissection of inguinal and femoral lymph nodes.

wound is closed in two layers. Postoperatively, the patient is kept at bed rest for 3–5 days, and minidose heparin or pneumatic calf compressors, together with active leg exercises, are used to prevent venous stasis.

Management of a Patient with Positive Groin Nodes

Pelvic lymphadenectomy was once considered standard treatment for all patients.[5, 29, 67] In the 1970s, several authors suggested that it could be omitted in patients with negative groin nodes,[27, 47, 68, 69] but should be performed on all patients with positive groin nodes.

In the 1980s, several papers have allowed a more rational approach to the patient with positive groin nodes. In 1980, Curry and colleagues from the M.D. Anderson Hospital reported on 52 patients with three or less unilaterally positive groin nodes; none had positive pelvic nodes, although 2 patients (8%) subsequently developed pelvic recurrences.[24] In 1983, Hacker and colleagues from UCLA reviewed 113 patients with invasive vulvar cancer and reported that all patients who had positive pelvic nodes, or developed a pelvic recurrence, had the following:

1. Three or more unilaterally positive groin nodes
2. Palpably suspicious (N2) groin nodes preoperatively[32]

All positive pelvic nodes were located on the same side as the multiple positive groin nodes. A similar experience was subsequently reported from the University of Michigan.[46] In the UCLA series, the 5-year survival for 16 patients with one positive node was 94%. Of 9 patients with three or more unilaterally positive groin nodes, 3 (33%) had recurrence in the groin, 4 (44%) had recurrence in the pelvis, and 6 (66%) experienced recurrence systemically.

In 1986, Homesley and colleagues reported the results of a phase III Gynecologic Oncology Group (GOG) Study, which randomized patients with one or more positive groin nodes between ipsilateral pelvic node dissection and bilateral groin and pelvic radiation.[52] Radiation therapy consisted of 4500–5000 cGy to the midplane of the pelvis at a rate of 180–200 cGy/day. There was a significant survival advantage at 2 years (68% vs. 54%; $P = .03$) for the group receiving radiation. The survival advantage was due to a significantly decreased incidence of groin recurrence in the irradiated group (5% vs. 23.6%; $P = .02$). There was no significant difference in the incidence of local, pelvic, or distant recurrence between the two groups. The significance was found only for patients with more than one positive groin node and clinically suspicious groin nodes preoperatively.

On the basis of the preceding studies, it would seem that patients with one microscopically positive groin node require no additional treatment.

Patients with two or more positive ipsilateral groin nodes, which is unusual with T1 tumors, are best treated with radiation therapy to the groin and pelvis. It is reasonable to observe the vulva carefully, without radical vulvectomy. If the patient has had bilateral groin dissection, it is tempting not to treat the contralateral groin or pelvis if these nodes are negative. However, if there is one or more large ipsilateral node completely replaced with tumor, retrograde lymphatic permeation can spread over a large distance, and the author has seen one such patient develop skin metastases in the contralateral lower abdomen and groin.

Management of Patients with T2 and Early T3 Tumors and N0 or N1 Nodes

In general, patients with T2 and early T3 tumors are treated with radical vulvectomy and bilateral inguinal-femoral lymphadenectomy. Two basic surgical approaches can be used:

1. The en bloc approach, using a trapezoid or butterfly incision.[68, 70]
2. The separate incision approach, using three separate incisions—one for the radical vulvectomy, and one for each groin dissection.[48, 49]

Technique for En Bloc Radical Vulvectomy and Groin Dissection

The operation can be performed with the patient in a low lithotomy position so that groin and vulvar dissection can proceed simultaneously, if appropriate. The original technique described by Stanley Way (Fig. 10–9) removed a large amount of skin and subcutaneous tissue over the mons pubis and femoral triangles, and closure was always under tension, if achievable at all.[5] Hence, delayed healing by granulation of open wounds was usual, and prolonged hospitalization was to be expected.

Most surgeons who perform an en bloc dissection have modified the incision to minimize the amount of skin resected, thereby improving primary healing (Fig. 10–10).

The groin dissection is accomplished initially, and this is best performed using a two-team approach to save operating time. The dissection is carried down to the aponeurosis of the external oblique and anterior rectus fascia, about 2 cm above the inguinal ligament. A skin flap is raised over the femoral triangle to allow dissection of the femoral triangle. To avoid skin necrosis, this flap should include all subcutaneous fat to the level of the superficial (Camper's) fascia. The technique for groin dissection has been described earlier (see Fig. 10–8).

The vulvar incision is carried posteriorly along each labiocrural fold, or within a 1–2 cm margin of the primary lesion. Posteriorly, the dissection may come across the perineum, if this gives adequate tumor clearance, or may extend in a V-shaped fashion onto each buttock if necessary. The incision extends down to the periosteum over the pubic symphysis, the fascia lata, and the inferior fascia of the urogenital diaphragm, and removes the bulbocavernosus, ischiocavernosus, and superficial transverse perineal muscles. Because of the vascularity, it is desirable to perform most of the dissection with the diathermy after the initial skin incision. In addition, the vessels supplying the clitoris should be clamped and tied, as should the internal pudendal vessels, which emerge from Alcock's canal at the 4 and 8 o'clock positions.

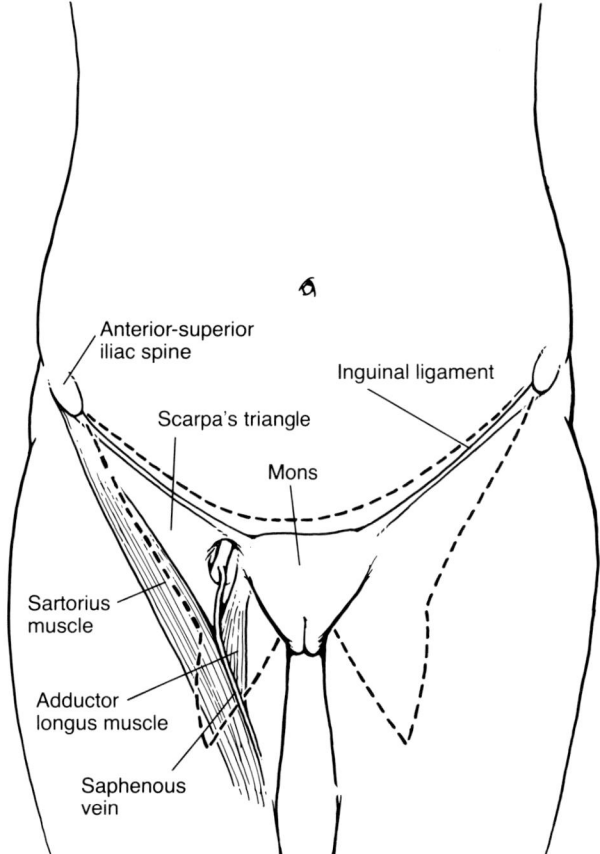

Figure 10–9
Stanley Way's incision for radical vulvectomy and bilateral groin dissection.

The vaginal incision normally circumscribes the introitus just outside the hymen. However, the distal third of the urethra or some distal vagina may need to be excised in order to achieve surgical clearance of at least 1 cm. If the tumor is close to the urethra or vagina, dissection around the tumor is greatly facilitated by transecting the vulva, thereby facilitating adequate exposure of the involved area.

Closure of the vulvar incision can usually be accomplished without tension, but if necessary, the thigh skin flaps and vaginal wall can be undermined to facilitate closure (Fig. 10–11). If distal urethra has been resected, a Silastic Foley catheter should be left in place for about 14 days to allow granulation and epithelialization of the tract. Large suction drains are placed in both parts of the groin prior to closure of the groin skin.

184 SURGERY FOR MALIGNANT TUMORS OF THE VULVA

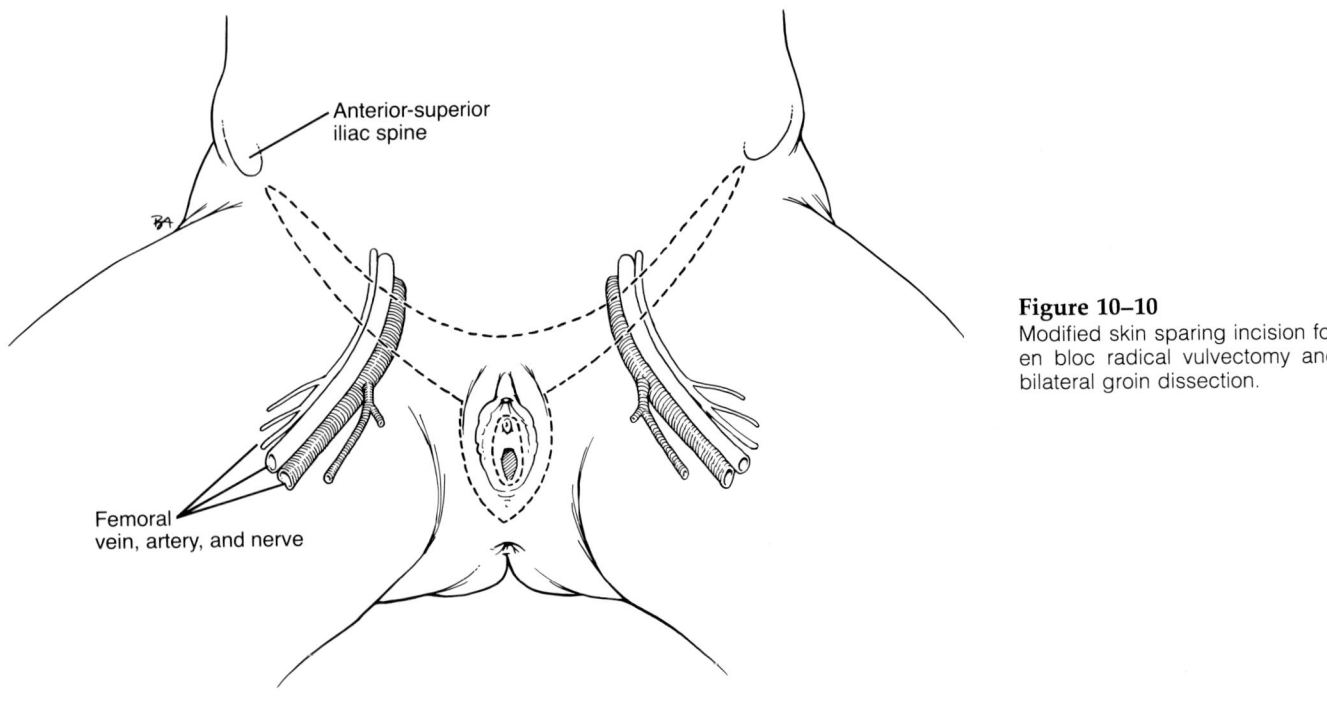

Figure 10–10
Modified skin sparing incision for en bloc radical vulvectomy and bilateral groin dissection.

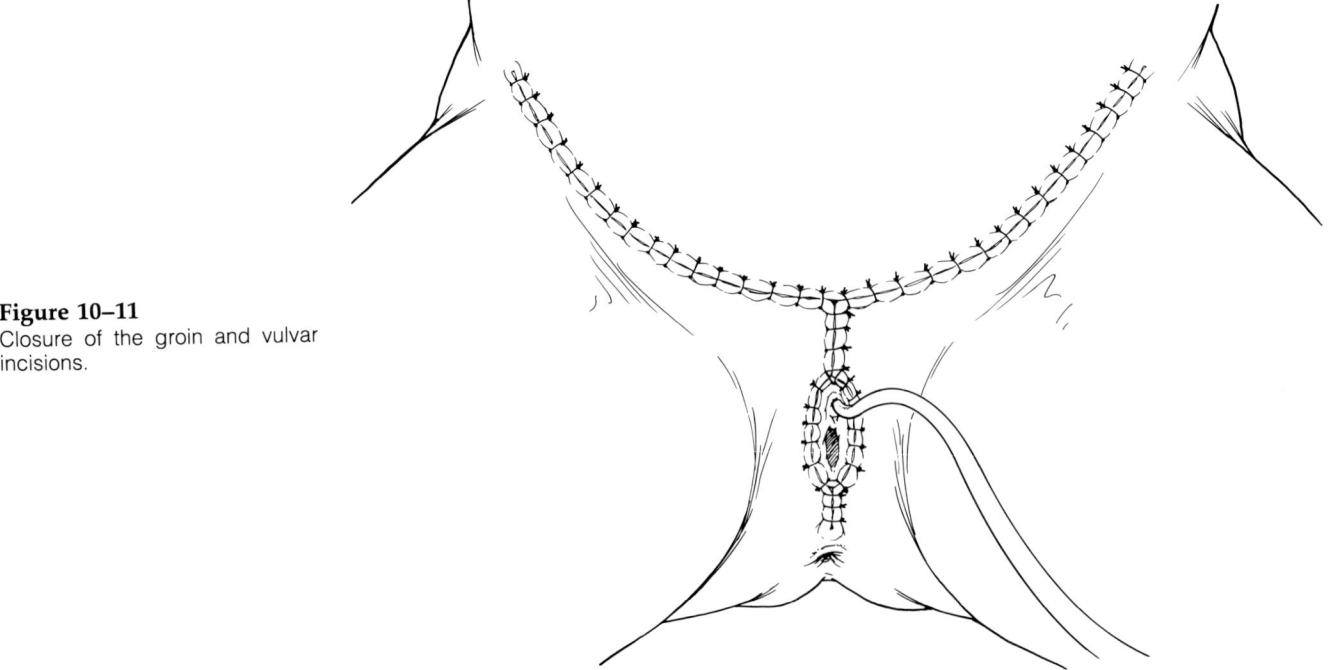

Figure 10–11
Closure of the groin and vulvar incisions.

Radical Vulvectomy and Groin Dissection Through Separate Incisions

The three-incision approach was initially described by Byron and associates in 1962[48] and has gained increasing popularity because of the improved rate of primary healing and decreased hospital stay. Byron worked at the City of Hope Hospital, which was part of the UCLA complex of hospitals. Therefore, this technique has been widely, though not exclusively, used by surgeons at UCLA since the early 1960s. In 1981, Hacker and colleagues reported the experience of the first 100 patients treated at UCLA and City of Hope Medical Centers by this technique.[49] Patients with Stages I, II, and III disease were treated in this manner, and survival was comparable for each stage with that achieved by the en bloc approach. Major wound breakdown occurred in only 14% of cases. Two patients developed a recurrence in the skin bridges, but both had clinically suspicious (N2) nodes, and multiple positive nodes histologically. These patients would now be offered postoperative radiation.

Technique. The groin dissection has been described earlier. The radical vulvectomy is also carried out in the manner previously described, except that the incision anteriorly is elliptical over the mons pubis to allow closure without distortion or tension.

Vulvar Conservation for T2 and Early T3 Tumors

In recent years, the indications for vulvar conservation have been extended to T2 and early T3 tumors by some surgeons, and although it is too early to determine whether or not this approach increases the rate of local invasive recurrence, preliminary results are promising.

Burrell and colleagues reported the use of a modified radical vulvectomy with bilateral inguinal-femoral lymphadenectomy in 14 patients with Stage II disease and in 3 patients with Stage III.[56] Five patients had postive nodes, but none developed recurrent disease.

Burke and colleagues at the M.D. Anderson Hospital reported on 32 patients with invasive squamous cell carcinoma of the vulva (depth of invasion > 1 mm) and clinically negative inguinal nodes, who underwent radical local excision for the primary tumor.[45] Seventeen patients had T1 tumors, and 15 had T2 tumors. Diameter of the tumors ranged from 5 to 65 mm (mean, 23 mm) and depth of invasion ranged from 1.5 to 13 mm (mean, 4.1 mm). With a mean postoperative follow-up of 36 months, only 2 patients (6%) developed a local invasive recurrence, and both were salvaged by additional resection.

The author has treated 6 patients with T2 tumors by radical local excision over the past 3 years, and no patient has experienced recurrence at the time of writing. In five cases, the clitoris, mons pubis, and anterior one-third of the labia were preserved.

Some validation for a more conservative vulvar resection has come from a clinicopathologic review of the UCLA experience by Heaps, Fu, and colleagues.[54] They reviewed 135 patients with invasive squamous cell carcinoma of the vulva treated between 1957 and 1985. Sixty-two patients had Stage I disease, 48 had Stage II, 18 had Stage III, and 7 had Stage IV. No patient with a histologically free margin greater than or equal to 8 mm developed a local recurrence, regardless of stage of disease. Forty-eight per cent of patients with margins less than 8 mm experienced recurrence locally. Allowing for about a 25% tissue shrinkage with fixation in formalin, this suggests that the risk of local recurrence is very low provided that the tumor-free surgical margin is at least 1 cm. Although stage of disease, depth of invasion, infiltrating growth pattern, and lymph-vascular space invasion were also significant risk factors for local recurrence on a univariate analysis, no combination of factors could improve on the significance of the tumor-free margin alone.

Management of Patients with TX, N2, or N3 Tumors

These patients differ from the previous group discussed in that they have a significant likelihood of having positive (frequently multiple positive) groin nodes. Prior to the GOG study showing the benefits of pelvic and groin irradiation for such patients, they would have been treated with en bloc radical vulvectomy, bilateral inguinal-femoral lymphadenectomy, and at least an ipsilateral pelvic lymphadenectomy. However, postoperative groin and pelvic radiation following full groin dissection often results in quite debilitating leg edema, and because radiation is quite capable of sterilizing microscopic metastases in lymph nodes, there seems to be little value to removing palpably normal nodes.

The author's present approach to patients with N2 or N3 groin nodes is as follows:

1. A preoperative CT scan is obtained of the pelvis, to determine whether or not there are any enlarged pelvic nodes.

2. All enlarged groin nodes are removed through a separate incision approach and sent for frozen section diagnosis. If metastatic disease is confirmed, full lymphadenectomy is not carried out.

3. Any enlarged pelvic nodes on CT scan are removed via an extraperitoneal approach, to be described.

4. Full pelvic and groin irradiation is given as soon as the groin incision(s) is healed.

5. If the frozen section reveals no metastatic disease in the removed nodes, full groin dissection is performed.

Technique for Extraperitoneal Pelvic Lymphadenectomy

If an extraperitoneal pelvic lymphadenectomy is required, the external oblique aponeurosis is opened 2 cm above the inguinal ligament, and the incision extended laterally and superiorly for about 10 cm. The incision is continued through the internal oblique and transversalis muscles, and the external iliac vessels are exposed by retracting the peritoneum medially. Sufficient exposure can be obtained to perform a complete pelvic lymphadenectomy, although it is preferable to remove enlarged nodes only and rely on postoperative radiation to destroy micrometastases. Following the lymphadenectomy, the abdominal wall muscles are closed in two layers.

Closure of Large Defects

Although it is usually possible to close the vulvar defect without tension, a large primary tumor will necessitate a more extensive dissection, and closure may be difficult. The following options have been advocated:

1. An area may be left open to granulate and epithelialize, which it will usually do over a period of 6–8 weeks.[10]

2. Full-thickness skin flaps may be devised.[71–73] An example is the rhomboid flap, which is particularly applicable to large posterior defects.

3. Unilateral or bilateral myocutaneous grafts may be developed, such as the gracilis, tensor fascia lata, or gluteus maximus. Because these grafts bring in a new blood supply to the area, they are particularly helpful if the vulva is poorly vascularized from prior surgery or radiation.

Technique for Rhomboid Flap

This technique has been well described by Barnhill and colleagues.[73] The medial incision should approximate the length of the perineal defect, whereas the lateral incision should be half the width of the defect. The incisions should be carried deeply into the subcutaneous tissues, then the flaps undermined to allow placement without tension.

Technique for Gracilis Myocutaneous Graft

This technique has been described by Ballon and colleagues.[75] The patient is placed in the "ski" position, and a line is drawn from the pubic tubercle to the medial femoral condyle. The superior incision is made about 1 cm below this line. The length and width of the graft to be taken are measured from the vulvar defect and are drawn on the medial thigh. The inferior incision is then made and carried down to the fascia lata, which is incised to isolate the gracilis muscle. The skin may be sutured to the edge of the fascia to prevent separation of the fat and skin from the muscle. The muscle is transected distally, and then it is mobilized, incising the fascia lata as the mobilization proceeds in a cephalad direction. The vascular pedicle, from the obturator artery, appears under the inferior border of the adductor longus muscle, about 6 cm below the pubic arch. Care must be taken to preserve this bundle as the entire graft is mobilized and rotated onto the vulva. If necessary, the muscle can be divided at its origin from the pubic arch to give more mobility. The thigh defect can be closed in two layers without undue tension (Fig. 10–12).

Technique for Tensor Fascia Lata Myocutaneous Graft

The procedure has been well described by Chafe and colleagues.[74] The vascular supply for the tensor fascia lata muscle comes from a terminal branch of the lateral circumflex femoral artery, and enters the muscle 6–8 cm below the anterior superior iliac spine. The length of the proposed flaps are judged by using a measuring tape held at the lateral thigh at the anatomic site of entry of the vascular pedicle, and measuring the distance to the perineum.

The anterior border of the flap is outlined by a line drawn from the anterior-superior iliac spine down to the lateral condyle of the tibia. The posterior border is a line from the greater trochanter of the hip, down to the knee. The distal border is about 5 cm above the knee. The width of the flap is dictated by the width of the defect.

After the vulva and groin have been dissected, the flap is raised from distal to proximal, in the plane below the fascia lata, that is, the plane above the vastus lateralis muscle, until the desired length has been obtained (Fig. 10–13). Damage to the vascular pedicle is avoided by staying deep to the fascia lata and identifying the pedicle at its point of entry into the tensor fascia lata. Once the flaps are raised, they are rotated and sutured into place. The donor site is then closed primarily. Occasionally, skin grafts may be necessary to cover the flap donor sites.

Technique for Gluteus Maximus Myocutaneous Graft

This has been well described by Achauer and by Knapstein.[76, 77] The gluteus maximus is supplied by

SURGERY FOR MALIGNANT TUMORS OF THE VULVA 187

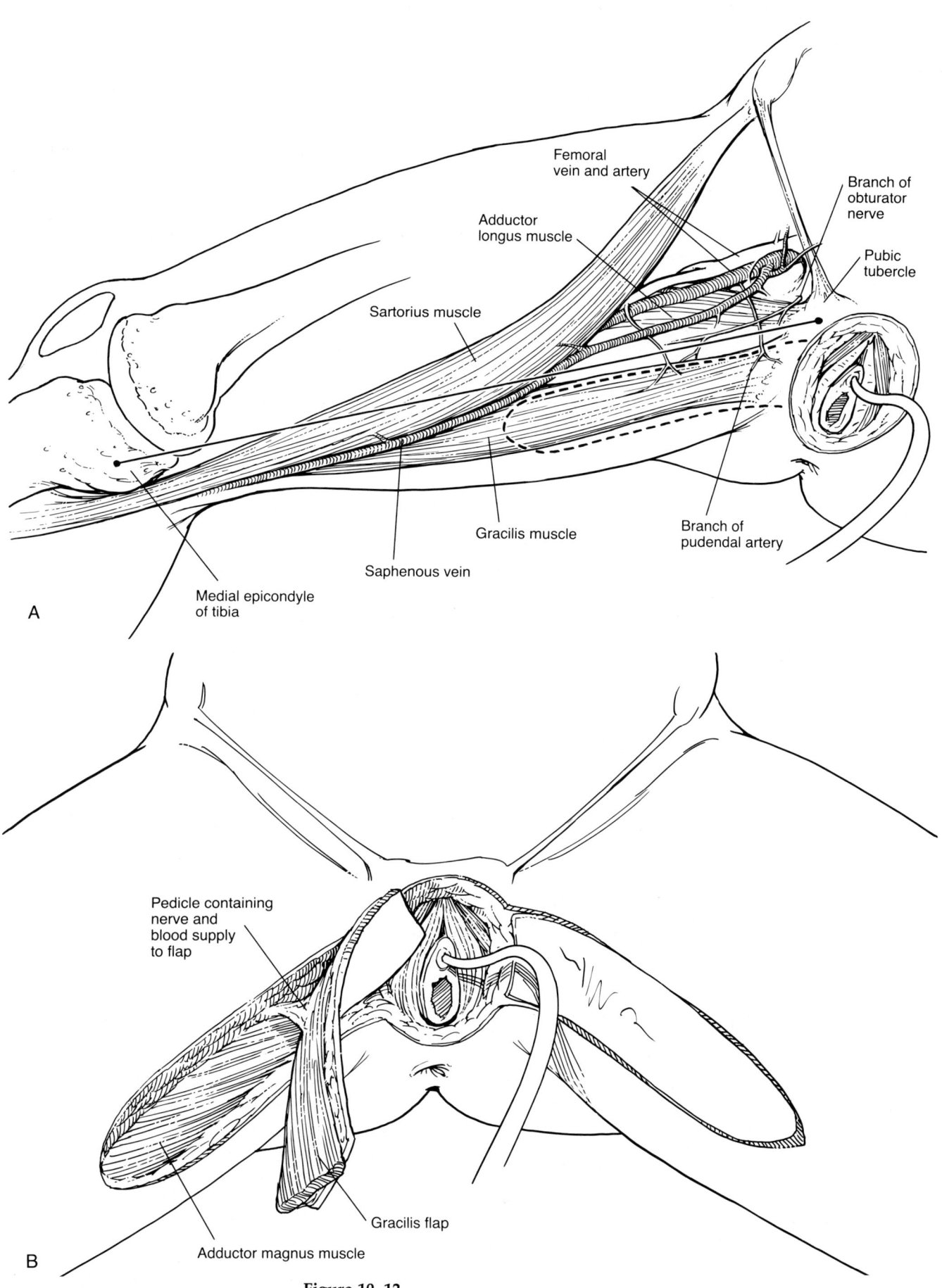

Figure 10–12
A to *C*, Technique for gracilis myocutaneous graft.

Illustration continued on following page

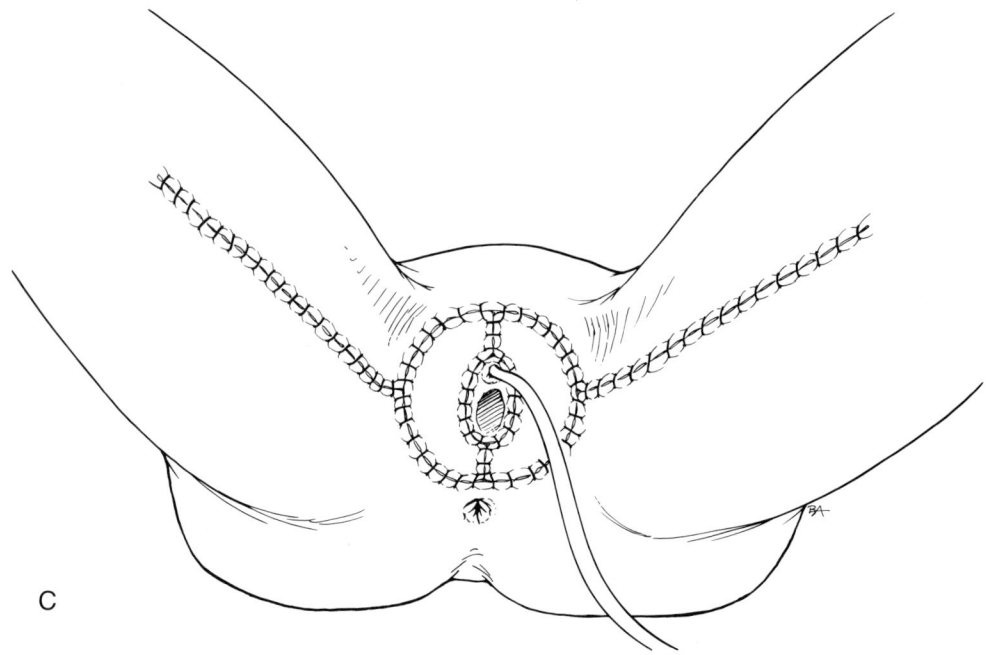

Figure 10–12 *Continued*

the inferior gluteal artery, the surface marking for which runs around the ischial tuberosity and passes towards the midpoint of the knee (Figure 10–14). It parallels the course of the posterior cutaneous nerve of the thigh, which lies deep to the fascia and the artery. The flap is centred around the neurovascular bundle. The width of the flap is determined by the defect to be covered, but should not exceed 12 cm. The flap is thick and reliable and can be extended to the mid-thigh. It is preferable to create an island flap and pass it through a subcutaneous tunnel to the vaginal area rather than use an incision connecting the two areas.

Postoperative Management

In spite of the advanced age of many patients with vulvar cancer, the surgery is usually remarkably well tolerated, and age alone should never be considered a contraindication to appropriate surgery. Bed rest is usually desirable for 3 or 4 days to immobilize the wounds and foster healing, but a low-residue diet can begin on the first postoperative day. Pneumatic calf compression or subcutaneous heparin should be given to help prevent deep venous thrombosis, and active, non–weight bearing leg movements should be encouraged. Support stockings help to decrease leg edema and venous stasis. Frequent wound dressings and perineal swabs are important. Suction drainage of each groin is continued for about 10 days to help decrease the risk of groin seromas. A Foley catheter is left in the bladder until the patient is walking around. Once the patient is fully ambulant, sitz baths or whirlpool therapy are helpful, followed by drying the perineum with a hair dryer.

Postoperative Complications

The major early complications are related to groin wound infection, necrosis, and breakdown. The latter has been reported in up to 85% of patients having an en bloc resection.[33] With the separate incision approach, major wound breakdown should be reduced to about 15% of cases.[49] Other early complications include urinary tract infection, seromas in the femoral triangle, deep venous thrombosis, pulmonary embolism, hemorrhage, and, rarely, osteitis pubis. Anesthesia of the anterior thigh from femoral nerve injury is common and usually resolves slowly. Seromas occur in 15–20% of cases and may require repeated sterile aspiration.

The major late complication is chronic leg edema, which has been reported in up to 69% of cases.[33] Recurrent lymphangitis or cellulitis of the leg occurs in about 10% of cases, as does urinary stress incontinence. Introital stenosis may cause dyspareunia and require surgical correction. A femoral hernia may occur if care is not taken to close the femoral canal by suturing the inguinal ligament to Cooper's ligament. Rare late complications include rectovaginal or rectoperineal fistulas and pubic osteomyelitis.

Advanced Disease

When the disease involves the anus, rectum, rectovaginal septum, or urethra, the standard radical

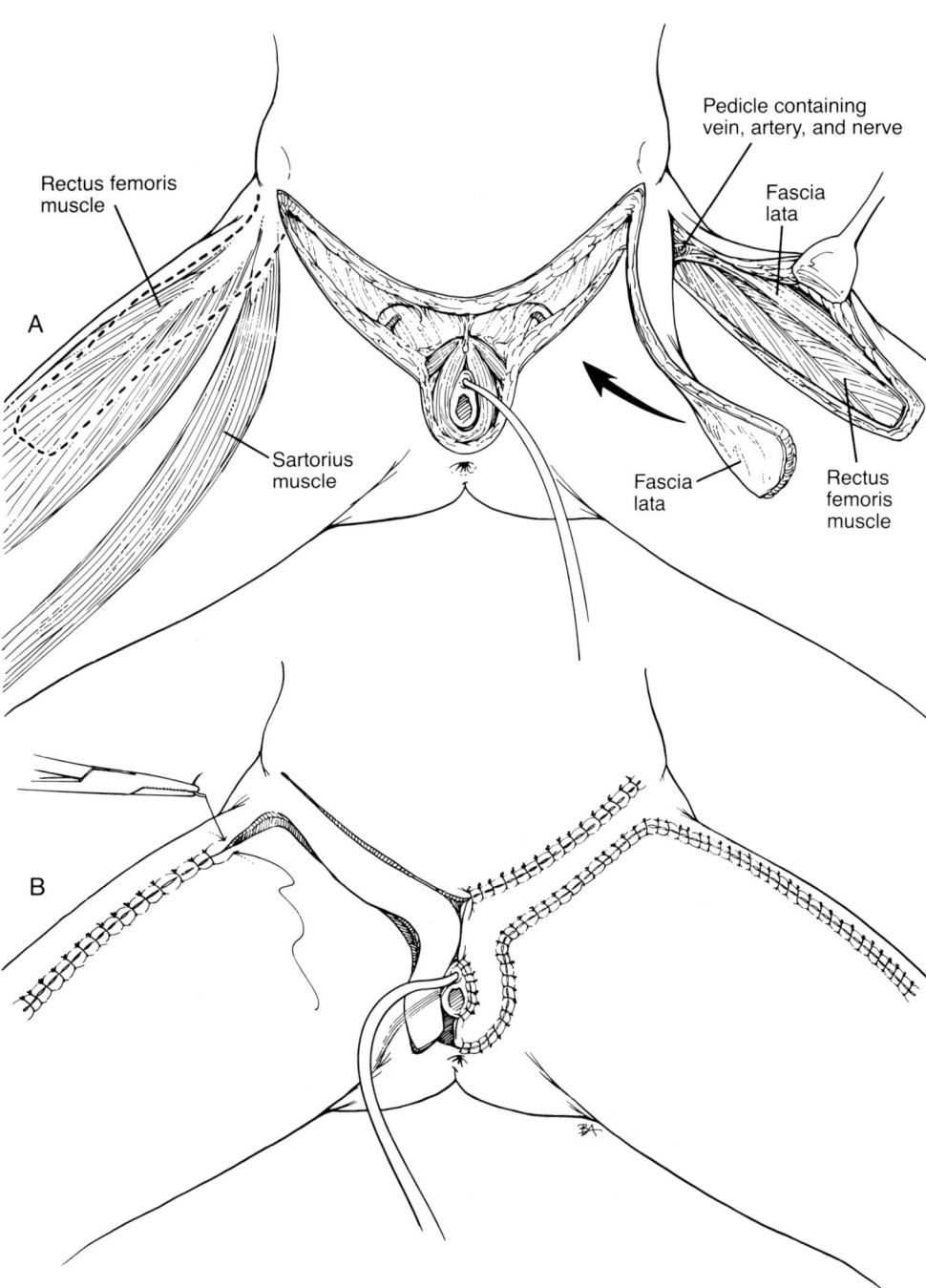

Figure 10–13
A and B, Technique for tensor fascia lata myocutaneous graft.

190 SURGERY FOR MALIGNANT TUMORS OF THE VULVA

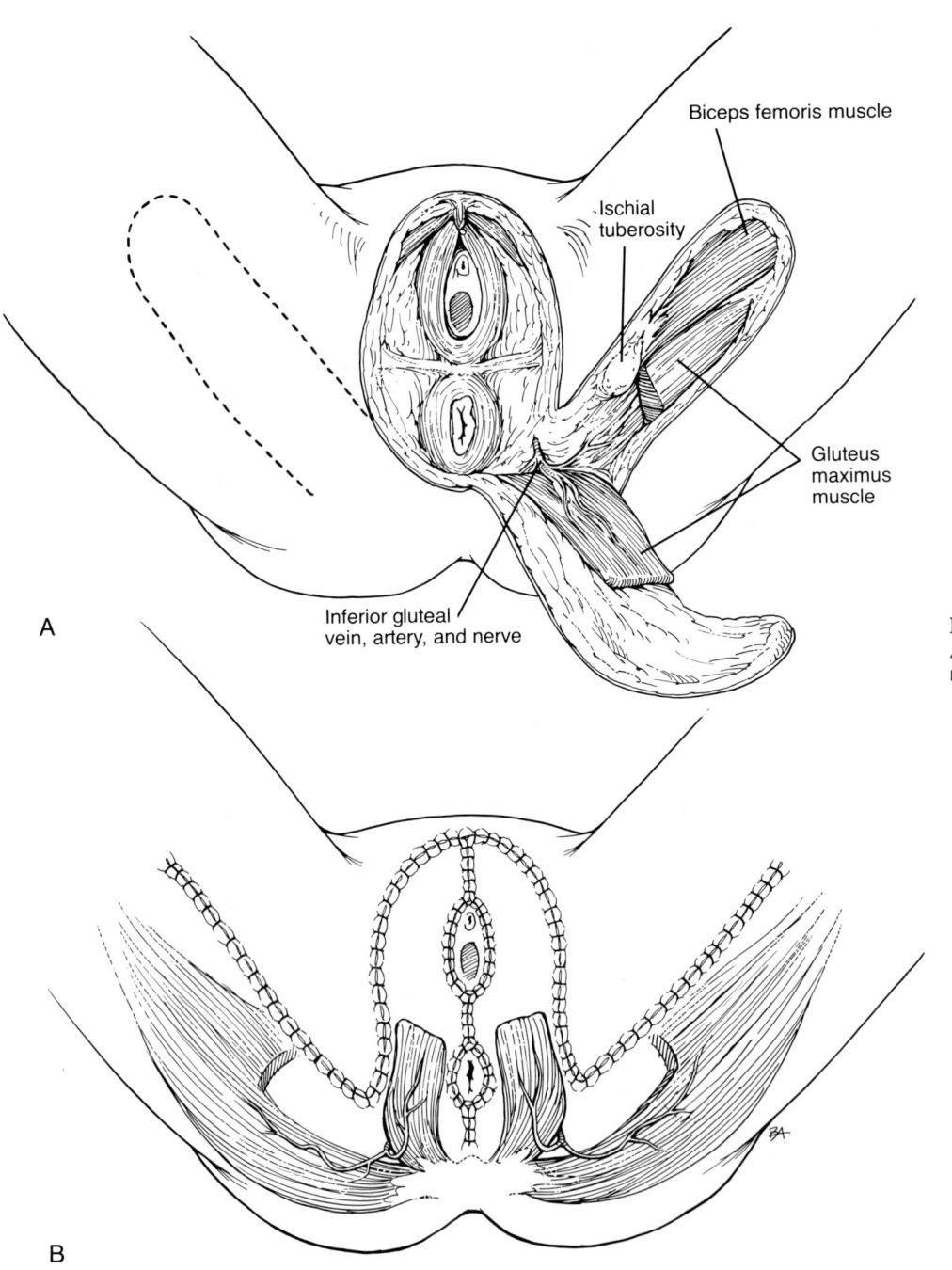

Figure 10–14
A and B, Technique for gluteus maximus myocutaneous graft.

vulvectomy will not encompass all of the disease. Early surgical attempts at extended radical vulvectomy, to encompass all gross disease, were associated with a high local failure rate;[67] therefore, pelvic exenteration, combined with radical vulvectomy and bilateral groin dissection, has become more popular in the last 30 years. Such radical surgery carries an operative mortality of about 10%, a high postoperative morbidity, and a high psychologic morbidity.[41, 78] Nevertheless, a 5-year survival of about 50% can be anticipated.[79–81]

When the tumor involves the anal canal and lower rectum, anoproctectomy is a simpler and less morbid procedure, which may be combined with radical vulvectomy and bilateral groin dissection.[82] The vulvectomy incision is extended around the anus and down to the level of the coccyx. Following the vulvectomy, the rectum is isolated by dissecting it from its surrounding fatty tissue, from the pubococcygeus muscles, and from the vagina. With traction on the surgical specimen, the rectum can be transected at the peritoneal reflection with a TA stapler, and the levator muscles approximated in the midline just distal to the rectal stump (Fig. 10–15). An end sigmoid colostomy can be performed, with the distal end of the sigmoid brought to the skin as a mucous fistula.

An alternative approach to these patients was first suggested by Boronow in 1973.[50] In his initial report, he recommended intracavitary radium, with or without external irradiation, to eliminate the internal genital disease, and subsequent surgery, usually radical vulvectomy and bilateral groin dissection, to treat the external genital disease.

In 1984, Hacker and colleagues reported the use of preoperative external irradiation for eight patients with advanced vulvar cancer.[51] Brachytherapy was reserved for patients with persistent disease that would otherwise necessitate exenteration. Rather than performing radical vulvectomy on all patients, these investigators resected only the tumor bed, on the assumption that any microscopic foci present in the vulva would have been sterilized by the radiation. Half of the patients had no residual disease in the specimen, and long-term morbidity was low with the predominant use of teletherapy. No patient developed a fistula. There were five long-term survivors, including two patients whose primary tumor was fixed to bone.

In 1987, Boronow and colleagues updated their experience with preoperative radiation for locally advanced vulvovaginal cancer.[83] They reported 37 primary cases and 11 cases of recurrent disease treated with preoperative radiation therapy. The 5-year survival for the primary cases was 75.6%, whereas a 62.6% survival was achieved for the recurrent cases. Seventeen of 40 vulvectomy specimens (42.5%) contained no identifiable residual disease. Eight patients (20%) developed a local recurrence, and 5 patients (12.5%) developed a fistula. However, only 2 of the 48 patients ultimately required exenterative surgery. As the experience of these investigators has evolved, their approach has been refined. They now recommend external radiation for all cases, with more selective use of intracavitary therapy. Also, the radicality of the surgery has been significantly modified. A more limited vulvar resection is now advocated. N0 nodes are not resected, and for patients with N2 and N3 nodes, the enlarged nodes are resected, but a formal groin dissection is not performed.

In 1989, Thomas and colleagues reported on the use of radiation with concurrent infusional 5-fluorouracil, with or without mitomycin-C, for 33 patients with vulvar cancer.[84] Median follow-up was 16 months. Of 9 patients receiving primary chemoradiation, 6 had an initial complete response in the vulva, but 3 of the 6 subsequently experienced relapse locally. This suggests that chemoradiation should always be combined with excision of the tumor bed.

In 1990, Rotmensch and associates reported a 45% 5-year survival for 13 patients with advanced vulvar cancer treated with a combined radiosurgical approach,[85] and it would seem that preoperative radiation, with or without concurrent chemotherapy, should be regarded as the treatment of first choice for patients with advanced vulvar cancer who would otherwise require some type of pelvic exenteration.

Recurrent Vulvar Cancer

Recurrence of vulvar cancer correlates most closely with the number of positive groin nodes.[32, 52] Patients

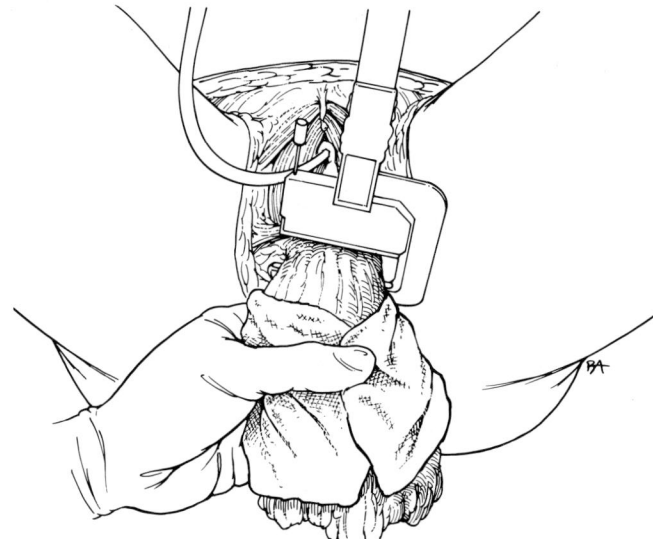

Figure 10–15
Radical vulvectomy combined with anoproctectomy.

with three or more positive nodes have a high incidence of local, regional, and systemic recurrence. Local recurrence correlates closely with surgical clearance, patients with surgical margins of 10 mm or greater having a very low likelihood of local recurrence.[54]

Local recurrences can usually be successfully treated by further wide surgical excision, which will probably necessitate the use of a myocutaneous graft to cover the defect. Alternately, radiation therapy, alone or in combination with surgery, may be successful.[83, 86] Prempree and Amornmarn (1984) reported successful treatment of 6 of 6 patients with recurrent vulvar cancer limited to the introitus and vagina with interstitial brachytherapy, with or without external beam therapy.[86]

Regional and distant metastases are difficult to manage.[87] Radiation and surgery may be used for groin recurrence,[86] whereas chemotherapy may be offered for distant metastases. Agents that have activity against squamous cell carcinomas include cisplatin, methotrexate, cyclophosphamide, bleomycin, and mitomycin-C. Response rates are low, and duration of response is usually disappointing.[87]

Prognosis

The overall prognosis for vulvar cancer is good, because the majority of patients now present with relatively early disease. The 5-year survival for operable cases is about 70% (Table 10–8). Patients with negative groin nodes have a 5-year survival of about 90%, but this falls to about 50% for patients with positive nodes.[35]

The number of positive groin nodes is the single most important prognostic variable.[32, 33, 46, 52] Patients with one microscopically positive node have a good prognosis regardless of the stage of disease,[32, 46, 52] whereas patients with three or more positive nodes have a poor prognosis.

Survival also correlates with the clinical status of the groin nodes. In the GOG Study, patients with

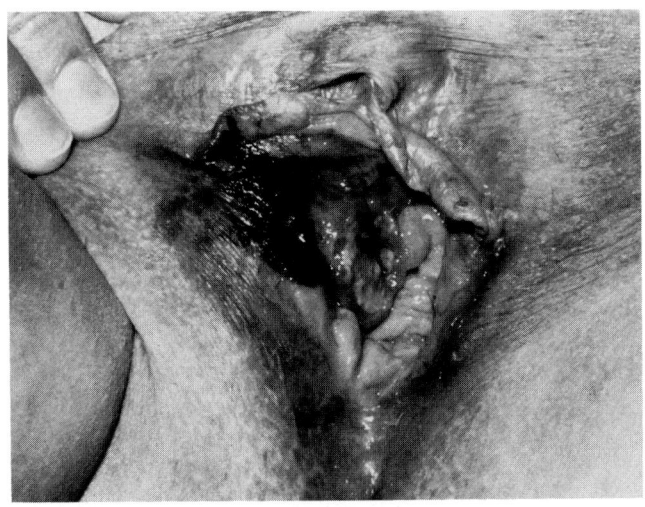

Figure 10–16
Melanoma of the vulva.

N0 or N1 nodes had a 2-year survival of 78%, compared with 52% for patients with N2 nodes and 33% for patients with N3 nodes ($P = .01$).[52] Survival for patients with positive pelvic nodes is about 15%.[41]

MELANOMA

In spite of their rarity, malignant melanomas are the second most common vulvar malignancy. They occur predominantly in white women between the ages of 50 and 80 years.[91, 92] Melanomas may arise de novo, or from a pre-existing junctional nevus, and occur mainly on the labia minora and clitoris (Fig. 10–16). The incidence of cutaneous melanomas worldwide is increasing significantly, but whether or not the incidence of vulvar melanomas conforms to this trend is unknown.[93] Morrow and DiSaia considered that the vulva may be predisposed to the development of melanomas, because it occupies only 2% of the body surface area but accounts for 3–5% of all melanomas.[94]

Most patients present because of a lump or tumor on the external genitalia, although complaints of itching, bleeding, or discharge are often volunteered.[92] Change in a pre-existing mole may also prompt some patients to seek attention.

For cutaneous melanomas, the emphasis now is on the recognition of persons with an increased risk of developing a melanoma by virtue of their family history or the presence of one or more precursor lesions. However, no single clinical feature or combination of clinical features is diagnostic of a dysplastic melanocytic nevus. In addition, the difficulty with adequately observing vulvar lesions will make it more desirable to excise pigmented lesions in this location, unless they have been present and unchanged for some years.[95]

Table 10–8

Five-Year Survival vs. Stage for Patients Treated with Curative Intent

FIGO Stage (1969)	Number	Dead of Disease	Corrected 5-Year Survival (%)
I	376	36	90.4
II	310	71	77.1
III	238	116	51.3
IV	111	91	18.0
Totals	1035	314	69.7

From Hacker NF: Vulvar cancer. In Berek JS, Hacker NF (eds.): Practical Gynecologic Oncology. © 1989, the Williams & Wilkins Co., Baltimore.

There are three basic histologic types. The most common is the superficial spreading melanoma, which tends to remain superficial in its early development but may penetrate more deeply if left untreated. The lentigo maligna melanoma is a flat freckle that tends to remain quite superficial, although it may become quite extensive. The most aggressive lesion is the nodular melanoma, which is a raised lesion that penetrates deeply and may metastasize widely. Amelanotic varieties may occasionally occur.

Staging

The FIGO system used for staging squamous cell carcinomas is not applicable for melanomas, because these lesions are usually much smaller and prognosis is mainly related to depth of penetration of the tumor.[92, 96, 97] The leveling system established by Clark and coworkers for cutaneous melanomas is less applicable for vulvar lesions because the papillary dermis is not well defined in vulvar skin.[98] Chung and colleagues proposed a modified system that retained Clark's definitions for Levels I and V but arbitrarily defined Levels II, III and IV using measurements in millimeters.[96] Breslow measured the thickest portion of the melanoma from the surface of the intact epithelium to the deepest point of invasion.[99] A comparison of these systems is shown in Table 10–9.

Treatment

The relatively recent identification of depth of invasion as the most important prognostic variable has allowed some individualization of treatment for vulvar melanomas. In addition, there has been a trend towards more conservative surgery for vulvar melanomas[93] in line with the trend towards more conservative surgery for cutaneous melanomas. Historically, margins of 5–15 cm have been advocated for cutaneous melanomas, but several studies have opposed this concept.[99–101] The World Health Organization's collaborative study reported on 281 patients with lesions with less than 2 mm of invasion. The local recurrence rate was only 1.8% and was not affected by margin sizes of 1–5 cm.[99]

Data are more limited for vulvar lesions. Rose and colleagues reported on 8 patients with a vulvar melanoma with less than 2 mm of invasion.[93] Radical local excision (with 2-cm margins) rather than radical vulvectomy produced a disease-free survival of 75%. Davidson and colleagues reported on 32 patients with vulvar melanoma treated with local excision (N = 14), simple vulvectomy (N = 7), or radical resection (N = 11). No group had a superior survival, but only one patient had a lesion with less than 0.75 mm of invasion, and the overall survival was only 25% at 5 years.[102]

There seems to be no justification for groin dissection in patients with less than 1 mm of invasion, because nodal metastases in such patients are rare.[96, 97] For more deeply penetrating lesions, the author still favors en bloc resection of the primary tumor and regional nodes, although radical vulvectomy will usually not be necessary. Podratz and colleagues reported recurrent groin disease in only 1 of 44 patients treated in this manner.[92] Although distant metastases may occur, local control remains important for quality of life. Because melanomas commonly involve the clitoris and labia minora, the vaginourethral resection margin is a common site of failure, and care must be taken to obtain an adequate "inner" resection margin.[103] Podratz demonstrated a 10-year survival of 61% for lateral lesions, compared with 37% for medial lesions ($P = 0.027$).[92]

Pelvic node metastases do not occur in the absence of groin node metastases.[103–105] Because the prognosis for patients with positive pelvic nodes is so poor, there seems to be no justification for pelvic lymphadenectomy.

Chemotherapy and immunotherapy for vulvar melanomas are disappointing, but estrogen receptors have been demonstrated in human melanomas,[106] and responses to tamoxifen have been reported.[107, 108]

Prognosis

Although the behavior of melanomas can be quite unpredictable, the overall prognosis is poor. The mean 5-year survival for reported cases of vulvar

Table 10–9

Microstaging of Vulvar Melanomas

	Clark's Levels[98]	Chung's[96]	Breslow's[99]
I	Intraepithelial	Intraepithelial	<0.76 mm
II	Into papillary dermis	≤1 mm from granular layer	0.76–1.50 mm
III	Filling dermal papillae	1–2 mm from granular layer	1.51–2.25 mm
IV	Into reticular dermis	>2 mm from granular layer	2.26–3.0 mm
V	Into subcutaneous fat	Into subcutaneous fat	>3 mm

melanoma is about 32%,[41] which is comparable with that for cutaneous melanomas. Patients with lesions invading up to 1 mm have an excellent prognosis. Chung and colleagues reported a corrected 5-year survival of 100% for patients with Level II lesions, 40% for Level III or IV lesions, and 20% for Level V lesions.[96] Tumor volume has been correlated with prognosis, patients whose lesions have a volume less than 100 mm^3 having an excellent prognosis.[105]

BARTHOLIN'S GLAND CARCINOMA

Primary carcinoma of Bartholin's gland accounts for about 5% of vulvar malignancies. About 280 cases have been reported in the literature.[25, 109] By definition, vulvar cancer should be considered a Bartholin's gland carcinoma if it fulfills Honan's criteria, which are as follows:

1. It is in the correct anatomic position.
2. It is located deep in the labium majus.
3. The overlying skin is intact.
4. There is some recognizable normal gland present.

Strict adherence to these criteria will underdiagnose some cases, because large lesions may ulcerate through the overlying skin and obliterate the residual gland. Although transition from normal to malignant glandular tissue is the most diagnostic criterion,[110] some cases will be appropriately diagnosed on the basis of their histology and anatomic location.

The duct of the gland is lined by stratified squamous epithelium, which gradually changes to transitional epithelium as the gland is approached. Hence, it is not surprising that several histologic variants have been reported. Adenocarcinomas and squamous cell carcinomas each constitute about 45% of cases, with the other 10% including such uncommon tumors as transitional cell carcinomas, undifferentiated carcinomas, adenosquamous carcinomas, sarcomas, and adenoid cystic carcinomas.[64]

Bartholin's gland carcinomas have been reported in patients as young as 18 years and as old as 91 years, but the mean age is about 52 years.[111] A history of inflammation of the gland may be obtained from about 10% of patients, and malignancies may be mistaken for benign cysts or abscesses. Physician and patient delay in diagnosis is common. Because the overlying skin will be intact until the tumor is advanced, biopsy of a mass in this area is often delayed because malignancy is not always suspected. The differential diagnosis of any pararectovaginal neoplasm should include cloacogenic carcinoma and secondary neoplasm.[109]

Treatment

Bartholin's gland carcinoma has traditionally been treated by radical vulvectomy, with bilateral groin and pelvic node dissection.[112] However, pelvic node metastases are rare in the absence of groin node metastases;[25] therefore, there seems to be no indication to manage the lymph nodes differently from squamous vulvar carcinomas.

Copeland and colleagues at the M.D. Anderson Hospital have questioned the need for radical vulvectomy on all patients.[109] Of a series of 36 patients, 12 had hemivulvectomy or wide excision, with or without radiation, as treatment for the primary lesion (Fig. 10–17). The local recurrence rate was 17% (2 of 12), which was comparable with the 21% local recurrence rate for the 24 patients treated with radical vulvectomy (5 of 24). Because these lesions may be deep in the vulva, extensive dissection is required in the ischiorectal fossa to obtain clear surgical margins. Postoperative vulvar radiation reduced the incidence of local recurrence in Copeland's series from 27% (6 of 22) to 7% (1 of 14). If the ipsilateral groin nodes are positive, bilateral groin and pelvic radiation may decrease regional recurrence.

If the tumor is fixed to the inferior pubic ramus or is involving adjacent structures, such as the anal sphincter or rectum, preoperative radiation should be used to try to avoid the need for exenterative surgery.

PAGET'S DISEASE OF THE VULVA

Extramammary Paget's disease of the vulva (adenocarcinoma in situ) was first described in 1901, 27

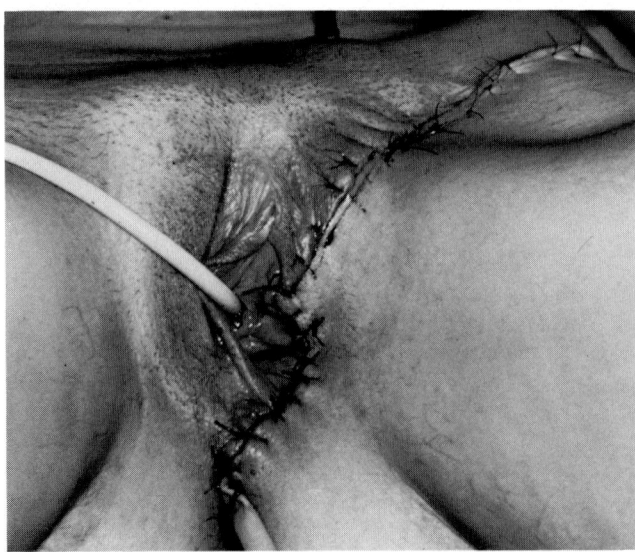

Figure 10–17
En bloc resection of left Bartholin's gland and left groin.

years after the initial report by Sir James Paget of the mammary lesion that now bears his name.[113] Unlike its counterpart in the breast, which is invariably associated with an underlying ductal carcinoma, only about 20% of patients with vulvar Paget's disease have an underlying adenocarcinoma. However, the lesion may be locally invasive, without a discrete underlying carcinoma, and the author has seen one such patient with 2 mm of stromal invasion and metastasis in an inguinal lymph gland.

Clinically, the disease predominantly affects postmenopausal white women. The presenting symptoms are usually pruritus and local soreness, and the lesion has an erythematous, scaly appearance. From the vulva, the disease may spread to the mons pubis, thighs, vagina, and buttocks, while extension to the mucosa of the rectum and urinary tract has also been described.[114] The author has seen a patient with true urinary incontinence necessitating urinary diversion caused by extension up the urethra, producing a lead-pipe effect. A second synchronous or metachronous primary neoplasm is associated with extramammary Paget's disease in about 30% of patients.[115] When the anal mucosa is involved, there is usually an underlying rectal adenocarcinoma.[116]

Treatment of Paget's disease requires wide local excision, because the disease usually extends well beyond the gross lesion.[117] The use of multiple frozen sections is desirable to ensure that the lesion has been completely excised.[116] If there is an underlying adenocarcinoma or underlying stromal invasion, a more radical local excision or radical vulvectomy is required, which should be combined with at least an ipsilateral inguinal-femoral lymphadenectomy. Because of the possibility of underlying invasive disease, laser therapy is inappropriate for primary Paget's disease.

OTHER ADENOCARCINOMAS

Apart from adenocarcinomas arising from the Bartholin's gland or underlying Paget's disease, adenocarcinomas may rarely arise from the skin appendages, paraurethral glands, minor vestibular glands, aberrant breast tissue, endometriosis, or a misplaced cloacal remnant.[64]

A particularly aggressive type of adenocarcinoma is the adenosquamous carcinoma, which has a propensity for perineural invasion, early lymph node metastasis, and local recurrence.[118] This tumor has a number of synonyms, including adenoid squamous carcinoma, pseudoglandular squamous cell carcinoma, cylindroma, and adenoacanthoma of the sweat gland of Lever. Underwood and colleagues reported a 5-year survival of 5.5% (1 of 18) for patients with this tumor, compared with 62.3% (48 of 77) for patients with squamous cell carcinomas.[118] Treatment should be by radical vulvectomy and bilateral groin dissection, and postoperative radiation therapy to the vulva may be appropriate.

BASAL CELL CARCINOMA

Basal cell carcinomas account for about 2% of all vulvar malignancies, and occur preponderantly in white, postmenopausal women. Most lesions are less than 2 cm in diameter, but giant lesions, up to 10 cm in diameter, have been reported.[119] They are usually situated on the anterior labia majora, and most present as a "rodent" ulcer with rolled edges. Other morphologic variants include nodules, plaques, and cystic lesions, while melanin pigmentation may be present.

Adequate biopsy is necessary for diagnosis, and the lesion must be differentiated from the more aggressive "basosquamous" carcinoma, a histologic variant of squamous cell carcinoma, and from a mixed basal and squamous cell carcinoma.[119] One of the subtypes of basal cell carcinomas—adenoid basal cell carcinoma—must be differentiated from the more aggressive adenoid cystic carcinoma arising in a Bartholin's gland or skin.[120]

These tumors are generally locally aggressive, and should be treated by radical local excision. The local recurrence rate is approximately 20%;[121] therefore, close follow-up is important. Metastasis to inguinal lymph nodes is rare, but has been documented.[120, 122, 123] Inguinal nodes should therefore be evaluated histologically by excisional biopsy or fine-needle aspiration cytology if palpable.

VERRUCOUS CARCINOMA

In 1948, Ackerman first reported a variant of squamous cell carcinoma, called verrucous carcinoma, in the oral cavity, and such tumors have subsequently been described in the larynx, nasal cavity, paranasal sinuses, penis, anorectum, and female genital tract.[64]

Grossly, the tumors are cauliflower-like in appearance (Fig. 10–18), while microscopically, they contain multiple papillary fronds that lack the central connective tissue core that characterizes condylomata acuminata.[124] The gross and microscopic features, as well as the natural history of these lesions, are very similar to those of the giant condyloma of Buschke-Löwenstein, and they probably represent the same disease entity.[64, 125] Adequate biopsy, to include the base of the lesion, is necessary to distinguish this lesion from a benign condyloma acuminatum, or a squamous cell carcinoma with a verrucous growth pattern.

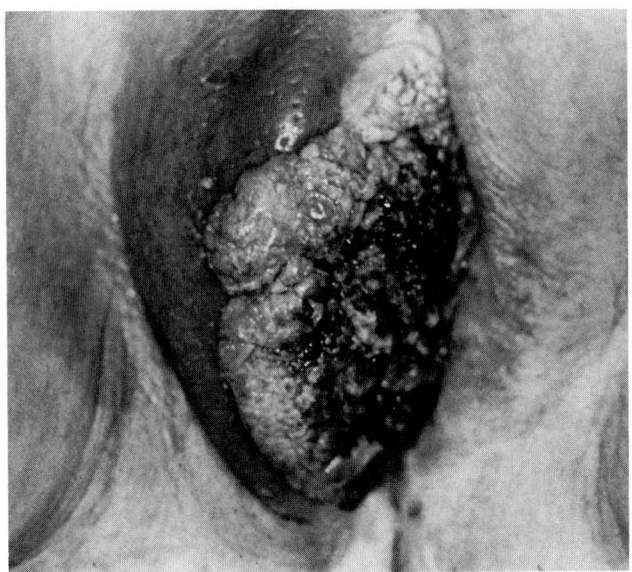
Figure 10-18
Verrucous carcinoma of the vulva.

Clinically, the lesions usually occur in postmenopausal women, and most patients present with a long-standing, slow-growing warty lesion. The tumors are locally destructive, and even bone may be invaded. Metastasis to regional lymph nodes has been reported but is rare.[126] Treatment should be by radical local excision. Palpably suspicious groin nodes should be evaluated by fine-needle aspiration cytology or excisional biopsy, but will usually show reactive hyperplasia only.[64, 127] Local recurrences are common if the tumor is incompletely excised, and some type of pelvic exenteration may be necessary to clear recurrent disease.

Radiation therapy is not useful, and may induce anaplastic transformation with subsequent regional and distant metastasis.[128] Japaze and colleagues reported a corrected 5-year survival of 94% for 17 patients treated by surgery alone, compared with 42% (4 of 7) for patients treated with surgery and radiation.[127] Metastases were found in 3 of the 7 patients treated with surgery and radiation, but in none of the 17 patients treated with surgery alone.

VULVAR SARCOMAS

Sarcomas represent 1-2% of vulvar malignancies, and many histologic types have been described. They include leiomyosarcomas, fibrosarcomas, neurofibrosarcomas, liposarcomas, rhabdomyosarcomas, angiosarcomas, and epithelioid sarcomas.[129]

Leiomyosarcomas are the most common vulvar sarcomas. Most patients present with an enlarging mass, which may be painful. Most are situated in the labium majus or in the area of Bartholin's gland. Tavassoli and Norris reviewed the clinical and pathologic features of 32 smooth muscle tumors of the vulva and reported that recurrence was associated with three main determinants: lesion size greater than 5 cm, infiltrating margins, and five or more mitotic figures per 10 high-power fields.[130] These investigators concluded that a tumor should be designated as a sarcoma when it has demonstrated aggressive behavior by metastasis or has an infiltrating margin. Radical local excision is the treatment of choice. Four of their 32 patients developed a local recurrence, which was re-excised, and all patients were alive and well at 11 months and at 1.2, 2.5, and 6 years after the last recurrence.

Epithelioid sarcomas usually occur in the labia majora of young women, but may occur in later life. Ulbright and colleagues described two cases and reviewed three other reported cases.[131] They concluded that vulvar epithelioid sarcomas behave more aggressively than the corresponding extragenital lesions. Four of the five patients died of metastatic sarcoma, and in three patients, the course of the disease was quite rapid. These authors suggested that complete initial excision was important, because all patients with a local recurrence died with distant metastases.

Rhabdomyosarcomas are the most common soft tissue sarcomas in childhood, and 20% of these cancers involve the pelvis or genitourinary system.[132] They are particularly aggressive tumors, and radical pelvic surgery, such as exenteration, was once considered standard treatment. Over the past 15-20 years, a combined modality approach has evolved using chemotherapy, radiotherapy, and less radical surgery. Survival rates have improved, and morbidity has been decreased.

Hays and colleagues reported the experience in Intergroup Rhabdomyosarcoma Study I and II (1972-1984), with patients with primary tumors of the vagina, uterus, and vulva.[133] There were nine patients with vulvar lesions, and their ages ranged from 1 to 19 years. They were managed with chemotherapy (vincristine, dactinomycin, ± cyclophosphamide, ± doxorubicin), with or without radiotherapy. Resection was carried out initially or after chemotherapy. Eight patients have been disease-free from 4 to 10 years (mean, 6.4 years), and one is alive with probable disease at 2.5 years.

RARE VULVAR MALIGNANCIES

In addition to the tumors discussed previously, a number of malignancies more commonly seen in other parts of the body may rarely present as isolated vulvar tumors. They include the following:

Dermatofibrosarcoma Protuberans of the Vulva. This is a rare tumor of low malignant potential, which has a marked tendency for local recurrence but a low risk of systemic metastasis. It can involve any skin surface except the palms and soles. Rarely the genital area may be involved.[134] Radical local excision should be sufficient treatment.

Endodermal Sinus Tumor (Yolk Sac Tumor). There have been four reported cases of endodermal sinus tumors involving the vulva, and three of these patients have died with distant metastases.[129] The patients ranged in age from 22 months to 26 years. None was treated with modern aggressive chemotherapy utilizing cisplatin, bleomycin, and etoposide. Addition of such adjuvant chemotherapy to local tumor excision may improve the prognosis for these tumors in the future.

Merkel Cell Carcinoma. Merkel cell tumors are primary small cell carcinomas of the skin that resemble oat cell carcinomas of the lung. Merkel cells are touch-sensitive receptor cells located in the basal layer of the epidermis.[64] The tumor cells contain membrane-bound neurosecretory granules and are reactive to neuron-specific enolase. They most frequently occur in the skin of the head, neck, and extremities of elderly people, and metastasize frequently to regional lymph nodes and visceral organs. Bottles and colleagues described a Merkel cell tumor in the labium majus of a 73-year-old woman.[135] The patient died following radical vulvectomy, and autopsy revealed metastases in the inguinal and para-aortic lymph nodes, vertebral bodies, liver, and pulmonary vessels. More recently, Husseinzadeh and colleagues reported on a 47-year-old woman with a Merkel cell tumor involving the right labium minus and clitoris.[136] She had positive inguinal lymph nodes at the time of surgery, and died about 6 months later with metastases in hilar lymph nodes, lung, liver, and pancreas.

Lymphomas. Malignant lymphomas may involve the genital tract as a primary tumor, but more commonly, genital tract involvement is part of a systemic disease. In the lower genital tract, the cervix is the most frequently involved site, followed by the vulva and vagina.[129] Most patients are in their third to sixth decade of life. Seventy to eighty per cent of primary lymphomas of the lower genital tract are diffuse large cell or histiocytic non-Hodgkin's lymphomas. The remainder are nodular or Burkitt's lymphomas.[137] They generally respond well to surgical excision followed by chemotherapy and/or radiation, with an overall 5-year survival rate of 73%.[137]

CONCLUSION

Before treating any vulvar lesion, all relevant pathologic information must be available. This will necessitate adequate biopsy and histologic examination by a gynecologic pathologist.

The modern management of vulvar malignancies should be individualized, with careful consideration given to the most appropriate operation for the primary lesion and the regional lymph nodes. In addition, the possible integration of radiation therapy, and in some instances chemotherapy, into the overall management should be considered before embarking on any surgery.

Radical vulvectomy should no longer be considered mandatory for most vulvar malignancies. Procedures that spare much of the vulva may be appropriate in many instances, thereby decreasing psychologic morbidity. When more conservative procedures are used, careful patient selection is critical to ensure that survival is not compromised.

References

1. Blair-Bell W, Datnow MM: Primary malignant diseases of the vulva, with special reference to treatment by operation. J Obstet Gynaecol Br Emp 1936; 43:755.
2. Way S: The anatomy of the lymphatic drainage of the vulva and its influence on the radical operation for carcinoma. Ann R Coll Surg Engl 1948; 3:187.
3. Basset A: Traitement chirurgical operatoire de l'epithelioma primitif du clitoris. Indications-technique-results. Rev Chir 1912; 46:546.
4. Taussig FJ: Cancer of the vulva: An analysis of 155 cases. Am J Obstet Gynecol 1940; 40:764.
5. Way S: Carcinoma of the vulva. Am J Obstet Gynecol 1960; 79:692.
6. Plentl AA, Friedman EA: Lymphatic System of the Female Genitalia. Philadelphia, WB Saunders Co., 1971.
7. Iversen T, Aas M: Lymph drainage from the vulva. Gynecol Oncol 1983; 16:179.
8. Figge DC, Tamimi HK, Greer BE: Lymphatic spread in carcinoma of the vulva. Am J Obstet Gynecol 1985; 152:387.
9. Cavanagh D, Roberts WD, Bryson SCP, et al.: Changing trends in the surgical treatment of invasive carcinoma of the vulva. Surg Gynecol Obstet 1986; 162:164.
10. Simonsen E, Johnsson JE, Trope C: Radical vulvectomy with warm-knife and open-wound techniques in vulvar malignancies. Gynecol Oncol 1984; 17:22.
11. Franklin EW, Rutledge FD: Epidemiology of epidermoid carcinoma of the vulva. Obstet Gynecol 1972; 39:165.
12. Newcomb PA, Weiss NS, Daling JR: Incidence of vulvar carcinoma in relation to menstrual, reproductive, and medical factors. J Natl Cancer Inst 1984; 73:391.
13. Mabuchi K, Bross DS, Kessler H: Epidemiology of cancer of the vulva. A case-control study. Cancer 1985; 55:1843.
14. Hay DM, Cole, FM: Primary invasive carcinoma of the vulva in Jamaica. J Obstet Gynaecol Br Commonw 1969; 76:821.
15. Kaufman RH, Dreesman GR, Burke J, et al.: Herpesvirus-induced antigens in squamous-cell carcinoma in situ of the vulva. N Engl J Med 1981; 305:483.
16. Pilotti S, Delle Torre G, Rilke F, et al.: Immunohistochemical and ultrastructural evidence of papilloma virus infection associated with in situ and microinvasive squamous cell carcinoma of the vulva. Am J Surg Pathol 1984; 8:751.

17. Gross G, Hagedorn M, Ikenberg H et al.: Bowenoid papulosis: Presence of human papillomavirus (HPV) structural antigens and of HPV 16–related DNA sequences. Arch Dermatol 1985; 121:858.
18. Friedrich EC Jr: Vulvar carcinoma in situ in identical twins: An occupational hazard. Obstet Gynecol 1972; 39:837.
19. Buscema J, Woodruff JD, Parmley TH, et al.: Carcinoma in situ of the vulva. Obstet Gynecol 1980; 55:225.
20. Rastkar G, Okagaka T, Twiggs LB, Clark BA: Early invasive and in situ warty carcinoma of the vulva: Clinical, histologic, and electron microscopic study with particular reference to viral association. Am J Obstet Gynecol 1982; 143:814.
21. Hacker NF, Nieberg RK, Berek JS, et al.: Superficially invasive vulvar cancer with nodal metastases. Gynecol Oncol 1983; 15:65.
22. Parker RT, Duncan I, Rampone J, et al.: Operative management of early invasive epidermoid carcinoma of the vulva. Am J Obstet Gynecol 1975; 123:349.
23. Chu J, Tamimi HK, Figge DC: Femoral node metastases with negative superficial inguinal nodes in early vulvar cancer. Am J Obstet Gynecol 1981; 140:337.
24. Curry SL, Wharton JT, Rutledge F: Positive lymph nodes in vulvar squamous carcinoma. Gynecol Oncol 1980; 9:63.
25. Leuchter RS, Hacker NF, Voet RL, et al.: Primary carcinoma of the Bartholin gland: A report of 14 cases and a review of the literature. Obstet Gynecol 1982; 60:361.
26. Piver MS, Xynos FP: Pelvic lymphadenectomy in women with carcinoma of the clitoris. Obstet Gynecol 1977; 49:592.
27. Rutledge F, Smith JP, Franklin EW: Carcinoma of the vulva. Am J Obstet Gynecol 1970; 106:1117.
28. Green TH Jr: Carcinoma of the vulva: A reassessment. Obstet Gynecol 1978; 52:462.
29. Krupp PJ, Bohm JW: Lymph gland metastases in invasive squamous cell cancer of the vulva. Am J Obstet Gynecol 1978; 130:943.
30. Benedet JL, Turko M, Fairey RN, et al.: Squamous carcinoma of the vulva: Results of treatment, 1938 to 1976. Am J Obstet Gynecol 1979; 134:201.
31. Iversen T, Aalders JG, Christensen A, et al.: Squamous cell carcinoma of the vulva: A review of 424 patients, 1956–1974. Gynecol Oncol 1980; 9:271.
32. Hacker NF, Berek JS, Lagasse LD, et al.: Management of regional lymph nodes and their prognostic influence in vulvar cancer. Obstet Gynecol 1983; 61:408.
33. Podratz KC, Symmonds RE, Taylor WF, et al.: Carcinoma of the vulva: Analysis of treatment and survival. Obstet Gynecol 1983; 61:63.
34. Monaghan JM, Hammond IG: Pelvic node dissection in the treatment of vulval carcinoma—is it necessary? Br J Obstet Gynaecol 1984; 91:270.
35. Hacker NF: Vulvar cancer. In Berek JS, Hacker NF (eds.): Practical Gynecologic Oncology. Baltimore, Williams & Wilkins, 1989.
36. Magrina JF, Webb MJ, Gaffey TA, et al.: Stage I squamous cell cancer of the vulva. Am J Obstet Gynecol 1979; 134:453.
37. Kneale B, Elliot P, Fortune D: Microinvasive carcinoma of the vulva. Proceedings of the International Society for the Study of Vulvar Disease, 6th World Congress, Cambridge, England, 1981.
38. Wilkinson EJ, Rico MJ, Pierson KK: Microinvasive carcinoma of the vulva. Int J Gynaecol Pathol 1982; 1:29.
39. Hoffman JS, Kumar NB, Morley GW: Microinvasive squamous carcinoma of the vulva: Search for a definition. Obstet Gynecol 1983; 61:615.
40. Hacker NF, Berek JS, Lagasse LD, et al.: Individualization of treatment for stage I squamous cell vulvar carcinoma. Obstet Gynecol 1984; 63:155.
41. Hacker NF, Berek JS: Vulvar cancer. In Haskell CM (ed.): Cancer Treatment, 3rd ed. Philadelphia, WB Saunders Co., 1990, pp. 351–361.
42. Andersen BL, Hacker NF: Psychological adjustment after vulvar surgery. Obstet Gynecol 1983; 62:457.
43. Iversen T, Abeler V, Aalders J: Individualized treatment of stage I carcinoma of the vulva. Obstet Gynaecol 1981; 57:85.
44. DiSaia PJ, Creasman WT, Rich WM: An alternative approach to early cancer of the vulva. Am J Obstet Gynecol 1979; 133:825.
45. Burke TW, Stringer CA, Gershenson DM, et al.: Radical wide excision and selective inguinal node dissection for squamous cell carcinoma of the vulva. Gynecol Oncol 1990; 38(3):328.
46. Hoffman JS, Kumar NB, Morley GW: Prognostic significance of groin lymph node metastases in squamous carcinoma of the vulva. Obstet Gynecol 1985; 66:402.
47. Morris JM: A formula for selective lymphadenectomy: Its application in cancer of the vulva. Obstet Gynecol 1977; 50:152.
48. Byron RL, Mishell DR, Yonemoto RH: The surgical treatment of invasive carcinoma of the vulva. Surg Gynecol Obstet 1965; 121:1243.
49. Hacker NF, Leuchter RS, Berek JS, et al.: Radical vulvectomy and bilateral inguinal lymphadenectomy through separate groin incisions. Obstet Gynecol 1981; 58:574.
50. Boronow RC: Therapeutic alternative to primary exenteration for advance vulvo-vaginal cancer. Gynecol Oncol 1973; 1:223.
51. Hacker NF, Berek JS, Juillard GJF, Lagasse LD: Preoperative radiation therapy for locally advanced vulvar cancer. Cancer 1984; 54:2056.
52. Homesley HD, Bundy BN, Sedlis A, Adcock L: Radiation therapy versus pelvic node resection for carcinoma of the vulva with positive groin nodes. Obstet Gynecol 1986; 68:733.
53. Dean RE, Taylor ES, Weisbrod DM, et al.: The treatment of premalignant and malignant lesions of the vulva. Am J Obstet Gynecol 1974; 119:59.
54. Heaps JM, Fu YS, Montz FJ, et al.: Surgical-pathologic variables predictive of local recurrence in squamous cell carcinoma of the vulva. Gynecol Oncol 1990; 38(3):309.
55. Buscema J, Stern JL, Woodruff JD: Early invasive carcinoma of the vulva. Am J Obstet Gynecol 1981; 140:563.
56. Burrell MO, Franklin EW III, Campion MJ, et al.: The modified radical vulvectomy with groin dissection. An eight-year experience. Am J Obstet Gynecol 1988; 159:715.
57. Wharton JT, Gallager S, Rutledge RN: Microinvasive carcinoma of the vulva. Am J Obstet Gynecol 1974; 118:159.
58. Microinvasive cancer of the vulva: Report of the ISSVD task force. J Reprod Med 1984; 29:454.
59. Atamdede F, Hoogerland D: Regional lymph node recurrence following local excision for microinvasive vulvar carcinoma. Gynecol Oncol 1989; 34:125.
60. Dvoretsky PM, Bonfiglio TA, Helmkamp F, et al.: The pathology of superficially invasive thin vulvar squamous cell carcinoma. Int J Gynecol Pathol 1984; 3:331.
61. Kabulski Z, Frankman O: Histologic malignancy grading in invasive squamous cell carcinoma of the vulva. Int J Gynaecol Obstet 1978; 16:233.
62. Sedlis A, Homesley H, Bundy BN, et al.: Positive groin lymph nodes in superficial squamous cell vulvar cancer. Am J Obstet Gynecol 1987; 156:1159.
63. Barnes AE, Crissman JD, Schellhas HF, et al.: Microinvasive carcinoma of the vulva: A clinicopathologic evaluation. Obstet Gynecol 1980; 56:234.
64. Fu YS, Reagan JW: Benign and malignant epithelial tumors of the vulva. In Fu YS, Reagan JW: Pathology of the Uterine Cervix, Vagina, and Vulva. Philadelphia, W.B. Saunders Co., 1989, pp. 138–192.
65. Chu J, Tamimi HK, Ek M, Figge D: Stage I vulvar cancer: Criteria for microinvasion. Obstet Gynecol 1982; 59:716.
66. Daly JW, Million RR: Radical vulvectomy combined with elective node irradiation for TxN0 squamous cell carcinoma of the vulva. Cancer 1974; 32:161.
66a. Stehman F, Bundy B, Bell J, et al.: Groin dissection versus groin radiation in carcinoma of the vulva. In press.
67. Green TH Jr, Ulfelder H, Meigs JV: Epidermoid carcinoma of the vulva: An analysis of 238 cases. Parts I and II. Am J Obstet Gynecol 1958; 73:834.
68. Morley GW: Infiltrative carcinoma of the vulva: Results of surgical treatment. Am J Obstet Gynecol 1976; 124:874.
69. Figge CD, Gaudenz R: Invasive carcinoma of the vulva. Am J Obstet Gynecol 1974; 119:382.
70. Abitbol MM: Carcinoma of the vulva: Improvements in the surgical approach. Am J Obstet Gynecol 1973; 117:483.

71. Trelford JD, Deer DA, Ordorica E, et al.: Ten-year prospective study in a management change of vulvar carcinoma. Am J Obstet Gynecol 1984; 150:288.
72. Julian CG, Callinson J, Woodruff JD: Plastic management of extensive vulvar defects. Obstet Gynecol 1971; 38:193.
73. Barnhill DR, Hoskins WJ, Metz P: Use of the rhomboid flap after partial vulvectomy. Obstet Gynecol 1983; 62:444.
74. Chafe W, Fowler WC, Walton LA, Currie JL: Radical vulvectomy with use of tensor fascia lata myocutaneous flap. Am J Obstet Gynecol 1983; 145:207.
75. Ballon SC, Donaldson RC, Roberts JA: Reconstruction of the vulva using a myocutaneous graft. Gynecol Oncol 1979; 7:123.
76. Achauer BM, Braly P, Berman ML, DiSaia PJ: Immediate vaginal reconstruction following resection for malignancy using the gluteal thigh flap. Gynecol Oncol 1984; 19:79.
77. Knapstein PG, Friedberg V: Reconstructive operations on the vulva and vagina. In Knapstein PG, Friedberg V, Seven B-U (eds.): Reconstructive Surgery in Gynecology. New York, Thieme Medical Publishers, 1990, pp. 40–52.
78. Andersen BL, Hacker NF: Psychosexual adjustment following pelvic exenteration. Obstet Gynecol 1983; 61:457.
79. Kaplan AL, Kaufman RH: Management of advanced carcinoma of the vulva. Gynecol Oncol 1975; 3:220.
80. Phillips B, Buchsbaum JH, Lifshitz S: Pelvic exenteration for vulvovaginal carcinoma. Am J Obstet Gynecol 1981; 141:1038.
81. Cavanagh D, Shepherd JH: The place of pelvic exenteration in the primary management of advanced carcinoma of the vulva. Gynecol Oncol 1982; 13:318.
82. Adams J, Daly JW: Proctectomy combined with vulvectomy for carcinoma of the vulva. Obstet Gynecol 1979; 54:643.
83. Boronow RC, Hickman BT, Reagan MT, et al.: Combined therapy as an alternative to exenteration for locally advanced vulvovaginal cancer. II. Results, complications, and dosimetric and surgical considerations. Am J Clin Oncol (CCT) 1987; 10(2):171.
84. Thomas G, Dembo A, DePetrillo A, et al.: Concurrent radiation and chemotherapy in vulvar carcinoma. Gynecol Oncol 1989; 34:263.
85. Rotmensch J, Rubin SJ, Sutton HG, et al.: Preoperative radiotherapy followed by radical vulvectomy with inguinal lymphadenectomy for advanced vulvar carcinomas. Gynecol Oncol 1990; 36:181.
86. Prempree T, Amornmarn R: Radiation treatment of recurrent carcinoma of the vulva. Cancer 1984; 54:1943.
87. Podratz KC, Symmonds RE, Taylor WF: Carcinoma of the vulva: Analysis of treatment failures. Am J Obstet Gynecol 1982; 143:340.
88. Boutselis JG: Radical vulvectomy for invasive squamous cell carcinoma of the vulva. Obstet Gynecol 1972; 39:827.
89. Japeze H, Garcia-Bunuel R, Woodruff JD: Primary vulvar neoplasia. A review of in situ and invasive carcinoma, 1935–1972. Obstet Gynecol 1977; 49:404.
90. Cavanagh D, Roberts WS, Bryson SCP, et al.: Changing trends in the surgical treatment of invasive carcinoma of the vulva. Surg Gynecol Obstet 1986; 162:164.
91. Karlen JR, Piver MS, Barlow JJ: Melanoma of the vulva. Obstet Gynecol 1975; 45:181.
92. Podratz KC, Gaffey TA, Symmonds RE, et al.: Melanoma of the vulva: An update. Gynecol Oncol 1983; 16:153.
93. Rose PG, Piver MS, Tsukada Y, Lau T: Conservative therapy for melanoma of the vulva. Am J Obstet Gynecol 1988; 159:52.
94. Morrow CP, Di Saia PJ: Malignant melanoma of the female genitalia: A clinical analysis. Obstet Gynecol Surv 1976; 31:233.
95. Fitzpatrick TB, Rhodes AR, Sober AJ: Prevention of melanoma by recognition of its precursors. (editorial). N Engl J Med 1985; 312:115.
96. Chung AF, Woodruff JW, Lewis JL Jr: Malignant melanoma of the vulva: A report of 44 cases. Obstet Gynecol 1975; 45:638.
97. Phillips GL, Twiggs LB, Okagaki T: Vulvar melanoma: A microstaging study. Gynecol Oncol 1982; 14:80.
98. Clark WH, From L, Bernardino EA, Mihm MC: The histogenesis and biologic behavior of primary human malignant melanomas of the skin. Cancer Res 1969; 29:705.
99. Breslow A: Thickness, cross-sectional area and depth of invasion in the prognosis of cutaneous melanoma. Ann Surg 1970; 172:902.
100. Aitkin DR, Clausen K, Klein JP, et al.: The extent of primary melanoma excision—a reevaluation. How wide is wide? Ann Surg 1983; 198:634.
101. Day CL, Mihm MC, Sober AJ, et al.: Narrower margins for clinical Stage I malignant melanoma. N Engl J Med 1982; 306:479.
102. Davidson T, Kissin M, Wesbury G: Vulvo-vaginal melanoma—should radical surgery be abandoned? Br J Obstet Gynaecol 1987; 94:473.
103. Morrow CP, Rutledge FN: Melanoma of the vulva. Obstet Gynecol 1972; 39:745.
104. Jaramillo BA, Ganjei P, Averette HE, et al.: Malignant melanoma of the vulva. Obstet Gynecol 1985; 66:398.
105. Beller U, Demopoulos RI, Beckman EM: Vulvovaginal melanoma: A clinicopathologic study. J Reprod Med 1986; 31:315.
106. Fischer RI, Neifeld JP, Lippman ME: Oestrogen receptors in human malignant melanoma. Lancet 1976; 2:337.
107. Masiel A, Buttrick P, Bitran J: Tamoxifen in the treatment of malignant melanoma. Cancer Treat Rep 1981; 65:531.
108. Nesbit RA, Woods RL, Tattersall MH, et al.: Tamoxifen in malignant melanoma. N Engl J Med 1979; 301:1241.
109. Copeland LJ, Sneige N, Gershenson DM, et al.: Bartholin gland carcinoma. Obstet Gynecol 1986; 67:794.
110. Chamlian DL, Taylor HB: Primary carcinoma of the Bartholin's gland. A report of 24 patients. Obstet Gynecol 1972; 39:489.
111. Trelford JD: Bartholin's gland carcinomas. Five cases. Gynecol Oncol 1976; 4:212.
112. Barclay DL, Collins CG, Macey HB: Cancer of the Bartholin gland. A review and report of 8 cases. Obstet Gynecol 1964; 24:329.
113. Debreuilh W: Pigmentation of the skin due to *Demodex folliculorum*. Br J Dermatol 1901; 13:403.
114. Lee RA, Dahlin DC: Paget's disease of the vulva with extension into the urethra, bladder, and ureters: A case report. Am J Obstet Gynecol 1981; 140:834.
115. Hart WR, Millman RB: Progression of intraepithelial Paget's disease of the vulva to invasive carcinoma. Cancer 1977; 40:2333.
116. Stacy D, Burrell MO, Franklin EW III: Extramammary Paget's disease of the vulva and anus. Use of intraoperative frozen-section margins. Am J Obstet Gynecol 1986; 155:519.
117. Gunn RA, Gallager HS: Vulvar Paget's disease. A topographic study. Cancer 1980; 46:590.
118. Underwood JW, Adcock LL, Okagaki T: Adenosquamous carcinoma of skin appendages (adenoid squamous cell carcinoma, pseudoglandular squamous cell carcinoma, adenoacanthoma of sweat gland of Lever) of the vulva. A clinical and ultrastructural study. Cancer 1978; 42:1851.
119. Dudzinski MR, Askin FB, Fowler WC: Giant basal cell carcinoma of the vulva. Obstet Gynecol 1984; 63:575.
120. Hoffman MS, Roberts WS, Ruffolo EH: Basal cell carcinoma of the vulva with inguinal lymph node metastases. Gynecol Oncol 1988; 29:113.
121. Palladino VS, Duffy JL, Bures GJ: Basal cell carcinoma of the vulva. Cancer 1969; 24:460.
122. Jimenez HT, Fenoglio CM, Richart RM: Vulvar basal cell carcinoma with metastasis: A case report. Am J Obstet Gynecol 1975; 121:285.
123. Sworn MJ, Hammond GT, Buchanan R: Metastatic basal cell carcinoma of the vulva: A case report. Br J Obstet Gynaecol 1979; 86:332.
124. Isaacs HJ: Verrucous carcinoma of the female genital tract. Gynecol Oncol 1976; 4:259.
125. Partridge EE, Murad R, Shingleton HM, et al.: Verrucous lesions of the female genitalia. II. Verrucous carcinoma. Am J Obstet Gynecol 1980; 137:419.
126. Gallousis S: Verrucous carcinoma: Report of three vulvar cases and a review of the literature. Obstet Gynecol 1972; 40:502.
127. Japaze H, Dinh TV, Woodruff JD: Verrucous carcinoma of the vulva: Study of 24 cases. Obstet Gynecol 1982; 60:462.

128. Demian SDE, Bushkin FL, Echevarria RA: Perineural invasion and anaplastic transformation of verrucous carcinoma. Cancer 1973; 32:395.
129. Fu YS, Reagan JW: Nonepithelial and metastatic tumors of the lower genital tract. In Fu YS, Reagan JW. Pathology of the Uterine Cervix, Vagina, and Vulva. Philadelphia, WB Saunders Co., 1989, pp. 336–379.
130. Tavassoli FA, Norris HJ: Smooth muscle tumors of the vulva. Obstet Gynecol 1979; 53:213.
131. Ulbright TM, Brokaw SA, Stehman FB, Roth LM: Epithelioid sarcoma of the vulva. Cancer 1983; 52:1462.
132. Bell J, Averette H, Davis J, Toledano S: Genital rhabdomyosarcoma: Current management and review of the literature. Obstet Gynecol Surv 1986; 41:257.
133. Hays DM, Shimada H, Raney RB, et al.: Clinical staging and treatment results in rhabdomyosarcoma of the female genital tract among children and adolescents. Cancer 1988; 61:1893.
134. Bock JE, Andreasson B, Thorn A, Holck S: Dermatofibrosarcoma protuberans of the vulva. Gynecol Oncol 1985; 20:129.
135. Bottles K, Lacy CG, Goldberg J, et al.: Merkel cell carcinoma of the vulva. Obstet Gynecol 1984; 63:61S.
136. Husseinzadeh N, Wesseler T, Newman N, et al.: Neuroendocrine (Merkel cell) carcinoma of the vulva. Gynecol Oncol 1988; 20:105.
137. Harris NL, Scully RE: Malignant lymphoma and granulocytic sarcoma of the uterus and vagina. Cancer 1984; 53:2530.

Surgery for Cancer of the Vagina

11

Michael P. Hopkins

Vaginal cancer is a rare malignancy and accounts for only 1–2% of all gynecologic malignancies. The International Federation of Gynecology and Obstetrics (FIGO) staging system determines that cancers involving the vulva or cervix and the vagina will be considered to be a primary malignancy of the vulva or cervix, not of the vagina. Thus, only those cancers in which the vagina is invaded without cervical or vulvar involvement are considered to originate from the vagina. This malignancy is usually of squamous cell origin (85% of all vaginal malignancies) and is most common in the elderly population with its peak incidence in the sixties.[1-9] However, malignancy has been reported in women from the age of 20 to their nineties. The exception to this is clear cell adenocarcinoma of the vagina in young women, which is often related to in utero diethylstilbestrol (DES) exposure. Clear cell adenocarcinoma has been reported in girls as young as 7 years of age. The peak incidence for clear cell adenocarcinoma of the vagina is age 19 and is rare beyond age 30. This chapter provides an overview of the etiology, symptoms, diagnosis, staging, and treatment of vaginal cancer.

ETIOLOGY

The etiology of vaginal cancer is unclear. It has been reported in association with vulvar and cervical cancer. Women who have been treated for a cervical or vulvar squamous cell malignancy are more likely to develop a squamous cell cancer of the vagina. This phenomenon has given rise to the "field effect."[10] This theory postulates that the entire genital tract is at risk of developing a squamous cell abnormality once an initial malignancy has occurred. The human papillomavirus (HPV) has been associated with cervical and vulvar cancer, and the viral theory is an attractive explanation for the observed field effect. The entire genital tract would be exposed to the virus, leading to the eventual development of abnormalities in the vagina. A previous hysterectomy does not appear to be a risk factor for developing vaginal cancer. Gallup reported that 46% of patients with vaginal cancer had their hysterectomy performed for benign disease, whereas Bell reported that 36% of patients had their hysterectomy performed for benign disease.[2, 11] Thus, the majority of patients who develop vaginal cancer have had their hysterectomy performed for a premalignant or malignant process on the cervix. The most common location for malignancy is the upper vagina, where the anterior or posterior walls are involved. The increased exposure to pooled semen or vaginal secretions in the upper vagina may be the reason that cancer commonly develops in this area.

Squamous cell carcinoma (SCC) is the most common pathologic type, and there appears to be a continuum of development. Squamous cell disease progresses from vaginal intraepithelial neoplasia (VAIN) or carcinoma in situ to microinvasion to invasion. However, the microinvasive stage of disease has seldom been reported. Peters reported on six patients with apparent microinvasive carcinoma of the vagina, all of whom did well without recurrence.[12] All of these microinvasive lesions arose in a field associated with carcinoma in situ. Eddy reported on an additional six patients, of whom one patient died of disease.[13]

SYMPTOMS AND DIAGNOSIS

The most common symptom is postmenopausal bleeding, which is present in 65% of patients with vaginal cancer. A chronic vaginal discharge is the presenting symptom in 30% of cases, whereas the remainder are asymptomatic. Patients with carcinoma in situ or very early invasive disease are usually asymptomatic, and their malignancy is diagnosed by cytologic examination. When the cervix is absent, cytologic studies will usually be positive. Bell reported that 65% of patients with invasive cancer had a positive cytologic smear and a further 25% had atypical smears leading to a tissue diagnosis. However, if the cervix is present, the diagnosis may be more difficult to establish. Cytologic examination of the cervix may be negative. Alternatively, positive cytologic findings thought to be cervical in origin may be from the vagina. When colposcopy and cone biopsy examination of the cervix are negative in the presence of positive cytologic findings, it is important to inspect the vagina. The lesions usually occur on the upper anterior and posterior walls of the vagina, and these are the areas commonly covered with the speculum. It is important, therefore, to include visual inspection of all walls of the vagina by rotation of the speculum. Careful palpation for raised, hardened areas during the bimanual examination is also important. Invasive cancer of the vagina will oftentimes be ulcerative or polypoid, and these visible lesions should be biopsied. A submucosal lesion suggests that the malignancy is metastatic via the vaginal lymphatics.

STAGING AND PROGNOSIS

Vaginal cancer is staged clinically utilizing the staging system of the International Federation of Gynecology and Obstetrics (FIGO). The staging system corresponds to the local extension of disease in the pelvis as well as the hematogenous and lymphatic spread (Table 11–1). Most patients are diagnosed with Stage I or II disease, with Stage II being the more frequently diagnosed. The distribution of patients according to the stage of disease is as follows: Stage I, 26%; Stage II, 40%; Stage III, 18%; Stage IV, 16%. Vaginal cancer spreads by local extension into the paravaginal tis-

Table 11–1

Clinical Staging System for Vaginal Cancer

Stage	
0	Carcinoma in situ
I	Early invasion to vaginal wall
II	Paravaginal tissue involved but not to the pelvic sidewall
III	Involvement to the pelvic sidewall
IVA	Involvement of the bladder or rectum
IVB	Distant metastases

sues and eventually extends to the pelvic sidewall. When the lesions are anterior or posterior, they can spread directly into the bladder or the rectum. With the extensive blood supply to the vagina, a hematogenous spread is also possible. Clinical staging of vaginal cancer, therefore, includes a chest x-ray, cystoscopy, and sigmoidoscopy. Prior to treatment, a computed tomographic (CT) scan of the abdomen and pelvis is usually performed to evaluate the possibility of metastatic disease to the lymph nodes. The lymphatic drainage of the upper and lower vagina is routed to different nodal areas. The lymphatic drainage of the upper two-thirds of the vagina drains to the pelvic lymph nodes, whereas the drainage from the lower vagina is directed to the inguinal area. The exact incidence of metastatic disease to lymph nodes is not well documented because the surgical staging of vaginal cancer with para-aortic, pelvic, and inguinal lymphadenectomy has not been routinely performed. Many of these patients are elderly, precluding extensive surgery prior to treatment. Rubin reported 40% incidence of metastatic disease to lymph nodes when a lymphangiogram was performed, and Pride reported that 16% of patients presented with node metastases.[3,5]

The overall prognosis is related to the stage of disease.[1-9] The 5-year survival for all patients with vaginal cancer is approximately 45% and decreases corresponding to the stage: Stage I, 72%; Stage II, 52%; Stage III, 28%; and Stage IV, 5% (Table 11–2).

TREATMENT: RADIATION VERSUS SURGERY

The usual method of treatment for vaginal cancer is radiation therapy. This is based on the age of the patient as well as the proximity of the bladder and the rectum. The elderly patient is usually not a good candidate for extensive radical surgery with its attendant anesthesia, blood loss, and postoperative recovery. Also, radiation allows for preservation of the bladder and the rectum when the cancer is extending close to these structures. When radiation therapy is utilized for treatment of vaginal cancer, the combined

Table 11–2

Survival for Patients with Cancer of the Vagina

	Per Cent Survival
All Stages	45
Stage I	72
Stage II	52
Stage III	28
Stage IV	5

modality of internal and external beam radiation is superior to external beam radiation therapy alone. Rubin reported on 15 of 29 patients who survived free of disease when treated by the combined method, whereas 3 of 13 survived when treated by external beam only.[3] Gallup reported on 7 of 17 patients who survived free of disease when treated by the combined modality, whereas only 1 of 6 survived when treated by external beam radiation only.[2] Peters also found the combined treatment more favorable, and when doses exceeded 7500 cGy, the survival was better.[1] When radiation is administered for vaginal cancer, the rectum and bladder are in very close proximity, leading to a high complication rate.[5] Rubin reported a 10% major and 15% minor complication rate, whereas Pride reported an 18% major and 23% minor complication rate.[3, 5] Complications include sigmoiditis, cystitis, enteritis, and vaginal stenosis. Interstitial radiation has also been used for vaginal cancer with good results. Proponents of this therapy consider it to be ideal for treatment of vaginal cancer. The interstitial needles can give a tailored dose of radiation to the neoplasm.[14] However, the interstitial radiation is more difficult to administer and must be given in centers specializing in this modality. Care must be taken when inserting the needles so that the bladder and rectum are not injured.

The surgical approach to vaginal cancer is limited by the proximity of the bladder and the rectum. The usual treatment is with radiation, and the number of reported patients treated by surgery is limited (Table 11–3). A total of 62 patients reviewed had a 56% survival. Survival, again, corresponds to the stage of disease: Stage I, 69%; Stage II, 38%; Stage III, 43%; and Stage IV, 25%. Peters reported on 12 patients treated with primary surgery.[1] Ten of these patients had superficial disease, and vaginectomy was performed. Three of these patients experienced a recurrence of their cancer, yielding a 70% survival. Gallup reported the use of vaginectomy for squamous cell disease; all 3 of the 3 reported patients survived free of disease.[2] Rubin studied a total of 15 patients treated by either exenteration or radical surgery.[3] Eight of these patients survived. Perez reported on 4 of 9 patients who survived,[9, 15] and Herbst recorded 13 of 25 patients who survived with radical surgery.[6] In general, when the surgical approach is utilized, the stage of the disease is critical. In Stage I disease, when malignancy is confined to the vagina, the radical surgical approach provides favorable results. If the upper vagina down to the mid-portion is involved, a radical hysterectomy, pelvic lymph node dissection with upper vaginectomy, or complete vaginectomy can be performed. Once again, the distance between the vesicovaginal septum and the rectovaginal septum usually results in a close margin. When the lower vagina is involved, especially the posterior vagina, a radical vulvovaginectomy with groin node dissection can be performed with the posterior vagina being removed. When disease extends anteriorly or posteriorly beneath the bladder or the rectum, consideration must then be given to an exenteration. Patients with this extent of disease are usually treated initially with radiation. Should the disease recur after radiation, exenteration is then the treatment of choice.[61] Reirradiation for vaginal cancer after previous radiation for cervical cancer can be attempted. Peters reported on 2 of 9 patients who survived with reirradiation.[1] However, 4 of the 9 patients who received reirradiation developed major fistula complications, and one of the patients died of these complications.

PATHOLOGY

A variety of pathologic cell types can involve the vagina (Table 11–4). The most common type is squamous cell, arising from the squamous epithelium that covers the müllerian epithelium of the vagina. The next most common type is adenocarcinoma, with clear cell adenocarcinoma being the best publicized.[16, 40] Melanoma can occur in the vagina, but fewer than 200 patients have been reported.[41] Sarcomas arise in the vagina, as do small cell neuroendocrine type carcinomas.[42–55] Carcinoma can also arise from the neovagina, and this is related to the type

Table 11–3

Survival for Patients with Vaginal Cancer Treated by Surgery

	Stage				
Author	I	II	III	IV	Total
Peters[1]	7/10				
Gallup[2]	3/3				
Rubin[3]	5/6	2/6	1/2	0/1	
Perez[9, 15]	1/3	1/2	1/1	1/3	
Herbst[6]	9/14*		4/11†		
Total	25/36	3/8	6/14	1/4	35/62
Per cent survival	69	38	43	25	56

*Stages I and II.
†Stages III and IV.

Table 11-4

Pathologic Cell Types of Vaginal Cancer

> Squamous cell
> > In situ
> > Microinvasive
> > Invasive
>
> Adenocarcinoma
> > Clear cell
> > Mucoid
> > Mesonephroid
>
> Sarcoma
> > Leiomyosarcoma
> > Endometrial stromal sarcoma
> > Rhabdomyosarcoma
> > Angiosarcoma
> > Schwannoma
> > Mixed müllerian sarcoma
> > Fibrosarcoma
> > Alveolar sarcoma
> > Neurofibrosarcoma
> > Synovial cell
>
> Granulocytic sarcoma/lymphoma
> Melanoma
> Small Cell neuroendocrine
> Neovagina
> Metastatic disease
> > Endometrial
> > Urothelial/renal
> > Trophoblastic
> > Cervix/vulva
> > Colon

of neovagina that was constructed.[56] Metastatic lesions occur in the vagina and are usually located in the submucosal tissues.

THERAPY

The treatment of vaginal cancer must be approached on an individual basis. A complete staging work-up should be performed, and the pathologic subtype is important in deciding treatment. An overview is presented in Table 11-5.

Squamous Cell

Early stage squamous cell cancer can be treated satisfactorily with the surgical approach. In situ disease can be treated with upper vaginectomy or complete vaginectomy. The vaginectomy can be tailored to the location and the extent of disease. For multifocal disease involving the entire vagina, a complete vaginectomy can be performed, starting at the hymenal ring and working to the apex (Fig. 11-1). Great care must be taken not to enter the bladder or the rectum while the dissection is being performed. When this dissection is performed, it is critical that the rectovaginal and vesicovaginal septum be identified with certainty. A uterine sound placed through the urethra into the bladder and the operator's finger

in the rectum can greatly assist in this dissection. There is usually scarring in the upper vagina after a hysterectomy, and this area requires sharp dissection (Fig. 11-2). A split-thickness skin graft can then be placed should the patient desire continued sexual function. In many patients the carcinoma in situ will involve only the upper vagina, and in these patients an upper vaginectomy can be performed after colposcopy has outlined the extent of the disease (Figs. 11-2 and 11-3). An alternative is ablation of the vaginal surface disease utilizing the carbon dioxide laser.[57-60] This provides satisfactory results with less operative time. The depth is critical, and when using the laser, care must be taken not to enter the rectum or bladder. An alternative to surgery is intravaginal 5-fluorouracil (5-FU) cream. This produces sloughing of the surface epithelium where the carcinoma in situ is present. The disadvantage of laser and 5-FU therapy is the lack of a surgical specimen, which may show an invasive process. Thus, great care and judgment are necessary to ensure that only in situ lesions are treated when using these methods. Preoperative evaluation with colposcopy and biopsy is mandatory.

Microinvasive and early Stage I invasive vaginal cancer can be treated with radical surgery. Wide excision of the lesions through the vagina may be satisfactory for very early microinvasive disease. Either radical hysterectomy with vaginectomy or radical vaginectomy with removal of the lateral parametrial tissue provides satisfactory results for invasive lesions (Fig. 11-4). When treating an invasive lesion with the surgical approach, a pelvic lymph node dissection is required to ensure that metastatic

Table 11-5

Therapy of Vaginal Cancer According to the Pathologic Cell Type

Cell Type	Therapy
Squamous cell	
In situ	Laser or 5-FU cream or vaginectomy
Microinvasive	Vaginectomy or radiation
Invasive	Radical vaginectomy or radiation
Recurrent after radiation	Exenteration
Adenocarcinoma	
Clear cell Stage I	Radical vaginectomy
Other	Radiation
Melanoma	Wide excision with radiation or exenteration
Sarcoma	
Adult	Radiation; exenteration for recurrence or persistence
Pediatric	Chemotherapy and wide excision with radiation for involved margins
Small cell	Wide excision with radiation and chemotherapy
Neovagina	Exenteration
Metastatic	Biopsy only

SURGERY FOR CANCER OF THE VAGINA

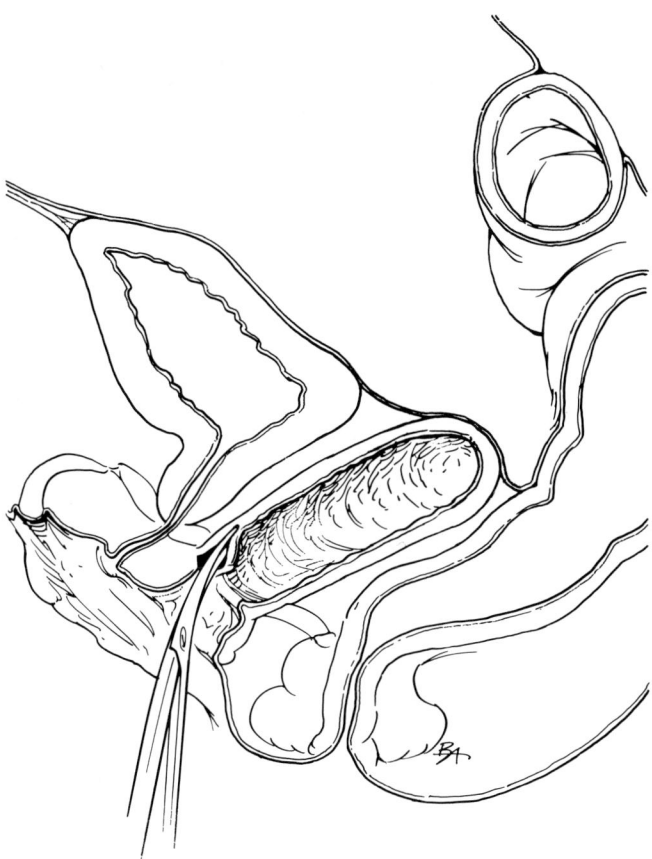

Figure 11–1
Dissection begins at the hymenal ring for a total vaginectomy. The vaginal mucosa is dissected from the underlying tissue.

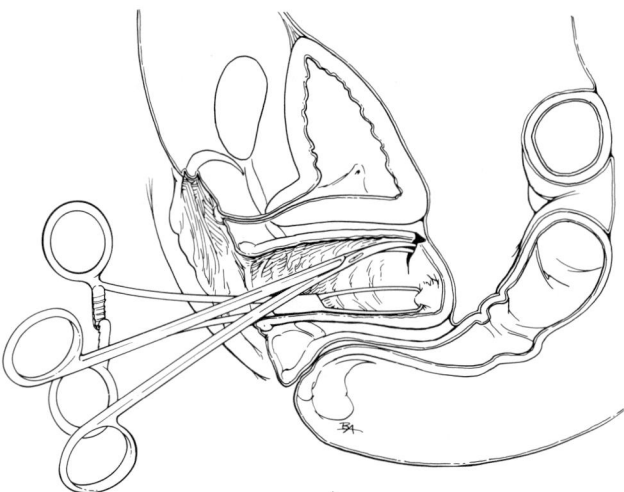

Figure 11–2
In the upper vagina, the bladder and rectum are in close proximity. It is important to identify the vesicovaginal and rectovaginal septums to avoid injury.

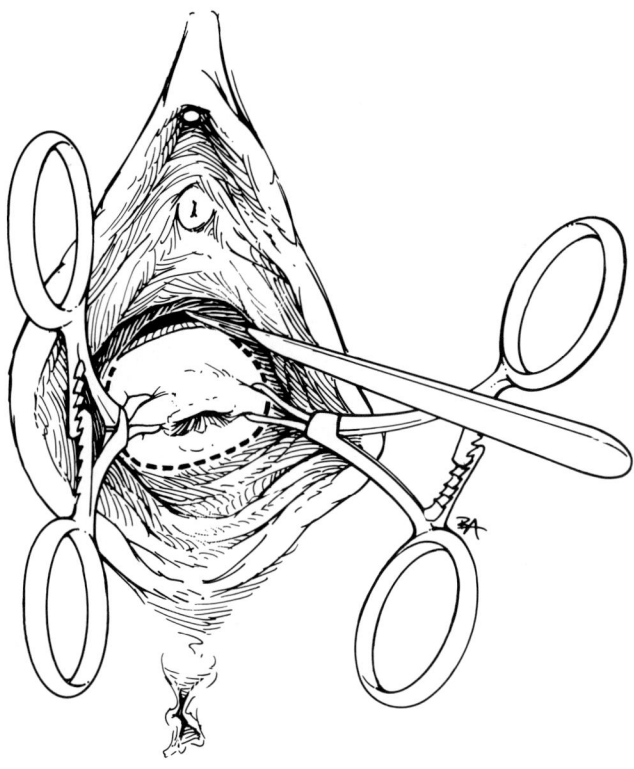

Figure 11–3
Upper vaginectomy is begun by retracting the upper vagina at the vaginal dimples, which are present after hysterectomy. The initial incision is made with the scalpel and then continued with the scissors in a similar fashion to that shown in Figure 11–2.

disease is not present. If the lesion extends to the lower one-third of the vagina, an inguinal node dissection may also be necessary. Lesions that involve the anteroposterior vagina will be closer to the bladder or rectum, and should there be a question as to the depth of invasion, intraoperative frozen sections may be necessary to determine if adequate margins are present. The upper posterior lesions are more amenable to the surgical approach because the sigmoid colon reflects away from the posterior vagina whereas the bladder is in close proximity to the entire length of the anterior vagina (Fig. 11–5). Multifocal vaginal lesions lend themselves to surgery, and this approach has the particular advantage of treating the disease in one setting. Radiation in this situation may be more difficult as a result of the multifocal lesions. Lesions that extend beyond Stage I are best treated with radiation therapy.

Occasionally, a patient with an invasive lesion in close proximity to the bladder can be treated by radical hysterectomy and vaginectomy with resection of the base of the bladder (Fig. 11–6). This procedure requires bilateral transection of the ureters followed by their reimplantation into the reconstructed bladder. However, patients with disease that would require this extent of surgery are usually treated by radiation. This approach can be utilized for recurrent disease after radiation as an alternative to exenteration. However, after a full course of pelvic radiation, the fistula rate is extremely high, precluding the widespread use of this procedure.

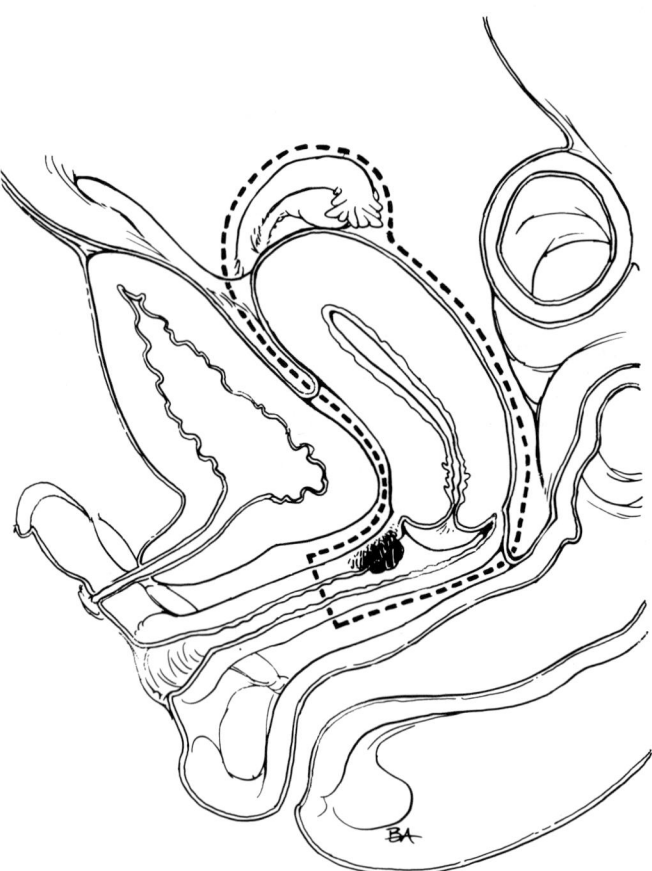

Figure 11–4
A small vaginal cancer in the upper vagina can be treated by radical hysterectomy with upper vaginectomy. The vaginectomy can be extended to a total vaginectomy if the disease is multifocal and involves the lower vagina.

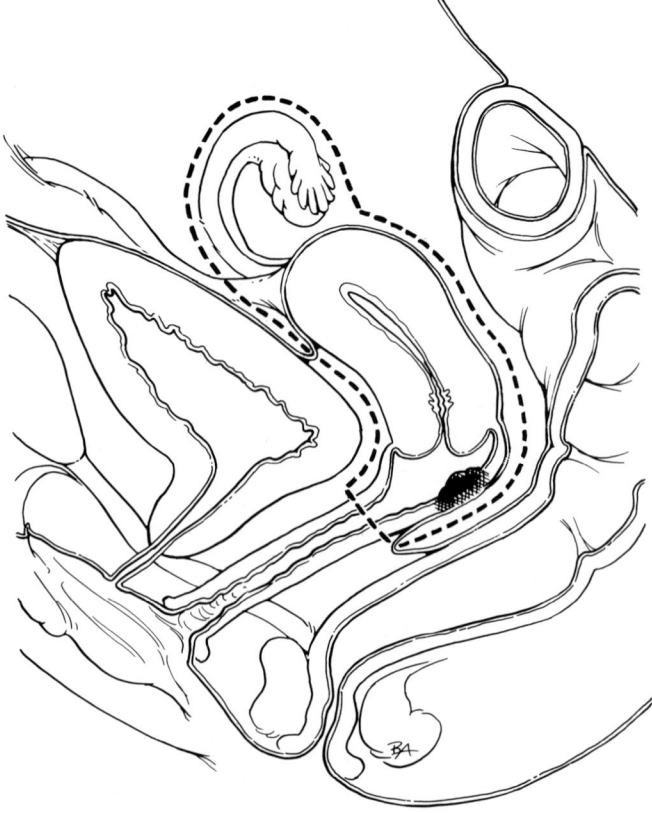

Figure 11–5
Posterior upper vaginal lesions are more amenable to the surgical approach because the sigmoid colon reflects lateral to the vagina at approximately the midpoint of the vagina. The bladder is in close proximity throughout the length of the vagina.

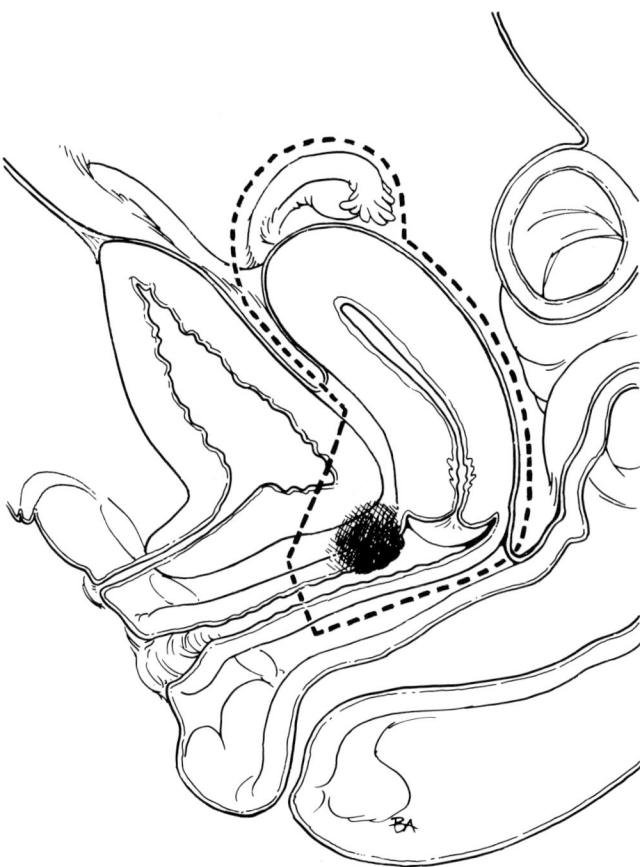

Figure 11–6
Resection of the base of the bladder can be performed to obtain adequate surgical margins in a lesion extending close to or into the bladder. Bilateral ureteral reimplantation is then required.

Lesions that are located in the lower vagina can be treated by radical vulvovaginectomy (Fig. 11–7). Lesions on the posterior wall require care to dissect them from the rectal mucosa and the anal sphincter. Occasionally, resection of a portion of the rectum with reconstruction of the sphincter will be necessary. Lesions on the lower anterior wall can be approached with resection of a portion of the urethra. However, any lesion that is extensive would require an anterior or posterior exenteration to ensure an adequate margin around the malignancy.

All invasive lesions that are approached with surgery require dissection of the nodal pathway. In the upper vagina the pelvic nodes are dissected, and in the lower vagina the inguinal area is examined. A bilateral dissection should be performed because there is extensive cross-over of vaginal lymphatics and the vaginal lesions are rarely completely unilateral.

Recurrent vaginal malignancy after radiation therapy should be approached with pelvic exenteration as the primary mode of therapy provided there is no evidence of metastatic disease.[61] If the recurrent malignancy is located on the anterior or posterior wall, an anterior or posterior exenteration can be performed (Figs. 11–8 and 11–9). When the recurrence is located at the vaginal apex after a previous hysterectomy, a total exenteration should be performed because the bladder and rectum will be contiguous with the upper vagina (Fig. 11–10).

Adenocarcinoma

Adenocarcinoma of the vagina usually presents in advanced stages and is treated with radiation therapy. The exception to this is clear cell adenocarcinoma, which typically presents in young women. This oftentimes presents as Stage I multifocal disease. In these young women, radical hysterectomy with radical vaginectomy and split-thickness skin grafting provides an excellent alternative to radiation therapy. An alternative to radical vaginectomy in very early clear cell adenocarcinoma is wide excision followed by local radiation. It is necessary to perform a pelvic lymph node dissection to ensure that metastatic disease to regional nodes is not present. Utilizing this approach, Senekjian reported 43 patients with a 92% five-year survival.[34] These patients had a much higher recurrence rate when radiation therapy was not utilized. Therefore, the investigators recom-

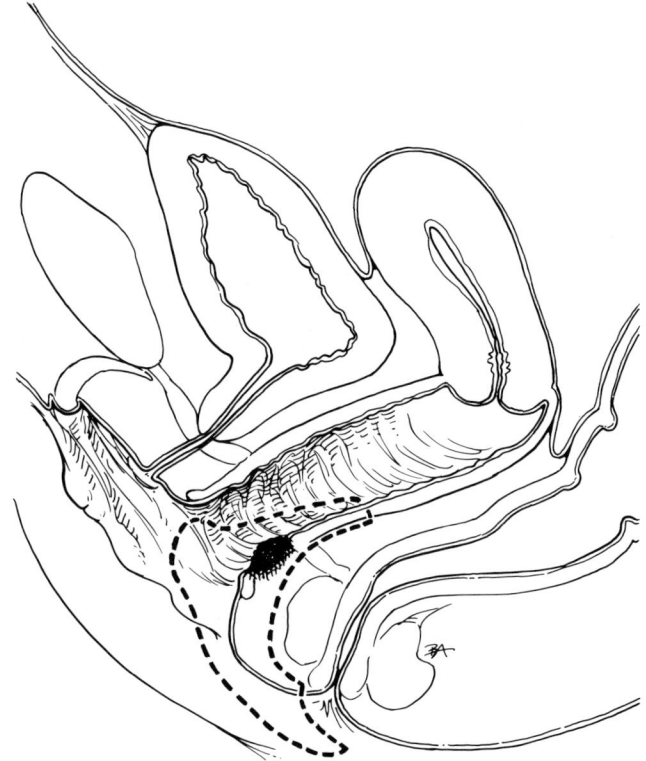

Figure 11–7
A lower posterior vaginal cancer can be treated with radical hemivulvectomy and lower vaginectomy with bilateral groin node dissection.

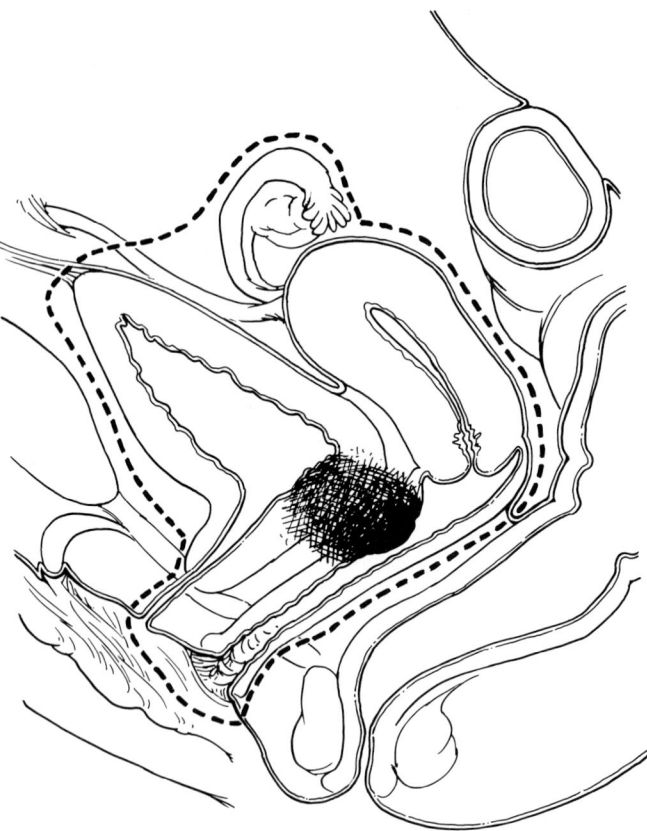

Figure 11–8
Anterior exenteration for anterior vaginal cancer involving the bladder removes the vagina and the bladder.

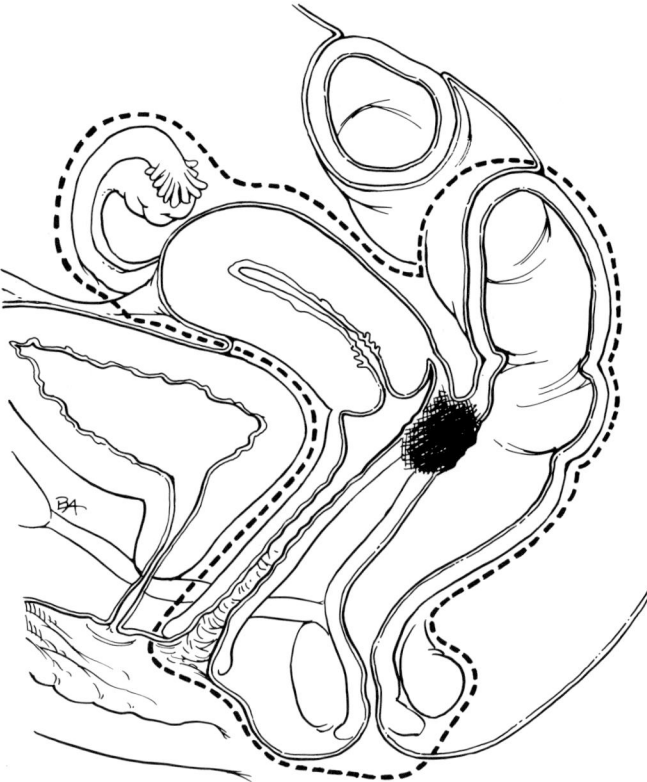

Figure 11–9
Posterior exenteration for posterior vaginal cancer involving the rectum removes the vagina and the rectum.

mended that local therapy should include local radiation.

Melanoma

Melanomas of the vagina have traditionally been treated with radical excision, usually exenteration. Reid, in a review of vaginal melanoma, reported no difference in survival when radical surgery was compared with radiation therapy or radical surgery and radiation.[41] In the review by Reid, the size of the melanoma was the significant factor predicting survival, whereas the thickness was a prognostic factor for the disease-free interval. Those patients with a melanoma less than 6 mm in thickness had an increased disease-free survival. In this review, the 5-year survival for melanoma was 17% regardless of treatment. In melanoma, radical wide excision with radiation therapy can preserve organ function, and exenteration should be reserved for recurrent disease.

Sarcoma

A variety of sarcomas can occur in the vagina. In the pediatric age group, embryonal carcinomas and rhabdomyosarcomas can occur. Prior to 1970, there was less than a 15% survival. After 1970, when radical surgery was combined with radiation and chemotherapy, the survival increased to 50% for all sites and stages, whereas survival for patients with localized disease has increased to 80–90%.[49] Importantly, in these young girls, sarcomas previously were treated by exenterative therapy, but now these tu-

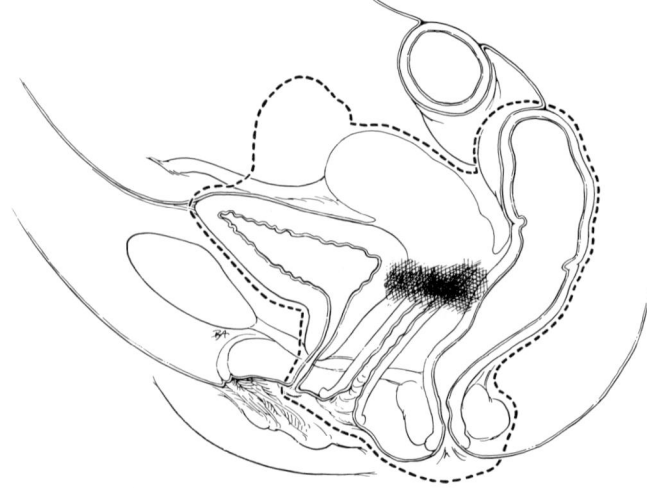

Figure 11–10
Total exenteration for apical vaginal cancer involving the bladder and the rectum removes the vagina, bladder, and rectum.

mors can be satisfactorily treated with an organ-sparing intent. Hays, in reporting the experience of the Inter Group Sarcoma Study, noted a local relapse rate of 18% when vincristine, actinomycin, and cytoxan chemotherapy was administered followed by resection of the tumor.[48] Even with a complete response to chemotherapy, resection should be performed because almost all of these specimens contained microscopic disease. Importantly, however, a limited resection can be performed, sparing the bladder and rectum. Copeland also reported an excellent survival, with only one of nine patients dying of disease when the sarcomas were treated by chemotherapy and limited surgery.[50] Radiation therapy should be added after surgery if the surgical margins are involved.

The adult vagina can be involved with leiomyosarcoma, mixed müllerian sarcoma, and endometrial stromal sarcoma. Peters, in reviewing the literature, reported a 36% survival for patients with leiomyosarcoma and a 17% survival for those with mixed müllerian sarcomas.[44] Sarcomas can be approached first with radiation therapy. This can be followed by exenteration if persistent or recurrent disease is present. Reid reported that patients with recurrent mixed müllerian sarcoma had a dismal outlook regardless of treatment and that exenteration did not add to this survival. Leiomyosarcomas, when localized to the vagina, are associated with a favorable survival when treated by exenteration.[62]

Small Cell

Small cell neuroendocrine carcinoma can involve the vagina, although these patients have only rarely been reported.[54, 55] Excellent local control can be achieved with excision and radiation therapy. Like the small cell carcinoma of the cervix and, more commonly, the lung, these tumors tend to metastasize early. The reported patients with disease arising in the vagina rapidly developed disseminated disease. Two of the three patients reported by Hopkins had an initial excellent response to chemotherapy.[54] Primary treatment for these patients includes wide excision of the lesion followed by radiation. This should achieve excellent local control, but adjuvant chemotherapy should be administered in an attempt to avoid widespread metastatic disease. The usual chemotherapy regimens are those that have shown activity in small cell cancer of the lung.

Neovagina

There are approximately 10 patients reported in the literature who have developed a carcinoma involving the neovagina. A variety of malignancies can involve the neovagina, depending on the tissue used for the vaginal reconstruction. When a portion of bowel is used, adenocarcinomas are the usual reported malignancy; when a split-thickness skin graft is utilized, a squamous cell carcinoma is the usual tumor. Radiation therapy has been used to treat these patients. As summarized by Hopkins, these patients appear to have a high rate of recurrence when treated by radiation therapy only.[56] The initial management of these patients should be based on the extent of the tumor. If the disease is extensive, radiation therapy should be followed by an exenterative type surgery. When the malignancy is small, exenteration can be the primary mode of treatment.

Metastatic

A variety of metastatic lesions can involve the vagina, and the only surgery required is for biopsy and diagnosis. The exception to this is squamous cell cancer of the cervix or vulva, which can involve the vagina. When this situation exists, the malignancy can be removed as part of an upper or lower vaginectomy when performing a radical hysterectomy or radical vulvectomy. Endometrial cancer can metastasize to the vagina through the vaginal lymphatics, and this usually signifies widespread intra-abdominal disease. Surgical exploration should be performed, but rarely would a vaginectomy be indicated to remove metastatic endometrial cancer. Gestational trophoblastic disease can metastasize to the vagina and is the second most common site of metastases after the lungs. In a patient with a known gestational trophoblastic disease, a biopsy must be undertaken with caution. Profuse hemorrhage can result, and if not critical to the management of the patient, biopsies are best not performed. Renal cell cancer can metastasize to the vagina, and occasionally this will be the only symptom.[63] Biopsy and pathology evaluation should lead to the primary source. Colon or rectal cancer can involve the vagina, usually by direct extension of the invading neoplasm into the vagina. Colorectal disease to this extent is usually metastatic to other organs, precluding an aggressive surgical approach. However, if the disease is localized, radiation followed by posterior exenteration can be curative.

Benign Tumor

A variety of benign tumors can involve the vagina (Table 11–6). These are usually removed for diagnosis with a wide excision. Nothing further is necessary after removal.[64–72]

Table 11–6
Benign Tumors That May Involve the Vagina

Gartner's duct cyst
Neurofibroma
Capillary hemangioma
Fibroepithelial polyp
Leiomyoma
Benign rhabdomyoma
Müllerian mixed tumor

SUMMARY

Vaginal cancer is a rare malignancy and accounts for only 1–2% of all gynecologic malignancies. The most common pathologic type is squamous cell, accounting for 85% of all vaginal malignancies. Survival depends upon the stage of the disease, and therapy should be individualized for each patient based on the stage of disease, the pathologic cell type, and the patient's age. Radiation therapy is the preferred treatment with the exception of early Stage I cancer of the vagina, in which surgery can provide excellent results in selected patients. In pediatric patients with sarcomas, a combination of chemotherapy, surgery, and radiation produces excellent survival results while preserving organ function.

References

1. Peters WA, Kumar NB, Morley GW: Carcinoma of the vagina. Cancer 1985; 55:892.
2. Gallup DG, Talledo OE, Shah KJ, Hayes C: Invasive squamous cell carcinoma of the vagina: A 14-year study. Obstet Gynecol 1987; 69:782.
3. Rubin SC, Young J, Mikuta JJ: Squamous carcinoma of the vagina: Treatment, complications, and long-term follow-up. Gynecol Oncol 1985; 20:346.
4. Benedet JL, Murphy KJ, Fairey RN, Boyes DA: Primary invasive carcinoma of the vagina. Obstet Gynecol 1983; 62:715.
5. Pride GL, Schultz AE, Chuprevich TW, Buchler DA: Primary invasive squamous carcinoma of the vagina. Obstet Gynecol 1979; 53:218.
6. Herbst AL, Green TH, Ulfelder H: Primary carcinoma of the vagina. Am J Obstet Gynecol 1970; 106:210.
7. Rutledge F: Cancer of the vagina. Am J Obstet Gynecol 1967; 97:635.
8. Whelton J, Kotmeier HL: Primary carcinoma of the vagina. Acta Obstet Gynecol 1962; 41:23.
9. Perez CA, Camel HM: Long-term follow-up in radiation therapy of carcinoma of the vagina. Cancer 1982; 49:1308.
10. Marcus S: Multiple squamous cell carcinomas involving the cervix, vagina, and vulva: The theory of multicentric origin. Am J Obstet Gynecol 1960; 80:802.
11. Bell J, Sevin BU, Averette H, Nadji M: Vaginal cancer after hysterectomy for benign disease: Value of cytologic screening. Obstet Gynecol 1984; 64:699.
12. Peters WA, Kumar NB, Morley GW: Microinvasive carcinoma of the vagina: A distinct clinical entity? Am J Obstet Gynecol 1985; 153:505.
13. Eddy GL, Singh KP, Gansler TS: Superficially invasive carcinoma of the vagina following treatment for cervical cancer: A report of six cases. Gynecol Oncol 1990; 36:376.
14. Puthawala A, Nisar-Syed AM, Nalick R, et al.: Integrated external and interstitial radiation therapy for primary carcinoma of the vagina. Obstet Gynecol 1983; 62:367.
15. Perez CA, Arneson AN, Dehner LP, Galakatos A: Radiation therapy in carcinoma of the vagina. Obstet Gynecol 1974; 44:862.
16. Ballon SC, Lagasse LE, Chang N, Stehman F: Primary adenocarcinoma of the vagina. Surg Gynecol Obstet 1979; 149:233.
17. Herbst AL, Anderson S, Hubby MM, et al.: Risk factors for the development of diethylstilbestrol-associated clear cell adenocarcinoma: A case-control study. Am J Obstet Gynecol 1986; 154:814.
18. Herbst AL, Cole P, Norusis MJ, et al.: Epidemiologic aspects and factors related to survival in 384 registry cases of clear cell adenocarcinoma of the vagina and cervix. Am J Obstet Gynecol 1979; 135:876.
19. Herbst AL, Ulfelder H, Poskanzer DC: Adenocarcinoma of the vagina. N Engl J Med 1971; 284:878.
20. Robboy SJ, Szyfelbein WM, Goellner JR, et al.: Dysplasia and cytologic findings in 4,589 young women enrolled in diethylstilbestrol adenosis (DESAD) project. Am J Obstet Gynecol 1981; 140:579.
21. Herbst AL, Cole P, Colton T, et al.: Age-incidence and risk of diethylstilbestrol-related clear cell adenocarcinoma of the vagina and cervix. Am J Obstet Gynecol 1977; 128:43.
22. Herbst AL, Hubby M, Azizi F, Makii M: Reproductive and gynecologic surgical experience in diethylstilbestrol-exposed daughters. Am J Obstet Gynecol 1981; 141:1019.
23. Robboy SJ, Kaufman RH, Prat J, et al.: Pathologic findings in young women enrolled in the National Cooperative Diethylstilbestrol Adenosis (DESAD) project. Obstet Gynecol 1979; 53:309.
24. O'Brien PC, Noller KL: Vaginal epithelial changes in young women enrolled in the National Cooperative Diethylstilbestrol Adenosis (DESAD) project. Obstet Gynecol 1979; 53:298.
25. Anderson B, Watring WG, Edinger DD, et al.: Development of DES-associated clear-cell carcinoma: The importance of regular screening. Obstet Gynecol 1979; 53:293.
26. Kaufman RH, Binder GL, Gray PM, Adam E: Upper genital tract changes associated with exposure in utero to diethylstilbestrol. Am J Obstet Gynecol 1977; 128:51.
27. Chanen W, Pagano R: Diethylstilboestrol (DES) exposure in utero. Med J Aust 1984; 141:491.
28. Paul C, Skegg DCG, Seddon RJ: Past use of oestrogens during pregnancy in New Zealand. NZ Med J 1984; 97:831.
29. Kinlen LJ, Badaracco MA, Moffett J, Vessey MP: A survey of the use of oestrogens during pregnancy in the United Kingdom and of the genito-urinary cancer mortality and incidence rates in young people in England and Wales. J Obstet Gynaec Br Emp 1974; 81:849.
30. Piver MS, Lele SB, Baker TR, Sandecki A: Cervical and vaginal cancer detection at a regional diethylstilbestrol (DES) screening clinic. Cancer Detect Prev 1988; 11:197.
31. Kjørstad KE, Bergstrøm J, Abeler V: Clear cell adenocarcinoma of the cervix uteri and vagina in young women in Norway. J Norv Med Assoc 1989; 109:1660.
32. Ruffolo EH, Foxworthy D, Fletcher JC: Vaginal adenocarcinoma arising in vaginal adenosis. Am J Obstet Gynecol 1971; 111:167.
33. Jones WB, Koulos JP, Saigo PE, Lewis JL: Clear-cell adenocarcinoma of the lower genital tract: Memorial Hospital 1974–1984. Obstet Gynecol 1987; 70:573.
34. Senekjian EK, Frey KW, Anderson D, Herbst AL: Local therapy in stage I clear cell adenocarcinoma of the vagina. Cancer 1987; 609:1319.
35. Robboy SJ, Keh PC, Nickerson RJ, et al.: Squamous cell dysplasia and carcinoma in situ of the cervix and vagina after prenatal exposure to diethylstilbestrol. Obstet Gynecol 1978; 51:528.
36. Wharton JT, Rutledge FN, Gallager HS, Fletcher G: Treatment of clear cell adenocarcinoma in young females. Obstet Gynecol 1975; 435:365.
37. Noller KL, Decker DG, Symmonds RE, et al.: Clear-cell adenocarcinoma of the vagina and cervix: Survival data. Am J Obstet Gynecol 1976; 124:285.
38. Lanier AP, Noller KL, Decker DG, et al.: Cancer and stilbestrol:

A follow-up of 1,719 persons exposed to estrogens in utero and born 1943–1959. Mayo Clin Proc 1973; 48:793.
39. Horwitz RI, Viscoli CM, Merino M, et al.: Clear cell adenocarcinoma of the vagina and cervix: Incidence, undetected disease, and diethylstilbestrol. J Clin Epidemiol l988; 41:593.
40. Kaminski PF, Maier RC: Clear cell adenocarcinoma of the cervix unrelated to diethylstilbestrol exposure. Obstet Gynecol 1983; 62:720.
41. Reid GC, Schmidt RW, Roberts JA, et al.: Primary melanoma of the vagina: A clinicopathologic analysis. Obstet Gynecol 1989; 74:190.
42. Crist WM, Garnesy L, Beltangady MS, et al.: Prognosis in children with rhabdomyosarcoma: A report of the intergroup rhabdomyosarcoma studies I and II. J Clin Oncol 1990; 8:443.
43. Davos I, Abell MR: Sarcomas of the vagina. Obstet Gynecol 1976; 47:342.
44. Peters WA, Kumar NB, Andersen WA, Morley GW: Primary sarcoma of the adult vagina: A clinicopathologic study. Obstet Gynecol 1985; 65:699.
45. Kasai K, Yoshida Y, Okumura M: Alveolar soft part sarcoma in the vagina: Clinical features and morphology. Gynecol Oncol 1980; 9:227.
46. Schram M: Leiomyosarcoma of the vagina. Obstet Gynecol 1958; 12:195.
47. Vawter GF: Carcinoma of the vagina in infancy. Cancer 1965; 18:1479.
48. Hays DM, Shimada H, Raney RB, et al.: Clinical staging and treatment results in rhabdomyosarcoma of the female genital tract among children and adolescents. Cancer 1988; 61:1893.
49. Bell J, Averette H, Davis J, Toledano S: Genital rhabdomyosarcoma: Current management and review of the literature. Obstet Gynecol Surv 1986; 41:257.
50. Copeland LJ, Gershenson DM, Saul PB, et al.: Sarcoma botryoides of the female genital tract. Obstet Gynecol 1985; 66:262.
51. Hilgers RD, Malkasian GD, Soule EH: Embryonal rhabdomyosarcoma (botryoid type) of the vagina. Am J Obstet Gynecol 1970; 107:484.
52. Andersen WA, Sabio H, Durso N, et al.: Endodermal sinus tumor of the vagina. Cancer 1985; 56:1025.
53. Harris NL, Scully RE: Malignant lymphoma and granulocytic sarcoma of the uterus and vagina. Cancer 1984; 53:2530.
54. Hopkins MP, Kumar NB, Lichter A, et al.: Small cell carcinoma of the vagina with neuroendocrine features. J Reprod Med 1989; 34:486.
55. Chafe W: Neuroepithelial small cell carcinoma of the vagina. Cancer 1989; 64:1948.
56. Hopkins MP, Morley GW: Squamous cell carcinoma of the neovagina. 1987; 69:525.
57. Jobson VW, Homesley HD: Treatment of vaginal intraepithelial neoplasia with the carbon dioxide laser. Obstet Gynecol 1983; 62:90.
58. Krebs HB: Treatment of vaginal intraepithelial neoplasia with laser and topical 5-fluorouracil. Obstet Gynecol 1989; 73:657.
59. Townsend DE, Levine RU, Crum CP, Richart RM: Treatment of vaginal carcinoma in situ with the carbon dioxide laser. Am J Obstet Gynecol 1982; 143:565.
60. Hernandez-Linares W, Puthawala A, Nolan JF, et al.: Carcinoma in situ of the vagina: Past and present management. Obstet Gynecol 190; 56:356.
61. Morley GW, Hopkins MP, Lindenauer M, Roberts JA: Pelvic exenteration: University of Michigan, 100 patients at 5 years. Obstet Gynecol 1989; 74:934.
62. Reid GC, Morley GW, Schmidt RW, Hopkins MP: The role of pelvic exenteration for sarcomatous malignancies. Obstet Gynecol 1989; 74:80.
63. DePrez DP, Hunter RE, Hopkins TB: A bleeding vaginal lesion as the presenting sign of hypernephroma. Am J Obstet Gynecol 1981; 140:709.
64. Deppisch LM: Cysts of the vagina. Obstet Gynecol l975; 45:632.
65. Chirayil SJ, Tobon H: Polyps of the vagina: A clinicopathologic study of 18 cases. Cancer 1981; 47:2904.
66. Davis GD, Patton WS: Capillary hemangioma of the cervix and vagina: Management with carbon dioxide laser. Obstet Gynecol 1983; 62:95s.
67. Burt RL, Prichard RW, Kim BS: Fibroepithelial polyp of the vagina. Obstet Gynecol 1976; 47:52s.
68. Dekel A, Avidan D, Barziu J, et al.: Neurofibroma of the vagina presenting with urinary retention: Review of the literature and report of a case. Obstet Gynecol Survey 1988; 43:325.
69. Quan A, Birnbaum SJ: Vaginal leiomyoma: Report of a case and review of the literature. Obstet Gynecol 1961; 18:360.
70. Gold HJ, Bossen EH: Benign vaginal rhabdomyoma. Cancer 1976; 37:2283.
71. Buntine DW, Henderson PR, Biggs JSG: Benign müllerian mixed tumor of the vagina. Gynecol Oncol 1979; 8:21.
72. Naves AE, Monti JA, Chichoni E: Basal cell–like carcinoma in the upper third of the vagina. Am J Obstet Gynecol 1980; 90:136.

Vaginal Fistulas: Operative Management

12

Ivan Jelen

Communications between the vagina and urinary or intestinal tracts, also called fistulas, create a miserable lifestyle for their bearers. Anatomically, these fistulas can develop in various portions of the vagina, and the terminology of the fistula will depend on the surrounding organs with which the vagina communicates. Figure 12–1 gives an anatomic classification of vaginal fistulas. The most common fistulas encountered in today's gynecologic practice are vesicovaginal and rectovaginal varieties.

VESICOVAGINAL FISTULA

By definition, *vesicovaginal fistula* means communication between the urinary bladder and the vagina. The bladder trigone, which lies directly against the vaginal wall, where anatomically the lack of rugae represents a trigonum of Pawlik, is mainly affected by fistula formation, but other parts of the bladder may be affected.

Although vesicovaginal fistulas have existed since time immemorial, judging by the findings on Egyptian mummies, the modern era of surgical repair started in 1849 when an Alabama country doctor, J. Marion Sims, achieved a successful closure of a vesicovaginal fistula using silver wire.[1] Many new approaches have been developed in later years, but the basic principles of fistula closure remain unchanged.

Etiology

Development of vesicovaginal fistula may be due to various causes.

Operative Injury

This is probably the most common etiologic factor today. Complications of abdominal hysterectomy and vaginal hysterectomy are mainly responsible, the former occurring more frequently.

Obstetric Injury

Fistulas can develop as a result of prolonged obstructed labor, trauma during instrument delivery, or as a complication of cesarean section.

Gynecologic Malignancy

These are most commonly due to carcinoma of the uterine cervix either as a sequela of disease progression or as a complication of radiotherapy or surgery.

Other Causes

The less common causes are as follows:

Inflammatory bowel conditions—for example, Crohn's disease
Trauma mainly from foreign vaginal bodies
Congenital abnormalities

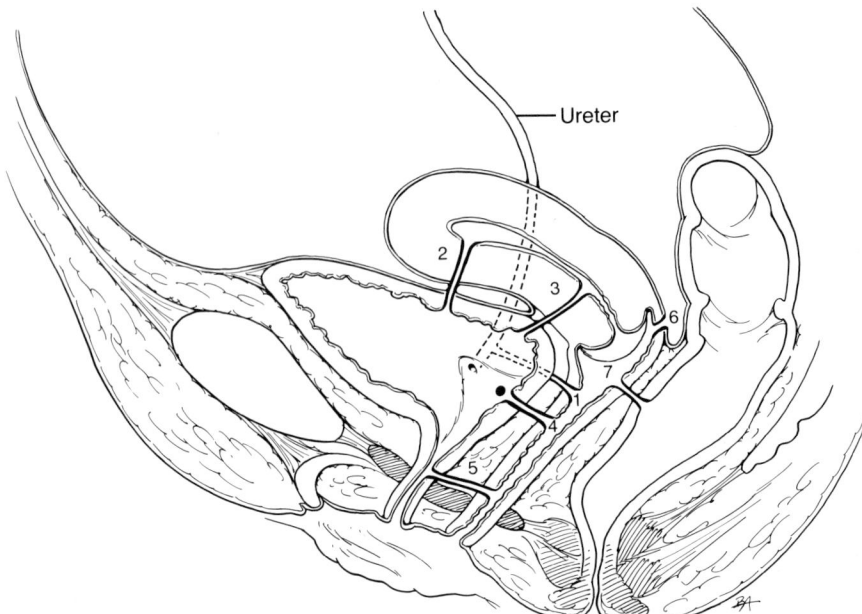

Figure 12-1
Anatomy of female genital fistulae: 1, ureterovaginal; 2, vesicouterovaginal; 3, vesicocervicovaginal 4, vesicovaginal; 5, urethrovaginal; 6, enterovaginal; 7, rectovaginal.

There are very few medical conditions in which the old dictum "The prevention is better than the cure" is more appropriate than in the management of vaginal fistulas. Recognition of bladder injury during gynecologic surgery and primary closure with 3–0 polyglycolic or chromic running sutures in two layers and subsequently postoperative bladder drainage are the most important preventive steps in modern gynecology.

Diagnosis and Preoperative Management

The most common symptom of vesicovaginal fistula is involuntary total incontinence. In instances in which the fistula is small, the urinary leakage will be slight or even intermittent. The latter will happen in cases of a small fistula in which the narrow track works as a valve. Following gynecologic surgery, the triad of watery vaginal discharge, abdominal pain, and elevated temperature is very suggestive of a developing fistula. The appearance of discharge as early as a few hours after the operation suggests fistula due to direct trauma of the urinary tract. Development of fistula a few days later suggests indirect injury with subsequent devascularization. The diagnosis is usually made by speculum examination in the dorsal lithotomy position. If the fistula is not easily visible, the bladder is filled with dilute methylene blue or sterile milk, which can be visualized in the vagina. The tampon Moir test can be utilized to distinguish between a small ureterovaginal and vesicovaginal fistula.[2] It consists of instilling 150–200 ml of diluted methylene blue into the bladder and placing three tampons in the vagina. The patient is then encouraged to walk for 10 minutes before the tampons are removed. If the lower tampon is blue, the patient presumably suffers from stress incontinence. If the middle tampon is wet and blue, the diagnosis is vesicovaginal fistula; if the upper tampon is just wet, but not blue, ureteric injury is most likely.

A good history and gynecologic examination with or without instillation of the dye will diagnose a fistula in the majority of cases. To complete the evaluation, cystoscopy and intravenous pyelogram are recommended. Ureteral dilatation on the affected side is not an uncommon finding. The greatest value of cystoscopy is in the assessment of the relationship between the fistula and the uterteric orifices. In cases of suspected ureterovaginal fistula, a retrograde pyelogram is indicated because it is more likely to visualize the leakage than the intravenous pyelogram.

Principles and Methods of Treatment

The treatment of vesicovaginal fistula is summarized in Table 12-1.

A small postoperative fistula in nonmalignant situations has a good chance of healing, provided that sufficient bladder drainage is maintained for 2–3 weeks. When a ureterovaginal fistula is diagnosed immediately postoperatively, a ureteral stent should be inserted and left in place for 2 weeks. Because of edema, the attempt at insertion may be unsuccessful and should be repeated a week later. The spontaneous healing of a ureterovaginal fistula is feasible provided that there is continuity of the ureteral lumen and the infralesional ureter is normal.[3]

Table 12–1

Treatment of Vesicovaginal Fistula

    Spontaneous closure
    Cautery of the fistulous tract
    Surgical repair
        Vaginal
            Primary closure
                Interposition of a flap
        Abdominal
            Primary closure
                Interposition of a flap
        Combination of both
    Diversion of urine
    Ureteric blockage by percutaneous techniques

Small fistulas, up to 2 mm in size, have been treated by fulguration or chemical cautery with subsequent bladder drainage.[4,5] However, this approach has a high failure rate with additional damage inflicted on surrounding tissues. The modern approach is to treat persistent fistulas surgically even when they are of small size.

Principles of Surgical Repair

1. *Timing* is important. The time-proven recommendation is to wait for 3–6 months until tissues are free of infection and edema. Early closure at the time of diagnosis is an accepted alternative, provided that the site is nonfriable and free of edema.[6,7]

2. *Good exposure* is essential, with the patient usually in the dorsal lithotomy position with Trendelenburg's tilt. The majority of the fistulas will be accessible this way. However, in some instances the knee-chest position is preferable, particularly for anterior vaginal lesions retracted behind the pubis. Assistants on both sides are essential, and good exposure is achieved by using the Sims, Breisky, or Wertheim retractors.

3. *Mobilization and dissection* of the fistulous tract and surrounding scar tissue are of utmost importance. Complete excision of vaginal mucosa close to the tract is recommended.

4. *Surgical closure* of the appropriate layers should be achieved without tension and preferably with the closures not overlapping each other. If the latter cannot be achieved, interposition of a tissue flap may be utilized. The bladder closure should be watertight, and this can be tested by instillation of diluted methylene blue or sterile milk into the bladder.

5. *Bladder drainage* postoperatively is best achieved by suprapubic catheterization for a period of 10–14 days. There are various catheters available, and the advantages of the suprapubic versus urethral catheters are mainly decreased urinary infection, improved patient comfort, and early voiding.

Surgical Repair by Vaginal Approach

Modified Sims-Emmet Technique. The principle of this technique is total excision of the fistulous tract with mobilization of surrounding tissues. It is usually suitable for small to moderate-sized fistulas up to 2 cm in diameter. The excision of a small fistulous tract may be helped by using a Foley catheter as shown in Figure 12–2. Excision of larger fistulas situated in the bladder trigone can endanger the ureters at their insertion. This complication can be greatly reduced by passing ureteric stents prior to surgery. In large fistulas, the plugging of the defect during cystoscopy may be a trial of the surgeon's ingenuity. However, with ureters clearly identified, the excision of the fistula can be safely performed (Fig. 12–3). It is the closure of the bladder wall rather than the vagina that determines the success of the procedure. The closure is performed using 3–0 polyglycolic or chromic sutures, excluding the bladder mucosa. Watertight closure should be achieved, using a second

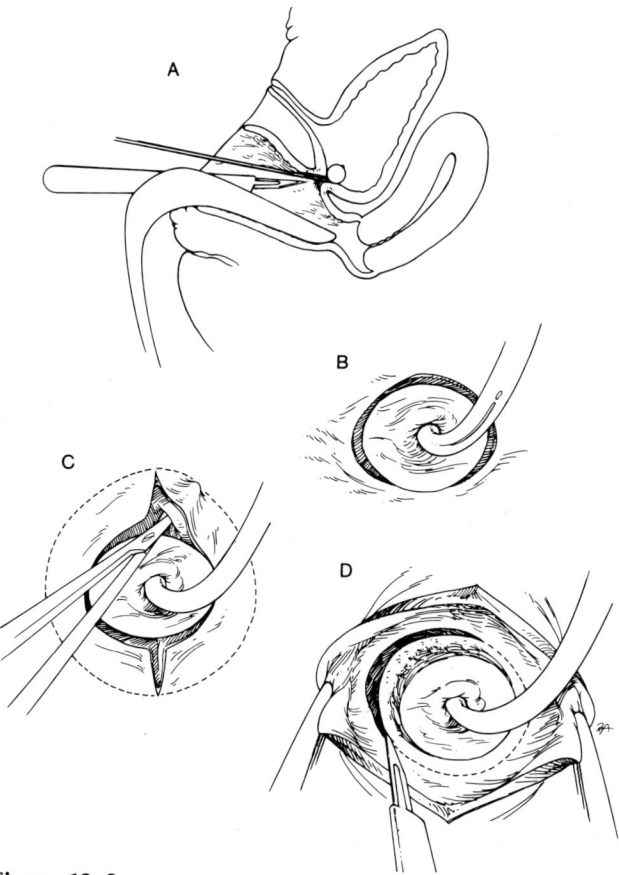

Figure 12–2
Modified Sims-Emmet technique. *A* and *B*, A small Foley catheter is passed through the fistula, and a circular incision is made through the vaginal wall. *C*, Two longitudinal incisions are made through the vaginal wall. *D*, The vaginal wall is undermined and separated from the bladder. The excision of the fistulous tract is completed by circular incision through the bladder wall.

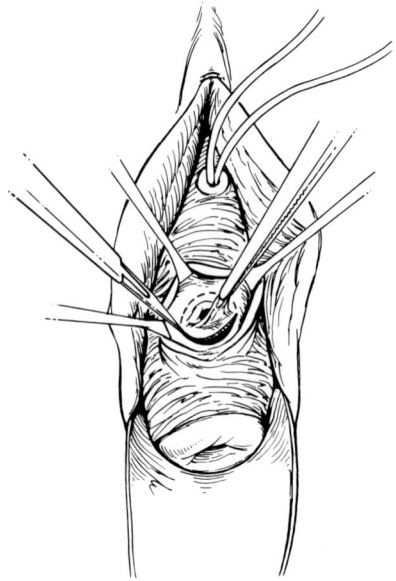

Figure 12–3
Modified Sims-Emmet technique. Larger fistula is excised without the help of a Foley catheter. Ureteric stents have been passed to prevent damage to the ureters.

layer if need be. There seems to be no clear advantage of interrupted over continuous sutures. The vagina is then closed using 2–0 polyglycolic or chromic mattress suture (Fig. 12–4). Running suture is also an acceptable alternative.

Füth-Mayo Technique. In this method, the fistula is circumcised through the vaginal wall, leaving a small vaginal cuff.[8] After careful mobilization of the centrifugal vaginal wall, the bladder wall is exposed. The fistula with the small cuff of attached vaginal epithelium is invaginated into the urinary bladder. The suture of the bladder fascia and muscularis layers is performed with 3–0 polyglycolic or chromic sutures, which close the defect. The vagina is closed using 2–0 polyglycolic or chromic sutures.

Latzko's Technique. This is the procedure of partial colpocleisis with the obliteration of the upper vagina. Its main use is to repair a fistula following total or radical abdominal hysterectomy.[9] The nature of the injury invariably places the defect in the upper vagina, and exposure may be difficult. The fistula can be pulled downward by placing tension sutures near the opening, or when the vagina is narrow a large episiotomy will provide adequate exposure. The technique requires a circular cut through the vaginal wall approximately 2 cm in diameter. The vaginal wall within the circle is then separated from the bladder and excised. The separation may be facilitated by infiltrating the tissues with saline or epinephrine in 1:200,000 dilution. The excision of the fistulous tract is controversial. Latzko did not feel it necessary,[9] but some authors recommend it to enable better healing.[10] The closure is accomplished by interrupted 3–0 polyglycolic or chromic sutures as shown in Figure 12–5, with a second layer inverting the previous suture line. After a test for leakage, the vagina is closed using 2–0 polyglycolic or chromic suture. The vagina is made shorter, but this usually does not create a social problem.

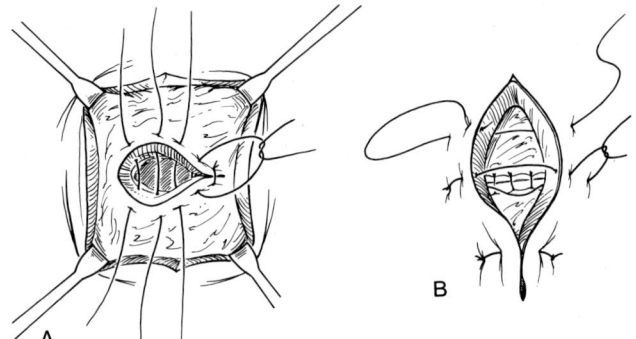

Figure 12–4
Closure of vesicovaginal fistula. *A*, Bladder is sutured in two layers, excluding the bladder mucosa. *B*, The vaginal closure is completed using mattress suture.

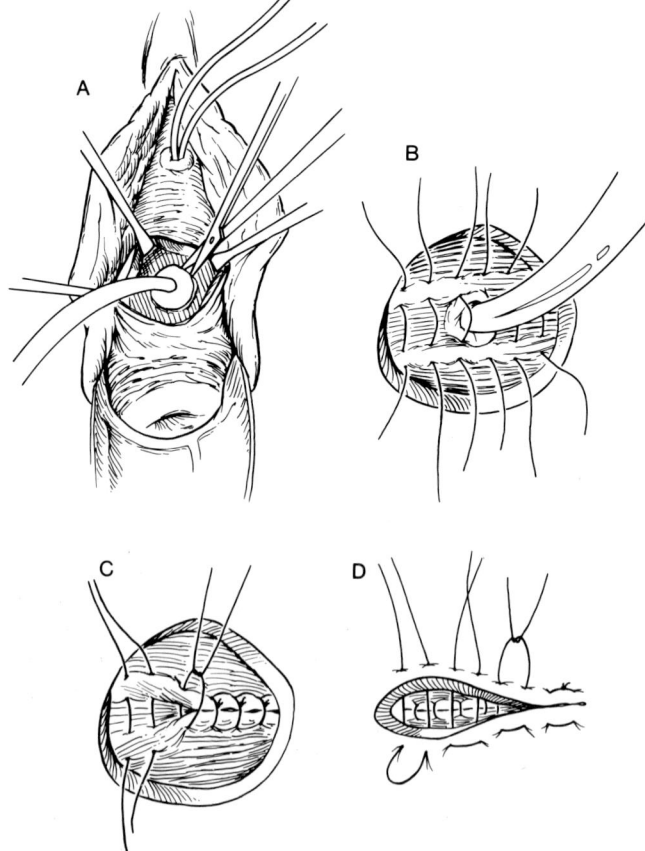

Figure 12–5
Latzko's technique. *A*, Disc of vaginal wall surrounding the fistula is excised. *B*, The first layer of sutures will invert the bladder wall. *C*, The second layer will ensure watertight closure. *D*, Closure of the vagina by simple or mattress sutures.

Martius' Bulbocavernous Flap Technique. At times the surgeon faces a fistula in an irradiated area, with poor vascularization and lack of surrounding healthy tissue. The repair can be supported by using pedicle grafts interposed between the bladder and the vagina. A fistula in the lower part of the vagina is well suited for the Martius flap technique shown in Figure 12–6. Large defects or defects in the upper vagina may be repaired with the help of gracilis or rectus abdominis pedicles. These techniques are beyond the scope of this text.

Abdominal Approach

The usual approach to vaginal problems for a gynecologist is by the vaginal route. There are very few fistulas that are not amenable to vaginal repair. If the patient is referred to a urologist, the abdominal approach will be chosen unless the fistula is positioned very low in the vagina. There are, however, certain situations in which a gynecologist is advised to adopt the abdominal approach:

1. Multiple failed previous repairs
2. Inadequate exposure due to narrow, scarred vagina
3. Other pelvic pathology or involvement of other organs—for example, bowel, ureter, or uterus
4. Ureteric orifice in close proximity to the fistula

The principles of abdominal closure of a fistula are identical to those described for the vaginal approach. The bladder wall has to be adequately mobilized, and watertight closure is accomplished using two layers of continuous 3-0 polyglycolic or chromic sutures. If the ureteric orifices are in close proximity to the fistula edge, passing ureteric stents is essential to prevent ureteric injury. In situations in which the ureter is involved in the fistula, it must be cut off and reimplanted away from the closure. In cases of severe inflammation or poor vascularization mainly due to previous irradiation, a "J" omental flap or paravesical peritoneal flap helps to achieve successful healing.

Urinary Diversion

In spite of improvements in the therapy of female genital cancer, large fistulas will continue to occur, mainly owing to complications of radiotherapy or recurrent disease. More often than not, the unfavorable tissue changes will prevent primary closure of the fistula. Uncontrolled leakage of urine makes the patient's life miserable, and urinary diversion brings much needed relief. The chosen technique for this procedure will depend on the surgeon's preference and experience as well as the patient's life expectancy. If the fistula is caused by necrosis rather than persistent or recurrent malignancy, the patient's life expectancy is good, and ileal or colonic conduits are suitable possibilities. The part of the bowel used for the conduit should come from an area that was not irradiated. More and more gynecologic oncologists use transverse colon as a suitable reservoir. Tech-

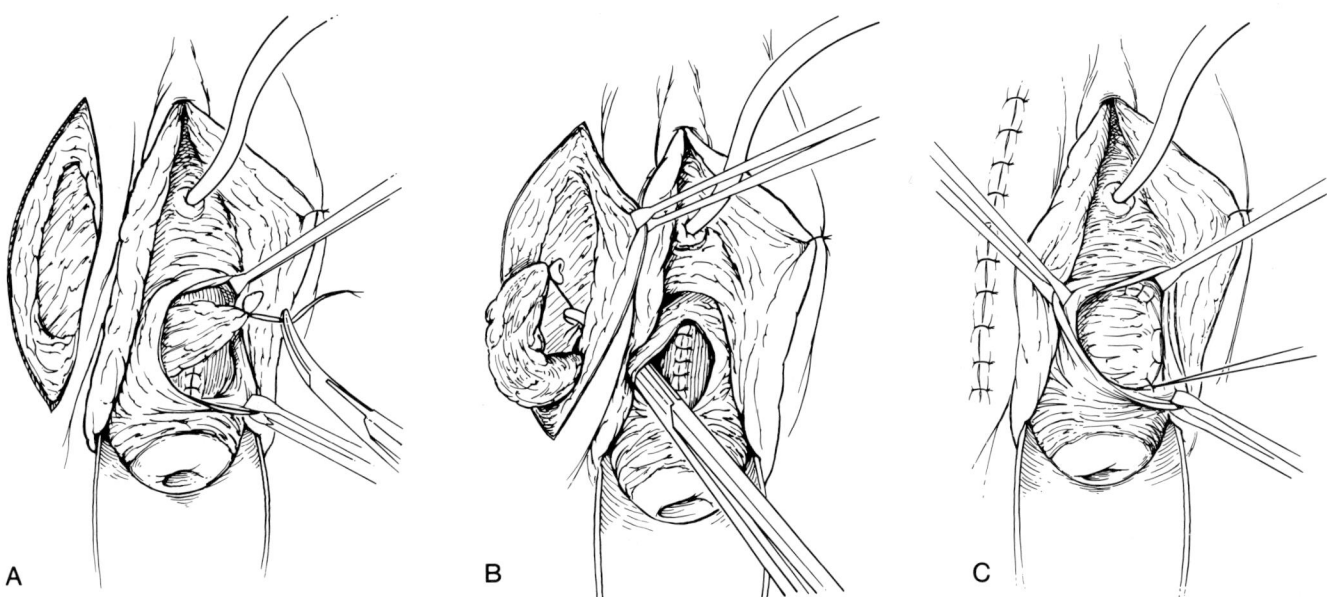

Figure 12–6
Martius bulbocavernosus pedicle graft. *A*, The urinary bladder closure is completed. An incision is performed through the labia majora and the pedicle is mobilized, leaving the attachment posteriorly. *B*, The pedicle is drawn to the operating field under the skin bridge. *C*, Flap is sutured to the paravaginal fascia; closure of the vagina (not shown) completes the procedure.

niques of "continent" conduits are preferred by some surgeons and can be found in standard urology texts.

In cases of persistent or recurrent disease, the same approach may be taken, although palliative cutaneous ureterostomy causes less operative trauma and may be preferable. The usual stenosis is not a problem, owing to the short life expectancy. With the development of invasive radiology, a suitable alternative may be offered without major surgery. Percutaneous nephrostomy is performed under ultrasound guidance, and the ureter is blocked in its distal part by nylon plugs and "glue" bucrylate,[11] electrocautery,[12] or percutaneous ureteral clips.[13] The small nephrostomy tube remains above the block and is easily taken care of by the patient. These methods are new and have many "teething problems," but they will be part of the incurable fistula management in the future.

RECTOVAGINAL FISTULA

By definition, *rectovaginal fistula* represents a communication between the vagina and rectum. Although much more talked about and often grouped together with anovaginal fistula, rectovaginal fistula accounts for only 5% of anorectal fistulas.[14] It is defined as a fistula adjacent to the external sphincter as far as 3 cm from the anal orifice. Anatomically, that division is represented by the dentate line. All fistulas occurring above the dentate line are truly rectovaginal. Although a few cases are asymptomatic, for most women the symptoms of rectovaginal fistula are extremely distressing, often converting them into social outcasts.

Etiology

Any hollow viscus may become malformed during embryologic development, and the rectum is not an exception. Congenital rectovaginal fistula usually develops as a sequel to imperforate anus when the rectum opens into the posterior vaginal fornix. It is a rare occurrence, with a frequency of approximately 1:5000 births. However, the majority of rectovaginal fistulas are a result of acquired disorders.

Obstetric Injury

Fistulas can develop as a result of prolonged, obstructed labor; trauma during vaginal delivery, particularly owing to instrumentation, leading to a fourth-degree perineal tear; or as a complication of cesarean section.

Gynecologic Malignancy

The formation of a fistula is mainly associated with carcinoma of the uterine cervix. It may be due to progression of disease or as a complication of radiotherapy. The incidence has been reported to range from 1% to 10%.[15, 16]

Inflammatory Bowel Disease

Crohn's disease as well as ulcerative colitis can cause rectovaginal fistulas. The former is more likely to be responsible when the full thickness of the wall is involved by the inflammatory process. Diverticular disease with abscess formation near the vagina and its subsequent discharge through the vagina can also result in fistula formation.

Trauma

The majority of these fistulas are caused by obstetric trauma, particularly when associated with inadequate repair and secondary infection.

Other Causes

The less common causes are as follows:

Trauma during abdominal gynecologic surgery or foreign body trauma causing a penetrating wound or pressure necrosis (e.g., supportive pessary).

Hematologic malignancies (e.g. leukemias or lymphomas).

Endometriosis.

Infection. Bartholin's gland abscess, rectal or perianal abscesses, and lymphogranuloma venereum can all penetrate through the vaginal wall and cause a fistula.

Classification

Rectovaginal fistulas are classified by their size and location. The fistula is small when it is less than 0.5 cm in diameter, medium when between 0.5 cm and 2.5 cm, and large when over 2.5 cm. By location, the fistula is described as high when it is situated near the uterine cervix in the area covered by peritoneum, and low when it is above the dentate line near the sphincter and perineal body. The mid-fistula fills the gap between high and low locations.

Diagnosis and Preoperative Management

The symptoms of rectovaginal fistula may vary from vaginal odor, with or without discharge, to passage of frank stool through the vagina. The symptoms are invariably exaggerated in the presence of diarrhea. The majority of rectovaginal fistulas can be visualized directly either by spreading the labia with the examiner's fingers or with the help of a vaginal speculum. The visualization of a small fistula may present a diagnostic challenge. The equivalent of the Moir tampon test (diagnosis of vesicovaginal fistula) is useful in the diagnosis.[17] Methylene blue is instilled into the rectum, and the sphincter is plugged with a tampon. Another tampon is placed in the vagina, and the patient is encouraged to walk for 10–15 minutes. Any methylene blue stain on the vaginal tampon is strongly suggestive of rectovaginal fistula. In case of suspicion of bowel inflammatory disease (weight loss, fistula painful to touch) barium enema and/or colonoscopy should evaluate the rest of the colon. Proctoscopy should conclude the diagnostic work-up. The repair of a fistula due to inflammatory bowel disease is notoriously unsuccessful.

Preoperative Bowel Preparation

Ideally, the surgical field should be clean and sterile. However, systemic antibiotics given for a short period of time seem to have little effect on intestinal bacterial flora. It is the mechanical clearance that is undoubtedly beneficial and, in combination with laxatives, enable the surgeon to operate in a relatively clean field. The preoperative bowel preparation as described in Chapter 21, should be used for all patients.

Principles and Methods of Treatment

The treatment of rectovaginal fistula is summarized in Table 12–2.

A small rectovaginal fistula that is due to operative injury or foreign body injury has a fair chance of spontaneous healing, provided that the foreign body has been removed and satisfactory treatment of a local infectious process has been accomplished. On the other hand, fistulas due to inflammatory bowel disease, neoplasm, or irradiation, however small, hardly ever heal spontaneously.

Principles of Surgical Repair

1. *Timing* is of vital importance to the success of surgical repair. Fistulas due to obstetric trauma have a 50% chance of healing spontaneously, and the usual recommendation is to wait 6 months before attempting repair. Generally, the surrounding tissues should be as healthy as possible, presenting as soft and pliable. There are no scientific rules about timing, but it is generally accepted to wait at least 3 months in case of trauma or infection and 6 months to a year in cases of post-irradiation fistula, usually with a proximal colostomy.

2. *Approach and exposure.* High fistulas are invariably approached via the abdominal route. However, fistulas in the lower part of the vagina are usually repaired vaginally by gynecologists and rectally by surgeons. The latter emphasize that the rectum presents the high-pressure area; its closure is essential to the success of the repair, and the exposure is better by this approach. There is no doubt that careful closure of the rectal wall is the cornerstone of success, and this must be kept in mind regardless of the approach.

3. Mobilization of tissues around the fistula and excision of scar tissue in and around the fistula are essential.

4. Layer-for-layer closure with broad approximation of the surrounding tissue should be accomplished without tension, and if direct overlap of the vaginal and rectal closures is a problem, flap interposition or flap advancement techniques may be utilized.

5. If drainage of the area is required, the vaginal side (low-pressure area) of the fistula should be left open, with or without insertion of a drain.

6. Prevention of constipation postoperatively is accomplished by administering stool softeners. Docusate sodium (Colace) is one of the possibilities and should be given for approximately 1 month. Delayed defecation is desirable, and patients may be started on a liquid diet postoperatively with advancement to a low-residue diet on the third postoperative day. Coitus should be avoided for a minimum of 2 months.

Surgical Repair by Vaginal Approach

Repair of a Low Fistula by Creating a Fourth-Degree Perineal Tear. Every obstetrician-gynecologist

Table 12–2
Treatment of Rectovaginal Fistula

Spontaneous closure
Surgical correction
  Vaginal approach
    Creation of fourth-degree perineal defect
    Repair of small fistula by inversion into the rectum
    Repair of large fistula by excision and layer closure
    Martius' bulbocavernous flap interposition
    Warren's flap for repair of healed complete fourth-degree tear
      Anterior rectal wall sliding flap advancement: Noble-Mengert-Fish procedure
      Partial colpocleisis: Latzko procedure
  Anorectal approach
    Transanal mucosal flap advancement
    Endorectal flap advancement
  Abdominal approach

220 VAGINAL FISTULAS: OPERATIVE MANAGEMENT

has sufficient training to repair obstetric perineal trauma, because fourth-degree tears are not infrequent in daily practice. The low-lying rectovaginal fistula can be successfully repaired by cutting through the sphincter to the fistula and creating a fourth-degree defect as shown in Figure 12–7. To enhance the likelihood of success, the fibrous edges of the fistula must be completely excised and the vaginal wall widely separated from the rectum. Soft, normal looking edges of rectal and vaginal mucosa with fresh bleeding are desirable. The closure starts at the apex of the rectal opening and continues through the anal mucosa, using 3–0 polyglycolic or chromic continuous suture. The full-thickness suture is the safest. The sphincter ends are identified and approximated with 0 polyglycolic or chromic inter-

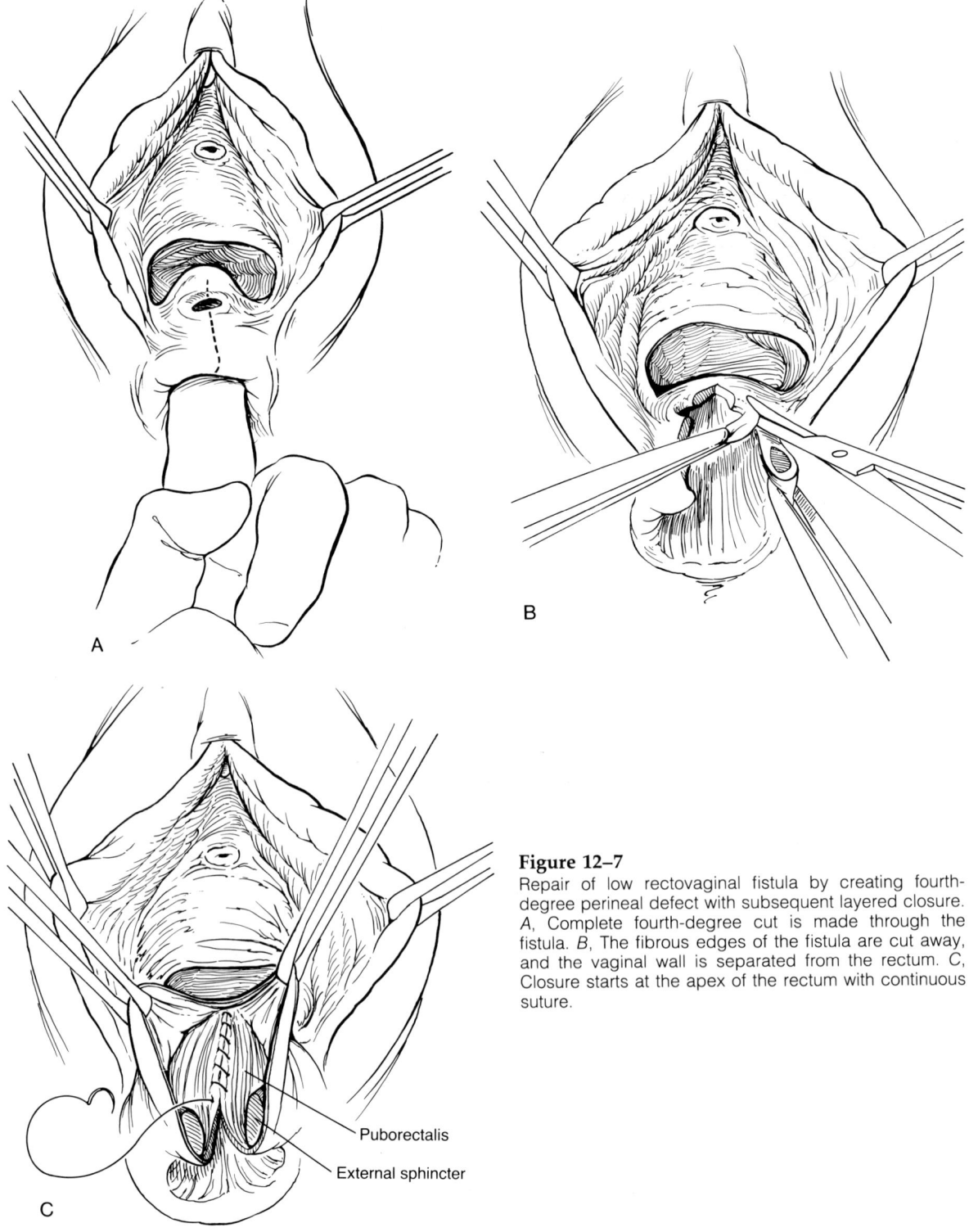

Figure 12–7
Repair of low rectovaginal fistula by creating fourth-degree perineal defect with subsequent layered closure. *A*, Complete fourth-degree cut is made through the fistula. *B*, The fibrous edges of the fistula are cut away, and the vaginal wall is separated from the rectum. *C*, Closure starts at the apex of the rectum with continuous suture.

VAGINAL FISTULAS: OPERATIVE MANAGEMENT 221

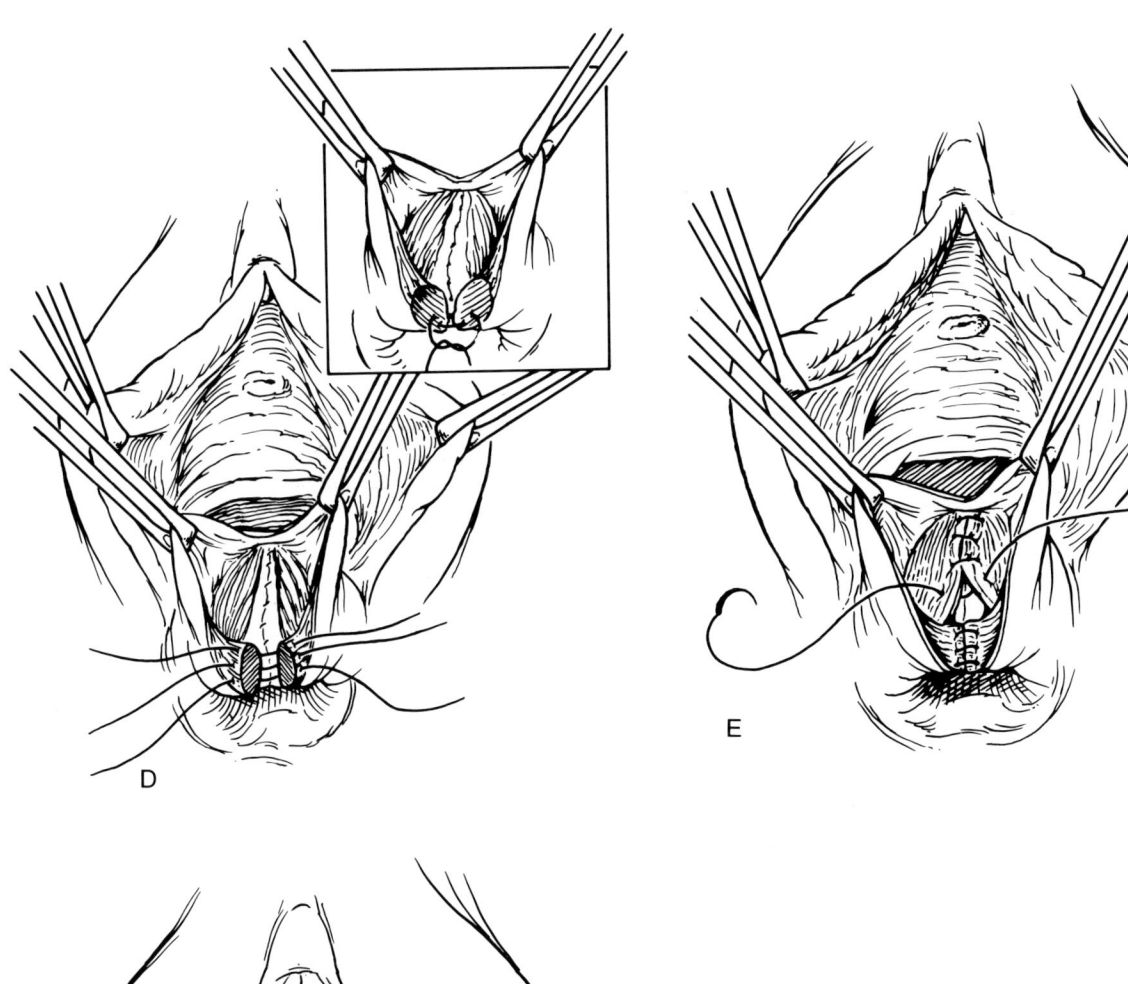

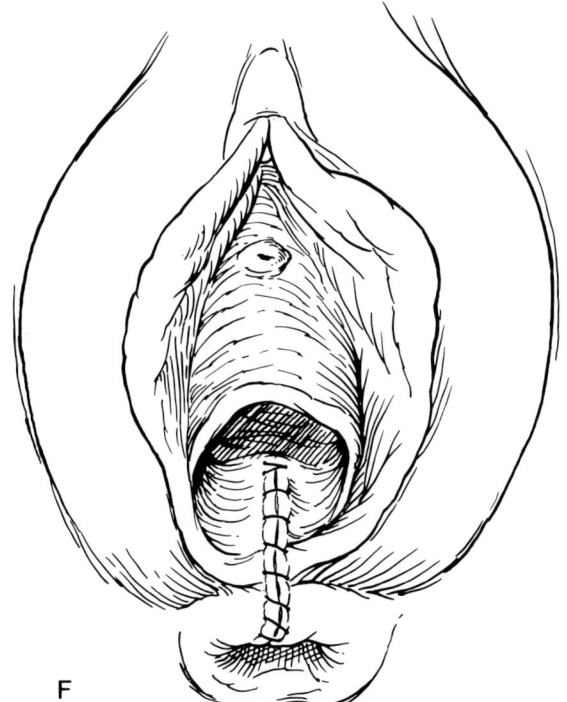

Figure 12–7 *Continued*
D, Sphincter is approximated using through-and-through or near-and-far techniques. *E*, The puborectalis muscles are approximated by interrupted suture. *F*, Closure of the vagina and perineal skin.

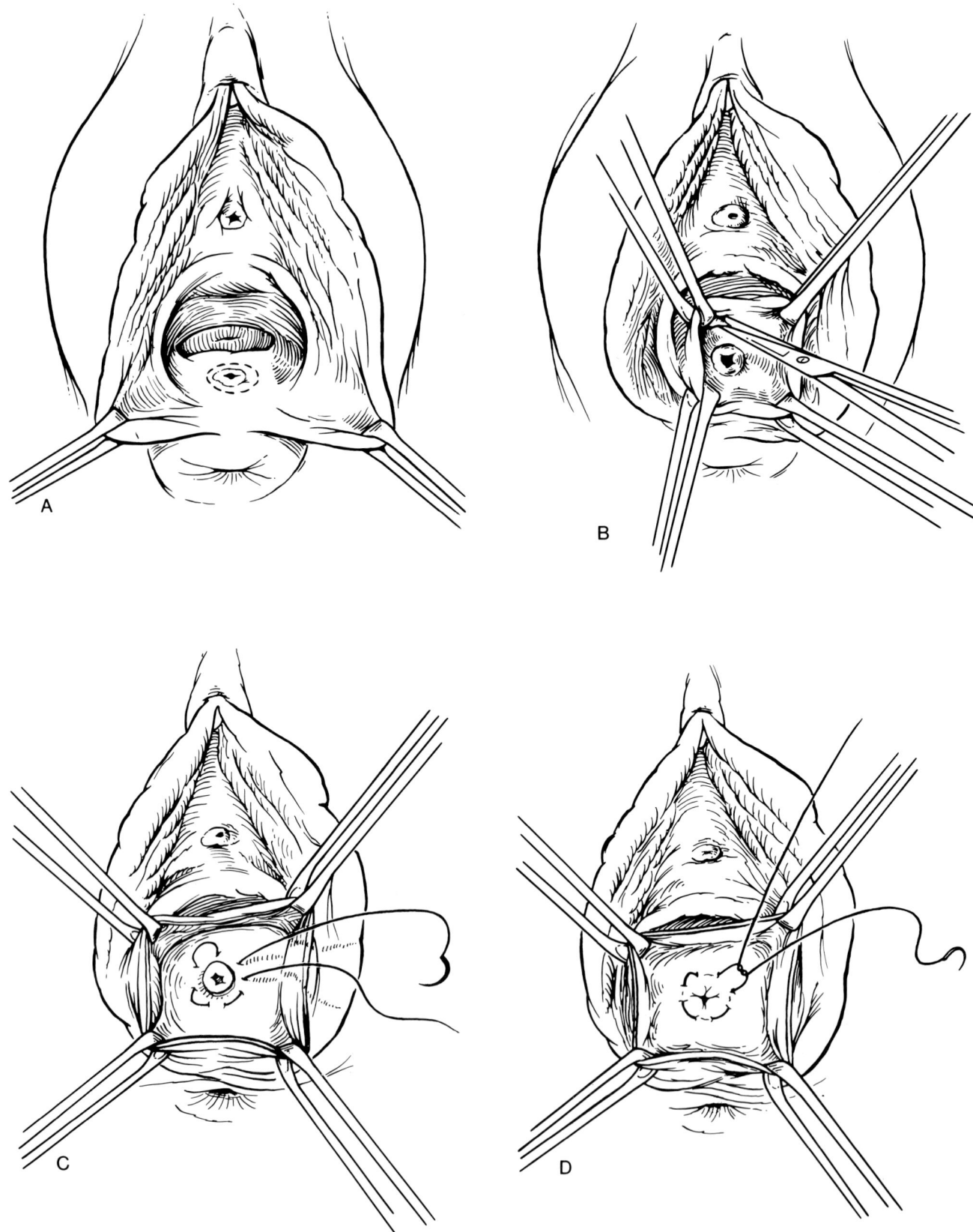

Figure 12–8
Repair of a small rectovaginal fistula. A, A circular incision is made through the vaginal mucosa 4–5 mm from the fistulous opening. B, Vaginal mucosa is undercut to approximately 2 cm around the opening. C, Pursestring stitch is placed around the opening, and the fistula is inverted into the rectum. D, Second pursestring stitch is placed.

rupted stitches, making sure that the suture brings the muscle ends together. In the case of frayed sphincter ends or sutures pulling through, the near-and-far suture technique is desirable as shown in Figure 12–7E.

The puborectalis (levator) muscles are approximated using 0 polyglycolic or chromic interrupted suture. Good support is obtained by bringing the muscle to the midline high up in the vaginal canal, while observing the diameter of the vagina. The procedure is then completed by a continuous 2–0 polyglycolic or chromic suture of the vagina (starting at the apex) and subsequent closure of the perineum.

Repair of a Small Fistula by Inversion into the Rectum. For a small rectovaginal fistula with a reasonably intact perineal body, the method of repair shown in Figure 12–8 may be used. A circular incision is made through the vaginal mucosa approximately 5 mm from the fistulous opening. The vaginal mucosa is then undercut for about 4–5 cm, freely mobilizing the bowel wall. A pursestring stitch of 3–0 polyglycolic or chromic suture is placed in the bowel submucosa around the defect. When this is tied, the fistula is inverted into the bowel lumen. A second pursestring stitch is placed a few millimeters beyond the first and tied. A third layer of 3–0 polyglycolic or chromic continuous suture provides closure of the rectovaginal space. The procedure is completed by closing the vagina with continuous 2–0 polyglycolic or chromic suture.

Repair of a Large Fistula by Excision and Layer Closure. An incision is made through the vaginal wall, below the fistula, and with a finger, the rectum is dissected from the vaginal wall. A longitudinal vaginal incision is performed, heading towards the fistula, and then the vaginal part of fistula is excised Figure 12–9. With traction on the fistula, the rectal wall immediately around it is excised, leaving a fresh, round defect. The rectal wall must be sufficiently mobilized to enable subsequent closure without tension. This is accomplished using 3–0 polyglycolic or chromic sutures. The goal is to invert the edges of the tract into the bowel lumen, and this can be achieved either by vertical mattress sutures (not entering the bowel lumen) or with a continuous suture (excluding the mucosa). To broaden the area of tissue apposition between the defects, a second layer of interrupted or continuous sutures, using the same material, is inserted a few millimeters beyond the first. The next layer depends on the position of the fistula in the vagina. In the upper vagina, the pararectal fascia is approximated with 2–0 polyglycolic or chromic interrupted sutures. In the lower vagina, the puborectalis muscles are approximated

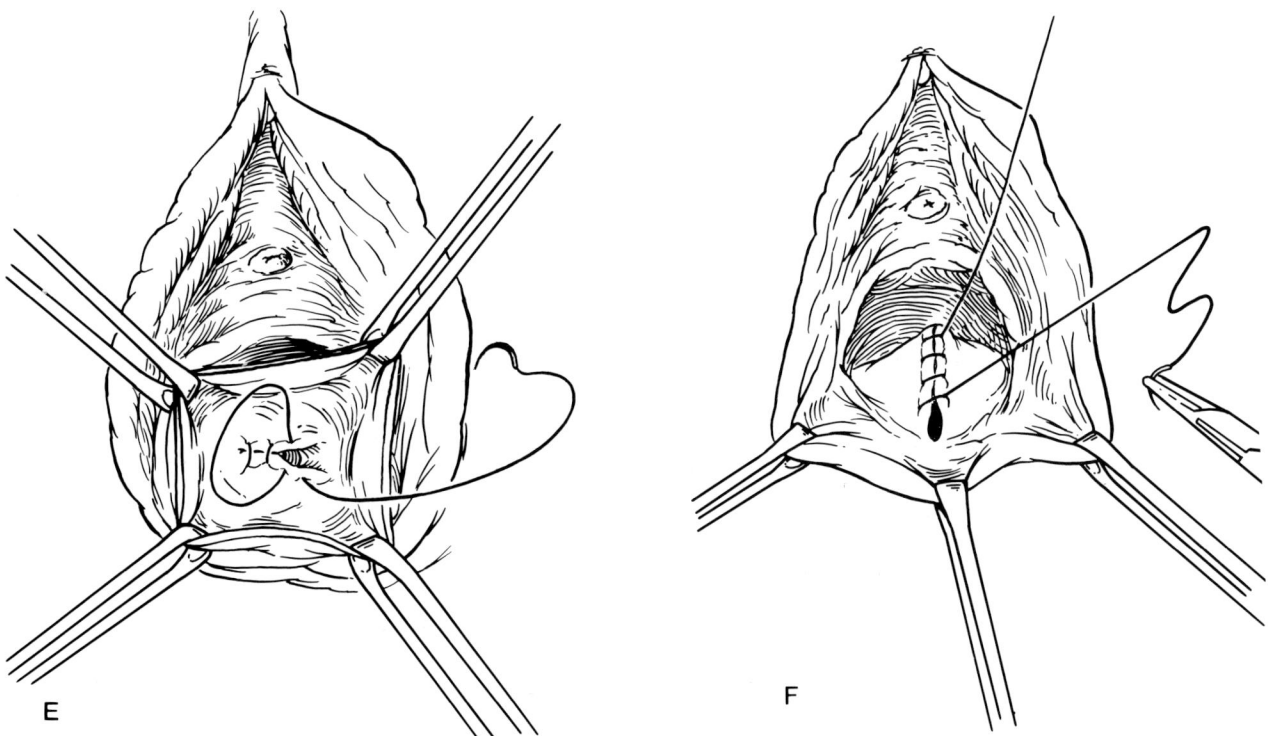

Figure 12–8 *Continued*
E, Third layer provides closure of rectovaginal space. F, Vagina is closed using continuous locking suture.

224 VAGINAL FISTULAS: OPERATIVE MANAGEMENT

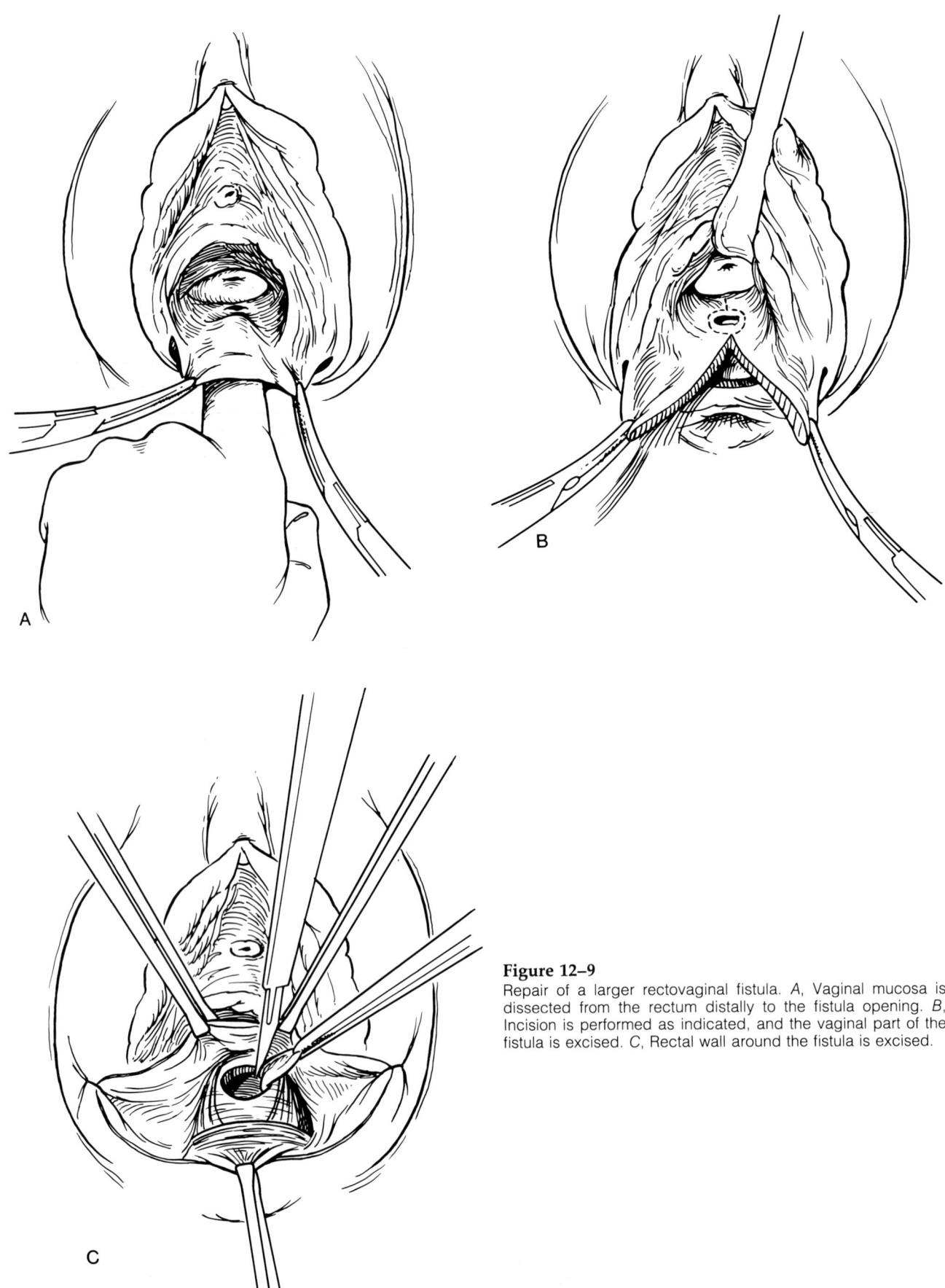

Figure 12–9
Repair of a larger rectovaginal fistula. *A*, Vaginal mucosa is dissected from the rectum distally to the fistula opening. *B*, Incision is performed as indicated, and the vaginal part of the fistula is excised. *C*, Rectal wall around the fistula is excised.

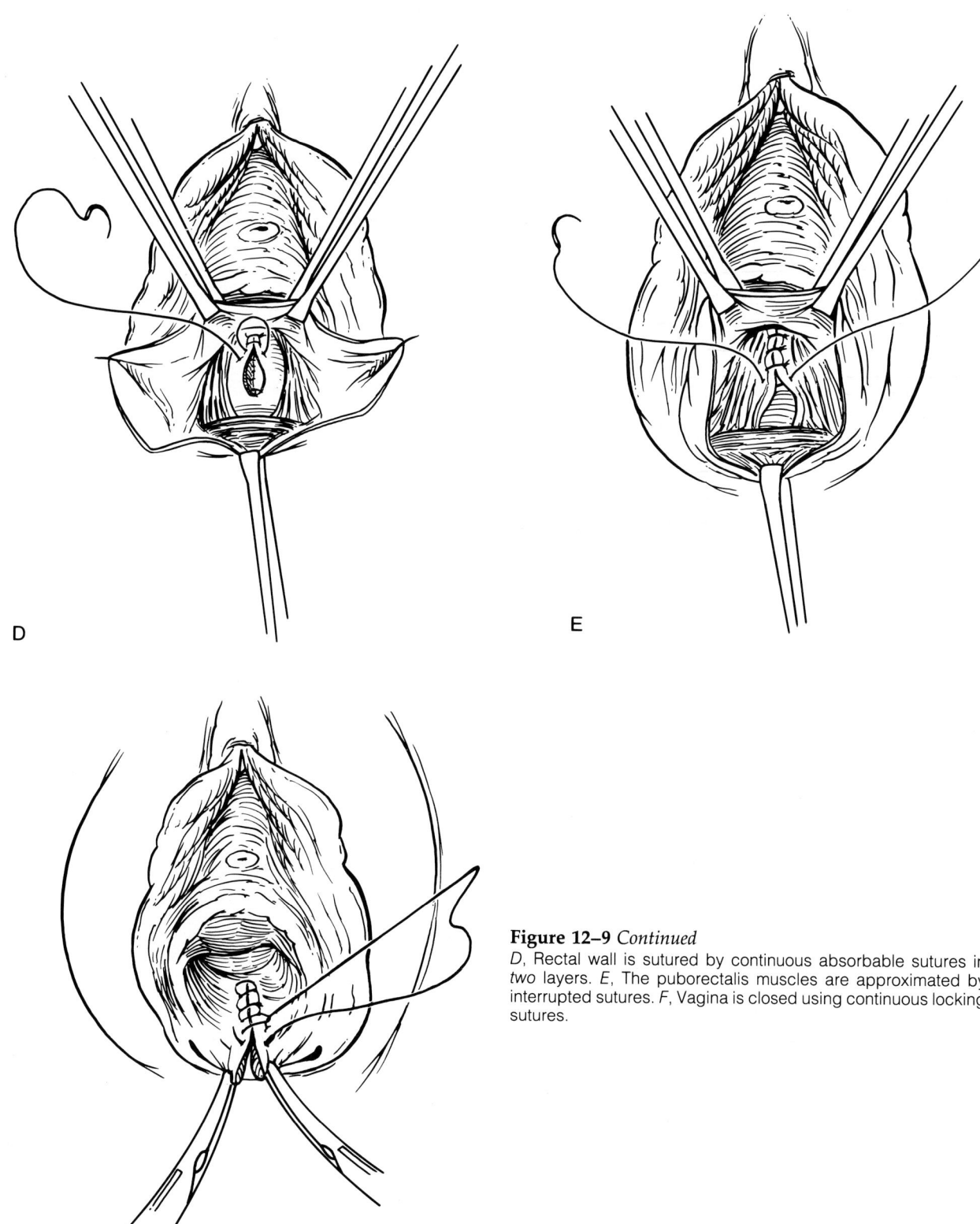

Figure 12–9 *Continued*
D, Rectal wall is sutured by continuous absorbable sutures in *two* layers. *E*, The puborectalis muscles are approximated by interrupted sutures. *F*, Vagina is closed using continuous locking sutures.

with 0 polyglycolic or chromic interrupted sutures. The procedure is completed by closing the vagina with 2–0 polyglycolic or chromic continuous suture.

Martius' Bulbocavernous Flap Interposition. When the rectovaginal fistula is located in the midvagina, the rectovaginal septum is very thin and vascularization in the area may be poor. A vascularized pedicle between the vaginal and rectal walls decreases the possibility of failure. The bulbocavernous flap technique, described by Martius in 1932,[18] can be used for repair of a vesicovaginal fistula, as shown in Figure 12–6, or, by swinging the flap posteriorly, for repair of a rectovaginal fistula.

Warren Flap for Repair of Healed Fourth-Degree Tear. This procedure, described originally by Warren in 1882,[19] consists of creating a flap from the posterior vaginal wall, the part of which becomes the anterior anal margin and the cover for the rebuilt perineum (Fig. 12–10). The incision is made in the shape of an inverted "V", connecting laterally the dimples of the retracted ends of anal sphincter with the apex of the flap approximately 3 cm above the rectovaginal margin. The vaginal flap is dissected and pulled downwards with great care, making sure that the underlying rectal wall is not damaged and the vaginal flap is not too thin. The sphincter ani ends are grasped, brought to the midline, and sutured with 0 polyglycolic or chromic suture. Three through-and-through or far-and-near sutures should suffice. The puborectalis muscles are then approximated with 0 polyglycolic or chromic sutures in the manner described previously for fourth-degree tears. The posterior vaginal wall is sutured with 2–0 polyglycolic or chromic continuous suture, starting at the apex. Redundant vaginal mucosa is trimmed, and the procedure is completed by closing the perineum with an absorbable subcuticular suture.

Noble-Mengert-Fish Procedure: Anterior Rectal Wall Sliding Flap Advancement. This procedure described by Noble in 1902[20] and later popularized by Mengert and Fish, consists of dissecting of rectovaginal septum and drawing the freed anterior anorectal wall outside the anal orifice (Fig. 12–11). An inverted "U" incision is made following the margin of the anal mucosa connecting the dimples of the retracted sphincter ani. The rectovaginal space is entered, and dissection is carried to approximately 4 cm above the line of inversion. The separation of the anal flap is facilitated by gentle traction with Allis' clamps. The main area of separation should be in the midline rather than laterally to avoid bleeding from the inferior hemorrhoidal vessels. The ends of the sphincter ani are then identified, freed as much as possible from scar tissue, brought to the midline, and sutured with 0 polyglycolic or chromic suture in the manner described previously.

The puborectalis muscles are plicated with 0 polyglycolic or chromic interrupted sutures, care being taken not to narrow the vaginal canal. In the case of vaginal narrowing, the proximal stitches may be removed. The vagina is closed from the apex with 2–0 polyglycolic or chromic continuous suture. The redundant vaginal and anal mucosae are trimmed, and the anterior anal wall is pulled over the reconstructed sphincter and sutured to the perineal edges using 2–0 polyglycolic or chromic mattress sutures, forming an inverted "Y" closure (Fig. 12–11*E*).

Latzko Procedure: Partial Colpocleisis. High vaginal fistulas, following hysterectomy or therapy for malignancy, can be treated by partial colpocleisis. The principles and technique are identical to those for the repair of vesicovaginal fistula as described in Figure 12–5. Utmost care must be taken to invert the bowel mucosa into the bowel lumen. The excision of part of the vaginal wall with subsequent closure will result in shortening of the vagina, but adequate function can usually be preserved.

Surgical Repair by Anorectal Approach

This approach is favored by general surgeons. The argument in its favor is that closure of the rectum is the cornerstone of successful repair by shutting off the anorectal source of infection and closing the higher pressure system (up to 80 cm H_2O pressure as opposed to atmospheric pressure in the vagina). To these surgeons, the vaginal closure is of secondary importance, but most gynecologists favor the vaginal approach.

The techniques of transanal mucosal and endorectal flap advancement are beyond the scope of this text and are described elsewhere.[21, 22]

Surgical Repair by Abdominal Approach

This approach may be necessary for two reasons. First, the fistula may be located too high to be accessible by the vaginal or rectal approach. Second, underlying abdominal disease, which led to the creation of the fistula, must be dealt with to facilitate subsequent repair healing. For example, fistula repair without treatment of bowel affected with Crohn's disease is doomed to failure. Rectovaginal fistulas that are the result of active inflammatory bowel disease cannot be treated by traditional layered repair only.

High rectovaginal fistulas not caused by active inflammatory disease or malignancy are best treated by dissection of rectal and vaginal walls in proximity to the fistula. The fistulous tract is excised, and the

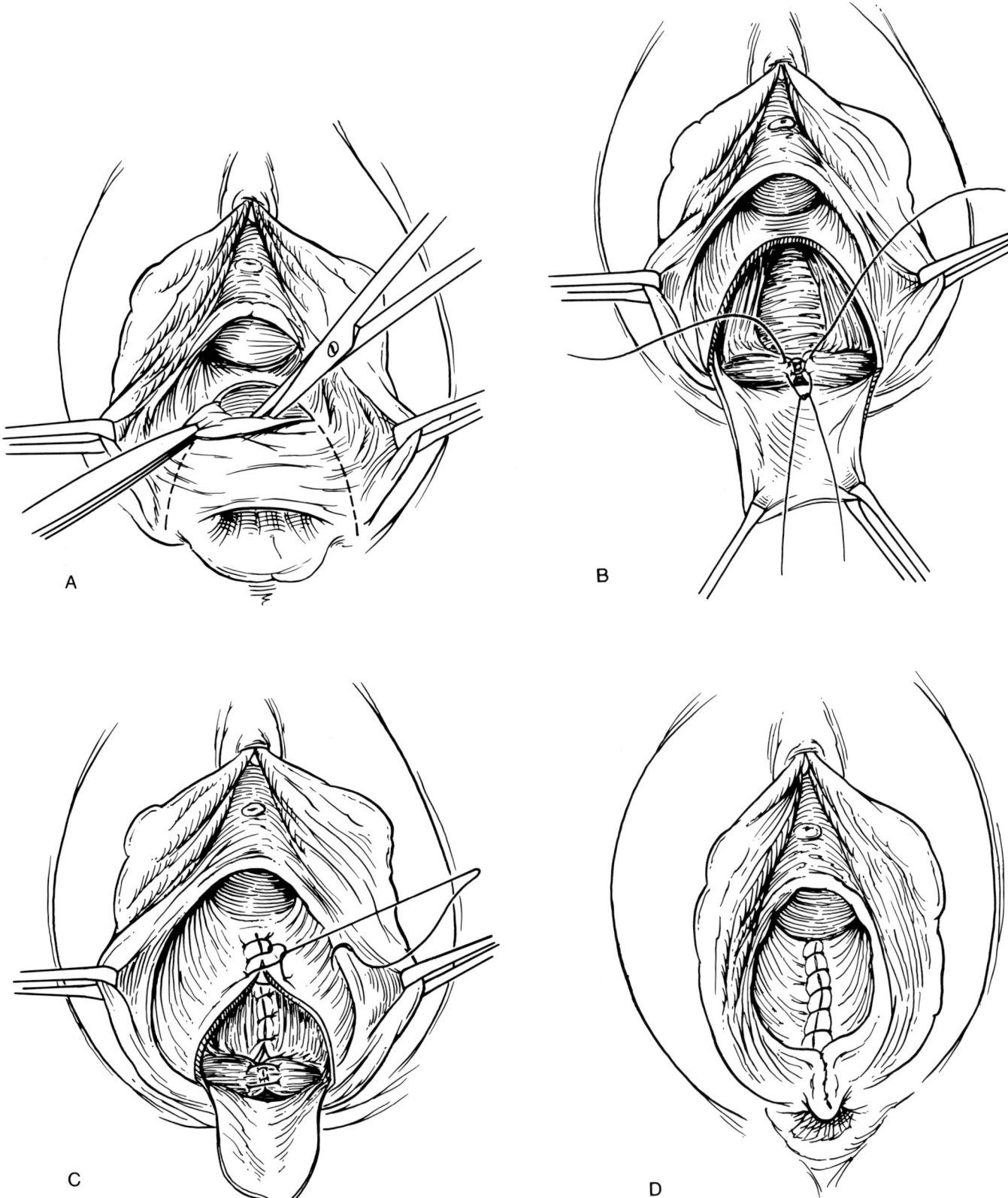

Figure 12–10
Warren flap procedure for repair of healed complete fourth-degree tear. *A*, Line of incision approximately 3 cm above the rectovaginal margin laterally to the dimples of sphincter ani. The vaginal flap is dissected and pulled downward. *B*, The sphincter ani ends are identified and sutured using through-and-through or far-and-near absorbable sutures. *C*, The puborectalis muscles are approximated by interrupted sutures, and the vagina is closed using continuous locking sutures. Redundant vaginal mucosa is trimmed. *D*, The perineal skin is closed using absorbable subcuticular sutures.

228 VAGINAL FISTULAS: OPERATIVE MANAGEMENT

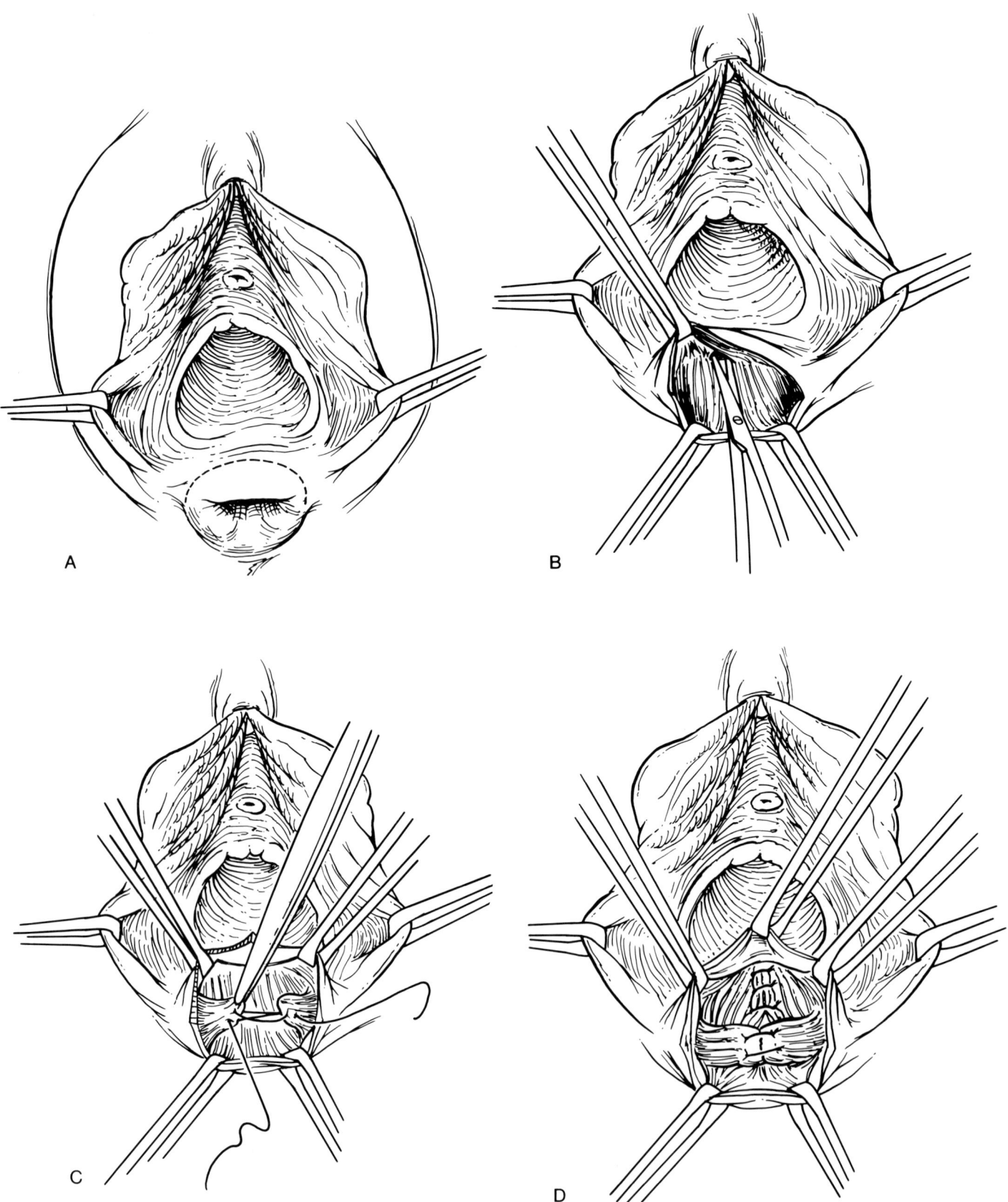

Figure 12–11
Noble-Mengert-Fish procedure. *A*, Line of mucocutaneous incision. *B*, Rectovaginal space is dissected to at least 4 cm from the incision. *C*, The sphincter ani ends are identified and united with absorbable sutures. *D*, The puborectalis muscles are approximated by interrupted sutures.

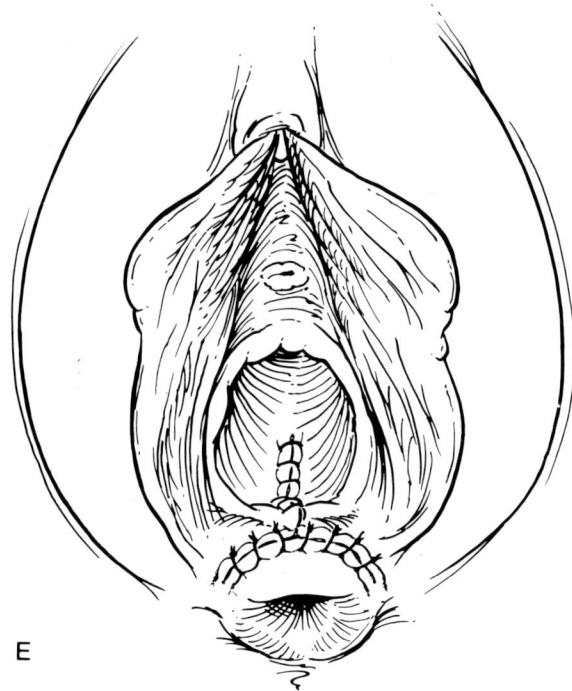

Figure 12–11 *Continued*
E, Vaginal and anal mucosae are closed, resulting in inverted Y suture.

defect in rectal and vaginal walls is closed by an inverting technique, using 3–0 polyglycolic or chromic continuous suture and 2–0 sutures, respectively. The close apposition of the defects in the rectal and vaginal walls in the final repair is not desirable, and separation can be achieved by the following:

1. Additional sutures in rectovaginal septum
2. Interposition of a "J" omental flap
3. Slight rotation of the rectum resulting in its intact wall lying under the vaginal repair

Role of Colostomy

There is a divergence of opinions about the role of colostomy in repair of rectovaginal fistulas ranging from routine to seldom use. The appearance of the rectal and vaginal mucosa is a useful guide to the need for colostomy. Simple fistulas due to trauma will heal without a colostomy. More complex fistulas caused by malignancy, irradiation, or inflammatory bowel disease may require a two-stage procedure—diverting colostomy and subsequent fistula repair. The time between the stages depends on the condition responsible for fistula formation and varies from 3 to 12 months. Following successful repair, the colostomy is closed in 2–3 months.

References

1. Sims JM: On the treatment of vesico-vaginal fistula. Am J Med Sci 1852; 23:59.
2. Moir JC: The Vesicovaginal Fistula, 2nd ed. London, Bailliere, Tindall and Cassell, 1957.
3. Hulse EA: Sawtelle WW, Nadig PW, Wolf HL: Conservative management of ureterovaginal fistula. J Urol 1968; 99:42.
4. Falk HC, Orkin LA: Nonsurgical closure of vesicovaginal fistulas. Obstet Gynecol 1957; 9:538.
5. Hyman RM: Coagulation therapy for small vesicovaginal fistulas. Clin Obstet Gynecol 1968; 8:465.
6. Persky L, Herman G, Guerrier K: Nondelay in vesicovaginal fistula repair. Urology 1974; 13:273.
7. Crinkshank SM: Early closure of posthysterectomy vesicovaginal fistulas. South Med J 1988; 81:1525.
8. Füth H: Zur Operation der Blasenscheidenfisteln. Arch Gynecol 1918; 109:489.
9. Latzko W: Postoperative vesicovaginal fistulas: Genesis and therapy. Am J Surg 1942; 58:211.
10. Mattingly RF, Thompson JD: TeLinde's Operative Gynecology, 6th ed. Vesicovaginal Fistula. Philadelphia, JB Lippincott, 1985.
11. Stern JL, Maroney TP, Lacey CG: Management of incurable urinary fistulas by percutaneous ureteral occlusion. Obstet Gynecol 1987; 70:958.
12. Kopecky KK, Sutton GP, Bihrle R, Becker GJ: Percutaneous transrenal endoureteral radio-frequency electrocautery for occlusion: Case report. Radiology 1989; 170:1047.
13. Darcy MD, Lund BB, Smith TP, et al.: Percutaneously applied ureteral clips: Treatment of vesicovaginal fistula. Radiology 1987; 163:819.
14. Laird DR: Procedures used in treatment of complicated fistulas. Am J Surg 1948; 75:701.
15. Alert J, Jimenes J, Beldarrain L, et al.: Complications from irradiation of carcinoma of the uterine cervix. Acta Radiol Oncol 1980; 19:13.
16. VanNagel JR, Parker JC, Maruyama T, et al.: Bladder or rectal injury following irradiation therapy for cervical cancer. Am J Obstet Gynecol 1974; 119:727.
17. Lesher TC, Pratt JH: Vaginal repair of the simple rectovaginal fistula. Surg Gynecol Obstet 1967; 124:1317.
18. Martius H: Über die Behandlung von Blasenscheidenfisteln insbesondere mit Hilfe einer Lappenplastik. Ztschr. f Geburtsch u Gynäk 1932; 103:22.
19. Warren JC: A new method of operation for the relief of rupture of the perineum through the sphincter of the rectum. Trans Am Gynecol Soc 1882; 7:322.
20. Noble GM: A new operation for complete laceration of the perineum designed for the purpose of eliminating danger of infection from the rectum. Trans Am Gynecol Soc 1902; 27:357.
21. Greenwald JC, Mouter B: Repair of rectovaginal fistulas. Surg Gynecol Obstet 1978; 146:443.
22. Russell TR, Gallagher DM: Low rectovaginal fistulas: Approach and treatment. Am J Surg 1977; 134:13.

Preinvasive Diseases of the Female Lower Genital Tract

13

Michele Follen Mitchell

Forty years ago, preinvasive diseases of the female lower genital tract were treated the same as their invasive counterparts. Today, however, it is known that these preinvasive diseases represent a spectrum of intraepithelial neoplasms ranging from mild dysplasia to carcinoma in situ. Although they have the potential to become invasive neoplasms, their natural history is often characterized by regression or persistence rather than progression. For these reasons, preinvasive diseases lend themselves to less morbid therapies. In recent years, more attention has been focused on the use of the colposcope to detect them and less morbid therapies to treat them.

The natural history of preinvasive lesions is not well understood. Although a great deal of work has been focused on the cervix,[1] little has been focused on vulvar, perianal, or vaginal intraepithelial lesions. Much of what is known about the cervix comes from four sources: (1) prospective studies of cervical intraepithelial neoplasia (CIN) in patients not treated; (2) cervical screening programs focusing on prevalence/incidence ratios; (3) studies focusing on patients who are lost to follow-up and return with invasive disease; and (4) studies of patients whose lesions recur after primary therapy.

Several researchers have focused their attention on prospective studies in which patients are observed either by cytology and colposcopy or by cytology, biopsy, and colposcopy. One of the largest studies is that by Nasiell and coworkers in which 1714 patients with grade 1 and grade 2 lesions were observed prospectively with cytology, endocervical curettage, and colposcopically directed biopsies.[2-4] These patients were observed for 39–78 months. The authors noted that in 1939 (55%) of the patients the lesions regressed, in 314 (18%) the lesions persisted at the same grade, and in 461 (27%) they progressed. The study indicates that less than one-third of the low-grade lesions progressed. This may not be true of higher grade lesions.

Several authors reported in the 1960s on patients with severe dysplasia or carcinoma in situ (CIS) who were evaluated with biopsy only. In these studies, progression to invasive cancer varied from as little as 13% in 67 patients reported by Koss to 74% in 34 patients reported by Kottmeier.[5,6] These numbers indicate that low-grade lesions are characterized by a high rate of persistence and regression and very little progression, whereas high-grade cervical lesions are probably characterized more often by progression.

The second source of data about the natural history of these lesions is derived from cervical cancer screening programs.[7-13] Studies in both the United States and British Columbia demonstrate that the peak age for CIN is between 25 and 30, whereas that for carcinoma in situ is 35, and that for invasive carcinoma is in the fifties. Because of this age-related progression, it has been assumed that one disease state leads to another. However, when the annual incidences for these various conditions are studied, there are many more cases of CIN than CIS, and far more cases of CIS than invasive carcinomas. There are so many more, in fact, that even correcting for treatment, it is impossible to prove that the majority of lesions progress from one state to another. When the incidences are subjected to mathematical modeling, it is possible to demonstrate only that approximately 10% of CIN lesions progress to CIS and that approximately 10% of CIS lesions progress to invasive cancer.[14] The weakness of projecting data based on screening programs is that the observations are of the entire population and do not follow the disease process in individuals. However, the data generated from these large screening programs provide a view of the natural history of the disease in the population. Once again, numbers do not support that all preinvasive lesions progress to invasive ones.

The third type of information about the natural history of CIN is derived from series in which patients with CIN were lost to follow-up but re-entered the health care system at a later time. Because they were untreated when lost to follow-up, they provide an excellent model for the natural history of the disease. Kinlen and Spriggs identified 60 of 101 patients with untreated CIN for whom follow-up information eventually became available.[15] The median follow-up interval for the group was 5.2 years. The lesions regressed in 19 (32%), persisted in 8 (13%), progressed to CIS in 20 (33%), and progressed to invasive cancer in 13 (22%). Gad similarly reported on the natural history of CIN grade 3 in 13 patients and of CIS in 17 patients who received no therapy and who were observed from 1–17 years.[16] Of the 13 patients with grade 3 CIN, 3 cases (23%) progressed to CIS and 2 (15%) progressed to invasive cancer. Of the 17 patients with CIS, 5 (29%) had persistent CIS and 7 (41%) had progression to invasive cancer. Because these studies are about noncompliant patients, they are biased in the direction of less favorable outcomes. Nonetheless, they confirm the invasive potential of high-grade lesions and justify our prompt attention to treatment.

Finally, a fourth source of information is retrospective series that focus on the recurrence of lesions after adequate primary therapy. Three authors (Boyes, Kolstad, and McIndoe) have published data on three such series.[17–19] In the study by Boyes, which details the therapy of 3688 patients with CIN, disease recurred in 55 (1.5%) of the patients as CIS, and in 12 (0.3%) as invasive cancer. In Kolstad's study of 1121 patients, disease recurred in 22 patients (2%) as CIS and in 15 (1.3%) as invasive cancer. McIndoe published a study of 948 patients, of whom 96 (10%) had recurrent CIS and 41 (4.3%) had invasive cancer. Higher percentages of patients in McIndoe's series had progression to both CIS and invasive cancer. In all three studies, patients were observed for more than 20 years.

From these four sources, one can see that the natural history of the preinvasive disease, at least in the cervix, is characterized by regression, persistence, and progression. Although progression rates differ in the various series, probably only a third of CIN lesions progress to a higher grade and only a very small percentage progress to invasive carcinomas. When restricted to high-grade lesions such as CIS, probably a third progress to invasion if untreated.

The caveat in evaluating these preinvasive lesions is the exclusion of an invasive neoplasm. It is important to review large retrospective series focusing on the treatment of these lesions. An ideal study about treatment should include a good description of the following: the population; the manner in which the patients were evaluated (i.e., how an invasive neoplasm was excluded); the details of their treatment and the experience of the physician; which patients experienced treatment failures; the length of follow-up; which patients dropped out of the study; the complications both short-term and long-term; the salvage therapies and how they work; and the cost. To judge treatment failure effectively, these factors must be known. Failure of therapy can be characterized by persistence of disease, recurrence of disease, or progression to an invasive neoplasm. In each case, it is best if the studies focus on these outcomes. Many of the studies listed address some of these topics but not all. There is a great need for innovative prospective studies in the area of preinvasive disease.

CERVICAL INTRAEPITHELIAL NEOPLASIA

Cervical intraepithelial neoplasia (CIN) is defined as the spectrum of intraepithelial changes beginning with a generally well-differentiated intraepithelial neoplasm, traditionally classified as mild dysplasia, and ending with invasive carcinoma.[20] These neoplastic changes are confined to the squamous epithelium. They include nuclear pleomorphism, loss of polarity, and presence of abnormal mitoses. When lesions break through the basement membrane, they are capable of spreading through the lymphatic and vascular system; thus they are called invasive neoplasms.[20] All cervical intraepithelial neoplasia is confined to the surface epithelium. These lesions are graded from 1 to 3, based on the amount of undifferentiated cells present from the basement membrane to the surface. When one-third of the distance from the basement membrane to the surface is involved, the lesions are called grade 1; when between one-third and two-thirds of the distance is involved, they are called grade 2, and when more than two-thirds of the distance is involved, they are called grade 3.[20] Carcinoma in situ (CIS) refers to full-thickness involvement by undifferentiated cells. In many modern series, CIS is included in the spectrum of severe dysplasia; in many older series, it is considered a separate entity.

Epidemiology

CIN is a relatively common preinvasive disease. Unfortunately, CIN is not a reportable condition. The National Cancer Institute maintains a cancer registry called The Surveillance Epidemiology and End Results (SEER) for the American population. The areas in the registry, which contain in some cases entire cities, entire regions, and entire states, represent about 10% of the American population. The areas chosen focus on different ethnic populations in the United States. This registry is used to predict the projected number of cases of neoplasms in the United States in a given year. According to the SEER data, approximately 55,000 cases of CIS were projected for 1992.[21] CIS and grade 3 CIN made up 8.4% of the total CIN incidence in a series of 1,045,059 women screened in the nationwide Planned Parenthood Program.[22] These figures indicate that the actual incidence of CIS in the United States is much higher and that the incidence of CIN is probably nine times that of CIS.

There is good evidence that CIN and CIS are occurring in younger and younger women. Data from the well-organized British Columbian cervical cytology screening program demonstrated an appreciable increase in the number of cases and rates of CIS in women between 20 and 30 years old. Similar findings arose from the Dundee and Angus screening program in Scotland. Reasons for the changes are unknown, however, but may have something to do with the commencement of sexual activity by women at earlier ages.[23, 24]

The risk factors for CIN have not been studied as extensively as have those for cervical cancer, but most studies confirm that the risk factors are similar.[25, 26] Age at first intercourse and multiple sexual partners increase the risk for the development of CIN, both independently and multiplicatively. Higher rates of CIN are seen in black and Hispanic women than in white women. Smoking adds significant risk for CIN, even when controlling for age at first intercourse and for multiple sexual partners. Oral contraceptives have been shown to increase slightly the risk for the development of CIN, even when the use of barrier contraception is controlled in the analysis. Sexually transmitted diseases such as herpes simplex virus type 2 also increase the risk of CIN.[26] Well-designed prospective studies looking at serum antibody levels to herpes have demonstrated that although herpes is associated with CIN and invasive cancers, it is not causal but may be a cofactor.[27, 28] Nutritional factors are thought to be important in the development of CIN, and case control studies have demonstrated that patients with CIN have low-normal levels of vitamin A, vitamin C, and folate, compared with non-CIN controls.[26] Prospective studies providing supplementary vitamins have been demonstrated to improve CIN. Immunodepression is another important risk factor for CIN. Higher rates of CIN have been demonstrated in patients who have had malignancies, organ transplants, AIDS, or are undergoing immunosuppressive therapy.[26]

One of the most important risk factors for CIN is thought to be human papillomavirus (HPV). Convincing molecular biologic evidence exists for HPV being a causal element in cervical carcinogenesis.[29] HPV has been demonstrated in biopsy specimens from invasive cervical cancers and CIN, and HPV has been seen in cervical cancer cell lines. Papillomaviruses have also been shown to act as a cocarcinogen in rabbits, cows, and humans. Cottontail rabbits develop squamous neoplasms in sun-exposed areas infected with papillomavirus. Cows develop neoplasms in areas exposed to bovine papillomavirus and bracken fern. Patients with epidermodysplasia verruciformis develop squamous cell neoplasms in sun-exposed areas infected with HPV types 5 and 8.[30, 31] Perhaps most importantly, HPV, in conjunction with oncogenes, is known to transform human cervical epithelial cell lines in vitro.[32, 33]

Despite the compelling biologic and molecular evidence for the transforming functions of HPV, the epidemiologic evidence of its carcinogenic potential in humans is, at present, minimal and somewhat contradictory. Many investigators believe this is the case because of the great difficulty in testing for the virus. Case reports and case series have demonstrated that HPV is found in many cervical biopsy specimens from patients with both CIN and invasive cancer. Screening studies demonstrate that HPV is more common in patients with abnormal Papanicolaou's smears than in those with normal smears. However, whereas data from the National Disease and Therapeutic Index show that there has been a great increase in the number of HPV infections,[34] the SEER data indicate that the rates of cervical cancer are decreasing slightly yearly.[21] Many investigators feel these rates are stabilizing and will increase in a decade when HPV has acted as a carcinogen in young women now exposed. Others feel that if HPV is causal in carcinogenesis, the rates of cervical cancer should be increasing explosively, as are the rates of HPV infection. Likewise, two large correlational studies failed to show that HPV infection is higher increased in areas where the rates of cervical cancer are highest,[35-37] yet two case control studies support the idea that HPV increases the risk for cervical neoplasia.[38, 39] The HPV testing methods used in the conventional studies were not as sensitive as the polymerase chain reaction (PCR), which is now widely utilized in such studies. Fortunately, several investigators have turned their attention to the seroepidemiology of HPV.[40] They are measuring serum antibodies to HPV in patients with CIN and invasive cancer and in controls. Some of these investigators have demonstrated a difference between the groups; others have not. Eventually, large-scale cohort studies that focus on risk factors as well as on the serum antibody response will probably clarify the role of HPV in cervical carcinogenesis. These studies will follow women without CIN who are HPV exposed and compare them with women without CIN who are not exposed and see if the development of CIN differs in these groups. With good measures of HPV and biological measures of other risk factors, the causal role of HPV will be more evident.

Clinical Management

Most patients with CIN are asymptomatic. The condition is brought to their attention when the screening Pap smear reveals an abnormality. These patients are referred for colposcopy, colposcopically directed biopsies, and endocervical curettage. Although the colposcope has been in use in Germany since 1925, it did not gain popularity in the United States until the 1970s.[41] It is a mounted magnifying lens that produces a view of the cervix enlarged 8–16 times (Figs. 13–1 and 13–2). After the application of 3–5% acetic acid, areas of the cervix with abnormal DNA content show a white color. Vessels beneath the surface can be easily seen through a green filter that makes them appear dark. Because CIN shows disordered growth and is usually accompanied by angiogenesis, CIN lesions often have vascular atypia. This vascular atypia takes many forms, including both fine and coarse punctuation, loose and tight mosaic patterns, and atypical vessels. Atypical vessels are the most worrisome and signal that an invasive lesion may be present.[42] Because the predictive capability of the colposcope is disputed, its main purpose should be to focus the site of biopsy. However, samples should be widely taken, in order to exclude invasion.

The colposcope has been a great aid in treating preinvasive lesions of the cervix. Because it helps to focus biopsies, it enables physicians to exclude invasive neoplasms in a great majority of cases. Once again, the caveat in the management of preinvasive lesions is exclusion of an invasive neoplasm. Several criteria have been proposed to help exclude any invasive neoplasm of the cervix: that the transformation zone in the squamocolumnar junction be completely visible through the colposcope, that the lesion be seen in entirety, that the endocervical curettage be negative, that there be no discrepancy between Pap smear and biopsy (in the direction of the Pap smear being higher grade than the biopsy), and that there be no suspicion of invasion of any specimen.[43]

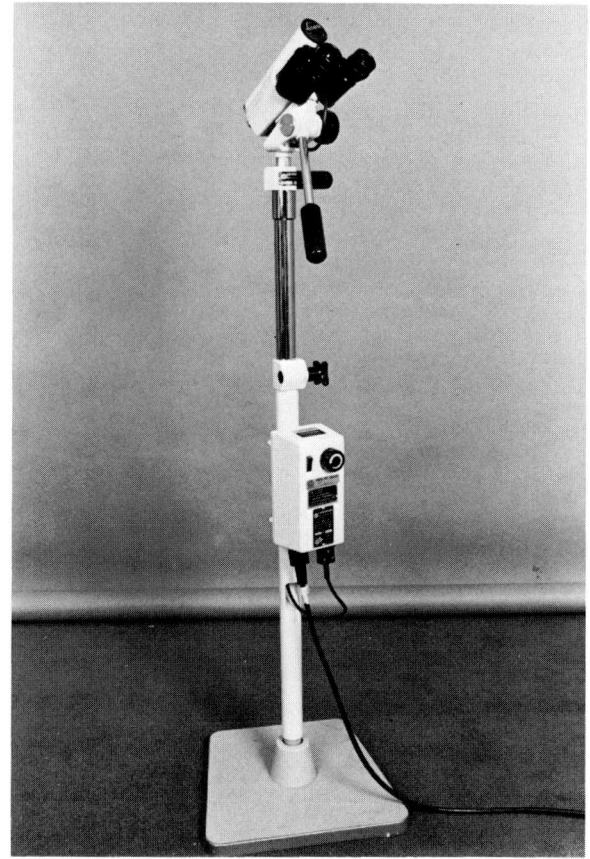

Figure 13–1
Leisegang colposcope on a tilt stand.

Although the usefulness of endocervical curettage was once debated, several series have shown that a weak point in the management of preinvasive conditions is the omission of this procedure. Endocervical curettage allows for the evaluation of the endocervical canal, where invasive lesions can arise without being easily seen. Omission of this procedure may lend to misdiagnosing an invasive cancer.

It is important to sample widely when performing cervical biopsies. The amateur colposcopist may sample all areas that appear to be suspicious. The senior colposcopist will be guided by experience. Atypical vessels signal carcinogenic growth, and these areas should always be sampled.

Treatment

The treatment of intraepithelial neoplasia depends on whether or not obtaining a larger specimen to

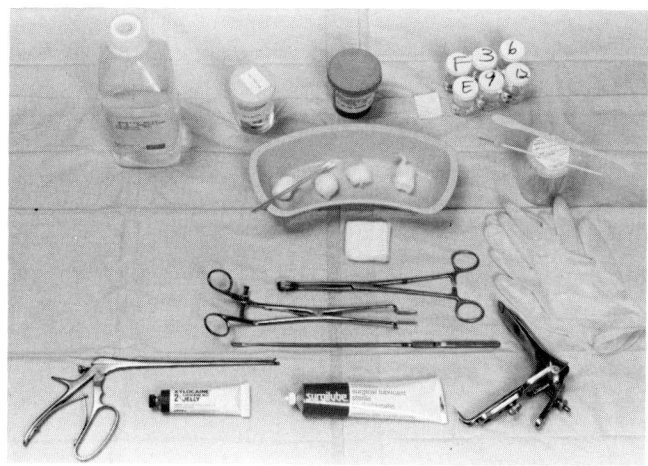

Figure 13-2
Colposcopy set-up. The necessary equipment for colposcopically directed biopsies include acetic acid (3-6%), alcohol fixative, Monsel's paste, specimen containers, basin with cotton balls and cotton swabs, the Ayre spatula and Cytobrush for Pap smear, a ring forceps, an endocervical speculum, a Kevorkian endocervical curette, a "Baby Tischler" biopsy forceps, lidocaine lubricant, unmedicated lubricant, a speculum, and gloves.

exclude invasion is necessary. If a specimen is needed, the patient must undergo cone biopsy or loop electrosurgical excision. If a specimen is not required, the patient may be treated by ablative therapies, which include cryotherapy, laser therapy, and loop electrosurgical excision procedure (LEEP). Although hysterectomy was often used in the past to treat this condition, now it is more commonly used to treat patients with recurrent intraepithelial neoplasia or those who need hysterectomy for another reason.

The choice between "ablative procedures" and "cone procedures" is an important one. If any of the previously mentioned criteria for excluding an invasive neoplasm are not met or invasion is suspected, a specimen must be obtained. Although the procedures that remove a specimen have higher cure rates than the ablative therapies, they are complicated by more bleeding and infection. In addition, cold knife cone biopsy is usually performed under general anesthesia. The ablative therapies, on the other hand, suffer from a lower cure rate, but they are performed on an outpatient basis, have fewer complications, and cost less. LEEP cone may be performed under local anesthesia in the outpatient setting and may revolutionize the management of CIN. Caution must be exercised, however, because a LEEP cone is not as deep a specimen as a cold knife cone. All of these factors must be taken into account when evaluating these procedures.

Cryosurgery

Cryosurgery was first used to treat CIN by Crisp in 1972.[44] Since then, numerous reports have certified the successful management of CIN by outpatient cryotherapy (Table 13-1). Cryotherapy controls the local destruction of tissue by applying subfreezing temperatures. There are two methods of refrigeration used for cooling the probes. One is through evaporating a liquid or solid, in which the resulting liquid gas is circulated through the probe. The second method involves expanding compressed gas through a small orifice (the Jewel-Thompson effect). The gases used for cryosurgery must have boiling points in the cryogenic range. For nitrogen, carbon dioxide, freon-22, and nitrous oxide, those gases most often used, the boiling points are in the $-80°$ C range.[45]

Kaufman and colleagues have, through the use of serial biopsies, studied the gross and histologic changes that follow cryosurgery.[51] They have demonstrated that extensive necrosis is noted 24 hours afterward. Granulation tissue is noted in 2 weeks; in 4 weeks, the surface of the cervix is covered with

Table 13-1

Cryotherapeutic Treatment of Cervical Intraepithelial Neoplasia (CIN)

Author	Ref. No.	Year	Total Patients	Patients Lost to Follow-Up	Evaluable Patients	Patients Failing Therapy (%)	Range of Follow-Up (Months)
Crisp	44	1972	123		123	*8 (6.5)	
Tredway	49	1972	118		118	*22 (18.6)	6-18
Underwood	50	1976	64	1 (1.5%)	63	4 (6.3)	6-25
Kaufman	51	1978	433	38 (8.7%)	395	44 (11)	24-96
Popkin	52	1978	208		208	*9 (4)	1-30
Ostergard	53	1980	344		344	*29 (8.4)	3-60
Walton	54	1980	152	14 (9.2%)	138	38 (25)	2-110
Hatch	55	1981	968	234 (24.2%)	734	78 (10.6)	3-95
Sedlis	56	1981	221	43 (19.4%)	178	18 (10.1)	6-80
Benedet	48	1987	1675	81 (4.9%)	1594	91 (5.7)	12
Levine	57	1985	279		279	*11 (3.9)	3-48
Creasman	58	1984	974	204 (20.9%)	770	78 (10.1)	6-48
Totals			**5559**		**4821**	**430 (8.9)**	

*These authors did not substract their patients lost to follow-up.

immature squamous epithelium; and in 6 weeks, a normal stratified squamous epithelium is found.

The lesion is usually re-identified colposcopically prior to freezing. A probe that is the correct size for the lesion is chosen, and a lubricant is applied to the probe. The probe is then applied against the cervix (Fig. 13–3). Care is taken to protect the vagina during the procedure. Many cryosurgical techniques have been described, including both single-freeze and double-freeze techniques. Some investigators emphasize the timing of the procedure, whereas others emphasize the size of the ice ball formed. Most series have used a freeze-thaw-freeze technique, in which the cervix is frozen for 3 minutes, allowed to thaw for 3–5 minutes, and frozen again for 3 more minutes. Other authors have emphasized that a 3–5 mm ice ball extending beyond the lesion is necessary for cure. The debate about single-freeze and double-freeze techniques started when Creasman demonstrated that failure rates were much higher when the single-freeze technique was used in the treatment of high-grade lesions.[47] The large British Columbia series by Benedet demonstrated that the single-freeze technique could be used successfully for all lesion grades.[48]

Although researchers may not agree on the better method, there is little doubt that cryosurgery shows a high degree of success. Out of 5559 patients (4821 of whom were evaluable) observed in 12 different series, only 430 (8.9%) had failed therapy. Many of these studies did not provide information on who was being studied, how they were evaluated, what the treatment entailed, who experienced treatment failure, how long the follow-up was, who dropped out, or why they dropped out. Reviewed together, however, the studies do provide valuable information on the success rates of cryotherapy in this population. One of the best series was that published by Benedet in 1987. The population was part of a large, well-described screening program. Participants were evaluated by experienced colposcopists and were treated with the single-freeze technique. Those patients with large lesions were treated multiple times during one session. The length of follow-up was explicitly stated. Those who were lost to follow-up were quantified. Of 1675 patients treated, 1594 were available for analysis. Treatment failed in only 91 (5.7%) at the end of 1 year. For the 5-year follow-up, 843 patients were available; 118 (14%) were lost to follow-up; therapy failed in only 77 of the remaining 725 (10.6%). One hundred twenty-five patients were available for the 10-year follow-up; of these, 36 (28.8%) were lost to follow-up, and therapy failed in 13 of the remaining 89 (14.6%). Because of the careful collection of data involved in this study, these numbers are very reliable.

Laser Therapy

Stafl introduced the use of the laser for the treatment of CIN in 1977.[59] The carbon dioxide laser is an instrument in which an electrical discharge mixed with carbon dioxide, helium, and nitrogen gives rise to an infrared laser beam with a wavelength of 10.6 microns. The laser beam travels from an articulated arm containing seven mirrors and rotary joints. This arm connects to the cabinet, where the laser tube and colposcope are housed. The narrow laser beam strikes a mirror located along the optical axis of the colposcope. The mirror is positioned so that the beam deflects along the viewing axis of the colposcope. Movement of the laser is controlled by a joystick, which is located on the micromanipulator. The laser beam can be produced in either a continuous or a pulsed fashion, but to treat the cervix, it is usually used continuously. Energy output can be changed

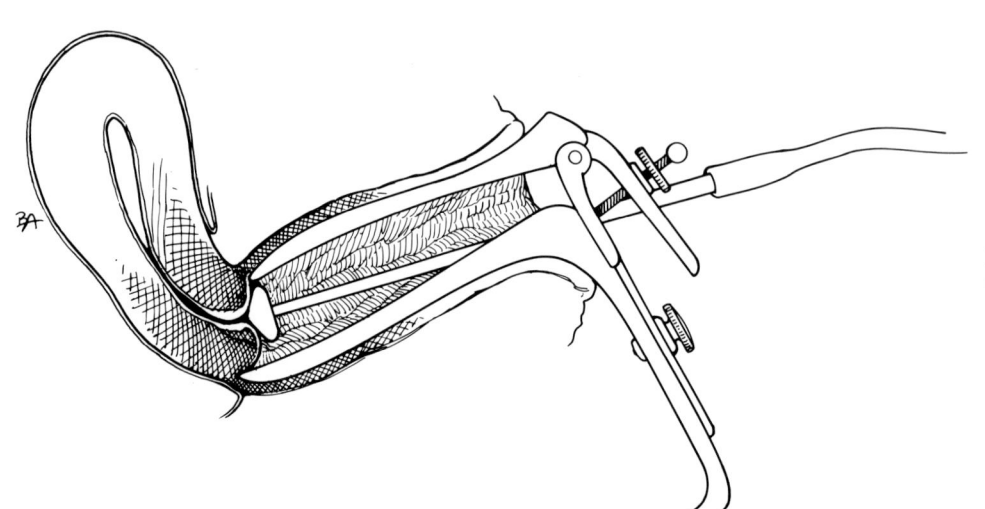

Figure 13–3
Cryotherapy of cervical intraepithelial neoplasia (CIN). Example of the cryotherapy probe applied to the cervix.

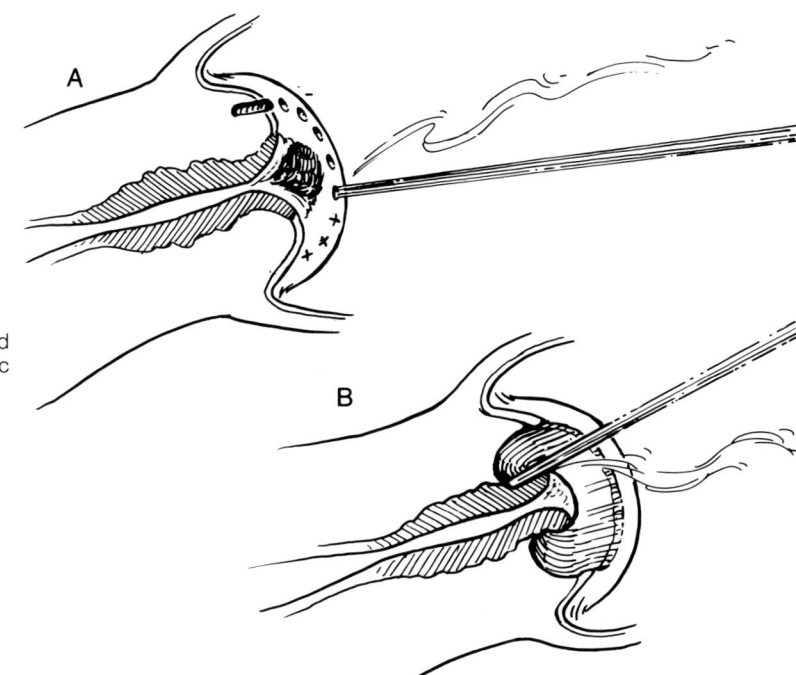

Figure 13–4
Laser ablation of CIN. *A*, The laser beam is being used to ablate to a depth of 8 mm. *B*, Ablation is hemostatic using the laser beam.

from 0 to 100 watts. Laser light differs from ordinary light in that it is monochromatic, coherent, and collimated; hence, it can be focused to a fine point via an interposed lens. By attaching the laser to a colposcope, true microsurgery can be performed. Power density is a concept that helps guide the clinician to use the correct amount of energy in treating a lesion.[60] The power density is measured in watts/cm^2:

$$\text{Power density (watts/cm}^2) = \frac{\text{watts}}{\text{spot size }(\pi r^2)}$$

Where r = radius of spot in centimeters.

Baggish has written a great deal about the use of the laser in treating intraepithelial neoplasia.[61] He demonstrates that critical points in achieving high cure rates relate to three factors: vaporizing the entire transformation zone, vaporizing to a depth of 7 mm, and vaporizing the peripheral extent of the lesion (Fig. 13–4). He recommends using a power density of 1000 watts/cm^2 to achieve this goal. He divides the cervix into quadrants starting on the posterior lip and vaporizing to a depth of 7 mm. Most of the patients in his series were able to undergo laser ablation without anesthesia.[61]

The failure rates of laser surgery are similar to those of cryotherapy. Table 13–2 lists the results of 10 series in which patients were treated with the laser. Of a total of 4934 patients, 4874 of whom were evaluable, there were 464 treatment failures (9.4%). However, because many of the patients were treated

Table 13–2

Laser Treatment of CIN

Author	Ref. No.	Year	Total Patients	Patients Lost to Follow-Up	Evaluable Patients	Patients Failing Therapy (%)	Range of Follow-Up (Months)
Stafl	59	1977	40		40	*4 (10)	3–12
Carter	62	1978	45	0	45	3 (6.6)	24–?
Bellina	63	1981	256		256	*18 (7)	3–13
Benedet	64	1981	192	13 (7%)	179	33 (18.4)	12–19
Masterson	65	1981	230		230	*41 (18)	1–60
Anderson	66	1982	441	5 (1%)	436	104 (23.5)	4–34
Burke	67	1982	131	0	131	17 (12.9)	3–32
Evans	68	1983	410	2 (0.5%)	408	46 (11.3)	12–24
Stanhope	69	1983	119	20 (16.8%)	99	9 (8.9)	3–39
Baggish	70	1989	3070	0	3070	189 (6.1)	12–120
Totals			**4934**		**4894**	**464 (9.4)**	

*Authors did not subtract their patients lost to follow-up.

two or three times before, their treatment was classified as a failure; therefore, comparing the studies is difficult.

Three retrospective nonrandomized studies comparing laser therapy with cryotherapy are detailed in Table 13–3. The fact that their failure rates are not significantly different lends support to the equivalence of these therapies. Definitive answers, however, cannot come until a number of prospective randomized trials are completed. One such trial was that by Kirwin and associates.[74] Although the authors state that the trial was truly randomized, only 35 patients underwent cryotherapy, compared with 71 who underwent laser therapy. As shown in Table 13–3, the failure rate for cryotherapy was 17% compared with 11% for laser therapy. A second, better-designed randomized trial, that of Berget, included 101 patients treated with cryotherapy and 103 treated with laser therapy.[75] The patients were stratified by grade. The failure rate for cryotherapy was 8.9%, whereas that for laser therapy was 9.7%. The patients were observed for 3–23 months. Of note, the squamocolumnar junction was scarred more often in the group treated with cryotherapy than in the other group. Following laser therapy, 79% of the squamocolumnar junctions could be visualized in entirety, compared with only 50% of the junctions in patients who received cryotherapy. The difference between the scarring in the two groups is statistically significant. Surprisingly, this scarring does not affect the results but does affect the choice of future treatment methods. If the squamocolumnar junction cannot be seen completely, patients whose lesions recur cannot be treated with ablative therapies. Although the number of patients who experienced treatment failure with these therapies is small, the necessity of performing cone biopsy for those who have treatment failure may make cryotherapy less desirable than laser therapy. Because treatment fails so rarely, a sample size of 1600 patients would be necessary to perform an adequate clinical trial to effectively study scarring.

Electrocautery

Electrocautery has been used to treat CIN since 1949. Electrocautery, which includes both hot cautery and electrocoagulation diathermy, was used at that time to ablate CIN lesions and the transformation zone. To fulgurate the lesions, these early electrosurgical treatment procedures used either a resistance-type heating element similar to a soldering iron or a "spark-gap" electrodiathermy generator and ball electrode. Table 13–4 outlines several of the studies using these techniques.[76] In the studies involving electrocautery, failure rates ranged from 5% to 25%. When lower grade lesions are treated more than once, cure rates of 100% can be achieved. The Semm cold coagulator also has high cure rates, as does electrocoagulation diathermy. Chanen and coworkers have published a great deal on the use of this technique.[82] After the patient is placed under general anesthesia, a needle electrode is inserted along the long axis of the cervix into the stroma. Then, the ball electrode is used to destroy the transformation zone in adjacent columnar epithelium (Fig. 13–5). The diathermy extends well up into the endocervical canal. In a 1983 study on the treatment of 1864 patients, Chanen[82] recorded 130 (6.9%) patients lost to follow-up; of the remaining 1734 patients, therapy failed in only 47 (2.7%). Of all the ablative therapies, then, this technique has the highest cure rate, the drawback being that it requires general anesthesia. Despite its high cure rates, electrocautery has largely been replaced by cryotherapy and laser therapy.

Table 13–3

Cryotherapy vs. Laser Therapy in the Treatment of CIN

Author	Ref. No.	Year	Total Patients	Treatment	Range of Follow-Up (Months)	Failure (%)
Nonrandomized Trials						
Wright	71	1981	334	152 cryo	12–42	22 (14.5)
				131 laser		4 (3.1)
Townsend	72	1983	200	100 cryo	12	7 (7)
				100 laser		11 (11)
Ferenczy	73	1985	294	147 cryo	12–48	13 (8.8)
				147 laser		6 (4.1)
Randomized Trials						
Kirwan	74	1985	98	35 cryo	17–24	6 (17.1)
				71 laser		8 (11.3)
Berget	75	1987	204	101 cryo	3–23	9 (8.9)
				103 laser		10 (9.7)

Table 13-4

Electrocautery-Type Treatment of CIN

Author	Ref. No.	Year	Total Patients	Patients Lost to Follow-Up	Evaluable Patients	Patients Failing Therapy (%)	Range of Follow-Up (Months)
Electrocautery							
Younge	76	1949	16	0	16	4 (25)	60–144
Richart	77	1968	182	12 (6.6%)	170	†1 Rx 19 (11.2)	12–16
						†2 Rx 9 (5.3)	
Ortiz	78	1973	148	—	148	*12 (8.1)	5–27
Deigan	79	1986	776	50 (6.4%)	726	73 (10.1)	3–60
Semm Cold Coagulator							
Staland	80	1978	71	0	71	2 (2.8)	12–84
Ducan	81	1983	598	—	598	*20 (4.7)	6–72
Electrocoagulation Diathermy							
Chanen	82	1983	1864	130 (6.9%)	1734	47 (2.7)	12–180

*Authors did not subtract for patients lost to follow-up.
†1 Rx, one treatment; 2 Rx, two treatments.

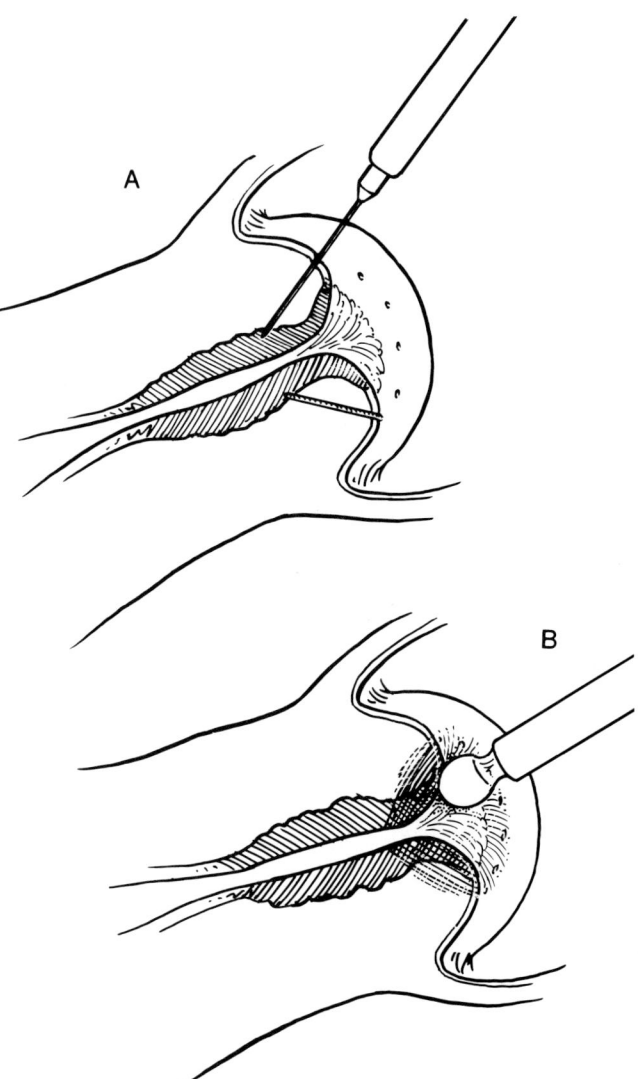

Figure 13-5
Electrocoagulation diathermy of CIN. *A*, Needle probe is used to desiccate the cervical tissue to depths of 8 mm to 1 cm. *B*, The ball electrode is then used to fulgurate remaining cervical tissue.

Interferon Chemotherapy

Three investigators looked at the effects of treating CIN with interferon. The results of their trials are summarized in Table 13–5. Moller and colleagues reported in a 1983 study the treatment of six patients with interferon gel.[83] They used human leukocyte interferon (alpha) in doses of 60,000 units twice weekly for 12 weeks. For the first 6 weeks of the trial, the interferon was applied with a swab; for the last 6 weeks, it was placed in the cervical cap and left in place overnight. The patients were monitored by biopsy. Three of the six patients were complete responders after 4 months. Three other patients were partial responders.

In 1986, Byrne and associates conducted a randomized, double-blind, placebo-based trial. Twenty-six patients were treated, and 13 were randomized to each arm. The investigators used human leukocyte interferon (alpha) in doses of 400,000 units. Each patient was treated twice weekly for 6–8 weeks for a total of 12 treatments. The cervical cap was left in place during each occasion for 24 hours. After the 12 treatments, the patients were followed with biopsies. Dysplasia regressed completely in two patients who had received interferon and in two patients who received the placebo. Because there was no statistically significant difference between the results for the two arms, Byrne concluded that the interferon gel was inactive. However, he used a much higher dose than did Moller.

Choo reported in 1986 on a single-arm trial in which 12 patients were treated with interferon. Seven were treated with interferon-alpha and five with interferon-beta. They were observed from 12–36 months. Doses of 200,000 units were applied twice weekly until the lesion completely regressed and then monthly for 3 months, after which a biopsy was performed to confirm disease remission. Six of seven patients (86%) treated with interferon-alpha and two of five patients (40%) treated with interferon-beta were complete responders. These studies indicate that interferon may indeed be effective to some degree in the treatment of CIN. At present, however, success rates are lower than those with other therapies. More work needs to be done to determine the correct dose and timing of treatment, a common problem with biologic response modifiers.

Loop Electrosurgical Excision Procedure

Another technique for treating CIN is the loop electrosurgical excision procedure (LEEP), which can be performed without general anesthesia. LEEP can be used to treat CIN with the same indications as those for ablative therapies: no suspicion of invasion, no discrepancy between Pap smear and biopsy, negative endocervical curettage, satisfactory colposcopic examination, and good patient compliance. When LEEP is used to replace other ablative therapies, one sample is taken. Later, the technique for LEEP cone is described, which includes two samples.

LEEP involves the use of an electrosurgical generator, the kind that is used in laparoscopic and urologic surgeries. Monopolar outputs are employed, and the alternating current, which ranges between 350,000 and 4,000,000 cycles/second, is used to sever the tissue and achieve hemostasis. At such a high frequency, cellular membrane depolarization does not occur, and there is no neuromuscular excitation or shock.[86, 87] The high-frequency alternating current produced by these generators imparts kinetic energy to cells. This energy raises the temperature and is responsible for the cutting effects of the current. The amount of heat imparted to the tissue depends on the tissue's resistance to current flow; the length of time the current is flowing; and the current density, which is defined as amps/cm^2. The tissue resistance is fairly constant, so that the heating effects can be controlled by changing the amount of current in the unit. The loops, which are made from a very thin stainless steel wire, have an insulated shaft and crossbar to prevent thermal damage. They come in various sizes and are used with power settings that depend on the size of the loop (Fig. 13–6).

The disadvantages of LEEP are few but include burns, bleeding, and infection. As with any type of cautery, burns can occur to an unintended area,

Table 13–5

Interferon Treatment of CIN

Author	Ref. No.	Year	No. of Patients	Type of Interferon and Dose in Units	Method of Administration	Range of Follow-Up (Months)	Complete Response (%)
Moller	83	1983	6	α 60,000	Gel	4	3 (50%)
Byrne	84	1986	26		Gel	4–8	
			13	Placebo			2 (15%)
			13	α 400,000			2 (15%)
Choo	85	1986	12			12–36	
			7	α 200,000	Intralesional injection		6 (86%)
			5	β 200,000			2 (40%)

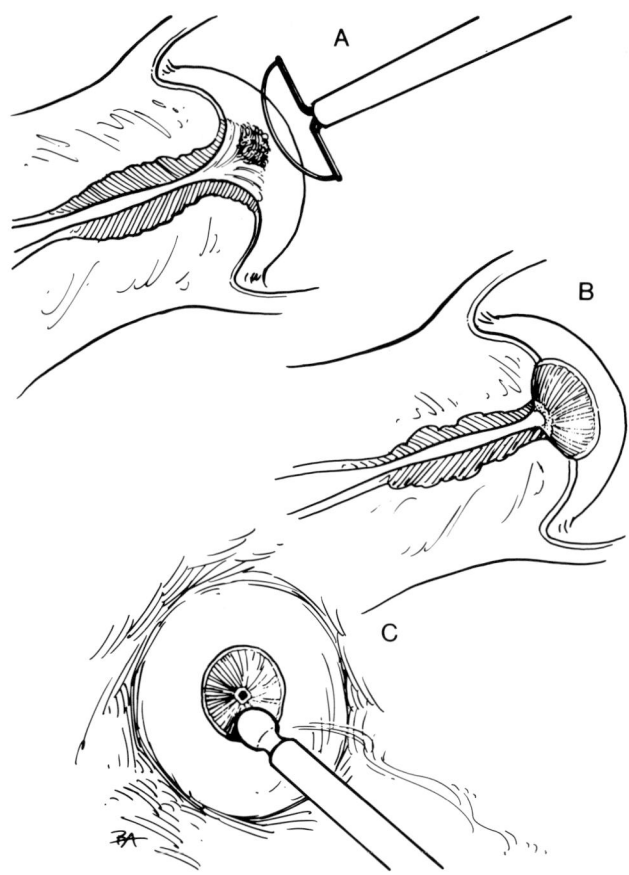

Figure 13-6
Loop excision of CIN. *A, B,* The 20 × 8 mm loop is used to excise a portion of the cervix. *C,* The bed has been electrocoagulated with the ball electrode.

through an alternative pathway from patient to ground that develops through a small contact point at a site other than the return electrode and under the grounding pad. As with all coning procedures, a certain amount of bleeding and infection are standard. In four series in which LEEP has been used to treat CIN (Table 13-6), the postoperative bleeding ranged from 2% to 7%. The response rates ranged from 89% to 96%. One major advantage of LEEP is that it can be performed in the clinic under paracervical block rather than general anesthesia.

LEEP needs to be compared in prospective trials with other forms of treatment for CIN, and the short- and long-term complications must be measured carefully. If LEEP is found to have as few complications as the ablative methods, it will probably replace them because the advantage of obtaining a specimen would be salutary.

Cone Biopsy

Cone biopsy is used to obtain a tissue sample when invasive cancer is suspected. Suspicion occurs when cytologic examination indicates invasive cells, when there is a discrepancy between the Pap smear and biopsy (in the direction of the Pap smear being higher grade than the biopsy), when the endocervical curettage is positive, when the extent of a lesion cannot be seen, when the entirety of the squamocolumnar junction transformation zone cannot be visualized, or when there is a question of microinvasion on cervical biopsy. The cone biopsy can be performed using three techniques: cold knife cone, laser cone, and loop electrosurgical excision cone.

According to Larsson, cone biopsies have been performed for centuries.[92] These operations were probably first performed on the uterine cervix in the sixteenth century. The first known use of this procedure to treat cancer was by Lisfranc in 1815.[94] Sims revised the procedure in 1861, using a technique in which the healthy vaginal mucosa was made to cover the denuded cervix, leaving a small opening just over the outlet of the cervical canal.[95] In 1916, Sturmdorf devised a technique that removed all the disease and did not complicate future pregnancies.[96]

Cold Knife Cone. After the patient is examined under anesthesia and the cervix is viewed through a colposcope, the endocervical canal is sounded to determine its direction and length. During the procedure, many surgeons first ligate the descending branch of the uterine arteries. Others use vasoconstrictive agents in the cervical stroma. A knife is then used to remove a conical specimen that includes the lesion, the transformation zone, and the endocervical canal (Fig. 13-7). The specimen itself is often tagged to identify the position of the cervix for the pathol-

Table 13-6

Loop Electrosurgical Excision Procedure (LEEP) as a Treatment for CIN

Author	Ref. No.	Year	Patients Treated	Patients Failing Treatment (%)	Range of Follow-Up (Months)	Complications	
						Bleeding	Stenosis
Boulanger	88	1989	88	10 (11.3%)	12–60	6 (7%)	3 (3%)
Prendiville	89	1989	102	5 (4.9%)	12–36	4 (4%)	—
Whiteley	90	1990	66	6 (7.5%)	1–12	1 (2%)	—
Luesley	91	1990	557	19 (3.4%)	6–12	29 (5%)	7 (1%)
Totals			813	40 (4.9%)		40 (4.9%)	10 (1.2%)

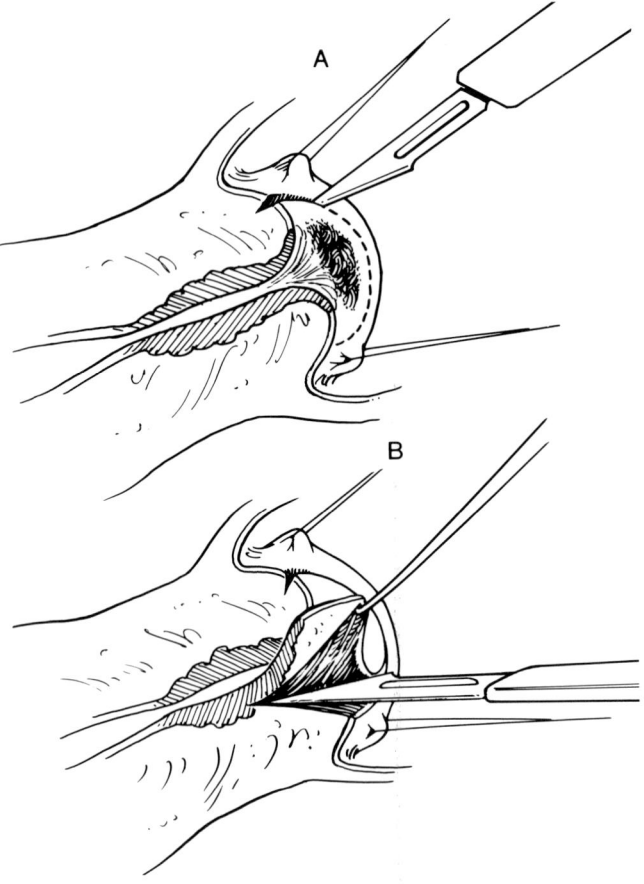

Figure 13-7
Cold knife cone biopsy. A and B, The knife is used to remove a conical piece of tissue. The bed is then sewn with a running locked suture or overlapping figure-of-eight sutures.

ogist. Some surgeons then recommend leaving the cone bed open to heal by secondary intention, whereas others provide hemostasis by suture ligation using either figure-of-eight sutures or continuous interlocking sutures.

A cold knife cone delivers an optimal specimen from which the pathologist is able to study multiple sections. Because of the nature of the specimen obtained, this procedure will stay in the armamentarium of operations used to diagnose carcinoma of the cervix. The procedure has a number of important short- and long-term complications. One short-term problem is bleeding. Retrospective analyses show that in many series, the rate of patients returning because of bleeding ranges from 5% to 15%. Another short-term complication is infection, which is in the 1–3% range in many series. Important long-term complications include cervical stenosis, which ranges from 3% to 5% in the series mentioned.[92] Incompetent cervix, another complication, is harder to find in retrospective series; thus, the rate is unknown. It probably occurs in patients who undergo more than one coning procedure.

There is no question that cold knife cone biopsy has a high cure rate, even in the treatment of high-grade lesions. Kolstad and Klem reported on 1121 cases of carcinoma in situ followed for 5–25 years.[97] Only 19 of 795 (2.3%) patients treated with cone biopsy had recurrent carcinoma in situ. Of the 238 patients treated with hysterectomy, 3 (1.2%) had a recurrence of the cancer. Thus, the cure rate achieved with hysterectomy was only 1% better than that achieved with cone biopsy in this retrospective series.

Laser Cone. The laser removes a conical specimen in a way similar to that of the cold knife. Baggish recommends placing lateral figure-of-eight stitches in the cervix at the 3 and 9 o'clock positions.[98] The cervix is then injected with a vasoconstrictive agent. The laser is used at a low power density of 500 watts/cm^2 to outline the area to be coned (Fig. 13–8). Power is then turned up to 8000–12,000 watts/cm^2 to remove the conical specimen. The laser will usually seal vessels up to 0.5 mm in diameter, so bleeding is not often a problem. Fine hooks are used to provide traction and countertraction as the laser beam cuts more deeply into the cervical stroma. The scalpel or the laser may be used to cut the cervix from its endocervical margin. Baggish recommends brushing the cone bed with the laser in order to prevent bleeding. He also recommends lasering the area around the endocervical canal to a slightly deeper level to evert the endocervical canal, a procedure he calls "button-holing."

The laser cone was compared with the cold knife cone in a prospective randomized trial by Larsson and colleagues.[99] One hundred ten consecutive women underwent conization of the cervix for either severe dysplasia or carcinoma in situ. All were prospectively randomized in one of the two groups: cold knife cone and laser cone. The mean intraoperative blood loss for the laser cone group was 1.6 ml, whereas that for the cold knife cone group was 16.3 ml. The range of blood loss for the laser cone group was 0–8 ml; that for the cold knife cone group was 1–98 ml. Only one of the patients treated with the laser returned with hemorrhaging 24 hours after this surgery, compared with four patients in the cold knife cone group. The authors reported that the quality of the specimens obtained with the laser was good. Other investigators will need to repeat this study in order to determine whether findings are comparable.

Loop Electrosurgical Excision Cone. LEEP has recently been used to treat patients with preinvasive disease (Fig. 13–9). Leep can be used for cone biopsies; two specimens are taken rather than one specimen, as for ablative therapy. The second specimen

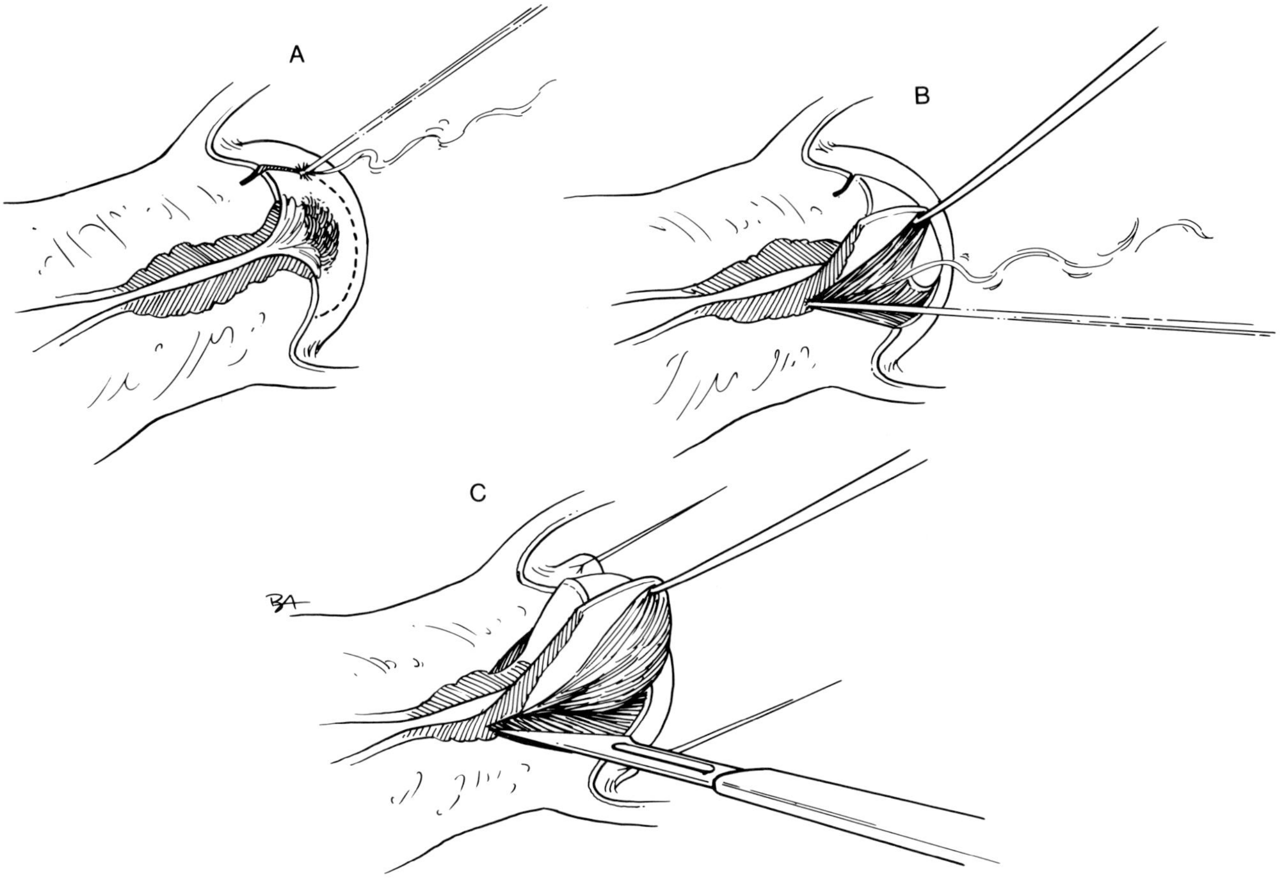

Figure 13–8
Laser cone. *A* and *B*, The laser beam is used to excise a conical piece of tissue. *C*, Either laser or knife will be used to extricate the specimen from the uterus.

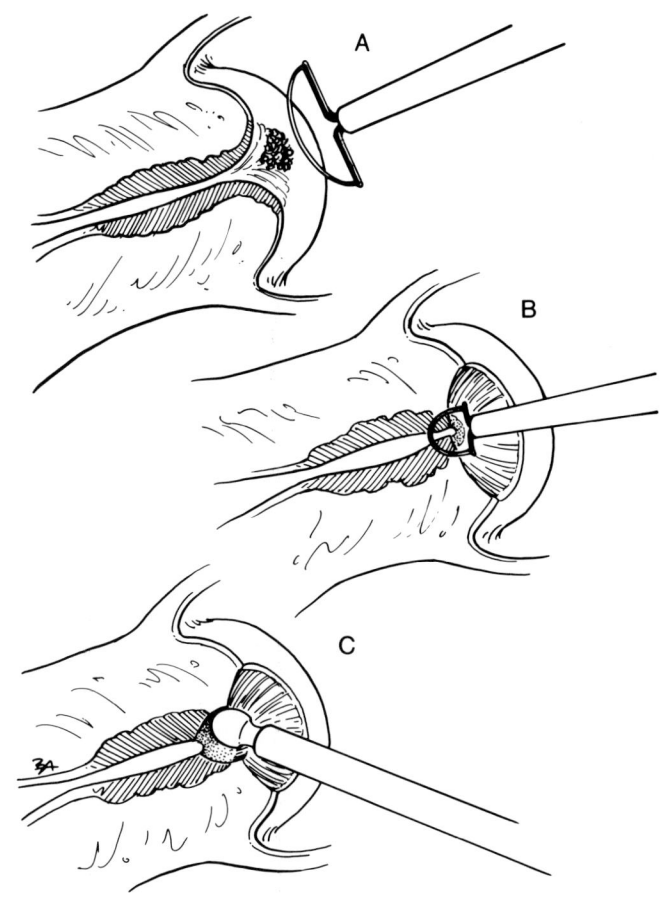

Figure 13–9
Loop electrosurgical excision procedure cone biopsy. *A*, The 20 × 8 mm loop is used to excise a piece of tissue. *B*, The 10 × 10 mm loop is then used to remove an endocervical specimen. *C*, The bed is electrocoagulated with a ball electrode.

is of the endocervical canal. Whiteley reported on 14 cone procedures performed with LEEP.[90] Two of the 14 were complicated by hemorrhage. None of the cases recurred. Mor-Yosef reported on 50 cones using the loop diathermy, of which 40 were performed under general anesthesia and 10 under local anesthesia with no supplemental or parenteral analgesia.[100] Two patients returned because of postoperative bleeding, one in the early postoperative period and one in the late postoperative period. Ten per cent of samples were considered inadequate. In this series, ball diathermy was used to coagulate the surface of the wound to control any active bleeding and to prevent bleeding in the future. The possible advantages of loop diathermy over cold knife cone or laser cone remain to be studied, but the obvious advantage is that it can be performed in the outpatient setting under local anesthesia. These cases are at least 2 cm in depth, which is not as deep as cold knife cones performed in the operating room. Caution should be exercised when they are used to exclude invasion, evaluate microinvasion, or evaluate adenocarcinoma in situ.

VAGINAL INTRAEPITHELIAL NEOPLASIA

Like CIN, vaginal intraepithelial neoplasia (VAIN) is characterized by neoplastic changes confined to the squamous epithelium and by nuclear pleomorphism, loss of polarity, and presence of abnormal mitoses. VAIN is graded similarly to CIN. Grade 1 involves one-third of the distance from the basement membrane to the surface epithelium; grade 2 involves more than one-third and up to two-thirds of that distance; and grade 3 involves from two-thirds of that distance to full thickness. Vaginal carcinoma in situ, defined as full-thickness involvement from the basement membrane to the surface epithelium, is often included in the classification of grade 3 VAIN. Like CIN, VAIN is considered a precursor of invasive vaginal carcinoma.[101]

Epidemiology

Neither VAIN nor vaginal carcinoma in situ is a reportable condition; thus, incidence and prevalence are unknown for either. Invasive vaginal carcinoma makes up only 1–2% of all gynecologic neoplasms.[21] The age range in most series is from 19 to 86 years,[102–121] and the median age is the mid-forties.

The risk factors for both vulvar carcinoma and VAIN are not well documented. They are believed to be similar to those for CIN. In the studies listed in Table 13–7, over 80% of vaginal carcinoma in situ is associated with the previous history of carcinoma in situ of the cervix, vulvar intraepithelial neoplasia, invasive vaginal cancer, or radiotherapy for any of the preceding. Three reported cases of vaginal CIS occurred in a graft after vaginectomy and skin grafting as treatment for vaginal carcinoma in situ.[122–124] One author noted the progression of vaginal CIS to invasive carcinoma.[117] These cases are usually associated with a previous history of squamous cell carcinoma of the cervix. It is unclear, therefore, whether they represent progression of vaginal carcinoma in situ to invasive vaginal carcinoma or rather the metastasis of cervical carcinoma to the vagina.

Clinical Management

VAIN may be detected with routine screening Pap smears. It is usually asymptomatic, although some authors have reported the concurrent presence of a clear, bloody vaginal discharge. Once VAIN is suspected, the diagnostic strategy is the same as for CIN. Patients undergo repeat Pap smear as well as colposcopy and colposcopically directed biopsies. One significant difference between VAIN and CIN is that there is less vascular atypia in the vagina than in the cervix.

Treatment

Several procedures have been devised for the treatment of VAIN. Lesions may be treated by surgery (either total or partial vaginectomy), local excision, radiation therapy, chemotherapy (intravaginal application of 5-fluorouracil) laser, or diathermy. The series of interest are tabulated in Table 13–7.[102–121] For the purpose of this table, all invasive procedures, whether they are local excisions and vaginectomies, are included under the surgery column.

Radiation Therapy

Rutledge was the first to report the use of radiotherapy for vaginal carcinoma in situ. He observed 31 patients, of whom 26 received vaginal radium. No treatment failures were noted, but treatment was complicated by vaginal stenosis and the resultant loss of sexual function. Rutledge recommended surgery for younger patients in order for them to maintain sexual function. He commented on the development of VAIN in patients for whom radiotherapy had been used to treat carcinoma of the cervix and on the potential for VAIN to progress to an invasive neoplasm.

Table 13-7

Treatment of Vaginal Intraepithelial Neoplasia (VAIN)

Author	Ref. No.	Range of Follow-Up (Months)	No. of Patients	XR Treatment	Failure	Surgical Treatment	Failure	5-FU Treatment	Failure	Laser Treatment	Failure	Diathermy Treatment	Failure
Rutledge	102	48–108	31	31	0	0	0	0	0	0	0	0	0
Gallup	103	12–144	25	2	0	24	5	0	0	0	0	0	0
Woodruff	104	1–72	9	0	0	0	0	9	1	0	0	0	0
Lee	105	1–288	66	12	0	54	2	0	0	0	0	0	0
Ballon	106	6–30	12	0	0	0	0	12	3	0	0	0	0
Oliver	107	6–216	22	4	0	17	2	1	0	0	0	0	0
Piver	108	13–83	8	0	0	0	0	8	2	0	0	0	0
Daly	109	24–60	0	0	0	0	0	17	3	0	0	0	0
Petrilli	110	3–60	41	0	0	0	0	15	3	10	1	0	0
Hernandez-Linares	111	24–264	35	29	0	6	0	0	0	0	0	0	0
Caglar	112	3–48	*27	0	0	0	0	27	4	0	0	0	0
Sillman	113	6–31	10	0	0	0	0	10	0	0	0	0	0
Capen	114	6–46	*15	0	0	0	0	0	0	15	3	0	0
Townsend	115	1–72	*36	0	0	0	0	0	0	36	3	0	0
Jobson	116	6–27	*24	0	0	0	0	0	0	24	0	0	0
Woodman	117	6–44	23	4	0	4	0	0	0	14	8	1	0
Lenehan	118	3–112	59	2	0	21	4	0	0	22	11	12	3
Stuart	119	6–38	*27	0	0	0	0	0	0	27	6	0	0
Krebs	120	12–84	59	0	0	0	0	37	7	22	6	0	0
Stafl	121	3–12	8	0	0	0	0	0	0	8	1	0	0
Totals			554	84	0 (0%)	126	13 (10%)	136	20 (15%)	178	39 (22%)	13	3 (23%)

*Authors did not subtract their patients lost to follow-up.

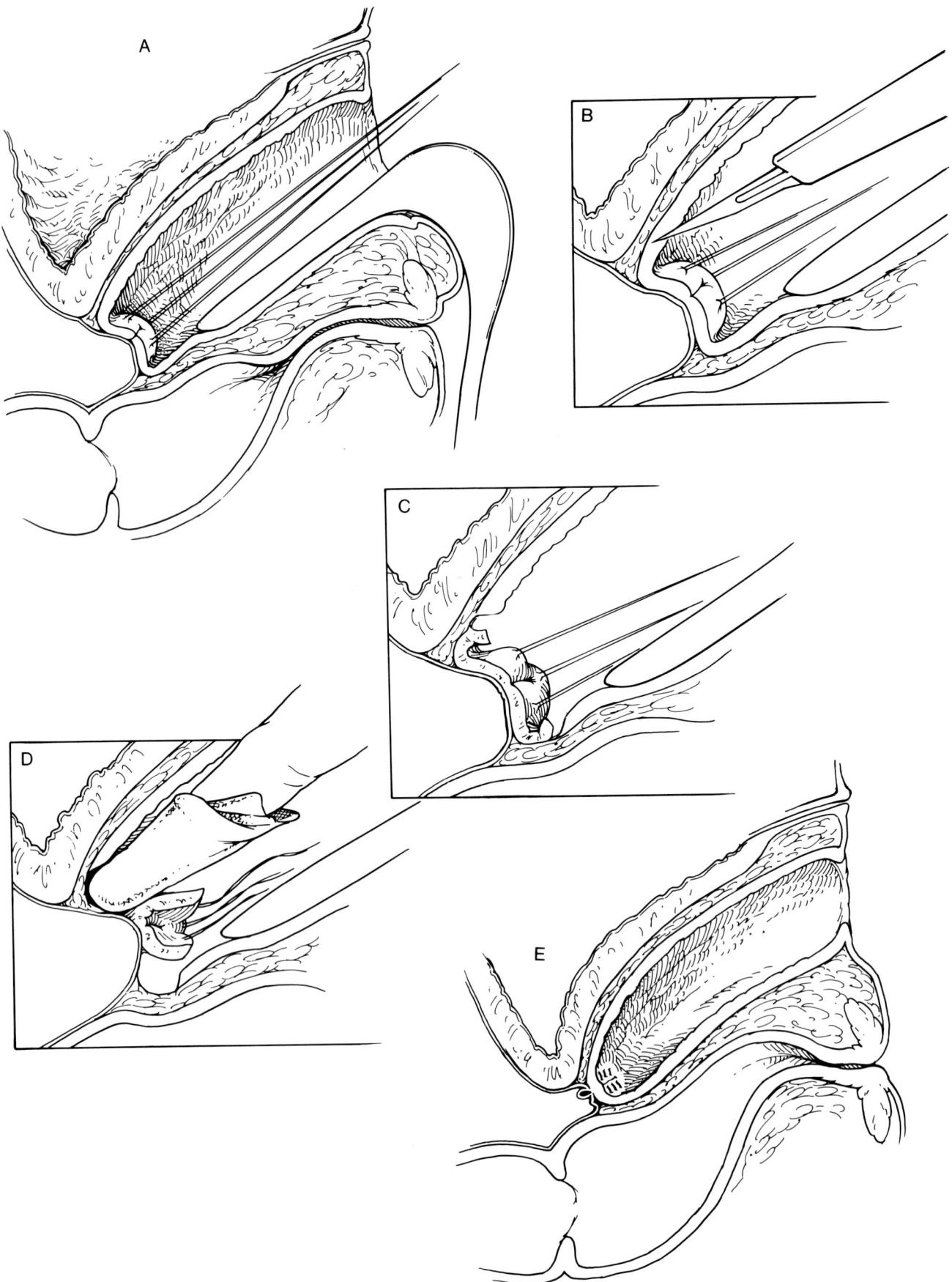

Figure 13–10
Vaginectomy. *A*, Sutures are used to place traction on the upper vagina, *B* and *C*, which is then excised using the knife. *D*, Blunt dissection is used to further remove the specimen. *E*, The vagina is closed with interrupted sutures of biodegradable material.

Surgery

Different types of surgery have been used to treat VAIN since the late 1950s, including wide local excisions and partial and total vaginectomies. Wide local excisions can be used for well-circumscribed lesions, whereas partial and total vaginectomies are used in two other circumstances (Fig. 13–10): Parial or total vaginectomies are used to obtain a tissue sample to exclude invasive vaginal carcinoma; total vaginectomies are also used for multifocal disease when lesser procedures would not be considered curative. Reported failure rates range from 0 to 20%. The average failure rate for surgery in 126 patients included in Table 13–7 was 10%.

Chemotherapy

The use of topical chemotherapy with 5% fluorouracil (5-FU) was first reported by Woodruff in 1975[104] (Fig. 13–11). Nine patients were treated twice a day for 1 month and then monthly. The patients were observed from 6 weeks to 6 years; only one experienced failed therapy. Since then, a wide variety of regimens have been described. Ballon recommended treating patients twice daily for 2 weeks.[106] Piver recommended treating for 2 hours a day for 5 days. Daly recommended a third of an applicator twice daily for 10 to 14 days. Petrilli recommended twice daily therapy for 5 days.[108] Capen recommended once-daily application for 5–10 days, repeating the procedure in 3 weeks.[114] He treated patients three times before evaluating them. Sillman recommended therapy once daily for 14 days.[113] Some authors treated patients for two or three cycles before evaluating them, whereas others treated for only one cycle. All authors noted vaginal ulceration, and some reported having to stop therapy because of denudation of the vaginal epithelium. Overall, the failure rates for 5-FU ranged from 12% to 15%.

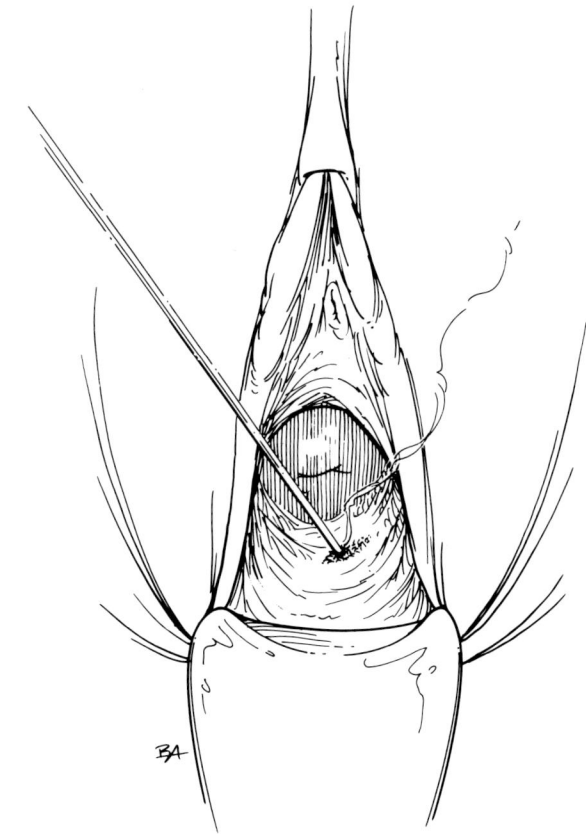

Figure 13–12
Laser diathermy of the vagina. The laser beam is used to ablate the vaginal lesions through the submucosal layers.

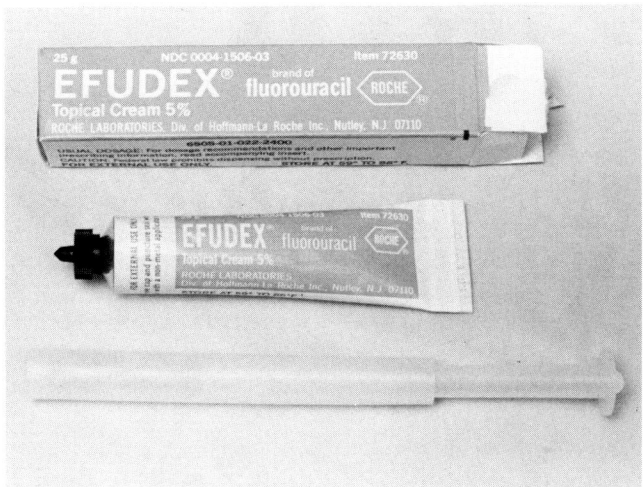

Figure 13–11
5-FU for treatment of vaginal intraepithelial neoplasia (VAIN). A 5% mixture of fluorouracil with vaginal applicator is shown.

Laser Therapy

In 1977, Stafl reported the successful use of the laser to treat VAIN[121] (Figs. 13–12 and 13–13). Eight patients were treated, and only one experienced failed therapy. Since then, the laser has been commonly used to treat VAIN. The laser is well suited to treating VAIN because the vagina can be distended and the laser used to precisely delineate the abnormal areas. Again, it is difficult to evaluate this series because, depending on the study, patients may have been treated one time or several times before their treatment was classified as a cure or a failure. In 178 cases reviewed for this table, 39 (22%) failed laser therapy, often after several treatments.

Electrocautery

A fifth technique, electrocautery, was used to treat 13 patients, with three failures noted. Because of the thermal burns associated with diathermy, and the proximity of the bladder and rectum to the vagina, this therapy is probably less desirable than the others.

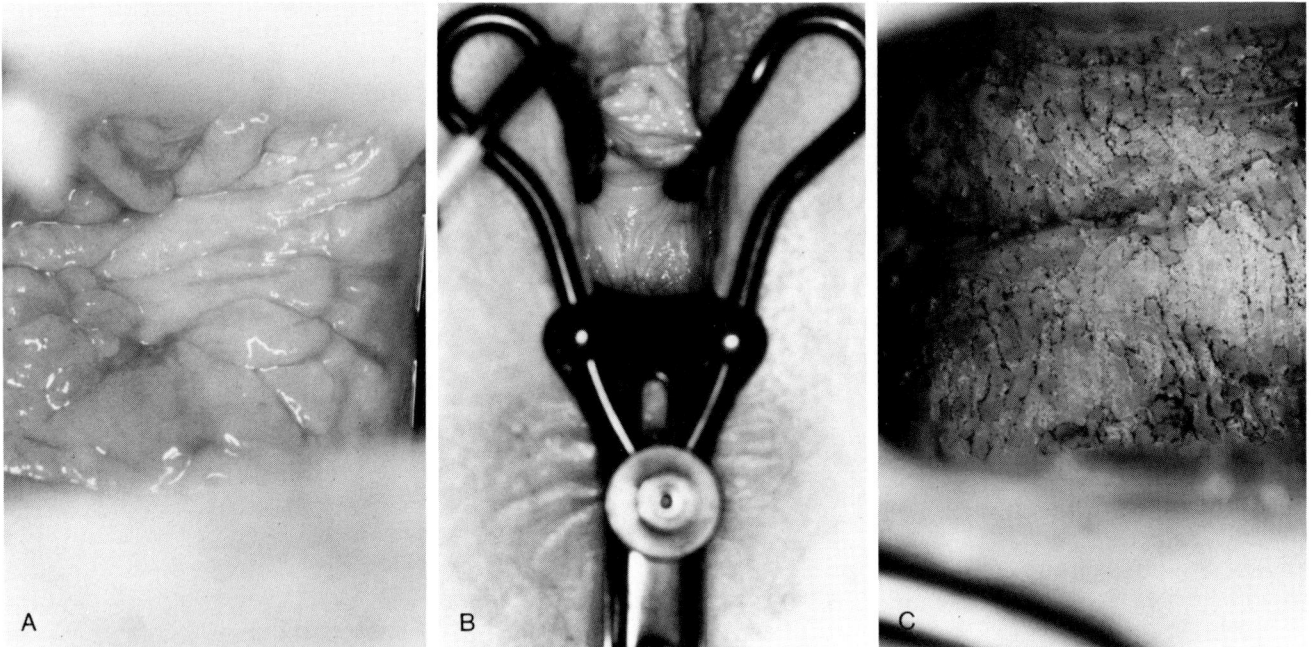

Figure 13-13
Laser in the treatment of VAIN. A VAIN lesion is shown (A), with the speculum in place (B), and after laser ablation (C).

VULVAR AND PERIANAL INTRAEPITHELIAL NEOPLASIA

Vulvar intraepithelial neoplasia (VIN) and perianal intraepithelial neoplasia (PAIN) are defined as neoplastic changes like those in CIN and VAIN, confined to the squamous epithelium. The neoplastic changes include nuclear pleomorphism, loss of polarity, and the presence of abnormal mitoses in cytogenetic analyses. These lesions are graded similarly to those in CIN and VAIN in that the grading is based on the amount of undifferentiated cells present from the basement membrane to the surface. Full-thickness involvement is termed vulvar carcinoma in situ. Bowenoid papillosis is indistinguishable from other forms of VIN and, therefore, is not recognized as a separate entity by the International Society for the Study of Vulvar Disease.[125]

Epidemiology

VIN and vulvar carcinoma in situ, like VAIN and vaginal CIS, are not reportable conditions. No reliable estimates of their instance or prevalence are available. Vulvar invasive cancer, although more frequent than vaginal cancer, makes up only a small percentage of invasive gynecologic neoplasms.[21] The age range in the series included in Table 13-8 is 14-90 years.[126-149] Many studies have suggested that the incidence of VIN is higher in the 1990s than in previous decades for women 18-35 years old.[130, 131, 145]

Risk factors for VIN have not been systematically studied, but they are thought to be similar to those for CIN. Of note, 36% of the patients being treated for VIN (Table 13-8) also had preinvasive or invasive disease of the cervix or vagina. Fifteen per cent were noted to have had associated condylomata, and immunodepressive disorders were noted in an additional 4%. The role of human papillomavirus in the development of VIN and PAIN is unknown but is thought to be important. Many authors have reported the presence of human papillomavirus in specimens taken from biopsies of VIN. Again, however, epidemiologic data that would show that the infection occurred before the development of VIN would be necessary to prove causality.

Clinical Analysis

Unlike CIN and VAIN, VIN often produces symptoms. Over 60% of patients present with pruritus. In addition, lesions are visible with the naked eye and are often highly pigmented; being erythematous, beige, brown, black, or white. The lesions are often raised and, after the application of acetic acid, turn white. There is less vascular atypia on the vulva than on the cervix, but fine punctation is often present. Both toluidine blue and the colposcope are useful in identifying areas for potential biopsy.

Table 13–8
Treatment of Vulvar Intraepithelial Neoplasia (VIN)

Author	Ref. No.	Range of Follow-Up (Months)	No. of Patients	Vulvectomy	Failure Rate	Wide Local Excision	Failure Rate	5-FU Treatment	Failure Rate	Laser Treatment	Failure Rate	Cryotherapy	Failure Rate	XRT Treatment	Failure Rate
Woodruff	126	1–72	44	14	3	17	2	13	5	0	0	0	0	0	0
Carson	127	24	1	0	0	0	0	1	0	0	0	0	0	0	0
Forney	128	6–48	27	11	1	11	1	6	6	0	0	4	0	0	0
Krupp	129	3–39	8	0	0	0	0	8	2	0	0	0	0	0	0
Hilliard	130	3–12	6	2	0	1	0	3	1	0	0	0	0	0	0
Buscema	131	12–180	102	28	8	63	20	11	8	0	0	0	0	0	0
Liftshitz	132	9–96	12	0	0	0	0	12	10	0	0	0	0	0	0
Friedrich	133	2–96	41	20	3	17	3	3	3	0	0	1	1	0	0
DiSaia	134	12–90	39	39	13	0	0	0	0	0	0	0	0	0	0
Kaplan	135	18–50	10	9	2	1	0	0	0	0	0	0	0	0	0
Baggish	136	12–30	35	0	0	0	0	0	0	35	3	0	0	0	0
Ulbright	137	1–156	14	2	1	12	2	0	0	0	0	0	0	0	0
Caglar	138	3–132	50	21	0	23	0	3	3	2	1	0	0	0	0
Townsend	140	?	33	0	0	0	0	0	0	33	2	0	0	0	0
Di Paola	141	3–120	28	12	0	11	1	0	0	0	0	0	0	3	0
Bernstein	142	6–108	65	18	3	16	2	0	0	18	1	0	0	0	0
Ferenczy	143	1–24	11	0	0	0	0	0	0	11	3	0	0	0	0
Leuchter	144	9–240	119	23	6	45	15	9	8	42	7	0	0	0	0
Wolcott	145	5–209	56	20	4	36	19	0	0	0	0	0	0	0	0
Crum	146	6–132	41	15	0	23	5	0	0	2	0	0	0	1	0
Andreasson	147	6–62	49	0	0	49	14	0	0	0	0	0	0	0	0
Jones	148	24–276	31	4	1	26	4	0	0	0	0	0	0	1	0
Wright	149	12–48	29	0	0	0	0	0	0	29	2	0	0	0	0
Rettenmaier	150	15–102	48	48	13	0	0	0	0	0	0	0	0	0	0
Totals			**899**	**286**	**58 (20%)**	**351**	**88 (25%)**	**69**	**46 (66%)**	**172**	**19 (11%)**	**5**	**1 (20%)**	**5**	**0 (0%)**

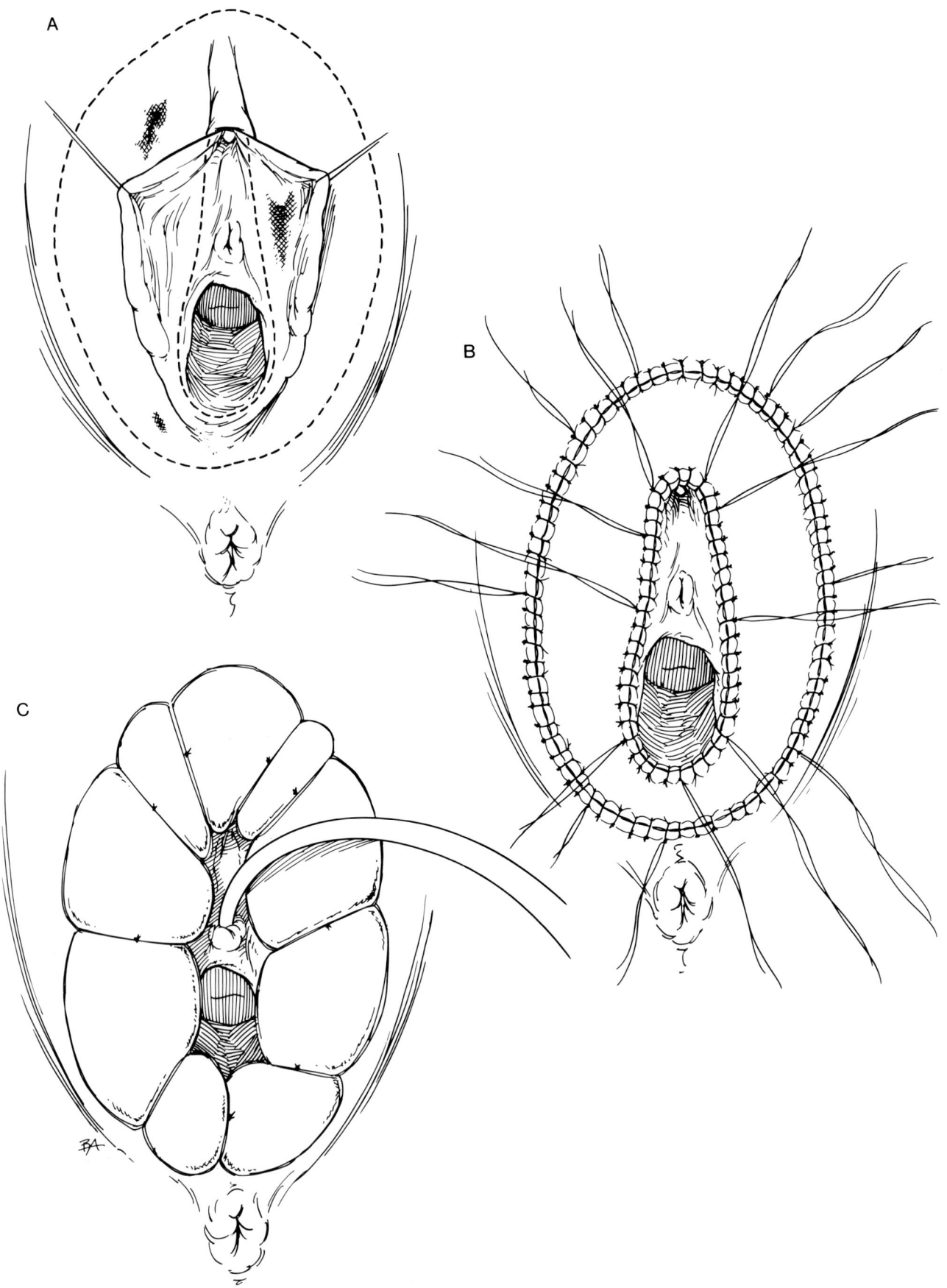

Figure 13–14
Superficial skinning vulvectomy. *A,* The skin of the labia majora and minora is removed, sparing the clitoris. *B,* A skin graft is sewn into place with *(C)* superficial padding for protection. A Foley catheter is placed for voiding.

Treatment

As for the other preinvasive conditions of the female lower genital tract, the treatment of VIN has become more conservative in recent years. Possible treatments include vulvectomy, either with or without split-thickness skin grafting, wide local excision, chemotherapy with 5-fluorouracil (5-FU), laser therapy, cryotherapy, and radiation.

Surgery

Vulvectomy is the treatment of choice if a sample is needed to exclude an invasive neoplasm. Rutledge and Sinclair reported in 1968 on the treatment of intraepithelial carcinoma of the vulva by skin excision and graft[151] (Fig. 13–14). The skin graft gave patients a more normal appearance and function than was possible with vulvectomy alone. In young patients for whom cosmesis is important, this therapy seemed ideal.

From a review of the literature, a total of 980 patients were found who had been treated for VIN. For the 332 treated with vulvectomy, the recurrence rate was 18%. Within this group, 104 were treated with split-thickness skin grafts. Their failure rate was 28 (27%).

Wide local excisions of various sizes have also been used to treat VIN (Fig. 13–15). An elliptical incision around the lesion is usually made in the direction of the skin lines. In the 393 patients reviewed, 88 (22%) had recurrences. This rate is not significantly different from that for vulvectomy. It is likely that wide local excision is just as curative as vulvectomy and is better suited to the young patient in whom scarring is a consideration. It is strongly suggested that absorbable suture be used for repair.

Chemotherapy

5-FU has also been used to treat VIN. Although it often leads to severe ulceration, it seems to work for some patients. The reported failure rate is 66%, so it should be reserved for patients for whom better treatments cannot be found.

Laser Therapy

VIN has also been treated with the laser. For the young patient in whom invasion is unlikely, the laser is probably the treatment of choice (Fig. 13–16).

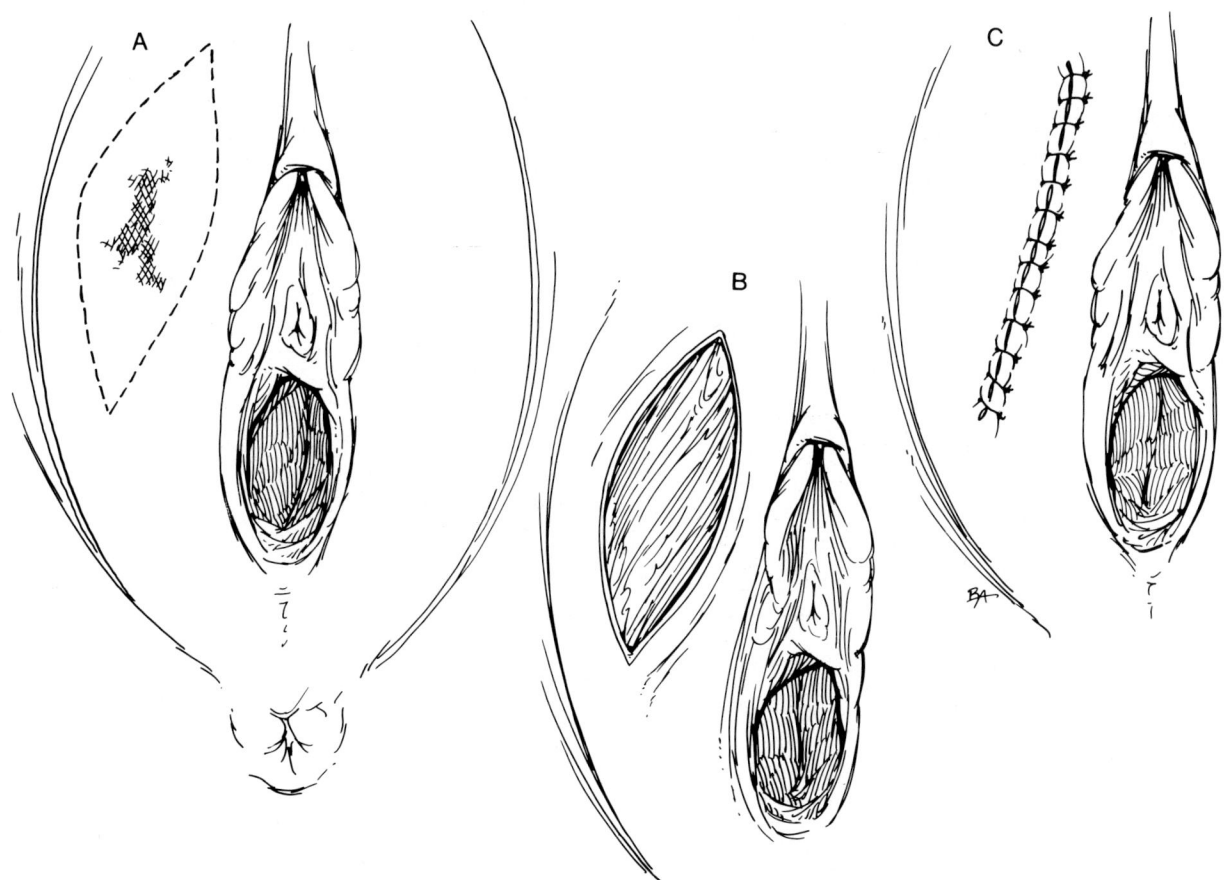

Figure 13–15
A to C, Wide local excision of the vulva. An epithelial section of vulva is removed. The defect is enclosed with interrupted sutures of biodegradable material.

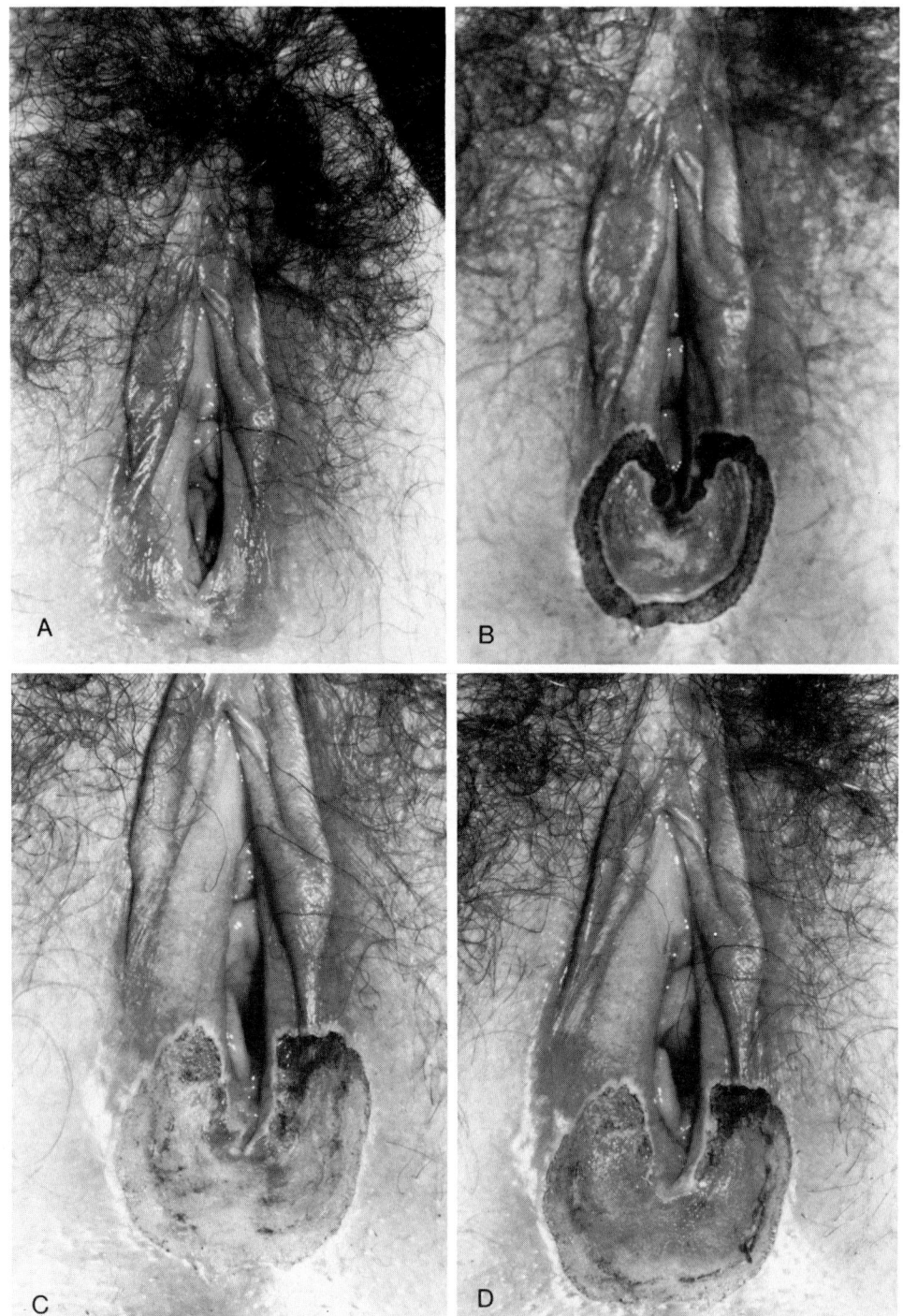

Figure 13–16
Laser in the treatment of vulvar intraepithelial neoplasia (VIN). A VIN lesion is shown. The laser is used to outline the lesion (*A*), ablate the surface epithelium to the level of the basement membrane (*B*), then to the level of the papillary dermis (*C*), and then to the level of the reticular dermis (*D*).

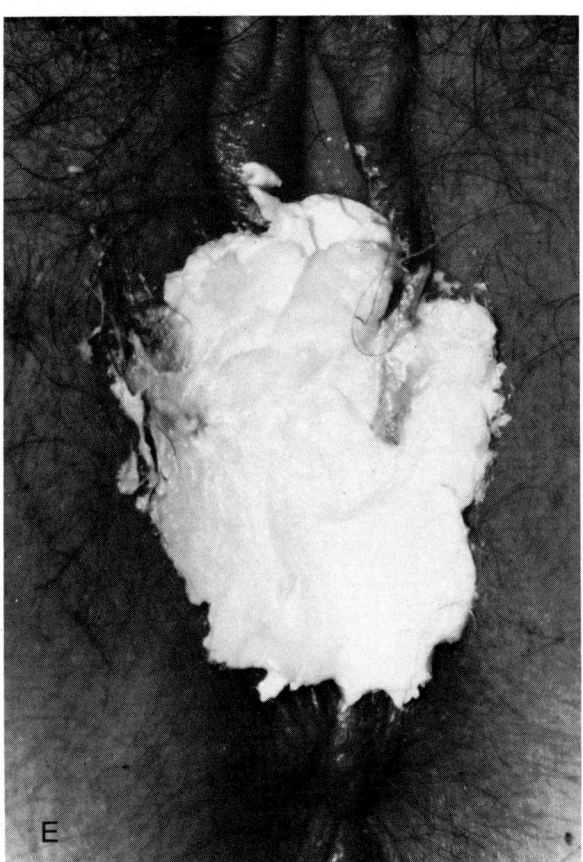

Figure 13–16 *Continued*
The vulva is then covered with Silvadene cream (*E*).

However, the laser must be used extremely carefully, because burns to this area can cause long-term dyspareunia. Mucosal areas of the vulva should be treated with the laser to a depth of 1 mm in non–hair-bearing areas and to a depth of 3 mm in hair-bearing areas. The failure rate for 172 cases was 11%.

Reid's description for using the laser is excellent. He recommends using power densities of less than or equal to 600 watts/cm² and an anatomic orientation to control the depth of the laser.[152, 153]

The problem with the laser treatment is that no surgical specimen is obtained. A few authors have noted microinvasion in young patients. One way to deal with this issue would be to combine wide local excision with the laser, as has been suggested by some authors.[154]

Other Therapies

Radiation has been successfully used in a few patients but would probably not be the treatment of choice at this time. Cryotherapy has also been used in a few patients, but apparently patients do not tolerate sloughing of the vulva as well as they do sloughing of the cervix. Although the cure rate is high, healing is slow, so this is not currently a therapy of choice.

SUMMARY

Not much is known about the incidence or prevalence of any of the preinvasive conditions. More is known about the risk factors for CIN than for VAIN or VIN, but they are presumed to be similar because of the multicentric nature of the lesions. The clinical presentation for CIN and VAIN is asymptomatic. For VIN, symptoms such as pruritus may be present. The caveat in evaluation of all the preinvasive lesions is the exclusion of an invasive neoplasm. For the cervix, an invasive neoplasm must be excluded with cone biopsy if a Pap smear indicates possible invasion, if there is a discrepancy between the Pap smear and biopsy, if the endocervical curettage is positive, or if the entire lesion or squamocolumnar junction cannot be seen colposcopically. For the vagina, an invasive neoplasm should be excluded, especially in the presence of cytologic findings suspicious for invasion, if there is a history of invasive carcinoma of the female genital tract, or if the woman is over 50. For the vulva, invasive lesions should be suspected in women over age 40–45, for thick lesions, or in women in whom a previous invasive neoplasm has been demonstrated. Diagnosis is expedited in all cases with the use of the colposcope, which is able to identify abnormal areas to be biopsied. Several treatment modalities are available for each of type of lesion. Few prospective clinical trials exist, however, that compare one therapy to another. Review of these studies is complicated because they lack information on several important points: a definition of the population being treated, a complete description of their evaluation, details about treatment, a description of who experienced treatment failure, how long these patients were observed, how many times they were treated before their therapy was classified a cure or failure, a mention of short- and long-term complications, and an assessment of costs. In addition, outcomes of interest, such as failure in both persistent and recurrent disease and the development of invasive disease, are not consistently mentioned in those series. Fortunately, as more of the natural history of these conditions has been understood, less morbid therapies have been implemented in treatment. Well-designed prospective studies that compare these therapies and the development of newer, less morbid therapies are imperative.

References

1. Mitchell MF: Natural history of cervical intraepithelial lesions. (In press.)
2. Nasiell K, Nasiell M, Vaclavinkova V, et al.: Follow-up studies of cytologically detected precancerous lesions (dysplasia) of the uterine cervix. In Bostrom H, Larsson T, Ljungstedt N (eds.): Health Control in Detection of Cancer. Skandia International Symposia, September 23–25, 1975, pp. 244–256.

3. Nasiell K, Roger V, Nasiell M: Behavior of mild cervical dysplasia during long-term follow-up. Obstet Gynecol 1986; 67:665.
4. Nasiell K, Nasiell M, Vaclavinkova V: Behavior of moderate cervical dysplasia during long-term follow-up. Obstet Gynecol 1983; 61:609.
5. Koss LG, Stewart FW, Foote FW, et al.: Some histological aspects of behavior of epidermoid carcinoma in situ and related lesions of the uterine cervix: A long-term prospective study. Cancer 1963; 16:1160.
6. Koss LG: Natural history of carcinoma in situ and related lesions of the cervix. In Koss LG (ed.): Diagnostic Cytology and Its Histopathologic Bases, 3rd ed. Philadelphia, JR Lippincott, 1979, p. 305.
7. Kashgarian M, Dunn JE Jr: The duration of intraepithelial and preclinical squamous cell carcinoma of the uterine cervix. Am J Epidemiol 1970; 92:211.
8. Dunn JE Jr: The relationship between carcinoma in situ and invasive cervical carcinoma. Cancer 1953; 6:873.
9. Dunn JE Jr: Relation of carcinoma in situ to invasive carcinoma of the cervix uteri. In Proceedings of the Fourth Berkeley Symposium on Mathematical Statistics and Probability, University of California Press, Berkeley, 1961, pp. 211–221.
10. Dunn JE, Martin PL: Morphogenesis of cervical cancer: Findings from San Diego County cytology registry. Cancer 1967; 20:1899.
11. Boyes DA, Fidler HK, Lock DR: Significance of in situ carcinoma of the uterine cervix. Br Med J 1962; 1:203.
12. Fidler HK, Boyes DA, Worth AJ: Cervical cancer detection in British Columbia: A progress report. J Obstet Gynaecol Br Cwlth 1968; 75:392.
13. Boyes DA, Morrison B, Knox EG, et al.: A cohort study of cervical cancer screening in British Columbia. Clin Invest Med 1982; 5:1.
14. Prorok PC: Mathematical models and natural history in cervical cancer screening. In Kahama M, Miller AB, Day NE (eds.): Screening for Cancer of the Uterine Cervix. Lyon, IARC Scientific Publications No. 76, 1986, pp. 185–198.
15. Kinlen LJ, Spriggs AI: Women with positive cervical smears but without surgical intervention. Lancet 1978; 2:463.
16. Gad C: The management and natural history of severe dysplasia and carcinoma in situ of the uterine cervix. Br J Obstet Gynaecol 1976; 83:554.
17. Boyes DA, Worth AJ, Fidler BK: The results of treatment of 4389 cases of pre-clinical cervical squamous carcinoma. J Obstet Gynaecol Br Cwlth 1970; 77:769.
18. Kolstad P, Klem V: Long-term follow-up of 1121 cases of carcinoma in situ. Obstet Gynecol 1976; 48:125.
19. McIndoe WA, McLean MR, Jones RW, Mullins PR: The invasive potential of carcinoma in situ of the cervix. Obstet Gynecol 1984; 64:451.
20. Ferenczy A: Cervical intraepithelial neoplasia. In Blaustein A (ed.): Pathology of the Female Genital Tract. New York, Springer-Verlag, 1982, pp. 157–158.
21. Cancer facts and figures. American Cancer Society, 1992.
22. Sadeghi SB, Sadeghi A, Robboy SJ: Prevalence of dysplasia and cancer of the cervix in a nationwide Planned Parenthood population. Cancer 1988; 61:2359.
23. Anderson GH, Boyes DA, Benedet JL, et al.: Organisation and results of the cervical cytology screening programme in British Columbia, 1955–85. Br Med J 1988; 296:975.
24. Duguid HLD, Duncan ID, Currie J: Screening for cervical intraepithelial neoplasia in Dundee and Angus 1962–81 and its relation with invasive cervical cancer. Lancet 1985; 2:1053.
25. Brinton LA, Fraumeni JF Jr: Epidemiology of uterine cervical cancer. J Chron Dis 1986; 39:1051.
26. Mitchell MF: Diagnosis and treatment of preinvasive disease of the female lower genital tract. Cancer Bull 1990; 42:71.
27. Vonka V, Kanka J, Jelinek J, et al.: Prospective study on the relationship between cervical neoplasia and herpes simplex type-2 virus. 1. Epidemiological characteristics. Int J Cancer 1984; 33:49.
28. Vonka V, Kanka J, Hirsch I, et al.: Prospective study on the relationship between cervical neoplasia papillomavirus infection and neoplasia of the cervix and anogenital region in women with Hodgkin's disease. Acta Cytol 1987; 31:845.
29. zur Hausen H: Human papillomaviruses and their possible role in squamous carcinoma. Curr Top Microbiol Immunol 1977; 78:1.
30. Gissman L: Papillomaviruses and their association with cancer in animals and man. Cancer Surv 1984; 13:161.
31. Galloway DA, McDougall JK: Human papillomavirus and carcinomas. Adv Virus Res 1989; 37:125.
32. zur Hausen H: Papillomaviruses in anogenital cancer as a model to understand the role of viruses in human cancers. Cancer Res 1989; 49:4677.
33. Wright TC Jr, Richart RM: Review: Role of human papillomavirus in the pathogenesis of genital tract warts and cancer. Gynecol Oncol 1990; 37:151.
34. Becker TM, Stone KM, Alexander ER: Genital human papillomavirus infection: A growing concern. Obstet Gynecol Clin North Am 1987; 14:389.
35. Acs J, Hildesheim A, Reeves WC, et al.: Regional distribution of human papillomavirus DNA and other risk factors for invasive cervical cancer in Panama. Cancer Res 1989; 49:5725.
36. Kjaer SK, de Villiers EM, Haugaard BJ, et al.: Human papillomavirus, herpes simplex virus and cervical cancer incidence in Greenland and Denmark. A population-based cross-sectional study. Int J Cancer 1988; 41:518.
37. Kjaer SK, Teisen C, Haugaard BJ, et al.: Risk factors for cervical cancer in Greenland and Denmark: A population-based cross-sectional study. Int J Cancer 1989; 44:40.
38. Reeves WC, Brinton LA, Garcia M, et al.: Human papillomavirus infection and cervical cancer in Latin America. N Engl J Med 1989; 320:1437.
39. Bosch FX: Personal communication (5-17-90).
40. Mitchell MF, Tortolero G: Epidemiology of human papillomas. (In press.)
41. Richart RM: The patient with an abnormal Pap smear: Screening techniques and management. N Engl J Med 1980; 302:332.
42. Colposcopic appearance of the atypical transformation zone. In Coppleson M, Pixley E, Reid B (eds.): Colposcopy: A Scientific and Practical Approach to the Cervix, Vagina and Vulva in Health and Disease, 3rd ed. Springfield, IL, Charles C Thomas, 1986, pp. 223–254.
43. Premalignant and related disorders of the lower genital tract. In Morrow CP, Townsend DE (eds.): Synopsis of Gynecologic Oncology, 3rd ed. New York, John Wiley & Sons, 1987, pp. 22–25.
44. Crisp WE: Cryosurgical treatment of neoplasia of the uterine cervix. Obstet Gynecol 1972; 39:495.
45. Charles EH, Savage EW: Cryosurgical treatment of cervical intraepithelial neoplasia. Obstet Gynecol Surv 1980; 35:539.
46. Sonek MG (coordinator), Acosta AA, Collins RJ, Crisp WE, et al. (correspondents): Cryosurgery in the treatment of abnormal cervical lesions: An invited symposium. J Reprod Med 1971; 7:14.
47. Creasman WT, Weed JC, Curry SL, et al.: Efficacy of cryosurgical treatment of severe cervical intraepithelial neoplasia. Obstet Gynecol 1973; 41:501.
48. Benedet JL, Miller DM, Nickerson KG, Anderson GH: The results of cryosurgical treatment of cervical intraepithelial neoplasia at one, five, and ten years. Am J Obstet Gynecol 1987; 157:268.
49. Tredway DR, Townsend DE, Hovland DN, Upton RT: Colposcopy and cryosurgery in cervical intraepithelial neoplasia. Am J Obstet Gynecol 1972; 114:1020.
50. Underwood PB Jr, Lutz MH, Fletcher RV Jr: Cryosurgery: Its use for the abnormal Pap smear. Cancer 1976; 38:546.
51. Kaufman RH, Irwin JF: The cryosurgical therapy of cervical intraepithelial neoplasia. Am J Obstet Gynecol 1978; 131:381.
52. Popkin DR, Scali V, Ahmed MN: Cryosurgery for the treatment of cervical intraepithelial neoplasia. Am J Obstet Gynecol 1978; 130:551.
53. Ostergard DR: Cryosurgical treatment of cervical intraepithelial neoplasia. Obstet Gynecol 1980; 56:231.
54. Walton LA, Edelman DA, Fowler WC Jr, Photopulos GJ: Cryosurgery for the treatment of cervical intraepithelial neoplasia during the reproductive years. Obstet Gynecol 1980; 55:353.
55. Hatch KD, Shingleton HM, Austin JM Jr, et al.: Cryosurgery of cervical intraepithelial neoplasia. Obstet Gynecol 1981; 57:692.

56. Sedlis A, Castadot M-J, Glatt B: Cryotherapy in cervical disease. NY State J Med 1981; 81:1757.
57. Levine RU, Carillo EJ, Crum CP: Outpatient management of cervical intraepithelial neoplasia. A summary of 279 cases. J Reprod Med 1985; 30:351.
58. Creasman WT, Hinshaw WM, Clarke-Pearson DL: Cryosurgery in the management of cervical intraepithelial neoplasia. Obstet Gynecol 1984; 63:145.
59. Stafl A, Wilkinson EJ, Mattingly RF: Laser treatment of cervical and vaginal neoplasia. Am J Obstet Gynecol 1977; 128:128.
60. Basic laser physics for the gynecologist. In McLaughlin DS (ed.): Lasers in Gynecology. Philadelphia, JB Lippincott, 1991, pp. 7–24.
61. Baggish MS: Laser management of cervical intraepithelial neoplasia. Clin Obstet Gynecol 1983; 26:980.
62. Carter R, Krantz KE, Hara GS, et al.: Treatment of cervical intraepithelial neoplasia with the carbon dioxide laser beam. Am J Obstet Gynecol 1978; 131:831.
63. Bellina JH, Wright VC, Voros JI, et al.: Carbon dioxide laser management of cervical intraepithelial neoplasia. Am J Obstet Gynecol 1981; 141:828.
64. Benedet JL, Nickerson KG, White GW: Laser therapy for cervical intraepithelial neoplasia. Obstet Gynecol 1981; 58:188.
65. Masterson BJ, Krantz KE, Calkins JW, et al.: The carbon dioxide laser in cervical intraepithelial neoplasia: A five-year experience in treating 230 patients. Am J Obstet Gynecol 1981; 139:565.
66. Anderson MC: Treatment of cervical intraepithelial neoplasia with the carbon dioxide laser: Report of 543 patients. Obstet Gynecol 1982; 59:720.
67. Burke L: The use of the carbon dioxide laser in the therapy of cervical intraepithelial neoplasia. Am J Obstet Gynecol 1982; 144:337.
68. Evans AS, Monaghan JM: The treatment of cervical intraepithelial neoplasia using the carbon dioxide laser. Br J Obstet Gynaecol 1983; 90:553.
69. Stanhope CR, Phibbs GD, Stuart GCE, Reid R: Carbon dioxide laser surgery. Obstet Gynecol 1983; 61:624.
70. Baggish MS, Dorsey JH, Adelson M: A ten-year experience treating cervical intraepithelial neoplasia with the CO_2 laser. Am J Obstet Gynecol 1989; 161:60.
71. Wright VC, Davies EM: The conservative management of cervical intraepithelial neoplasia: The use of cryosurgery and the carbon dioxide laser. Br J Obstet Gynaecol 1981; 88:663.
72. Townsend DE, Richart RM: Cryotherapy and carbon dioxide laser management of cervical intraepithelial neoplasia: A controlled comparison. Obstet Gynecol 1983; 61:75.
73. Ferenczy A: Comparison of cryo- and carbon dioxide laser therapy for cervical intraepithelial neoplasia. Obstet Gynecol 1985; 66:793.
74. Kirwan PH, Smith IR, Naftalin NJ: A study of cryosurgery and the CO_2 laser in treatment of carcinoma in situ (CIN III) of the uterine cervix. Gynecol Oncol 1985; 22:195.
75. Berget A, Andreasson B, Bock JE, et al.: Outpatient treatment of cervical intraepithelial neoplasia: The CO_2 laser versus cryotherapy, a randomized trial. Acta Obstet Gynecol Scand 1987; 66:531.
76. Younge PA, Hertig AT, Armstrong D: A study of 135 cases of carcinoma in situ of the cervix at the free hospital for women. Am J Obstet Gynecol 1949; 58:867.
77. Richart RJ, Sciarra JJ: Treatment of cervical dysplasia by outpatient electrocauterization. Am J Obstet Gynecol 1968; 101:200.
78. Ortiz R, Newton M, Tsai A: Electrocautery treatment of cervical intraepithelial neoplasia. Obstet Gynecol 1973; 41:113.
79. Deigan EA, Carmichael JA, Ohlke IE, Karchmar J: Treatment of cervical intraepithelial neoplasia with electrocautery: A report of 776 cases. Am J Obstet Gynecol 1986; 154:255.
80. Staland B: Treatment of premalignant lesions of the uterine cervix by means of moderate heat thermosurgery using the SEMM coagulator. Ann Chir Gynaecol 1978; 67:112.
81. Duncan ID: The SEMM cold coagulator in the management of cervical intraepithelial neoplasia. Clin Obstet Gynecol 1983; 26:996.
82. Chanen W, Rome RM: Electrocoagulation diathermy for cervical dysplasia and carcinoma in situ: A 15-year survey. Obstet Gynecol 1983; 61:673.
83. Moller BR, Johannesen P, Osther K, et al.: Treatment of dysplasia of the cervical epithelium with an interferon gel. Obstet Gynecol 1983; 62:625.
84. Byrne MA, Moller BR, Taylor-Robinson D, et al.: The effect of interferon on human papillomaviruses associated with cervical intraepithelial neoplasia. Br J Obstet Gynaecol 1986; 93:1136.
85. Choo YC, Seto WH, Hsu C, et al.: Cervical intraepithelial neoplasia treated by perilesional injection of interferon. Br J Obstet Gynaecol 1986; 93:372.
86. Atkinson K: Symposium on cervical neoplasia IV. Diathermy loop excision. Colposcopy Gynecol Laser Surg 1985; 1:285.
87. Wright TC Jr, Gagnon S, Ferenczy A, Richart RM: Excising CIN lesions by loop electrosurgical excision procedure. Contemp Obstet Gynecol, March 1991.
88. Boulanger J-C, Vitse M, Gondry J, Thomas E: L'electroconisation du col uterin. Rev Fr Gynecol Obstet 1989; 84:663.
89. Prendiville W, Cullimore J, Norman S: Large loop excision of the transformation zone (LLETZ): A new method of management for women with cervical intraepithelial neoplasia. Br J Obstet Gynaecol 1989; 96:1054.
90. Whiteley PF, Olah KS: Treatment of cervical intraepithelial neoplasia: Experience with the low-voltage diathermy loop. Am J Obstet Gynecol 1990; 162:1272.
91. Luesley DM, Cullimore J, Redman CWE, et al.: Loop diathermy excision of the cervical transformation zone in patients with abnormal cervical smears. Br Med J 1990; 300:1690.
92. Larsson G: Conization for preinvasive and early invasive carcinoma of the uterine cervix. Acta Obstet Gynecol Scand 1983; 114(Suppl):7.
93. Leonard VN: Post-operative results of amputation of the cervix. Surg Gynecol Obstet 1913; 16:390.
94. Lisfranc MJ: Memoire sur l'amputation du col de l'uterus. Gaza Med de Par 1834; 2.S ii:385.
95. Sims M: Amputation of cervix. Tr Med Soc NY, 1861.
96. Sturmdorf A: Tracheloplastic methods and results. A clinical study based upon the physiology of the mesometrium. Surg Gynecol Obstet 1916; 22:93.
97. Kolstad P, Klem V: Long-term followup of 1121 cases of carcinoma in situ. Obstet Gynecol 1976; 48:125.
98. Baggish MS, Dorsey JH: Carbon dioxide laser for combination excisional-vaporization conization. Am J Obstet Gynecol 1985; 151:23.
99. Larsson G, Gullberg B, Grundsell H: A comparison of complications of laser and cold knife conization. Obstet Gynecol 1983; 62:213.
100. Mor-Yosef S, Lopes A, Pearson S, Monaghan JM: Loop diathermy cone biopsy. Obstet Gynecol 1990; 75:884.
101. Sedlis A, Robboy SJ: Diseases of the vagina. In Kurman RJ (ed.): Blaustein's Pathology of the Female Genital Tract, 3rd ed. New York, Springer-Verlag, 1987, pp. 111–112.
102. Rutledge F: Cancer of the vagina. Am J Obstet Gynecol 1967; 97:635.
103. Gallup DG, Morley GW: Carcinoma in situ of the vagina: A study and review. Obstet Gynecol 1975; 46:334.
104. Woodruff JD, Parmley TH, Julian CG: Topical 5-fluorouracil in the treatment of vaginal carcinoma in situ. Gynecol Oncol 1975; 3:124.
105. Lee RA, Symmonds RE: Recurrent carcinoma in situ of the vagina in patients previously treated for in situ carcinoma of the cervix. Obstet Gynecol 1976; 48:61.
106. Ballon SC, Roberts JA, Lagasse LD: Topical 5-fluorouracil in the treatment of intraepithelial neoplasia of the vagina. Obstet Gynecol 1979; 54:163.
107. Oliver JA Jr: Severe dysplasia and carcinoma in situ of the vagina. Am J Obstet Gynecol 1979; 134:133.
108. Piver MS, Barlow JJ, Tsukada Y, et al.: Postirradiation squamous cell carcinoma in situ of the vagina: Treatment by topical 20 percent 5-fluorouracil cream. Am J Obstet Gynecol 1979; 135:377.
109. Daly JW, Ellis GF: Treatment of vaginal dysplasia and carcinoma in situ with topical 5-fluorouracil. Obstet Gynecol 1980; 55:350.
110. Petrilli ES, Townsend DE, Morrow CP, NaKao CY: Vaginal

intraepithelial neoplasia: Biologic aspects and treatment with topical 5-fluorouracil and the carbon dioxide laser. Am J Obstet Gynecol 1980; 38:321.
111. Hernandez-Linares W, Puthawala A, Nolan JF, et al.: Carcinoma in situ of the vagina: Past and present management. Obstet Gynecol 1980; 56:356.
112. Caglar H, Hertzog RW, Hreshchyshyn MM: Topical 5-fluorouracil treatment of vaginal intraepithelial neoplasia. Obstet Gynecol 1981; 58:580.
113. Sillman FH, Boyce JG, Macasaet MA, Nicastri AD: 5-Fluorouracil/chemosurgery for intraepithelial neoplasia of the lower genital tract. Obstet Gynecol 1981; 58:356.
114. Capen CV, Masterson BJ, Magrina JF, Calkins JW: Laser therapy of vaginal intraepithelial neoplasia. Am J Obstet Gynecol 1982; 142:973.
115. Townsend DE, Levine RU, Crum CP, Richart RM: Treatment of vaginal carcinoma in situ with the carbon dioxide laser. Am J Obstet Gynecol 1982; 143:565.
116. Jobson VW, Homesley HD: Treatment of vaginal intraepithelial neoplasia with the carbon dioxide laser. Obstet Gynecol 1983; 62:90.
117. Woodman CBJ, Jordan JA, Wade-Evans T: The management of vaginal intraepithelial neoplasia after hysterectomy. Br J Obstet Gynecol 1984; 91:707.
118. Lenehan PM, Meffe F, Lickrish GM: Vaginal intraepithelial neoplasia: Biologic aspects and management. Obstet Gynecol 1986; 68:333.
119. Stuart GCE, Flagler EA, Nation JG, et al.: Laser vaporization of vaginal intraepithelial neoplasia. Am J Obstet Gynecol 1988; 158:240.
120. Krebs HB: Treatment of vaginal intraepithelial neoplasia with laser and topical 5-fluorouracil. Obstet Gynecol 1989; 73:657.
121. Stafl A, Wilkinson EJ, Mattingly RF: Laser treatment of cervical and vaginal neoplasia. Am J Obstet Gynecol 1977; 128:128.
122. Gallup DG, Castle CA, Stock RJ: Recurrent carcinoma in situ of the vagina following split-thickness skin graft vaginoplasty. Gynecol Oncol 1987; 26:98.
123. Imrie JEA, Kennedy JH, Holmes JD, McGrouther DA: Intraepithelial neoplasia arising in an artificial vagina. Case report. Br J Obstet Gynaecol 1986; 93:886.
124. Lathrop JC, Ree HJ, McDuff HC Jr: Intraepithelial neoplasia of the neovagina. Obstet Gynecol 1985; 65:91S.
125. Wilkinson EJ, Friedrich EG Jr: Diseases of the vulva. In Kurman RJ (ed.): Blaustein's Pathology of the Female Genital Tract, 3rd ed. New York, Springer-Verlag, 1987, pp. 66–70.
126. Woodruff JD, Julian C, Puray T, et al.: The contemporary challenge of carcinoma in situ of the vulva. Am J Obstet Gynecol 1973; 115:677.
127. Carson TE, Hoskins WJ, Wurzel JF: Topical 5-fluorouracil in the treatment of carcinoma in situ of the vulva. Obstet Gynecol 1976; 47(Suppl):59S.
128. Forney JP, Morrow CP, Townsend DE, DiSaia PJ: Management of carcinoma in situ of the vulva. Am J Obstet Gynecol 1977; 127:801.
129. Krupp PJ, Bohm JW: 5-Fluorouracil topical treatment of in situ vulvar cancer: A preliminary report. Obstet Gynecol 1978; 51:702.
130. Hilliard GD, Massey FM, O'Toole RV Jr: Vulvar neoplasia in the young. Am J Obstet Gynecol 1979; 135:185.
131. Buscema J, Woodruff JD, Parmley TH, Genadry R: Carcinoma in situ of the vulva. Obstet Gynecol 1980; 55:225.
132. Lifshitz S, Roberts JA: Treatment of carcinoma in situ of the vulva with topical 5-fluorouracil. Obstet Gynecol 1980; 56:242.
133. Friedrich EG Jr, Wilkinson EJ, Fu YS: Carcinoma in situ of the vulva: A continuing challenge. Am J Obstet Gynecol 1980; 136:830.
134. DiSaia PJ, Rich WM: Surgical approach to multifocal carcinoma in situ of the vulva. Am J Obstet Gynecol 1981; 140:136.
135. Kaplan AL, Kaufman RH, Birken RA, Simkin A: Intraepithelial carcinoma of the vulva with extension to the anal canal. Obstet Gynecol 1981; 58:368.
136. Baggish MS, Dorsey JH: CO_2 laser for the treatment of vulvar carcinoma in situ. Obstet Gynecol 1981; 57:371.
137. Ulbright TM, Stehman FB, Roth LM, et al.: Bowenoid dysplasia of the vulva. Cancer 1982; 50:2910.
138. Caglar H, Tamer S, Hrechchyshyn MM: Vulvar intraepithelial neoplasia. Obstet Gynecol 1982; 60:346.
139. Benedet JL, Murphy KJ: Squamous carcinoma in situ of the vulva. Gynecol Oncol 1982; 14:213.
140. Townsend DE, Levine RU, Richart RM, et al.: Management of vulvar intraepithelial neoplasia by carbon dioxide laser. Obstet Gynecol 1982; 60:49.
141. Di Paola GR, Rueda-Leverone NG, Belardi MG, Vighi A: Vulvar carcinoma in situ: A report of 28 cases. Gynecol Oncol 1982; 14:236.
142. Bernstein SG, Kovacs BR, Townsend DE, Morrow CP: Vulvar carcinoma in situ. Obstet Gynecol 1983; 61:304.
143. Ferenczy A: Using the laser to treat vulvar condylomata acuminata and intraepidermal neoplasia. Can Med Assoc J 1983; 128:135.
144. Leuchter RS, Townsend DE, Hacker NF, et al.: Treatment of vulvar carcinoma in situ with the CO_2 laser. Gynecol Oncol 1984; 19:314.
145. Wolcott HD, Gallup DG: Wide local excision in the treatment of vulvar carcinoma in situ: A reappraisal. Am J Obstet Gynecol 1984; 150:695.
146. Crum CP, Liskow A, Petras P, et al.: Vulvar intraepithelial neoplasia (severe atypia and carcinoma in situ): A clinicopathologic analysis of 41 cases. Cancer 1984; 54:1429.
147. Andreasson B, Bock JE: Intraepithelial neoplasia in the vulvar region. Gynecol Oncol 1985; 21:300.
148. Jones RW, McLean MR: Carcinoma in situ of the vulva: A review of 31 treated and five untreated cases. Obstet Gynecol 1986; 68:499.
149. Wright VC, Davies E: Laser surgery for vulvar intraepithelial neoplasia: Principles and results. Am J Obstet Gynecol 1987; 156:374.
150. Rettenmaier MA, Berman ML, DiSaia PJ: Skinning vulvectomy for the treatment of multifocal vulvar intraepithelial neoplasia. Obstet Gynecol 1987; 69:247.
151. Rutledge F, Sinclair M: Treatment of intraepithelial carcinoma of the vulva by skin excision and graft. Am J Obstet Gynecol 1968; 102:806.
152. Reid R: Superficial laser vulvectomy. III. A new surgical technique for appendage-conserving ablation of refractory condylomas and vulvar intraepithelial neoplasia. Am J Obstet Gynecol 1985; 152:504.
153. Reid R, Elfont EA, Zirkin RM, Fuller TA: Superficial laser vulvectomy. II. The anatomic and biophysical principles permitting accurate control over the depth of dermal destruction with the carbon dioxide laser. Am J Obstet Gynecol 1985; 152:261.
154. Bornstein J, Kaufman RH: Combination of surgical excision and carbon dioxide laser vaporization for multifocal vulvar intraepithelial neoplasia. Am J Obstet Gynecol 1988; 158:459.

Dilatation and Curettage and Cervical Conization

14

Steven R. Bayer
José A. Soto-Hunnicutt

Dilatation and curettage (D & C) and conization of the cervix are two fundamental procedures of gynecologic surgery that have both diagnostic and therapeutic capabilities. Since the introduction of these procedures over a century ago, the indications have changed but are now better defined. This chapter provides a thorough review of the technique of these surgical procedures. In addition, the basic pathophysiology of the underlying disease states and the decision making process leading up to the performance of these procedures are also discussed.

DILATATION AND CURETTAGE

Introduction and Historical Aspects

Probing of the uterine cavity was practiced by the ancient Egyptians to insert various substances into the uterus. In the early 1800s, the uterine sound was used to probe the uterine cavity for diagnostic purposes. In the past, the cervix was dilated with rubber dilators, sponge tents, or laminaria. These techniques were not optimal, and the use of laminaria was associated with a high rate of infection. Hegar (1879) is credited with the development of graduated metal dilators that could safely and effectively dilate the cervix. Cervical dilatation by itself was commonly used for the treatment of dysmenorrhea. The uterine curette was introduced in 1842 by Récamier but initially was not well accepted because the inventor reported complications with its use, including two deaths following uterine perforation with resultant peritonitis. The procedure finally gained acceptance when it was reintroduced almost 30 years later. Over the past century, the combination of cervical dilatation and uterine curettage has become one of the most commonly performed surgical procedures in all of medicine.

Indications

In the past, the D & C was the only means the gynecologist had to study the contents of the uterine cavity. Other diagnostic techniques to evaluate the uterus have emerged and include hysterosalpingography, hysteroscopy, ultrasonography, and the office endometrial biopsy. These tools, together with the D & C, allow a more accurate assessment and determination of the etiology of the patient's symptoms. In addition to its diagnostic capabilities, the D & C is a therapeutic modality that is commonly used to empty the uterus in cases of incomplete abortion and pregnancy termination. These and other indications for performing this procedure are discussed in the following sections.

Abnormal Pregnancy

Vaginal bleeding in the first trimester of pregnancy is a common occurrence, and in most patients the bleeding will resolve and the pregnancy will progress to term. However, if the bleeding increases and is associated with lower abdominal cramping, the overall prognosis for the pregnancy is worse. The pelvic examination will help to identify the source of the bleeding, and one cannot assume that all bleeding during pregnancy is uterine in origin; it may be secondary to vaginal infection, cervicitis, or even cervical cancer. If, on examination, the cervix is dilated with tissue, the presumptive diagnosis of incomplete abortion can be made. In the presence of heavy uterine bleeding, cramping and a closed cervical os, the most likely diagnosis is an inevitable abortion. For these presentations, a D & C will correct the problem and in some situations can be a lifesaving procedure. However, not all first-trimester pregnancy losses have to be treated with surgical intervention. Many times, the entire pregnancy will pass spontaneously, the bleeding and cramping will abate, and the patient will require no further treatment. In other instances, the simple removal of the intact products of conception from the cervical os will suffice for treatment. It is imperative that all tissue be subjected to histologic examination to confirm the presence of placental villi. Heavy vaginal bleeding and the passage of a decidual cast can be associated with an ectopic pregnancy and be misdiagnosed as an incomplete abortion.

A hydatidiform mole is an uncommon complication of pregnancy that is also managed by a D & C. It complicates approximately 1 out of 1200 pregnancies. Any patient who develops pre-eclampsia during the first trimester or has severe hyperemesis gravidarum should be considered at risk for a molar pregnancy. On physical examination, the uterus can be smaller, larger, or appropriate size for gestational age. In the past, the diagnosis was established by amniography, which displays the typical honeycomb appearance; this diagnostic tool has now been replaced by the ultrasound. Ultrasound examination will fail to demonstrate the presence of a fetus, and the uterine cavity will be filled with multiple echoes demonstrating a "snowflake" pattern. Once the diagnosis is established, a suction curettage should be performed. It is important after the procedure, that patients avoid pregnancy for at least 1 year so that serum beta–human chorionic gonadotropin (β-hCG) levels can be monitored to rule out persistent or recurrent disease.

A D & C is also useful when one is trying to rule out the presence of an ectopic pregnancy. During the first trimester of pregnancy, the serum β-hCG titer should double every 2–3 days and an intrauterine gestational sac can be identified by pelvic ultrasound once the titer has reached a level of 6500 mIU/ml.[1] With vaginal ultrasonography, an intrauterine gestational sac can be seen earlier once the β-hCG titer has risen to 2000 mIU/ml. In any institution, the β-hCG titer at which an intrauterine gestational sac can be identified will depend on the type of ultrasound used, the expertise of the ultrasonographer, and the hCG standard used in the radioimmunoassay. If the β-hCG titers fail to rise appropriately or an intrauterine gestational sac is not identified once the critical titer is reached, the diagnostic possibilities include a missed abortion and an ectopic pregnancy. These can be differentiated with a D & C, and if the histologic examination of the curettings fails to document placental villi, an ectopic pregnancy needs to be ruled out and a laparoscopy performed.

Abnormal Uterine Bleeding

The normal menstrual cycle length ranges between 22 and 35 days. The duration of menses can last from 3 to 7 days, and the average blood loss is 30 ml. The frequency, duration, and amount of blood loss during menses may vary from woman to woman; however, in any individual, these parameters should remain stable from cycle to cycle. Only when the woman experiences a deviation from her norm does she present for evaluation.

When a patient presents with complaints of abnormal uterine bleeding, one must first determine if it is ovulatory or anovulatory in nature. If there are regular intervals between the bleeding episodes and the patient experiences premenstrual symptoms prior to the bleeding, this is presumptive evidence that ovulation is occurring. A biphasic basal body temperature chart or a serum progesterone level greater than 3.0 ng/ml is confirmatory of ovulation. If there is still question regarding the patient's ovulatory status, an endometrial biopsy can be performed during the onset of a bleeding episode. If secretory changes are seen histologically, this provides absolute confirmation that ovulation has occurred.

Anovulatory bleeding results from chronic unopposed estrogen that increases the thickness of the endometrium to an unstable height, making it prone to bleeding. The pattern of bleeding in the anovulatory patient can be variable. Some patients have only light spotting that occurs every few weeks, whereas others can present with heavy bleeding and clotting that follows a long duration of amenorrhea. If the acute bleeding episode is not excessive, a progestational agent will stabilize the endometrium and the bleeding will resolve. If the patient fails to respond to medical treatment within 24–48 hours or if the initial bleeding episode is excessive, a D & C should be performed.

Unopposed estrogen also puts the patient at increased risk for adenomatous hyperplasia, which can lead to endometrial cancer. For this reason, endometrial sampling is indicated and can easily be accomplished by an endometrial biopsy performed in the office. Medical treatment with oral contraceptives or a progestational agent administered on a monthly basis will induce a normal, regular menstrual flow and give protection against the development of uterine cancer.

If the clinician determines that the abnormal bleeding is occurring in the presence of ovulation, another etiology must be sought. The pelvic examination may give further insight into a possible cause. As stated previously, one cannot assume that all vaginal bleeding is uterine in origin, and a complete inspection of the genital tract is indicated. On bimanual examination, uterine enlargement is suggestive of uterine fibroids, adenomyosis, or a possible pregnancy. A rectal examination with a stool guaiac test is also important and will rule out a rectal cause of the bleeding. Particularly in older women, rectal bleeding may be misconstrued as vaginal bleeding.

Initial laboratory work-up includes a β-hCG determination to rule out pregnancy. A complete blood count should be obtained to assess the degree of anemia, if present, and to rule out thrombocytopenia as a cause of the menorrhagia. In addition, many patients with leukemia can first present to the gynecologist with menstrual irregularities. Clotting studies will help to rule out a coagulopathy as a cause of the abnormal bleeding. A hysterosalpingogram may demonstrate an abnormal uterine cavity suggesting the presence of a submucous uterine fibroid, endometrial polyp, or adenomyosis.

In every patient, one must always consider the possibility of endometrial cancer as a cause of the abnormal bleeding even if a more obvious cause is present (i.e., uterine fibroids, adenomyosis). Therefore, endometrial sampling is indicated.

Abnormal Pap Smear

Following an abnormal Pap smear, a colposcopic examination of the cervix should be performed. In some instances, the colposcopic examination of the cervix and vagina is negative and the source of the abnormal cells cannot be identified. An occult lesion may exist high in the cervical canal, or the abnormal cells may be arising from a uterine or ovarian cancer. Following this presentation, a cone biopsy of the cervix and a D & C are indicated.

Postmenopausal Bleeding

In the United States, the average age of menopause is 50 years, and the diagnosis can be made once the patient has been amenorrheic for 1 year. Anovulatory bleeding during the perimenopausal period is common. These patients should be evaluated and treated as previously described with a 10-day course of a progestational agent each month.

When does postmenopausal bleeding necessitate endometrial sampling to rule out endometrial cancer? If the patient is on estrogen replacement, withdrawal bleeding following completion of the progestational agent is common and does not need to be evaluated. However, if the bleeding occurs at other unexpected times during the month, endometrial sampling is indicated. Any vaginal bleeding in the menopausal patient who is not taking hormonal replacement should be considered abnormal and needs to be investigated.

Dysmenorrhea

Pain associated with menses can begin prior to or with the onset of menstrual flow. If the physical examination demonstrates no abnormalities, a trial of oral contraceptives or prostaglandin synthetase inhibitors may resolve the symptomatology. If this proves to be unsuccessful, further investigation is warranted. Some patients' symptomatology may be caused by cervical stenosis that does not allow egress of the menstrual fluid, causing uterine distention. Patients at risk for cervical stenosis are those previously exposed to diethylstilbestrol, or those who have been treated with cryosurgery or conization of the cervix. The combination of a D & C and a laparoscopy may be useful not only from a therapeutic standpoint but also to help rule out other causes of dysmenorrhea, including endometriosis and chronic pelvic inflammatory disease.

Surgical Technique

Anesthesia

Most of the discomfort experienced by the patient during the procedure results from the cervical dilatation, but any instrumentation in the uterine cavity produces moderate to severe lower abdominal cramping. General anesthesia provides the best relaxation and comfort for the patient. However, if the patient has recently eaten prior to the procedure, regional or local anesthesia is a safer alternative. The paracervical block usually provides enough anesthesia to allow the procedure to be performed. A 1% lidocaine solution is used, and 5–10 ml is injected at the junction of the vagina and cervix at the 5 o'clock and 7 o'clock positions at a depth of 0.5 cm. It is imperative that prior to the injection, the plunger of the syringe is pulled back to ensure that the needle is not in an intravascular position. Lidocaine toxicity can result if the medication is injected intravenously or if the maximal dose administered exceeds 7.0 mg/kg.

Patient Positioning and Preparation

The patient is placed in the dorsal lithotomy position. It is important that her buttocks are brought just beyond the break in the table to allow adequate placement of vaginal retractors. The perineum and vagina are prepped with a povidone-iodine or hexachlorophene solution. Next a bimanual examination is performed to examine the adnexa and to determine the size, shape, consistency, and position of the uterus. A full bladder may interfere with the determination of the uterine position, and catheterization of the bladder may be necessary. Knowledge of uterine position is of utmost importance; otherwise, the chance of uterine perforation with the procedure will increase.

The next step is to choose the method of vaginal retraction. If there is a only a single operator present, a weighted vaginal speculum can provide the necessary exposure. A Graves speculum can also be used, but the exposure can be somewhat confining once the instrumentation is begun. Otherwise, an assistant, if present, can retract the vagina posteriorly with a Sims retractor and anteriorly with a Dever retractor. The cervix is visualized, and the anterior lip is grasped with a single-tooth tenaculum. If one cannot get a good hold of the cervix with this instrument, a four-pronged tenaculum/straight Jacob clamp should be used instead (Fig. 14–1). For patients who present with an incomplete abortion, the cervix may already be dilated enough to allow placement of a ring forceps on the cervix, which is less traumatic than a tenaculum. Next the cervix is pulled toward the introitus and slight pressure is maintained. This will help to align the cervix and the uterus in the same axis. This maneuver is especially important if the uterus is sharply anteverted or retroverted, when the risk of perforation is greater. Next a uterine sound is inserted and the depth of the uterine cavity is measured. In the older woman at risk for endometrial cancer, an endocervical curet-

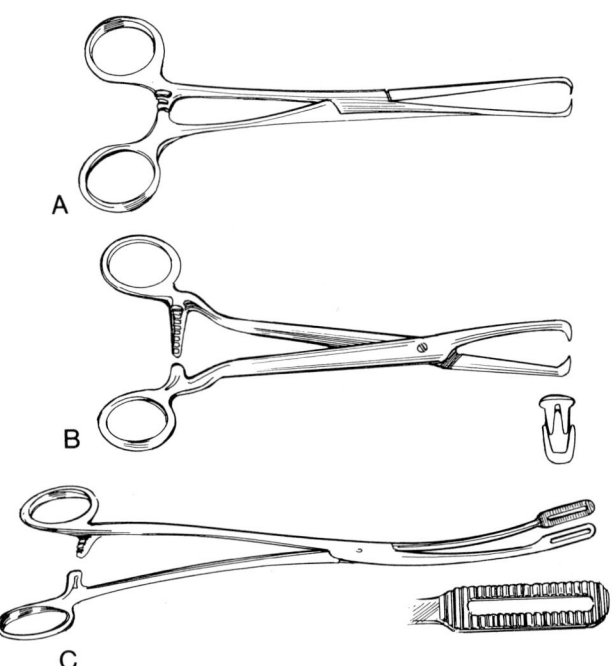

Figure 14–1
A, Single-tooth tenaculum. B, Straight Jacob's double-tooth tenaculum. C, Uterine polyp forceps.

tage is performed next with a Kevorkian curette. A vigorous curettage of the endocervix is usually necessary to obtain an adequate tissue specimen, which is sent separately for pathologic study.

Cervical Dilatation

Active Cervical Dilatation. The cervix has to be dilated to allow insertion of the uterine curette. Cervical dilatation can be the most arduous and time-consuming part of the procedure, and one must proceed with patience. For active dilatation of the cervix, one has the choice of Hegar, Pratt, or Hank-Bradley graduated metal dilators (Figs. 14–2 and 14–3; Table 14–1). The different types of dilators vary somewhat in their design. The ends of the Hegar

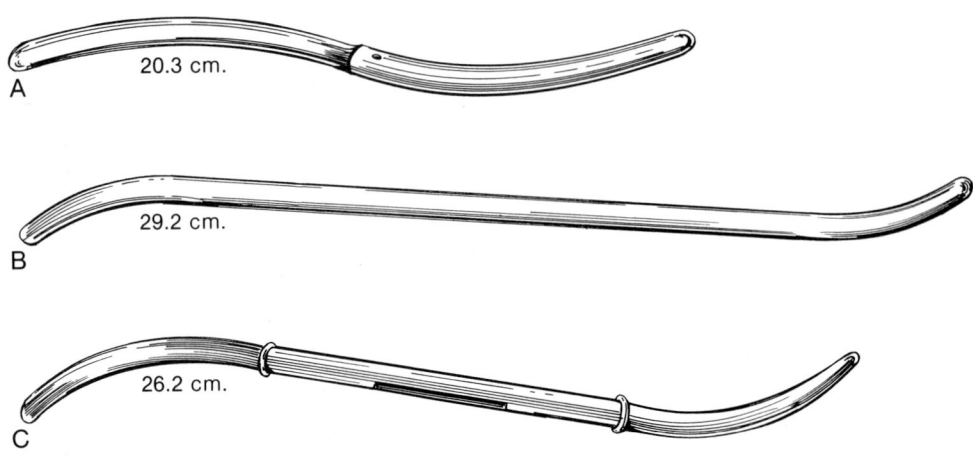

Figure 14–2
Cervical dilators. A, Hegar: blunt ends; solid steel or hollow shafts; available sizes, 1–26 mm in diameter. B, Pratt: tapered ends; available sizes, 17–43 French scale. C, Hank-Bradley: tapered ends; cannulated shaft; available in sizes 9–20 American scale.

Table 14-1

Gauge Conversion for French, American, and English Scales

Diameter (mm)	Scale		
	French	*American*	*English*
0.33	1	—	—
0.50	—	1	—
0.66	2	—	—
0.99	3	2	—
	—	—	1
1.32	4	—	—
1.50	—	3	—
1.65	5	—	—
1.98	6	4	2
2.32	7	—	—
2.50	—	5	3
2.64	8	—	—
2.97	9	6	4
3.33	10	—	5
3.50	—	7	—
3.63	11	—	6
3.96	12	8	—
4.29	13	—	—
4.50	—	9	7
4.62	14	—	—
4.95	15	10	8
5.28	16	—	—
5.50	—	11	9
5.61	17	—	—
5.94	18	12	10
6.27	19	—	—
6.50	—	13	11
6.60	20	—	—
6.93	21	14	12
7.26	22	—	—
7.50	—	15	13
7.59	23	—	—
7.92	24	16	14
8.25	25	—	—
8.50	—	17	15
8.58	26	—	—
8.91	27	18	16
9.24	28	—	—
9.50	—	19	17
9.57	29	—	—
9.90	30	20	18
10.56	32	21	—
11.00	33	22	19
11.55	35	23	—

technique will help to reduce the chance of uterine perforation. Initially, the smallest dilator is inserted into the cervical canal just beyond the internal os. The direction of the curve and angle of insertion of the dilator are adjusted according to the position of the uterus. The greatest resistance during the dilatation is encountered at the level of the internal os, and once the os has admitted the dilator, the operator will feel a sudden decrease in resistance. After the internal os has accommodated the dilator, it is left in place for several seconds before the next larger dilator is introduced. The cervical canal can be tortuous, which can create difficulty with the dilatation. Initially, if difficulty is encountered, simply changing the angle of insertion should allow entry of the dilator. If this proves unsuccessful, a small probe can be gently inserted to better identify the location and direction of the cervical canal. However, if difficulty continues to persist after these simple maneuvers, the procedure should be stopped or performed under ultrasound guidance. Forceful cervical dilatation without a sense of direction of the cervical canal will result in the creation of a false passage and/or perforation of the uterus. Dilation of the cervix to a No. 8 Hegar dilator should be adequate for the passage of the uterine curette. If the procedure is performed for cervical stenosis, it is advised not to dilate past a No. 10 Hegar because of the possibility of producing an incompetent cervix.

Passive Cervical Dilatation. Mechanical dilatation of the cervix can be difficult and potentially traumatic. For over a century, laminaria has been used to achieve a gradual passive dilatation of the cervix that eliminates or decreases the overall force needed for further active dilatation. Laminaria cervical tents are made from the stems of dried seaweed (*Laminaria japonica* and *Laminaria digitata*), formed into a cylindrical shape and then sterilized. The processed laminaria can contain residual spores that are resistant

dilators are more uniform in their diameter, whereas the ends of the Pratt dilators are tapered, allowing an easier cervical dilatation. The Hank-Bradley dilators have the same shape and contour as the Hegar dilators, but they are more tapered and contain an open channel throughout the shank of the dilator, which allows egress of air, preventing the dilator from acting as a piston forcing air up into the uterine cavity. When performing cervical dilatation, one has the best control of the instrument if it is held like a pen and the fourth and fifth digits are extended so that when the operator has overcome the resistance of the cervix during the dilatation, the extended digits will halt the movement of the instrument once they come in contact with the introitus (Fig. 14-4). This

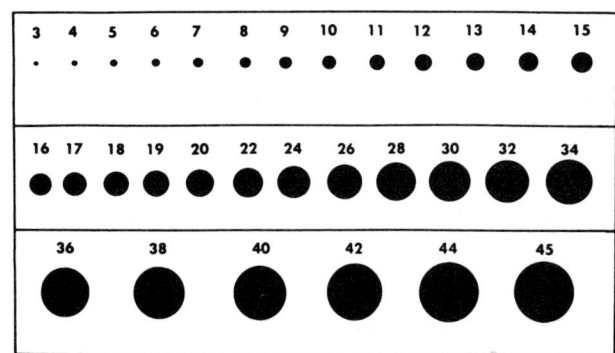

Figure 14-3
The standard French scale is used in the size calibration of catheters and other tubular instruments. It is based on the metric system, and each unit is approximately 0.33 mm; there is a difference of 0.33 mm between consecutive sizes.

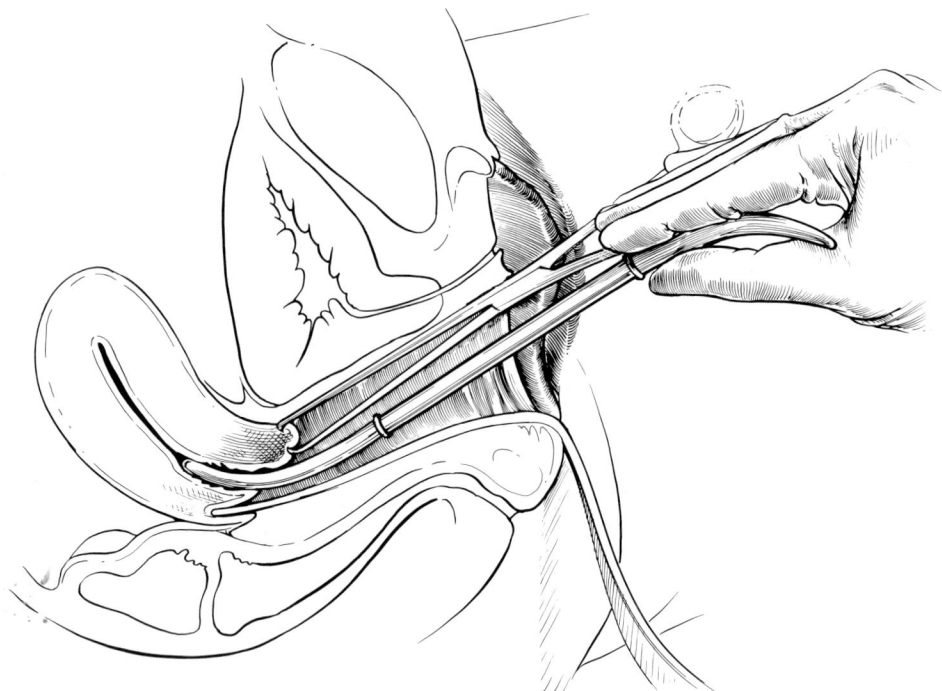

Figure 14–4
Technique of cervical dilatation. The tenaculum is placed on the anterior lip of the cervix and is then pulled out to the introitus, which aligns the cervix and uterine cavity in the same axis. When performing the cervical dilatation, the dilator is placed in the hand as shown with the fourth and fifth fingers extended so that once the resistance of the internal cervical os has been overcome, the extended fingers will come in contact with the vulva and halt the movement of the instrument, decreasing the chance of uterine perforation.

to sterilization techniques and may increase the chance of infection. The hygroscopic laminaria will absorb water from the surrounding tissues, which will increase its diameter by fourfold. For placement of the laminaria, the cervix is first cleansed with povidone-iodine solution and the anterior lip of the cervix is grasped with a tenaculum for countertraction. The proximal end of the laminaria is grasped with a ring forceps and is inserted into the cervical canal just beyond the internal os. A sponge is placed in the vagina and packed up against the cervix to prevent early dislodging of the laminaria. The laminaria are available in different diameters, ranging from 2 to 6 mm. Maximal dilatation occurs 12–24 hours after placement, but most of the swelling of the laminaria occurs in the first 4–6 hours. The segment of the laminaria above the internal cervical os will swell to a greater degree, because it is not directly opposed by any barrier. This causes the laminaria to assume a dumbbell shape, which may create difficulty with its removal. This complication can be avoided if one places several smaller laminaria into the cervix instead of a single large one.

A disadvantage of laminaria is that it takes several hours before it achieves its maximal diameter. Synthetic cervical dilators containing hydrophilic polymers have been produced. They are more uniform in shape and achieve their maximal diameter in a shorter time span. One such device is Lamicel, which is a cylindrical polyvinyl alcohol surgical sponge impregnated with magnesium sulfate. Like laminaria, this device absorbs water but at a much quicker rate, and maximal dilatation is achieved within 2 hours.[2] Another technique to aid in cervical dilatation is the direct application of prostaglandin E_1 analogues, which induce softening of the cervix.[3] Preoperative cervical dilatation is safer but does increase the cost and inconvenience to the patient, because additional office visits are necessary.

Curettage of the Uterine Cavity

Following cervical dilatation, the uterine sound can be reinserted into the uterus to ensure that perforation has not occurred. The choice of curette will depend on the clinical presentation (Fig. 14–5). For diagnostic purposes, a No. 2 Sims uterine curette will be sufficient. The curette is inserted into the uterine cavity in the same fashion as the cervical dilator. When inserting the curette, careful attention is paid to the position of the uterus and one keeps in mind the depth of the cavity measured on the previous sounding. Most curettes have a malleable shank, allowing the operator to adjust the curve according to the degree of flexion of the uterus. The curette is inserted until it comes in contact with the upper aspect of the uterine cavity. If one does not feel this resistance after continued insertion of the instrument, uterine perforation must be suspected, the instrument should be slowly removed, and the procedure stopped. Otherwise, when the curette encounters the upper aspect of the cavity, upward force is generated and the curette is withdrawn, scraping the uterine wall. The curettage is performed in a systematic fashion to ensure that all walls of the uterine cavity have been sampled. The curette is

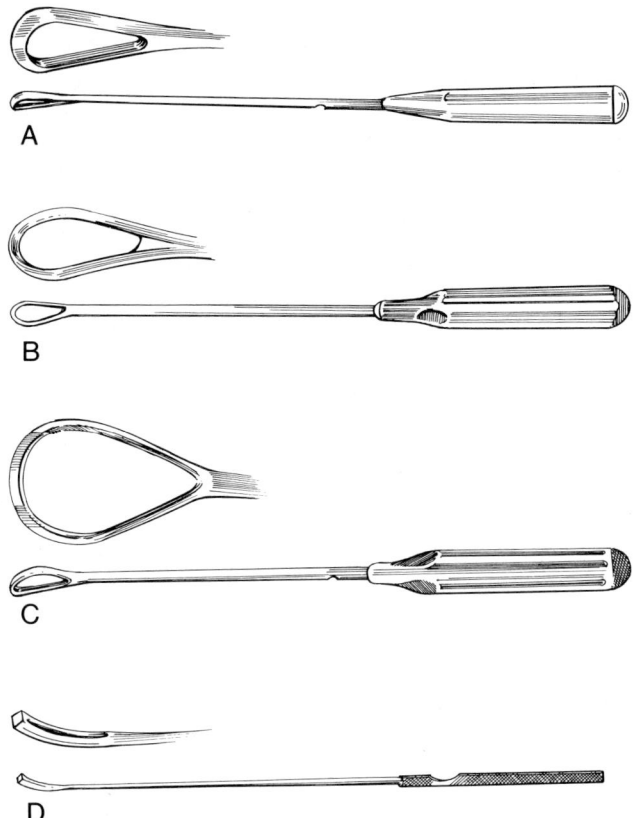

Figure 14–5
Curettes. *A*, Sims uterine curette: sharp blade on malleable shank with a hollow handle; available in six widths ranging from 8 to 14 mm. *B*, Thomas uterine curette: blunt blade on malleable shank with a hollow handle; curette is available in six widths ranging from 10 to 15 mm. *C*, Hunter large uterine curette: width of 3 cm. *D*, Kevorkian-Younge endocervical biopsy curette.

removed periodically to collect the endometrial curettings, which at the end of the procedure are placed in formalin and sent to Pathology. After the curettage is completed, polyp forceps are inserted into the uterine cavity, opened, closed, and withdrawn to ensure that all endometrial polyps have been removed.

Uterine curettage may be necessary in the postpartum patient with retained placental fragments. The pregnant uterus is soft and prone to perforation. For this reason, one should avoid probing the uterine cavity with the uterine sound. The curettage should be performed as previously described, but the widest curette available should be used (see Fig. 14–5).

Suction curettage is the best method to evacuate the uterus in cases of incomplete abortion or pregnancy termination up to 12 weeks. The straight or curved suction curettes are made of plastic and are available in different sizes ranging from 4 to 16 mm in diameter. The larger suction curettes are associated with greater suction and increased chance of perforation. As a general rule, the size of the suction curette used should be equivalent to or one size less than the gestational age in weeks. Uterine sounding should not be performed. After the cervix has been dilated, the curette by itself is inserted into the uterine cavity until the top of the uterine cavity is encountered. The suction tubing is then attached to the curette, and the suction machine is turned on. Once a pressure of 60 mm Hg has been attained, the curettage is begun. In contrast to the sharp curettage, the suction curettage is performed in a circular rotary fashion. The curette is slowly withdrawn as the circular rotation is continued to ensure that the entire uterine cavity is suctioned. The curettage is repeated until no further tissue is aspirated into the tubing. At this point, a light sharp curettage is then performed.

Special care should be taken when evacuating the uterus of a molar pregnancy. Because of the increased chance of hemorrhage, all patients should be typed and crossmatched for possible transfusion. If the uterus is significantly enlarged, the operating room should also be set up to perform a laparotomy if uncontrollable hemorrhage is encountered. The uterine cavity is emptied with suction curettage using a large curette. After the procedure is begun, intravenous oxytocin (Pitocin) is started to help contract the uterus. At the end of the procedure, a sharp curettage is performed and the specimen should be sent for pathologic study separately.

The Use of Ultrasound Guidance

The intraoperative use of ultrasound has demonstrated its utility in aiding the surgeon in the placement of intrauterine tandems,[4] the aspiration of placental tissue for chorionic villus biopsy,[5] and the performance of a uterine curettage[6] (Fig. 14–6). In a previous report, Hunter and colleagues performed a

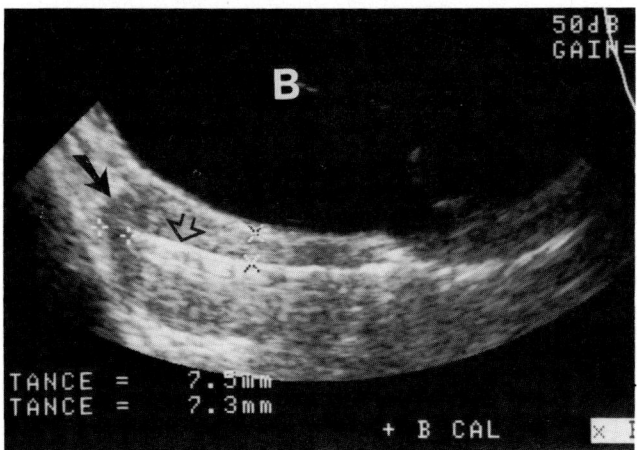

Figure 14–6
Transabdominal ultrasonography can help in the proper placement of instruments up into the uterine cavity. In this longitudinal view, the bladder (*B*) and top of the uterine fundus (*closed arrow*) can be seen. An intrauterine tandem inserted into the uterine cavity can be visualized (*open arrow*). (Courtesy of Dr. Frederick Doherty, Boston, MA.)

D & C under ultrasound guidance in postmenopausal women with cervical stenosis, a group at significant risk for uterine perforation.[7] In all 21 patients studied, the cervical canal and the uterine cavity were easily visualized and the procedure was completed without any complications. This study suggests that ultrasound guidance may be useful in those patients undergoing D & C who are at greater risk for uterine perforation, including those with cervical stenosis and patients with a markedly retroverted or anteverted uterus. In addition, ultrasound guidance would improve the safety and efficiency of suction curettage performed on the postpartum patient with retained placenta.

Complications

The technique for performance of a D & C is relatively basic, but potential serious complications can result and must be identified and managed appropriately. The complications following the procedure are discussed in the following sections.

Uterine Perforation

The most common complication of a D & C is uterine perforation, and its incidence ranges from 0.04 to 1.5%[8-11] (Fig. 14–7). Most perforations occur during the cervical dilatation, and the diagnosis can be made when no resistance is encountered with continued insertion of any instrument into the uterine cavity. Risk factors for this complication include cervical stenosis and a retroverted uterus. In a previous study, 14 of 17 patients who suffered uterine perforation following a D & C had a retroverted uterus.[12] This finding is even more impressive when one considers that only 30% of patients subjected to the procedure had a uterus in this position. The risk of perforation is also related to the experience of the operator. In one study, 75% of uterine perforations were caused by physicians in training.[10]

Management of uterine perforation is dependent on the perforating instrument and the indication for the D & C. If during a diagnostic D & C the perforation occurs with insertion of the uterine sound, cervical dilator, or a uterine curette, the procedure should be terminated and the patient admitted overnight for observation. If omentum or bowel is noted with the removal of a curette, an immediate exploratory laparotomy should be performed. Most perforations through the uterine fundus will be uncomplicated and heal spontaneously. However, if the perforation site is through the lateral uterine wall, there is the possibility of injury to the uterine vessels. Bleeding from this area can be concealed and result in the development of a broad ligament hematoma. Any evidence of intra-abdominal hemorrhage necessitates an immediate laparotomy.

The management of uterine perforation differs if

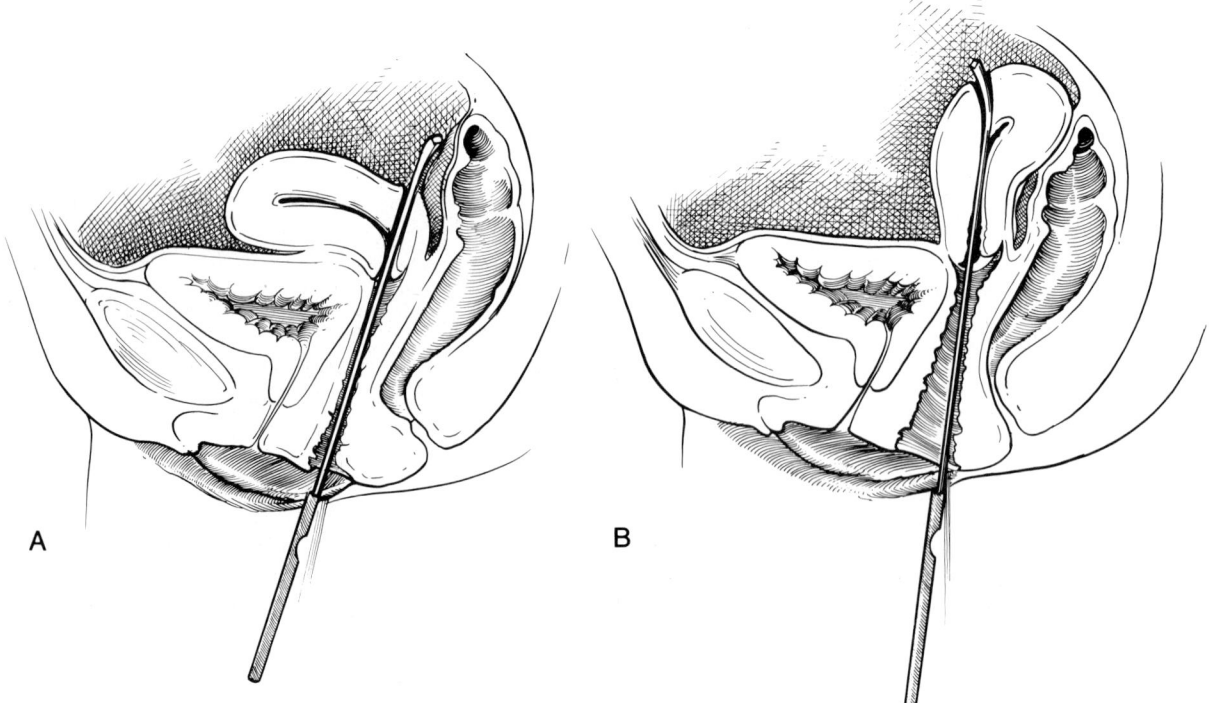

Figure 14–7
A markedly retroverted (A) or anteverted (B) uterus will increase the risk for uterine perforation. Ways to prevent this complication include (1) knowing the uterine position, (2) adjusting the angle of insertion of the instruments according to uterine position, and (3) maintaining constant outward traction on the cervix with the tenaculum.

it occurs in the patient undergoing the procedure for an incomplete or therapeutic abortion. If the perforation occurs with the uterine sound or cervical dilator, a laparoscopy should be performed to examine the perforation site and the procedure should be completed under laparoscopic visualization. If the perforation is noted after the suction curette has been used, an exploratory laparotomy is indicated and any injury to the intra-abdominal organs is managed accordingly.

Infections

The overall rate of infectious morbidity following a D & C ranges from 0.3 to 3.0%.[8, 9, 13–16] This complication is higher when the D & C is performed for an incomplete abortion, because placental tissue and blood provide an excellent growth medium for bacteria. Preoperatively, any mucopurulent cervical discharge that is noted should first be cultured and treated before performing the procedure. In addition, adherence to good aseptic technique will also help to minimize this complication.

Hemorrhage

Postoperative bleeding following the procedure can be secondary to a cervical laceration at the tenaculum site or may result from overaggressive dilatation of the cervix. If the D & C was performed to empty the uterus of a pregnancy, postoperative bleeding may signify the incomplete removal of the pregnancy or the development of a hematometra, and in these circumstances a repeat curettage will correct the problem.

Asherman's Syndrome

Asherman's syndrome is the result of partial or complete obliteration of the uterine cavity by intrauterine adhesions. The syndrome can follow a cesarean section, myomectomy, or diagnostic D & C. The postpartum patient undergoing a D & C for retained, infected placental parts is at greatest risk for this complication. Depending on the extent and location of the intrauterine adhesions, the patient can present with a history of habitual abortion, hypomenorrhea, or amenorrhea. A hysterosalpingogram will help to establish the diagnosis, and hysteroscopic lysis of the adhesions is the treatment of choice.

The Role of the Endometrial Biopsy

For diagnostic purposes, the D & C has probably been overutilized. In the United States between 1979 and 1983, almost 1 million procedures were performed each year at a cost of close to a billion dollars.[17] An excellent review and reappraisal of the role of the D & C for diagnostic purposes was published by Grimes.[18] He summarized previous studies that compared the diagnostic capability of the outpatient endometrial biopsy (Vabra aspirator) with the D & C. A general misconception is that the D & C results in a curettage of the entire uterine cavity. Less than half of the endometrial cavity is usually sampled following this procedure.[19] The Vabra aspirator samples even less of the cavity, but its diagnostic accuracy for identifying adenocarcinoma of the endometrium is 96%.[18] The D & C is more efficient in the removal of endometrial polyps. Another argument in support of the D & C is that it may be effective treatment for those patients with menorrhagia secondary to benign conditions of the uterus. Even though most patients experience improvement in their bleeding pattern following the procedure, the effect is only temporary and the menorrhagia returns within a few months.[20] The outpatient endometrial biopsy is less expensive and safer, because it can be done without anesthesia. In addition, it is also associated with a lower incidence of uterine perforation, infection, and hemorrhage.

There are several endometrial biopsy instruments that can be used in the office setting, including the Vabra aspirator and the Novak and Miegs curettes. These metal instruments are rigid and produce moderate discomfort with their use. A disposable, plastic endometrial suction curette is currently available (Pipelle; Unimar, Wilton, CT). After this instrument is inserted into the cavity, the plunger is pulled back and creates a suction, drawing endometrial tissue into the open cannula. This instrument, as compared with the other endometrial biopsy curettes, is reasonably inexpensive, associated with less discomfort, and provides an adequate tissue specimen for examination.[21–23]

For diagnostic purposes, any patient with abnormal bleeding should first be evaluated with an endometrial biopsy. This is the only assessment that is needed in the anovulatory patient with unopposed estrogen when one is trying to rule out adenomatous hyperplasia or adenocarcinoma, which should be a diffuse process throughout the endometrial cavity. If adenocarcinoma is diagnosed, there is no need for a D & C as long as an office endocervical curettage can be performed. In other patients, if the endometrial biopsy fails to identify a cause of the abnormal bleeding or if the abnormal bleeding continues, a formal D & C should be performed.

CONIZATION OF THE CERVIX

Introduction and Historical Aspects

In the 1800s, the most common indication for cervical conization was chronic cervicitis that festered in cervical lacerations from traumatic childbirth. Because chronic cervicitis was thought to be a forerunner of cervical cancer, removal of the inflamed cervix not only was therapeutic but also provided a tissue specimen for histologic examination. In 1815 Lisfranc was one of the first to describe a surgical technique that resulted in the removal of a cone-shaped specimen that included the entire cervix to the junction of the vagina and the cervical canal up to the internal os.[24] This procedure essentially resulted in the amputation of the cervix, and the exposed area was allowed to heal by granulation, which could take up to 6 weeks. Secondary to the scarring, there was a high incidence of cervical stenosis resulting in dysmenorrhea and infertility. In 1861, Sims and Emmet described a procedure called a trachelorrhaphy.[25] The cone biopsy specimen was taken as previously described, but an important difference was that the cone bed was covered with adjacent vagina, leaving a small opening at the cervical os. With this modification, these investigators noted improved healing with a reduced incidence of cervical stenosis. In 1915, Sturmdorf refined the trachelorrhaphy and described his technique of mobilization of adjacent vagina to cover over the cone bed.[26] His suturing technique and plastic repair of the cervix have remained popular ever since.

Chronic cervicitis is no longer an indication for conization. In 1943, the Papanicolaou (Pap) smear was introduced and in the presence of abnormal cytology a cone biopsy was obtained to rule out microscopic lesions of the cervix. In the 1970s, colposcopy was introduced and superseded cervical conization for this purpose. In addition to its diagnostic capabilities, the cone biopsy in the past was used as primary treatment for cervical dysplasia, but other, more conservative treatment modalities (i.e., cryosurgery, laser vaporization) have emerged and proved their effectiveness.

Since cervical conization was first described, there are fewer indications to perform this procedure, but the indications are now better defined and this procedure continues to be an important part of gynecologic surgery. Although it is considered a minor procedure, cervical conization has one of the highest complication rates of any gynecologic surgery.

Indications

A Pap smear should be performed annually on any woman over the age of 20, or sooner if she becomes sexually active. If dysplastic cells are seen on the Pap smear, colposcopy is indicated. During the colposcopic examination, the entire transformation zone must be examined and any suspicious lesions are biopsied. At the termination of the examination, an endocervical curettage should be performed. In most cases, the colposcopic examination is adequate for diagnostic purposes; however, approximately 5.0% of patients will have an inadequate examination and a cone biopsy will be indicated for further diagnostic evaluation.[27, 28] Even if the colposcopy is adequate, cervical conization may be indicated if there is discordancy between the degree of dysplasia noted on the Pap smear and the biopsy or if the biopsy demonstrates microinvasive cancer. Other indications for a cone biopsy are shown in Table 14–2.

Table 14–2

Indications for Conization of the Cervix

Inadequate colposcopy
    Lesion extends up the cervical canal
    Entire transformation zone not visualized
Biopsy demonstrates microinvasive disease
Discordancy of cervical biopsy specimens with previous cytologic findings
A positive endocervical curettage
Treatment for carcinoma in situ

Surgical Technique

The objective of cervical conization is to obtain a cone-shaped tissue specimen that includes the entire transformation zone and the cervical canal up to the level of the internal cervical os (Fig. 14–8). The

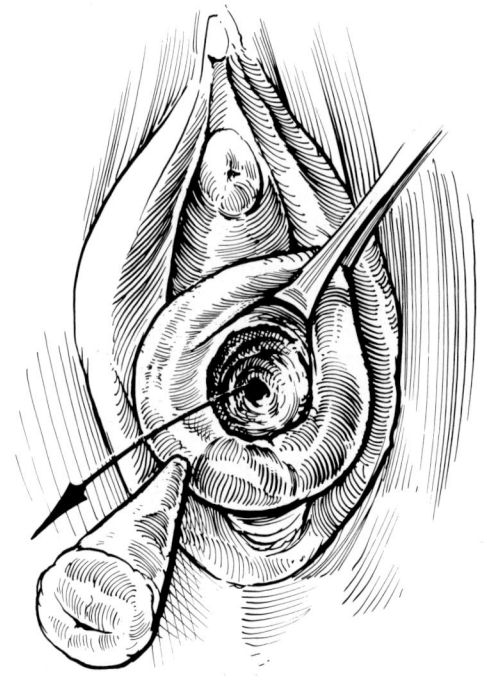

Figure 14–8
The cone biopsy specimen includes the entire transformation zone and the endocervical canal up to the level of the internal cervical os.

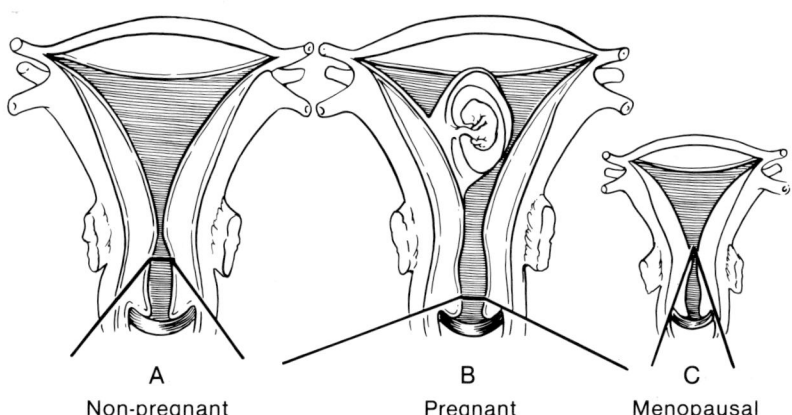

Figure 14–9
The location of the transformation zone varies during a woman's lifetime. The shape of the cone biopsy taken will depend on whether the patient is (A) of childbearing years and not pregnant, (B) pregnant, or (C) postmenopausal.

A Non-pregnant   B Pregnant   C Menopausal

anatomic position of the transformation zone changes during a woman's lifetime. In the postmenopausal woman, it assumes a higher location in the cervical canal as compared with the premenopausal woman. The transformation zone in the pregnant woman is farther out on the portio of the cervix. This is important information that will allow the surgeon to tailor the shape of the cone biopsy accordingly (Fig. 14–9). Furthermore, prior knowledge of the location and extent of the lesion in question will result in further modification of the biopsy specimen.

The anesthesia used and patient positioning are the same as for a D & C. However, an important difference is that the vagina is not prepped, because it would disrupt the integrity of the cervical epithelium and interfere with the histologic examination.

Cold Knife Cone Biopsy

Traditionally, the scalpel has been used to obtain the cone biopsy. This technique is referred to as a cold knife cone. To identify the outer margins of the biopsy, the vagina is painted with Lugol's (5%) iodine solution; this solution stains glycogen, which is present in normal vaginal epithelium but lacking in dysplastic and endocervical tissue. The paracervical area is then circumferentially infiltrated with a vasoconstrictive agent that will help to control the blood loss from the procedure. Hemostatic agents available for this use include phenylephrine hydrochloride (Neo-Synephrine), lidocaine (Xylocaine) with epinephrine, and vasopressin. The authors have found vasopressin to be most effective for this purpose and inject up to 10 ml of a 1:30 dilution. Because it is a potent vasoconstrictor, one must be certain that the injection is not intravascular. To further control blood loss, sutures can be placed at the 3 o'clock and 9 o'clock positions at the lateral walls of the cervix to ligate the descending branches of the uterine artery. The sutures are placed at the level of the internal os, but one must be careful not to place the sutures too high, for fear of injury to the ureters that course nearby. A straight knife handle with a No. 11 blade can be used to cut the cone biopsy, but inadequate exposure or a deep vagina may make it difficult to cut the desired cone-shaped specimen. An angled knife handle is better suited for this purpose (Fig. 14–10). The outer border of the cone biopsy should be just outside the unstained areas on the cervix. The cone biopsy is cut in a circular fashion, and following removal of the specimen a suture is placed at the 12 o'clock location and the specimen is then fixed in formalin. At the end of the procedure, an endocervical curettage is performed with a Kevorkian curette. In the past, an endometrial curettage was routinely performed following the cone biopsy, but unless there is a good indication to perform this procedure, it should not be done.

The technique of the cold knife cone is basic and really has not changed since it was introduced. However, what *has* changed over the years is the management of the exposed cone bed. Previously, surgeons advocated a plastic closure of the cone bed to recreate a normal appearing, functional cervix and, more importantly, to aid in achieving hemostasis. Traditionally the Sturmdorf type of closure has been used, and mattress sutures are placed to approximate

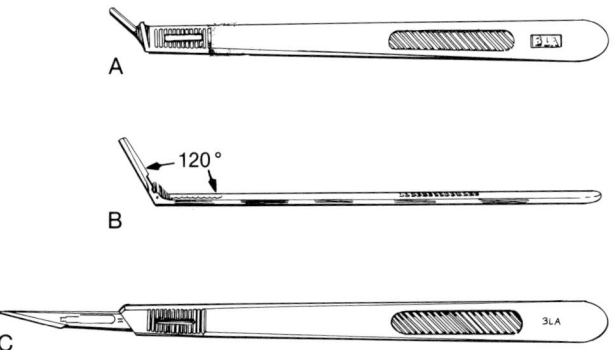

Figure 14–10
A and B, The angled knife handle with a No. 11 knife blade is shown. Compared with the straight knife (C), this instrument allows an easier means to obtain the desired cone-shaped specimen.

the anterior and posterior lips of the cervix separately to the cut edges of the endocervical canal. Other methods of suturing that have been described include the use of a running interlocking suture around the circumference of the cone bed and the placement of interrupted sutures. However, the authors' approach is to coagulate the cone bed, place a piece of Gelfoam in the cervix, and allow it to heal by second intention. The cosmetic result is excellent, and this technique is associated with less blood loss than the suture techniques.[29]

Laser Cone Biopsy

Since its introduction, the laser has been applied to many aspects of gynecologic surgery in hopes that it may offer a potential advantage over more conventional techniques. It has proved its effectiveness in surgery on the cervix, including the destruction of dysplastic lesions and as a method to incise a cervical cone biopsy. Cervical conization with the laser was first reported by Dorsey in 1979,[30] and the technique was later modified by Baggish.[31]

The objective of the laser cone is the same as that of the cold knife cone, but the technique is somewhat different. First a colposcopic examination of the cervix is performed and the transformation zone is identified. The CO_2 laser, controlled by either a free handpiece or a joy stick attached to the colposcope, is used to trace the outer extent of the cone, which should be 3 mm outside the transformation zone. Bleeding can be kept to a minimum with the placement of sutures in the lateral margins of the cervix at 3 and 9 o'clock and a paracervical infiltration with vasopressin. When performing the conization, the laser spot size is adjusted to 0.5–1.5 mm and the power density is set at 25–50 watts. The laser is then used to cut the cone biopsy while an assistant aspirates the flume from the vagina. Titanium hooks placed in the cervical stroma can be used for traction and countertraction as the specimen is taken. Before the cervical canal is entered, the apex of the cone biopsy is cut with a scalpel to avoid thermal damage to the tissue that could interfere with histologic examination. The cone bed is coagulated with a defocused laser beam and is then allowed to heal by second intention.

The laser is an expensive instrument and not available to all surgeons, but it does seem to offer some distinct advantages over the traditional cold knife cone. There is a decreased incidence of all postoperative complications, including cervical stenosis and postoperative hemorrhage.[32] Another distinct advantage of the laser cone is that it can be performed in an office setting under local anesthesia, which would eliminate the risk of general anesthesia and decrease the overall cost of the procedure. Nevertheless, one must achieve a certain level of expertise with the laser before he or she can perform this procedure in the office.

Interpretation of the Biopsy and Follow-up

Once the specimen arrives in the laboratory, the cone biopsy is cut at the 12 o'clock position and then laid out in a lengthwise fashion. The specimen is fixed and then cut into as many pieces as possible, usually 12 or more. Each separate piece is then embedded, and then multiple slices are taken from each specimen. It is important that the surgeon be assured that the pathologist is taking enough sections of the cone specimen. The overall error rate of interpretation of the cone biopsy is about 5%. If the histologic examination of the cone biopsy confirms the presence of invasive or microinvasive cancer, appropriate therapy should be instituted. If the cone biopsy confirms dysplasia contained within the margins of the specimen and the endocervical curettings are negative, a repeat Pap smear should be performed in 4 months and then repeated every 4 months for the next 2 years. During the follow-up period, if cervical dysplasia is noted on any cytologic smear, a repeat colposcopy is indicated.

There is greater concern when the final pathology report states that dysplasia extends to the margin of the biopsy specimen or the endocervical curettage is positive for dysplastic cells. In a previous study, 47% of those patients who had disease extending to the margin of the cone were found to have residual disease in the hysterectomy specimen.[33] Patients who were at greater risk for residual disease were those who had positive margins at the endocervical border. In another study, it is reassuring that all patients with residual disease had abnormal Pap smears during the follow-up period.[34] Unless there is a high index of suspicion of cervical cancer, a patient who has a cone biopsy with positive margins is followed with Pap smears and endocervical curettages every 4 months for a total of 2 years. At any time, if the sampling demonstrates dysplastic cells, a repeat colposcopy and/or cervical conization is indicated.

Complications

The most frequent complication following conization of the cervix is immediate or delayed hemorrhage, which can occur up to several weeks after performing the procedure. The average incidence of postoperative hemorrhage is 12%, and about 5% of all patients subjected to this procedure will require a blood transfusion.[32, 35–38] Postoperative hemorrhage can be managed by packing the cervix or application of ferric subsulfate (Monsel's solution). However, if these conservative measures prove unsuccessful, the patient may have to return to the operating room for further treatment, which may include cauterization of the bleeding site or suture placement. If these measures prove unsuccessful in the presence of heavy bleeding, ligation of the hypogastric arteries or hysterectomy may be in order. The latter procedure had to be performed in less than 1% of cases.[36, 38] Because of the risk of bleeding, all patients should be counseled on the possibility of requiring a transfusion and be given the option to bank autologous blood preoperatively.

The reduction of this frequent complication has been the object of continued investigation. One study reported a reduced incidence of hemorrhage when the cone was performed with the laser as compared with the cold knife cone (1.8% vs. 14%).[32] The placement of Sturmdorf sutures was thought to decrease bleeding complications, but most studies have failed to show any benefit of this technique when compared with allowing the cone bed to heal by second intention. One study reported on two groups of patients who underwent cone biopsies that were left to heal secondarily.[37] The first group had placement of sutures at the 3 and 9 o'clock positions for hemostasis, and the other group had the cone bed packed with gauze soaked in Monsel's solution. It was of interest that the latter group was found to have a lower incidence of postoperative bleeding and other complications.

Delayed complications result from the scarring at the cone biopsy site. If there is extensive scarring, cervical stenosis may occur and the patient can complain of dysmenorrhea. This complication can be reduced if the cervical canal is sounded 3–4 weeks after the surgery is performed. The cervix also plays an important role in reproduction, and its production of a thin, watery mucus at the time of ovulation is important for the storage of sperm after coitus. Therefore, the cone biopsy can compromise the functional capacity of the cervix and be a cause of infertility. Those patients who do achieve pregnancy following a cone biopsy must be watched carefully for the development of an incompetent cervix. In addition, secondary to the scarring there is an increased chance of cervical dystocia and cervical lacerations with vaginal delivery.

The Cone Biopsy and the Pregnant Patient

Management of an abnormal Pap smear during pregnancy is the same as in the nonpregnant patient and requires colposcopy. The primary goal of colposcopy during pregnancy is simply to rule out the presence of invasive cancer. During pregnancy, the vascularity of the cervix is enhanced and performing cervical biopsies can result in significant bleeding. For this reason, the colposcopic examination should be performed by an expert colposcopist, who may be able to determine the severity of the dysplastic lesions by visualization, which would reduce the number of biopsies that are necessary. The only indication for a cone biopsy in pregnancy is to rule out invasive cancer after a previous biopsy has demonstrated microinvasive cancer. There are several modifications in the technique of cervical conization in the pregnant patient. A shallower cone biopsy is taken, because the transformation zone during pregnancy migrates out onto the portio of the cervix. A deeper cone is unnecessary and could rupture the membranes or result in the development of an incompetent cervix. During pregnancy, an endocervical curettage is not performed because of the risk of rupturing the membranes. Conization of the cervix during pregnancy results in a greater blood loss, and in one study 10% of patients had a blood loss greater than 500 ml, requiring a transfusion.[39] Therefore, these patients should be given the option of autologous blood donation if it is feasible.

Conclusion

The cone biopsy continues to be an important diagnostic test in gynecology but must always be preceded by colposcopy. In the past, cervical conization was used for the treatment of dysplasia, but more conservative treatment modalities (i.e., cryosurgery, laser vaporization) are now available and have proved their effectiveness. However, a cone biopsy may be indicated treatment for the patient with a diffuse dysplastic lesion or carcinoma in situ. Nevertheless, women of the reproductive age group must be counseled on the long-term complications of this procedure (i.e., cervical stenosis, infertility).

References

1. Romero R, Kadar N, Jeanty P, et al.: Diagnosis of ectopic pregnancy: Value of the discriminatory human chorionic gonadotropin zone. Obstet Gynecol 1985; 66:357.
2. Nicolaides KH, Welch CC, MacPherson MBA, et al.: Lamicel: A new technique for cervical dilatation before first trimester abortion. Br J Obstet Gynaecol 1983; 90:475.
3. Chen JK, Elder MG: Preoperative cervical dilatation by vaginal pessaries containing prostaglandin E_1 analogue. Obstet Gynecol 1983; 62:339.
4. Granai CO, Allee P, Doherty F, et al.: Intraoperative real time ultrasonography during intrauterine tandem placement. Obstet Gynecol 1986; 67:112.

5. Liu DTY, Morman S, Richardson R, et al.: Experience with real time ultrasound directed transcervical chorionic villus biopsy. Asia Oceania J Obstet Gynaecol 1985; 11:515.
6. Romero R, Copel JA, Jeanty P, et al.: Sonographic monitoring to guide the performance of postabortal uterine curettage. Am J Obstet Gynecol 1985; 151(1):51.
7. Hunter RE, Reuter K, Kopin E: Use of ultrasonography in the difficult postmenopausal dilation and curettage. Obstet Gynecol 1989; 73;813.
8. Lilaram D, Basu S, Khan PK, et al.: Evaluation of 496 menstrual regulation and abortion patients in Calcutta. Int J Gynaecol Obstet 1978; 15;503.
9. Menstrual Regulation Update: Population report series F, No. 4. Washington, Department of Medical and Public Affairs, George Washington University Medical Center, 1974.
10. Beric BM, Kupresanin M: Vacuum aspiration, using pericervical block, for legal abortion as an outpatient procedure up to the 12th week of pregnancy. Lancet 1971; 2: 619.
11. Courtney LD: Methods and dangers of termination of pregnancy. Proc Roy Soc Med 1969; 62:834.
12. Nathanson BN: Management of uterine perforations suffered at elective abortion. Am J Obstet Gynecol 1972; 114:1054.
13. McElin TW, Bird CC, Reeves BD, Scott RC: Diagnostic dilatation and curettage: A 20-year survey. Obstet Gynecol 1969; 33:807.
14. MacKenzie IS, Bibby JG: Critical assessment of dilatation and curettage in 1029 women. Lancet 1978; 2:566.
15. Brenner WE, Edelman DA: Menstrual regulation: Risks and abuses. Int J Gynaecol Obstet 1977; 15:177.
16. Landesman R, Kaye RE, Wilson KH: Menstrual regulation: Review of 400 procedures at Woman's Services, New York, New York. Contraception 1973; 8:527.
17. Rutkow IM: Obstetric and gynecologic operations in the United States, 1979 to 1984. Obstet Gynecol 1986; 67:755.
18. Grimes DA: Diagnostic dilation and curettage: A reappraisal. Am J Obstet Gynecol 1982; 142:1.
19. Stock RJ, Kanbour A: Prehysterectomy curettage. Obstet Gynecol 1975; 45:537.
20. Haynes PJ, Hodgson H, Anderson ABM, Turnbull AC: Measurement of menstrual blood loss in patients complaining of menorrhagia. Br J Obstet Gynaecol 1977; 84:763.
21. Koonings PP, Moyer DL, Grimes DA: A randomized clinical trial comparing Pipelle and Tis-u-trap for endometrial biopsy. Obstet Gynecol 1990; 75:293.
22. Kaunitz AM, Masciello A, Ostrowski M, Rovira EZ: Comparison of endometrial biopsy with the endometrial Pipelle and Vabra aspirator. J Reprod Med 1988; 33:427.
23. Hill GA, Herbert CM, Parker RA, Wentz AC: Comparison of late luteal phase endometrial biopsies using the Novak curette or Pipelle endometrial suction curette. Obstet Gynecol 1989; 73:443.
24. Lisfranc J: Memoire sur l'amputation du col de l'uterus. Gaz Med de Par 1834; 2S, ii, 385.
25. Sims JM: Amputation of the cervix. Trans Med Soc State of New York, 1861.
26. Sturmdorf A: Tracheloplastic methods and results. Surg Gynec Obstet 1916; 22:93.
27. Stafl A, Mattingly RF: Colposcopic diagnosis of cervical neoplasia. Obstet Gynecol 1973; 41:168.
28. Talebian F, Shayan A, Krumholz BA, et al.: Colposcopic evaluation of patients with abnormal cervical cytology. Obstet Gynecol 1977; 49:670.
29. Chao S, McCaffrey RM, Todd WD, Moore JG: Conization in evaluation and management of cervical neoplasia. Am J Obstet Gynecol 1969; 103:574.
30. Dorsey JH, Diggs ES: Microsurgical conization of the cervix by carbon dioxide laser. Obstet Gynecol 1979; 54:565.
31. Baggish MS: Laser management of cervical intraepithelial neoplasia. Clin Obstet Gynecol 1983; 26:980.
32. Larsson G, Gullberg BO, Grundsell H: A comparison of complications of laser and cold knife conization. Obstet Gynecol 1983; 62:213.
33. Lubicz S, Ezekweche C, Allen A, Schiffer M: Significance of cone biopsy margins in the management of patients with cervical neoplasia. J Reprod Med 1984; 29:179.
34. Buxton EJ, Luesley DM, Wade-Evans T, Jordan JA: Residual disease after cone biopsy: Completeness of excision and follow-up cytology as predictive factors. Obstet Gynecol 70:529.
35. Bjerre B, Eliasson G, Linell F, et al.: Conization as only treatment of carcinoma in situ of the uterine cervix. Am J Obstet Gynecol 1976; 125:143.
36. Luesley DM, McCrum A, Terry PB, et al.: Complications of cone biopsy related to the dimensions of the cone and the influence of prior colposcopic assessment. Br J Obstet Gynaecol 1985; 92:158.
37. Gilbert L, St G Saunders NJ, Stringer R, Sharp F: Hemostasis and cold knife cone biopsy: A prospective randomized trial comparing a suture versus non-suture technique. Obstet Gynecol 1989; 74:640.
38. Villasanta U, Durkan JP: Indications and complications of cold conization of the cervix. Obstet Gynecol 1966; 27:717.
39. Hannigan EV, Whitehouse HH, Atkinson WD, Becker SN: Cone biopsy during pregnancy. Obstet Gynecol 1982; 60:450.

Surgical Therapy for Cervical Cancer

15

J. R. van Nagell, Jr.
P. D. DePriest
R. V. Higgins
D. E. Powell

With the increased use of regular cervical cytologic screening throughout the world, more patients with invasive cervical cancer are being diagnosed with early stage disease. In the United States, for example, it is estimated that there will be approximately 7000 new cases of invasive cervical cancer diagnosed each year, and that 70% of these patients will have Stage I disease. As a result of this trend in early diagnosis, an increasing number of cervical cancer patients will be candidates for primary treatment with surgery. This chapter discusses the major operative procedures used in the therapy of patients with invasive cervical cancer. Indications for specific methods of surgical treatment as well as complications related to their use are reviewed.

MICROINVASIVE CANCER

During the past two decades, there has been marked interest in identifying a group of patients with early invasive cervical cancer who have minimal risk for extracervical disease. Such patients could then be treated by conservative surgery without incurring the risks of radical surgery or radiation therapy.

The concept of microinvasive cervical cancer was first proposed by Mestwerdt in 1947. Since that time, there have been a number of definitions of this entity, with the reported frequency of lymph node metastases varying from 0 to 6%. In order for the concept of microinvasive cervical cancer to be clinically meaningful, patients with this diagnosis should have no lymph nodal spread. In addition, the histologic criteria used to define microinvasion should be readily adaptable for use by practicing pathologists. In this regard, the authors prefer the definition of microinvasive cervical cancer proposed in 1974 by the Committee on Nomenclature of the Society of Gynecologic Oncologists (SGO). According to this definition, microinvasive cancer is a lesion that invades the cervical stroma to a depth of 3.0 mm or less below the base of the epithelium and in which there is no evidence of lymph vascular space invasion. It should be emphasized that the diagnosis of microinvasive cancer can be made only after a cervical conization has been performed and the conization specimen has been properly sectioned. A minimum of 12 sections should be taken from each conization specimen, and additional step sections should be taken when necessary (Fig. 15–1). Each section should be examined using an ocular micrometer to determine the maximum penetration of the tumor beneath the basement membrane (Fig. 15–2). Likewise, each section should be examined for lymph vascular space invasion by a pathologist who is experienced in making this diagnosis. Lymph vas-

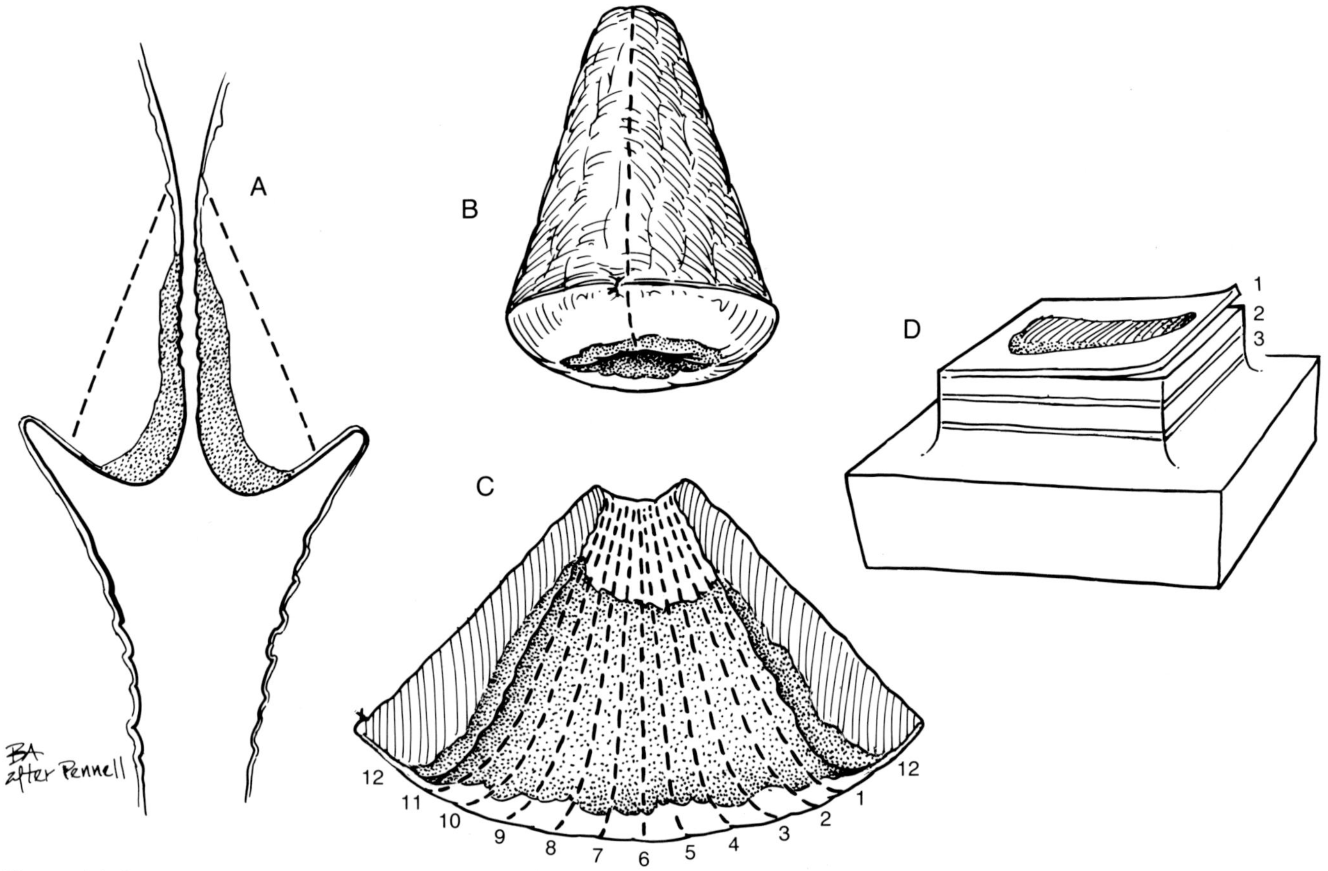

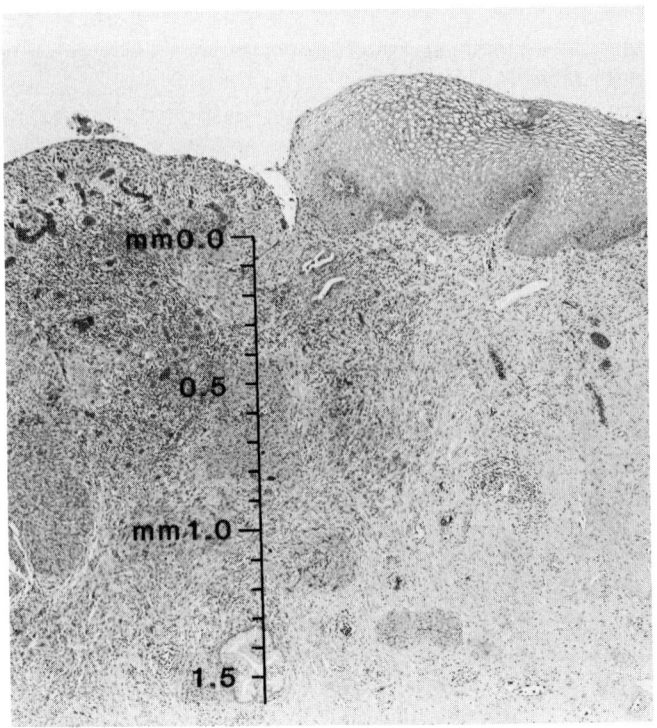

Figure 15–1
Processing the conization specimen. *A*, The surgical specimen, tagged with a suture at 12 o'clock, is opened along the longitudinal axis. *B* and *C*, The opened conization specimen is fixed and sectioned into 12 equal slices. *D*, Sections of the paraffin blocks are cut 6 μ thick at three different levels of the block. If initial sections do not adequately show the transformation zone, step sections may be required.

Figure 15–2
Microinvasive cervical cancer. Nests of tumor extend into the cervical stroma in the mid portion of the photomicrograph. An ocular micrometer is used to measure the depth of stromal invasion from the base of the epithelium (H&E × 40).

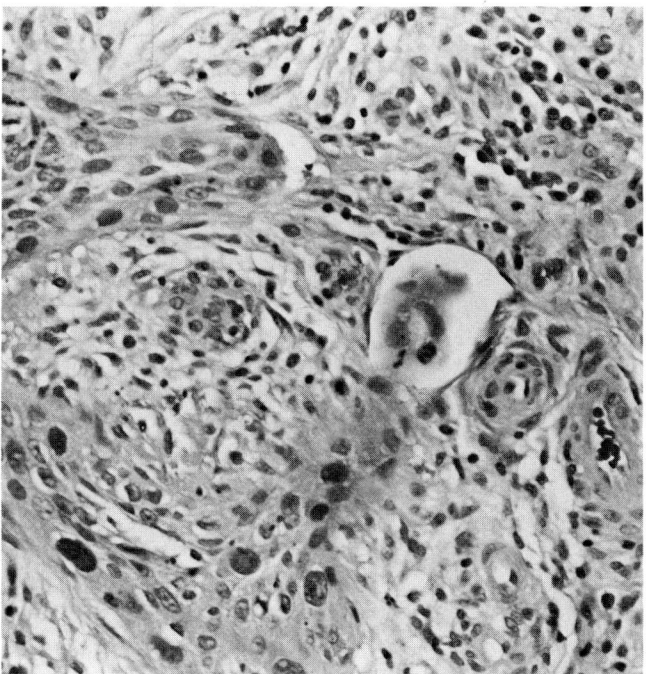

Figure 15–3
Lymph vascular space invasion. This invasive squamous cell carcinoma illustrates lymph vascular invasion. A nest of tumor cells is seen in the center of the photomicrograph within an endothelial-lined space. (H&E × 264).

cular space invasion is considered positive when tumor cells are observed within or attached to a space lined by flattened endothelial cells (Fig. 15–3).

Data concerning the frequency of pelvic lymph node metastases according to depth of stromal invasion are presented in Table 15–1. In over 500 patients with stromal invasion of less than 3.0 mm and no lymph vascular space invasion, there were no cases of lymph nodal metastases. In contrast, the incidence of lymph nodal spread in patients with cervical carcinoma invading the stroma to a depth of 3.1–5.0 mm was 7%. The presence of lymph vascular space invasion confers the potential for lymph nodal spread independent of the depth of stromal penetration.[11]

Once the definition of microinvasive cervical cancer has been established, the patient can be treated safely with either total abdominal hysterectomy or total vaginal hysterectomy. Van Nagell and coworkers reported the results of therapy in 145 patients with microinvasive cervical cancer (SGO definition) who were treated as follows: radical hysterectomy with pelvic lymphadenectomy, 52; total abdominal hysterectomy, 42; and total vaginal hysterectomy, 51.[8] In patients treated with radical hysterectomy and pelvic lymphadenectomy, 984 lymph nodes were examined histologically and none contained tumor metastases. Following surgery, patients were examined clinically at regular intervals from 2 to 14 years (mean, 7.2 years). There were no invasive recurrences in any of these patients, and the morbidity and hospital stay were significantly reduced in women treated by conservative hysterectomy when compared with those treated by more radical surgery. Colposcopy should be performed on all patients with microinvasive cancer prior to treatment so that any area of vaginal extension can be identified and excised at the time of hysterectomy.

Theoretically, cervical conization should be adequate therapy for patients with microinvasive cervical cancer provided that the SGO definition is used and the margins of the conization specimen are free of disease. However, the authors are hesitant to recommend this method of therapy until data are available on a large number of patients treated in this fashion who have been followed for an adequate time period.

Unfortunately, the FIGO* definitions of early invasive cervical cancer (Stages Ia1 or Ia2) do not take into consideration the presence of lymph vascular space invasion. Therefore, it is more difficult to relate specific types of treatment to these definitions. If

Table 15–1

Frequency of Lymph Node Metastases Related to Depth of Stromal Invasion in Patients with Stage I Cervical Cancer

Depth of Stromal Invasion*	No. of Patients	Patients with Lymph Node Metastases
≤3.0 mm	569	0 (0.0%)
3.0–5.0 mm	124	9 (7.3%)

*Measured by ocular micrometer from conization specimen.
Data from refs. 1–9.

*International Federation of Gynecology and Obstetrics.

there is any doubt as to whether the depth of stromal invasion exceeds 3.0 mm or whether lymph vascular space invasion is present, the patient should be treated by radical hysterectomy and pelvic lymphadenectomy or radiation therapy.

INVASIVE CERVICAL CANCER

Primary surgery is most effective as a therapeutic method in patients with invasive cervical cancer when the disease is confined clinically to the cervix itself. There have been few randomized trials comparing the efficacy of radical surgery with radiation therapy in patients with various stages of cervical cancer. However, there is considerable retrospective data that are helpful in identifying those patients who are optimal candidates for surgical therapy. Webb and Symmonds, for example, reported that 5-year survival following radical hysterectomy and pelvic lymphadenectomy decreased from 83% to 59% in the presence of lymph node metastases.[12] Therefore, the best candidates for primary radical surgery are those patients who have a relatively low incidence of lymph node metastases.

Histomorphologic findings directly related to the frequency of lymph node metastases in cervical cancer include lesion size, cell type, and depth of stromal penetration. Piver and Chung, for example, reported that 21% of patients with Stage IB lesions less than or equal to 3 cm in diameter had lymph node metastases, as opposed to 35% of patients with larger lesions.[13] These observations have been confirmed by other investigators.[14,15] Cell type has also been shown to be related to the frequency of lymph node metastases. Small cell cancers, although rare, are highly aggressive tumors with a propensity for early lymph nodal spread. The frequency of lymph node metastasis in patients with Stage IB small cell cancers less than or equal to 3 cm in diameter is 40%, and the majority of these patients die rapidly of widespread disease.[16] In contrast, large cell squamous tumors have a significantly lower incidence of lymph node metastases and are therefore more amenable to surgical therapy. Depth of stromal invasion has also been shown to be an important prognostic variable in patients with Stage IB cervical cancer. Cervical cancers invading the stroma to a depth of greater than or equal to 1.5 cm have been reported to have a significantly higher recurrence rate than more superficial lesions treated by radical surgery.[17] Until recently, there has been no effective method to assess depth of stromal invasion prior to surgery. However, preliminary studies suggest that the accuracy of magnetic resonance imaging (MRI) in determining depth of stromal invasion by cervical cancer is as high as 90%. If these early studies are confirmed in large numbers of patients, MRI could become a valuable method of assessing tumor volume and could be beneficial in selecting those patients who are optimal candidates for surgical therapy. At the present time, radical hysterectomy with pelvic lymphadenectomy is the treatment of choice in healthy patients with large cell squamous cancers less than or equal to 3 cm in diameter.

All potential candidates for radical hysterectomy should undergo a thorough medical evaluation prior to surgery. Careful attention should be taken to elicit any history of thromboembolic disease. A CT scan should be performed to rule out parametrial spread or para-aortic lymph node metastases. Intravenous pyelography should also be performed to identify occult ureteral obstruction. Ureteral obstruction has been reported to occur in approximately 2% of patients whose tumors are confined to the cervix on clinical examination.[18]

On the evening prior to surgery, all patients undergoing radical hysterectomy should be given a mechanical bowel preparation and intravenous hydration. Prophylactic heparin (5000 U every 12 hours subcutaneously) is also begun at that time and continued until the patient is fully ambulant. Prophylactic antibiotics in the form of a broad-spectrum cephalosporin or a semisynthetic penicillin are given 2 hours prior to surgery so that tissue antibiotic concentrations will be adequate prior to initiation of the operation.

Surgical Procedure

1. The patient is placed in the dorsal lithotomy position and is prepped both vaginally and abdominally. A No. 16 Foley catheter is placed in the bladder and connected to a drainage system that also allows the bladder to be filled with saline.

2. A midline abdominal incision is made from the symphysis pubis to a point approximately 3 cm above the umbilicus.

3. The upper abdomen is carefully inspected, and all major lymph nodal groups are palpated. Any enlarged or suspicious para-aortic lymph nodes are excised and sent for frozen section histologic examination.

4. A self-retaining retractor is placed in the incision, and the rectus abdominis muscles are retracted laterally.

5. The intestine is packed into the upper abdomen, and a thyroid clamp is placed in the uterine fundus.

6. The right round ligament is clamped, cut, and ligated at the right lateral pelvic wall (Fig. 15–4A). The anterior leaf of the right broad ligament is incised inferiorly along the lateral pelvic wall for a distance of approximately 3 cm.

7. The posterior leaf of the right broad ligament is incised superiorly along the lateral wall to the level of the infundibulopelvic ligament (Fig. 15–4B).

8. If the right ovary is to be preserved, the posterior leaf of the right broad ligament is further incised parallel and inferior to the infundibulopelvic and utero-ovarian ligaments. The right utero-ovarian ligament is then clamped, cut, and ligated, and the ovary is packed superiorly into the iliac fossa (Fig. 15–4C).

9. If the right ovary is to be excised, the right infundibulopelvic ligament is clamped, cut, and doubly ligated at the lateral pelvic wall. The right ovary and fallopian tube are then suspended to the thyroid clamp previously placed in the uterine fundus.

10. Steps 6–9 are repeated on the left side.

11. The right retroperitoneal space is then entered along the lateral pelvic wall, thereby exposing the common iliac artery, external iliac artery, and internal iliac artery and associated lymph nodal tissue.

12. The ureter is identified, and two silk sutures are placed in the adjacent peritoneum, thereby pulling the ureter medially away from the iliac vessels (Fig. 15–4D).

13. The lymph node dissection is begun by sharply excising all lymph nodal tissue surrounding the right common iliac and external iliac arteries. The lateral extent of this dissection is the right genitofemoral nerve (Fig. 15–E). The external iliac and common iliac arteries are retracted laterally, and lymph nodal tissue surrounding the common iliac and external iliac veins is removed by sharp dissection (Figs. 15–4F and G). Lymph nodal tissue from each of the major anatomic sites (i.e., common iliac, external iliac, internal iliac, and obturator) is placed in separate containers and submitted to the Pathology Department for histologic analysis.

14. The anterior division of the internal iliac artery is identified, ligated with 2–0 silk, and then suture ligated with 3–0 Prolene (Fig. 15–4H).

15. A vein retractor is placed on the external iliac artery and vein, and the obturator nerve is identified. All lymph nodal tissue is removed from the obturator fossa by sharp dissection (Fig. 15–4I).

16. Steps 10–14 are repeated on the left side.

17. The right pararectal and paravesical spaces are defined by blunt dissection, and the lateral aspect of the cardinal ligament containing the vascular web is clamped, cut, and ligated with 2–0 silk suture (Figs. 15–4J and K). Ligation of the left vascular web is completed in the same fashion.

18. The right ureter is dissected from the medial peritoneum at the level of the uterosacral ligament, and a 3/8-inch Penrose drain is placed around the ureter (Fig. 15–4L). The ureter is dissected laterally from the parametrial tunnel using right angle clamps (Figs. 15–4M and N). The parametrium is ligated, and the ureter is rolled laterally out of the tunnel. The right ureter is dissected free of surrounding tissue until its entrance into the bladder (Fig. 15–4O). The left ureter is then dissected free of parametrial tissue in the same fashion.

19. The bladder is sharply dissected from the anterior vagina, and the peritoneum between the uterus and the rectum is incised (Fig. 15–4P). The anterior rectal wall is reflected away from the posterior vagina.

20. The uterus is elevated, and the uterosacral ligaments are clamped, cut, and tied (Fig. 15–4Q). The anterior, posterior, and lateral attachments of the uterus and parametrium have now been ligated. The paravaginal tissue at the inferior margin of the dissection is clamped, cut, and tied using curved Haney clamps (Fig. 15–4R).

21. The vagina is transected approximately 3 cm below the cervix and is closed using a continuous interlocking 1 chromic suture (Fig. 15–4S).

22. Following removal of the surgical specimen, the bladder is filled with 300 ml sterile saline and carefully inspected. If any lacerations of the bladder wall are present, they are repaired at this time.

23. The anterior vesical space is developed by blunt dissection, and a No. 16 Silastic Foley catheter is inserted into the bladder through an anterior cystotomy incision. The Foley catheter is sutured in place using a running inverting suture of 0 chromic in the anterior bladder wall (Fig. 15–4T).

24. Hemovac drains are placed in both retroperitoneal spaces and are brought out through stab wounds in each lower abdominal quadrant. These drains are sutured to the skin with 2–0 silk (Fig. 15–4T).

25. The pelvis is then reperitonealized using a continuous running 2–0 chromic suture (Fig. 15–4U).

26. Both ovaries are sutured to the iliac fossa peritoneum with 2–0 Prolene, and titanium clips are placed on the suture site and fimbria ovarica for future identification (Fig. 15–4V).

27. The abdomen is then closed in layers, using the interrupted Smead-Jones method. The skin is closed using an interrupted subcuticular suture of 4–0 Dexon and a running 5–0 nylon suture.

Following surgery, the patient should be closely monitored for fluid, electrolyte, and protein losses. The volume and protein and electrolyte concentration of retroperitoneal suction drainage following radical hysterectomy and pelvic lymphadenectomy were initially studied by Roddick and coworkers.[19] These investigators noted that the volume of retroperitoneal drainage was greatest on the first postoperative day (200–400 ml) and decreased progressively thereafter to approximately 50 ml/24 hours on the fifth postoperative day. Because protein and electrolyte content of drainage fluid closely approximates that of serum, an accurate estimate of daily losses can be calculated. These losses can then be replaced, thereby avoiding postoperative electrolyte imbalance or abnormalities in intravascular colloid oncotic pressure. Retroperitoneal suction drains should be kept in place until their total output is less than or equal to 50 ml/24 hours.

Text continued on page 281

276 SURGICAL THERAPY FOR CERVICAL CANCER

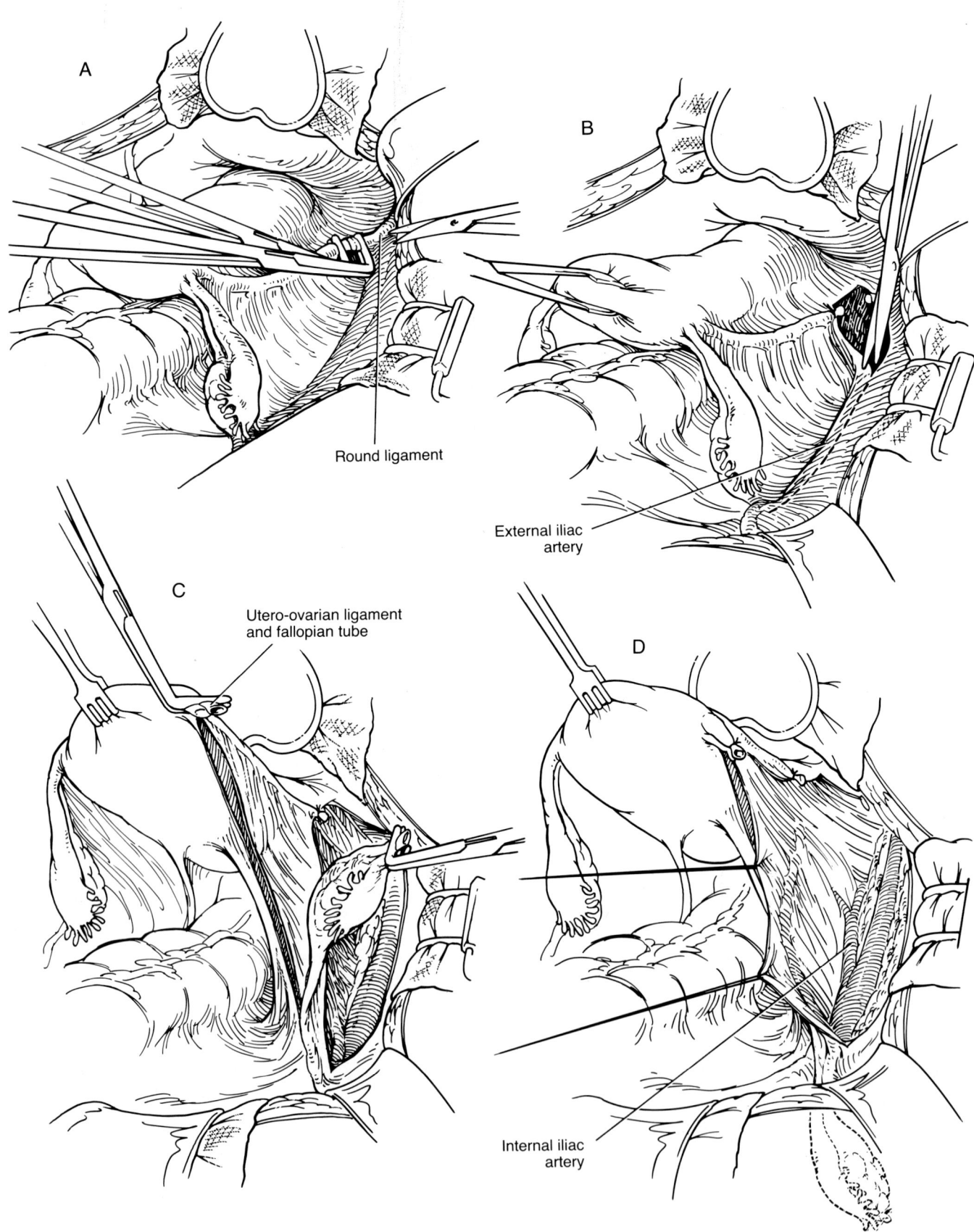

Figure 15–4

SURGICAL THERAPY FOR CERVICAL CANCER 277

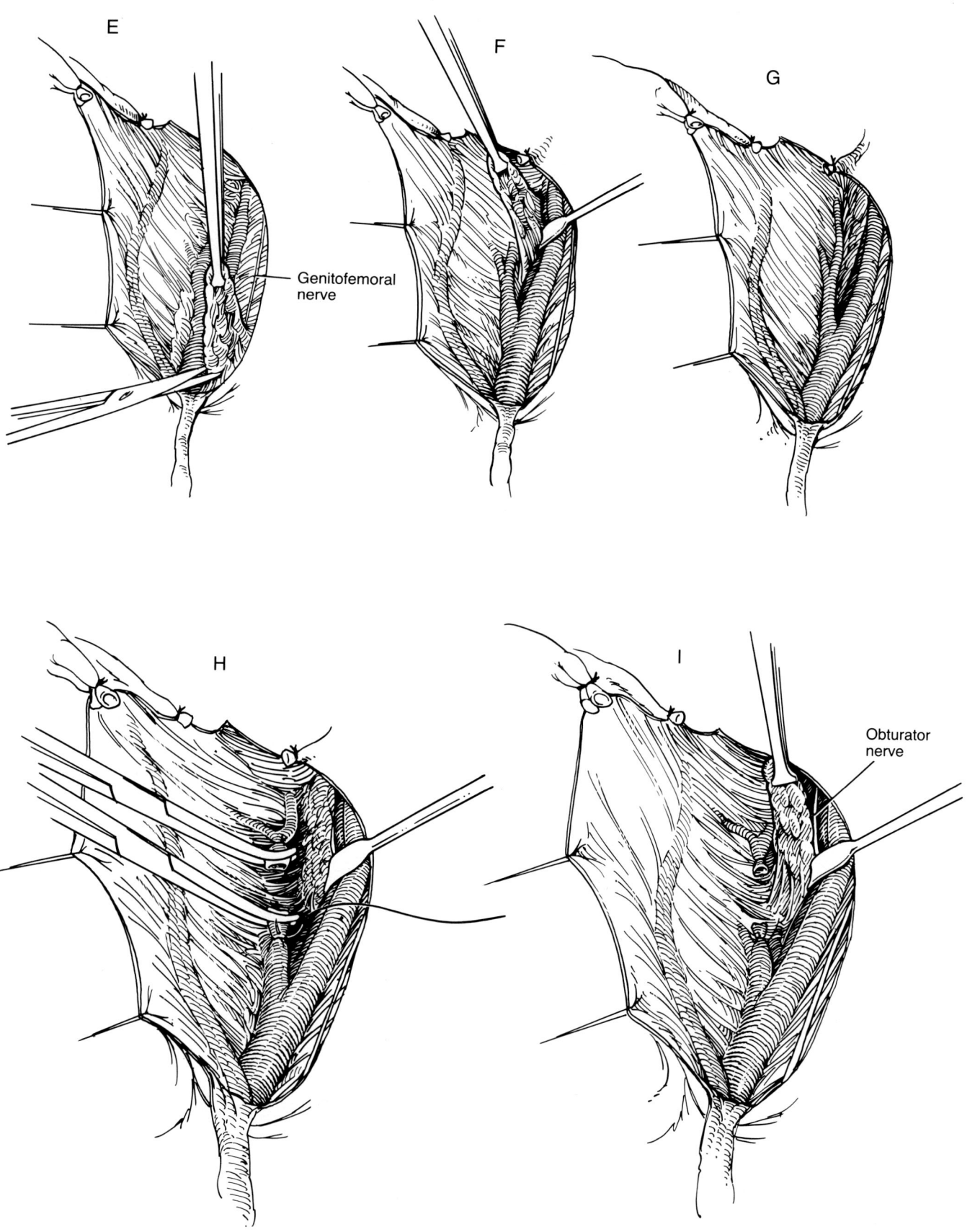

Figure 15–4 *Continued*

Illustration continued on following page

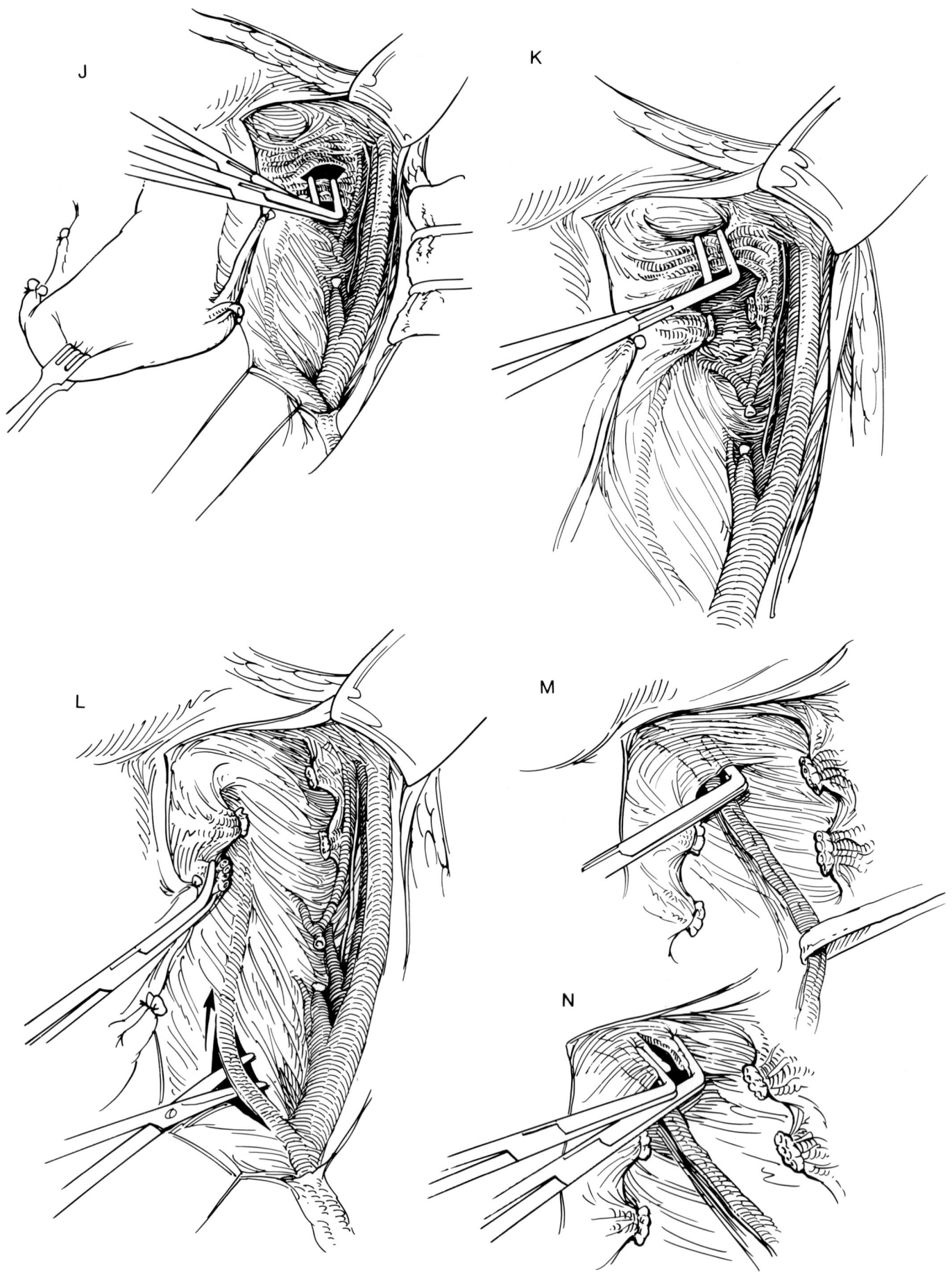

Figure 15–4 Continued

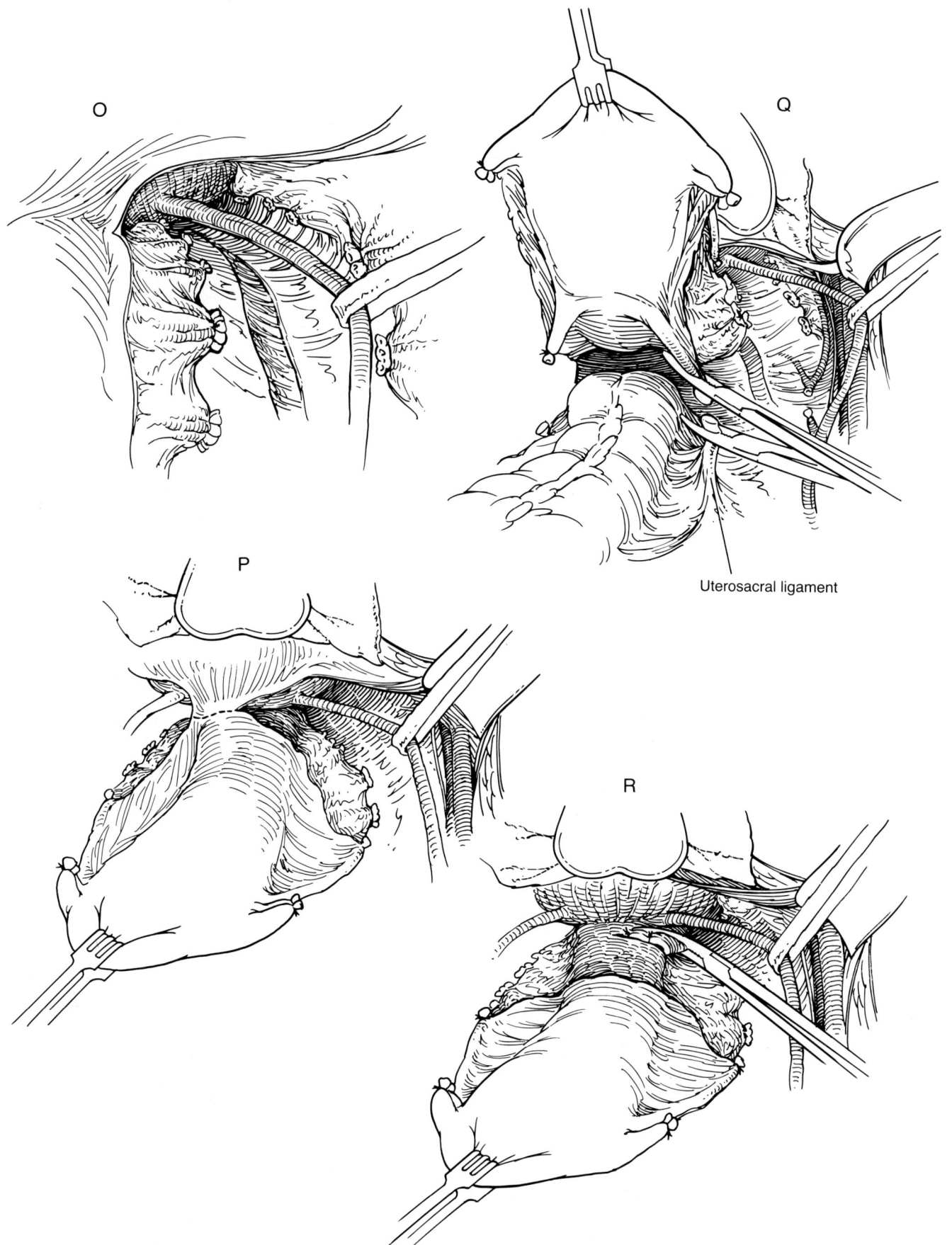

Figure 15–4 *Continued*

Illustration continued on following page

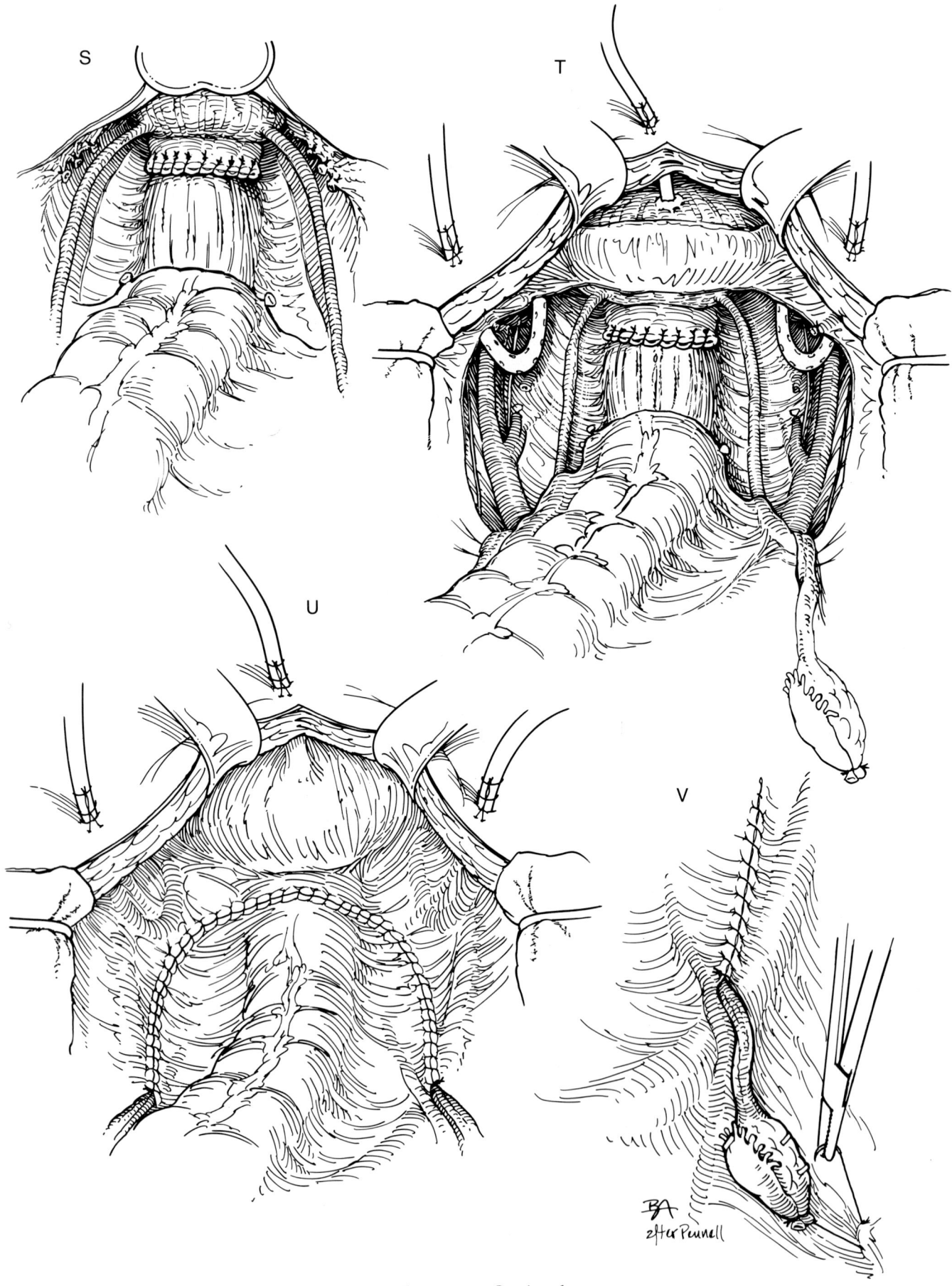

Figure 15–4 Continued

Complications following radical hysterectomy and pelvic lymphadenectomy are summarized in Table 15–2. The most frequent of these complications are related to the urinary tract. Extensive dissection of the bladder base and transection of the uterosacral ligaments at the time of radical hysterectomy often produce interruption of the sympathetic beta-adrenergic nerve supply to the bladder.[31] This causes an initial phase of bladder hypertonicity,[32] which is followed by a hypotonic phase secondary to interruption of parasympathetic nerve fibers.[33] During the hypotonic phase, bladder sensation is diminished and residual urine volume is increased. As a result, there is an increased risk of urinary tract infection and fistula formation.

The use of suprapubic bladder drainage was initially reported by van Nagell and coworkers.[34] These authors reported that the frequencies of urinary tract infection and fistula formation were significantly reduced when suprapubic bladder drainage was utilized. Generally, intermittent clamping of the suprapubic catheter is begun 3–4 days after radical hysterectomy and residual urine volumes are measured. Suprapubic bladder drainage is maintained until the post-voiding residual urine volume is consistently less than 50 ml. In a large series of patients undergoing radical hysterectomy and suprapubic bladder drainage, the mean time to normal voiding was 25 days (range, 4–77 days).[30] Forney has reported that normal bladder function can be restored more rapidly if the cardinal ligaments are only partially transected at the time of radical hysterectomy.[33] This technique may be possible in some cases, but it may also result in incomplete tumor removal and a higher rate of local recurrence. Patients with persisting long-term bladder hypotonicity following radical hysterectomy are taught periodic urethral self-catheterization.

The frequency of urinary tract fistulas following radical hysterectomy has progressively decreased over the past decade. Ureterovaginal fistula is more common than vesicovaginal fistula, but the combined fistula rate in most recent series is less than 3%.[27, 28] This reduction in fistula rate is attributable to (1) careful inspection of the bladder and distal ureters after removal of the surgical specimen, (2) intraoperative repair of bladder or ureteral lacerations, and (3) suprapubic bladder drainage. Should a ureterovaginal or vesicovaginal fistula be diagnosed in the immediate postoperative period, cystoscopy with retrograde ureteral dye studies should be performed to identify the location of the fistula. Ureterovaginal fistulas should be repaired immediately, and ureteral stents should be placed to prevent stenosis and subsequent loss of renal function. Patients with vesicovaginal fistulas will often require treatment with antibiotics and peroxide vaginal washes prior to surgical repair of the fistula. The relationship of the fistula to the ureteral orifices should always be known prior to attempted surgical repair.

The most serious life-threatening complication following radical hysterectomy with pelvic lymphadenectomy is pulmonary embolism. Approximately 1% of patients undergoing radical pelvic surgery will experience this complication. There has been increasing interest concerning the role of prophylactic heparin in the prevention of pulmonary embolism. There are a large number of prospective studies comparing low-dose heparin to placebo in patients undergoing thoracic or abdominal surgery. The majority of these studies have demonstrated a significant reduction in venous thrombosis and fatal pulmonary embolism in

Table 15–2

Complications of Radical Hysterectomy (N = 3892)

Author	No. of Patients	Urinary Fistula		Bladder Atony (%)	Thrombophlebitis (%)	Pulmonary Embolism (%)	Lymphocysts (%)	Intestinal Obstruction (%)
		Vesicovaginal (%)	Ureterovaginal (%)					
Hoskins et al., 1976[20]	224	0.4	1.3	—	—	0.4	—	—
Christensen et al., 1976[21]	670	0.4	5.7	6.9	1.9	0.3	—	—
Webb et al., 1979[12]	423	0.7	1.4	—	5.0	2.1	4.3	0.5
Sall et al., 1974[22]	349	0.9	2.0	0.9	1.1	0.3	1.7	0.9
Underwood et al., 1979[23]	178	1.1	2.8	—	—	—	—	—
Langley et al., 1980[24]	284	1.4	5.6	3.5	—	—	—	—
Lerner et al., 1980[25]	108	—	0.9	5.6	0.9	0.9	0.9	1.9
Powell et al., 1984[26]	255	1.6	0.8	2.7	2.7	2.0	0.8	1.2
Artman et al., 1987[27]	153	1.3	1.3	—	0.7	1.3	1.3	—
Lee et al., 1989[28]	954	1.3	1.3	—	0.2	—	—	1.0
Kenter et al., 1989[29]	213	2.8	3.3	6.1	1.4	.47	6.6	—
DePriest et al., in press	81	0.0	0.0	1.2	0.0	0.0	1.2	0.0
Total	3892	1.0	2.3	4.2	1.6	1.0	2.6	1.1

patients treated by low-dose heparin.[35, 36] Generally, heparin is given in a dose of 5000 U every 12 hours beginning prior to surgery and continuing until the patient is fully ambulant. External pneumatic calf compression has also been shown to reduce the frequency of thromboembolic complications following radical hysterectomy. Clarke-Pearson and co-workers reported that the use of calf compression, intraoperatively and for the first 5 postoperative days, reduced the frequency of deep venous thrombosis from 34% to 13% in patients undergoing radical pelvic surgery.[37] It is the authors' present policy to use prophylactic low-dose heparin in all patients undergoing radical hysterectomy with pelvic lymphadenectomy.

Although pelvic lymphocysts were once a significant complication following radical hysterectomy, the use of retroperitoneal suction drainage has virtually eliminated their occurrence. Similarly, the incidence of postoperative pelvic infections has been significantly reduced by use of prophylactic antibiotics.[38]

EXTRAFASCIAL HYSTERECTOMY WITH PARA-AORTIC LYMPH NODE SAMPLING

Evidence would suggest that the combination of radiation therapy followed by extrafascial hysterectomy and para-aortic lymph node sampling is the treatment of choice in bulky (>4 cm diameter), barrel-shaped cervical cancers.[39–41] These tumors contain a large volume of poorly perfused, hypoxic cells that are characteristically noncycling and therefore resistant to gamma radiation. In addition, many of these lesions spread superiorly to involve the lower uterine segment and therefore extend beyond the curative isodose of radiation (Fig. 15–5).

The addition of extrafascial hysterectomy following radiation allows removal of this central core of theoretically resistant tumor cells. Para-aortic lymph node sampling is performed to assess occult extrapelvic lymph nodal spread beyond the conventional pelvic field of external radiation. Durrance and coworkers were the first to report improved treatment results using combined radiation and surgery for bulky Stage IB cervical cancer.[42] In general, 4000 cGy external therapy and one intracavitary implant were followed 6 weeks later by extrafascial hysterectomy. Using this therapeutic approach, Rutledge and coworkers reported a 5-year survival of 93% for patients with bulky Stage IB cervical cancer.[43] This was significantly higher than that observed when these large-volume tumors were treated either by radiation therapy alone or by radical surgery. These observations were confirmed by Gallion and associates, who

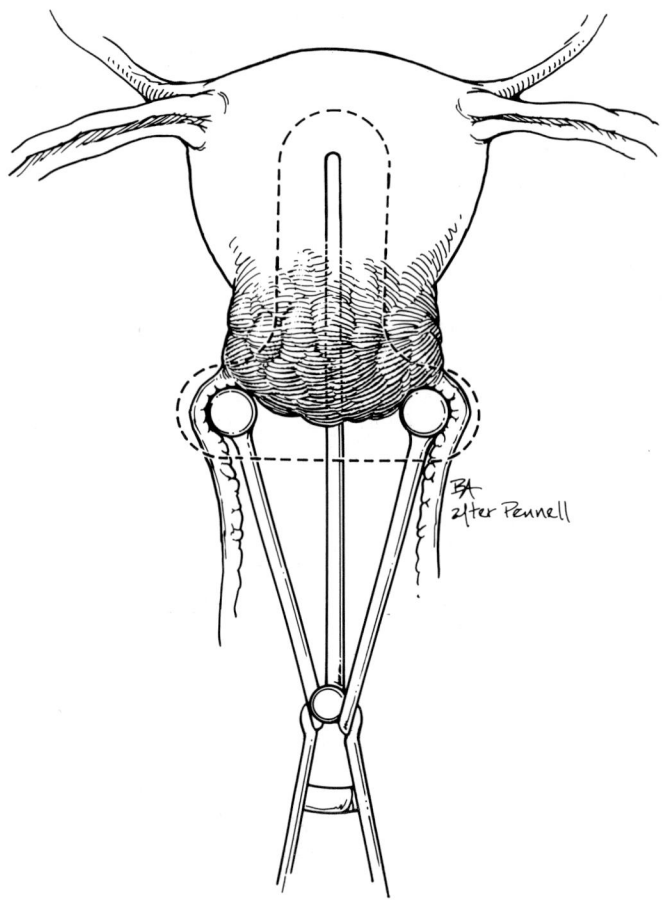

Figure 15–5
Barrel-shaped cervical cancer. The superior lateral aspects of this tumor are often beyond the illustrated curative isodose curve for radiation.

noted a significant reduction in the recurrence rate of patients with bulky (≥ 4 cm diameter), barrel-shaped tumors from 47% to 16% with the addition of extrafascial hysterectomy.[44] Residual invasive cervical cancer was documented in surgical specimens of 32% of these cases. In assessing the pattern of recurrence in patients with bulky, barrel-shaped Stage IB tumors treated by radiation therapy alone, it was noted that many of these tumors first recurred locally and then 5–7 months later spread to extrapelvic sites. It is postulated that combined therapy not only decreases local tumor recurrence but also reduces distant metastases by removing a major source of viable tumor cells that subsequently would spread to other sites.

A second indication for the use of post-radiation extrafascial hysterectomy is the failure of a Stage IB cervical cancer to regress during radiation therapy. Marcial and Bosch carefully observed cervical tumors throughout external and intracavitary radiation and related treatment response to prognosis.[45] Patients whose tumors had disappeared by completion of radiation therapy had a 96% 3-year survival compared with only 2% survival in patients whose tumors never regressed during treatment. In a similar investigation, Hardt and coworkers noted that patients with no palpable or visible evidence of disease 1 month following completion of therapy had a 5-year survival of 95%.[46] In contrast, patients with obvious persistent disease at this time had a recurrence rate of 80%. Patients with Stage IB cervical cancer whose disease has not regressed within 1 month following completion of radiation therapy should be evaluated for extrafascial hysterectomy. Ideal candidates for this procedure should have histologic confirmation of persistent disease confined to the central cervix by magnetic resonance or CT imaging and no evidence of extracervical metastases.

Surgical Procedure

1. The patient is placed in the dorsal lithotomy position and is prepped both vaginally and abdominally. A No. 16 Foley catheter is placed in the bladder.

2. A midline abdominal incision is made from the symphysis pubis to a point approximately 3 cm above the umbilicus.

3. A self-retaining retractor is placed in the incision, and the rectus abdominis muscles are retracted laterally.

4. The intestine is packed into the upper abdomen, and a thyroid clamp is placed in the uterine fundus.

5. The round ligament on the right is clamped, cut, and ligated 2 cm medial to the pelvic sidewall.

6. The anterior leaf of the right broad ligament is incised inferiorly and medially to transect the vesicouterine peritoneum. This incision is then extended superiorly to the level of the infundibulopelvic ligament.

7. The posterior leaf of the right broad ligament is incised to the level of the infundibulopelvic ligament.

8. After identification of the right ureter, the right infundibulopelvic ligament is clamped, cut, and doubly ligated at the lateral pelvic wall. The right ovary and fallopian tube are then suspended to the thyroid clamp previously placed in the uterine fundus.

9. Steps 5–8 are repeated on the left side (Fig. 15–6A).

10. A curved Haney clamp is placed on the right cardinal ligament adjacent to the uterus, and a curved 8-inch Kelly clamp is placed medially to prevent back bleeding. The cardinal ligament is then cut and suture ligated using the Haney technique (Fig. 15–6B). This step is repeated on the left side.

11. The right and left uterosacral ligaments are then clamped, cut, and suture ligated and the bladder is sharply dissected from the anterior vagina (Figs. 15–6C and D).

12. The uterine specimen is excised from the upper vagina, and the vaginal cuff is closed using a continuous interlocking suture (Figs. 15–6E and F).

13. The posterior abdominal peritoneum overlying the aorta is incised from the aortic bifurcation superiorly for approximately 8 cm. The exposed para-aortic lymph nodes are excised (Figs. 15–6G and H).

14. The pelvic and para-aortic peritoneum is reapproximated using a continuous suture of 2–0 chromic (Fig. 15–6I).

15. The abdomen is then closed using the Smead-Jones method with interrupted delayed absorbable sutures. The skin is closed using an interrupted subcuticular suture of 4–0 Dexon and a continuous running suture of 5–0 nylon.

The frequency of complications following combination therapy with radiation and extrafascial hysterectomy is presented in Table 15–3. Urinary tract infection is the most common complication following this procedure, occurring in approximately 4% of patients. Severe complications are rare, and the incidence of vesicovaginal or ureterovaginal fistulas is less than or equal to 1 per cent.

SURGICAL STAGING WITH SELECTIVE PARA-AORTIC LYMPHADENECTOMY

In order to plan effective treatment for cervical cancer, it is essential to document sites of extrapelvic spread so that they can be included in the field of therapy. Cervical carcinoma spreads laterally through the parametrial lymphatics to involve the pelvic and para-aortic lymph nodes. The frequency of pelvic and para-aortic lymph node metastases varies directly with tumor volume and stage of disease (Table 15–4). The presence of para-aortic lymph node metastases is particularly important because these nodes are not included in the traditional pelvic fields of radiation therapy.

Table 15–3

Complications Following Combined Radiation and Extrafascial Hysterectomy

Author	No. of Patients	Vaginal Vault Necrosis	Vesicovaginal Fistula	Small Bowel Obstruction	Urinary Tract Infection	Wound Separation	Pneumonia
O'Quinn et al., 1980[39]	78	1	1	1	0	0	0
Gallion et al., 1985[44]	43	0	0	0	0	2	1
van Nagell et al., 1986[40]	32	0	0	0	4	2	0

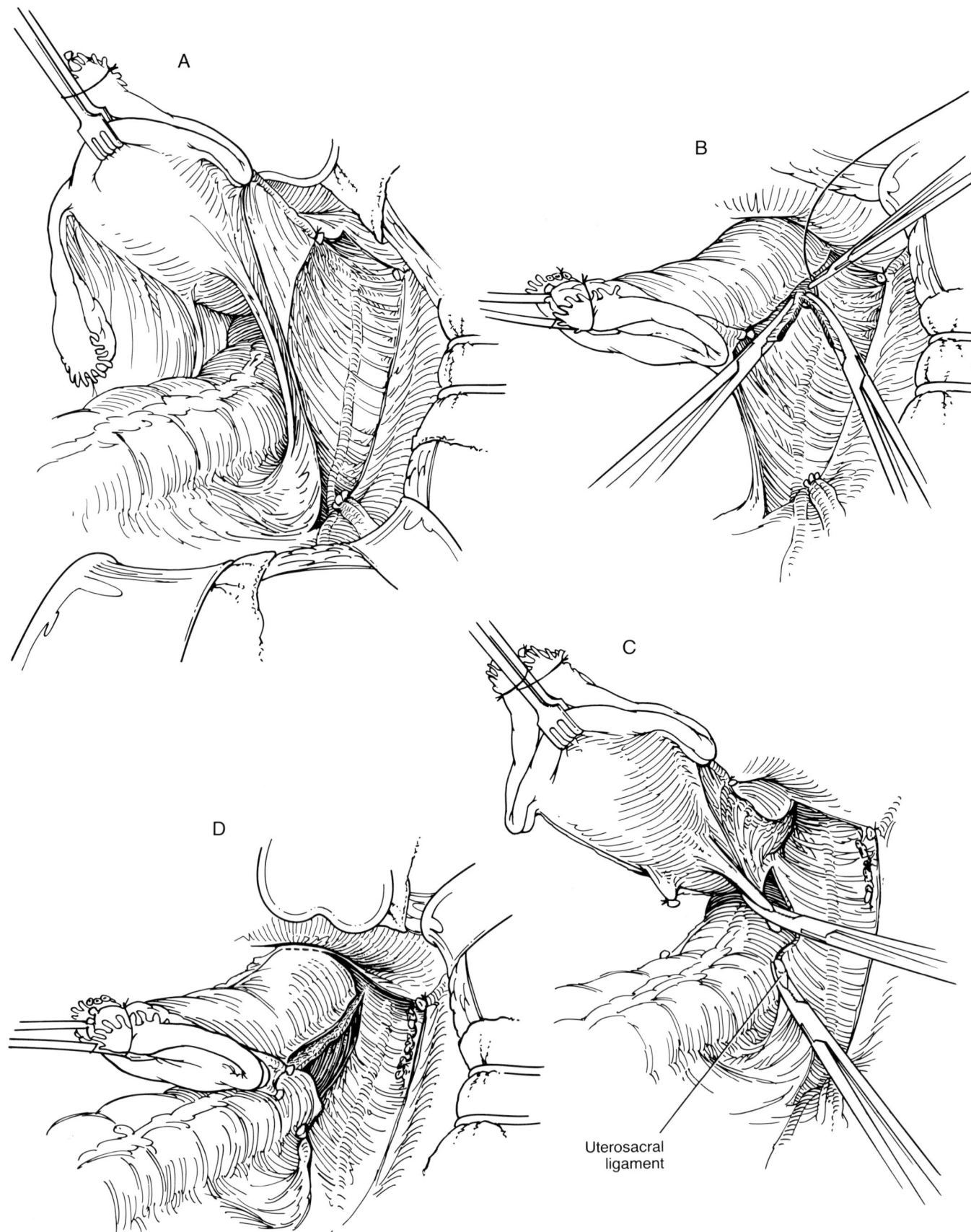

Figure 15–6

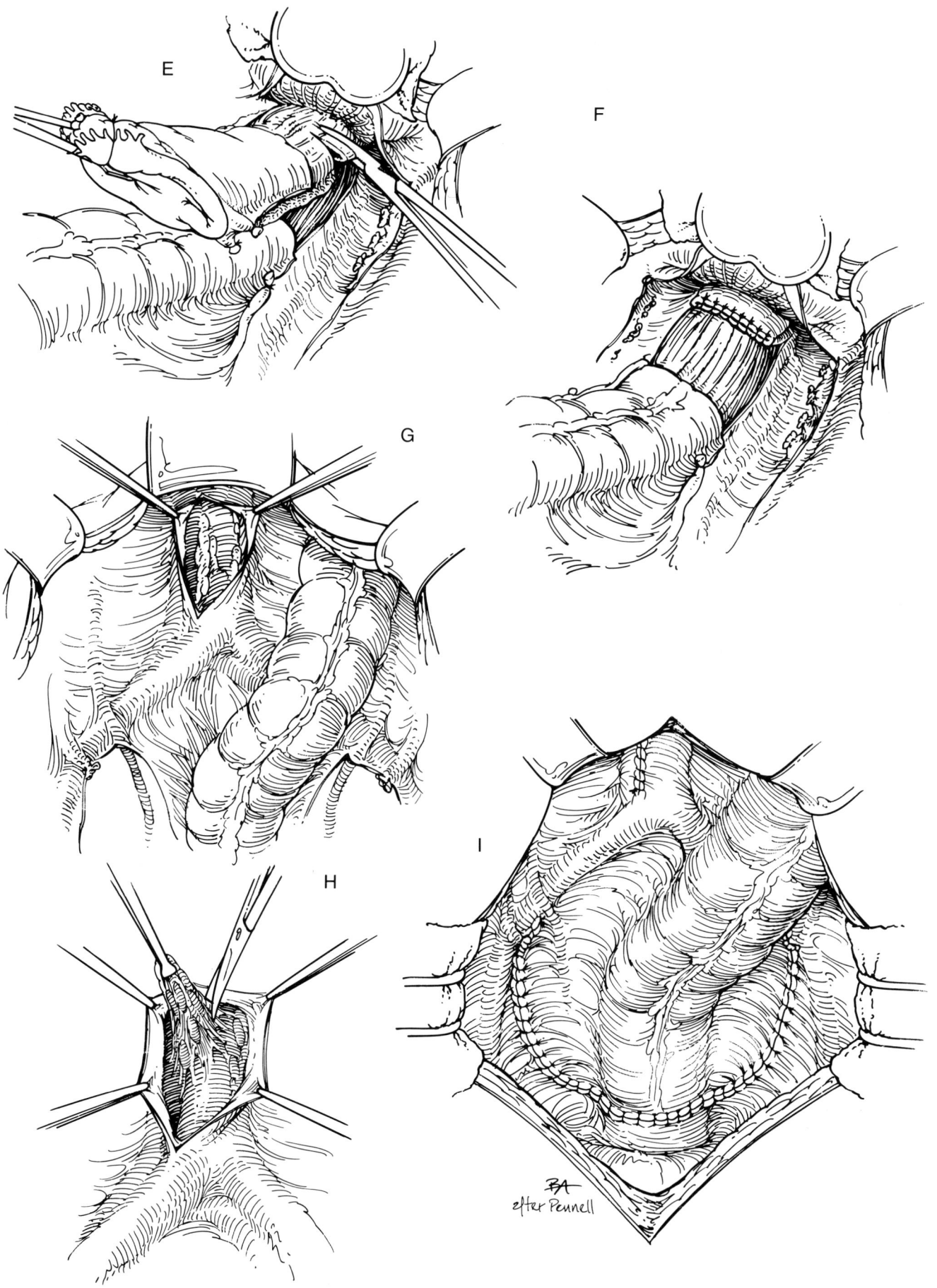

Figure 15-6 Continued

Table 15–4
Para-aortic Lymph Node Metastases by Stage

Stage	No. of Patients	Positive Para-aortic Nodes
IB	2026	118 (5.8%)
IIA	269	30 (11.2%)
IIB	743	76 (10.2%)
III	600	167 (27.8%)
IVA	84	26 (31.0%)

Data from refs. 17, 47–64.

The two methods most commonly used to detect para-aortic lymph nodal metastases are CT-directed fine-needle biopsy and selected retroperitoneal lymphadenectomy. The accuracy of CT-directed fine-needle biopsy in the diagnosis of para-aortic lymph node metastases is approximately 87%.[65] However, metastatic disease in normal sized (≤ 1.0 cm diameter) lymph nodes is undetectable by this method. The most accurate means to assess the status of para-aortic lymph nodes is by exploratory laparotomy with selected lymphadenectomy. Para-aortic lymphadenectomy can be performed through either a transperitoneal or an extraperitoneal approach, but the authors prefer the latter because it is associated with fewer enteric complications when combined with subsequent radiation therapy. Weiser and colleagues[66] compared the efficacy of extraperitoneal versus transperitoneal lymphadenectomy in 288 patients with predominantly Stage IIB or Stage IIIB cervical carcinomas. Although both techniques were of similar sensitivity in detecting lymph nodal metastases, transperitoneal lymphadenectomy was associated with a significantly higher rate of enteric injury than extraperitoneal lymphadenectomy (11.5% vs. 3.9%, $P = .03$). Another prognostically significant finding at exploratory laparotomy is the presence of malignant peritoneal cytology. Podczaski and colleagues, for example, noted that 11 of 155 patients with cervical cancer had positive peritoneal cytology at the time of pretreatment laparotomy.[62] The majority of these patients had advanced stage disease, and 73% died of recurrent cancer from 5 to 60 months after radiation. Although the optimal therapy for cervical cancer patients with positive peritoneal cytology has not been determined, it is beneficial to perform pelvic washings for cytology at the time of pretreatment laparotomy.

Surgical Procedure

1. The patient is placed in the dorsal lithotomy position and prepped both vaginally and abdominally. A No. 16 Foley catheter is placed in the bladder.

2. A midline abdominal incision is made from a point 8 cm below the umbilicus to a point 4 cm above the umbilicus (Fig. 15–7A). The incision is carried down to the posterior rectus sheath, which is separated from the right rectus abdominis muscle (Fig. 15–7B).

3. All perforating branches of the inferior epigastric artery anterior to the deep rectus sheath are cauterized. An incision is made in the posterior rectus sheath at the lateral aspect of the anterior abdominal wall, thereby exposing the underlying peritoneum (Figs. 15–7C and D).

4. The peritoneum is reflected medially, exposing the retroperitoneal structures (Fig. 15–7E). The ureter remains attached to the peritoneum and is also reflected medially.

5. The right para-aortic lymph nodes are excised from the bifurcation of the aorta superiorly to the level of the renal artery (Fig. 15–7F). If iliac lymph node sampling is required, these nodes can also be removed through this approach.

6. Steps 2–5 are repeated on the left side, and the left para-aortic and left iliac lymph nodes are excised.

7. A right paramedian incision approximately 4 cm in length is then made in the anterior abdominal peritoneum. Saline washes of the pelvis and abdomen are taken and submitted for cytologic analysis. The surgeon's right index finger is inserted intraperitoneally, and palpation of the tumor and parametria is performed. The peritoneal incision is closed using a running 3–0 chromic suture.

8. The abdomen is closed using the Smead-Jones method and interrupted delayed absorbable sutures. The skin is closed using an interrupted subcuticular suture of 4–0 Dexon and a continuous running suture of 5–0 nylon.

The complications of extraperitoneal selective para-aortic lymphadenectomy are presented in Table 15–5. Wound infection and vascular injury are the most common complications, occurring in approximately 2–3% of the cases. When this procedure is

Table 15–5
Complications of Extraperitoneal Selective Para-aortic Lymphadenectomy

Author	No. of Patients	Arterial Injury	Venous Injury	Ureteral Injury	Wound Infection	Pelvic Cellulitis
LaPolla et al., 1986[61]	34	2	2	0	2	2
Weiser et al., 1989[66]	128	2	1	0	2	2
Podczaski et al., 1989[62]	104	0	3	0	5	0
Total	266	4 (1.5%)	6 (2.2%)	0 (0%)	9 (3.4%)	4 (1.5%)

SURGICAL THERAPY FOR CERVICAL CANCER 287

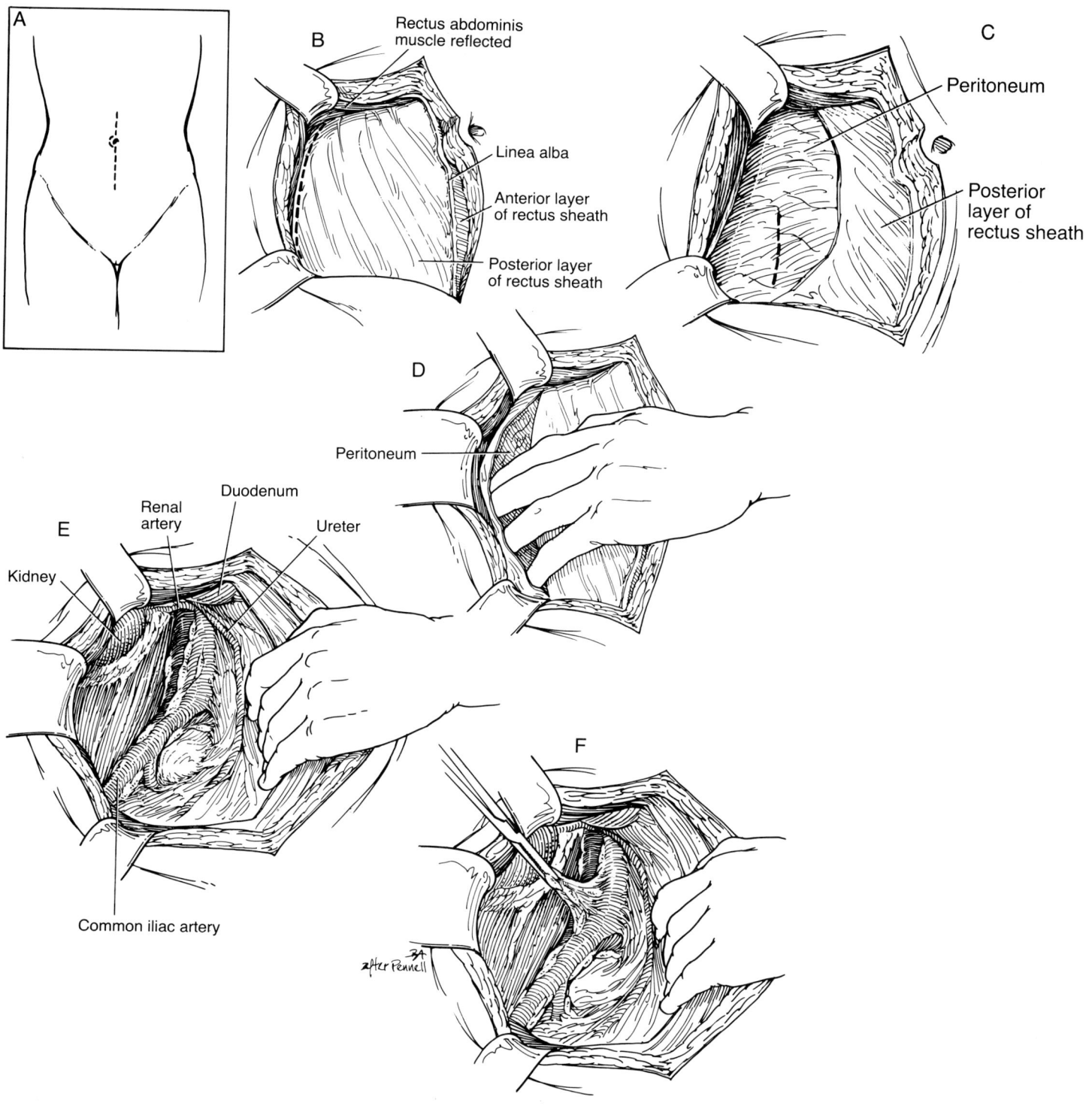

Figure 15–7

followed by a full course of external and intracavitary radiation, approximately 4% of patients experience small bowel obstruction or other types of enteric injury. An additional 1% of patients develop retroperitoneal fibrosis.[66]

The outcome of patients treated with extended field radiation for histologically confirmed para-aortic lymph node metastasis is presented in Table 15–6. The 5-year survival of this group varied from 14 to 50% (mean, 27%).

SCALENE FAT PAD BIOPSY

Biopsy of scalene lymph nodes is indicated in those patients with histologically confirmed para-aortic lymph node metastases. Although not apparent clinically, approximately 15% of patients with para-aortic lymph nodal disease will also have scalene lymph node metastases.

Patients with scalene lymph node metastases should be treated with systemic therapy rather than with extended-field radiation. In the absence of a palpably enlarged scalene lymph node, it is preferable to perform this operation on the left side. The purpose of this operation is to remove the fat pad and associated lymph nodal tissue from the subclavian triangle. This triangle is delineated by the subclavian vein inferiorly, the internal jugular vein medially, and the omohyoid muscle superolaterally.

Surgical Procedure

1. The patient is placed in the supine position, with a sandbag underneath the left scapula and the head turned to the right side.

2. The left supraclavicular area is prepped, and 10 ml of 0.5% lidocaine is injected subcutaneously along the site of the planned incision.

3. An incision is made 2 cm above the clavicle at the anterior border of the clavicular head of the sternocleidomastoid muscle (Fig. 15–8A). This incision is extended laterally for a distance of 5 cm.

4. The platysma and underlying fascia are divided, exposing the pre-scalene area between the sternocleidomastoid muscle and the external jugular vein (Fig. 15–8B).

5. The sternocleidomastoid muscle is retracted medially, and the omohyoid muscle is retracted superiorly. Superolateral traction is placed on the scalene fat pad, and it is dissected away from the internal jugular vein (Fig. 15–8C).

6. The incision is then retracted inferiorly, and the dissection of the medial border of the fat pad is continued down to the confluence of the internal jugular and subclavian veins.

7. The fat pad is mobilized superiorly to the level of the omohyoid muscle and is dissected free of the fascia overlying the scalenus anterior muscle (Fig. 15–8D).

8. The platysma is closed with interrupted sutures of 4–0 Dexon, and the skin is closed with interrupted sutures of 5–0 nylon.

The frequency of complications following scalene lymph node biopsy is low. Brantigan and coworkers,[71] for example, reported three complications (0.9%) in 341 consecutive patients undergoing scalene lymph node biopsy.[71] The most common complications reported are wound hematoma and infection. Despite this low complication rate, scalene lymph node biopsy should be performed in a meticulous fashion after thorough review of the anatomy of the subclavian triangle. Both the phrenic nerve and the thoracic duct are adjacent to the operative site, and care must be taken to avoid their injury.

PELVIC EXENTERATION

Pelvic exenteration is the treatment of choice in patients with recurrent cervical cancer confined to the central pelvis. Most of these patients have received a full course of external and intracavitary radiation, so that less radical methods of tumor removal are associated with an unacceptable complication rate. Symmonds and co-workers, for example, reported on 49 patients who underwent radical hysterectomy for recurrent cervical cancer.[72] Twenty-five patients (51%) were cured of disease, but 19% developed enteric or urinary tract fistulas. For this reason, most oncologists recommend exenterative surgery for recurrent cervical cancer following radiation therapy.

The one-stage pelvic exenteration as a treatment method for cervical cancer was initially described by Alexander Brunschwig in 1948.[73] There are three types of pelvic exenteration. Anterior pelvic exenter-

Table 15–6

Five-Year Survival for Patients Treated with Extended Field Radiation for Para-aortic Nodal Metastases from Cervical Carcinoma

Author	No. of Patients	Radiation Dose (cGy)	5-Year Survival (%)
Hughes et al., 1980[52]	38	4500–5100	30
Piver et al., 1981[67]	21	6000	14
Tewfik et al., 1982[68]	23	5000–5500	22
Rubin et al., 1984[59]	14	4000–5000	43
Nori et al., 1985[69]	27	5000–5200	30
Podczaski et al., 1989[62]	24	5000	27
Gaspar et al., 1989[70]	18	4000–6000	17
Lovecchio et al., 1989[64]	36	4500	50

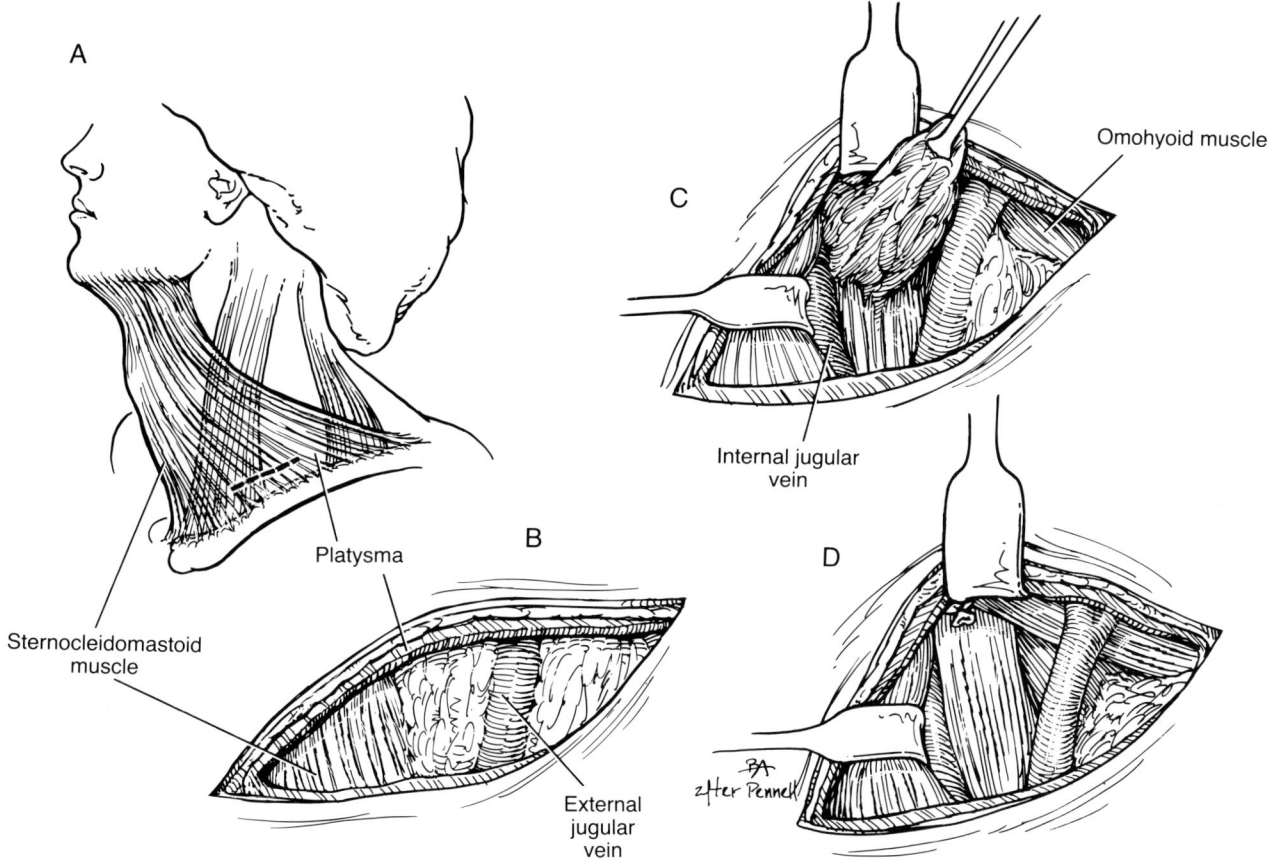

Figure 15–8

ation is a combination of radical cystectomy, radical hysterectomy, and vaginectomy and is indicated in the treatment of recurrent cervical cancer limited to the cervix, anterior vagina, or bladder. Posterior pelvic exenteration is a combination of abdominal perineal resection of the rectosigmoid, radical hysterectomy, and vaginectomy and is performed for tumor recurrence involving the posterior vagina and the rectovaginal septum. Total pelvic exenteration involves the en bloc excision of the bladder, uterus, fallopian tubes, ovaries, vagina, and rectum and is the type of exenteration most often required for recurrent cervical cancer.

Technical advances in this operation include the performance of continent vesicostomy, low rectal anastomosis, and vaginal reconstruction. Since Bricker[74] first described the use of an isolated segment of terminal ileum as a urinary conduit, a number of techniques for urinary diversion have been described in patients undergoing pelvic exenteration. These include use of both the sigmoid colon[75] and the transverse colon[76] as urinary reservoirs. Most recently, the use of continent vesicostomy has been proposed in patients undergoing cystectomy as part of pelvic exenteration. The ascending and transverse colon are used to form a urinary pouch that can be catheterized by the patient. Penalver and colleagues performed continent vesicostomy in 7 patients undergoing exenterative surgery for recurrent cervical cancer.[77] Postoperative urodynamic studies indicated that all patients were continent, and there was no evidence of urinary reflux in any case. The subject of urinary diversion is reviewed in more detail in Chapter 22.

Low rectal anastomosis has also been used successfully in patients undergoing pelvic exenteration. The invention of the end-to-end circular stapling device has allowed primary reanastomosis of the proximal sigmoid colon to the rectum in patients requiring excision of the distal sigmoid colon. In a review of 20 patients undergoing low rectal anastomosis at the time of exenteration, Hatch and colleagues reported that primary healing occurred in 70% of cases.[78] Anastomotic leaks were more common when the length of the rectal stump was less than or equal to 6 cm. The authors emphasized the importance of using an omental wrap as a source of blood supply to the anastomotic site. When an omental wrap could be used, the complete healing rate of the low rectal anastomosis was 85%.[79] In patients with inadequate omental length, a myocutaneous graft using the rectus abdominis muscle can be used as a source of neovascularization and pelvic support.

Because many patients are sexually active prior

to pelvic exenteration, every effort should be made to preserve sexual function after exenteration. Split thickness skin grafts can be used to create a neovagina, but this technique requires a base of granulation tissue that is often difficult to establish after total pelvic exenteration. Wheeless has reported the successful construction of a neovagina using an omental cylinder to provide the blood supply for split thickness skin grafts.[80] However, most surgeons favor the use of bilateral gracilis myocutaneous grafts for vaginal reconstruction following exenteration. These grafts not only form a functional vagina but also provide support and blood supply to the pelvis. Techniques for vaginal reconstruction are discussed in Chapter 32.

Despite the previously mentioned technical advances, pelvic exenteration remains a formidable operation that is often associated with significant long-term complications. For this reason, it is imperative that every effort be made to select those patients who are optimal candidates for this procedure. Exenterative surgery should be performed only when there is a reasonable chance for long-term survival, and not for palliation. The most obvious contraindication to pelvic exenteration is the presence of extrapelvic metastases. A CT scan of the pelvis, upper abdomen, and para-aortic lymph nodes should be performed on all patients being considered for pelvic exenteration, and any suspicious areas should be biopsied using fine-needle aspiration. A CT scan can be particularly helpful in determining the presence of tumor invasion of lateral pelvic wall structures. Likewise, hepatic or pulmonary lesions should be biopsied prior to exenterative surgery. Additional contraindications to pelvic exenteration include the following:

1. Ureteral obstruction by cervical cancer
2. Unilateral leg edema
3. Sciatic pain suggesting neural involvement by recurrent cancer
4. Metastatic disease involving lateral pelvic lymph nodes
5. Invasion of the lateral pelvic muscles by recurrent cancer

Psychologic evaluation is also necessary prior to the performance of pelvic exenteration. The extensive nature of this operation and the resultant changes in physiology and self-image require a stable personality and a supportive family environment. The authors remain hesitant to perform this operation on a patient who is psychologically unstable or who has minimal social support from family or friends.

Using these criteria, approximately 20% of patients evaluated will undergo exploratory laparotomy with intent to perform pelvic exenteration.[81]

Patients undergoing exploratory laparotomy for possible exenteration should undergo a thorough nutritional assessment prior to surgery. This should include anthropometrics, evaluation of secretory protein status (total serum protein, serum albumin, and serum transferrin), and immunologic function.[82] Total parenteral nutrition and intravenous hydration should be instituted at least 2 days prior to exenteration.

On the day before surgery, patients should have a mechanical and antibiotic bowel preparation and should be placed on mini-dose heparin (5000 U subcutaneously every 12 hours) to reduce the risk of thromboembolic disease.

Surgical Procedure

1. The patient is placed in the modified lithotomy or "ski" position with the hips abducted to expose the perineum. A No. 16 Foley catheter is placed in the bladder and connected to straight drainage. The optimal skin location for the continent vesicostomy is marked.

2. A midline abdominal incision is made from the symphysis pubis to a point approximately 3 cm above and to the left of the umbilicus.

3. The liver, omentum, and abdominal peritoneum are carefully inspected, and areas suspicious for malignancy are biopsied.

4. A self-retaining retractor is placed in the incision, and the rectus abdominis muscles are retracted laterally.

5. The peritoneum overlying the para-aortic lymph nodes is incised, and any enlarged lymph nodes are removed and sent for frozen section examination. If these lymph nodes contain metastatic cervical cancer, the procedure is terminated.

6. The round ligaments are then clamped, cut, and tied, and the anterior and posterior leaves of the broad ligament are opened (Fig. 15–9A). The lateral pelvic wall peritoneum is then incised superiorly to the level of the common iliac artery (Fig. 15–9B).

7. The paravesical, pararectal, and presacral spaces are all developed, and enlarged lymph nodes from the internal iliac, external iliac, common iliac, obturator, or presacral chains are removed and sent for histologic examination (Fig. 15–9C, and D).

8. If all submitted lymph nodes are negative and the tumor is not fixed to either lateral pelvic wall, the ureters are transected below the level of the common iliac arteries (Fig. 15–9E). The anterior divisions of the internal iliac arteries are identified, ligated with 2–0 silk, and suture ligated with 3–0 Prolene.

9. The sigmoid colon is transected proximal to the area of tumor recurrence using the GIA stapling device, and the presacral space is further developed by blunt dissection (Fig. 15–9F). The uterosacral ligaments are then clamped, cut, and ligated at the posterior pelvic wall.

10. The bladder is separated from the retropubic space, and the lateral vesicle attachments are sharply incised (Fig. 15–9G).

SURGICAL THERAPY FOR CERVICAL CANCER   291

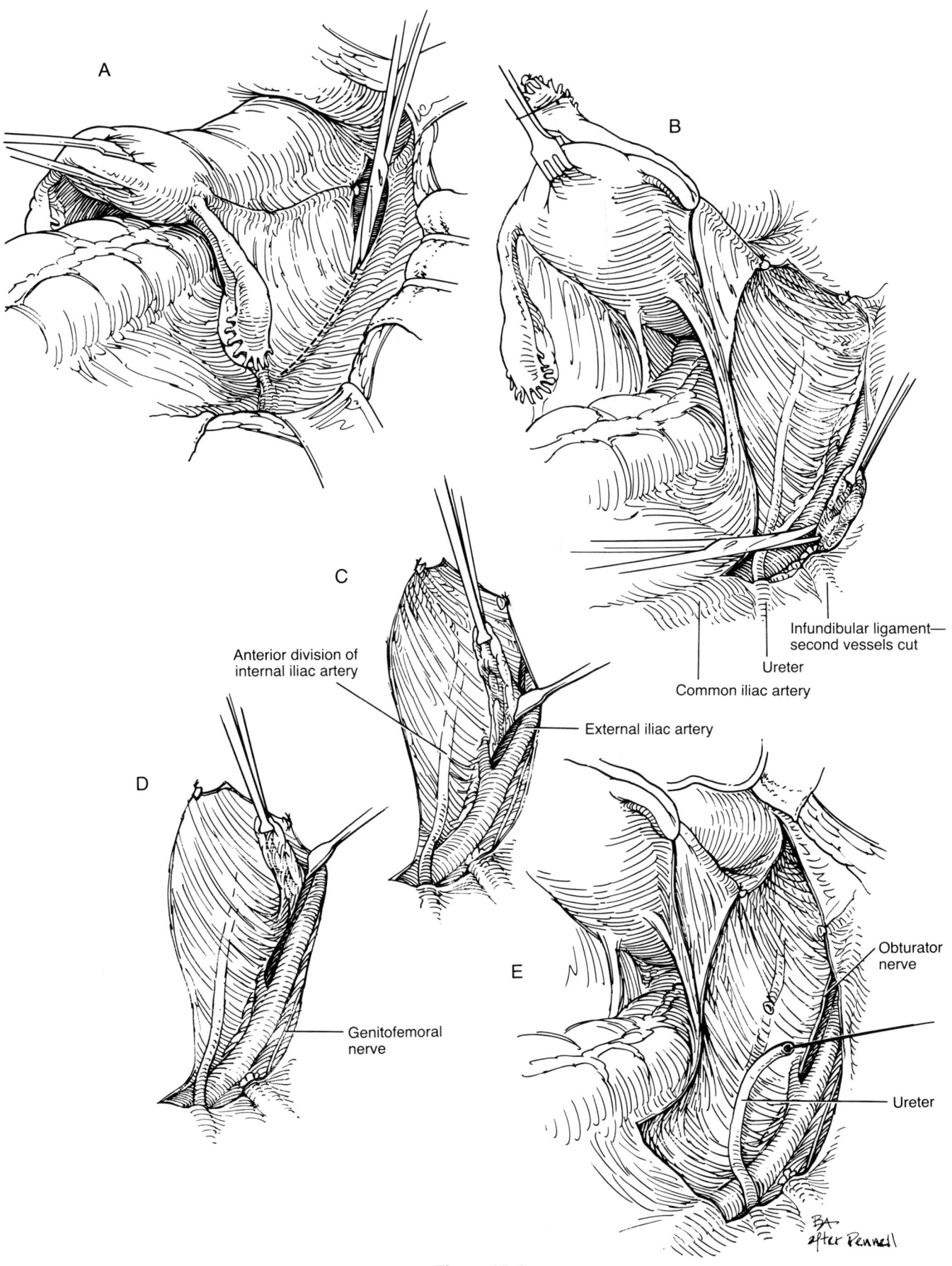

Figure 15–9

Illustration continued on following page

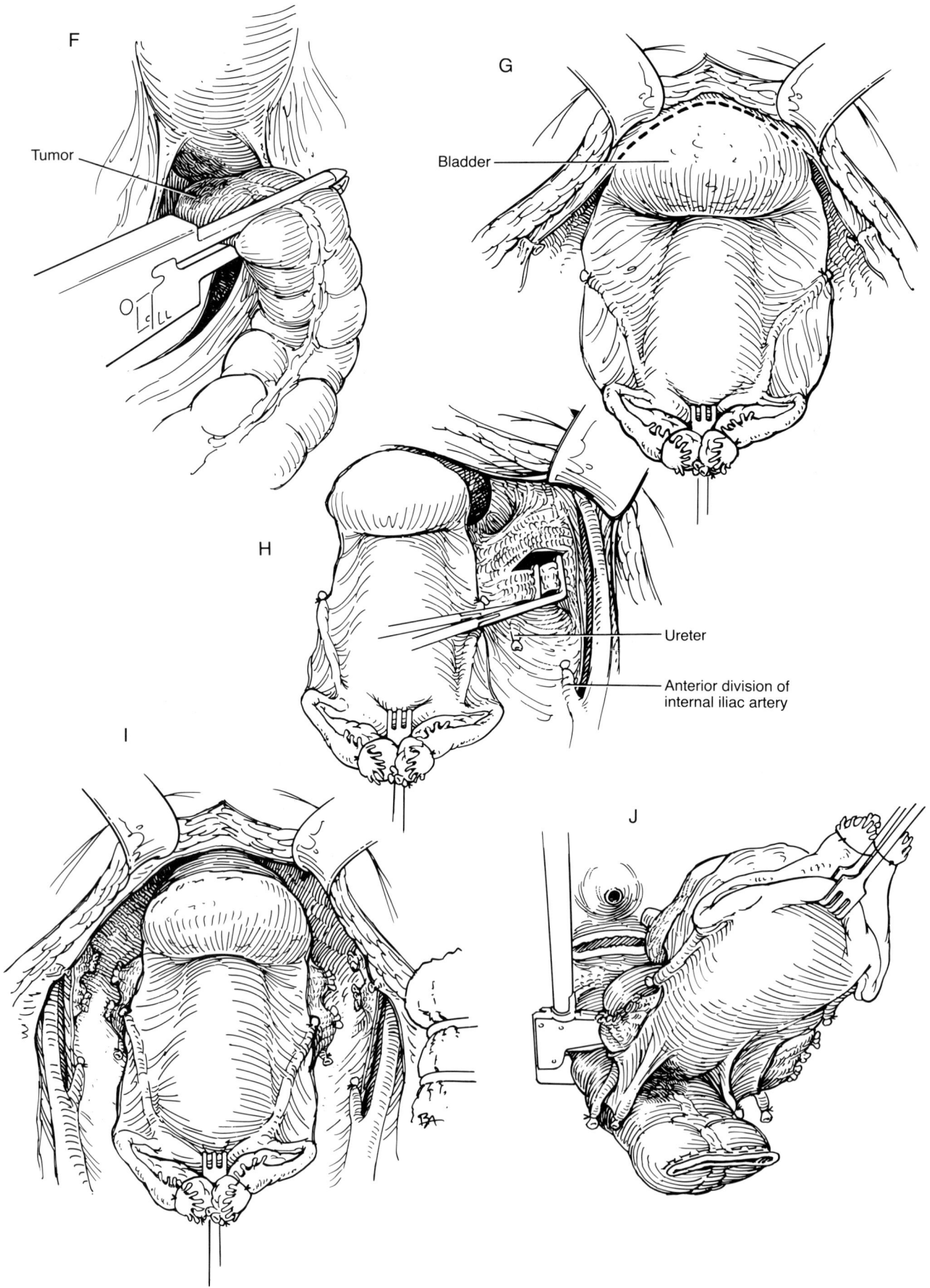

Figure 15–9 Continued

SURGICAL THERAPY FOR CERVICAL CANCER   293

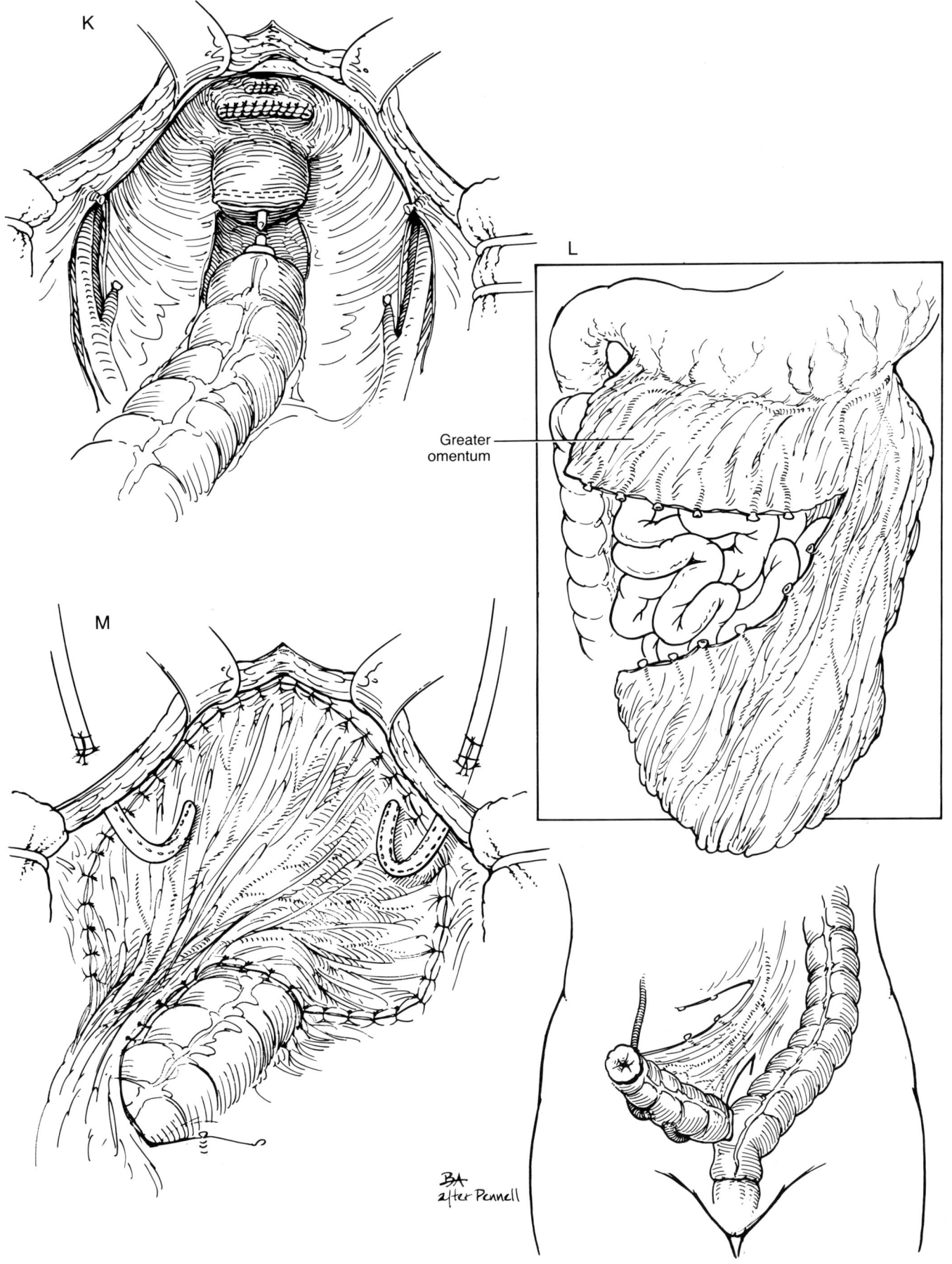

Figure 15–9 *Continued*

11. All lateral aspects of the specimen containing the vascular web are clamped, cut, and ligated using 2–0 silk suture (Fig. 15–9H). Transection of the vascular web is continued inferiorly to the level of the levator ani muscle (Fig. 15–9I).

12. The urethra and vagina are incised at the level of the levator sling, and the vaginal cuff is closed. The rectum is then transected following stapling with a TA-55 device at the level of the levator ani muscle or higher if an adequate proximal margin of normal tissue is identified (Fig. 15–9J).

13. Anastomosis of the proximal sigmoid colon to the rectum is performed using the EEA stapling device (Fig. 15–9K).

14. An omental J-flap is constructed by incising the attachments of the omentum to the colon, from the hepatic flexure medially to the mid-portion of the stomach (Fig. 15–9L). The left gastroepiploic artery is preserved as a source of blood supply for this pedicle.

15. The omental flap is used to cover the denuded pelvis and to provide blood supply to the site of low rectal anastomosis. This flap is sutured to the pelvic floor, and Hemovac drains are placed in the pelvis (Fig. 15–9M).

16. A continent vesicostomy is created as described in Chapter 22, and vaginal reconstruction is completed as illustrated in Chapter 32.

Following pelvic exenteration, careful measurement of Hemovac drainage should be instituted so that proper replacement of protein and electrolyte losses can be achieved. The volume of peritoneal suction drainage may be as great as 1000 ml/24 hours during the first several days after exenteration. Because the protein and electrolyte content of suction drainage following exenteration closely approximates that of serum, losses of these components can be accurately determined and replaced.

Operative complications of patients undergoing pelvic exenteration are summarized in series by Averette and coworkers[83] and Morley and colleagues.[81] The most common complications remain small bowel obstruction or fistula formation, which occurs in approximately 5% per cent of cases. However, the use of an omental lid, free peritoneal grafts, or myocutaneous pedical grafts to cover the pelvic floor has markedly reduced the frequency of these complications. Likewise, the use of prophylactic antibiotics has resulted in a significant reduction in the frequency of pelvic and wound infections following exenteration. Approximately 1% of patients undergoing pelvic exenteration continue to experience pulmonary embolism. For this reason, prophylactic mini-dose heparin and pneumatic compression stockings are continued until the patient is fully ambulant.

Table 15–7

Pelvic Exenteration: Operative Mortality and 5-Year Survival

Author	Total Cases	Cervical Cancer	Operative Mortality (%)	5-Year Survival (%)
Brunschwig et al., 1967[84]	312	312	17.3	18
Bricker, 1970[85]	207	207	7.7	35
Ketcham et al., 1970[86]	162	162	7.4	38
Symmonds et al., 1975[87]	198	117	8.1	33
Rutledge et al., 1977[88]	296	196	13.5	37
Averette et al., 1984[83]	92	70	23.9	37
Kraybill et al., 1988[89]	99	66	14.1	45
Shingleton et al., 1989[90]	143	143	6.3	50
Morley et al., 1989[81]	100	66	2.0	61

During the past decade, improved hemodynamic monitoring, nutritional support, and advances in surgical technique have resulted in a marked reduction in the operative mortality of pelvic exenteration (Table 15–7). In two series of patients undergoing pelvic exenteration, for example, the operative mortality was less than 7% and the 5-year survival was in excess of 50%.[81, 90] In addition, the use of low rectal anastomosis, continent vesicostomy, and vaginal reconstruction has obviated the severe changes in body image previously associated with this operation. The number of suitable candidates for pelvic exenteration continues to decline because the frequency of central pelvic recurrence following modern radiation therapy is low. Nevertheless, this operation remains an effective therapeutic method when applied to properly selected patients with recurrent cervical cancer.

As has been emphasized in this discussion, it is apparent that surgery remains an integral part of therapy for the majority of patients with cervical cancer. It is only by a thorough understanding of these surgical procedures and the indications for their use that therapy can be individualized to the needs of each patient.

References

1. Fouchee JH, Greiss FC, Loch FR: Stage IA squamous cell carcinoma of the uterine cervix. Am J Obstet Gynecol 1969; 105:46.
2. Roche WD, Norris HJ: Microinvasive carcinoma of the cervix: The significance of lymphatic invasion and confluent patterns of stromal growth. Cancer 1975; 36:180.
3. Averette HE, Nelson JH, Ng AG, et al.: Diagnosis and management of microinvasive (stage IA) carcinoma of the uterine cervix. Cancer 1976; 38:414.
4. Leman MH, Benson WL, Kurman RJ, Park RC: Microinvasive carcinoma of the cervix. Obstet Gynecol 1976; 48:571.

5. Seski JC, Abell MR, Morley GW: Microinvasive squamous carcinoma of the cervix: Definition, histologic analysis, late results of treatment. Obstet Gynecol 1977; 50:410.
6. Taki I, Sugimori H, Matsuyama T, et al.: Treatment of microinvasive carcinoma. Obstet Gynecol Surv 1979; 34:839.
7. Yajima A, Noda K: The results of treatment of microinvasive carcinoma (stage IA) of the uterine cervix by means of simple and extended hysterectomy. Am J Obstet Gynecol 1979; 135:685.
8. van Nagell JR Jr, Greenwell N, Powell DF, et al.: Microinvasive carcinoma of the cervix. Am J Obstet Gynecol 1983; 145:981.
9. Simon NL, Gore H, Shingleton HM, et al.: Study of superficially invasive carcinoma of the cervix. Obstet Gynecol 1986; 68:19.
10. Tsukamoto N, Kaku T, Matsukuma K, et al.: The problem of stage Ia (FIGO, 1985) carcinoma of the uterine cervix. Gynecol Oncol 1989; 34:1.
11. Nelson JH, Averette HE, Richart RM: Cervical intraepithelial neoplasia and early invasive cervical carcinomas. Cancer 1989; 39:157.
12. Webb MJ, Symmonds RE: Wertheim hysterectomy: A reappraisal. Obstet Gynecol 1979; 54:140.
13. Piver MS, Chung WS: Prognostic significance of cervical lesion size and pelvic node metastases in cervical carcinoma. Obstet Gynecol 1975; 46:507.
14. van Nagell JR Jr, Donaldson ES, Parker JC, et al.: The prognostic significance of cell type and lesion size in patients with cervical cancer treated by radical surgery. Gynecol Oncol 1977; 5:142.
15. Boyce JG, Fruchter RG, Nicastri AD, et al.: Vascular invasion in stage I carcinoma of the cervix. Cancer 1984; 53:1175.
16. van Nagell JR Jr, Powell DE, Gallion HH, et al.: Small cell carcinoma of the uterine cervix. Cancer 1988; 62:1586.
17. Gauthier P, Gore I, Shingleton HM, et al.: Identification of histopathologic risk groups in stage IB squamous cell carcinoma of the cervix. Obstet Gynecol 1985; 66:569.
18. van Nagell JR Jr, Sprague AD, Roddick JW Jr: The effect of intravenous pyelography and cystoscopy on the staging of cervical cancer. Gynecol Oncol 1975; 3:87.
19. Roddick JW, van Nagell JR Jr, Bell RM: Protein and electrolyte content of retroperitoneal suction drainage after radical hysterectomy and pelvic lymphadenectomy. Gynecol Oncol 1973; 1:149.
20. Hoskins WJ, Ford JH, Lutz MH, Averette HE: Radical hysterectomy and pelvic lymphadenectomy for the management of early invasive cancer of the cervix. Gynecol Oncol 1976; 4:278.
21. Christensen A, Foglmann R: Cervical carcinoma stage I and II treated by primary radical hysterectomy and pelvic lymphadenectomy, 320 cases by the method of Meigs-Taussig and 350 by the method of Okabayaschi. Acta Obstet Gynecol Scand Suppl 1976; 58:1.
22. Sall S, Rini S, Pineda A: Surgical management of invasive carcinoma of the cervix in pregnancy. Am J Obstet Gynecol 1974; 118:1.
23. Underwood PB Jr, Wilson WC, Kreutner A, et al.: Radical hysterectomy: A critical review of twenty-two years' experience. Am J Obstet Gynecol 1979; 134:889.
24. Langley II, Moore DW, Tarnasky JW, Roberts PH: Radical hysterectomy and pelvic lymph node dissection. Gynecol Oncol 1980; 9:37.
25. Lerner HM, Jones HW III, Hill EC: Radical surgery for the treatment of early invasive cervical carcinoma (stage IB): Review of 15 years' experience. Obstet Gynecol 1980; 56:413.
26. Powell JL, Burrell MO, Franklin EW III: Radical hysterectomy and pelvic lymphadenectomy. South Med J 1984; 77:596.
27. Artman LE, Hoskins WJ, Bibro MC, et al.: Radical hysterectomy and pelvic lymphadenectomy for stage IB carcinoma of the cervix: 21 years' experience. Gynecol Oncol 1987; 28:8.
28. Lee YN, Wang KL, Lin MH, et al.: Radical hysterectomy with pelvic lymph node dissection for treatment of cervical cancer: A clinical review of 954 cases. Gynecol Oncol 1989; 32:135.
29. Kenter GG, Ansink AC, Heintz AP, et al.: Carcinoma of the uterine cervix stage I and IIA: Results of surgical treatment: Complications, recurrence and survival. Eur J Surg Oncol 1989; 15:55.
30. DePriest PD, Gallion HH, van Nagell JR Jr: The efficacy of radical hysterectomy with pelvic lymphadenectomy as a treatment method in patients with stage IB cervical cancer ≤3 cm in diameter. Gynecol Oncol (in press).
31. Scotti RJ, Bergman A, Bhatia N, Ostergard DR: Urodynamic changes in urethrovesical function after radical hysterectomy. Obstet Gynecol 1986; 68:111.
32. Low JA, Mauger GM, Carmichael JA: The effect of Wertheim hysterectomy upon bladder and urethral function. Am J Obstet Gynecol 1981; 139:826.
33. Forney JP: The effect of radical hysterectomy on bladder physiology. Am J Obstet Gynecol 1980; 138:374.
34. van Nagell JR Jr, Penny R, Roddick JW Jr: Suprapubic bladder drainage following radical hysterectomy. Am J Obstet Gynecol 1972; 113:849.
35. Genton E, Turpie AGG: Venous thromboembolism associated with gynecologic surgery. In Pitkin RM (ed.): Clinical Obstetrics and Gynecology. Hagerstown, MD, Harper & Row, 1980, pp. 209–241.
36. International Multicentre Trial: Prevention of fatal postoperative pulmonary embolism by low doses of heparin. Lancet 1975; 2:45.
37. Clarke-Pearson DL, Synan I, Henshaw M, et al.: Prevention of postoperative venous thromboembolism by external pneumatic calf compression in patients with gynecologic malignancy. Obstet Gynecol 1984; 63:92.
38. Miyazawa K, Hernandez E, Dillon MB: Prophylactic topical cefamandole in radical hysterectomy. Int J Obstet Gynecol 1987; 25:133.
39. O'Quinn AG, Fletcher GH, Wharton JT: Guidelines for conservative hysterectomy after irradiation. Gynecol Oncol 1980; 9:68.
40. van Nagell JR Jr, Maruyama Y, Yoneda J, et al.: Treatment of bulky stage IB and IIB cervical cancers with outpatient neutron brachytherapy, external pelvic radiation and extrafascial hysterectomy. Nuc Sci Appl 1986; 2:483.
41. Maruyama Y, van Nagell JR Jr, Yoneda J, et al.: Dose-response and failure pattern by combined photon radiation and extrafascial hysterectomy for bulky, barrel stage IB cervical cancers. Cancer 1989; 63:70.
42. Durrance FY, Fletcher GH, Rutledge FN: Analysis of central recurrent disease in stages I and II squamous cell carcinomas of the cervix on intact uterus. Am J Roentgenol Rad Nucl Med 1968; 126:831.
43. Rutledge FN, Wharton JT, Fletcher GH: Clinical studies with adjunctive surgery and irradiation therapy in the treatment of carcinoma of the cervix. Cancer 1976; 38:596.
44. Gallion HH, van Nagell JR Jr, Donaldson ES et al.: Combined radiation therapy and extrafascial hysterectomy in the treatment of Stage IB barrel-shaped cervical cancer. Cancer 1985; 56:262.
45. Marcial VA, Bosch A: Radiation-induced tumor regression in carcinoma of the uterine cervix: Prognostic significance. Am J Roentgenol 1970; 108:113.
46. Hardt N, van Nagell JR Jr, Hanson MB, et al.: Radiation-induced tumor regression as a prognostic factor in patients with invasive cervical cancer. Cancer 1982; 49:35.
47. Averette HE, Ford JH Jr, Dudan RC, et al.: Staging of cervical cancer. Clin Obstet Gynecol 1975; 18:215.
48. Delgado G, Chun B, Caglar H, Bepko F: Para-aortic lymphadenectomy in gynecologic malignancies confined to the pelvis. Obstet Gynecol 1977; 50:418.
49. Wharton JT, Jones HW, Day TG, et al.: Preirradiation celiotomy and extended field irradiation for invasive carcinoma of the cervix. Obstet Gynecol 1977; 49:333.
50. Buchsbaum HJ: Extrapelvic lymph node metastases in cervical carcinoma. Am J Obstet Gynecol 1979; 133:814.
51. Chung C, Nahhas W, Stryker J, Curry S: Analysis of factors contributing to treatment failures in stage IB and IIA carcinoma of the cervix. Am J Obstet Gynecol 1980; 138:550.
52. Hughes RR, Brewington KC, Hanjani P, et al.: Extended field irradiation for cervical cancer based on surgical staging. Gynecol Oncol 1980; 9:153.
53. Lagasse LD, Creasman WT, Shingleton HM, et al.: Results and complications of operative staging in cervical cancer experience of the Gynecologic Oncology Group. Gynecol Oncol 1980;9:90.

54. Ballon SC, Berman ML, Lagasse LD, et al.: Survival after extraperitoneal pelvic and para-aortic lymphadenectomy and radiation therapy in cervical carcinoma. Obstet Gynecol 1981; 57:90.
55. Welander CE, Pierce VK, Nori D, et al.: Pretreatment laparotomy in carcinoma of the cervix. Gynecol Oncol 1981; 12:336.
56. Martinbeau PW, Kjorstad KE, Iversen T: Stage IB carcinoma of the cervix, the Norwegian Hospital. II. Results when pelvic nodes are involved. Obstet Gynecol 1982; 60:215.
57. Berman ML, Keys H, Creasman W, et al.: Survival and patterns of recurrence in cervical cancer metastatic to para-aortic lymph nodes. Gynecol Oncol 1984; 19:8.
58. Inoue T, Okumura M: Prognostic significance of parametrial extension in patients with cervical carcinoma stages IB, IIA, and IIB. A study of 628 cases treated by radical hysterectomy and lymphadenectomy with or without postoperative irradiation. Cancer 1984; 54:1714.
59. Rubin SC, Brookland R, Mikuta J, et al.: Para-aortic nodal metastases in early cervical carcinoma: Long-term survival following extended field radiotherapy. Gynecol Oncol 1984; 18:213.
60. Twiggs LB, Potish RA, George RJ, Adcock LL: Pretreatment extraperitoneal surgical staging in primary carcinoma of the cervix uteri. Surg Gynecol Obstet 1984; 158:243.
61. LaPolla JP, Schlaerth JB, Gaddis O Jr, Morrow CP: The influence of surgical staging on the evaluation and treatment of patients with cervical cancer. Gynecol Oncol 1986; 24:194.
62. Podczaski ES, Palombo C, Manetta A, et al.: Assessment of pretreatment laparotomy in patients with cervical carcinoma prior to radiotherapy. Gynecol Oncol 1989; 33:71.
63. Downey GO, Potish RA, Adcock LL, et al.: Pretreatment surgical staging in cervical carcinoma: Therapeutic efficacy of pelvic lymph node resection. Am J Obstet Gynecol 1989; 160:1055.
64. Lovecchio JL, Averette HE, Donato D, Bell J: Five-year survival of patients with periaortic nodal metastases in clinical stage IB and IIA cervical carcinoma. Gynecol Oncol 1989; 34:43.
65. van Nagell JR Jr, Higgins RV: Invasive cancer of the cervix: Clinical features, diagnosis, staging, and pretreatment evaluation. In Coppleson M (ed.): Gynecologic Oncology. London, Churchill Livingstone, 1992, pp. 663–671.
66. Weiser EB, Bundy BN, Hoskins WJ, et al.: Extraperitoneal versus transperitoneal selective para-aortic lymphadenectomy in the pretreatment surgical staging of advanced cervical cancer (a Gynecologic Oncology Group Study). Gynecol Oncol 1989; 33:283.
67. Piver MS, Barlow JJ, Krisnamsetty R: Five-year survival in patients with biopsy confirmed aortic node metastasis from cervical carcinoma. Am J Obstet Gynecol 1981; 139:575.
68. Tewfik HH, Buchsbaum HJ, Latourette HB, et al.: Para-aortic lymph node irradiation in carcinoma of the cervix after exploratory laparotomy and biopsy proven positive aortic nodes. Int J Radiat Oncol Biol Phys 1982; 8:13.
69. Nori D, Valentine E, Hilaris BS: The role of paraaortic node irradiation in the treatment of cancer of the cervix. Int J Radiat Oncol Biol Phys 1985; 11:1469.
70. Gaspar LE, Cheung AY, Allen HH: Cervical carcinoma: Treatment results and complications of extended-field irradiation. Radiology 1989; 172:271.
71. Brantigan JW, Brantigan CO, Brantigan OC: Biopsy of nonpalpable scalene lymph nodes in carcinoma of the lung. Am Rev Resp Dis 1973; 107:962.
72. Symmonds RE, Pratt JH, Welch JS: Extended Wertheim operation for primary, recurrent, or suspected recurrent carcinoma of the cervix. Obstet Gynecol 1964; 24:15.
73. Brunschwig A: Complete excision of the pelvic viscera for advanced carcinoma. Cancer 1948; 1:177.
74. Bricker EM: Bladder substitution after pelvic evisceration. Surg Clin North Am 1950; 30:1511.
75. Symmonds RE, Jones IV: Sigmoid conduit urinary diversion after exenteration. In Taymor ML, Green TH Jr (eds.): Progress in Gynecology, Vol. VI. New York, Grune & Stratton, 1975, p. 729.
76. Schmidt JD, Buchsbaum HJ, Jacobo EC: Transverse colon conduit for supravesical urinary tract diversion. Urology 1976; 8:542.
77. Penalver MA, Bejany DE, Averette HE, et al.: Continent urinary diversion in gynecologic oncology. Gynecol Oncol 1989; 34:274.
78. Hatch KD, Shingleton HM, Potter ME, Baker VV: Low rectal resection and anastomosis at the time of pelvic exenteration. Gynecol Oncol 1988; 32:262.
79. Hatch KD, Gelder MS, Soong SJ, et al.: Pelvic exenteration with low rectal anastomosis: Survival, complications, and prognostic factors. Gynecol Oncol 1990; 38:462.
80. Wheeless CR: Neovagina constructed from omental J-flap and a split thickness skin graft. Gynecol Oncol 1989; 35:224.
81. Morley GW, Hopkins MP, Lindenauer SM, Roberts JA: Pelvic exenteration, University of Michigan, 100 patients at 5 years. Obstet Gynecol 1989; 74:934.
82. Mullen JL, Buzby GP, Matthews DC, et al.: Reduction of operative morbidity and mortality by combined preoperative and postoperative nutritional support. Ann Surg 1980; 192:604.
83. Averette HE, Lichtinger M, Sevin BU, Girtanner RE: Pelvic exenteration: A 15-year experience in a general metropolitan hospital. Am J Obstet Gynecol 1984; 150:179.
84. Brunschwig A: Surgical treatment of carcinoma of the cervix, recurrent after irradiation or combination of irradiation and surgery. Am J Roentgenol 1967; 99:365.
85. Bricker EM: Pelvic exenteration. Adv Surg, 1970; 4:13.
86. Ketcham AS, Deckers PJ, Sugarbaker EV et al.: Pelvic exenteration for carcinoma of the uterine cervix. Cancer 1970; 26:513.
87. Symmonds RE, Pratt JH, Webb MJ: Exenterative operations: Experience with 198 patients. Am J Obstet Gynecol 1975; 121:907.
88. Rutledge FN, Smith JP, Wharton JT, O'Quinn AG: Pelvic exenteration: Analysis of 296 patients. Am J Obstet Gynecol 1977; 129:881.
89. Kraybill WG, Lopez M, Bricker EM: Total pelvic exenteration as a therapeutic option in advanced malignant disease of the pelvis. Surg Gynecol Obstet 1988; 166:259.
90. Shingleton HM, Soong SJ, Gelder MS, et al.: Clinical and histopathologic factors predicting recurrence and survival after pelvic exenteration for cancer of the cervix. Obstet Gynecol 1989; 73:1027.

Operations for Stress Incontinence and Benign Conditions of the Urethra

16

Raymond J. Reilly

Urinary incontinence occurs in approximately 20% of the female population in the United States. It is medically benign, socially malignant, and surgically problematic. One common form of incontinence is known as stress incontinence because of the uncontrollable loss of urine when pressure is exerted upon the bladder. An enormous amount of attention has been paid to diagnostic procedures, described elsewhere in this text, and surgical modifications that are often initiated with enthusiasm and modified with disappointment. This chapter reviews major established procedures for stress incontinence as well as those more recently developed.

In addition, treatment of some other benign surgical conditions of the bladder and urethra is presented.

STRESS INCONTINENCE

Regardless of complex cystometric, radiologic, ultrasonic, and other procedures, stress incontinence is most commonly and most definitively diagnosed by history when the patient complains to her physician that she is embarrassed often because she loses urine when she laughs, coughs, sneezes, climbs stairs, or otherwise stresses the bladder-urethral axis.[1] If there is no neurologic or infectious reason for the incontinence, it is usually assumed to have an anatomic basis. The therapy for anatomically based stress incontinence is surgery.

It is clear, however, that stress incontinence can occur in the absence of cystocele or urethrocele; conversely, cystocele and/or urethrocele can be seen with or without uterine descensus and without stress incontinence.

Two philosophies have formed the basis of the surgical approach. One earlier approach relied upon modifying the bladder descensus and enhancing the bladder supports; the other attempts to correct the cystourethral angle by supporting the urethra.

The history of the development of various procedures confirms the lack of unqualified success with treatments of this condition. There is a large body of papers on diagnostics, therapies, and modifications, but no method has been without failure and none without complications. The operations for true stress incontinence can be broadly categorized into three approaches: vaginal operations; abdominal operations, including slings; and a variety of extra-abdominal, extravaginal procedures often termed "needle suspensions." The enormous body of literature attests to the fact that the technical problems are not yet resolved. What follow are simplified descriptions by operative approach. Limited descriptions of the well-established procedures for repairing cystoceles and the Marshall-Marchetti-Krantz procedure are presented because they are well described in many other sources. The reader who wishes to review the techniques for established procedures as well as for the newer procedures would be well advised to purchase the video tapes available at the American College of Obstetricians and Gynecologists[18] and elsewhere. More recent procedures are described in detail.

Vaginal Procedures

When stress incontinence is associated with vaginal wall prolapse, the vaginal approach is logical. The normal anatomy of the bladder should be restored and the urethrovesical angle returned to its normal position within the pelvis. The correction of the urethrovesical angle by lateral sutures and the correction of urethral funneling in the bladder by plication of the cystocele can be readily achieved by the established Kennedy-Kelly procedure first described by Kelly in 1913 and modified by Kennedy in 1937.[2, 3] If it appears that the angle cannot be advanced high enough, the Marshall-Marchetti-Krantz procedure, Burch procedure, or one of the newer endoscopic needle procedures should be performed.

Kelly-Kennedy Procedure (Fig. 16–1)

Many minor modifications of the original procedures have been described, but the following is a fairly conventional procedure used by the author.

Preoperative Preparation. No unusual preoperative preparation is necessary in healthy women. Because it is almost always an elective procedure, surgery can usually be postponed until the patient is in good health. Nevertheless, many patients with stress incontinence are elderly or obese or have medical complications such as diabetes. These women are at risk for any surgery. The procedures should be as short and as noninvasive as possible.

Procedure. The vaginal approach necessitates opening the anterior vaginal wall longitudinally (Fig. 16–1). A Metzenbaum scissors is used to undermine the anterior vaginal wall from the cervix to 1 cm from the urethral meatus and divides it in the midline. The overlying vaginal mucosa is separated from the bladder and urethra laterally to the pubic rami by blunt finger dissection using a sponge. Then, the urethrovesical junction is easily visualized. The paraurethral tissue from both sides—referred to by some gynecologists as paraurethral ligaments—is brought across the midline by interrupted sutures. Some gynecologists use 0 chromic catgut with the intention of enhancing the scarring effect; others advocate the use of longer-lasting suture material such as polypropylene or even nonabsorbable materials. In the author's experience, the results are similar.

The objective of this dissection and repair is to advance the urethrovesical angle to the correct position intra-abdominally. A common cause of failure is insufficient dissection and placement of the "Kelly sutures" too far below the angle. The junction of the urethra and bladder can be defined by insertion of a Foley cather and palpation of the inflated bulb, if necessary. This is rarely required, because it is easily visualized if the dissection is adequate. Care must be taken not to overcorrect the bladder advancement, which results in diminishing the urethrovesical angle. The cystocele is then repaired by interrupted sutures, the excess skin is excised, and the vaginal wall is reapproximated with interrupted sutures. Common errors are the excessive plication of the bladder and the excesssive excision of skin. A vaginal pack is left in place for hemostasis as well as a Foley catheter.

Postoperative Care. In procedures involving hysterectomy or invasion into the peritoneal space, the author and his colleagues customarily use perioperative antibiotics. Treatment is continued as long as the catheter is used. The vaginal pack is removed on the next day, and the Foley catheter is removed on the fifth day. The patient can usually be discharged as soon as she can void spontaneously after the catheter is removed. A post-void residual urine after the third void ought to be obtained. If the residual volume is greater than 150 ml, the catheter is replaced. If the suburethral repair is tight, some patients may have difficulty voiding initially. The author considers this a good sign that the repair is successful. Conversely, women who have no trouble voiding immediately after the catheter is removed cause the author to consider if the repair was adequate.

Early success is gratifying—as high as 90%. However, after several years, the failure rate increases, so that success rates as low as 60% have been reported. The rates, however, are affected by time, interpretation of subjective improvement, and even the context of publication. For example, gynecologists or urologists reporting on a second procedure may accumulate a larger number of unsuccessful cases by the nature of their referral practices. In contrast, primary surgeons may have a better follow-up success rate because unsuccessful cases have gone elsewhere.

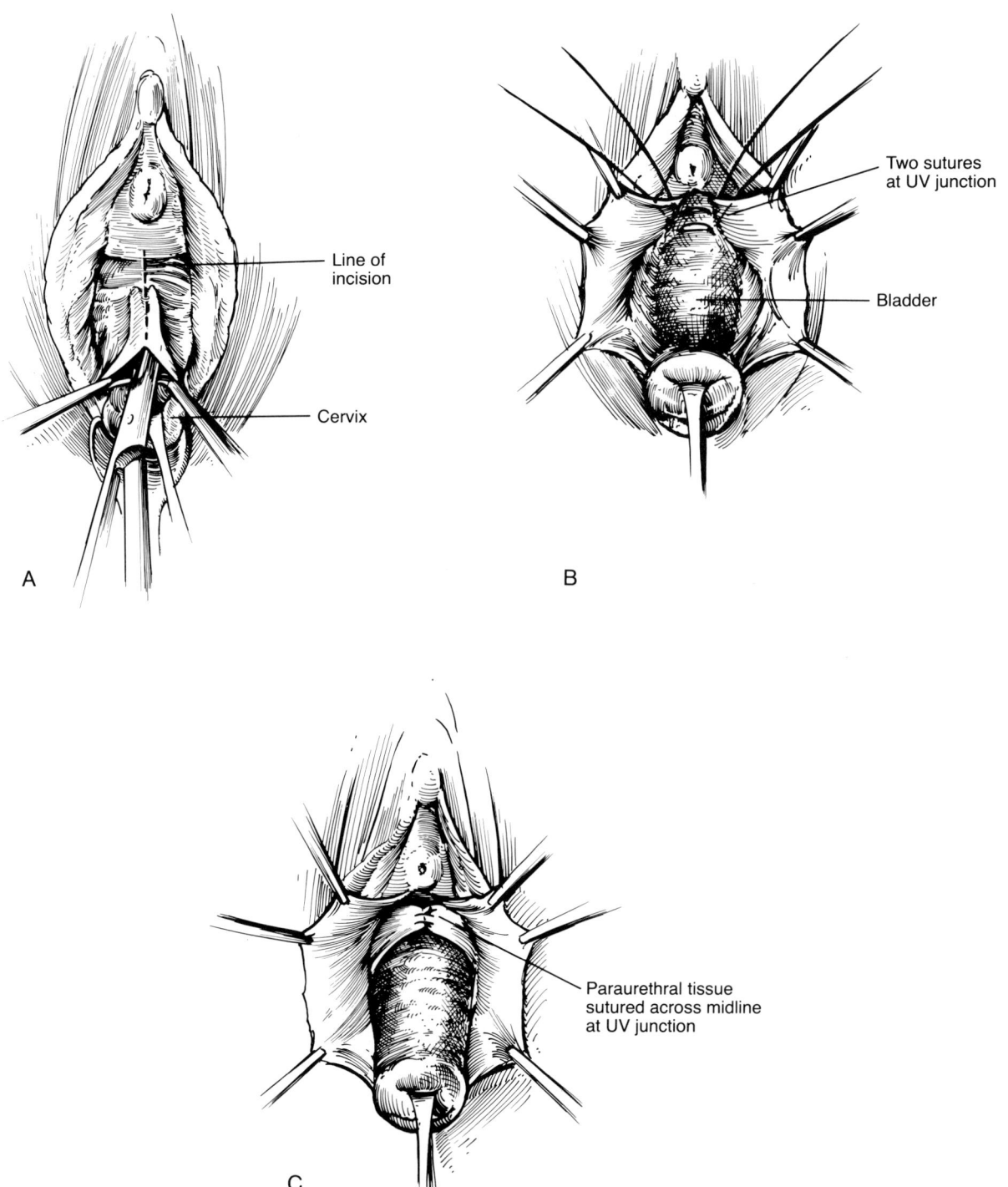

Figure 16–1
The Kelly-Kennedy procedure. A, A small transverse incision is made just above the cervix. Using downward traction with Kelly clamps on the vaginal angle, the anterior vaginal wall is undermined with a Metzenbaum scissors. The wall is then opened longitudinally to about 1 cm below the urethral orifice. B, The paraurethral tissue lateral to the urethrovesical junction is sutured with a generous bite on each side of the urethra. A second, reinforcing stitch is necessary. C, If the procedure is done properly, a firm bar of tissue supports the urethrovesical junction.

Operations by the Abdominal Approach

The Marshall-Marchetti-Krantz and Burch procedures are the common operations of choice if an intra-abdominal operation is indicated for other reasons such as a pelvic mass or abdominal hysterectomy. Until recent years, these two procedures have been the methods of choice to correct stress incontinence after failure with a vaginal procedure. Indeed, the patients noted in the original paper by Marshall, Marchetti, and Krantz were mostly women with histories of failed primary procedures. Many gynecologists (and more urologists who do not perform vaginal surgery) believe that these are the preferred primary procedures, especially in the absence of vaginal relaxations. At one time, it was thought that hysterectomy would enhance the cure rate; that view is no longer credible. On the other hand, there is no reason to retain the uterus if it should be removed for other reasons such as myomas or prolapse.

Marshall-Marchetti-Krantz Procedure
(Fig. 16–2)

This procedure, originally described in 1949, was the first completely different approach to stress incontinence.[4] Because of the technical difficulty in anchoring the sutures adequately to the symphysis pubis, it has been modified, most notably by the Burch procedure. It should be recognized that not only was this procedure a surgical innovation, but also it lent support to the theory that the etiology of stress incontinence is the displacement of the urethrovesical angle and not the relaxation of the vaginal tissues as evidenced by the cystocele.

Preoperative Preparation. No unusual preparations are necessary.

Procedure. The patient is placed on the operating table in the modified lithotomy position so that the surgeon can place his or her fingers in the vagina during the procedure. A 30-ml Foley catheter is inserted into the bladder to delineate the urethrovesical junction. A transverse or midline incision is made in the lower abdomen in accord with any other procedure that is required. It is extended to the symphysis to enable the operator to enter the space of Retzius retropubically by blunt dissection. Hemostasis is secured.

The operator then inserts his or her fingers into the vagina to identify the urethrovesical angle and elevates the angle towards the abdomen. This facilitates the placing of about two or three sutures on each side of the urethra from about mid-urethra to the angle. Occasionally, the needle will penetrate the vaginal wall; the error is not important. These sutures are then secured one by one to the periosteum on the back of the symphysis pubis. This is the most difficult step in the procedure because the periosteum tends to tear. A 5/8-inch urologic needle makes this step easier, because it seems to get a better purchase on the periosteum. Needless to say, good exposure and good retraction facilitate this procedure because the surgeon has one hand in the vagina. All types of suture, including chromic catgut and nonabsorbable types, have been used; there are no data to make a case for any particular type.

It is important to administer antibiotics perioperatively in order to avoid the complication of osteitis pubis. Careful hemostasis is desired. The abdomen is closed by conventional procedure in accordance with the type of incision made. A catheter is left in place.

Postoperative Care. Postoperative care is simply directed towards maintaining good catheteral flow and symptomatic comfort. If the procedure is accompanied by an intraperitoneal operation, most care will be directed towards the needs resulting from the other procedure. If the peritoneum has not been entered, the patient may complain of a little suprapubic pain, but ordinarily she is quite comfortable and mobile.

Follow-up. Within the first few months, results are excellent. Longer follow-up may be complicated by release of the sutures and the rare serious complication of osteitis pubis. Another complication that may arise from this and similar procedures that pull the anterior wall forward is the potential for subsequent enterocele formation.[5, 6] If the peritoneal cavity has been opened, the cul-de-sac should be obliterated to help prevent this problem.

Burch Procedure (Fig. 16–3)

Because of the difficulty in placing the periosteal sutures, Burch modified the Marshall-Marchetti-Krantz procedure by using Cooper's ligament (iliopectineal ligament) to anchor the urethrovesical angle.[5] When the urethrovesical angle is mobile, it will easily reach Cooper's ligament and can be fixed to it. It is easier and safer to drive the needle into the ligament than through the periosteum.

Preoperative Preparation. The preparations are the same as for the previously described procedures.

Procedure. The patient is positioned and the space of Retzius entered as described previously. The point of decision is when the bladder neck is elevated by

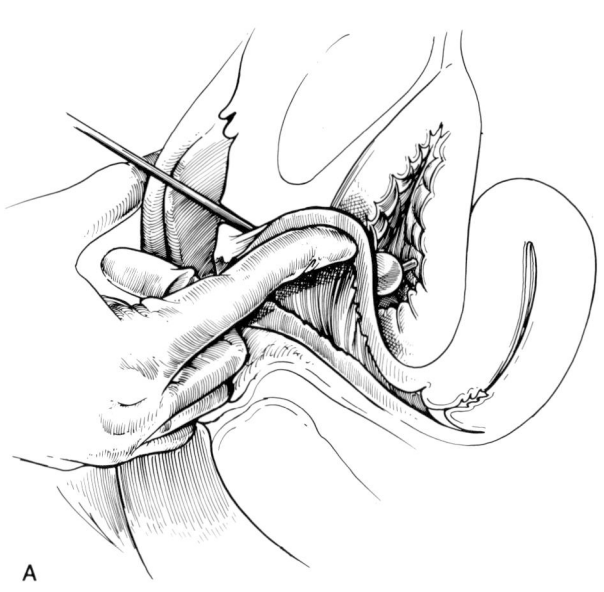
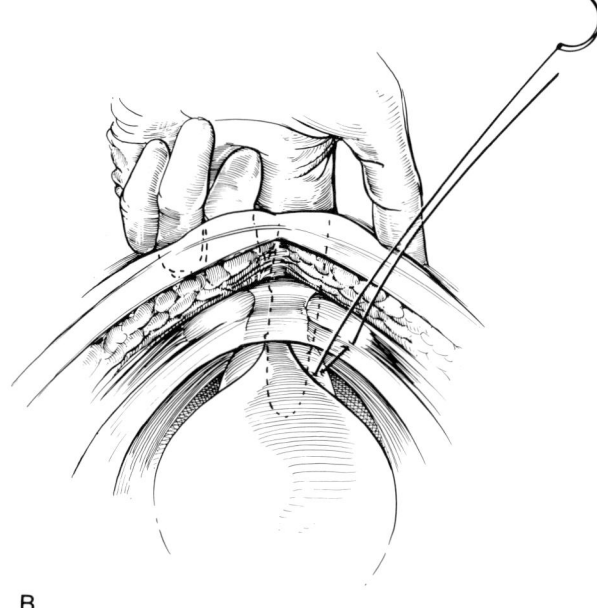
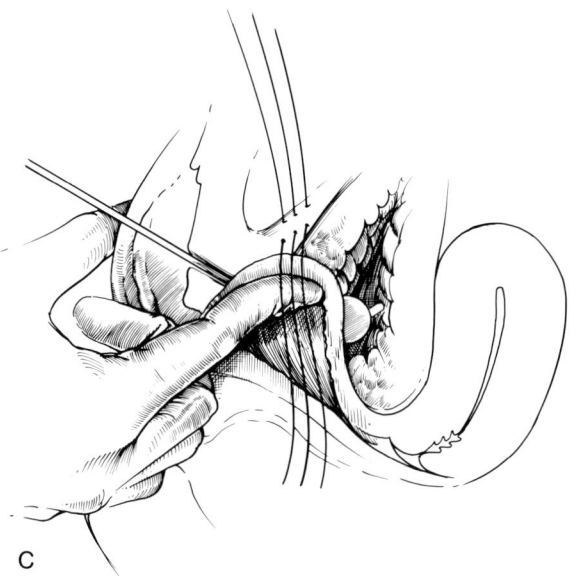

Figure 16–2
The Marshall-Marchetti-Krantz procedure. *A,* The surgeon's index finger is placed in the vagina near the urethrovesical junction, and the tissue is elevated. This enables the surgeon to place the sutures correctly in either the Marshall-Marchetti-Krantz or the Burch procedure. *B,* A suture placed in the periurethral area on the patient's right side is driven into the periosteum with a urologic 5/8-inch needle. Two or three sutures are placed on either side. *C,* The urethra is advanced upwards to an intra-abdominal position, thereby creating a urethrovesical angle posteriorly.

Figure 16–3
The Burch procedure. The tissue near the urethrovesical angle is sutured to the iliopectineal ligament (Cooper's ligament) on the right side. Usually, two sutures are used on each side.

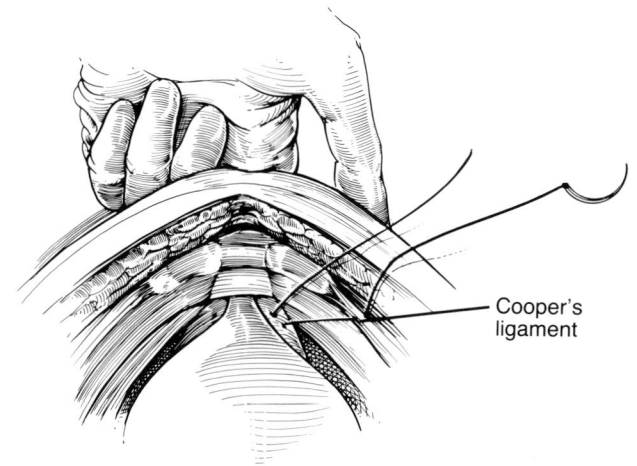

the vaginal finger to ascertain if it can be attached to Cooper's ligament. If it will not reach, a Marshall-Marchetti-Krantz procedure must be performed. If it does reach, two nonabsorbable 0 sutures are placed on each side of the bladder neck and stitched to Cooper's ligament. When the supporting hand is removed from the vagina, it can be seen that the bladder neck remains securely elevated. Closure and postoperative care are as described earlier, as are complications and follow-up, except that the hazard of osteitis is removed. The potential for enterocele formation, first mentioned by Burch himself, is described previously.

Sling Procedures

Sling procedures have tended to be reserved for patients who have had a failure of one or more of the conventional operations because they are associated with a higher complication rate than the standard procedures (see Fig. 16–4). However, as occurred historically with abdominal procedures for stress incontinence, sling procedures are being used more frequently to correct primary stress incontinence.

All of these procedures utilize some form of strap-like support to elevate the urethrovesical junction. The materials most commonly used are fascia lata, abdominal wall aponeurosis, and artifical substances such as Mersilene mesh or Gore-Tex mesh.[7] These procedures are technically more difficult than the conventional procedures described earlier because of the importance of applying the correct amount of tension to secure the sling. If the sling is too loose, it will be useless. If it is too tight, it may result in complete retention of urine or worse—transection of the urethra or bladder neck. Postoperatively, intermittent catheterization will be required for a variable interval of time. The apparent simplicity of these procedures is deceptive; results are consistent with the experience of the operator. The two traditional procedures are the Goebell-Frangenheim-Stoeckel, described by those authors independently in the second decade of the twentieth century,[8] and the Aldridge modification of it, described in 1942.[9]

Goebell-Frangenheim-Stoeckel Procedure
(Fig. 16–4)

The ideal placement of the patient for these procedures is the modified dorsal lithotomy position as for laparoscopy. Supporting the legs with skis is even better. A Foley catheter must be placed in the bladder. A midline incision is made from the umbilicus to the symphysis. The incision is extended to the fascia lata, which is cleared of fat. A 1–2 cm strip of fascia lata is mobilized but left attached at the lower end of the incision (Fig. 16–4A). If the length of fascia that would be obtained from the umbilicus-symphysis segment is judged to be too short to be placed around the urethra and carried back, the length of fascia must be extended above the umbilicus or an alternative operation used. Clearly, using a strip of fascia lata or the Aldridge sling approach would be better. Using a scissors to separate the rectus muscle fibers 2 cm lateral to the attached end of the fascial strip on both sides, the operator's finger is pushed through the muscle into the retropubic space and by gentle dissection reaches the urogenital diaphragm on both sides of the urethra. The rectus fascia can now be closed with interrupted sutures of nonabsorbable material to decrease the possibility of an incisional hernia.

The anterior vaginal wall is then opened as described for the anterior colporrhaphy. If the patient has a cystocele, the entire anterior vaginal mucosa is opened. If stress incontinence is the problem, only the mucosa over the urethrovesical junction need be opened. With the urethrovesical junction exposed and with the operator's fingers in the space of Retzius suprapubically, a uterine dressing forceps with the curvature oriented towards the posterior aspect of the symphysis is "popped" through the urogenital diaphragm from the vaginal side and guided on the fingertip of the left hand through the space of Retzius to the abdominal incision. The fascial strip is fed into the open forceps and pulled down into the vagina. The reverse process is then done. The uterine forceps is then directed from the abdominal approach behind the symphysis on the right side of the urethra to meet the operator's finger in the right urethrovesical angle and then "popped" into the vagina. The end of the fascia is then drawn up to the abdomen, making sure that it is not twisted. Correct placement under the urethrovesical angle is also ensured.

The most important part of the procedure is to obtain proper tension at this time. It should be neither too tight nor too loose, but if one is to err, it ought to be on the side of being too loose. By observing the urethrovesical angle from the vagina, one can generally judge the correct amount of tension that gives a good angle. The fascia is then sewn to the rectus fascia to stabilize the angle. The vaginal and abdominal incisions are then closed.

Aldridge Sling Modification (Fig. 16–5)

Aldridge modified the procedure by excising the fascial strip from the rectus fascia transversely instead of longitudinally.[9] This modification overcame the disadvantage of finding that the strip was too short to pass around the urethra and back to the abdominal wall and also permitted the use of the more cosmetically desirable transverse skin incision.

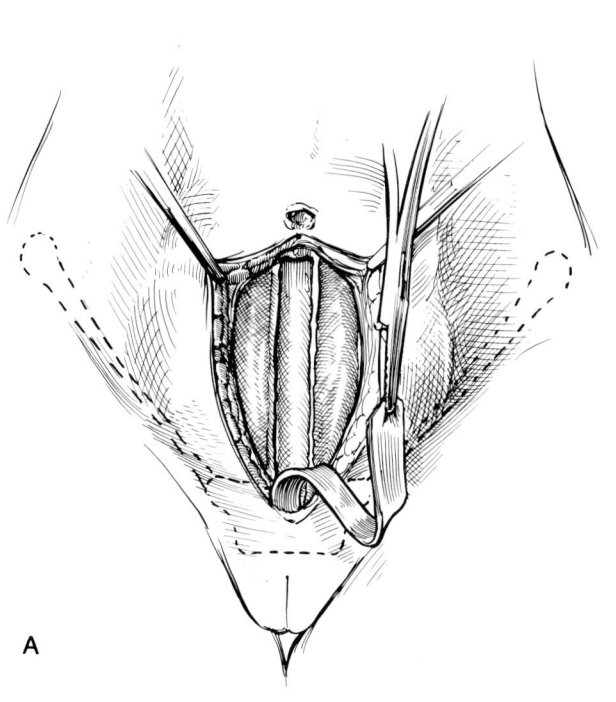
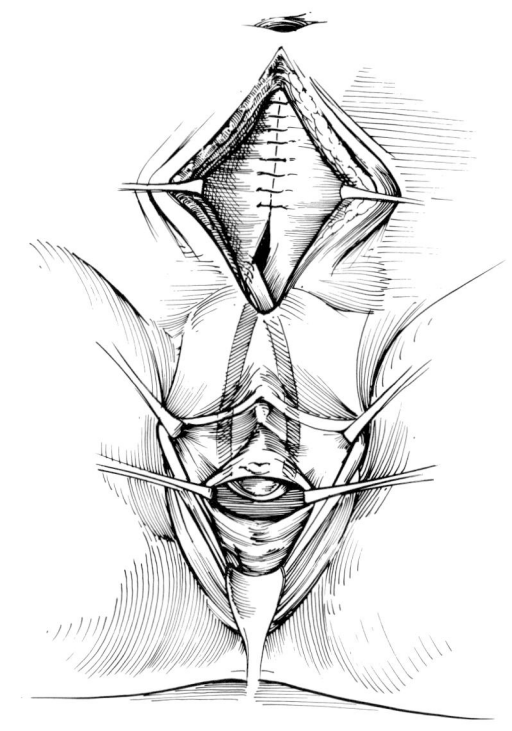
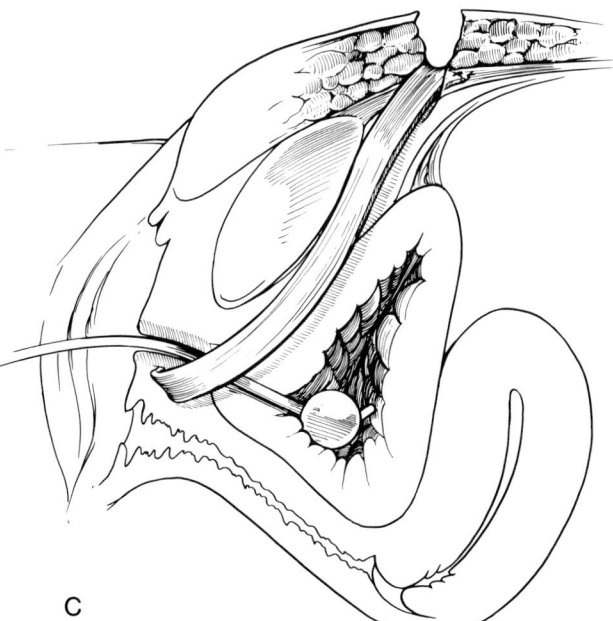

Figure 16–4
The Goebell-Frangenheim-Stoeckel procedure. *A*, A 1–2 cm strip of fascia is cut and left attached at its lower end. *B*, After proper placement and adjustment of the tension under the urethra, the fascia is sewn back to the abdominal wall aponeurosis. *C*, The fascia, without being twisted, is correctly placed at the urethrovesical angle.

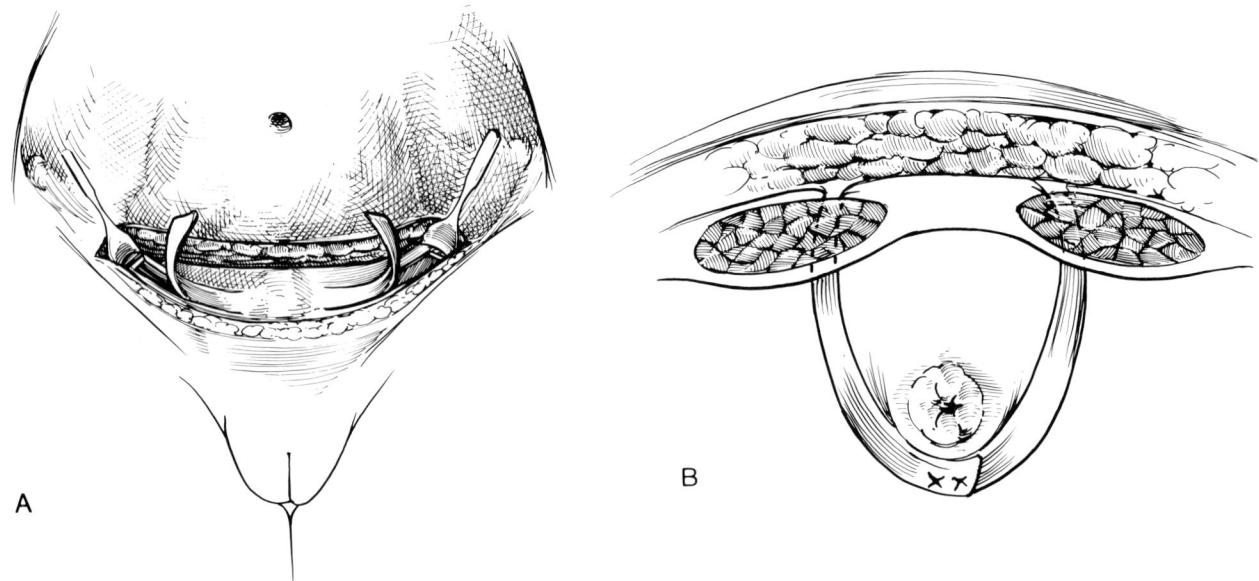

Figure 16–5
The Aldridge sling procedure. *A*, Transverse strips of abdominal aponeurosis, 1–2 cm wide, are cut and left attached at their medial ends about 2 cm from the midline. *B*, The fascial strips are sewn together under the urethrovesical junction with enough tension to obtain a proper angle. Excess fascia has been trimmed.

Through a Pfannenstiel incision, the fascia is exposed and cleared of fat as far laterally as necessary to obtain two fascial strips of sufficient length to encircle the urethra. These are dissected from the lateral ends and left attached medially 2 cm from the midline. They should be about 1.5 cm in width. The lateral ends of the abdominal incision can now be closed except for the midline area, or left open until the procedure is terminated. If open, the incision should be covered with a sterile, moist towel.

The vaginal wall is opened and the urethrovesical angle exposed as described previously. In this procedure, the curved uterine dressing forceps is passed from the vagina to the abdominal incision with the guidance of the operator's fingers to capture the fascial strips. This is done on both sides of the urethra, and the two fascial strips are brought into the vaginal incision. The strips are sewn together and the excess fascia cut off. Again, it is important to have the correct amount of tension to obtain optimal urethral angulation. The vaginal and abdominal incisions are then closed.

Of the modifications that have been proposed, the use of Stamey or Raz-Pereyra needles to facilitate the passage retropubically of the fascial strips makes the procedures technically easier. A suture is attached to the ends of the fascial strips and threaded onto the needles for the pass-through to the vagina. One advantage of these needles is that if the bladder should be perforated, the damage from the needle instrument is much less than from uterine forceps. Bladder perforations are more likely to occur from use of the retropubic space as in the Marshall-Marchetti-Krantz operation, which can cause retroperitoneal scarring. However, in the event of recognized perforation of the bladder, drainage with a Foley or suprapubic catheter until healing has occurred is all that is necessary.

Sling Procedures Using Fascia Lata or Artificial Materials (Fig. 16–6)

The established operations have been modified to use either fascia lata or Gore-Tex mesh for the sling. The fascia lata is obtained from the thigh with a Masson fascial stripper before the patient is placed in the semi-lithotomy position. Obtaining the fascia is uncomplicated. Both Gore-Tex and fascia lata have advantages of convenience and decreased potential for incisional hernias, but the fascia lata may be favored in not being a foreign body perhaps subject to rejection or other immune responses. More long-term studies are needed to evaluate the synthetics properly.

Needle Suspension Procedures
(Figs. 16–7 and 16–8)

The next innovation in the search for better and simpler procedures to cure stress incontinence was introduced by Pereyra in 1959 and modified by Raz in 1981 (Fig. 16–7).[10, 11] In this procedure, the urethrovesical angles are exposed and anchored to the abdominal wall with supporting sutures. In 1980, Stamey modified the procedure further by using a

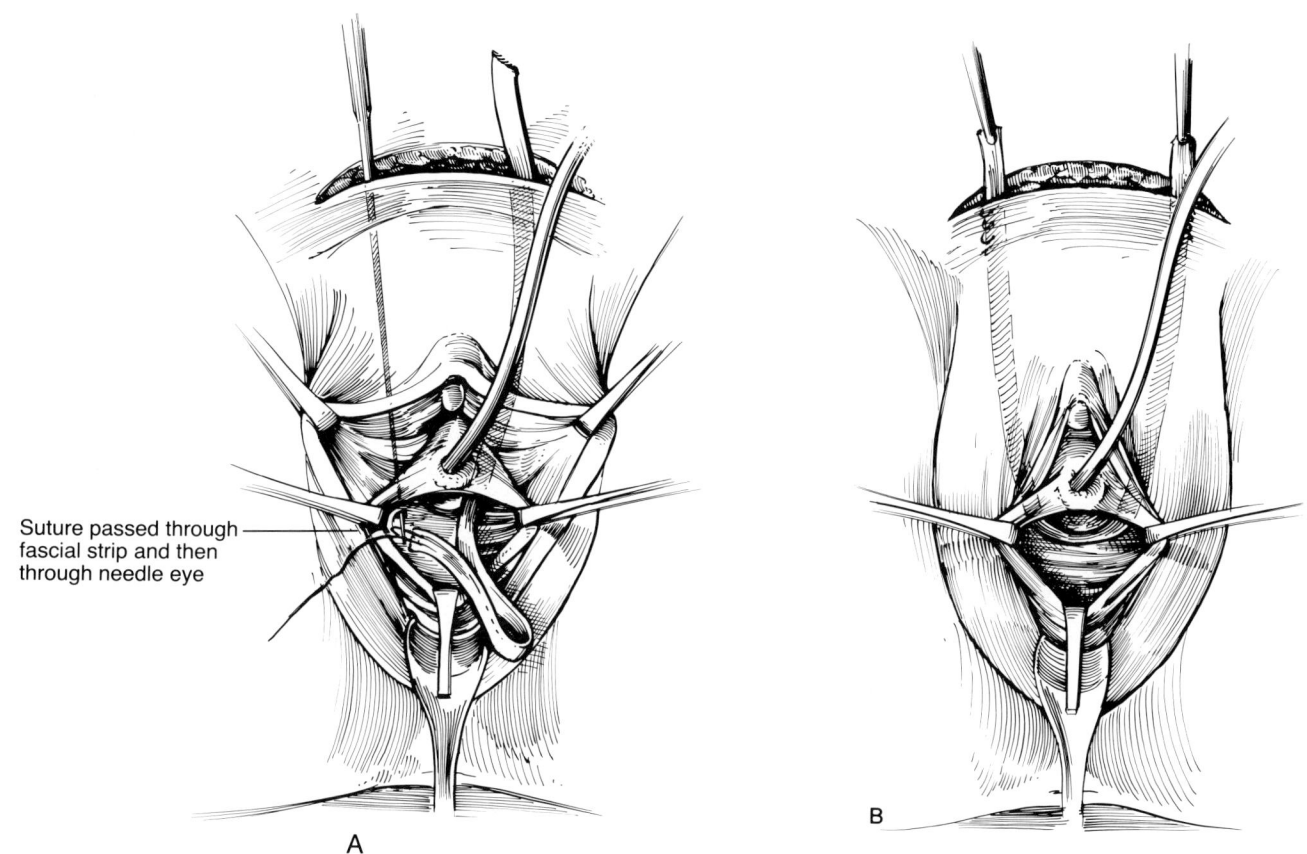

Figure 16–6
Sling procedures using needles. *A*, The strip of material (fascia, fascia lata, Gore-Tex mesh, or Mersilene mesh), after being brought into the vaginal incision on the left side, is now being threaded onto the Stamey needle eye for transfer back to the abdominal incision. *B*, The ends of the strip will be attached to the abdominal aponeurosis to effect the correct amount of angulation and tension at the urethrovesical junction.

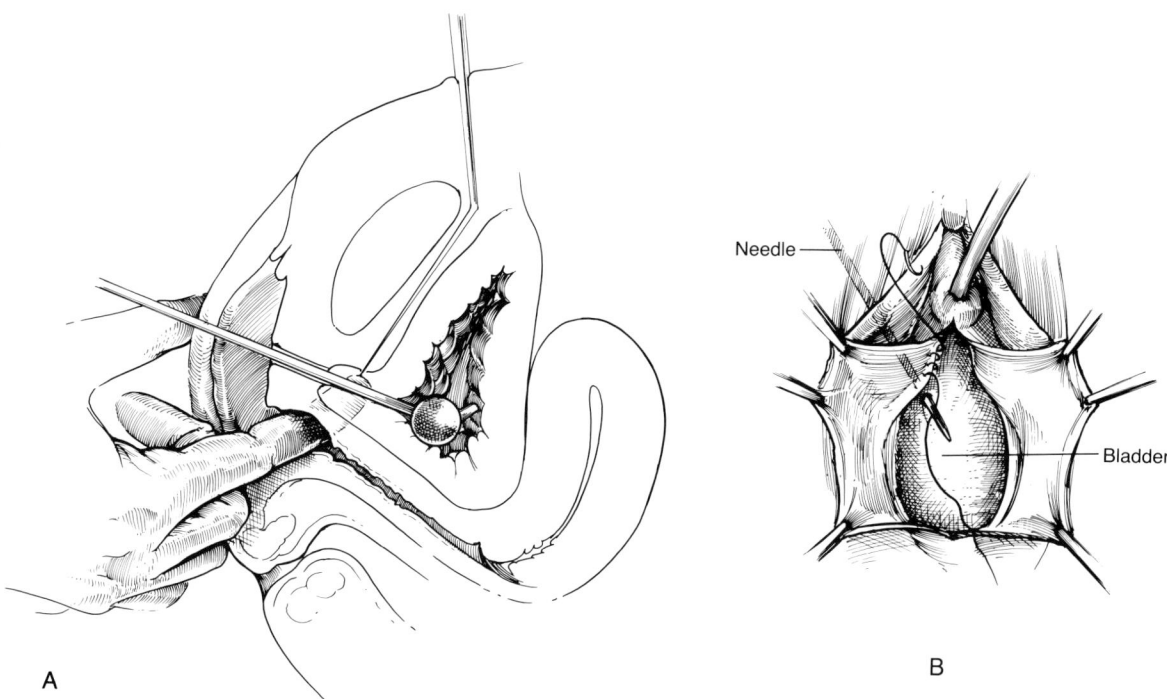

Figure 16–7
Pereyra-Raz procedure. *A*, The Pereyra needle is guided from its abdominal site of entry along the posterior surface by keeping the tip of the needle at the operator's fingers. *B*, The needle tip is pushed into the vagina. It is threaded with the free end of the helical stitch. This is repeated on the other side. By withdrawing the Pereyra needle, the suture is brought out through the suprapubic incision, where the two ends can be tied.

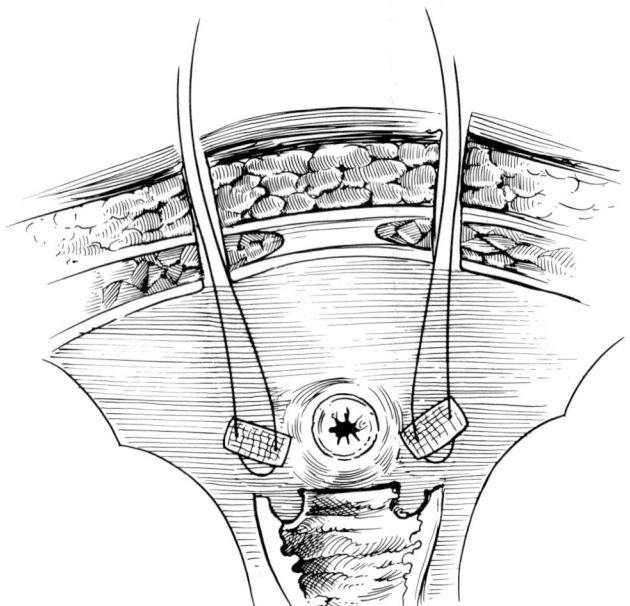

Figure 16–8
Stamey procedure. The Dacron support material prevents the sutures from tearing out by buttressing the paraurethral tissue.

buttress of Dacron to suspend the urethrovesical angle (Fig. 16–8).[12] Further simplification was achieved by Gittes and Loughlin in 1987 when they reported on their procedure, which uses the vaginal mucosa for support instead of the Dacron buttress.[13] It is also simpler to perform. All of the needle suspension operations are very effective in elevating the urethrovesical angle, equal to the more invasive abdominal procedures, with equivalent success rates of over 85%. Most important, their simplicity decreases the operative time as well as the invasiveness for elderly and other compromised patients.

Pereyra-Raz Procedure

The Pereyra-Raz procedure requires both abdominal and vaginal access (Fig. 16–7). The preoperative preparations are similar to those of the prior procedures.

Procedure. The patient is positioned in the modified lithotomy position as for a laparoscopy. A Foley catheter is introduced to empty the bladder and delineate the urethrovesical junction. If an anterior colporrhaphy is to be performed, the exposure to the urethrovesical junction is through the classic midline incision. If the only objective is to treat the stress incontinence, an inverted U-shaped incision described by Raz is preferable. This incision provides good visualization of the urethrovesical junction and the retropubic space. The vaginal mucosa is dissected laterally off the urethrovesical junction by blunt dissection with the index finger of the operator kept close to the rami of the symphysis pubis. The urogenital diaphragm is transgressed into the retropubic space until the dissection ends at the posterior aspect of the anterior abdominal wall. A helical stitch of three or four loops of 0 polypropylene suture is placed in the floor of the pubourethral ligament and the floor of the urogenital diaphragm near the urethrovesical junction. The opposite side is treated in exactly the same manner.

A 3–4 cm suprapubic incision is made transversely just above the superior aspect of the symphysis pubis. The Pereyra needle is pushed through the abdominal wall just behind the symphysis. The operator's finger in the space of Retzius guides the needle at its point into the vaginal incision. The sutures are threaded through to the needle carrier and brought out through the abdominal wall. The procedure is repeated on the contralateral side. At this point, cystoscopy will ensure that the bladder has not been transfixed. If so, the suture is removed and replaced without consequence. The operator must remember to close the vaginal epithelium before the sutures are tied abdominally because the elevation of the anterior vaginal wall after the ligatures are tied makes it extremely difficult to get adequate exposure to complete the closure. The suture ends are finally tied across the midline with care being taken that the correct amount of tension has been applied to adequately but not excessively elevate the ureterovesical angle. Either a suprapubic or a Foley catheter is inserted.

Postoperative. Postoperative care is not different from that of the previously described procedures.

Follow-up. Long-term successes for all suspension methods are about equivalent. In terms of symptomatology, it has been reported to be about 90% in premenopausal women but only about 70% in postmenopausal women.[14] There have been reports of voiding dysfunction after cystourethropexy leading to take-down of the repair and substitution with an obturator shelf or other repair.[15]

Stamey Procedure

The Stamey procedure is similar to the Pereyra-Raz procedure except for the use of Dacron support material (Fig. 16–8).

Procedure. A small (2 cm) incision is made just above the symphysis on each side of the midline and extended down to the fascia. With a Foley catheter in place, the urethrovesical junction area is opened either longitudinally or transversely as in the Pereyra procedure. A Stamey needle is passed down one side of the symphysis along its posterior aspect until the needle is brought out at the urethrovesical angle just in front of the Foley catheter bulb. A 70-degree cystoscope is introduced into the urethra and bladder to confirm that the needle has not entered the bladder and is properly located. A No. 2 nylon monofilament suture is threaded into the eye of the Stamey needle and brought out through the abdominal incision. Then the needle is passed again 2 cm lateral to the first site on the same side and brought out lateral to the free suture end near the urethrovesical junction. A pledget of Dacron about 1.5 cm × 1.5 cm is threaded onto the suture; the Stamey needle is loaded with the suture and withdrawn out through the abdominal wall. The Dacron buttresses the paraurethral tissues and prevents the suture from tearing through the soft tissues. The procedure is then repeated on the contralateral side. The panendoscope is inserted to verify placement of the suture and to monitor the angle as the sutures are approximated (but not tied). A suprapubic Stamey catheter can be placed while the bladder is visualized. The vaginal mucosa is closed while the vault is relaxed; the Stamey sutures are tied. Care must be taken not to overtighten the urethrovesical junction, as may occur if it is elevated too much.

Postoperative care and follow-up are described previously.

Simplified Cystourethropexy (Gittes)
(Fig. 16–9)

In 1985, Gittes suggested that the urethrovesical angle could be adequately suspended by passing the needle directly through the vaginal mucosa at the

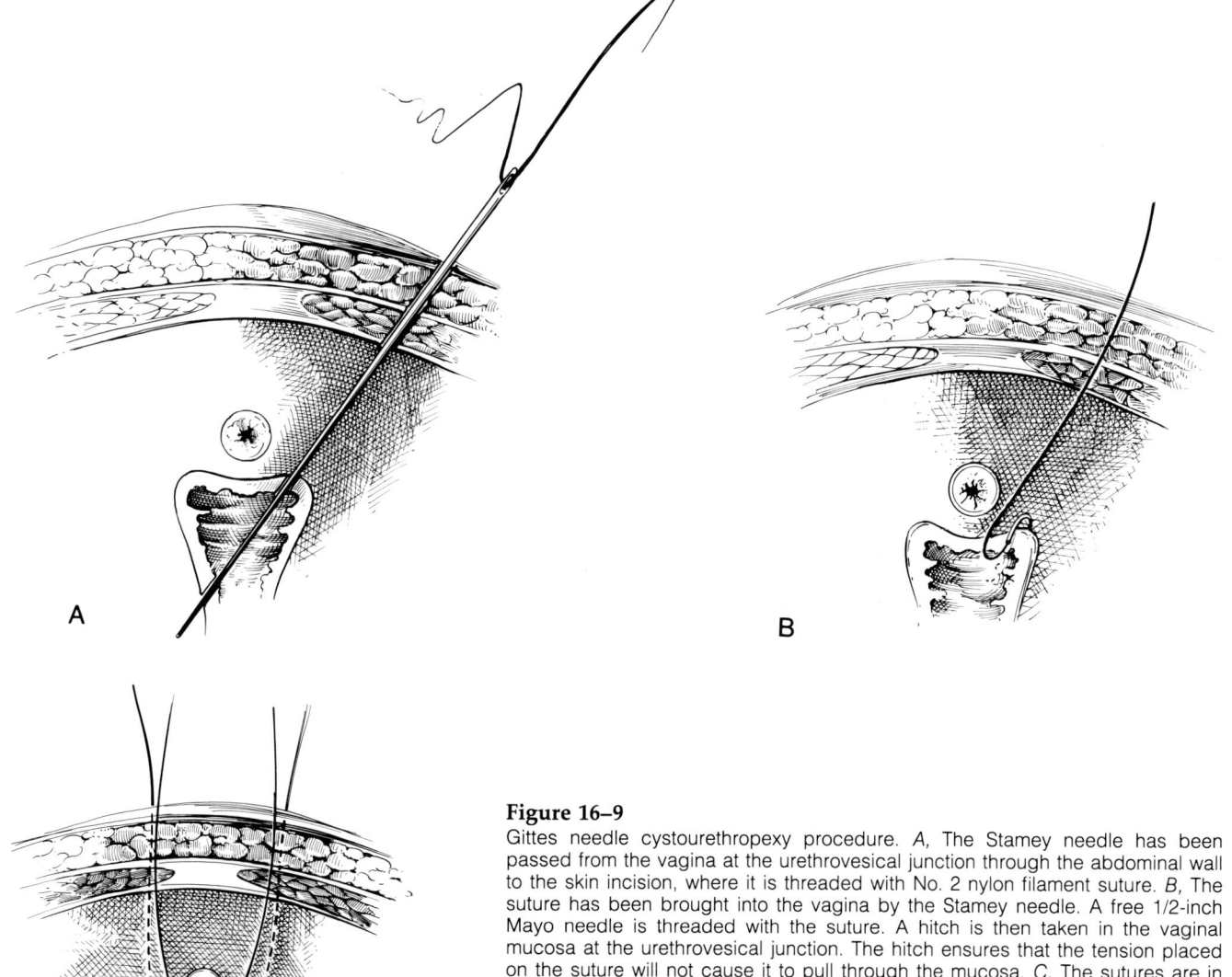

Figure 16–9
Gittes needle cystourethropexy procedure. A, The Stamey needle has been passed from the vagina at the urethrovesical junction through the abdominal wall to the skin incision, where it is threaded with No. 2 nylon filament suture. B, The suture has been brought into the vagina by the Stamey needle. A free 1/2-inch Mayo needle is threaded with the suture. A hitch is then taken in the vaginal mucosa at the urethrovesical junction. The hitch ensures that the tension placed on the suture will not cause it to pull through the mucosa. C, The sutures are in place for tying. When that is done, the urethrovesical junction will be pulled up behind the symphysis.

bladder neck. This procedure avoids opening the anterior vaginal wall, as described by Pereyra, Raz, and Stamey; eliminates the need for a Dacron patch, as described by Stamey; and greatly simplifies and accelerates the operation. Because the vagina is left intact, this operation incorporates the approach of the Marshall-Marchetti-Krantz and Burch procedures but uses the abdominal wall for support. Several years later, it was modified by looping the vaginal suture to gain tissue support. The author has favored this procedure for the last 7 years and presents his version of it (Fig. 16–9).

Procedure. The patient is placed in the dorsal lithotomy position with both abdominal and vaginal access. Two incisions about 2 cm long are made suprapubically and carried down to the fascia. The bladder is emptied, but the Foley catheter is not left in place because by removing it, there is less chance of transgressing the bladder. The author has found it better to pass the Stamey needle from the vagina up behind the symphysis to the abdominal incision because this facilitates that the suture be properly sited at the urethrovesical junction. Because gynecologists are familiar with the urethrovesical area from the vaginal aspect, the proper placement is ensured. The needle is guided to the abdominal incision. In Gittes' original procedure, the needle was passed from the abdominal incision to the urethrovesical junction and then through the vaginal mucosa as in the Pereyra and Stamey methods. A No. 2 nylon monofilament suture is threaded into the eye of the needle and drawn down through the abdominal incision. A 1/2-inch Mayo needle is attached to the vaginal end of the suture, and a hitch of vaginal mucosa is taken at the urethrovesical angle. The free end of the suture is again threaded into the Stamey needle and passed up to the abdominal incision. It should exit about 2 cm from the original puncture to ensure sufficient fascia to support the angle when the suture ends are tied. If sufficient support fascia is not included, the repair could break down. The procedure is repeated on the opposite side.

Before the sutures are tied, a 70-degree panendoscope is inserted into the bladder to verify the absence of intravesicular sutures. If a suture is found, it is removed and the procedure is repeated. A Stamey suprapubic catheter is placed into the bladder under direct vision through the endoscope. The sutures can now be tied. The proper tension on the suture is determined with vaginal palpation to ensure the correct advancement of the angle. A single subcuticular suture closes the incisions.

Postoperative Care. The suprapubic catheter is left in place for 2–5 days until the post-void residual urine is less than 150 ml.

Follow-up. Immediate follow-up is excellent. The procedure requires about 15 minutes, so that anesthesia effects are minimal. There is minimal blood loss. In long-term follow-up, Gittes and Loughlin in 1987[13] and Gittes himself (personal communication) found an 87% cure rate at 5 years. Benson and colleagues reported an objective cure rate of 91% and a subjective cure rate of 97% at 9 months.[16] The author has used this procedure exclusively for cases with stress incontinence without prolapse or without abdominal indications for standard methods of suspension. With over 50 cases in the last 5 years, the author's cure rate for this period is about 85%. The anticipated complication of the suture material in the vagina has not materialized. The nonabsorbable inert suture tends to bury itself in the epithelium, and the suture area becomes re-epithelialized. Neither the author nor Gittes (personal communication) has had to remove or loosen the sutures in any patients, as was reported for the Stamey procedure.[15, 17] A detailed video of this procedure is available from the American College of Obstetricians and Gynecologists.[18]

Comparison of Various Procedures

In 1989, Bergman and associates published a randomized study of patients who had undergone one of three surgical procedures for stress incontinence—anterior colporrhaphy, revised Pereyra, or Burch procedure.[19] The type of surgery and the surgeon were selected at random. Follow-up was performed 1 year later by strict clinical and urodynamic criteria. The results indicated that the Burch procedure had a success rate of 87%, whereas the Pereyra and anterior colporrhaphy success rates were 70% and 69%, respectively. Although long-term results might be different, experience indicates that the latter two methods will deteriorate more with time than will the Burch procedure.

The Gittes procedure does basically what the Burch procedure does except that the technique is simplified. One would expect, therefore, that the results would be equally good.

A less well-known procedure, called the paravaginal defect repair for the correction of anterior vaginal wall prolapse and stress incontinence, should not be overlooked. The operation is performed abdominally, and by opening the space of Retzius as in the Burch procedure, the paravaginal tissue is reattached to the lateral pelvic wall. The author has not performed the procedure and has no experience with it. However, Richardson reported a 6-year follow-up of 149 patients that showed 97% of the patients had excellent functional results and no postoperative complaints of stress incontinence. The reader is referred to the original publication.[20]

An emerging special interest group of gynecologists is appearing, with specific focus on the underlying cause of incontinence. These individuals are being referred to as urogynecologists, and they will greatly increase our knowledge of this subject. The broadening of our understanding by urodynamic studies of the entire subject will make it easier to choose the correct procedure for each patient, thereby improving results.

OPERATIONS FOR BENIGN CONDITIONS OF THE URETHRA

Several lesions that are commonly brought to the attention of the gynecologist are considered, with emphasis on those that can be treated surgically.

Caruncle (Fig. 16–10)

Generally, caruncles are relatively asymptomatic and do not require attention (Fig. 16–10). The two most common symptoms of those that do require treatment are pain and bleeding. Caruncles can be extremely sensitive to touch, and, as a result of sensitivity to local irritation, even by clothing, the patient can present with urinary symptoms of frequency or urgency. Obviously, dyspareunia is also a common complaint. Because caruncles are very vascular lesions, bleeding is often noted by the patient. This is presented as postcoital or postmenopausal bleeding.

The treatment of this lesion is its surgical removal. This can be accomplished by cauterizing the base.

The two most important lesions that should be

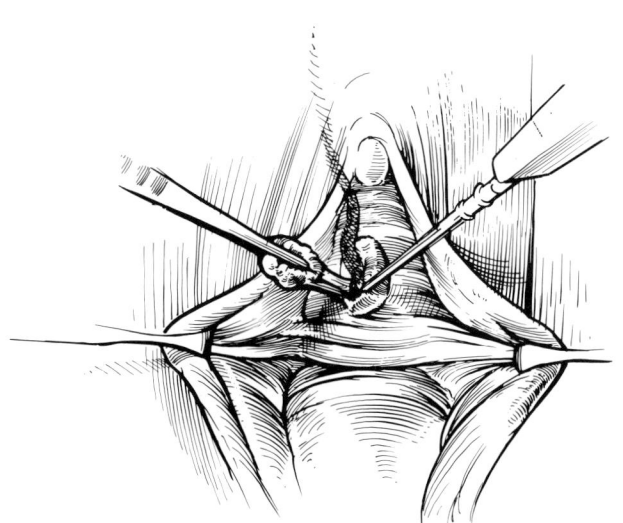

Figure 16–10
Urethral caruncle. The base of the caruncle arising from the posterior lip of the urethral meatus is cauterized at its base. The tissue is sent for pathologic examination.

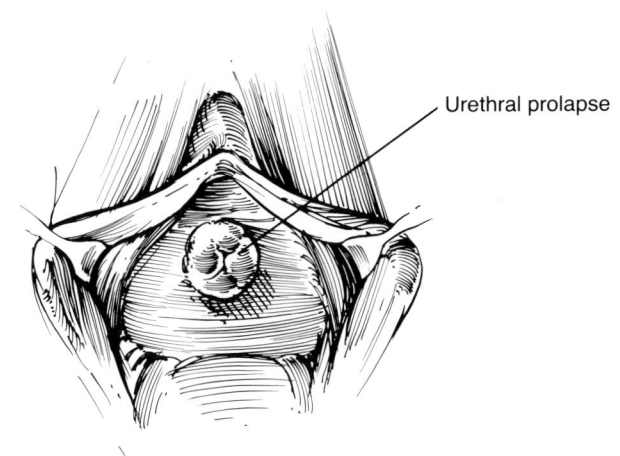

Figure 16–11
Urethral prolapse. The entire circumference of the meatal orifice has prolapsed.

distinguished from the caruncle are urethral prolapse and carcinoma. The caruncle arises from the posterior lip of the urethral orifice, whereas urethral prolapse involves the entire circumference of the urethral opening. On the other hand, the appearance of a caruncle can be similar to the early stages of urethral carcinoma; those tissues should always be sent for pathologic diagnosis.

Urethral Prolapse (Fig. 16–11)

Urethral prolapse is a relatively common condition that generally causes little or no problem (Fig. 16–11). In addition to the differences from the caruncle described previously, the prolapsed mucosa is less sensitive and does not bleed easily. If it is symptomatic, however, it should be excised.

Excision is accomplished by removing the excess mucosa and suturing the edges together with absorbable fine material such as 3-0 or 4-0 chromic catgut. A catheter is left in place for a few days until healing is established.

Urethral Diverticulum (Fig. 16–12)

Most urethral diverticula arise in the middle third of the urethra in its posterior aspect.[21] These are thought to be caused by chronic infection involving the paraurethral glands.[22] They are often asymptomatic and can be ignored. If symptomatic, the most likely complaints are frequency, dysuria, dyspareunia, and post-voiding dribbling. Microscopic examination of urinary sediment shows leukocytes and often erythrocytes unexpectedly, especially if stones are present. Definitive diagnosis is made by insertion of a Davis catheter. This very useful tool tamponades the blad-

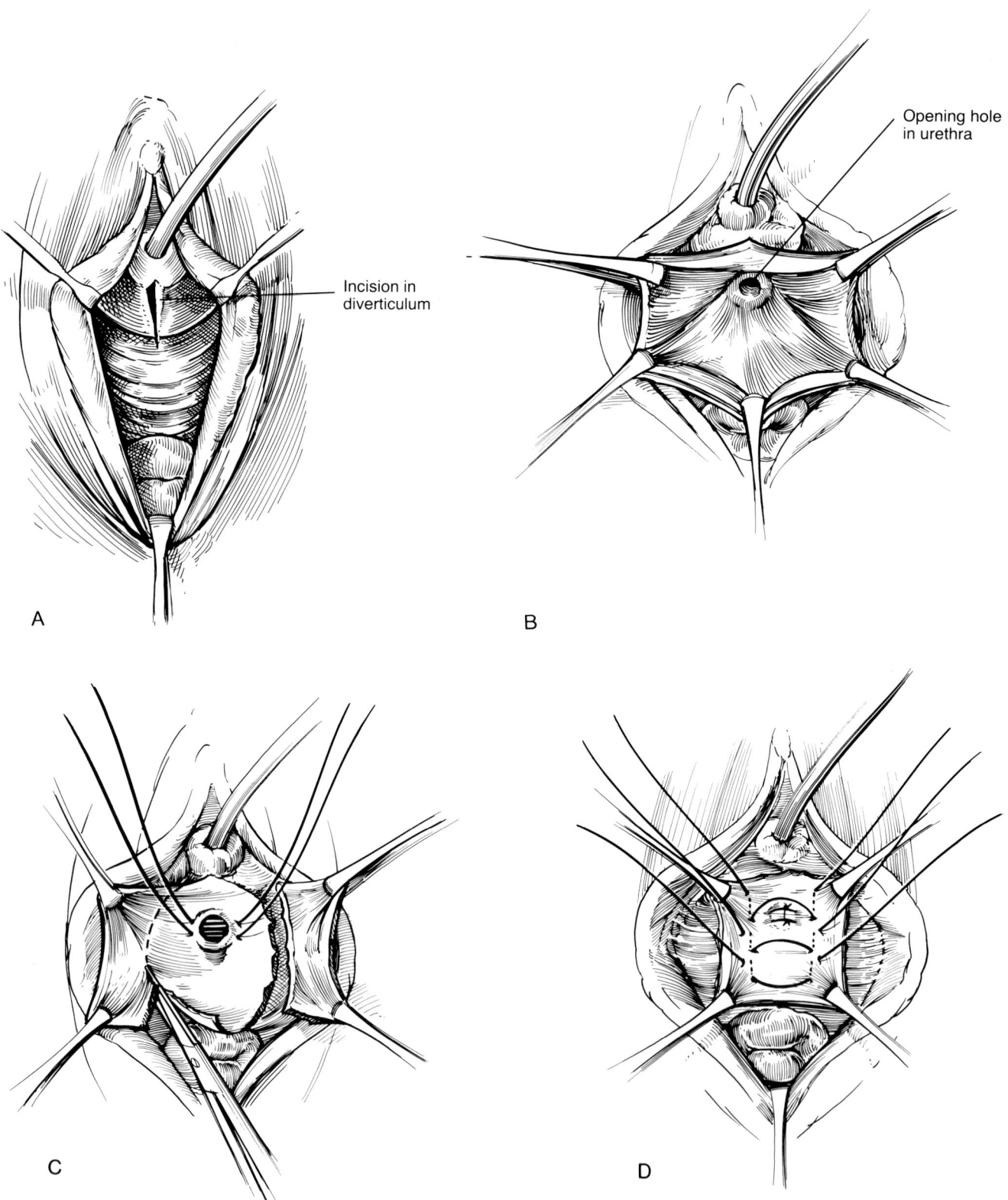

Figure 16–12
Urethral diverticulum. *A*, The vagina is excised over the diverticulum, exposing the underlying sac. *B*, The sac has been opened and the urethral opening visualized. *C*, The sac has been excised. The urethral opening is closed with 3-0 chromic catgut sutures. *D*, A second layer of sutures is placed over the meatal closure. The vagina is resutured.

der neck and the external urethral opening, permitting intraurethral injection of dye for visualization of the diverticulum. It should be emphasized that more than one diverticulum may be present; obviously, it is important to ascertain this possibility. Endoscopic visualization of the urethra while stripping the anterior vaginal wall will demonstrate pus extruding from the orifice of the sac, usually on the posterior wall of the urethra.

Treatment is surgical if the patient is symptomatic (Fig. 16–12). A Foley catheter in the bladder helps delineate the urethra. A longitudinal incision is made in the anterior vaginal wall. It is important to mobilize the plane between the sac and the overlying vaginal wall in all directions. This can be difficult if infection has been a factor in the formation of the diverticulum. In this situation, opening the sac intentionally can be helpful. The sac is then trimmed and the urethral opening closed with 3-0 chromic catgut suture. A second layer is placed over the closure, and the vaginal mucosa is closed in routine fashion. The Foley catheter is left in place for about 5 days.

Marsupialization was the most common surgical procedure in over 100 cases of urethral diverticula reported by Lichtman and Robertson.[23] Complications were reported to be only 4% but included recurrence, especially if multiple diverticula were present and not appreciated. In addition, urethral strictures and fistulas are possible. On the other hand, Nichols and Randall did not recommend marsupialization because of troublesome postoperative incontinence.[24]

References

1. LeCoutour X, Jung-Faerber S, Klein P, Renaud R: Female urinary incontinence: Comparative value of history and urodynamic investigations. Eur J Obstet Gynecol Reprod Biol 1990; 37:279.
2. Kelly HA: Incontinence of urine in women. Urol Cutan Rev 1913; 17:289.
3. Kennedy WT: Incontinence of urine in women: Some functional observations of the urethra illustrated in roentgenograms. Am J Obstet Gynecol 1937; 33:19.
4. Marshall VF, Marchetti AA, Krantz KE: The correction of stress incontinence by simple vesicourethral suspension. Surg Gynecol Obstet 1949; 88:509.
5. Burch JA: Cooper's ligament urethro-vesical suspension for stress incontinence. Am J Obstet Gynecol 1968; 100:764.
6. Stanton SL, William JE, Ritchie B: The colposcopic operation for urinary incontinence. Br J Obstet Gynaecol 1976; 83:890.
7. Parker RT, Addison WA, Wilson CJ: Fascia lata urethrovesical suspension of recurrent stress incontinence. Am J Obstet Gynecol 1979; 135:843.
8. Goebell R: Zur operativen beseitigung der angeboren Incontinentia vesicae. Ztschr Gynak Urol 1910; 2:187.
9. Aldridge AH: Transplantation of fascia for relief of urinary stress incontinence. Am J Obstet Gynecol 1942; 44:398.
10. Pereyra AJ: A simplified procedure for correction of stress incontinence in women. West J Surg Obstet Gynecol 1959; 67:223.
11. Raz S: Modified bladder neck suspension for female stress incontinence. Urology 1981; 17:82.
12. Stamey TA: Endoscopic suspension of the vesical neck for urinary incontinence in females: Report on 203 consecutive patients. Am Surg 1980; 192:465.
13. Gittes RF, Loughlin KR: No-incision pubovaginal suspension for stress incontinence. 3. Urology 1987; 138:568.
14. Langer R, Golan A, Ron-El R, et al.: Colposuspension for urinary stress incontinence in premenopausal and postmenopausal women. Surg Gynecol Obstet 1990; 171:13.
15. Webster GD, Kreder KJ: Voiding dysfunction following cystourethropexy: Its evaluation and management. J Urol 1990; 144:670.
16. Benson JT, Agosta A, McClellan E: Evaluation of a minimal incision–pubovaginal suspension as an adjunct to other pelvic floor surgery. Obstet Gynecol 1990; 75:844.
17. Araki T, Takamoto H, Hara T, et al.: The loop-loosening procedure for urination difficulties after Stamey suspension of the vesical neck. Urology 1990; 144:319.
18. Reilly RI: Needle Cystourethropexy. Washington and Boston, American College of Obstetricians and Gynecologists (ACOG) Film Library, 1990. (1–800–762–2264.)
19. Bergman A, Koonings DD, Rallard CA: Primary stress incontinence and pelvic relaxation: Prospective randomized comparison of three different procedures. Am J Obstet Gynecol 1989; 161:97.
20. Richardson AC, Edmonds PB, Williams NL: Treatment of stress incontinence due to paravaginal fascial defect. Obstet Gynecol 1981; 57:351.
21. Davis HL, Cian LG: Positive pressure urethrography: A new diagnostic method. J Urol 1958; 80:34.
22. Huffman JW: The detailed anatomy of the paraurethral ducts in the adult female. Am J Obstet Gynecol 1948; 55:86.
23. Lichtman AS, Robertson JR: Suburethral diverticula treated by marsupialization. Obstet Gynecol 1976; 47:203.
24. Nichols DH, Randall C: Urethral diverticulum and fistula. In Vaginal Surgery. Baltimore, Williams & Wilkins, 1989, pp. 358–368.

Operations for Pelvic Relaxation

17

Robert A. Starr
Bruce H. Drukker

Pelvic relaxation disorders comprise a heterogeneous yet common group of problems afflicting women. Although almost never life-threatening, these relaxation disorders become symptomatic, often disrupting a woman's lifestyle and adversely affecting her general comfort. Genital prolapse may result in a variety of patient complaints ranging from general feelings of aching pelvic pressure to marked abnormalities of urinary, gastrointestinal, and sexual function.

Historically, the earliest recorded reference to female genital prolapse as a distinct malady can be traced to approximately 2000 B.C. In a thorough review, Emge and Durfee note that in an Egyptian papyrus of that time, several references were made to "falling of the womb" (uterine prolapse).[1] Their comprehensive historical summary of the treatment of pelvic relaxation provides a fascinating account for the interested reader.

Nearly four millennia have passed since the earliest writings on pelvic relaxation. To a great extent, treatment approaches have mirrored the prevailing knowledge of the etiology of genital prolapse. For example, during the Hippocratic era, succussion represented one treatment for irreducible prolapse. Other remedies included the widespread use of different astringents, douches, and pleasant and malodorous fumigations, as well as the use of pessaries made of various organic and inorganic materials.[1]

Beginning around the sixteenth century, knowledge of the anatomic and clinical aspects of pelvic relaxation began evolving more significantly, leading to surgical treatment. During the nineteenth century, the advent of aseptic technique and the refinement of surgical instruments and materials led to the development of many operations to treat genital prolapse. It was also during this time that clear terminology and an anatomic classification of specific relaxation defects surfaced.

During the last century, a plethora of surgical techniques have been described to treat prolapse disorders. New descriptions often resembled or modified pre-existing techniques, incorporating new suture materials or changing technical aspects in an effort to eliminate the possible shortcomings of earlier approaches.

Certainly, the surgical management of genital prolapse will continue to evolve. Emge and Durfee very aptly point out that 40 centuries of writing on this topic has still not led to a treatment panacea. In fact, because genital prolapse disorders are heterogeneous, no one surgical approach can ever be expected to be universally useful. The goal of this chapter is to provide an overview of the etiology and classification of genital prolapse, along with various descriptions of specific surgical corrective procedures.

REGIONAL ANATOMY AND PELVIC SUPPORT

As with all surgical procedures, a detailed knowledge of the related anatomy is critical to both safe and effective outcomes. Pelvic organ prolapse results from the injury of supportive structures, most often through the tearing and attenuating forces first encountered during childbirth, and later amplified with aging. Surgical therapy focuses on reparative measures, and the primary goal is to alleviate symptoms while restoring and maintaining normal anatomic relationships. In order to achieve these goals, a thorough understanding of pelvic anatomy and support is necessary. Although many anatomic descriptions appear precise and complete, much of this information has been based upon study of cadaveric specimens. Nichols and Randall caution the pelvic surgeon to recognize that the anatomic relationships in the living, upright, unanesthetized female are often quite different.[2] Optimizing surgical repairs for genital prolapse demands a complete understanding of pelvic support and anatomic relationships.

Knowledge of vaginal anatomy is also very important, because the majority of pelvic reparative procedures are performed transvaginally. An overview of vaginal structure is found in the earlier chapter on pelvic anatomy (Chapter 2). The following description serves to highlight the inter-relationships between the vagina and surrounding structures.

The Vagina

The vagina is a tubular organ, and in its relaxed state the anterior and posterior walls appose each other. Along its length can be found varying anatomic supports collectively contributing to the maintenance of normal vaginal depth and axis. The adult vagina varies in length from 7 to 9 cm with the anterior wall generally shorter on average by 2 cm.[3] The cervix fuses with the upper vagina such that it occupies more of the anterior than the posterior vaginal wall, which accounts for the length discrepancy. The vagina is lined by a layer of nonkeratinized, stratified, squamous epithelium that is continuous with the mucosal lining of the cervix. A rich layer of elastin and collagen underlies the vaginal mucosa, and smooth muscle encloses these layers. This involuntary muscle is loosely arranged in an inner circular and outer longitudinal orientation. External to the smooth muscle layer is a capsule of elastin-rich fibrous tissue. The adventitial smooth muscle and fibroelastic tissues of the vagina are continuous with those of the cervix and lower uterus.

The vascular supply to the vagina derives from several sources, including the vaginal arteries from the internal iliac, branches from the inferior vesical and uterine vessels, and perhaps some branches from the internal pudendal artery. A rich anastomotic network makes this organ highly vascular, as evidenced by sometimes brisk blood loss during reconstructive vaginoplastic surgery. The blood vessels, along with lymphatics and some nerve fibers, course through the submucosal layer of the vagina.

Several components compose the overall structural support system of the vagina and uterus. Injury and alteration to these structural elements, either singularly or in combination, may result in symptomatic changes in the vagina and uterus.[4]

The upper vagina and cervix are principally supported by the cardinal and uterosacral ligament complex. Mengert demonstrated this through the use of his mechanical model of uterine support.[5] He showed that with traction applied to the cervix of a cadaver, significant uterine prolapse occurred only after the paracervical and upper paravaginal tissues were bisected. These tissues correspond to what we know as the cardinal and uterosacral ligaments.

Cardinal Ligaments

The cardinal ligaments join the cervix and upper vagina as lateral thickenings of the endopelvic fascia and house vascular and lymphatic structures. The latter are ensheathed within a meshwork of fibrous connective tissue. This collagen-rich tissue is more dense immediately lateral to the vagina and cervix. Histologically, Range and Woodburne found that these structures were not "ligaments" per se, but rather blood vessels, lymphatics, and nerves richly invested in smooth muscle fibers and areolar tissue.[6] At rest, no palpable ligament is detected within this tissue. However, with the uterus on stretch, a "ligament" is formed by tension along the neurovascular bundles.

Uterosacral Ligaments

Extending as posterior condensations of the endopelvic fascia, the uterosacral ligaments contribute to the support of the upper vagina and cervix. Thorough study of these structures by Campell revealed their composition as smooth muscle and fibroelastic tissue containing vascular and nervous structures.[7] The uterosacral ligaments course from their attachment to the posterolateral cervix and lateral aspects of the upper vagina to the sacrum, where they flare out and attach to the presacral fascia. The posterior cul-de-sac of Douglas is demarcated at its superior and lateral borders by these ligaments.

Based upon separate works by previous authors,[8–11] it is clear that in the erect woman the upper vaginal axis is horizontally oriented. This portion of the vagina lies upon the rectum, and in turn these two organs lie upon and parallel to the levator plate, thus being supported by the latter. The cardinal and uterosacral ligaments serve the important function of helping to maintain the upper vagina and cervix in position over the levator plate while maintaining the uterus in an anteverted position. A weakening in this supportive complex may lead to uterovaginal prolapse. Conversely, identification of these important structures allows for their incorporation and utilization in the reconstructive repair of specific prolapse disorders.

Pelvic Diaphragm

The pelvic diaphragm represents another key component of support for the vagina and other pelvic, as well as abdominal, viscera. It forms the floor of the spherical abdominopelvic cavity, consequently bearing considerable and variable forces, both gravitational and active. The pelvic diaphragm consists of the levator ani muscle group and its associated superior and inferior fascia. The constitution of the levator ani complex has been variably described but basically consists of paired muscle groups divided into the pubococcygeus, the puborectalis, and the iliococcygeus. Beginning anteriorly and moving posteriorly, the levator ani arises continuously from the pubic bone, the arcus tendineus levatoris ani, and finally the ischial spine. Insertion is into the perineal body, the external anal sphincter, the anococcygeal raphe, and the coccyx.

The levator plate is formed by the fusion of the medial aspects of the levator ani muscles just posterior to the rectum as they course towards their attachment to the coccyx. As previously mentioned, the normally supported rectum, upper vagina, and uterus rest upon this horizontal shelf. The levator ani are not fused between the anterior margin of the levator plate and the posterior pubic bone. A midline opening exists, known as the levator or genital hiatus, through which the urethra, vagina, and rectum pass (Fig. 17–1). Anatomic and histologic study by DeLancey and Starr has demonstrated clear attachments between the laterally situated pubococcygeus muscles and the vagina in the area of the paraurethral vaginal sulci.[12] These musculofascial attachments add further support directly to the vagina and indirectly to the urethra. Similarly, Lawson describes other supportive fibers of the levator ani muscle inserting circumferentially into the anal canal, contributing to the external anal sphincter.[13]

The pelvic diaphragm forms the floor of the pelvis

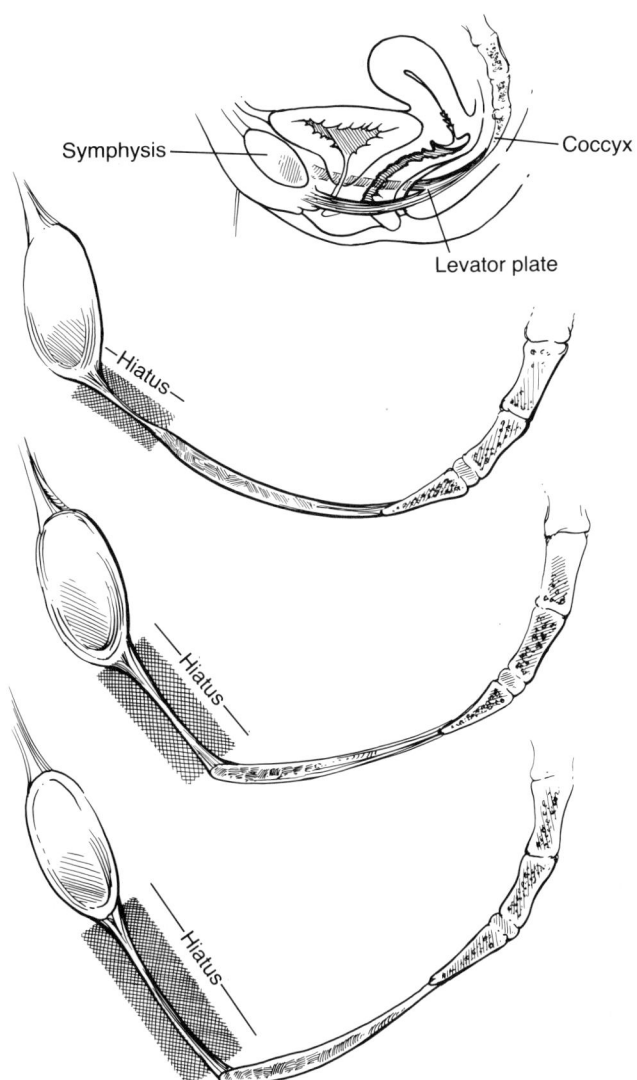

Figure 17–1
The levator plate and genital hiatus are shown. Under conditions of normal support, the levator plate is horizontal, supporting the rectum, upper vagina, and uterus. As support is impaired, the genital hiatus widens and the levator plate elongates, resulting in prolapse of pelvic organs.

and is generally slightly concave on its superior aspect. The pelvic diaphragm musculature, although striated, is in a tonic state of contraction.[14] Additional contractile strength can be generated by the levator group, either voluntarily or by reflex. In the case of the latter, stronger contractions occur simultaneously with abdominal muscle activity. These reciprocal contractions between the abdominal wall and the pelvic floor muscles serve to evenly distribute any increases in intra-abdominal pressure. When the levator ani contract, the levator plate elevates along with the genital hiatus. The genital hiatus is narrowed, thereby preventing the prolapse of pelvic viscera. Weakening of the pelvic diaphragm may occur as a consequence of childbirth or through the long-term, repetitive increases in intra-abdominal pressure seen with certain medical disorders. Whatever the cause, weakening of these support structures leads to a downward displacement and elongation of the generally strong levator plate and a widening of the genital hiatus. Loss of the horizontal support of the vagina and uterus as a result of excess funneling of the pelvic floor may displace these organs anteriorly and lead to their gradual prolapse through the genital hiatus.

Urogenital Diaphragm

The urogenital diaphragm is another component of the overall support mechanism of the pelvic viscera. Structurally, it is not truly a diaphragm and is sometimes referred to as the perineal membrane. Its shape is triangular, and it consists of a musculomembranous sheath attached anterolaterally to the paired ischiopubic rami and posteriorly to the perineal body. The urethra and vagina pass through it. Fibers of the urogenital diaphragm, particularly smooth muscle, are thought to insert into the outer layers of the urethra and vagina.[15] Multiple authors have independently described the pubourethral ligaments that provide additional support to the urethra.[16-19] Milley and Nichols[18] showed that histologically the pubourethral ligaments are composed of fibrous tissue and elastin arising from around the urethra and vagina, a finding later corroborated by DeLancey[20] in his study of paraurethral anatomy. Together, the urogenital diaphragm and pubourethral ligaments provide localized support to the urethra and vagina.

Perineal Body

The pelvic diaphragm is slightly conical and forms the floor of the abdominopelvic cavity. The perineal body is the most dependent point of the pelvic floor. It is situated between the distal vaginal and anal canals and is bordered laterally by the ischial tuberosities. The perineal body is a pyramidally shaped wedge of fibromuscular tissue into which insert fibers of the levator ani, along with the superficial and deep perineal muscles. The apex of the perineal body extends inward, and its fibers meld with the rectovaginal septum. A large amount of elastic and smooth muscle fibers, along with its firm attachment to the rectovaginal septum, allow the perineal body to support the distal vagina and rectum. Consequently, when these tissues become damaged during childbirth or attenuated with advancing age, loss of support may lead to the development of a rectocele.

Bony Pelvis

Finally, the bony pelvis, which was described in Chapter 2, provides the ultimate support to the pelvic viscera. The various muscular and fascial supports attach to the pelvic bones and then to the viscera as described.

Pelvic Connective Tissue Spaces

Prerequisite to the safe and effective repair of genital prolapse disorders is a thorough understanding of the subperitoneal connective tissue spaces within the pelvis. These spaces are filled by loose areolar tissue and fat, thus separating the pelvic organs. In their undisturbed state, they are really potential spaces, which are easily delineated using blunt dissection. The spaces are free of blood vessels and nervous structures and are themselves separated by septa of endopelvic fascia. By nature of these connective tissue spaces, the various pelvic viscera are able to change volume independently while moving freely upon each other. That free mobility may become compromised, however, in the face of certain pathologic changes that may lead to scarring, fibrosis, or replacement of the spaces. Examples of such processes may include radiation exposure, malignancy, or previous surgery.

The connective tissue spaces are most easily understood diagrammatically (Fig. 17-2). Basically, there are four midline spaces and two paired lateral spaces, all separated by tissue septa. The midline spaces include the prevesical space (space of Retzius), the vesicovaginal space, the rectovaginal space, and the retrorectal space. The paired lateral spaces are the anterior paravesical and posterior pararectal spaces. It is essential for the gynecologic surgeon to thoroughly understand these pelvic tissue planes and spaces and their inter-relationships, particularly when operating vaginally. This knowledge will help avoid inadvertent trauma to the individual organs and excessive blood loss as a result of vascular damage. Accessing these avascular spaces allows one to approach the individual organ supports and will help to optimize reconstructive repairs. A comprehensive review of pelvic connective tissue planes and spaces is beyond the scope of this chapter. The interested reader is directed to a thorough discussion of the topic by Lansman.[21]

CLASSIFICATION OF GENITAL PROLAPSE

Broadly applied, the concept of pelvic relaxation includes all degrees of uterine prolapse, cystourethrocele, rectocele, enterocele, vaginal vault prolapse, and deficient perineal body. It implies a loss of support of the pelvic viscera whereby normal anatomic relationships are altered. The classification of pelvic prolapse disorders is based upon the type of

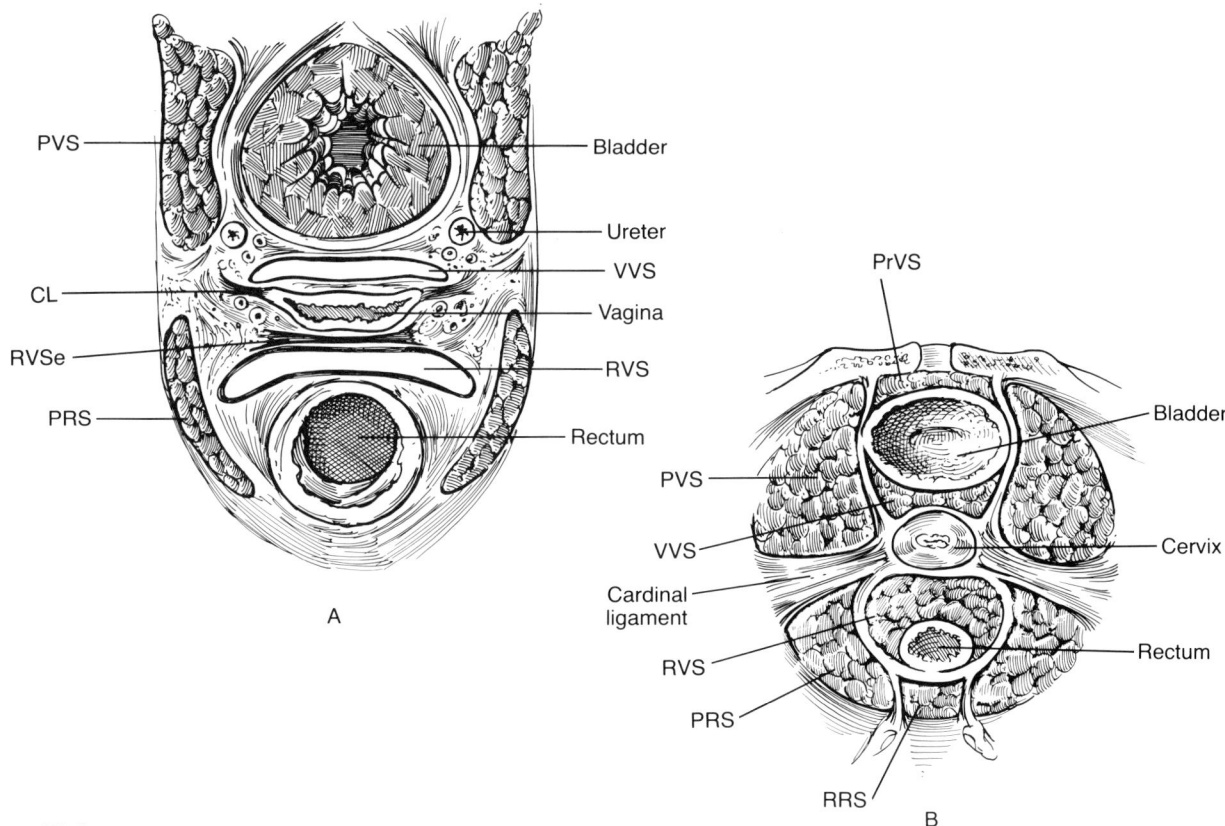

Figure 17–2
A, The connective tissue spaces and planes of the female pelvis are shown in this frontal section. Lateral to the bladder are the paravesical spaces *(PVS)*. The vesicovaginal space *(VVS)* and the rectovaginal space *(RVS)* separate the vagina from the bladder and rectum, respectively. Lateral to the rectum are the pararectal spaces *(PRS)*. The rectovaginal septum *(RVSe)* is seen between the vagina and the rectovaginal space. The anterolateral vaginal sulci are formed by connective tissue attachments of the vagina to the pelvic side wall in the region near the cardinal ligaments *(CL)*. The ureter is shown. B, Another view of these same connective tissue spaces and planes is shown with this cross-sectional diagram of the pelvis through the level of the uterine cervix. Two additional midline spaces are shown: the prevesical space *(PrVS)*, anterior to the bladder; and the retrorectal space *(RRS)*, posterior to the rectum.

herniation noted (Fig. 17–3). Specifically, the organ involved as well as the site of damaged support is considered.

Cystocele and Cystourethrocele

Anterior vaginal wall prolapse may involve herniation of the bladder with or without relaxation of the urethra, and these defects are specified as cystocele and cystourethrocele, respectively. A cystocele is the protrusion of the bladder downward into the vaginal canal. It results from damage to the normally supportive vesicovaginal septum. The urinary trigone, bladder neck, and urethra compose the most susceptible structures if the weakening is a byproduct of vaginal delivery. The bladder base is more likely to be pulled out of the pelvis during labor, owing to its attachment to the anterior uterus. Consequently, the bladder base is damaged relatively less often. When the bladder base does prolapse because of damaged support, the cystocele is often referred to as a posterior type, distinct from an anterior type, when only the anterior anatomy is altered. Urethrocele as an isolated finding remains very uncommon and probably has no clinical significance.

Rectocele and Enterocele

Posterior vaginal defects include rectocele and enterocele and are named according to the prolapsing organ. A rectocele is a herniation of the rectum into the vagina. Damage to posterior support, which involves the rectovaginal septum, the levator ani and associated fascia, and the perineal body, leads to rectocele formation. Deficient support of the perineal body may fail to channel stool out the anal canal, and the forces of defecation can lead to bulging of the distal posterior vagina with low rectocele formation. Loss of integrity of the rectovaginal septum permits the levator muscle bundles to regress laterally, opening a defect in the posterior vagina and allowing further development of low, mid, or high rectoceles.

An enterocele is a herniation of the posterior cul-

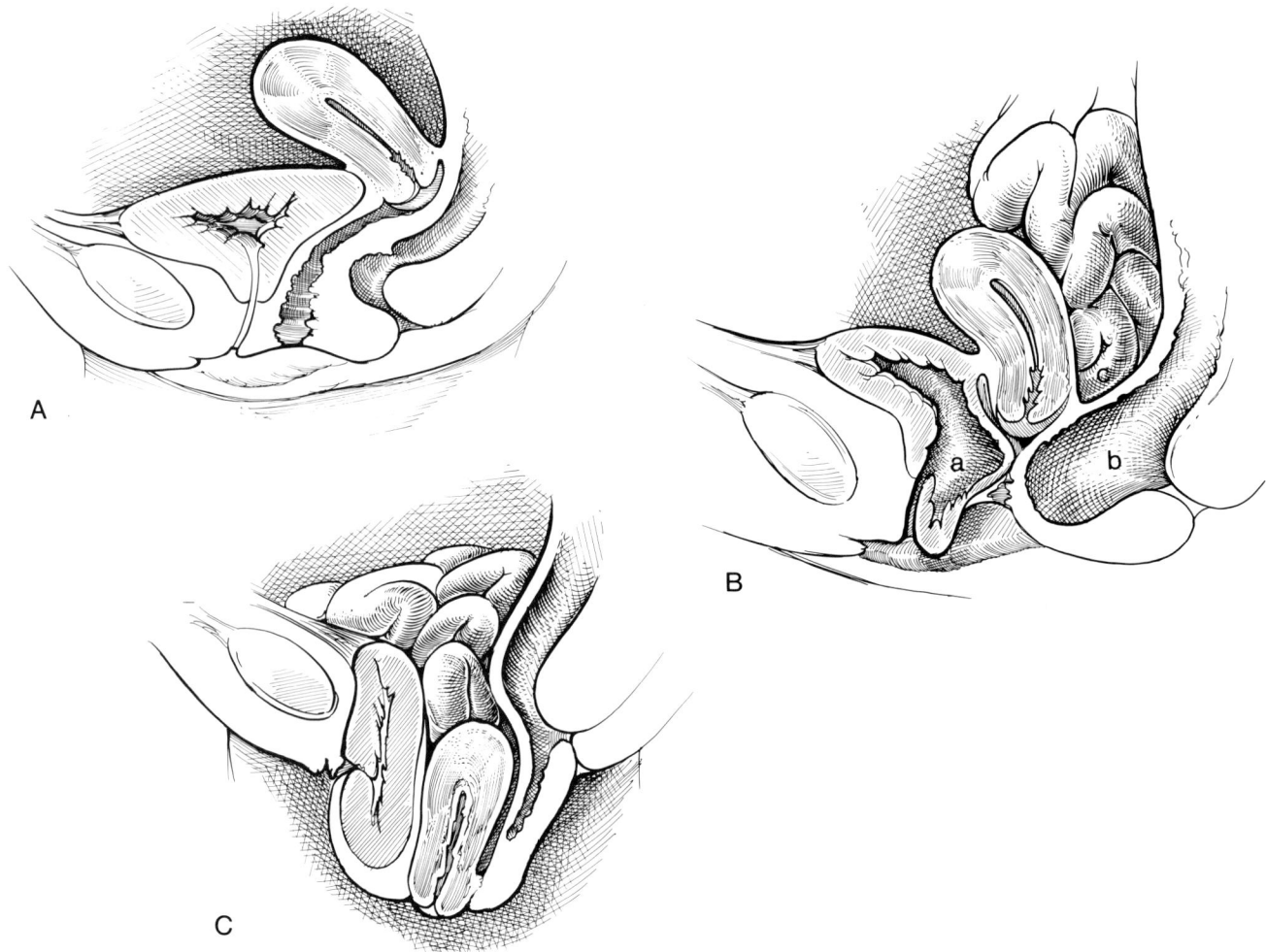

Figure 17–3
Types of genital prolapse are diagramatically shown. *A*, Sagittal section of a normally supported pelvis. *B*, Incomplete uterine prolapse is noted along with specific types of herniation: *(a)* cystocele, *(b)* rectocele, and *(c)* enterocele. *C*, Complete uterine prolapse (procidentia) is shown.

de-sac peritoneum between the uterosacral ligaments and down into the rectovaginal space. Enterocele is more often seen in women with congenitally deep cul-de-sacs, and once formed it contains loops of bowel that can often be palpated through the posterior vagina.

Uterine and Vaginal Vault Prolapse

Uterine and vaginal vault prolapse occurs secondary to weakening of the cardinal and uterosacral ligament complex. These strong structures provide the greatest support to the vagina and uterus, and their tearing or attenuation leads first to a posterior shift in the uterine axis. The uterine axis normally lies at a right angle to the vaginal axis, but once its support slackens the two axes become more closely aligned. A widening in the genital hiatus as a result of compromised vaginal wall or levator support may allow the now poorly supported upper vagina and uterus to begin prolapsing. Over time, repetitive increases in intra-abdominal pressure further exacerbate the degree of uterovaginal prolapse, pushing the uterus down through the vagina.

Currently, no one classification schema of pelvic relaxation is generally accepted. If classifying the extent of prolapse aids the communication on this topic, the system proposed by Beecham is uncomplicated and useful.[22] He describes first-degree prolapse as the prolapsing organ at the hymenal ring but within the introitus. Second-degree prolapse is present when the organ descends beyond the introitus; and third-degree prolapse occurs when the organ protrudes entirely outside the introitus.

SIGNS AND SYMPTOMS

Historically, women with symptomatic genital prolapse will complain variably of pelvic pressure, a feeling of heaviness, or of "bearing down." Often, there may be associated low back pain and, to a lesser degree, pulling groin pain. It is not uncommon for the first or primary complaint to be that of altered urinary or bowel function. Prolapse defects involving the anterior vaginal wall may result in various symptoms, which include urinary urgency, frequency, and incontinence. Cases of profound cystocele or uterovaginal prolapse may cause paradoxical kinking of the urethrovesical junction with resultant urinary retention. Rectocele may lead to altered bowel function. Constipation can occur, or the patient may find it necessary to apply digital pressure to the bulging posterior vagina to facilitate defecation. Commonly, the principal complaint with prolapse is that of a noticeable bulge or protrusion of vaginal tissues. When such a bulge is noted, an accompanying complaint may be that of coital discomfort. Also, if the prolapse is third-degree in magnitude, the overlying nonkeratinized vaginal epithelium becomes exposed, which may lead to drying, cracking, and ulceration with resultant bleeding.

Thorough history taking will reveal the chief and secondary complaints. The history should be focused in such a way that it helps clarify the patient's perceived magnitude of the problem and her expectations and motivation for treatment. Other areas to focus upon include the duration of the symptoms and their severity as well as any identifiable predisposing factors found in the obstetric, family, and past surgical and medical history.

Although the history is helpful and important in evaluating the patient for prolapse disorders, ultimately the diagnosis is made through careful physical examination. Both Porges[23] and TeLinde[24] wrote thoughtful accounts of how one should systematically examine the unanesthetized patient with genital prolapse in order to fully document the sites of pelvic injury and the overall support of the pelvis.

PATHOPHYSIOLOGY

Multiple etiologic factors may contribute to the development of genital prolapse, some of which have already been alluded to in this text. Most commonly, events during vaginal childbirth account for damage to the pelvic floor. Pregnancy-induced changes soften and stretch pelvic supports, perhaps mediated by such hormones as relaxin. The enlarged uterus provides a constant source of downward pressure upon the pelvic diaphragm.

Intrapartum structural changes in the pelvic floor are numerous and have been detailed by Power.[25] The elongation, tearing, and detaching of pelvic tissues occur with fetal passage through the birth canal. Other intrapartum events may further compromise pelvic tissues, such as precipitous or prolonged fetal descent, fetal macrosomia, or an ill-executed operative delivery. Resultant structural damage can be detected with careful postpartum examination.[26] It is likely that even following an uncomplicated vaginal birth, there is ultimately some compromise of pelvic support. This knowledge has led some authors to advocate episiotomy in all nullipara and any multipara lacking evidence of pelvic support defects.[27, 28]

Denervation injuries to the pelvic floor during parturition must be added to the more traditional explanations for pelvic organ prolapse. In an earlier study, 50% of women with genital prolapse exhibited abnormal pelvic floor electromyographic patterns when compared with normal controls.[29] More recently, Smith and colleagues, performing single-fiber electromyography of the pubococcygeus muscle, showed a greater nerve fiber density in women with genital prolapse compared with asymptomatic nulliparous controls.[30] These findings suggest an etiologic role for pelvic muscle damage secondary to denervation injuries during childbirth.

Nonobstetric factors that may contribute to the overall severity of pelvic relaxation include congenital weakness of pelvic tissues and chronic causes of increased intra-abdominal pressure such as pulmonary disease, obesity, chronic ascites, or abdominopelvic tumors. Certain repetitive exercises experienced recreationally or occupationally may also lead to chronic intra-abdominal pressure increases that jeopardize pelvic support.

Epidemiologically, genital prolapse disorders are seen more commonly with increasing parity and age. In the postmenopausal period, the salutary effects of estrogen are absent and, without adequate hormonal replacement, progression of relaxation defects may be hastened.

Iatrogenic causes of genital prolapse nearly always revolve around previous pelvic surgery. Failure to adequately support the upper vagina following hysterectomy may lead to prolapse. Also, if care is not taken to maintain the proper vaginal axis or if the vagina is abnormally foreshortened, normal pelvic support relationships can be altered and enterocele or vault prolapse results. In some instances, certain prolapse disorders are overlooked during repair of other defects and consequently remain unrepaired. Poor tissue handling and suturing may lead to ischemic changes in newly repaired tissue and lead to necrosis with redevelopment of support defects.

CHOICE OF OPERATION

The hallmark of effective and rational surgical repair of genital prolapse is adherence to the principle of individualization. Each surgery must be undertaken with a view towards tailoring the procedure to the specific defects. The natural prerequisite to surgery is the clear and precise identification of both the primary and, if present, secondary sites of damage within the pelvic support complex. Identifying these defects in the awake, unanesthetized patient requires a thorough physical examination with careful attention given to all areas of pelvic support. Therefore, examination may need to be performed with the woman in both the supine and standing positions; with a full bladder, followed by a post-voiding examination. Any specific urologic complaints that accompany the general signs and symptoms of genital prolapse should be thoroughly explored through appropriate urodynamic assessment.

In screening patients preoperatively, the patient's perception of the magnitude of her problem as well as her expectations of and motivation for treatment should be fully discussed. This information, in combination with the physical examination findings and assessment of risk factors, will allow the surgeon to candidly discuss the operative plan along with the issue of the risk/benefit ratio of treatment.

Once the decision to proceed with surgery has been made, the choice of operation is governed by the specific type of anatomic defect present. Damage to the urogenital diaphragm often occurs in tandem with anterior vaginal wall injury. Cystocele or cystourethrocele follows, and anterior colporrhaphy is indicated. Because these defects often alter bladder neck support and result in urinary incontinence, the repair may need to combine anterior colporrhaphy with a specific type of anti-incontinence procedure.

Posterior vaginal wall damage predisposes the patient to mid to high rectocele formation and/or enterocele formation. The differentiation of these two lesions is often difficult to make clinically. Consequently, the surgeon must be prepared to proceed with posterior colporrhaphy and, if enterocele is encountered, perform the appropriate repair as described later in this chapter. If the supportive damage is within the perineal body, the resultant defect is most times a low rectocele requiring posterior colporrhaphy and possibly a perineorrhaphy.

It is reasonable to consider the question of whether concurrent hysterectomy should be performed at the time of repairing pelvic prolapse disorders. If uterine relaxation is demonstrated and damage to the upper vaginal and cervical supports is present, hysterectomy should be completed as part of the overall repair. A vaginal approach is the clear choice for hysterectomy in the face of uterine prolapse, because it allows the entire repair to be completed by a single route.

Beyond the decision of which operation to perform lie several important surgical issues. First, if the patient desires further children, reparative surgery should be delayed until childbearing is complete to avoid the compromise of an adequate repair and the greater risk of recurrent prolapse. Second, after discussing the patient's attitudes about sexual intercourse, the concept of preservation of vaginal depth and caliber should be considered with the goal to maintain both should the patient desire coital activity. Third, the issue of ovarian conservation needs to be discussed preoperatively. If the patient is climacteric or postmenopausal, the prudent approach is to perform bilateral salpingo-oophorectomy. Finally, the pelvic surgeon must always bear in mind the concept of complete repair of all defective supports while maintaining normal anatomic relationships and function.

CYSTOCELE AND REPAIR

Cystocele, or protrusion of the bladder down into the anterior vaginal wall, is a relatively common defect in parous women. As many as 50% of multiparous women may suffer some mild to moderate degree of cystocele, with only 10–20% experiencing symptoms.[31] Although the anatomic defect may be commonly observed during clinical examination, the degree of symptomatology will vary from the nonexistent to the very severe, depending on the degree of bladder prolapse. Another factor that may impact upon the magnitude of symptoms is the duration of onset of the defect. If the cystocele has occurred insidiously, as is often the case, the patient may have few complaints.

Many of the signs and symptoms experienced with cystocele are common to women with other forms of pelvic relaxation. With first- or second-degree cystoceles, pelvic pressure or heaviness may be present. Less often, there is associated pain or perhaps discomfort while walking or during coitus. As the degree of prolapse worsens, the patient may feel a protrusion or bulging of tissues beyond the introitus. Although not uniformly so, stress urinary incontinence commonly coexists with milder degrees of cystocele, particularly when there is rotational descent of the bladder neck with loss of a well-supported urethrovesical angle. In cases of severe prolapse, the patient may be stress continent, presumably owing to an alteration of the normal continence mechanism and obstruction at the bladder neck. With such a severe cystocele, distention of the upper collecting system is not uncommon. This may result in hydroureter or even hydronephrosis.[32] Other urinary symptoms in women with anterior vaginal wall relaxation may include frequency and urgency. Finally, when the cystocele is severe, the exposed vaginal mucosa may become chronically irritated, ulcerate, and bleed.

Previously, the anatomy and supports of the

vagina were reviewed. Recollection of this information is important in understanding the anatomy of cystocele and its repair. Cystocele occurs as a result of aberrations of the vaginal wall or its supports.

The bladder rests upon the anterior vaginal wall, as does the urethra. The urethra, however, has the added support of the well-described pubourethral ligaments.[18, 19, 33]

The anterior vaginal wall is separated from the bladder by the potential vesicovaginal space and the pubocervical fascia. The normally supported upper vagina, upon which the bladder rests, is situated over the levator plate, and both are horizontally oriented in the erect female. The vagina draws its support from the cardinal ligament complex and through its attachments to the levator ani muscle. Although previous opinions regarding the existence of a direct attachment between the vaginal wall and the levator ani muscle have conflicted,[8, 13, 16] Delancey and Starr histologically demonstrated that an important musculofascial attachment is present.[12] This connection of the vagina to the levator ani occurs at the level of the paraurethral vaginal sulcus bilaterally. The paired sulci delineate the lateral margins of the anterior vaginal wall and are prominent when the vaginolevator attachment is intact.

Cystocele formation may result from damage to the anterior vaginal wall or any of its supports. These injuries most often follow childbearing and are aggravated by conditions causing chronic increases in intra-abdominal pressure. Estrogen deficiency may lead to atrophy of already attenuated tissue supports and a worsening of the cystocele. Specifically, cystocele may follow the stretching and damaging forces of vaginal delivery upon the musculoconnective tissues of the vescicovaginal septum. The overlying vaginal mucosa will generally distend with the cystocele symmetrically. The normal rugal folds may become attenuated or even flat, giving the anterior vaginal wall a smooth appearance. With repeated increases in intra-abdominal pressure, there is progressive stretching of supporting tissues, allowing the bladder and urethra to further descend, rotating posteriorly and inferiorly. As the relaxation progresses to permit descent of the urethra and bladder base below the pelvic and urogenital diaphragms, the bladder neck is now out of the sphere of the intra-abdominal cavity. Consequently, increases in intra-abdominal pressure are now unequally transmitted to the bladder and the urethra. A pressure gradient results when proportionately more pressure is transmitted to the bladder than the urethra. This forces the bladder neck open, resulting in urine flow or stress urinary incontinence.

If the support defect is lateral in the region where the vagina attaches to the levator ani muscle, the paraurethral sulcus may be blunted or lost on either one or both sides. This is the so-called paravaginal defect described by Richardson and coworkers.[34] Because the vagina and urethra are intimately related in this region,[17] loss of vaginal support through a paravaginal fascial defect also leads to urethral relaxation and a combined cystourethrocele. The urethral hypermobility that is seen with this defect may lead to unfavorable pressure transmission as described earlier, again with stress urinary incontinence resulting. Such an anatomic defect requires a specific repair for optimal results.

Any patient presenting with the finding of cystocele or related symptoms deserves a full and careful assessment. A thorough history and physical examination will help to clarify whether any intervention is necessary. Not every perturbation of the anterior vaginal wall requires surgical repair, and, in fact, it is generally inappropriate to undertake surgery unless the patient is distinctly symptomatic.

Techniques for examination are described previously in this chapter. As with any prolapse disorder, it is critical to determine whether other forms of prolapse coexist, including uterine descensus, rectocele, enterocele, or vaginal vault eversion. Mapping out the entire extent of relaxation allows one to carefully plan the proper surgical repair. In addition to taking a history and completing an examination, an appropriate urodynamic evaluation is necessary when urinary incontinence is part of the symptom profile. Documenting the exact type of urinary incontinence will aid the treatment planning and help to maximize the patient's chance of improvement or cure. It is particularly important to evaluate urinary function in the presence of severe cystocele. Although these patients may not complain of involuntary urine loss, as previously mentioned, this may be due to paradoxical kinking at the bladder neck. Bergman and colleagues describe a modification of preoperative urodynamic testing that screens patients for this phenomenon of urethrovesical obstruction that is due to severe prolapse.[35] They utilize a pessary to displace the prolapse followed by testing for urethra/bladder pressure transmission ratios. This technique allows them to identify occult stress urinary incontinence that may otherwise have not expressed itself until after the primary repair of cystocele had been accomplished.

The principal objectives of the anterior colporrhaphy are to correct the symptomatic cystourethrocele and to restore continence if stress urinary incontinence is present and due to hypermobility at the bladder neck. If the bladder base is merely surgically displaced anteriorly, coexistent stress urinary incontinence will probably not resolve and may be exacerbated. When stress urinary incontinence does accompany a cystourethrocele, the surgical objective is to differentially support and elevate the proximal urethra more than the bladder base. This relationship will situate the proximal urethra cephalad to the bladder base, thereby increasing the transmission of intra-abdominal pressure to the urethra during episodes of exertion with the goal of achieving urinary continence.[36]

Technique of Anterior Colporrhaphy

After a patient has been completely and carefully evaluated and a decision to proceed with anterior colporrhaphy has been made, the operation must be performed with care and precision, remaining mindful of the surgical objectives. Anterior colporrhaphy can be done as a separate procedure or more commonly with vaginal hysterectomy and/or rectocele or enterocele repair. In some situations when a retropubic urethropexy is performed for stress urinary incontinence, a minimal anterior colporrhaphy may be warranted to reduce a symptomatic cystocele. In this situation, it is important not to overcorrect the defect. Doing so may unfavorably alter pressure relationships between the bladder and urethra and actually negate the corrective effects of the urethropexy.

The operative procedure is accomplished with the patient in the dorsal lithotomy position following appropriate prepping and draping of the surgical field. The authors prefer using the Beaver scalpel and blade. It is a lightweight, long instrument that permits precise dissection, not only with the traditional side portion of the blade but also with the rounded front end. Submucosal injection of normal saline solution helps to delineate tissue planes through hydrodistention. A dilute solution (1:1000) of epinephrine in normal saline can be used as a combined distending medium and hemostatic agent. When anterior colporrhaphy immediately follows vaginal hysterectomy, the anterior vaginal wall incision is started at the upper free cut edge of the vagina where ultimately the vaginal cuff will be closed. If, on the other hand, cystocele repair does not accompany hysterectomy, the incision is started high on the anterior vaginal wall near the apex. The vaginal apex is drawn down towards the introitus using Allis clamps.

After the point of initial incision has been made, the incision is extended vertically from the apex of the vagina to the area underlying the urethra. The incision progresses stepwise, dissecting approximately 3–4 cm with each advance. The incision is made by first undermining the full thickness of the vaginal mucosa in the midline using the scissors. This allows entry into the vesicovaginal space. The full thickness of the mucosa is opened in the midline to a point corresponding to the urethrovesical junction (Fig. 17–4). With the cut edges of the vaginal mucosa elevated using Allis clamps, the vesicovaginal space is further opened bilaterally as the bladder and vaginal wall are separated. This generally begins as a sharp dissection, and, once the proper cleavage plane is delineated, further separation of tissues can usually be accomplished bluntly. Extensive scarring from previous surgery may preclude easy blunt dissection. Separation of the vaginal mucosa from the pubovesical fascia is done along the entire length of the incision and carried out bilaterally until all the vaginal mucosa is free. Occasional bleeding points can be ligated, but generally blood loss is minimal if the appropriate tissue plane is entered.

After the dissection has been completed, a Foley urethral catheter is placed into the bladder and the urine is drained. The bulb of the catheter helps to identify the urethrovesical junction by placing mild traction on the catheter and palpating where the bulb stops. If a urethrocele and stress urinary incontinence are present, specific separate supporting sutures will need to be placed to elevate the bladder neck. For this reason, further dissection of the bilateral paraurethral spaces is necessary and can be achieved

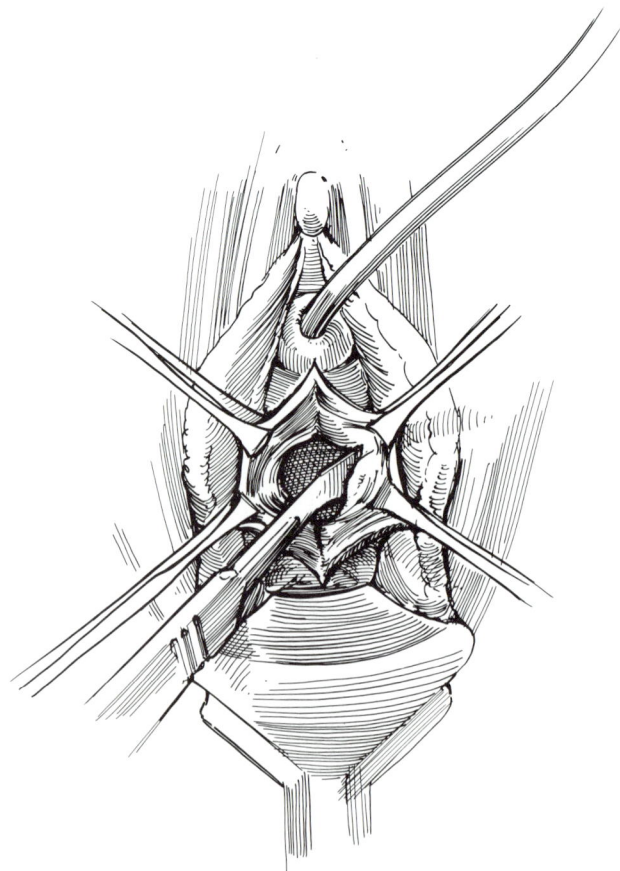

Figure 17–4
The anterior vaginal wall has been opened along a midline incision. The vesicovaginal space is being further developed using sharp technique. The vaginal mucosa is separated from the underlying pubovesical fascia.

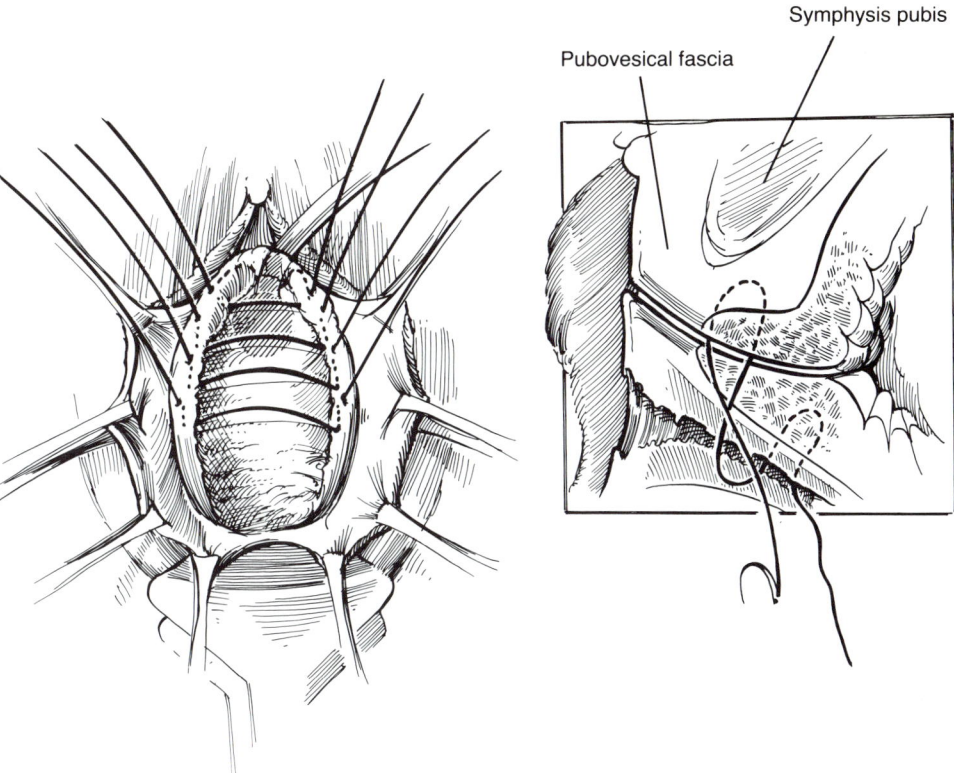

Figure 17–5
A specific supporting suture or two is placed at the level of the urethrovesical junction and anchored to the fibromuscular tissue of the underside of the pubic ramus bilaterally. The bladder neck is elevated when these sutures are tied. The cystocele is then reduced by placement of a series of plicating sutures along the bladder base.

through blunt and sharp technique. Care should be exercised not to overdissect the urethra while mobilizing this area. Doing so threatens to compromise the neurovascular supply of the urethra, which could produce scarring and rigidity of the urethra and predispose to poor function and closure pressure. In some patients, this step is unnecessary and may, in fact, destroy existing adequate urethral support.

To begin the reconstruction, the urethrovesical junction is elevated by placing plicating sutures into the paraurethral tissues. The fibromuscular tissue of the posteroinferior aspect of the pubic symphysis is grasped with an Allis clamp bilaterally. Traction on the Allis clamp will give immediate information about the integrity of the tissue as judged by the amount of resistance detected. Access to this tissue is through the paraurethral spaces previously dissected. Utilizing 0 or 2-0 polyglycolic acid suture material, a large bite of the tissue within the Allis clamp is taken with the needle on one side, attached to the pubourethral tissues in the midline at the level of the urethrovesical junction, and finally secured to the opposite side through the corresponding tissue marked by the other Allis clamp (Fig. 17–5). As this suture is tied, the urethrovesical junction is slowly elevated and maintained in this position. Judgment is required at this point to determine whether a second similar stitch is needed to further support the bladder neck.

Once the urethrovesical junction is supported, the cystocele is reduced by plicating the attenuated pubovesical fascia (bladder capsule) in the midline using interrupted 2-0 polyglycolic acid sutures (Fig. 17–6). This technique obliterates the cystocele and requires careful judgment. One does not want to overcorrect the cystocele by elevating the bladder too

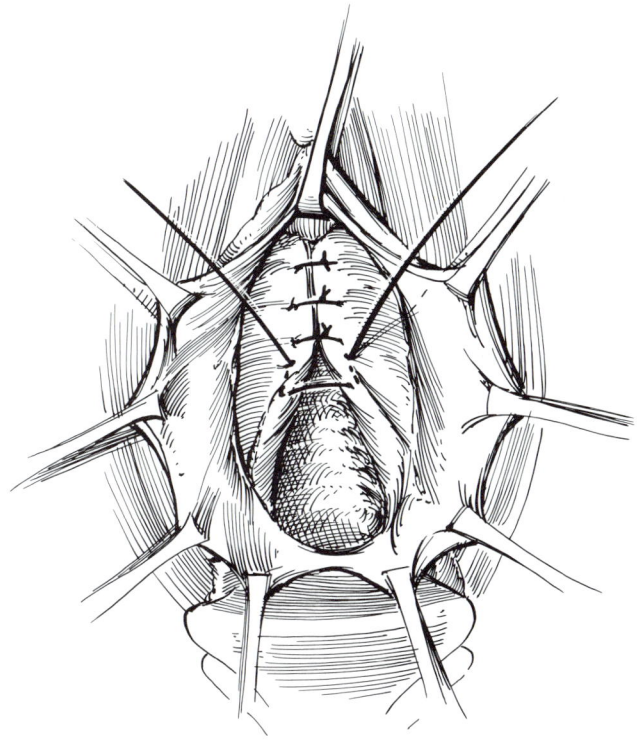

Figure 17–6
The pubovesical fascia is plicated to the midline, reducing the cystocele.

high. Particularly in the face of coexistent stress urinary incontinence, the urethra must be differentially better supported than the bladder base in order to correct the incontinence. Finally, the redundant vaginal mucosa is trimmed and the edges reapproximated with a continuous 3-0 suture (Fig. 17–7). After the operation, bladder drainage is accomplished either transurethrally or suprapubically, depending on the surgeon's preference. A vaginal pack is generally placed and then removed after approximately 24 hours.

The complications that can occur during anterior colporrhaphy are few when care is taken and adequate knowledge of regional anatomy is applied. Occasionally, a vesical laceration occurs. Once recognized, its margins should be noted and the defect immediately repaired. Closure is ideally in two or three layers using 3-0 absorbable material on the mucosa and 2-0 polyglycolic acid suture on the outer layers. If this injury does occur, bladder drainage should last 7–10 days. The integrity of the bladder repair can be evaluated by injecting a dilute solution of sterile infant formula into the bladder and observing whether there is any seepage of this whitish solution through the repair site.

Hemorrhage also can occur but is generally not a problem with careful dissection. Occasionally a vessel from the periurethral venous plexus bleeds, and although the blood flow can be brisk, hemostasis can be achieved by either suture-ligating the bleeding point or obliterating the dead space through closure of the vaginal mucosa.

Postoperative management of these patients is usually straightforward. The authors believe that the catheter should be left in place until the third postoperative day with continuous drainage. At that time, the patient has post-void residual urine volumes checked using the appropriate means. Once the residual volumes are below 100 ml, they are no longer monitored. If the patient develops postoperative urinary retention, the suprapubic catheter is reopened and a trial of voiding is periodically attempted until successful. The post-void residuals are checked until sufficiently low. If the postoperative urinary retention follows use of a transurethral catheter, the patient is taught the technique of intermittent self-catheterization and discharged home. A prophylactic dose of an oral antibiotic effective against urinary pathogens should be prescribed for as long as the patient is using the catheter. The patient continues self-catheterization until she is voiding spontaneously with acceptably low residual urine volumes.

RECTOCELE AND REPAIR

Rectocele is a protrusion of the rectum and posterior vaginal wall into the vaginal lumen. Rectocele is often a late consequence of childbirth injury, in which the musculofascial supports of the rectovaginal septum tear and separate, allowing the levator ani muscle bundles to retract laterally. The result of such damage is the thinning and weakening of the posterior vaginal wall support. With repetitive increases in intra-abdominal pressure during times of upright posture or while straining to defecate, the rectal contents no longer are deflected towards the anus, but rather protrude through the weakened rectovaginal septum into the posterior vaginal lumen.

Rectocele may occur along varying sites of the posterior vaginal wall and thus is referred to as low, mid, or high. The low rectocele may or may not be associated with a deficient perineal body, and either of these entities may result from failure to repair an obstetric laceration. The gaping of the lower vagina and introitus is seen with the avulsion and retraction of the bulbocavernosus and levator ani muscles from their usual attachments to the perineal body.

Mid-site rectocele, probably the most common type, is also the delayed product of tissue injury suffered during parturition. Unlike a low rectocele, a mid-vaginal defect is less likely due to separation of the levator ani and more likely the consequence of damage to the supporting rectovaginal septum. This rectocele type is more likely to cause symptoms, particularly abnormal bowel function.

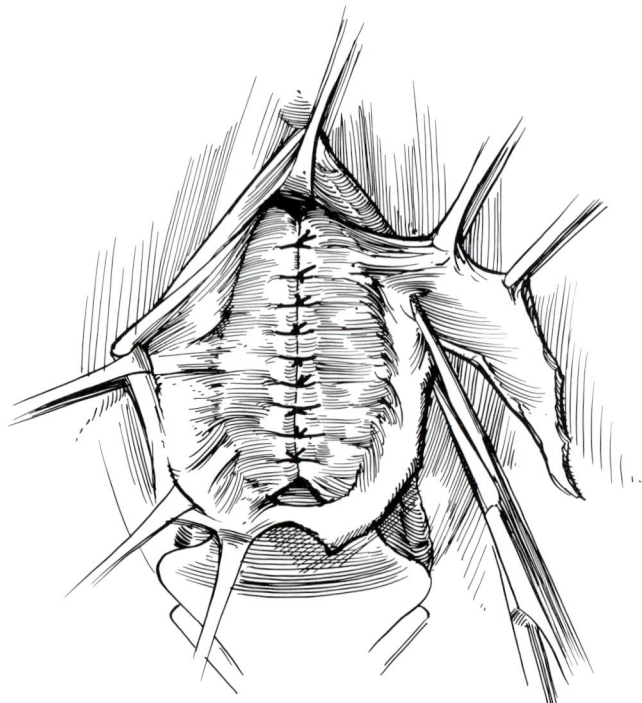

Figure 17–7
Redundant vaginal mucosa is trimmed and the incision then closed.

High rectocele is the bulging of the rectum into the upper vaginal wall. The pathogenesis may be marked overdistention of the upper vagina during labor or the traction effects of a prolapsing uterus. High rectocele often coexists with an enterocele, and the clinical distinction of the two is important but not always easy.

Small rectoceles will most times be asymptomatic. In the case of the larger defects, the predominant symptoms relate to altered bowel function. As the posterior vaginal wall defect enlarges, an abnormal pocket forms and fecal material fails to pass directly towards the anus. Instead, stool is forced into the rectocele pouch and the patient may find herself applying digital counterpressure to the posterior vagina in order to redirect the stool. If the rectocele is large enough, the patient may complain of a pressure sensation or a feeling of having to bear down. These specific sensations are often amplified while upright, owing to the added gravitational force bearing upon the prolapse. Like any vaginal defect that is severe enough to cause protrusion beyond the introitus, mucosal irritation and possibly ulceration may occur and lead to complaints of pain and/or bleeding.

The diagnosis of rectocele is generally made by inspection. While the patient is in the dorsal lithotomy position, the anterior vaginal wall is retracted using a Sims speculum and the rectocele is seen as a protrusion of the posterior vagina. During a cough or Valsalva maneuver, the rectocele is usually accentuated. A rectovaginal examination allows palpation of the defective area, and with gentle upward pressure of the rectal finger, the rectocele pocket is demonstrated. At times, distinguishing between a high rectocele and an enterocele is difficult and may necessitate examination of the patient in an upright position as well. Although somewhat awkward and perhaps embarrassing for the patient at first, a rectovaginal examination while the patient stands with legs parted and one foot elevated on a low stool proves invaluable at times in diagnosing coexistent enterocele and rectocele. The rectal and vaginal examining fingers are gently inserted to the top of the vagina and opposed while slowly withdrawing towards the introitus. The patient is asked to bear down. If an enterocele is present, the enterocele sac and its bowel contents can be felt slipping between the examiner's fingers.

It is essential to examine the patient in the unanesthetized state when normal muscular tone is present. Only then are the exact anatomic relationships of the pelvis unaltered, allowing a more accurate assessment of posterior vaginal support and vaginal and introital caliber. Clear operative objectives can be established as a result. However, even with such exact objectives established, TeLinde reminds us that there is great variation in the defects of the posterior vagina, necessitating flexibility and individualization intraoperatively when correcting these defects.[24]

Technique of Posterior Colporrhaphy

Whether the posterior colporrhaphy is to also include a perineorrhaphy will dictate the configuration of the initial incision. In either case, a thoughtful assessment of the existing caliber of the vaginal introitus is important. If the postoperative caliber is to be smaller, care must be taken not to overconstrict the introitus. As a basic guide to the appropriate caliber, the ultimate vaginal orifice should comfortably admit three fingers.

To delineate the lateral margins of the initial incision, Allis clamps are placed at the lateral aspects of the upper perineal body at the mucocutaneous junction. These clamps are then brought together in the midline to simulate a new introital diameter, and the examiner's fingers are inserted to test for proper size. To initiate a posterior colporrhaphy without perineorrhaphy, a horizontal incision through the skin of the perineal body is made, connecting the points marked by the Allis clamps (Fig. 17–8). The rectovaginal space is entered by dissecting parallel to and between the rectum and posterior vagina. Initially, sharp dissection is required, particularly if the lower vagina and perineum are scarred from previous surgery or obstetric laceration. Once the dissection extends above the level of scar tissue, the rectovaginal space is usually easily developed using blunt technique (Fig. 17–9). This potential space now developed should be relatively avascular and free of any major neurovascular structures. If adhesions

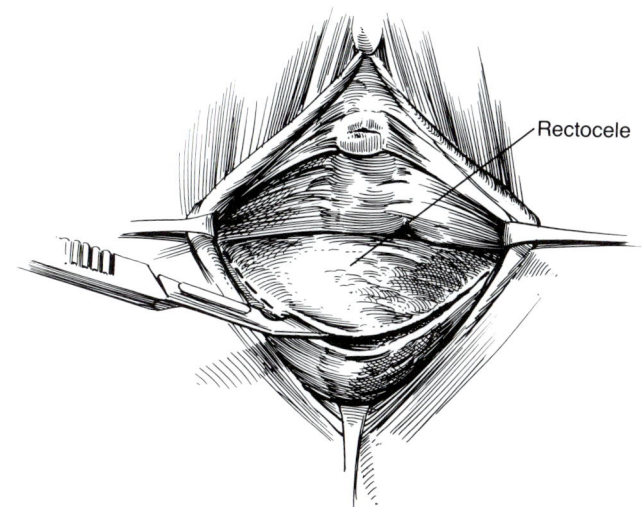

Figure 17–8
The rectocele repair is initiated by incising the skin of the perineal body along the mucocutaneous junction.

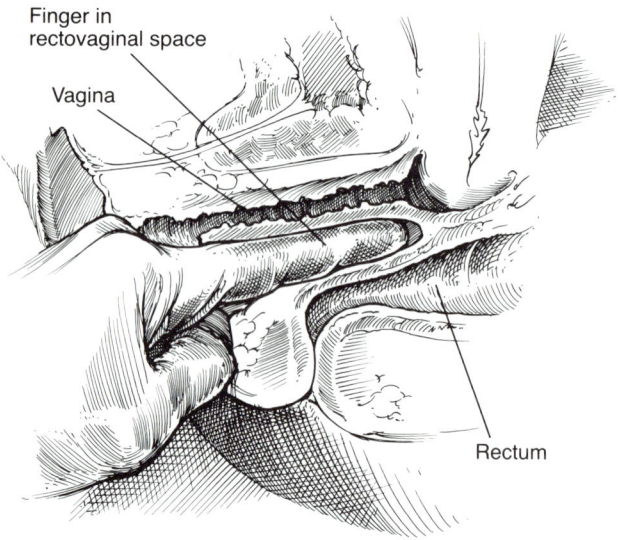

Figure 17–9
The rectovaginal space is bluntly developed once any scar tissue has been incised. The space is developed to a point above the site of the rectocele.

exist between the posterior vaginal wall and the anterior rectum, careful sharp dissection is necessary. The anterior rectal wall may be abnormally thinned in these areas of scar tissue. Therefore, if any doubt exists regarding cleavage planes, the surgeon's doubly gloved finger should be inserted into the rectum to help guide the dissection and to help avoid inadvertent puncture of the rectum.

Following the opening of the rectovaginal space to a point well above the rectocele, the full thickness of the posterior vaginal wall is transected along the midline. The tissue incised will include the vaginal mucosa and subtissues, along with the fused connective tissue of the rectovaginal septum. The posterior vaginal wall should be opened adequately along its length to correspond with the level to which the rectovaginal space was opened. The next step is to further open the rectovaginal space bilaterally using the necessary blunt and sharp technique to clearly expose the perirectal fascial tissues (Fig. 17–10). In the event of a high rectocele or coexistent enterocele, the attachment of the upper vagina to the posterior cul-de-sac peritoneum may need to be transected and the cul-de-sac entered. As described later in this text, this step allows the surgeon to identify the uterosacral ligaments for possible inclusion into the repair. The lateral margins of the lower vaginal cut edge may need to be separated sharply from the underlying levator ani (pubococcygeus) muscles bilaterally. This step is important and allows the perineal body to be built up by plicating the levators to the midline in this region prior to closing the vaginal mucosa.

Now that the operative field is fully dissected, reduction of the rectocele begins by approximating the perirectal fascia over the rectum from side to side. Using delayed-absorbable 0 or 2-0 suture material, a generous bite of perirectal fascia is taken on opposite sides of the rectum and tied in the midline using simple or mattress type interrupted sutures (Fig. 17–11). This plication of the fascia begins at the superior limit of the exposed tissue, and the rectum is depressed in the midline by the operative assistant while the surgeon ties. Care is taken not to strangulate the tissue or to create tension on the knots. Doing so may lead to tissue necrosis and excessive scarring. Jeffcoate cautioned that the rigidity that often results from such scarring may lead to dyspareunia and even complete avoidance of sexual intercourse owing to severe pain.[37] When this error is recognized, the involved sutures should immediately be removed and replaced, incorporating smaller amounts of tissue in order to avoid the creation of an artificial shelf of tissue held together by overly taut sutures.

The perirectal fascia is plicated in the midline over the rectum throughout its entire length. Only then should the amount of excess posterior vaginal mucosa be determined and excised. If this estimation is done before the rectocele is reduced by plicating the perirectal fascia, there exists the risk of excising too much mucosa, which may lead to undesirable narrowing of the vaginal vault.

Prior to closure of the vaginal mucosa, the perineal body is assessed and, if in need of support, the levators can be plicated to the midline using one or

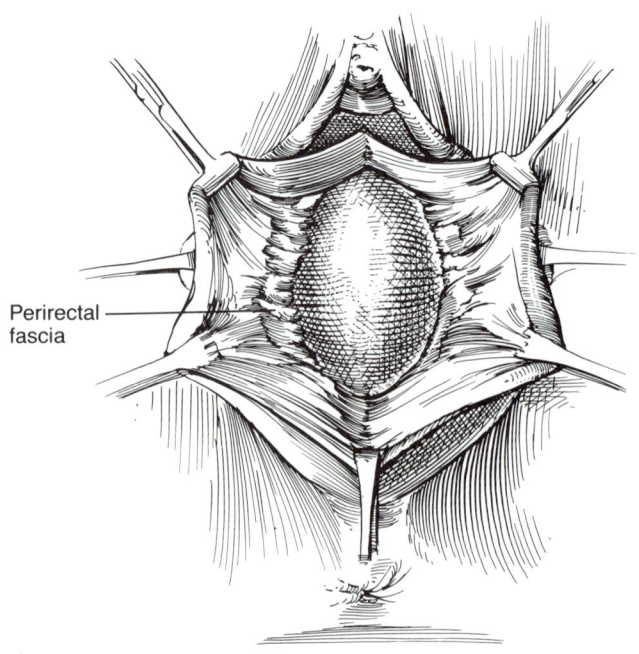

Figure 17–10
The posterior vaginal wall and rectovaginal septum are incised and reflected. The underlying rectum and perirectal fascia are exposed.

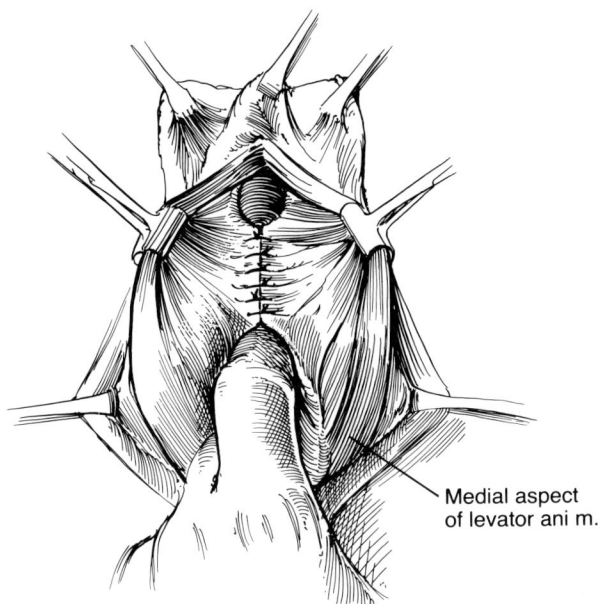

Figure 17–11
The rectocele is reduced by plicating the perirectal fascia to the midline. As the distal vagina is reached, the medial bodies of the levator ani are incorporated into the plicated tissues for additional support.

two interrupted sutures. The posterior vaginal mucosa is then closed using a running, nonlocked suture of 2-0 delayed-absorbable material (Fig. 17–12). While closing the posterior vaginal incision, the temptation to include the perirectal fascial layer into the mucosal closure should be avoided. Although it is argued that doing so closes any "dead space," it is precisely that space which should be maintained to allow the rectum and vagina to independently move upon each other during their separate functions. Lastly, the perineal incision is closed using a subcuticular stitch of fine delayed-absorbable suture material.

Technique of Perineorrhaphy

Deficiencies of the perineal body are often visualized as a gaping introitus and at times may appear as a low rectocele. Defects in the perineal body result from obstetric injury or poorly repaired lacerations or episiotomies. Correcting the deficient perineal body at the same time as other relaxation defects are repaired is essential, because adequate support of the perineal body contributes to the overall integrity of not only the lower posterior vagina and anus, but also the anterior vaginal wall and urethra. Recalling previous anatomic descriptions, the perineal body, along with the vagina, urethra, and rectum, receives portions of muscle fibers from the medial aspect of the levator ani. Re-establishing support to a gaping perineal body adds overall strength to surrounding structures and improves repairs to other areas of relaxation.

Perineorrhaphy begins by creating a triangular incision of the perineal skin. The skin is then raised and excised, exposing the underlying connective tissue. The posterior vaginal mucosa is freed in the area overlying the perineal body. Sharp technique is usually required, owing to scar tissue, which is commonly present. Mobilization of the perineal body bilaterally is often necessary in order to identify and locate the detached muscle bundles of the levator ani, transverse perinei, and bulbocavernosus.

Once dissection is complete, reconstruction of the superior portion of the perineal body is achieved by plicating the medial margins of the levator ani to the midline, utilizing interrupted sutures through the medial aspects or fascia of the muscle. Care should be taken to tie these sutures so as to loosely approximate the tissue to avoid necrosis. The perineal body is now further supported by approximating the identified separated ends of the transverse perinei and bulbocavernosus muscles using interrupted sutures. The more superficial connective and smooth muscle tissues of the perineal body are reapproximated in the midline with a running or interrupted fine suture.

Any redundant mucosa of the lower posterior vagina is now excised. The mucosa is then reapproximated using an absorbable fine suture. Finally, the perineal skin is closed using a fine subcuticular stitch.

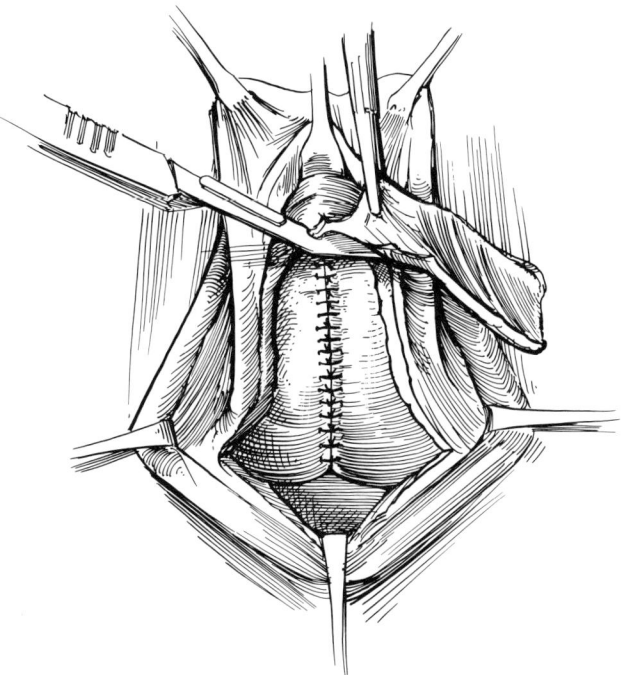

Figure 17–12
Excess vaginal mucosa is excised from the posterior vagina, and the vaginal incision is closed.

ENTEROCELE AND REPAIR

Enterocele is a herniation of the posterior cul-de-sac peritoneum into the rectovaginal space. Enterocele may occur as an isolated defect, although it can be accompanied by cystocele and rectocele. Enterocele is always present when significant uterine prolapse exists as a result of the traction forces upon the posterior cul-de-sac. Vaginal vault prolapse may or may not coexist with enterocele.

Being true hernias, all enteroceles characteristically are covered on their cephalad surface by peritoneum, whereas the caudad surface is vaginal mucosa. Enteroceles are typically classified as traction or pulsion, depending on the etiologic mechanism. Traction enterocele is associated with the prolapse of other pelvic organs as a result of the primary failure of upper vaginal and uterine support structures. Pulsion enterocele occurs most frequently as a late complication following hysterectomy. It involves pronounced damage to the upper vaginal support apparatus and is more commonly related to chronically elevated intra-abdominal pressure.

Etiologic factors leading to enterocele formation are several and are not unlike those associated with other forms of genital prolapse. Aside from a congenitally deep cul-de-sac, these etiologic factors include multiparity, obesity, and estrogen deficiency.

One cannot discuss the etiology of enterocele without devoting some comments to its prevention. It is commonly thought that the most frequent cause of posthysterectomy enterocele formation is failure to adequately obliterate the posterior cul-de-sac, either because pre-existing relaxation of this area is not recognized or the importance of closing the redundant tissue is overlooked.[24, 38, 39] Anytime hysterectomy or a procedure to correct genital prolapse is performed, the cul-de-sac should be thoughtfully assessed. If a deep defect is noted, even in the absence of symptoms referable to the area, preventive obliteration should be considered. Techniques for closing this area have been described. They include the McCall culdeplasty,[40] useful during vaginal cases; and the Moschowitz procedure,[41] which can be employed during abdominal surgery.

Another situation that requires approaching enterocele from a preventive perspective is the case of the surgical procedure that alters the axis of the vagina and thereby exposes the posterior cul-de-sac to greater pressure forces. Certain retropubic urethropexy procedures alter the vaginal axis by displacing it anteriorly to varying degrees. Burch helped to sensitize the gynecologic surgeon to this problem in his report of retropubic urethropexy using Cooper's ligament as a point of fixation.[42] In that report, 7.6% of patients treated with a Burch procedure developed postoperative enterocele, leading the author to advocate exploration of the posterior cul-de-sac and obliteration when indicated. That opinion has since been corroborated.[38] It therefore seems logical to consider taking specific intraoperative measures to obliterate the posterior cul-de-sac when performing abdominal approach urethropexy.

Diagnosing enterocele is not always easy. The first step is to suspect enterocele any time a posterior vaginal defect is either large or located high on the vaginal wall, perhaps even involving the apex. The time to diagnose an enterocele is preoperatively when the patient is awake and can be examined while erect. Distinguishing between a high rectocele and an enterocele is critically important, because the surgical approach to each is different. Even with this comment in mind, the preoperative distinction is not always possible. However, to help determine whether an enterocele is present, a rectovaginal examination is performed while the patient is standing, according to the technique described earlier in this chapter.

The signs and symptoms of enterocele overlap considerably with those seen in other prolapse disorders. These complaints and findings have been outlined earlier in this chapter. The pressure and bearing-down sensation experienced by women with prolapse may be accentuated with enterocele. This is felt to be due to drag on the bowel contents of the hernia sac and the stretch on the mesentery.[2]

Technique of Enterocele Repair

It has been pointed out that correction of a small enterocele encountered at the time of hysterectomy is important and may prevent subsequent formation of a larger symptomatic enterocele. In this situation, the techniques of McCall[40] or Moschowitz[41] may be employed if it is judged that the size of the enterocele does not warrant isolation and excision of the hernia sac. If, however, the enterocele is larger, the peritoneal sac must be carefully dissected away from the vaginal wall. Once the sac has been isolated, a pursestring ligature of delayed-absorbable or permanent suture is placed high on the inner surface of the sac and tied down to ligate the hernia sac's neck (Fig. 17–13). Preferably, a second ligature is used to help distribute the pressure over a larger area. If the upper portion of the uterosacral ligaments can be identified, they should be incorporated into the pursestring sutures. Care should be exercised to avoid occlusion or angulation of the closely juxtaposed ureters running lateral to the uterosacral ligaments at this level.

Larger pulsion enteroceles following hysterectomy can be repaired vaginally. In this case, the posterior vaginal wall is opened in a manner similarly

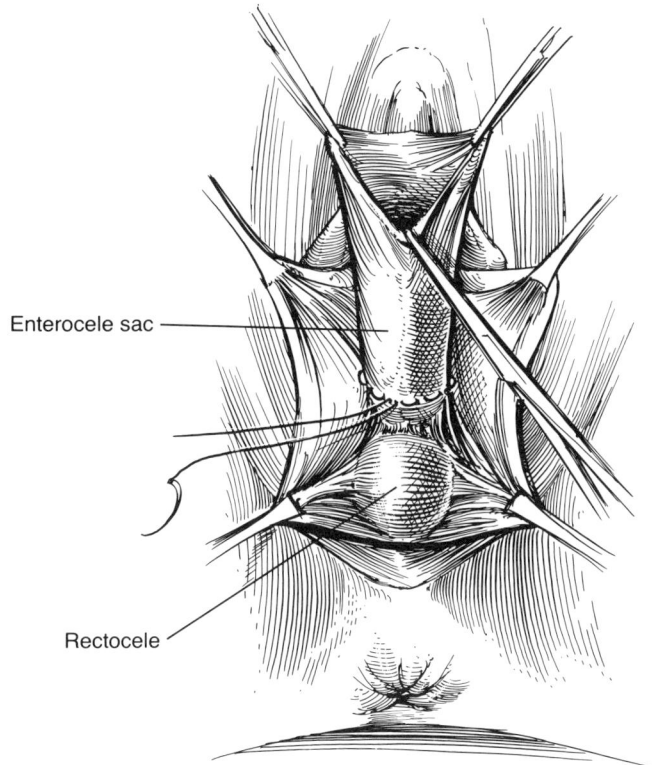

Figure 17–13
Enterocele repair involves opening the posterior vaginal wall much as is done during rectocele repair. The enterocele sac is then dissected free, opened, and its base ligated, taking care to avoid incorporating the bowel into the suture.

described for posterior colporrhaphy. The posterior vaginal wall is opened all the way to the apex. The enterocele sac is isolated, opened, and ligated as described earlier. If possible, the remnants of the cardinal and uterosacral ligaments are identified distal to the closed enterocele sac and plicated to the midline to further support the vaginal apex. Any coexistent rectocele is then reduced, and the posterior vaginal closure proceeds as for posterior colporrhaphy.

An alternative approach, and the one favored by the authors, is to begin the procedure by drawing the enterocele defect to the introitus using Allis clamps. The overlying vaginal mucosa is incised in a cruciate fashion, dissecting the vaginal mucosa back both anteriorly and posteriorly until the enterocele sac is identified. By careful dissection laterally and cephalad, the attenuated uterosacral ligaments can be identified on the inner surface of the vaginal wall. Sutures are placed through the upper portion of these ligaments and held. Again, care should be taken to avoid incorporating the ureters in these sutures. Further dissection is undertaken to free the enterocele sac. Once isolated, it is entered and a high ligation performed using pursestring sutures. After the sac has been ligated, the remaining posterior vaginal wall is opened. The tagged uterosacral ligament sutures are then tied in the midline. The enterocele sac has now been obliterated and the vaginal apex further supported below the defect. Rectocele repair and perineorrhaphy are then completed as indicated.

Large enterocele defects associated with vaginal eversion can be corrected by similar means or by utilizing the sacrospinous ligament fixation or abdominal sacral colpopexy procedures described later in this chapter. In addition, Zacharin and Hamilton achieved excellent curative results with an extensive abdominoperineal procedure, as treatment for severe pulsion enterocele.[43] All of these approaches have merit, and long-term success rates have been excellent.

VAGINAL VAULT PROLAPSE AND REPAIR

Prolapse of the vaginal vault or vaginal eversion is a complex and uncommon disorder. Incidence rates are not well established. Published reports help estimate that vaginal eversion occurs far less than 1% of the time following major gynecologic procedures.[44–46]

The degree of vaginal prolapse may be incomplete or complete. With the former, the vaginal apex is at or above the introitus; the latter represents prolapse of the apex beyond the introitus. Vaginal eversion may occur singularly, in which case there is always an enterocele behind the prolapsed vault. Alternatively, cystocele and/or rectocele may coexist. Determining the entire extent of pelvic defects is essential to the planning and optimization of reparative surgery. Examination of the patient should occur while the patient is awake, and inspection of the vagina is performed while the patient is first supine, then erect. By supporting the vaginal apex, the vagina can be examined for the presence of cystocele and rectocele. In addition, appropriate testing to document or exclude the presence of stress urinary incontinence is important, because this problem often coexists in the face of massive pelvic relaxation.

Women with vaginal eversion bear complaints similar to those found with other prolapse defects. They may note problems with pelvic pressure or difficulties with bowel or urinary function. Discomfort from vaginal tissues protruding through the introitus is common.[38] Inquiring about a previous history of untreated stress urinary incontinence is important, because following the surgical repositioning of the vaginal apex, recurrent stress incontinence may occur. Ideally, if stress urinary incontinence is detected preoperatively, added measures can be taken to correct the incontinence with some form of urethropexy.

Multiple procedures have been described to treat vaginal eversion. In 1976, Ridley reported that at least 40 operations had been described to address this malady, and that "no one surgical procedure has yet been fully accepted as satisfactory enough to exclude all others."[47] This remains true today. Currently, the operations for treating vaginal vault prolapse can generally be categorized as either obliterative or reconstructive.

Obliterative procedures, although more commonly performed in the past, remain an appropriate surgical choice in some patients. In general, the decision to perform such a procedure must be made only after thorough discussion of the patient's attitudes and desires, along with careful consideration of the patient's age, symptoms, and general health status. A full discussion of obliterative procedures such as partial or complete colpocleisis is found later in this text.

Along with the emergence of a greater sensitivity towards geriatric health issues has been a candor regarding the importance of preserving sexuality and vaginal function in the woman. Birnbaum has been one champion of these important concerns, and along with others supported the reconstructive approach to correcting the prolapsed vaginal vault.[46, 48-50] Earlier reconstructive techniques have included resuspension of the vaginal vault using the uterosacral ligaments,[45, 51] or by attaching the vaginal apex to the anterior abdominal wall.[47] Two reconstructive procedures commonly used today are the sacrospinous ligament fixation and the abdominal sacral colpopexy. Each of these procedures has its variations. In the case of the sacrospinous ligament fixation, the differences lie in the described technique and to some extent the suture material most often used.[52-54] The abdominal sacral colpopexy also has its variations in technique.[46, 55, 56] Differences also exist in the material used to attach the vaginal apex to the sacrum. These materials have been both naturally occurring and synthetic and include rectus muscle fascia,[57, 58] dura mater,[59] Teflon,[46, 60] Mersilene,[50] Marlex,[56] and Gore-Tex.[61]

Both the sacrospinous ligament suspension and the abdominal sacral colpopexy procedures have associated advantages and disadvantages. Irrespective of the technique employed, the challenge and goals of the surgical treatment for vaginal eversion are to relieve symptoms, to re-establish a coitally functional vagina by restoring adequate vaginal length and a normal vaginal axis, and to produce a long-lasting repair.

Technique of Sacrospinous Ligament Suspension

The sacrospinous ligament fixation operation was introduced and later popularized in the United States by Randall and Nichols[48] after earlier being described in Europe.[62] The procedure involves fixation of the vaginal apex directly to the coccygeus muscle–sacrospinous ligament complex. Of necessity, the vaginal vault must be of adequate length to reach this complex. Suspension can be either unilateral or bilateral, but experience has shown that one-sided attachments suffice. Generally, the right sacrospinous ligament is used, owing to the greater ease for the right-handed surgeon. The technique described herein has been previously detailed by Morley and DeLancey.[53]

The patient is adequately anesthetized, positioned, and prepped. The dimpled corners of the everted vaginal apex are identified and grasped with Allis clamps. The overall extent of prolapse and an estimation of desired length for the reconstructed vagina are determined. The limits of the "new" vaginal apex can be demarcated with additional Allis clamps followed by a delineating circumferential incision through the vaginal mucosa. Care is required to avoid overly excising the excess vaginal length. The final length should allow the vagina to easily reach the sacrospinous ligament without creating tension on the organ.

Once the apical incision is made, the underlying enterocele sac is dissected free, utilizing both blunt and sharp technique. The right sacrospinous ligament is then palpated through the vaginal mucosa, and the dissection is continued retroperitoneal toward the ligament in a posterolateral direction. Blunt dissection generally suffices, and overexuberance should be avoided to minimize the chance of traumatizing vascular structures in this area. Maintaining an intact enterocele sac with its overlying vaginal mucosa may help with retraction of these tissues during the retroperitoneal dissection.

The sacrospinous ligament is within the body of the coccygeus muscle, and it often fuses with the sacrotuberous ligament along its medial half. The ligament is firm and extends from the laterally palpable ischial spine medially to the sacrum. Directly beneath the ischial spine are the pudendal vessels and nerve, and the sciatic nerve is closely juxtaposed. Knowledge of these anatomic relationships is critical in avoiding trauma to them during the placement of the sacrospinous ligament stitches.

Precise placement of the ligament sutures is aided by establishing a reference point on the ligament. To achieve this, the right ischial spine is palpated with the left hand. At a point approximately two fingerbreadths medial to the spine, a long Allis clamp is placed on but not around the ligament. Traction on the clamp confirms proper placement, because firm resistance will be met. Using two or three medium-sized retractors, the ligament and attached Allis clamp are carefully exposed. Two long, swaged-on, No. 1, delayed-absorbable sutures are placed through the sacrospinous ligament near the Allis clamp. Again, so as to avoid trauma to surrounding vascular and nervous structures, care must be taken to place the sutures through and not around the ligament. With adequate exposure, suture placement can be safely executed with a long straight or curved needle driver. The suture ends are brought out through the vagina and tagged.

The enterocele sac is then opened and further isolated up to the neck of the sac. The neck of the sac is then closed using two pursestring sutures of permanent or delayed-absorbable material. The excess peritoneal tissue and overlying vaginal mucosa are excised. An anterior colporrhaphy is now performed if a cystocele coexists. Excising the excess vaginal mucosa as part of the colporrhaphy helps to narrow an overly wide upper vaginal vault.

To complete the sacrospinous ligament suspension, the upper free margin of the new vaginal apex is whipstitched with an absorbable suture. This also helps to narrow the caliber of the upper vagina. The ends of the sacrospinous sutures are now attached to the upper vagina with through-and-through placement. The vaginal apex is resuspended by tying the sutures, which slowly draws the apex toward the ligament. To maximize the durability of the repair, the vaginal apex must come into contact with the sacrospinous ligament. Contact with the ligament and prevention of a suture bridge between tissues allow fibrosis to develop, thus maintaining the vaginal apex in a suspended position. Immediately following suspension of the apex, the vagina is noted to be slightly deviated to the right. This fact is of no consequence.

Finally, if a rectocele or deficient perineal body is present, a posterior colporrhaphy and appropriate repair are performed. A vaginal pack is used for 48 hours along with the operator's choice of bladder drainage.

Technique of Abdominal Sacral Colpopexy

Following the induction of satisfactory anesthesia, the patient is prepared for surgery by placing her supine on the operating table with her legs positioned so as to allow simultaneous access to the abdomen and vagina. Sterile prepping and draping must include the abdomen, upper thighs, vulva, and vagina. An indwelling urinary catheter is inserted.

The entire extent of pelvic relaxation is reassessed to confirm the preoperative impression. If a significant cystocele or rectocele is present, the appropriate colporrhaphy procedure(s) is performed at this time. Waiting until after the abdominal sacral colpopexy is done before performing the necessary vaginal procedures may markedly limit exposure to the upper vagina, risking inadequacy of the vaginal repair.

The lower abdomen is opened through either a midline or a transverse incision. The pelvis is explored, and the bowel is packed out of the pelvis. A self-retaining retractor will generally prove useful. Prior to opening the abdomen, it is helpful to distend the vagina with vaginal packing or a firm stent, such as a large Hegar cervical dilator. The latter not only will help to identify and manipulate the vaginal apex, but also will eliminate the possibility of inadvertently incorporating a soft vaginal pack into the sutures that are later placed into this area.

Once the upper vagina is identified, the corners are grasped with Allis clamps and put on stretch. Carefully, a transverse peritoneal incision is made and the bladder is reflected anteriorly and the rectum posteriorly. An area of approximately 3–4 cm of vagina is exposed and denuded of peritoneum. This is the area to which the bridging material will be sewn.

The cul-de-sac is now obliterated using the culdeplastic technique of Moschowitz.[41] Care must be taken not to kink or otherwise compromise the ureters during placement of the culdeplasty sutures. Also, closure must be meticulous enough to prevent the bowel from dissecting into any small defects caused by incomplete closure of the cul-de-sac. Failure to perform adequate culdeplasty has been felt to contribute to failed sacral colpopexy.[63]

Following the culdeplasty, the overlying peritoneum of the sacrum is incised in the midline and parallel to the rectosigmoid mesentery. The incision should extend from the sacral promontory to the area of the culdeplasty. The sigmoid colon is now retracted to the left, and the anterior sacral ligament is exposed. Cautious dissection will help avoid trauma to nearby vessels and nerves as well as the ureter, which lies lateral to the incision.

Approximately four to six anchoring sutures of 2-0 monofilament permanent material are placed into the vagina, each one incorporating a double bite of full-thickness tissue. Using the same suture material, four stitches are transversely placed into the sacral ligament at the level of the S2–S3 vertebrae. A sterile segment of either Mersilene or Gore-Tex synthetic material is fashioned. Its approximate dimensions should be 2.5 × 12–14 cm. The bridging material is first secured to the upper vagina by placing the previously positioned sutures through the synthetic material and tying them down. The sacral sutures are then secured to the material and tied down. The length of material used should hold the upper vagina in an elevated position, while lying in the hollow of the sacrum free of tension. Excess tension on the strap of material may lead to failure as a result of pulling away of the vaginal apex. Tension may also overly flatten the anterior vaginal wall, which may predispose the patient to postoperative stress urinary incontinence.

Now that the vaginal vault has been suspended, any excess synthetic material is excised and the synthetic bridge is extraperitonealized by closing the peritoneal defects with a running stitch of absorbable material. If stress urinary incontinence was documented preoperatively, a retropubic urethropexy can be accomplished at this time.

CONCLUSION

In considering the surgical treatment of pelvic relaxation, one must remain mindful of several important points. Prolapse disorders as a group are characterized by heterogeneity. Consequently, what naturally follows is that surgical treatment must be individualized. This individualization involves repairing all of the specific anatomic support defects, as well as bearing in mind the individual patient and her needs as the process of repair and reconstruction is undertaken. To be effective and safe in the operative treatment of genital prolapse, a complete understanding of normal pelvic anatomy and support is necessary. Finally, the pelvic surgeon's operative armamentarium should be broad enough to allow him or her to capably tailor the surgery precisely and comprehensively, according to the constellation of findings in any given patient.

References

1. Emge LA, Durfee RB: Pelvic organ prolapse: Four thousand years of treatment. Clin Obstet Gynecol 1966; 9:997.
2. Nichols DH, Randall CL: Vaginal Surgery. Baltimore, Williams & Wilkins, 1989.
3. Krantz KE: The human vagina. J Clin Prac Sexual, special ed., 1990.
4. Bonney V: The sustentacular apparatus of the female genital canal, the displacements that result from the yielding of its several components, and their appropriate treatment. J Obstet Gynaec Br Emp 1914; 45:328.
5. Mengert WF: Mechanics of uterine support and position. Am J Obstet Gynecol 1936; 31:775.
6. Range RL, Woodburne RT: The gross and microscopic anatomy of the transverse cervical ligament. Am J Obstet Gynecol 1964; 90:460.
7. Campbell RM: The anatomy and histology of the sacrouterine ligaments. Am J Obstet Gynecol 1950; 59:1.
8. Dickinson RL: Studies of the levator ani muscle. Am J Obstet 1889; 22:897.
9. Berglas B, Rubin EC: Study of the supportive structures of the uterus by levator myography. Surg Gynecol Obstet 1953; 97:677.
10. Nichols DH, Milley PS, Randall CL: Significance of restoration of normal vaginal depth and axis. Obstet Gynecol 1970; 36:251.
11. Funt MI, Thompson JD, Birch H: Normal vaginal axis. South Med J 1978; 71:1534.
12. DeLancey JOL, Starr RA: Histology of the connection between the vagina and levator ani muscles. J Reprod Med 1990; 35:765.
13. Lawson JON: Pelvic anatomy. Ann R Coll Surg Eng 1974; 54:244.
14. Parks AG, Porter NG, Melzak J: Experimental study of the relaxation mechanism controlling muscles of the pelvic floor. Dis Colon Rectum 1962; 5:407.
15. Oelrich TM: The striated urogenital sphincter muscle in the female. Anat Rec 1983; 205:223.
16. Curtis AH, Anson BJ, McVay CB: The anatomy of the pelvic and urogenital diaphragms, in relation to urethrocele and cystocele. Surg Gynecol Obstet 1939; 68:161.
17. Krantz KE: The anatomy of the urethra and anterior vaginal wall. Am J Obstet Gynecol 1951; 62:374.
18. Milley PS, Nichols DH: The relationship between the pubourethral ligaments and the urogenital diaphragm in the human female. Anat Rec 1971; 170:281.
19. Zacharin RF: The suspensory mechanism of the female urethra. J Anat 1963; 97:423.
20. DeLancey JOL: Correlative study of paraurethral anatomy. Obstet Gynecol 1986; 68:91.
21. Lansman HH: The statics of the female pelvic viscera. South Caribb J Obstet Gynecol Spring and Summer 1989, Vol. 5, Nos. 3 and 4.
22. Beecham CT: Classification of vaginal relaxation. Am J Obstet Gynecol 1980; 136:957.
23. Porges RF: A practical system of diagnosis and classification of pelvic relaxations. Surg Gynecol Obstet 1963; 117:769.
24. TeLinde RW: Prolapse of the uterus and allied conditions. Am J Obstet Gynecol 1966; 94:444.
25. Power RMH: The pelvic floor in parturition. Surg Gynecol Obstet 1946; 83:296.
26. Gainey HL: Postpartum observation of pelvic tissue damage. Am J Obstet Gynecol 1943; 45:457.
27. Willson JR: Prophylactic episiotomy to minimize soft tissue damage. Infect Surg, July 1987; 399.
28. Gainey HL: Postpartum observation of pelvic tissue damage: Further studies. Am J Obstet Gynecol 1955; 70:800.
29. Sharf B, Zilberman A, Sharf M, Mitrani A: Electromyogram of pelvic floor muscles in genital prolapse. Internat J Gynecol Obstet 1976; 14:2.
30. Smith ARB, Hosker GL, Warrell DW: The role of partial denervation of the pelvic floor in the aetiology of genitourinary prolapse and stress incontinence of urine. A neurophysiological study. Br J Obstet Gynaecol 1989; 96:24.
31. Beck RP: Pelvic relaxational prolapse. In Kase NG, Weingold AB (eds.): Principles and Practice of Clinical Gynecology. New York, John Wiley & Sons, 1983; pp. 677–685.
32. Harris TA, Bent AE: Genital prolapse with and without urinary incontinence. J Reprod Med 1990; 35:792.
33. Zacharin RF: The anatomic supports of the female urethra. Obstet Gynecol 1968; 32:754.
34. Richardson AC, Edmonds PB, Williams NL: Treatment of urinary incontinence due to paravaginal fascial defect. Obstet Gynecol 1981; 57:357.
35. Bergman A, Koonings PP, Ballard CA: Predicting postoperative urinary incontinence development in women undergoing operation for genitourinary prolapse. Am J Obstet Gynecol 1988; 158:1171.
36. Beck RP: Vaginal vs. abdominal surgery for genuine stress incontinence. Obstet Gynecol Rep 1990; 2:322.
37. Jeffcoate TNA: Posterior colpoperineorrhaphy. Am J Obstet Gynecol 1959; 77:490.
38. Addison WA, Livengood CH, Parker RT: Posthysterectomy vaginal vault prolapse with emphasis on management by transabdominal sacral colpopexy. Postgrad Obstet Gynecol 1988; 8:1.
39. Ranney B: Enterocele, vaginal prolapse, pelvic hernia: Recognition and treatment. Am J Obstet Gynecol 1981; 140:53.
40. McCall ML: Posterior culdeplasty: Surgical correction of enterocele during vaginal hysterectomy, a preliminary report. Obstet Gynecol 1957; 10:592.
41. Moschowitz AV: The pathogenesis, anatomy and cure of prolapse of the rectum. Surg Gynecol Obstet 1912; 15:7.
42. Burch JC: Cooper's ligament urethrovesical suspension for stress incontinence. Am J Obstet Gynecol 1968; 100:764.
43. Zacharin RF, Hamilton NT: Pulsion enterocele: Long-term results of an abdominoperineal technique. Obstet Gynecol 1980; 55:141.

44. Phaneuf LE: Inversion of the vagina and prolapse of the cervix following supracervical hysterectomy and inversion of the vagina following total hysterectomy. Am J Obstet Gynecol 1952; 64:739.
45. Symmonds RE, Pratt JH: Vaginal prolapse following hysterectomy. Am J Obstet Gynecol 1960; 79:899.
46. Birnbaum SJ: Rational therapy for the prolapsed vagina. Am J Obstet Gynecol 1973; 115:411.
47. Ridley JH: A composite vaginal vault suspension using fascia lata. Am J Obstet Gynecol 1976; 126:590.
48. Randall CL, Nichols DH: Surgical treatment of vaginal inversion. Obstet Gynecol 1971; 38:327.
49. Soichet S: Surgical correction of total genital prolapse with retention of sexual function. Obstet Gynecol 1970; 36:69.
50. Addison WA, Livengood CH, Sutton GP, Parker RT: Abdominal sacral colpopexy with Mersilene mesh in the retroperitoneal position in the management of posthysterectomy vaginal vault prolapse and enterocele. Am J Obstet Gynecol 1985; 153:140.
51. Miller NF: A new method of correcting complete inversion of the vagina. Surg Gynecol Obstet 1927; 44:550.
52. Nichols DH: Sacrospinous fixation for massive eversion of the vagina. Am J Obstet Gynecol 1982; 142:901.
53. Morley GW, DeLancey JOL: Sacrospinous ligament fixation for eversion of the vagina. Am J Obstet Gynecol 1988; 158:872.
54. Robertson E, Lansman HH: Vaginal prolapse repair with sacrospinous ligament fixation. Contemp Obstet Gynecol, May 1990; 71.
55. Robertson EG, Lansman HH: Sacral colpopexy with a dura mater graft. Contemp Obstet Gynecol, April 1990; 58.
56. Drutz HP, Cha LS: Massive genital and vaginal vault prolapse treated by abdominal-vaginal sacropexy with use of Marlex mesh: Review of the literature. Am J Obstet Gynecol 1987; 156:387.
57. Hendee AE, Berry CM: Abdominal sacropexy for vaginal vault prolapse. Clin Obstet Gynecol 1981; 24:1217.
58. Maloney JC, Dunton CJ, Smith K: Repair of vaginal vault prolapse with abdominal sacropexy. J Reprod Med 1990; 35:6.
59. Lansman HH: Posthysterectomy vault prolapse: Sacral colpopexy with dura mater graft. Obstet Gynecol 1984; 63:577.
60. Angulo A, Kligman I: Retroperitoneal sacrocolpopexy for correction of prolapse of vaginal vault. Surg Gynecol Obstet 1989; 169:319.
61. Hurt WG: Postreproductive Gynecology. New York, Churchill Livingstone, 1990, pp. 413–440.
62. Richter K: Die chirurgische anatomie der vaginaefixatio sacrospinalis vaginalis. Ein Beitrag zur operativen Bechandlung des Scheidenblindsach prolapses. Geburtshilfe Fravenheilkd 1968; 28:321.
63. Addison WA, Timmons MC, Wall LL, Livengood CH 3rd: Failed abdominal sacral colpopexy: Observations and recommendations. Obstet Gynecol 1989; 74:480.

Abdominal and Vaginal Hysterectomy

18

Raymond Lui

By virtue of sheer numbers, hysterectomy is an important health issue in the United States. Data collected from the National Hospital Discharge Survey reveal that it was the most common major surgery until 1981, when it was supplanted by the rising cesarean section rate.[1] The number of hysterectomies peaked in 1975 at 725,000. Since then, the annual number and rate have leveled off at about 650,000 per year or 7 per 1000 women, age 15 or more.

Uterine fibroids (27%), uterine prolapse (21%), endometriosis (15%), and cancer (11%) are the most common indications for hysterectomy.

ABDOMINAL VERSUS VAGINAL HYSTERECTOMY

Abdominal hysterectomy is performed three times more frequently than vaginal hysterectomy. The increased exposure that the abdominal approach offers makes it the preferred route in situations of a large pelvic mass, pelvic infection, malignancy, adnexal pathology, or evidence of extensive adhesive disease.

As one might expect, pelvic relaxation is a frequent indication for vaginal hysterectomy. Others include recurrent abnormal uterine bleeding unresponsive to hormones and dilation and curettage (D & C), small symptomatic leiomyomas, and cervical intraepithelial neoplasia in patients who have no interest in future pregnancy. When appropriately chosen, the vaginal route is preferred over the abdominal route because it is associated with fewer complications,[2] an easier and shorter convalescence, and lack of a visible scar.

PREOPERATIVE CONSIDERATIONS

History and Physical Examination

Prior to any surgery, a complete history and physical examination are mandatory. Particular attention is made not only to the gynecologic and obstetric history, but also to the parts of the gastrointestinal and urologic systems that are in the immediate operative field. Anesthesia considerations also require thorough inquiry about the patient's cardiorespiratory status and current usage of medications.

Physical examination is especially focused upon the lower abdominal and pelvic regions that are involved in surgery. The pelvic examination includes inspection of the vulva, vagina, and cervix. The uterus and adnexa are evaluated by bimanual and rectal examination for size, shape, and consistency. Again, the cardiorespiratory system needs full evaluation from both surgical and anesthesia perspectives.

Laboratory Evaluation

Laboratory evaluation is individualized, with the surgeon deciding which tests are indicated based upon the patient's age, history, and physical examination. Blood count and cytologic smear of the cervix are necessary, but all other tests, including chemistry panels, ECG, and sonographic studies, are ordered as deemed appropriate. Women 35 years of age or older with postmenopausal or abnormal uterine bleeding should undergo some type of endometrial sampling prior to their scheduled hysterectomy. However, routine endometrial sampling prior to hysterectomy to detect an unsuspected or asymptomatic endometrial carcinoma does not appear to be warranted.[3-5]

Autologous Blood

The possibility of blood transfusion is a reality for any patient undergoing major surgery. Transfusion-associated hepatitis is commonly estimated to occur in 5–10% of recipients. However, the true incidence is difficult to estimate accurately, because it may range from as low as 1% when reporting only clinically apparent cases to as high as 18% when reporting those individuals with abnormal liver function tests. Of even greater concern is the risk of transmission of the human immunodeficiency virus. At worst, the incidence of transfusion-related infection has been estimated at 1 in 250,000.[6] Other risks include that of alloimmunization, malaria, and cytomegalovirus transmission. Given these real concerns, the surgeon should consider the use of autologous blood transfusion. With predeposit autologous blood transfusion, blood is collected 72 hours to 6 months prior to surgery and then is reinfused into the same patient at a later time. When the guidelines established by the American Association of Blood Banks are followed, autologous transfusion is the safest type of blood transfusion.[7]

GnRH Agonists

Gonadotropin-releasing hormone (GnRH) agonists may be useful as a presurgical adjuvant agent in those individuals with large uterine leiomyomas. The agonists effectively create a hypoestrogenic state by reducing pituitary gonadotropin secretion, which then results in ovarian suppression.[8] Because leiomyoma growth is linked to ovarian hormone production, the use of GnRH agonists for 3–6 months has been found to be effective in reducing the mean uterine volume by 40–60%.[9-13] This decrease in size may make performance of the hysterectomy easier or perhaps allow one to perform a previously planned abdominal hysterectomy through the vaginal route.[14] In addition, the amenorrhea that accompanies successful GnRH agonist treatment will improve the anemia in those individuals with menometrorrhagia related to their leiomyomas. The improved blood count may also decrease the need for blood transfusion as well as permit the patient to participate in predeposit autologous blood donation. Operative blood loss may be decreased after treatment as well.[15]

The side effects of the medication are primarily related to the hypoestrogenic state. Almost all patients will experience vasomotor symptoms and amenorrhea. Other less common symptoms can include a decrease in breast size, vaginal spotting or dryness, decreased libido, and insomnia.[10,11] Generally, treatment with these agents is not recommended beyond 6 months, owing to concerns about the development of osteoporosis, but longer-term use has been studied.[16]

PROPHYLAXIS

Antibiotic

Patients undergoing vaginal hysterectomy without antibiotic prophylaxis have a 40–50% febrile morbidity.[17-19] Use of prophylactic antibiotics can significantly reduce this morbidity (to 15%).[20] Single- and multiple-dose cephalosporins have been used most frequently for this purpose. Single-dose first-, second-, and third-generation cephalosporins, although different with respect to bacterial coverage and serum half-life, have been similarly efficacious in reducing the febrile morbidity.[21]

The use of prophylactic antibiotics in abdominal hysterectomy is controversial. Some studies seem to show no significant difference between treated and untreated patients, whereas other studies have shown significant reductions in the infection rate.[22-26] Individual determination is suggested to ascertain whether or not prophylaxis should be used.[26] Those surgeons who have a population with a low major infection rate may not wish to subject their patients to prophylaxis that may have no proven value. On the other hand, those surgeons with significant infection rates should consider evaluating the effectiveness of prophylactic antibiotics in their patient population.

Oophorectomy

Prophylactic oophorectomy at the time of hysterectomy for benign disease is a controversial topic in obstetrics and gynecology. In women less than 40 years old, the ovaries are almost always left in place if grossly normal in appearance. Over the age of 40, concerns about the development of a future ovarian malignancy has led to the frequent recommendation that the ovaries be removed. The rationale behind this thinking is related to the fact that epithelial ovarian cancer peaks in the 40–60 year age range.[27]

Furthermore, the residual ovary syndrome has been described, consisting of chronic pelvic pain, an asymptomatic pelvic mass, or dyspareunia.[28,29] It has been estimated that 2–7% of patients with retained ovaries will subsequently develop a lesion requiring a second operation.[30] Most individuals at the time of re-exploration are found to have extensive pelvic adhesive disease or cystic ovaries, but up to 3% may have a malignancy present.[31]

On the other hand, the actual incidence of ovarian cancer is only about 0.9% and is no greater in those individuals with retained ovaries. It is estimated that if prophylactic oophorectomy was performed on all women undergoing laparotomy, the incidence of ovarian carcinoma would be reduced from 8 to 7 cases per 1000 women.[32] In fact, evaluation of case-controlled studies of ovarian cancer in relation to prior hysterectomy suggests a decreased risk of subsequent ovarian cancer.[33]

From a hormonal perspective, premenopausal hysterectomy with bilateral oophorectomy would necessitate hormone replacement therapy to treat vasomotor symptoms as well as protect against the development of osteoporosis and cardiovascular disease. Although estrogen replacement therapy is effective, compliance is always an issue with any long-term medication. In addition, the postmenopausal ovary is not quiescent. The ovarian stromal tissue has been shown to produce measurable amounts of androstenedione, estrone, and estradiol, all of which may support the well-being and general health of the older woman.[34]

In summary, there is a very small risk of developing subsequent ovarian carcinoma after hysterectomy, but routine prophylactic oophorectomy to reduce this risk would not seem to outweigh the beneficial effects of continued hormone production, especially in the premenopausal patient. The exception to this practice of conservation may be those individuals with the rare familial ovarian carcinoma syndrome.[35] Although there is a somewhat larger risk of reoperation for the residual ovary syndrome, it tends to occur more frequently in those individuals who have undergone hysterectomy at a younger age, in whom, most would agree, that the benefits of long-term ovarian function favor preservation. Nevertheless, these issues should be freely discussed between the patient and surgeon so that each case is individualized and a decision mutually agreed upon.

TECHNIQUE OF ABDOMINAL HYSTERECTOMY

After general anesthesia has been administered, the patient is placed in the frog-leg position so that a careful examination under anesthesia can be performed. This examination is important to confirm the preoperative findings as well as to alert the examiner to possible difficulties that may be encountered at the time of surgery. If the choice of abdominal opening has not yet been made, the examination may also help to finalize this decision.

The patient's skin is prepared for surgery by use of a separate abdominal and vaginal povidine-iodine scrub. An indwelling transurethral catheter and electrocautery ground are placed after the surgical scrub. The patient is then repositioned and draped in a sterile fashion. Generally, the right-handed surgeon stands on the left side of the patient so that the dominant hand has an easier plane of approach to the pelvic organs.

Choice of Incision

There are multiple factors to consider regarding the choice of abdominal incision. Adequate exposure for the surgery required is of utmost importance. Generally, when there is a large uterus or when there is any suspicion of malignancy, a low midline vertical incision that can be subsequently extended if necessary is recommended.

A low transverse incision (Pfannenstiel) is commonly used in gynecologic surgery for benign disease. Anatomically, the transverse incisions produce a strong scar because the nerves and blood vessels are oriented in the same direction. Limitations of exposure can be overcome by use of a muscle cutting (Maylard) or tendon cutting (Cherney) type of incision. In fact, high transverse Maylard incisions have effectively allowed removal of very large pelvic-abdominal masses. The transverse incisions do require more time to open and close the abdomen but are cosmetically better accepted by the patients. Finally, all other factors being equal, the choice of incision may be determined by a pre-existing scar.

Abdominal Exploration

Upon entry into the peritoneal cavity, peritoneal fluid or washings should be obtained if malignancy is suspected. The abdominal cavity is explored in a systematic fashion. Beginning in the right upper quadrant, the right kidney, undersurface of the diaphragm, liver, gallbladder, pancreas, stomach, left kidney, and para-aortic lymph node chain are palpated. A self-retaining abdominal wall retractor can be placed at this time. After placing the patient in a moderate Trendelenburg position, the surgeon can obtain additional exposure to the pelvic organs by packing the bowel away into the upper abdomen. Any intestinal adhesions should be lysed prior to packing. Three abdominal packs are usually adequate; one pack is placed in the midline, and one is placed in each of the paracolic gutters.

Uterine Traction

The operation begins with placement of a clamp or suture on or adjacent to the uterus. Ideally, traction on the uterus lifts the entire corpus, tubes, and ovaries out of the pelvis (Fig. 18–1). In addition, steady upward traction facilitates dissection of the surgical planes, hemostasis, and placement of the clamps a safe distance from the ureter and bladder.

Round Ligament

Generally, the first incision on the uterus begins with clamping, cutting, and ligating the round ligament at a point one-third to one-half way lateral to its insertion on the uterus. Transection of the round ligament permits access to both the anterior and posterior leaves of the broad ligament. The incision into the broad ligament is then extended anteriorly down to the point of reflection of the bladder onto the midline of the uterus (Fig. 18–2). This dissection can be performed in an avascular fashion if care is taken to incise only the peritoneum and to avoid the underlying areolar tissue. A similar procedure is performed on the opposite side to complete dissection of the vesicouterine peritoneal fold.

Adnexal Management

If the tubes and ovaries are to be conserved, the posterior leaf of the broad ligament is opened beneath the adnexa (Fig. 18–3). The tube and utero-ovarian ligament are then triply clamped as close as possible to the uterine corpus so as not to disrupt the blood supply (Fig. 18–4). An incision is made between the clamp closest to the uterus and the middle clamp. This technique permits control of back-bleeding as well as allows double clamping of the ovarian vessels, which have a tendency to retract. A free tie ligature of 2-0 delayed absorbable suture is placed around the clamp most lateral to the uterus, and a transfixion suture is placed around the middle clamp.

If the adnexa are going to be removed with the uterus, the posterior leaf of the broad ligament is incised 1–2 cm lateral to the infundibulopelvic ligament with the incision extending upward toward the pelvic brim. The <u>ureter is then identified on the medial leaf of the broad ligament</u>. Once the ureter is located, the posterior leaf of the broad ligament is opened beneath the infundibulopelvic ligament and above the ureter (Fig. 18–5). The ligament is triply clamped and cut so that again, one clamp controls back-bleeding and two clamps remain on the ovarian vessel pedicle. The pedicle is doubly ligated by using a free tie followed by a transfixion suture.

Bladder Mobilization

With upward traction being applied on the uterus, the bladder peritoneum is elevated and sharp dissec-

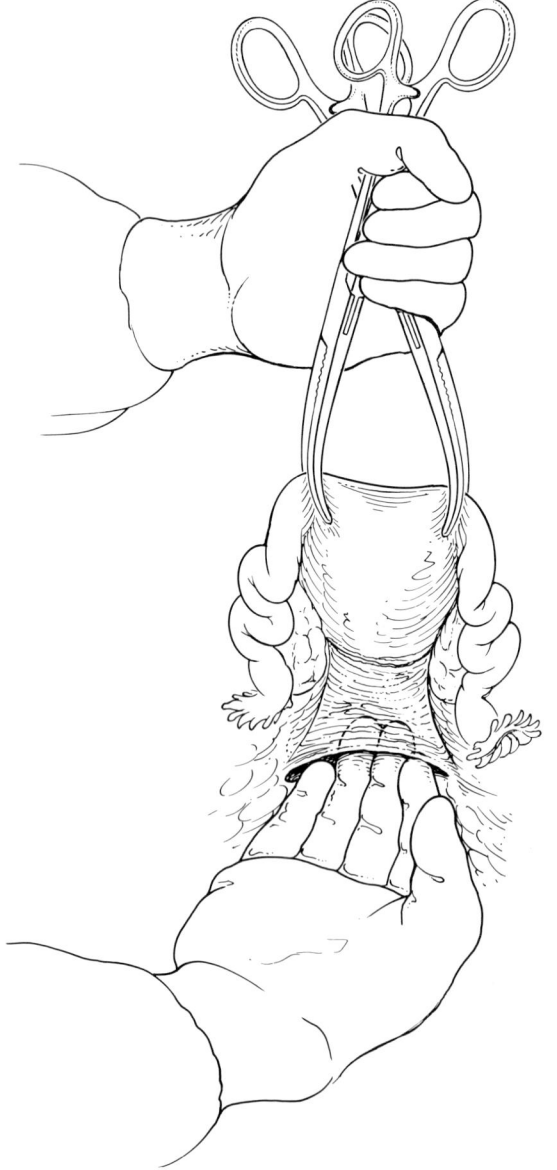

Figure 18–1
Clamps placed on the cornual region of the uterus allow the surgeon to lift the entire corpus, tubes, and ovaries out of the pelvis. Upward traction throughout the procedure facilitates dissection of the surgical planes and placement of future clamps a safe distance from the bladder and ureter.

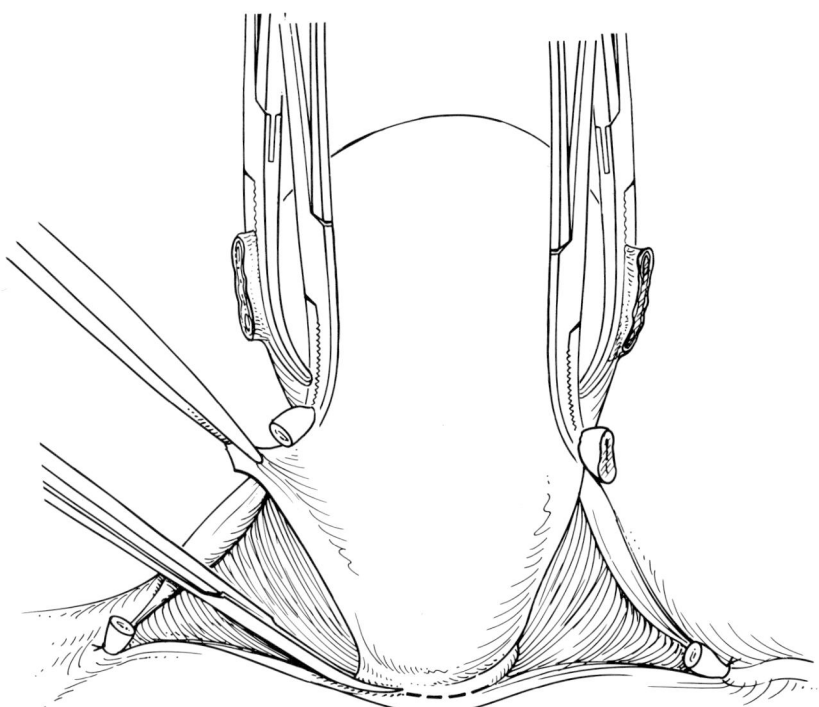

Figure 18–2
The round ligament has been clamped, cut, and ligated, allowing access to the anterior and posterior leaves of the broad ligament. Anteriorly, the incision is extended down to the point of reflection of the bladder onto the midline of the uterus on both sides, thus creating the vesicouterine peritoneal fold.

tion with Metzenbaum scissors cuts through the loose, avascular, fibroareolar tissue between the bladder and lower uterine segment (Fig. 18–6). The tips of the scissors should point towards the uterus to guard against injury to the bladder base; however, if one incises too far posteriorly on to the uterus, troublesome venous bleeding can be encountered.

Once the immediate areolar tissue has been lysed, additional mobilization of the bladder is accomplished by the placement of a thumb in the anterior vesicovaginal space and the second and third fingers behind the uterus to further compress the cervix and push away the remaining bladder fibers (Fig. 18–7). The blunt dissection should remain in the midline,

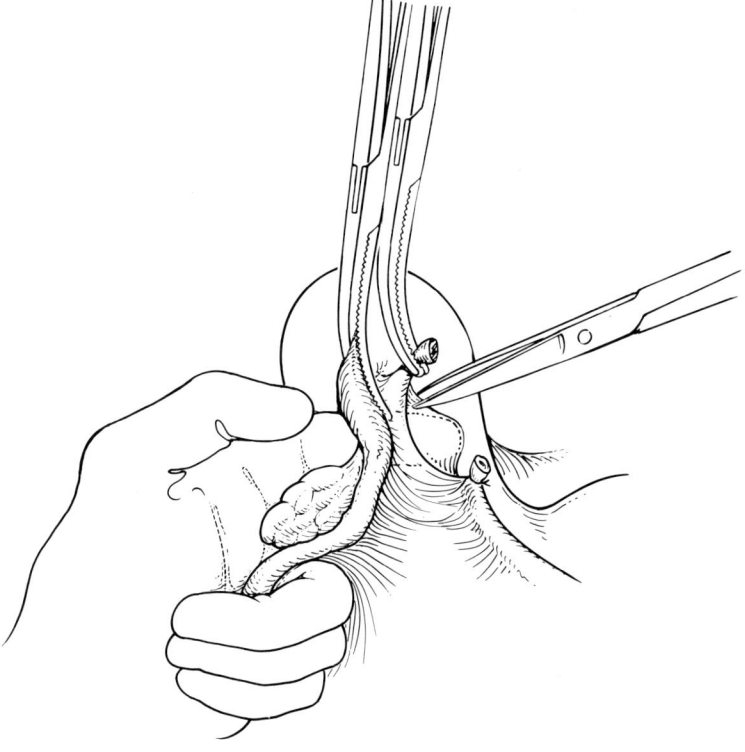

Figure 18–3
If the tubes and ovaries are conserved, the posterior leaf of the broad ligament is opened in the avascular plane beneath the adnexa.

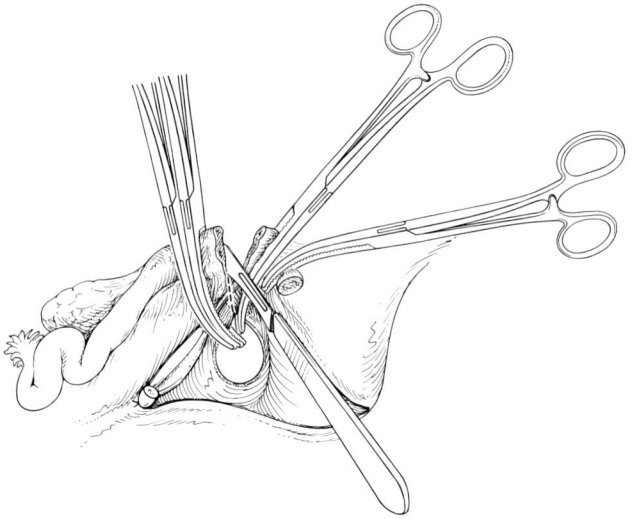

Figure 18–4
The tube and utero-ovarian ligament are then triply clamped as close as possible to the uterine corpus so as not to disrupt the blood supply. The ovarian vessels are then divided so that there are two clamps on the pedicle and one to control troublesome back-bleeding.

because lateral dissection can lead to bleeding from paracervical and paravaginal veins.

Uterine Vessel Ligation

The uterine vessels, which arise as a branch of the internal iliac or superior vesical artery, run anteriorly across the top of the cardinal ligament over the ureter and divide into corporal, cervical, and vaginal branches. Sharp dissection of the anterior and posterior peritoneum and associated areolar connective tissue will expose the uterine vessels. Prior to clamping the vessels, the pelvic ureter is routinely palpated as it courses beneath the artery, lateral to the internal

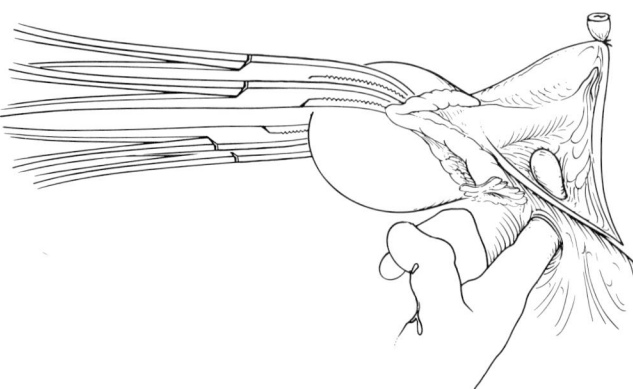

Figure 18–5
If the tube and ovary are to be removed with the uterus, the broad ligament is opened lateral to the infundibulopelvic ligament. The ureter should be identified on the medial leaf of the broad ligament. The posterior leaf of the broad ligament can then be opened beneath the ovarian vessels and above the ureter.

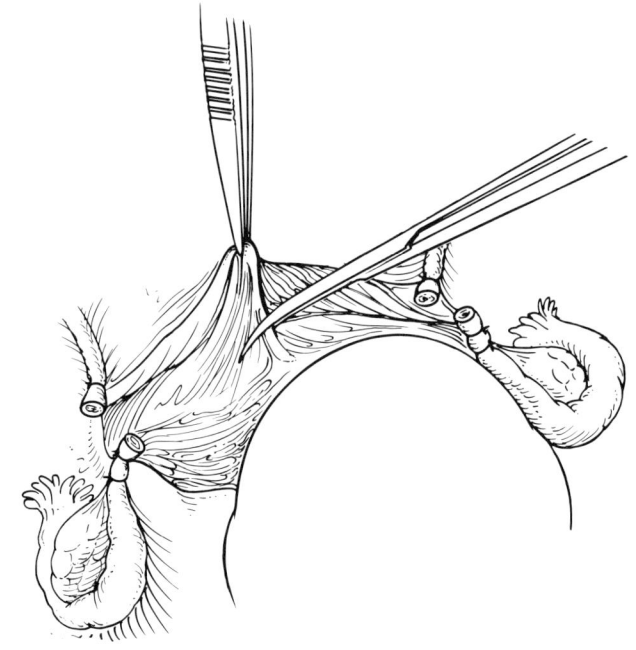

Figure 18–6
The bladder is mobilized by sharply dissecting the fibroareolar tissue between the bladder base and lower uterine segment. The tips of the scissors point down towards the uterus to avoid injury to the bladder.

cervical os (Fig. 18–8). Unless distorted by pelvic pathology, the combination of upward uterine traction and downward mobilization of the bladder base should place the ureters approximately 2 cm below

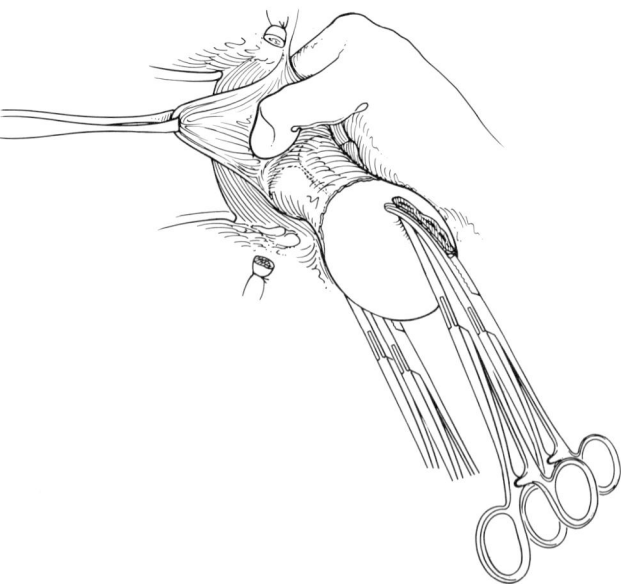

Figure 18–7
After lysing the immediate areolar tissue in the midline, additional mobilization of the inferior margins of the bladder can be accomplished bluntly by placement of the thumb in the anterior vesicovaginal space and the second and third fingers behind the uterus. Compression of the cervix in a downward fashion frees the remaining bladder fibers.

as it is closed. The lowest clamp should be applied first and none placed below it. Attention to these details should ensure that the vessels are completely within the clamps and placed above the ureters.

The artery is then divided between the upper and middle clamp and ligated with 0 delayed absorbable suture. Double clamping and ligation are wise precautions here, because <u>loss of this pedicle can result in ureteral injury if the clamps are reapplied blindly into a bloody field.</u>

Cardinal and Uterosacral Ligaments

The cardinal ligament and branches of the vaginal artery are subsequently clamped, cut, and ligated together by placing a straight clamp between the pedicle of the uterine vessels and the side of the uterus. Generally, two or three successive bites placed extrafascially on the cardinal ligaments are adequate to reach the junction of the upper vagina and lowermost cervix.

Some surgeons may prefer to use an <u>intrafascial technique</u> in operations for benign disease.[36, 37] Prior to clamping the cardinal ligaments, a <u>"V" or transverse incision is made on the</u> endopelvic fascia of the anterior cervix just below the level of the internal os. The fascia envelopes the cervix and contains many small arterioles and venous plexuses, which can be segregated to the base of the cardinal ligament with this maneuver. <u>Once incised, pushing down on this fascia with a sponge or end of a scalpel will help</u> to further drop the bladder and ureter away from the clamp. Only the fascia should be incised, because a deeper incision will result in unnecessary bleeding.

The uterosacral ligaments can be clamped, cut, and ligated individually or included with the clamping of the cardinal ligaments if they are in close proximity to each other. If there are adhesions in the posterior cul-de-sac, it is particularly helpful to ligate these ligaments individually so that the pararectal space can be developed to ensure the safety of the anterior rectal wall.

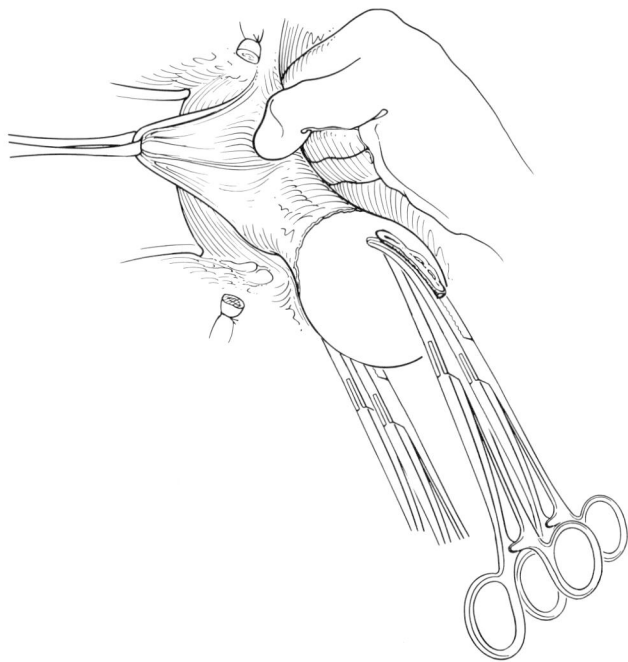

Figure 18–8
After mobilizing the bladder inferiorly (see Fig. 18–7), one should routinely palpate the pelvic ureter as it courses beneath the uterine artery lateral to the internal cervical os.

and lateral from the point of uterine artery ligation. Because the uterine artery runs along the vertical axis of the uterus, correctly placed clamps are applied perpendicular to this axis at the level of the internal cervical os (Fig. 18–9). If possible, the vessels are triply clamped, with each clamp sliding off the cervix

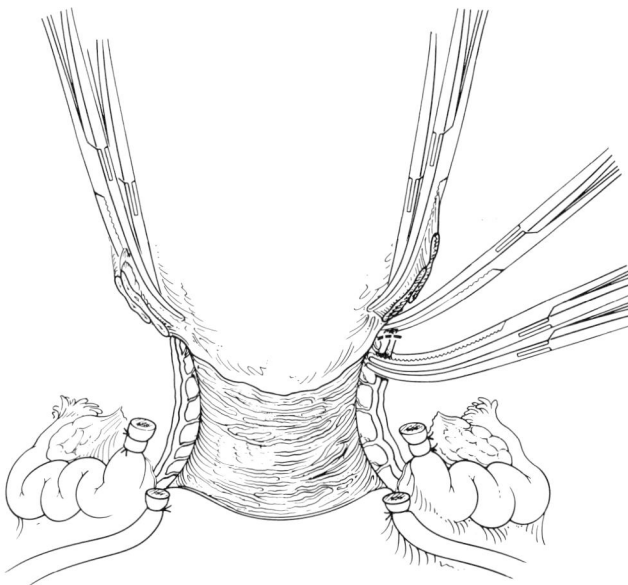

Figure 18–9
The uterine vessels are triply clamped at the level of the internal cervical os. The clamps are placed perpendicular to the uterine vessels that run along the vertical axis of the uterus and should actually slide off the cervix as they are placed to ensure that the vessels are grasped completely.

Vaginal Cuff

The surgeon compresses the cervix and vaginal walls together with his or her thumb and forefinger to determine that the bladder and rectum are free from the cervix prior to opening the vagina. The vagina is then entered anteriorly with the scalpel or scissors (Fig. 18–10). The incision is extended circumferentially around the vagina and close to the cervix in order to preserve vaginal depth. Straight clamps are placed at the lateral vaginal cuff angles and the anterior and posterior cuff as they are opened. These

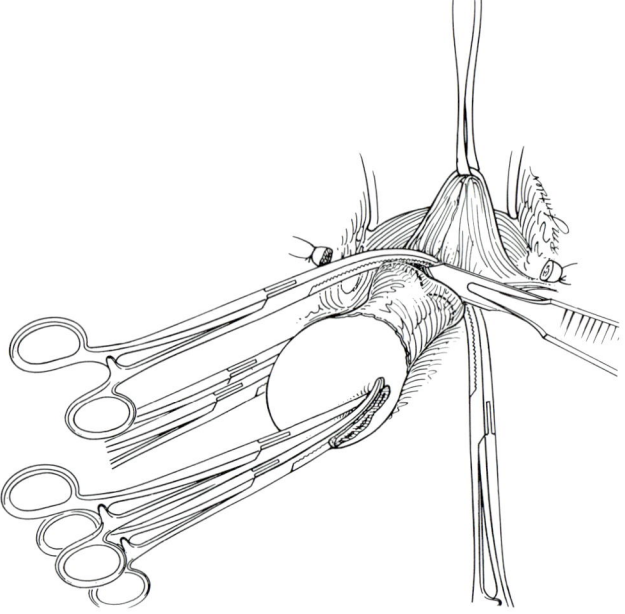

Figure 18–10
After compressing the cervix and vaginal walls together with the thumb and forefinger to determine that the bladder and rectum are completely free from the cervix, the vagina is opened anteriorly. A circumferential incision around the vagina frees the uterine specimen.

clamps facilitate the removal of the uterus and help to maintain hemostasis. Once the specimen has been removed, the general principles of cuff management involve closure of each vaginal angle separately to control bleeding from the vaginal arteries. The angles are attached to the cardinal and uterosacral ligaments in order to support the vaginal vault. This attachment can be performed simply by placing a suture through the anterior and posterior vagina, then incorporating the cardinal and uterosacral ligaments (Fig. 18–11).

Depending on the surgeon's preference, the vaginal cuff can be closed or left open. Closure of the cuff can be completed with an interrupted or a continuous running 0 or 2–0 delayed absorbable suture. If the cuff is to be left open, a continuous locking suture is placed circumferentially around the vaginal margin. Regardless of the method of closure, the entire denuded surface of the posterior endopelvic fascia is included in the suture to avoid troublesome oozing, and the anterior vagina is inspected to be certain that the bladder is not included. In situations of persistent oozing or when there is obvious infection, the cuff is generally left open for drainage.

Pelvic Hemostasis and Reperitonealization

Prior to closing the abdomen, one should again examine the vaginal cuff, adnexal pedicles, bladder base, and peritoneal edges for hemostasis. The pelvis can be reperitonealized with a single running suture beginning at the level of the pelvic brim where the round ligament was initially ligated. In proceeding with the reperitonealization suture, one should be conscious of the course of the ureter, which can often lie very close to the the peritoneal edge.

TECHNIQUE OF VAGINAL HYSTERECTOMY

On the evening prior to surgery, it is helpful to empty the rectum by giving an enema or oral cleansing solution, especially if a posterior repair is planned. Preoperative antibiotics are also given to the patient in the holding area to ensure that adequate levels are in the extravascular compartment prior to the initial incision.

After adequate anesthesia has been administered, the patient is placed in the dorsal lithotomy position with the hips in full flexion and the legs in almost full extension (Fig. 18–12). The hips should be located just past the end of the table and are in proper alignment when a line drawn between the two femoral heads are in line with the stirrups. Placing the table in a 10-degree Trendelenburg position will help to keep the bowel out of the operative field and the weighted speculum in place.

The vulva, perineum, vagina, and cervix are thoroughly prepared with a povidone-iodine solution and the bladder catheterized as necessary.

Examination under anesthesia prior to the initial incision is important to confirm previous office findings and to evaluate the likely success of the proce-

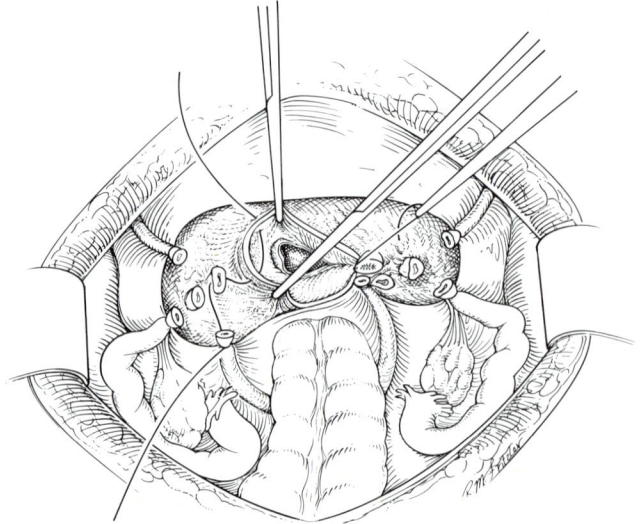

Figure 18–11
The vaginal angles are closed separately to maintain hemostasis and are attached to the corresponding cardinal and uterosacral ligaments for support.

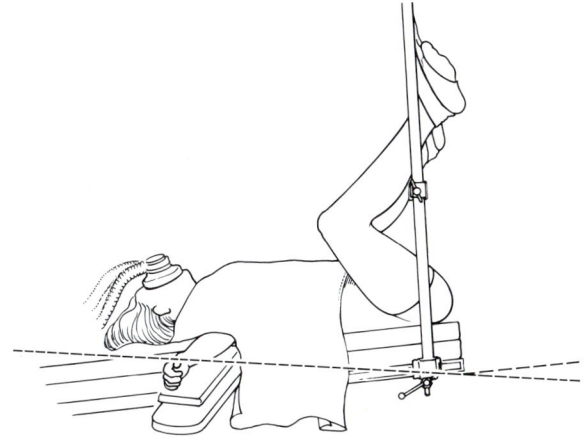

Figure 18–12
The patient should be placed in the proper dorsal lithotomy position with the hips in full flexion, located just past the end of the table; the legs in almost full extension; and the table placed in a moderate Trendelenburg position.

dure. The uterus is evaluated for size, shape, and, most importantly, mobility. The posterior vaginal fornix should be wide, deep, and free of thickening. One should evaluate the mobility, length, and strength of the supporting ligaments by grasping the cervix with a double-toothed tenaculum and pulling firmly on it in an upward and downward fashion. The vast majority of the time, the uterosacral–cardinal ligament complex is adequate to provide support of the vaginal vault; however, if it is found to be grossly inadequate, one should be prepared to use other tissues to support the vaginal vault so that the prolapse can be repaired primarily.

Cervical Circumcision

The vagina is infiltrated at its junction with the cervix with 10–30 ml of a dilute vasoconstrictor solution of 1:200,000 epinephrine or phenylephrine. Injection of this solution helps to decrease blood loss and enhance the development of the appropriate surgical planes. Normal saline alone has also been recommended by other investigators, because the vasoconstrictor agents may lead to an increased risk of cuff infection.[38]

The initial circumferential incision is made on the vagina, just above its junction with the cervix (Fig. 18–13). In patients who have a significant cystocele or prolapse, the surgeon should be certain that the incision is made beneath the bladder. Placement of a uterine sound transurethrally may help to delineate the lower limits of the bladder. It is important to incise the full thickness of the vaginal mucosa so that it can be completely pushed back from the connective tissue below.

Posterior Peritoneum

The cervix is pulled upward, and the posterior vaginal mucosa is pushed back. The posterior peritoneum is generally easy to identify. The exposed peritoneum is grasped with forceps and opened sharply with scissors, tips pointing up towards the uterus to avoid rectal injury (Fig. 18–14). A finger is placed in the cul-de-sac to confirm entry into the peritoneal cavity. Digital palpation can also determine the presence of intestinal adhesions, posterior wall leiomyomas, and fundal location. The posterior peritoneal incision is extended laterally on each side until impinging upon the uterosacral ligaments. A long weighted speculum is then placed in the posterior cul-de-sac.

Uterosacral and Cardinal Ligaments

The uterosacral ligaments on each side are clamped, cut, and ligated with a delayed absorbable No. 0 transfixion suture (Fig. 18–15). One should be certain to grasp the full thickness of the uterosacral ligament, including the peritoneum posterior to the ligament. Including this posterior peritoneum will help to ensure that the posterior leaf of the broad ligament will be included in successive bites. After ligation, the suture is kept long for future use and identification.

The lower portion of the cardinal ligament is clamped, cut, ligated, and held in a similar fashion as the uterosacral ligaments.

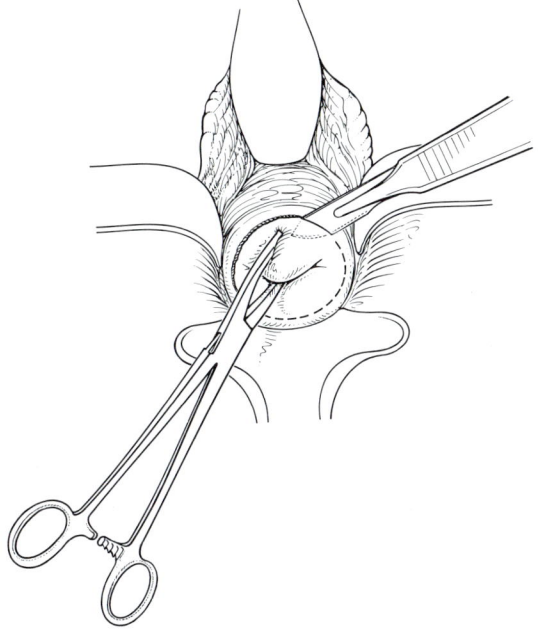

Figure 18–13
The initial incision is made circumferentially on the vagina, just above its junction with the cervix.

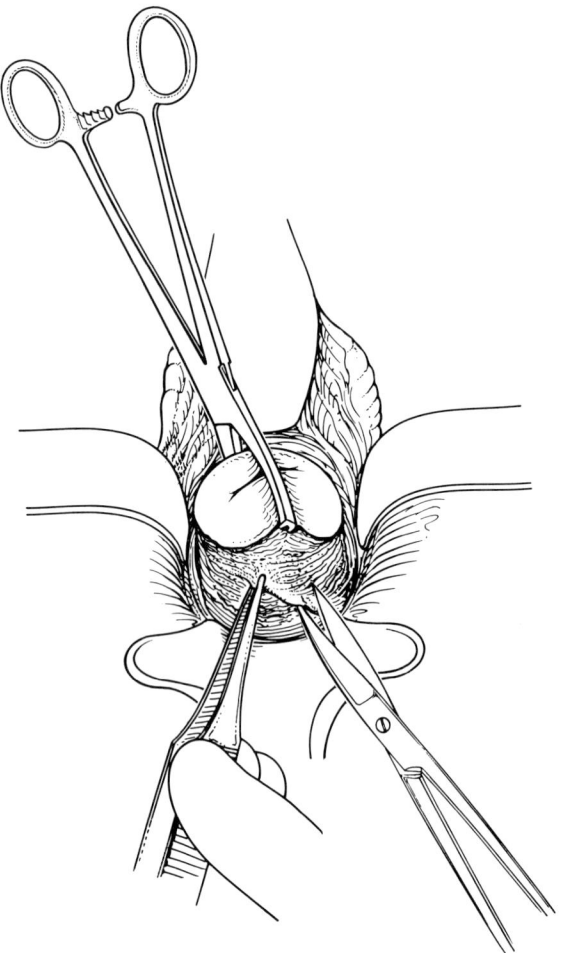

Figure 18–14
After the posterior peritoneum is exposed, it should be grasped and opened sharply with the scissors, tips pointing up towards the uterus to avoid rectal injury.

secting the tissues so that the bladder base is not torn. It is more prudent to proceed with the Mayo scissors to lyse the fibrous bands of tissue. Once visualized, the peritoneum can be grasped and opened. Similar to entry into the posterior peritoneum, the anterior peritoneal opening is explored with a finger to confirm entry into the peritoneal cavity and to assess the uterine contour and fundal location. A narrow retractor is then placed in the anterior cul-de-sac to keep the bladder and ureters out of the operative field.

Alternatively, if there is difficulty in visualizing the anterior peritoneal fold, one should place the index and middle fingers through the posterior cul-de-sac and hook them around the fundus in order to tent the anterior peritoneum from behind. One can then cut down directly on the anterior peritoneal fold, which is located between the operator's fingers (Fig. 18–17).

Uterine Vessels

Having entered the anterior and posterior cul-de-sac, one can proceed with ligation of the upper portion

Anterior Peritoneum

The bladder must be dissected free of its fascial attachments to the anterior surface of the uterus before the anterior peritoneum can be visualized. Holding the uterus on steady downward traction, the anterior vaginal mucosa and bladder are picked up with a forceps. By using a combination of blunt and sharp dissection, a plane is developed between the bladder and uterus. During the dissection, the handles of the scissors are held high above the horizontal plane, with the curves of the scissors pointing down toward the uterus to avoid injury to the bladder base (Fig. 18–16). The correct cleavage plane is relatively bloodless. The dissection is continued upward until the anterior peritoneal reflection is reached. The peritoneum can be palpated as the typically smooth, thin, easy gliding tissue plane. If there has been a history of previous surgery such as cesarean section, the surgeon should be especially careful not to use excessive force while bluntly dis-

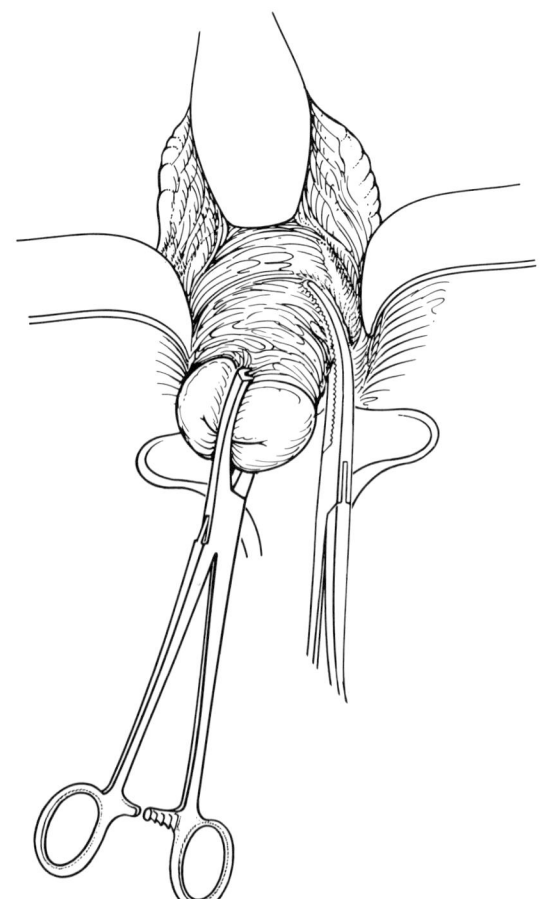

Figure 18–15
The uterosacral and cardinal ligaments are each clamped, cut, and ligated and held.

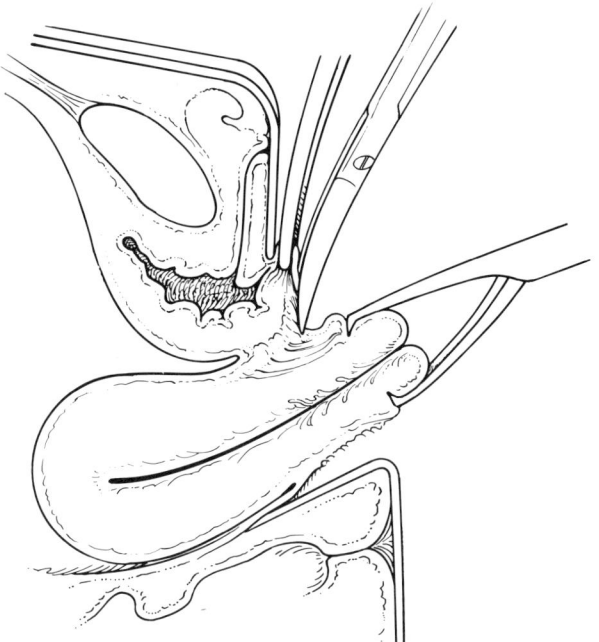

Figure 18–16
Entry into the anterior peritoneum is accomplished by a combination of sharp and blunt dissection until the fold of peritoneum between the bladder and uterus is exposed. Pointing the tips of the scissors down towards the uterus will help to avoid bladder injury during the dissection.

of the cardinal ligament and lower portion of the broad ligament, which contain the uterine vessels. Both the anterior and posterior leaves of peritoneum should be included in the clamps to ensure that all

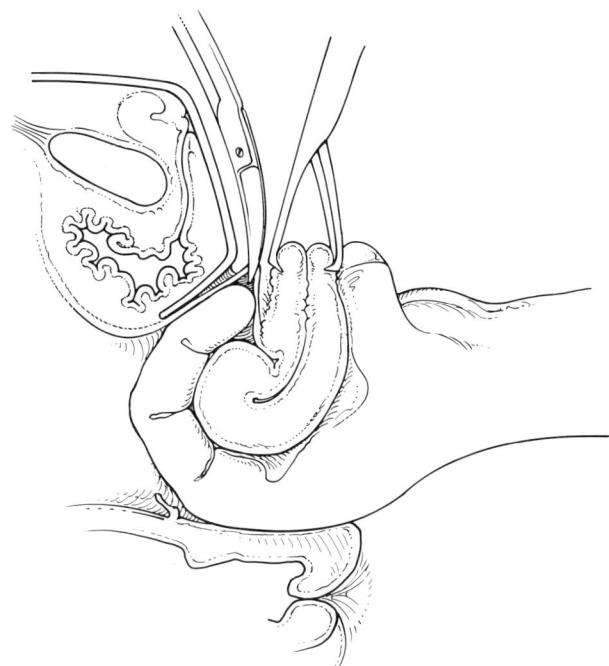

Figure 18–17
On occasion, the anterior peritoneal fold can be identified by hooking the fingers around the fundus and tenting the peritoneum from behind.

major vessels are grasped. The tissues are cut and are not ligated with a transfixion type suture unless the vessels are directly visualized; otherwise, blind fixation of the pedicle may result in the perforation of a vessel and the subsequent development of a broad ligament hematoma.

Adnexal Management

In a similar fashion, progressive clamping, cutting, and ligating of the broad ligament are performed up to and including the upper portion of the broad ligament, which includes the fallopian tubes, utero-ovarian ligament, and round ligament. This adnexal pedicle should be doubly clamped and ligated when possible, owing to the tendency of the ovarian vessels to retract. The distal ligature is kept long for later identification.

If the uterus does not descend easily or if there is difficulty in visualizing the upper broad ligament, an attempt is made to deliver the uterus through the anterior or posterior cul-de-sac. Once it is delivered, the tube, utero-ovarian ligament, and round ligament can be doubly clamped on both sides (Fig. 18–18). When inverting the uterus, one must remember that excessive traction can tear it from its remaining supports with the subsequent retraction of the ovarian vessels high up in the peritoneal cavity.

The surgeon inspects both adnexal pedicles. If the tubes and ovaries are to be removed, a pack is first placed in the peritoneal cavity to keep the intestines out of the field. The distal adnexal ligature is identified, and an atraumatic clamp is placed on the ovary or other adnexal structures. By applying downward traction, the infundibulopelvic ligament can be identified, doubly clamped, cut, and ligated (Fig. 18–19).

Intramyometrial Coring

Occasionally, after ligating the uterine vessels, one may reach a point in the surgery when the uterus no longer descends. At this point, one should reevaluate the pelvis to be certain there are no adhesions or adnexal masses prohibiting further uterine descent. If failure of descent is due to mechanical obstruction secondary to a large myomatous uterus, it can be morcellated or bisected. A particularly effective alternative to morcellation is the technique of intramyometrial coring.[39–41] An incision is made beneath the uterine serosa parallel to the axis of the uterus (Fig. 18–20). This incision is continued circumferentially at the same time that the cervix is being pulled outward. The net effect is to core out the body of the uterus. As the uterus lengthens, the fundal dimensions decrease, which permits further descent

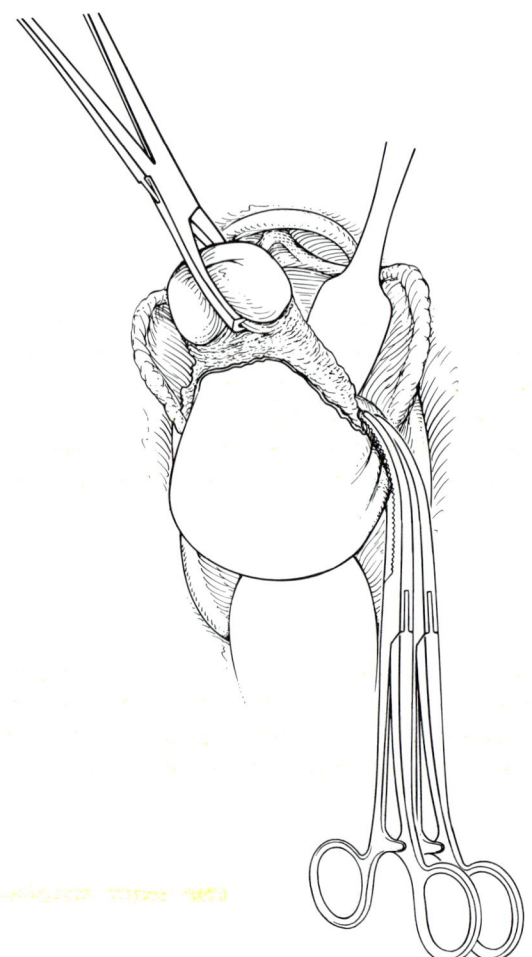

Figure 18–18
The uterus has been inverted and delivered through the posterior cul-de-sac, allowing access to the tube, utero-ovarian ligament, and round ligament, which are doubly clamped on both sides.

of the uterus and access to the adnexa. Steady outward traction on the uterus keeps blood loss to a minimum. Again, one must be certain to remain beneath the serosal surface of the uterus to ensure that no harm comes to the previously ligated uterine vessels laterally, or the intestines superiorly.

Enterocele Prevention

The posterior and anterior cul-de-sac should be closely examined prior to peritoneal closure (Fig. 18–21). If an enterocele sac is encountered, it can be lifted from the underlying connective tissue with sharp and blunt dissection and the excess peritoneum trimmed away up to the level of the anterior surface of the rectum. Alternatively, a small enterocele or potential enterocele can be treated by placement of posterior culdeplasty sutures, which serve to obliterate the cul-de-sac and plicate the uterosacral ligaments.[42] A stitch is placed through the left uterosacral ligament 1–2 cm from its cut edge, and several bites of redundant peritoneum are incorporated in the

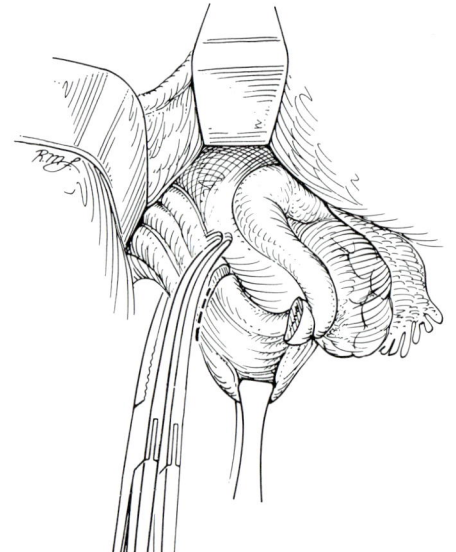

Figure 18–19
If the tubes and ovaries are to be removed, an atraumatic clamp is placed on the adnexa and downward traction is applied until the infundibulopelvic ligament is identified. The ovarian vessels can then be doubly clamped, cut, and ligated.

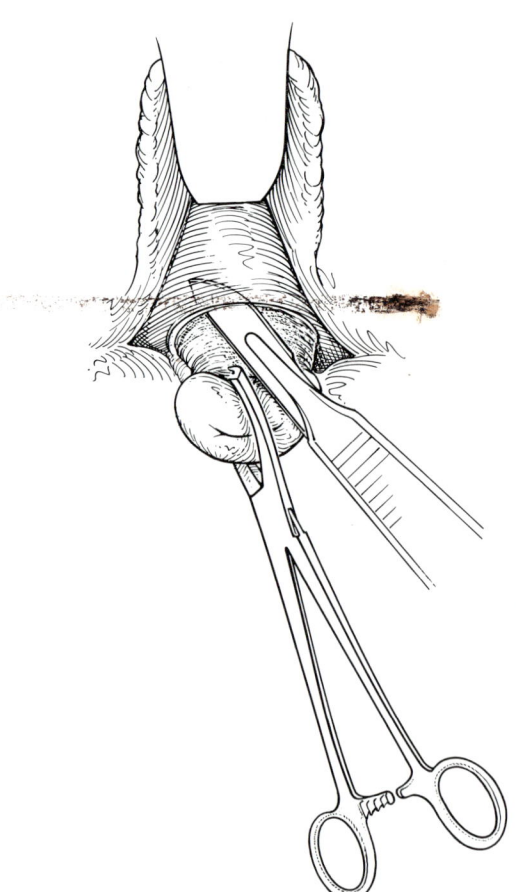

Figure 18–20
After the uterine vessels have been ligated, intramyometrial coring permits further descent of an enlarged uterus causing obstruction. The incision is carried circumferentially beneath the uterine serosa and parallel to the axis of the uterus, at the same time that the cervix is being pulled outward.

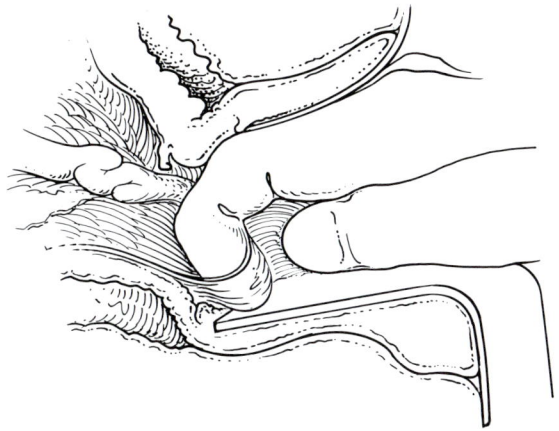

Figure 18–21
The anterior and posterior cul-de-sac should be examined prior to peritoneal closure. An enterocele sac is illustrated in this figure and should be excised.

suture before being placed through the right uterosacral ligament. One or two additional sutures can be placed above the initial suture to ensure reduction of the redundant peritoneum. The uterosacral ligaments are then plicated by placing a suture just to the right of the midline of the vagina and posterior peritoneum about 2 cm above the cut posterior edge. The right and then the left uterosacral ligament are grasped and the ligature brought out through the posterior peritoneum and vagina (Fig. 18–22). These sutures are kept until after the peritoneal closure suture is placed. When they are tied, they will help to lengthen the vagina as well as restore a horizontal upper axis, which is more physiologic.[43]

Vault Suspension and Peritoneal Closure

When there is an adequate uterosacral–cardinal ligament complex, the vaginal vault is suspended by placement of a suture through the full thickness of the posterior vagina, into the posterior peritoneum through the uterosacral ligament, cardinal ligament, peritoneum, and back through the full thickness of the vagina lateral to the initial site of tissue penetration (Fig. 18–23). A similar suspension suture is placed on the opposite side.

A high pursestring peritoneal closure suture is placed beginning anteriorly. After a hemostat is attached to one end, the closure is continued in a clockwise fashion to include the left round ligament, peritoneum of the broad ligament, cardinal ligament, uterosacral ligament, posterior peritoneum, and the corresponding structures on the opposite side (Fig. 18–24). This suture should be placed above the previous sutures in the peritoneal cavity to ensure that any bleeding that may occur from the major pedicles will remain extraperitoneal. The vault suspension

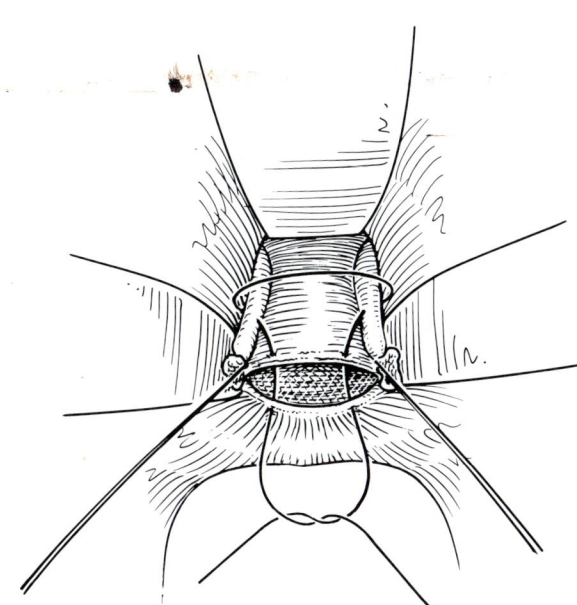

Figure 18–22
Prevention of enterocele formation can be accomplished by plication of the uterosacral ligaments. A suture is placed just to the right of the midline of the vagina and through the posterior peritoneum. The right and left uterosacral ligaments are incorporated into the suture, which is then brought out through the posterior peritoneum and vagina.

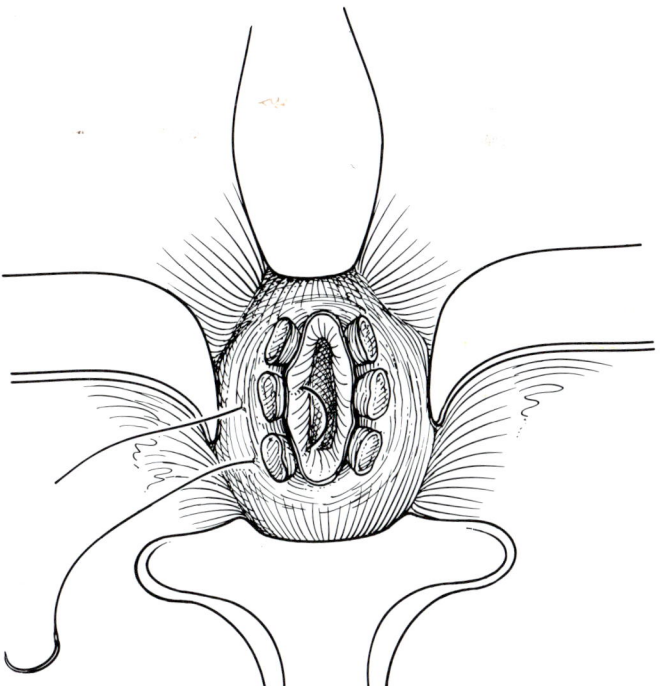

Figure 18–23
The vaginal vault is supported by placement of a suture through the full thickness of the posterior vagina, into the posterior peritoneum through the uterosacral ligament, cardinal ligament, peritoneum, and back through the vagina lateral to the initial site of tissue penetration.

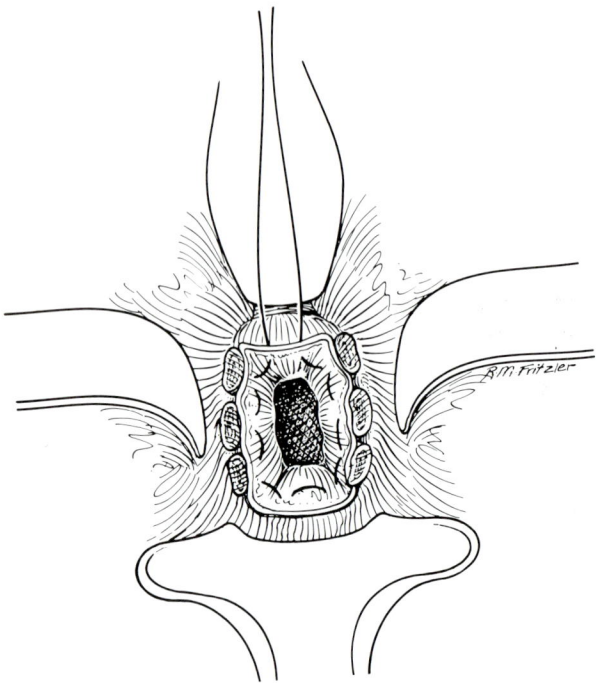

Figure 18–24
A high pursestring peritoneal closure above the previous sutures in the peritoneal cavity ensures that any bleeding that may occur from the major pedicles remains extraperitoneal.

ligatures are now tied, followed by the culdeplasty sutures, and, finally, the peritoneal closure suture.

Vaginal Vault Closure

The vaginal vault can be closed with either running or interrupted sutures. If vaginal depth is of concern, closing the vagina in a longitudinal fashion will help to preserve length. Otherwise, closure of the vault in a transverse fashion will help to preserve the lateral expanse of the vaginal apex. Alternatively, one can leave the vaginal cuff open for drainage by placing a continuous running lock suture around the vaginal mucosa. The vagina will then come together transversely.

COMPLICATIONS OF HYSTERECTOMY

Hemorrhage

One of the areas of greatest concern to the surgeon is postoperative hemorrhage within the first 24 hours after surgery. This may manifest itself as acute hypotension with oliguria, or it may be noted only as a dramatic fall in hematocrit greater than expected from the estimated intraoperative blood loss. One should generally repeat the blood count to rule out laboratory error while evaluating the need for re-exploration. If the bleeding is obviously vaginal in nature and an isolated site is discovered on examination, the bleeding may be controlled with a few hemostatic sutures placed at the vaginal cuff. If the bleeding is intraperitoneal and seemingly remains active, one has no choice but to stabilize the patient and re-explore the abdomen to search for a bleeding source. One should carefully inspect all vascular pedicles at the time of reoperation. Frequently the site of bleeding is at the vaginal cuff or angle, but at times no active source of bleeding is discovered. Double ligation of the vascular pedicles at the time of initial surgery as previously described should help to decrease the risk of intraperitoneal hemorrhage.

Late-onset bleeding occurring from the vagina is usually cuff related. On examination, a general ooze is noted from the vault. If isolated bleeding points are identified, they should be sutured. Otherwise, the bleeding may frequently be controlled with hemostatic agents such as Monsel's solution. At times, when there is a nonspecific cuff ooze, one may need to resort to mechanical compression of the vaginal vault by packing it with gauze for 24–48 hours. A tight vaginal pack will also require the use of a transurethral catheter.

Postoperative Fever

Febrile morbidity is the most common postoperative complication of hysterectomy. During the first 24 hours, fever is most likely related to pulmonary congestion. Excluding the first 24 hours after surgery, a temperature 38° C or greater was discovered on two other postoperative days in about 30% of patients undergoing abdominal and 15% of patients undergoing vaginal hysterectomy.[2] Once febrile morbidity has been documented, evaluation of the source of the fever should include other sites in addition to the surgical wound. The pulmonary system is evaluated again for signs of persistent atelectasis, pneumonia, or embolus. The extremities are evaluated for signs of thrombophlebitis. The urinary tract system is not usually a source of fever unless there is an accompanying pyelonephritis or obstruction related to ureteral injury. Urinalysis should be obtained to evaluate this possibility or an intravenous pyelogram (IVP) ordered if the history and examination are suggestive of ureteral injury. If there is an abdominal incision, it is inspected for erythema or fluctuance. Abdominal and pelvic examination is performed to feel for a mass that may represent the development of a cuff hematoma or abscess. At times, use of an ultrasound, CT, or MRI scan is helpful to diagnose a pelvic collection, especially when the patient is not responding to appropriate antibiotic treatment.

Urinary Tract Injury

The bladder is the most common site of urinary tract injury during hysterectomy, injury occurring in about 1% of cases.[44] During abdominal hysterectomy, the bladder is most likely to be damaged as the abdomen is being opened or during dissection of the bladder off the lower uterine segment. In both situations, scarring from previous surgeries makes bladder injury more likely. Techniques to avoid this injury during abdominal hysterectomy include correct transurethral catheter placement to avoid kinking and high entry into the peritoneal cavity with careful layer-by-layer dissection. When the bladder base is adherent to the lower uterine segment, sharp dissection in the midline is required. Forceful blunt dissection will only increase the likelihood of tearing the bladder. Finally, one should be certain that the bladder is mobilized well away from the anterior vaginal mucosa during cuff closure so that a vesicovaginal fistula can be avoided.

During vaginal hysterectomy, the bladder is most likely to be entered as it is being dissected off the lower uterine segment. Bladder injury is recognized by the leakage of urine or visualization of the catheter bulb. Injection of sterile milk or methylene blue through the urethral catheter can also help to identify the location of a small leak. Again, to avoid injury, one should keep the scissors tips directed toward the uterus, handles held high, and advance the dissection under direct vision.

When injury occurs to the base of the bladder, one should be certain to obtain a watertight closure. The first layer of closure includes the mucosa, and the second layer reinforces the first layer and includes only the muscularis and bladder fascia. The sutures are placed in a continuous or interrupted fashion using 2–0 or 3–0 absorbable suture, because permanent suture material can lead to stone formation. One should check the suture line for leakage by instilling sterile saline or methylene blue through the catheter. A third layer of suture is placed if necessary. On the other hand, injuries to the dome of the bladder are much more forgiving, owing to its generous blood supply, and will heal when closed in almost any fashion.

The course of the ureter is such that it is liable to injury during hysterectomy. The incidence of ureteral injury is estimated at 0.5–2.5%.[44, 45] There are three sites where the ureter is more likely to be damaged during hysterectomy: (1) the ureterovesical junction, (2) the junction of the uterine artery and the ureter, and (3) the level of the infundibulopelvic ligament (Fig. 18–25). Injury to the ureter is also more likely in the setting of a large uterus, pelvic mass, severe prolapse, pelvic inflammatory disease, or extensive endometriosis. In these situations, a preoperative IVP may be helpful.[46]

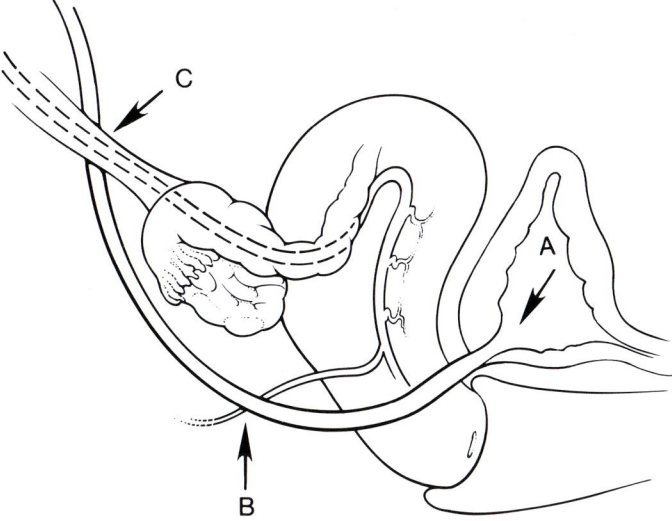

Figure 18–25
During hysterectomy, the most likely sites of ureteral injury are the ureterovesical junction (A), the junction of the uterine artery and ureter (B), and the level of the infundibulopelvic ligament (C).

The most effective way to avoid ureteral injury during hysterectomy is to identify the ureter by visualization and palpation when approaching the likely sites of ureteral injury or when performing any dissection along the pelvic sidewalls. During vaginal hysterectomy, when extensive prolapse is encountered, the surgeon must remember that downward traction on the cervix brings the ureter into the operative field. One should identify the cervicovaginal junction before cutting and clamping. Finally, when there is bleeding in the operative field, one should be cautious about applying the hemostatic clamps blindly. The ureter can even be identified during vaginal hysterectomy if necessary.[47]

Gastrointestinal Injury

Injury to the intestine during hysterectomy occurs most commonly when opening the abdomen, lysing adhesions, or when attempting to open the posterior cul-de-sac. A history of previous abdominal surgery, pelvic inflammatory disease, or endometriosis makes injury more likely. To avoid injury at the time of opening, the tissue above the peritoneum should be incised in layers and, if possible, the peritoneum itself opened away from the site of previous surgery. Once the abdominal cavity is entered, intestinal adhesions should be released by sharp, not blunt, dissection to avoid tearing the mesentery or serosa. An incision into the small bowel can be recognized by the leakage of the characteristic yellow contents.

A small incision can be repaired by closing the initial mucosal layer with a delayed 3–0 absorbable suture, which is then reinforced by an additional layer of suture. The laceration should be closed transversely so that the intestinal lumen is not narrowed.

Similarly, a small incision into the anterior rectal wall can usually be closed primarily with a double-layered closure. With rectal injury, the patient should be placed on a broad-spectrum antibiotic if it has not already been started. If the injury is large or the surgeon is uncomfortable with the repair, consult should be made with a surgeon experienced in bowel repair such as a gynecologic oncologist or general surgeon.

Vaginal Vault Prolapse

Fortunately, vaginal vault prolapse is a rare complication of hysterectomy. Although frequently thought of as a complication of vaginal hysterectomy, just as many patients give a history of previous abdominal hysterectomy.[48]

One can guard against the development of future prolapse by paying attention to the adequacy of support of the vaginal vault at the time of hysterectomy. The integrity of the uterosacral–cardinal ligament complex must be evaluated and, if adequate, these ligaments must be attached to the vaginal vault during vaginal and abdominal hysterectomy. In addition, the cul-de-sac must be evaluated and an enterocoele sac excised or obliterated with culdeplasty sutures as previously described during vaginal hysterectomy. During abdominal hysterectomy, the cul-de-sac can be obliterated with circumferential Moschowitz[49] or longitudinal type Halban[40] sutures. Occasionally, one may encounter no adequate ligament supports, and a primary colpopexy procedure should be performed at the time of hysterectomy.

Psychologic Response to Hysterectomy

All women undergoing hysterectomy undergo a psychologic response to the surgery. Most are able to adapt to the stress of surgery, but others may have adverse reactions that can result in severe depression. For some, hysterectomy may signal loss of reproductive capacity and, along with it, loss of their femininity and sexuality. On the other hand, hysterectomy can have important beneficial effects such as releasing the woman from previously troublesome bleeding, concerns about pregnancy or medical complications of contraception, and fears of malignancy of the organ.

The surgeon can attempt to minimize the adverse reactions to surgery by taking the time, preoperatively, to educate the patient and spouse about the risks and benefits of surgery. A thorough discussion about the surgery will help to allay many of the anxieties and misconceptions that she may have. Warning signals the surgeon should be alert to include those women with a previous psychiatric history, medically unnecessary operations, marital disruption, lack of any preoperative anxiety, or presence of misconceptions and fears about the effect of the operation.[50] When appropriate, additional preoperative and postoperative consultation is made for the patient with a mental health professional.

References

1. Pokras R, Hufnagel VG: Hysterectomy in the United States, 1965–84. AJPH 1988; 78:852.
2. Dicker RC, Greenspan JR, Strauss MS, et al.: Complications of abdominal and vaginal hysterectomy among women of reproductive age in the United States. Am J Obstet Gynecol 1982; 144:841.
3. Stovall TG, Solomon SK, Ling FW: Endometrial sampling prior to hysterectomy. Obstet Gynecol 1989; 73:405.
4. Smith JJ, Schulman H: Current dilation and curettage practice: A need for revision. Obstet Gynecol 1985; 65:516.
5. Lerner HM: Lack of efficacy of prehysterectomy curettage as a diagnostic procedure. Am J Obstet Gynecol 1984; 148:1055.
6. Bove JR: Transfusion-associated hepatitis and AIDS. New Engl J Med 1987; 317:242.
7. Council Report: Autologous blood transfusions. JAMA 1986; 256:2378.
8. Yen SSC: Clinical applications of gonadotropin-releasing hormone and gonadotropin-releasing hormone analogs. Fertil Steril 1983; 39:257.
9. Coddington CC, Collins RL, Shawker TH, et al.: Long-acting gonadotropin hormone releasing hormone analog used to treat uteri. Fertil Steril 1986; 45:624.
10. Friedman AJ, Barbieri RL, Benaceraf BR, et al.: Treatment of leiomyomata with intranasal or subcutaneous leuprolide, a gonadotropin-releasing agonist. Fertil Steril 1987; 48:560.
11. Friedman AJ, Barbieri RL, Doubilet PM, et al.: A randomized, double blind trial of gonadotropin-releasing hormone agonist (leuprolide) with or without medroxyprogesterone acetate in the treatment of leiomyomata uteri. Fertil Steril 1988; 49:404.
12. Maheux R, Guilteau C, Lemay A, et al.: Luteinizing hormone–releasing hormone agonist and uterine leiomyomata: A pilot study. Am J Obstet Gynecol 1985; 152:1034.
13. Schlaff WD, Zerhouni EA, Huth JAM, et al.: A placebo-controlled trial of depot gonadotropin-releasing hormone analogue (leuprolide) in the treatment of uterine leiomyomata. Obstet Gynecol 1989; 74:856.
14. Schneider D, Golan A, Bukovsky I, et al.: GnRH analogue–induced uterine shrinkage enabling a vaginal hysterectomy and repair in large leiomyomatous uteri. Obstet Gynecol 1991; 78:540.
15. Lumsden MA, West CP, Baird DT: Goserelin therapy before surgery for uterine fibroids (letter). Lancet 1987; 1:36.
16. Friedman AJ: Treatment of leiomyomata uteri with short-term leuprolide followed by leuprolide plus estrogen-progestin hormone replacement therapy for 2 years: A pilot study. Fertil Steril 1989; 51:251.
17. Cambell ZB: A report on 2798 vaginal hysterectomies. Am J Obstet Gynecol 1946; 52:598.
18. Copenhaver EH: Vaginal hysterectomy: An analysis of indications and complications among 1000 operations. Am J Obstet Gynecol 1962; 84:123.

19. Ohm MJ, Galask RP: The effect of antibiotic prophylaxis on patients undergoing vaginal operations. 1. The effect on morbidity. Am J Obstet Gynecol 1975; 123:590.
20. Faro S: Prevention of infections after obstetric and gynecologic surgery. J Reprod Med 1988; 33:154.
21. Hemsell DL, Heard MC, Nobles BJ, et al.: Single-dose prophylaxis for vaginal and abdominal hysterectomy. Am J Obstet Gynecol 1987; 157:498.
22. Ohm M, Galask R: The effect of antibiotic prophylaxis on patients undergoing total abdominal hysterectomy. I. Effect on morbidity. Am J Obstet Gynecol 1976; 125:442.
23. Grossman J, Greco, T, Minkin MJ, et al.: Prophylactic antibiotics in gynecologic surgery. Obstet Gynecol 1979; 53:537.
24. Duff P: Antibiotic prophylaxis for abdominal hysterectomy. Obstet Gynecol 1982; 60:25.
25. Allen JL, Rampone JF, Wheeless CR: Use of a prophylactic antibiotic in elective major gynecologic operations. Obstet Gynecol 1972; 39:218.
26. Hemsell DL, Reisch J, Nobles B, Hemsell PG: Prevention of major infection after elective abdominal hysterectomy: Individual determination required. Am J Obstet Gynecol 1983; 147:520.
27. Smith JP, Day TG: Review of ovarian cancer at the University of Texas Systems Cancer Center, MD Anderson Hospital and Tumor Institute. Am J Obstet Gynecol 1979; 135:984.
28. Grogan RH: Residual ovaries. Obstet Gynecol 1958; 12:329.
29. Christ JE, Lotze EC: The residual ovary syndrome. Obstet Gynecol 1975; 46:551.
30. Montgomery JB: On discussion of the frequency of oophorectomy at the time of hysterectomy. Am J Obstet Gynecol 1968; 100:724.
31. Aravantinos DJ: Keeping or removing the ovaries at the time of hysterectomy. Eur J Obstet Gynecol Reprod Biol 1988; 28:140.
32. Randall CL: Ovarian function and women after the menopause. Am J Obstet Gynecol 1957; 73:1000.
33. Weiss NS, Harlow BL: Why does hysterectomy without bilateral oophorectomy influence the subsequent incidence of ovarian cancer? Am J Epidemiol 1986; 124:856.
34. Garcia C-R, Cutler WB: Preservation of the ovary: A reevaluation. Fertil Steril 1984; 42:510.
35. Lynch HT, Albano WA, Lynch JF, et al.: Surveillance and management of patients at high genetic risk for ovarian carcinoma. Obstet Gynecol 1982; 59:5589.
36. Richardson EH: A simplified technique of abdominal panhysterectomy. Surg Gynecol Obstet 1929; 48:248.
37. Jaszczak SE, Evans TN: Intrafascial abdominal and vaginal hysterectomy: A reappraisal. Obstet Gynecol 1982; 59:435.
38. England GT, Randall HW, Graves WL: Impairment of tissue defenses by vasoconstrictors in vaginal hysterectomies. Obstet Gynecol 1983; 61:271.
39. Lash AF: A method for reducing the size of the uterus in vaginal hysterectomy. Am J Obstet Gynecol 1941; 42:452.
40. Nichols DH, Randall CL: Vaginal Surgery, 3rd ed. Baltimore, Williams & Wilkins, 1989.
41. Kovac SR: Intramyometrial coring as an adjunct to vaginal hysterectomy. Obstet Gynecol 1986; 67:131.
42. McCall ML: Posterior culdeplasty. Surgical correction of enterocele during vaginal hysterectomy: A preliminary report. Obstet Gynecol 1957; 10:595.
43. Nichols DH, Milley PS, Randall CL: Significance of normal vaginal depth and axis. Obstet Gynecol 1970; 36:251.
44. Holloway HJ: Injury to the urinary tract as a complication of gynecological surgery. Am J Obstet Gynecol 1950; 60:30.
45. Solomons E, Levin EJ, Bauman J, et al.: A pyelographic study of ureteric injuries sustained during hysterectomy for benign conditions. Surg Gynecol Obstet 1960; 111:41.
46. Piscitelli JT, Simel DL, Addison WA: Who should have intravenous pyelograms before hysterectomy for benign disease? Obstet Gynecol 1987; 69:541.
47. Cruikshank SH: Surgical method of identifying the ureters during total vaginal hysterectomy. Obstet Gynecol 1986; 67:277.
48. Symmond RE, Williams TJ, Lee RA, Webb MJ: Posthysterectomy enterocoele and vaginal vault prolapse. Am J Obstet Gynecol 1981; 140:852.
49. Moschowitz AV: The pathogenesis, anatomy, and cure of prolapse of the rectum. Surg Gynecol Obstet 1912; 15:7.
50. Polivy J: Psychologic reactions to hysterectomy: A critical review. Am J Obstet Gynecol 1974; 118:417.

Uterine Surgery

19

Jeffrey B. Russell

HISTORY

The history of knowledge of the uterine corpus is a very interesting one, with the evolution of information spanning over many centuries. The earliest reports arose from superstition, speculation, and tradition passed from one generation to the next. Because religion and early law forbade physicians from dissecting human bodies, most of the information obtained was extrapolated from animal dissection. Thus, most of the early knowledge centers around the vertebrate duplication of the reproductive system, which consistently expresses a duplex or bicornuate uterus.

The early developments surfaced during the Golden Age of Greece from the Father of Medicine, Hippocrates.[1, 2] Hippocrates (460–377 B.C.) believed that the uterus had a number of cavities, allowing only one gestation within each cavity.[3] Each cavity was lined with "tentacles" or "suckers." Surprisingly, Aristotle, who we think of as a philosopher rather than a scientist, was actually one of the greatest biologists of his time. Aristotle's work and theories about reproduction dealt with implantation, early embryo development, and ovulation within the uterine cavity. Aristotle's information came from his work with animals and discussed the concept of the uterus as a bicornuate anatomic structure.

Herophilus of Chalcedon (fourth century B.C.) and Rufus and Soranus of Ephesus (second century A.D.) continued the notion of the uterus as a duplicate entity or bicornuate.[3] They each noticed that the uterus and the tubes were separate entities and identified the ovaries but were not sure of their function. Unlike most of the early works and drawings from Aristotle's era (382–324 B.C.), which have been lost, Soranus (110 B.C.) was able to piece together some of the early thoughts from his predecessors and had them organized in a text fashion. In Soranus's *Gynecology*, unfortunately not illustrated, the uterus is described as a "cupping vessel with two folds that disappear with pregnancy."[3, 4] Soranus' writings clearly are some of the greatest works of science in the early Christian era. A similarity was established between the ovary and the testes. His objectivity and directness, which excluded superstition, was more compassionate with the nineteenth century writers than through all of the second century A.D. He was quoted and copied extensively by his students until the seventeenth century.

The historical focus during the Roman Empire changed from the educational and learning to the radical with surgical instruments and operative procedures prevailing. In 1350, a major advancement in the knowledge of human anatomy was achieved at the University of Bologna, where Mondino dei Luzzi had authorization for the dissection of a human body.[3, 5] This allowed Mondino to compose drawings that are similar to our present-day understanding of human anatomy.

From 1452 to 1519, Leonardo Da Vinci and his famous sketches revealed the uterus to contain only one cavity. A contemporary of Leonardo Da Vinci was Berenjario, who studied the reproductive system and found that the uterus contained a single chamber.[3, 7] Another major advancement in the elucidation of the uterine corpus came from Vesalius.[3, 6] Vesalius was born in Brussels, educated in Louvain, and settled in Padua. Vesalius prepared his work *(De Humani Corporis Fabrica)* and was sought by students from all over Europe, Britain, and Russia. Vesalius was a very popular gentleman during his lifetime. Many people who heard about Vesalius flocked to hear his lectures as well as observe his numerous eloquent human dissections. The term "uterus pelvis" was used for the first time in his teachings, and the ovaries were called "female testicles."

By the end of the sixteenth century and early seventeenth century, the uterus had been sectioned and studied extensively. Attention had turned to other components of the reproductive tract, such as the work by Graaff on the follicle and William Hunter's work on the placenta.

From 1801 to 1858, Johannas Peter Müller of London collaborated on the embryology of the genitalia and vertebrates in his *Bildungsgeschichteder Genitalien* (1830), describing clearly the development of the müllerian system comprising the uterus. Müller, the eldest of five children, wrote 20 books and 250 scientific papers illustrated with 350 hand-drawn plates.[3] This established Müller as the foremost German physiologist and one of the most prolific illustrious authors of the nineteenth century. Müller's success came from his direction towards concrete ideas with experiments and research rather than the typical abstract thought, speculation, and philosophy that was rampant during his time.[3]

During the twentieth century, a rapid growth and change in our ability to investigate and understand anatomy, physiology, and molecular biology have rapidly improved our knowledge of the uterus. The evolution of the uterine corpus, fallopian tubes, and ovary combined with the subjects of anatomy, embryology, and implantation has shown a rapid continuum of change and given us a new direction.

ANATOMY

The uterus is composed of two main parts—the cervix and the fundus uteri. The cervix, which protrudes into the vagina, is covered with a squamous epithelium and a number of mucus-secreting glands. The external os, which opens to the vaginal cavity, is approximately 2 cm long and is lined with squamous epithelium and endocervical glands. At the end of this canal is a transformation area with the uterine cavity, called the internal os. The endocervical canal is lined with mucus-secreting glands and is arranged in a series of folds called plicae palmatae. The uterine cavity, which lies above the internal cervical os, is triangular and approximately 3.5 cm in length. In a mature woman, the uterus is 7.5 cm long, 5 cm wide, and 2.5 cm thick, and weighs approximately 40 grams. The anterior and posterior walls of the uterus approximate each other, and potential space within the uterine cavity is minuscule if any.

The position of the uterus within the pelvic cavity may be from anteflexed and anteverted to retroflexed and retroverted. The most common position in a nulliparous woman would be a uterus that is slightly inclined toward the symphysis against the bladder or moderate anteflexion. Approximately 25–33% of women have a uterus that reflects posteriorly or is retroflexed towards the sacrum. The short area of constriction of the lower uterine segment is the isthmus, with the dome shape of the uterus turned to the fundus.

The uterus is divided into three layers, covered by a thin external serosal layer that is comprised from the visceral peritoneum. This is attached firmly to the uterus except anteriorly at the level of the internal os of the cervix. The wide middle muscular layer is composed of three indistinct layers of smooth muscle: the outer longitudinal layer, which is continuous with the muscle layers of the oviduct and vagina; the middle layer, which is interlacing spiral bundles of smooth muscle and large venous plexus; and the intermuscularis layer, which is longitudinal. The glands of the uterus are tubular and composed of columnar epithelium. The endometrium, which lines the intermuscularis layer, is composed of the interstratum basale and the outer stratum functionale. The stratum functionale, which is the only layer that responds to fluctuating hormonal levels, may be further divided into inner compact stratum and a more superficial spongy stratum.

The arterial blood supply to the uterus is provided by the ovarian and uterine arteries. The uterine arteries arise from the hypogastric artery and swing midline for insertion into the uterus at the level of the internal os. The ovarian arteries, on the other hand, originate directly from the aorta. The venous drainage from the uterine fundus travels to the inferior vena cava. Blood from the uterine corpus exits through the uterine veins into the iliac veins. The uterine artery divides into descending and ascending limbs. The descending limb courses downward towards the cervix and the lateral wall of the vagina. The ascending limb passes upwards along the uterus and continues below the fallopian tubes. The blood supply that enters the uterus is on the lateral margins. This is clinically important during uterine surgical procedures such as myomectomy or removal of a large leiomyomatous uterus during vaginal or abdominal surgery.

The vascular anatomy of the uterus reveals numerous branches running both centrifugally towards the serosa and centripetally towards the endometrium. There is an abundance of small arterial vessels immediately below the serosal surface. The inner two-thirds of the myometrium is supplied by tortuous radical branches of the arcuate arteries. At the basal layer of the endometrium with the subjacent myometrium, an abrupt change in the density of the arterial pattern is noted. The endometrial vessels are relatively sparse when compared with those of the myometrium during all different hormonal stages of the menstrual cycle.

The peritoneum that covers the uterus is separated from the uterine musculature by a thin layer of periuterine fascia. The periuterine fascia is a continuation of the transversalis fascia.

The uterus is principally supported by three pairs of ligaments. The most important are the paired cardinal or transverse cervical ligaments. These are also called Mackenrodt's ligaments. Mackenrodt's ligaments arise from the anterior posterior marginal walls of the cervix and fan out laterally to insert into the fascia overlying the obturator muscles and to levator ani muscles of the pelvic floor. The cardinal ligaments form the base of the broad ligament that surrounds the uterine blood vessels as well as accompanies nerves and the lymphatic supply.

The second pair of ligamentous support for the uterus arises from the anterior superior surface of the uterus through the inguinal rings. These are called the round ligaments, which travel through the inguinal rings and through the inguinal canals to end in the labia majora. The third pair of ligaments are the uterosacral ligaments; they insert into the sacral fascia over the second and third sacral vertebrae and arise from the posterior wall of the uterus at the level of the internal cervical os. These three sets of ligaments contain muscle fibers, connective tissue, blood vessels, nerves, and lymphatic drainage.

The endometrium is composed of three layers—the pars basalis, zona spongiosa, and superficial zona compacta. Sinus-like dilatations of the capillaries, which can be seen on ultrasound evaluation, are sometimes called lakes. These vascular lakes are drained by small veins.

UTERINE SURGERY

Conservative uterine surgery is essential for preservation of menstrual cycles and reproductive function. The two most commonly performed uterine procedures are the removal of a leiomyoma, or myomectomy, and correction of congenital müllerian anomalies. Occasionally, surgical indications are clear-cut when to operate, but many are somewhat controversial when related to the ability to conceive or subsequent pregnancy loss.

Myomectomy

Although the correlation between leiomyoma and infertility is lacking, myomectomy may be indicated for those patients attempting to maintain their reproductive potential. A well-circumscribed, nonencapsulated, benign tumor arising from smooth muscle cells from the cervix or uterine corpus is called a uterine leiomyoma. The cell origin of a leiomyoma is from immature smooth muscle cells in the myometrium or from smooth muscle cells surrounding neighboring blood vessels. Leiomyomas may also contain thick connective tissue. The classification of a leiomyoma is derived from its location. Leiomyomas may arise from the myometrium or interstitial or intramural portion and may remain intramural or extend internally, externally, submucosal, or subserosal. All uterine leiomyomas arise from the myometrium, and those that are subserous can be classified as either interligamentous or pedunculated. Submucous leiomyomas can also be classified as pedunculated. Leiomyomas that are pedunculated may become parasitic, obtaining their blood supply from other sources such as the omentum or bowel. Submucosal leiomyomas may occupy the entire uterine cavity and even extend through the cervical os.

The term leiomyoma is preferred to other terms such as myofibroma, fibroid, leiomyofibroma, fibroleiomyoma, and fibromyoma. In 1955, Miller and colleagues described smooth muscle cells within the uterus as the origin of the leiomyoma,[8] but Townsend and coworkers in 1970 proposed a unicellular histogenesis of uterine leiomyomas.[9] Leiomyomas are the most frequent tumors within the female pelvis and are three times more prevalent in black than in white women. The growth of leiomyomas is clearly dependent upon the estrogen environment. Leiomyomas grow with pregnancy and oral contraception use and regress during the menopausal period. Early reports by Spellacy and associates and by Goodman showed a decrease in fibroid size in women using antiestrogen preparations or with the utilization of progesterone.[10, 11] Although the estradiol levels in patients with fibroids are similar to those levels in women without these tumors, estrogen receptors and binding are much higher in women with leiomyoma, combined with a decrease in the conversion of estradiol to estrone.[12] A decrease or lack of 17-beta hydroxydehydrogenase may stimulate cellular growth at the molecular level.[13] Other endocrine abnormalities have been identified, both locally and centrally, to be associated with leiomyomatous growth. Centrally, lower follicle-stimulating hormone with a diminished response to gonadotropin-releasing hormones and thyroid-releasing hormones stimulates an excessive prolactin response, it has been reported.[14] In addition, growth hormone was found to be twice as high in patients with leiomyoma.[10] Leiomyomatous tissue has also been identified as having a higher 5-alpha reductase activity when compared with myometrium without leiomyomatous tissue.[15]

Histologic examination of a leiomyomatous uterus reveals a whirl-like arrangement of fibrous and muscular tissue, and a common change within this tissue is hyaline degeneration. Other changes have been noted to occur in leiomyomatous tissue, but the most serious changes are sarcomatous.

Indications

Leiomyomas are usually small and asymptomatic with less than 50% of patients having symptoms.[16] The symptoms that do arise are related to the size and location of the leiomyoma. Degeneration may account for only a small percentage of symptoms involving torsion, infarction, or infection. Possible symptoms include abnormal bleeding, pressure, pain, abdominal distention, and rapid growth during pregnancy. Problems such as miscarriage and pregnancy-related complications are due to the location and the size of the leiomyoma. Abnormal heavy menstrual bleeding (menorrhagia) or prolonged (metrorrhagia) periods may necessitate treatment. Chronic depletion of blood supplies is inapparent to the patient and may be detected only by sophisticated studies such as serum ferritin levels. Iron stains of the bone marrow or indices indicative of hypochromatic microcytic anemia may also be indications of the chronic anemia.

Any leiomyoma may cause heavy bleeding, but submucous leiomyomas are notoriously known for the increase in menstrual blood flow due to poor mucosal synchrony and decreased contractibility, thus cessating menstrual blood loss. The bleeding may be disguised as a pink or blood-tinged discharge and not associated specifically with menstrual blood loss. The surface area of a submucous leiomyoma increases 10-fold, and the specific histologic picture may vary from atrophy to hyperplasia.[17] The proximal congestion and obstruction of the uterus may cause thrombosis and sloughing, initiating heavy prolonged bleeding periods. Another symptom of leiomyomatous uterus is pressure. Rapid or continual growth of the leiomyoma may obstruct the pelvic brim, impinging upon the ureter, and must be closely watched for signs of hydronephrosis and hydroureter. Left unattended, irreversible kidney parenchymal damage may occur, causing uremia.

Pain from a leiomyomatous uterus is a common symptom and usually necessitates operative intervention such as myomectomy or hysterectomy. Rapid growth of a leiomyoma is reason for exploration with subsequent removal. Although rapid growth has attempted to be defined, a definitive method of documentation without a large intraobserver variation is very difficult.[18] Ultrasound and, more recently, vaginal ultrasound provide excellent methods of documenting uterine growth. The new technology of magnetic resonance imaging for leiomyomatous uterus may not be cost effective except in very selected cases for differentiating a pedunculated leiomyoma versus adnexal masses, but clearly can document rapid growth or leiomyomatous enlargement.

Asymptomatic leiomyoma in an infertile patient presents many issues and unanswerable questions. Is the cause of infertility related to the size of the leiomyomatous uterus? Does the location of the leiomyoma in a patient who is infertile with adequate cervical mucus, sperm transport, capacitation, fertilization, and implantation have any implication for subsequent fertility, requiring surgical intervention?

When to Treat Leiomyomas

The main focus of treating leiomyomas concentrates around the conservation of reproductive function. Most importantly, the interaction with the patient must include a thorough history and physical examination and a discussion about possible complications. Although rare, the possibility of a hysterectomy during the myomectomy must be discussed with the patient desperately seeking conservative reproductive surgery to maintain future fertility. A preoperative hysterosalpingogram for a submucosal leiomyoma and ultrasound occasionally combined with magnetic resonance imaging should provide the surgeon with an excellent approach to the uterine cavity and the knowledge about the leiomyoma (Fig. 19–1).

A large uterine leiomyoma may compromise fertility by decreasing the uterine cavity sperm transport time as well as impairing implantation. Anatomically, distortion of the fallopian tube by a pedunculated or intraligamentous leiomyoma may interfere with sperm and egg transport as well as embryo transfer back to the uterine cavity. Venous stasis or vascular congestion of the endometrium and/or myometrium can result in a deleterious effect by the tumor causing vascular compromise. Cervical compression of cervical glands changing the position of the canal and/or the composition of the cervical mucus may interfere with cervical gland production and sperm transport. Histologic changes from intramural fibroids may cause pathologic changes consisting of atrophy to hyperplasia, preventing nidation or implantation. Uterine irritability with the release of prostaglandins from the leiomyoma may change the implantation environment to one of diminishing receptivity.

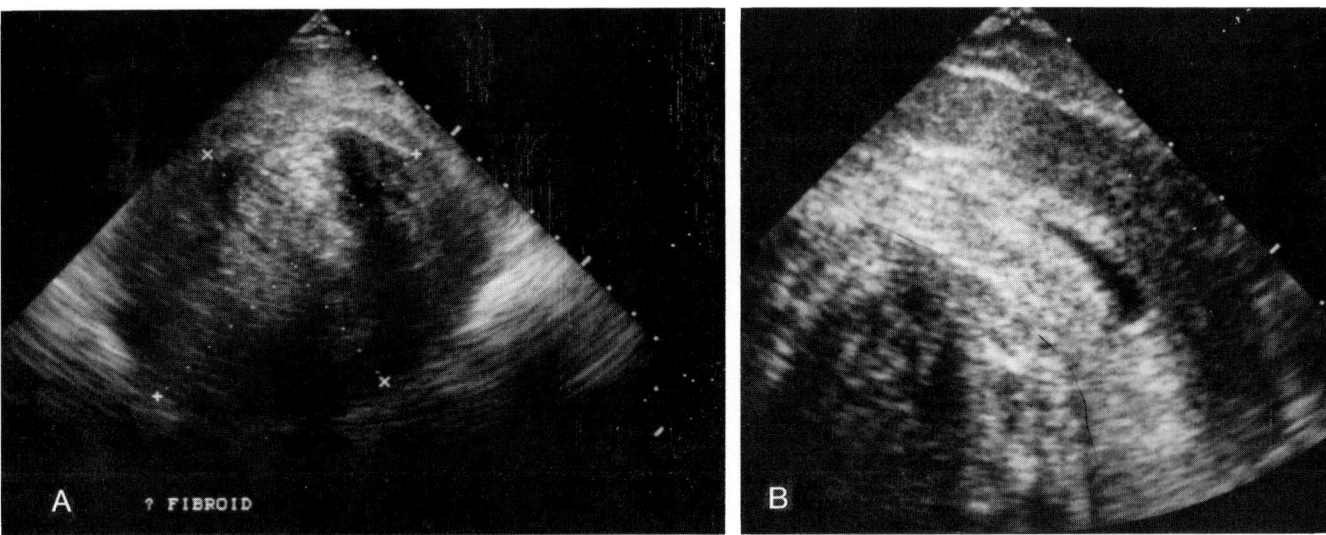

Figure 19–1
A, Large posterior leiomyoma 8.4 cm in widest diameter identified by transvaginal ultrasound. B, Edge of leiomyoma adjacent to endometrium.

Clearly, all factors must be excluded prior to performing a myomectomy for fertility purposes. The location, size, or number of leiomyoma must be evaluated as well as the fertility status of the woman undergoing the procedure. The actual procedure itself has been shown by Berkeley and associates to decrease fertility through postoperative adhesions.[19]

A difficult decision is encountered when the patient between the ages of 38 and 42 seeks advice about her infertility treatment and has been identified as having a leiomyomatous uterus. All options must be considered by the patient. An association with infertility to a leiomyomatous uterus is identified when a cornual obstruction or cervical impedance is discovered. Whether infertility is hindered or the incidence of a spontaneous abortion is increased must be discussed with the patient with all available information, including risks, complications, outcome, and results.

Techniques of Myomectomy

The techniques of surgical myomectomy probably date back to the middle of the nineteenth century, but it was not until the first half of the twentieth century and the reports by Kelly and Noble, Mayo, Bonney, and Rubin that the procedure became popularized.[20–23] The focus by various textbooks on gynecologic surgery today specifically addresses the surgical technique with strict adherence to microsurgical principles through gentle tissue handling, minimalization of blood loss, and meticulous approximation after perpendicular dissection of tissue planes as the hallmarks of conserving reproductive function and decreasing adhesion formation. Conception rates following myomectomy vary significantly, from 6 to 100%. When the leiomyoma was the prime cause of infertility, the relationship to conception following myomectomy ranged from 16% to 88%.[18, 19, 21–23]

In 1978, Babaknia and colleagues followed 46 patients retrospectively over a 24-year period who had been identified as having a leiomyomatous uterus as the only cause of their infertility.[24] Of those 46 patients whose only treatment was myomectomy, 22 (48%) conceived, and 19 patients carried to term. When the infertility was separated into primary versus secondary, 34 patients had primary infertility with 14 (41%) of these patients conceiving, and 13 (96%) carrying to term. Only 8 of the other 12 patients with secondary infertility had a 66% conception rate, and only 6 of the 8 carried to term. One year later (1979), Ranney and Frederick noted that 8 of 9 patients in whom uterine leiomyomas were reported as the major cause of infertility delivered a total of 15 infants.[25] Although their data are confusing, Ranney and Frederick also looked at 16 patients in whom there were other causes of infertility and identified such conditions as endometriosis, tubal disease, a cystadenoma, and polycystic ovarian disease and found that 13 of 16 patients (81%) who underwent a subsequent myomectomy conceived after the surgical procedure was performed for the leiomyoma. In 1981, Buttram and Reiter retrospectively reviewed 1193 patients and found an overall pregnancy rate of 40%, which was increased to 54% by performing a myomectomy among 76 patients in whom no other cause was found.[18] More recently, Berkeley and associates reported a 42% conception rate in patients undergoing any other reconstructive infertility procedures for conditions that were correctable at the time of the myomectomy.[19] However, when Berkeley compared those patients who underwent a surgical procedure for a myomectomy alone, only a 16% conception rate was attributed to the myomectomy.

In 1986, D.L. Rosenfeld showed that 15 of 23 patients (65.2%) conceived after abdominal removal of subserosal or intramural leiomyomas.[26] None of these leiomyomas were submucosal in their location, nor did their number, size, preoperative hysterosalpingogram, or presence of menorrhagia necessarily predict the success from the procedure. Starks reported on 20 of 32 infertility patients with unexplained infertility who conceived after a CO_2 laser myomectomy.[27] Seventeen of these women ultimately delivered a viable term infant. Of the 20 patients who had conceived, 14 had previously been categorized as having primary infertility and 6 as having secondary infertility. Gatti and colleagues evaluated 30 patients undergoing abdominal myomectomy with subsequent conception and term pregnancy.[28] Of the 30 patients who had a myomectomy performed, 13 conceived and 10 had a term infant delivered. Of the other 17 patients who did not conceive, 10 had other causes of their infertility. Most studies confirm that the age of the patient and the size of the leiomyoma does not significantly influence the subsequent pregnancy rate after myomectomy. Gatti did show that the most important correlation related to subsequent infertility was the duration of infertility prior to myomectomy, and a higher term pregnancy rate appears to be associated with a positive previous obstetric history.

The relationship of the location of the leiomyoma to subsequent outcome has been inferred by all reproductive surgeons, although little data in a controlled fashion have been utilized to confirm this hypothesis. Brown and coworkers reported on 28 patients in an uncontrolled series who underwent removal of a submucous leiomyoma; only 6 of these patients conceived. Of these 6 patients, 3 later aborted.[29] Brown compared this to the overall 42% conception rate. In a study by Finn and Muller in 1950, no alteration in the conception or obstetric prognosis was noted in terms of the location of the leiomyoma.[30] The relationship of the size of the uterine cavity with its influence on conception is also without convincing information. In a study performed by Babaknia, the preoperative hysterosalpingogram had no correlation associated with the subsequent ability for a term delivery.[24] In contrast, a review by Buttram and Reiter noted that in 10 patients who had a preoperative uterine size of 8 weeks' gestation or less, a 100% conception rate occurred, whereas in those patients with a uterine size greater than 10 weeks' gestation, no pregnancy occurred.[18]

Preoperative Evaluation

The preoperative evaluation prior to myomectomy may include ultrasound, computed tomography (CT scan), or magnetic resonance imaging (MRI). When the masses are very large, an intravenous pyelogram may help delineate the course and any possible anomalies of the ureters. The more complex masses may require higher resolution such as a CT scan or MRI. Preoperatively, the placement of a pediatric Foley catheter inside the uterine cavity will immediately alert the surgeon that the uterine cavity has been opened. The pediatric Foley catheter also keeps the cervical os open for postoperative bleeding or drainage.

Abdominal myomectomy may be performed through a transverse Pfannenstiel incision for a small leiomyomatous uterus or by using a larger muscle splitting incision called a Maylard incision. The procedure is initiated by opening the abdomen, and the adhesions to the peritoneal surface are lysed or removed. The pelvis is explored, and the upper abdomen is checked for any abnormalities; the kidneys, liver, spleen, and any periaortic masses are identified at this time. The intestines are packed up into the upper abdominal cavity. Lap sponges are placed in sterile plastic bags soaked in Ringer's lactate solution to reduce abrasion and subsequent adhesion formation. The field is kept moist with Ringer's lactate. The initial incision into the uterine cavity should maximize the amount of leiomyomatous tissue to be removed, which subsequently decreases blood loss and the amount of raw surface area for postoperative adhesion formation.

Blood loss from the procedure can be extensive. Routinely, the patient donates two units of blood within 2 weeks of the procedure for the possibility of an autologous transfusion. In addition to having autologous blood available, several methods of decreasing blood loss during the procedure are useful, including meticulous and delicate dissection. Occlusion of the uterine arteries with a clamp, forceps, or tourniquet will decrease uterine blood flow. A 0.25-inch Penrose drain secure enough to occlude arterial flow may be placed around the uterine arteries through an avascular area created in the broad ligament. Another Penrose drain may be placed around the infundibular pelvic ligament using the same opening in the broad ligament. The use of one ampule of vasopressin combined with 10 ml of injectable saline along the incision decreases the initial blood loss from the uterine corpus. Venous pools and arterial bleeding should be coagulated individually or tied during the operative procedure. Atraumatic vascular clamps can be placed on the ovarian vessels bilaterally, which will also decrease uterine blood loss.

If several incisions are required to remove the leiomyomas, an anterior incision is preferred so as not to interfere with oocyte pickup from the fallopian tubes. Anteriorly, the adhesions may attach to the posterior aspect of the bladder and provide a "pseudo" uterine suspension.

Once the initial incision is made, as many leiomyomas as possible should be removed through this incision. Sharp and blunt dissection using the Metzenbaum scissors, CO_2 laser, or the knife handle may be used to separate the leiomyomas from surrounding tissues. Occasionally, finger dissection may aid in enucleating the leiomyoma from the uterus in conjunction with countertraction with a single-tooth tenaculum or Lahey thyroid clamp. The base of the leiomyoma may be coagulated or suture ligated with a 2-0 to 4-0 polyglactin suture.

Special attention should also be employed when removing a leiomyoma from the interstitial portion of a cornu in close proximity to the ostium of a fallopian tube. The ostium may be disrupted, compromising the patency of the tube. If the leiomyoma is near the insertion of the fallopian tube lumen, a small flexible guide wire or ureteral stent may be easily passed through the lumen to maintain the patency of the fallopian tube. Once the leiomyoma is removed, it is important to understand that dead space must be approximated and the anatomy of the uterine myometrium restored as much as possible to its original shape. If the cavity is entered, the myometrium must be approximated so as not to invaginate or incorporate endometrium into the myometrial portion of the uterine corpus. This will avoid the possibility of adenomyosis and its associated problems.

The serosal surface of the uterine cavity is approximated with 4-0 to 6-0 polyglactin suture, and all bleeding should be secured before closing the incision. A baseball or external-to-internal stitch, covering the knot within the incision, is very helpful in decreasing adhesion formation. The use of high-molecular-weight dextran intraabdominally along with removing any clots or residual blood from the peritoneal cavity will also aid in decreasing the adhesion formation. Meticulous dissection and gentle tissue handling are hallmarks for successful adhesion-free removal of leiomyomas.

Preoperative Medical Treatment

Gonadotropin-releasing hormone (GnRH) agonists have been used as a pretreatment to decrease blood loss during the enucleation and dissection of the leiomyoma from the uterine cavity. In a randomized, placebo-controlled study evaluating use of the GnRH agonist before a myomectomy, Friedman and colleagues revealed that the mean total intraoperative blood loss was significantly less in those treated with a long-acting GnRH agonist prior to the myomectomy.[31] The initial experience with long- and short-acting GnRH was very promising. All patients showed a rapid reduction in uterine size; unfortunately, once the analogue was discontinued, the leiomyomas returned to their original size. Myomectomy should be scheduled at the peak of the reduction of uterine size, which is 3 to 4 months after the drug is initiated.

Transcervical Hysteroscopic Myomectomy

Neuwirth described the use of a urologic resectoscope to remove pedunculated or submucous intrauterine leiomyomas.[32, 33] He initially used a cutting loop powered by a transistorized unit with approximately 70 watts of continuous cutting power. His distending media was high-molecular-weight dextran to visualize and distend the intrauterine cavity. The depth of the burn using the cutting loop was not believed to be more than 2 mm even at such an elevated wattage. Occasionally, the resectoscope may be used to first morcellate a submucous leiomyoma by several passes of the resectoscopic loop until the surface is contiguous with the surrounding endometrium.

The resectoscope is introduced into the uterine cavity, and the leiomyoma is identified. The position of the leiomyoma in reference to the uterine wall and the tubal ostium is also noted. Concurrently, diagnostic laparoscopy is performed to decrease the possibility of uterine perforation with bowel or bladder injury. The resectoscope is then advanced to the fundus and withdrawn until the leiomyoma is resected. Occasionally, large parcels of resected leiomyoma may be removed through the hysteroscopic sheath to allow adequate visualization. If hemostasis is not adequately maintained during the procedure, the resectoscopic loop may be transferred to the coagulating mode and bleeders coagulated. Occasionally, a Silastic or pediatric Foley balloon catheter may be placed inside the uterine cavity if bleeding does not readily stop with electrocoagulation.

Hallez and Perino also reported their experience with the transcervical resection of 61 submucous leiomyomas.[34] They clearly showed the advantages of this technique by demonstrating precise hemostasis, complete and controlled uterine evacuation, minimal postoperative infection, and precise histologic diagnosis without the complications associated with hysterectomy or abdominal myomectomy. Lin and colleagues also expressed their favorable experience in 13 women with chief complaints of menorrhagia and metrorrhagia who underwent transcervical resection of pedunculated submucous leiomyomas.[35] Eight of those thirteen women subsequently were resolved of their chief complaints without any further surgical procedures. Brooks and coworkers performed a transcervical hysteroscopic myomectomy on 90 women with uncontrollable uterine bleeding due to submucous leiomyomas or large polyps.[36] These investigators revealed a 91% resumption of normal menses in those patients with submucous leiomyomas and a term pregnancy rate of 33% in 15 patients who had uncontrollable uterine bleeding combined with infertility. Brooks and colleagues reported only two complications—uterine perforation and endometritis—but overall believed that transcervical hysteroscopic myomectomy was a safe and highly effective alternative to the abdominal surgical procedure. Grainger and DeCherney reported pretreatment with a GnRH agonist to shrink tumors prior to performing transcervical hysteroscopic resection.[37] The size of the leiomyoma after 3–4 months' use of a GnRH agonist facilitated easier hysteroscopic removal.

The introduction of fiberoptic lasers for infertility surgery has also affected the area of transcervical hysteroscopic myomectomy. Initial experience revealed that small leiomyomas can be vaporized using the KTP or argon laser, although larger lesions require the larger cutting surface diameter employed by the resectoscopic wire loop. The Nd:YAG laser, which has been introduced primarily for endometrial ablation, appears to promote charring in the uterine cavity without actual vaporization of the submucous fibroid. The combination of both fiberoptic and resectoscopic techniques appears to maximize the surgical ability of both instruments.

Obstetric Management

The obstetric management of patients who undergo abdominal myomectomy should be routine in nature unless other confounding obstetric indications require abdominal delivery. Several studies have reported successful vaginal delivery without uterine rupture. Davids, in a series of 1150 patients, and Brown and colleagues described vaginal delivery even when the endometrial cavity was entered at the time of myomectomy.[29, 38] Typically, the rupture of a post-myomectomy gravid uterus usually occurs in the third trimester or during labor. In an unusual case, Golan and coworkers reported spontaneous rupture at 20 weeks' gestation in a post-myomectomy uterus.[39] Although most studies report a 60–70% vaginal delivery rate, patients who are status post–abdominal myomectomy should be observed closely during their third trimester and during labor for possible signs or symptoms of uterine rupture.

Recurrence

One must always discuss with the patient undergoing a myomectomy the potential for recurrence. Owing to the conservative nature of the surgical procedure, future myomectomy or subsequently uterine removal may be required. Patients more prone to recurrence are those with multiple leiomyomas at the time of the initial operative procedure. Those patients with one or two contiguous leiomyomas, no matter what the size, appear to do very well without subsequent recurrence.

Müllerian Anomalies

The absence of müllerian-inhibiting factors (MIF) produced by the functioning testes allows the müllerian ducts to develop. The human uterus is derived from the paramesonephric or müllerian ducts. The müllerian ducts arise as an invagination of the embryonic coelomic mesothelium somewhere around the sixth to seventh week of gestation. The ducts grow inferiorly and medially towards the urogenital sinus with the superior portions becoming the fallopian tubes and the inferior portions fusing to form the uterus, cervix, and upper two-thirds of the vagina. The ducts are initially solid and later undergo invagination with resorption of the tissue between the two pairs of ducts. The resorption of tissue between the two ducts gives rise to a normal upper vagina, uterus, and single uterine cavity. Any degree of failure of migration or fusion or subsequent failure of resorption results in a wide variety of clinical müllerian abnormalities.

The early description of müllerian anomalies by Jarcho in 1946 has been modified and expounded on by many authors over the years.[40] Considering the two pairs of paramesonephric ducts with the failure of fusion and regression of the solid portions, the uterine malformations may be symmetrical or asymmetrical as well as obstructive or nonobstructive. Asymmetrical uterine malformations occur when one paramesonephric duct develops normally while the other duct is imperfect or completely absent. The unicornuate uterus with or without any rudimentary horns falls in this category of asymmetrical uterine malformations.

Because the reproductive and urinary tracts are so closely related embryologically, a thorough investigation of malformed reproductive organs is incomplete unless a radiologic investigation of the urinary tract is performed. The congenital absence of one kidney in patients with genital or müllerian abnormalities was found by Rock and Jones to be present in 9% of patients.[41] Thompson and Lynn found a solitary kidney in 40% of those patients with genital abnormalities.[42] The occurrence of total agenesis of the müllerian ducts is incompatible with life, because neither would likely develop.

Uterine Anomalies Associated with the Need for Surgery

The most common uterine anomalies are those from various degrees of failure of fusion of the müllerian ducts. The exact determination of the frequency of these anomalies is difficult, owing to the extensive variability. An estimate of their incidence varies from 0.13 to 0.40% and can be detected only by direct visualization or radiographic studies. The reason for the variability in müllerian abnormalities is due to pregnancies that proceed without any evidence that a uterine abnormality is present.

Green and Harris reviewed approximately 32,000 deliveries and detected müllerian anomalies only in 0.25%.[43] Most authors report the incidence of congenital uterine malformations to range between 0.1 and 1.0%. Pregnancy occurs in many of these women despite anomalies with a slightly higher increase in complications such as abortion, prematurity, hemorrhage, retained placenta, breech deliveries, and abnormal fetal presentations. Any patient with a history of reproductive failure, including repeat fetal wastage, premature labor, or fetal malpresentation, must be evaluated for the possibility of a congenital uterine abnormality.

Prior to performing any uterine septum unification or uterine müllerian abnormality procedures, it is essential to completely understand the anatomic communication and the absence or presence of the uterine cavities.

Congenital anomalies of the müllerian ducts associated with lateral fusion include septate uterus, bicornuate uterus, didelphys uterus, unicornuate uterus, and longitudinal vaginal septum with or without obstruction (Fig. 19–2). Complete failure of the medial fusion of the two müllerian ducts may result in a complete duplication of the vagina, cervix, and uterus. The first reported excision of a uterine septum was performed by Schroder in 1884 in a woman who had two previous abortions. The patient recovered from the procedure and subsequently went on to deliver a child at term. Paul Strassman of Berlin and later his son Erwin Strassman were strong advocates of uterine surgery and specifically unification operations.[44]

The extensive work by Howard and Georgianna Jones has aided greatly in our understanding and management of patients with congenital müllerian abnormalities.[45, 46] A wide variety of uterine abnormalities may occur but escape the attention or detection of the attending physician if the patient does not have any gynecologic difficulties or decreased reproductive performance. The anomalies associated with obstruction come to the attention of the gynecologist shortly after menarche.

Preoperative Evaluation

Occasionally on physical examination, a heart-shaped fundus or a rudimentary horn may be palpated, but the majority of müllerian abnormalities are discovered by curettage, hysterosalpingogram,

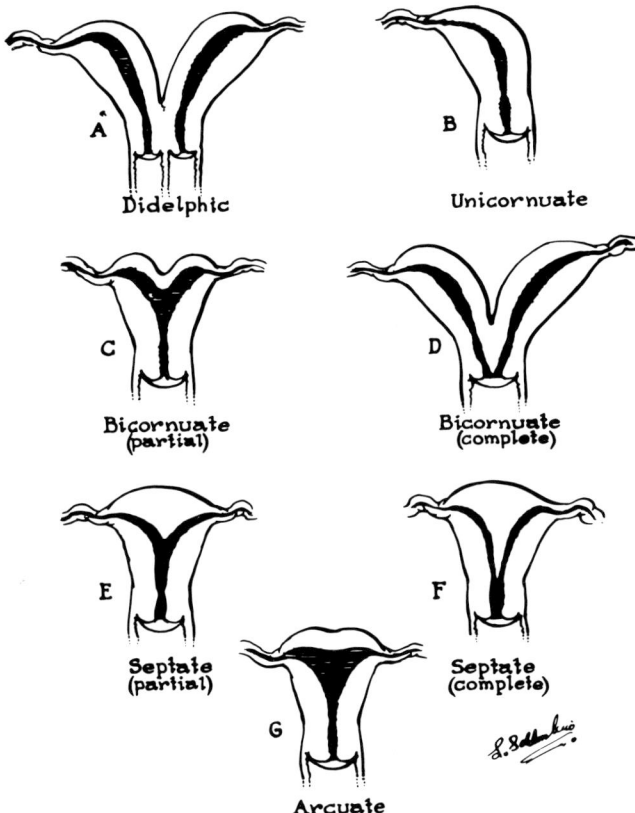

Figure 19–2
A to G, Congenital anomalies of the müllerian ducts associated with lateral fusion. (From Jones H Jr: Reproductive impairment and the malformed uterus. In Wallach E, Kempers R (eds.): Modern Trends in Infertility and Conception Control, Vol. 2. Philadelphia, JB Lippincott (Harper Medical), 1982, pp. 282–293.)

hysteroscopy, ultrasonography, and pelvic endoscopy. A hysterosalpingogram is the most commonly used procedure to diagnose or detect uterine anomalies but is limited to the delineation of the internal contour of the uterine cavity. The hysterosalpingogram fails to show any external abnormalities or the number of uterine horns, thus not being able to differentiate a bicornuate from a septate uterus. Although many classifications and explanations for uterine anomalies exist, the American Fertility Society classification of müllerian anomalies may standardize the wide variety of anatomy with some consistency (Fig. 19–3).

Pelvic ultrasound may identify müllerian anomalies and, with the introduction of transvaginal ultrasound, can delineate the number of uterine corpora without hysteroscopy combined with laparoscopy (Fig. 19–4). Pelvic ultrasound can also identify obstructive abnormalities by the presence of hematometria, hematocolpos, and hematosalpinx. Although not always cost-effective, magnetic resonance imaging can provide additional diagnostic information to ascertain the type of uterine abnormality. The most optimal view of the endometrial cavity is during the midluteal phase, when the menstrual endometrium is thicker and easily identifiable. Occasionally an

362 UTERINE SURGERY

THE AMERICAN FERTILITY SOCIETY CLASSIFICATION OF MULLERIAN ANOMALIES

Patient's Name _____ Date _____ Chart # _____

Age _____ G _____ P _____ Sp Ab _____ VTP _____ Ectopic _____ Infertile Yes _____ No _____

Other Significant History (i.e. surgery, infection, etc.) _____

_____

HSG _____ Sonography _____ Photography _____ Laparoscopy _____ Laparotomy _____

EXAMPLES

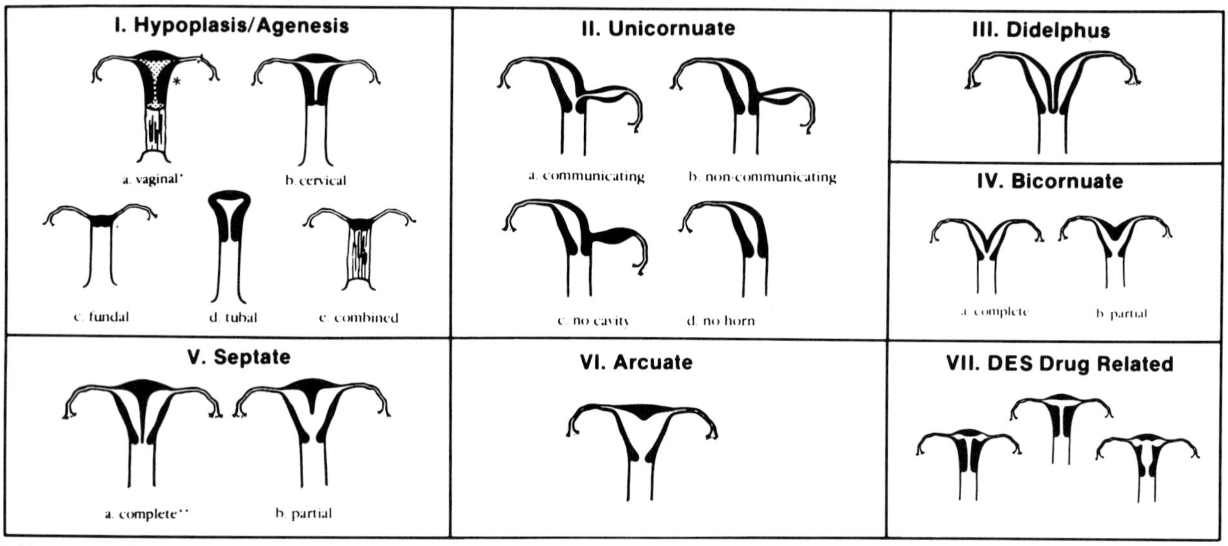

I. Hypoplasis/Agenesis
a. vaginal*
b. cervical
c. fundal
d. tubal
e. combined

II. Unicornuate
a. communicating
b. non-communicating
c. no cavity
d. no horn

III. Didelphus

IV. Bicornuate
a. complete
b. partial

V. Septate
a. complete**
b. partial

VI. Arcuate

VII. DES Drug Related

* Uterus may be normal or take a variety of abnormal forms.
** May have two distinct cervices

Type of Anomaly

Class I _____   Class V _____
Class II _____   Class VI _____
Class III _____   Class VII _____
Class IV _____

Treatment (Surgical Procedures): _____

_____

Prognosis for Conception & Subsequent Viable Infant*

_____ Excellent (> 75%)

_____ Good (50-75%)

_____ Fair (25%-50%)

_____ Poor (< 25%)

*Based upon physician's judgment.

Recommended Followup Treatment: _____

_____

Property of
The American Fertility Society

Additional Findings: _____

_____

Vagina: _____
Cervix: _____

Tubes: Right _____ Left _____
Kidneys: Right _____ Left _____

DRAWING
L   R

For additional supply write to:
The American Fertility Society
2140 11th Avenue, South
Suite 200
Birmingham, Alabama 35205

Figure 19-3
The American Fertility Society classification of müllerian anomalies. (From Fertil Steril 1988; 49:944.)

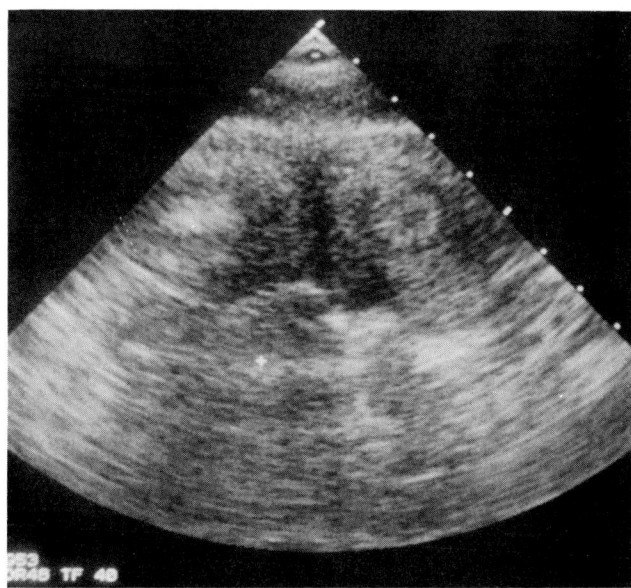

Figure 19–4
Two uterine corpora in a patient with a bicornuate uterus.

arcuate uterus, which is a minor malformation of the failure of the complete fusion of the müllerian ducts, may be confused with a septate or a bicornuate uterus. Perino and coworkers studied 40 women with a suspected septate uterus with ultrasonography.[47] The condition was confirmed by laparoscopy in 95% of those suspected of having a septate uterus.

The surgical correction of a bicornuate uterus must be performed abdominally with the septate uterus being amenable to hysteroscopic metroplasty. The septum in a septate uterus may have variable thickness, be complete or partial, and may even have a small opening to connect the two cavities. Pregnancy wastage indicates the need for a metroplasty or removal of the uterine septum. When a septum is identified initially on an infertility evaluation by the hysterosalpingogram, the question of metroplasty is always entertained. If any other cause is present, it should be corrected first before hysteroscopic septum removal is considered. If all of the infertility factors are within normal limits and a diagnostic laparoscopy is performed, the septum may be removed at the time of the procedure.

Reproductive Performance

Patients with a septate uterus are twice as likely to abort than patients with a bicornuate uterus. The incidence of abortion appears to be higher in those women who have a complete septum versus an incomplete septum. Although information pertaining to the decreased likelihood of conception in those patients with a septate uterus is lacking, Buttram and Gibbons reported 88% of pregnancies in patients who had a complete septum that ended in a fetal loss versus only 70% with a partial septum.[48] Perino and colleagues found 37 of 52 patients who had a previous pregnancy ended in a spontaneous abortion when evaluated for a uterine septum.[47] In a large study by March and Israel, 240 pregnancies in 57 women before a metroplasty was performed resulted in 212 pregnancies ending in the first or second trimester.[49] Only 7 pregnancies (3%) went to term, with 21 pregnancies ending in premature delivery. Only 12 of the 21 premature infants who were delivered survived.

One of the conflicting reports about the reproductive function in women with uterine anomaly comes out of Finland. Heinonen studied the reproductive histories of 182 women with uterine abnormalities.[50] He found a better pregnancy outcome in patients with septate versus complete bicornuate or unicornuate uteri. The septate uterus had an 86% infant survival versus a bicornuate uterus of a 50% or unicornuate uterus of 40%. Jewelewicz, on the other hand, estimated the spontaneous abortion rate in women with a bicornuate uterus to be 33.8% versus 22.2% in those with a septate uterus.[51] Capraro and associates found a preoperative fetal salvage rate for septate uterus to be 33.3%, 10% for bicornuate uterus, and 0% for a didelphys uterus.[52] The presence of a double uterus or a uterine didelphys is more often than not associated with reproductive problems. Only one-third of the patients with a double uterus have important reproductive problems, according to Jones and Seeger-Jones.[53] A didelphys uterus has two uterine corpora and is easily diagnosed because these patients will be found to have two hemicervices visible on a speculum examination or a longitudinal vaginal septum. The experience of Rock and Jones revealed that of the 43 patients who underwent the Jones metroplasty, 77% of those patients had a term delivery.[41]

Capraro and colleagues and Strassman reported that cases of dysmenorrhea and menometrorrhagia found in conjunction with uterine anomalies are relieved by unification procedures combining the two cavities.[44, 52, 54] Although two isolated reports reveal similar findings, it is highly questionable that the unification procedure can alleviate such problems as dysmenorrhea or menorrhagia.

The diagnosis of infertility in conjunction with a müllerian anomaly is not a reason for a metroplasty procedure. Although there have been isolated reports of infertility being corrected by metroplasty procedures, nonuterine causes of infertility must be eliminated and only as a last resort should a metroplasty be performed.

Most of the patients with recurrent pregnancy loss and who have an anatomic abnormality are found to have a septate uterus. Several theories are working when discussing etiology of pregnancy loss with a uterine septum. Many investigators believe that the blood supply from the septum is inadequate for implantation and the gestational sac to develop, whereas others think that the septum impinges upon uterine growth mainly during the second trimester, causing second-trimester fetal loss as well as prematurity.[55-58]

A noncommunicating rudimentary horn with or without an endometrial cavity may warrant surgical intervention to avoid the risk of endometriosis or the complication of an ectopic pregnancy. The overall expectation of fertility and pregnancy outcome in those uteri that are unicornuate with a rudimentary horn is similar to that of a unicornuate uterus. Buttram and Gibbons provide information about 13 pregnancies in 9 patients with a unicornuate uterus who had a rudimentary horn. Only two full-term pregnancies were reported in the patients with a communicating cavity.[48] Although this is a very convincing report, there are no consistent data to suggest that surgical removal of the rudimentary horn would improve fertility or fetal salvage. For obstructed rudimentary horns, O'Leary and O'Leary reviewed 327 gestations and noted that 89% of the uteri had ruptured by the end of the second trimester and that only 1% of the pregnancies resulted in live term births.[59]

Pregnancy outcome with a didelphys uterus appears to be similar to that of the unicornuate uterus. There are only scattered reports of primary infertility, pregnancy loss, or premature labor associated with the didelphys uterus. There are some reports that reflect fetal wastage of up to 40%, but the consensus substantiated by Musick and Behrman confirms a successful pregnancy rate of 57% without any surgical intervention.[60] Only patients with a poor obstetric history should be considered for the metroplasty procedure with a 75% term pregnancy rate.[60]

Prior to a patient undergoing hysteroscopic metroplasty, the patient must have other causes of spontaneous abortion ruled out. A timed endometrial biopsy, cervical cultures, thyroid and prolactin studies, chromosome studies of both parents, screening partial thromboplastin time, antinuclear antibodies, lupus anticoagulant, and anticardiolipin antibodies must be added to the preliminary evaluation before surgery is scheduled.

Abdominal Metroplasty Uterine Unification Procedures

The two types of metroplasty procedures depend upon whether the uterine corpora are separate or a single cavity. The Tompkins or Jones procedure (Fig. 19–5) is used for a septate uterus with two cavities and one uterine corpus.[61, 62] The Strassman procedure is used for unification of a bicornuate or didelphys uterus[44] (Fig. 19–6). Performing the wrong surgical

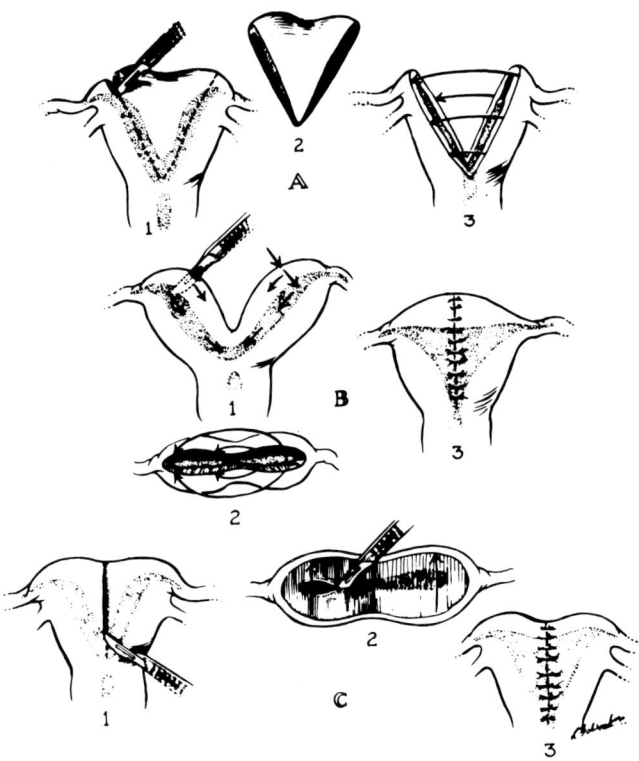

Figure 19–5
A, Jones' procedure. B, Strassman's procedure. C, Tompkins' procedure. (From Jones H Jr: Reproductive impairment and the malformed uterus. In Wallach E, Kempers R (eds.): Modern Trends in Infertility and Conception Control, Vol. 2. Philadelphia, JB Lippincott (Harper Medical), 1982, pp. 282–293.)

procedure in a septate uterus may be disfiguring as well as causing excessive blood loss to the patient.

The Jones procedure is used for a septate uterus. Once the abdomen is opened and the uterine and ovarian arteries are tied, a Penrose drain is placed around the cervix to tamponade the uterine arteries and an outline is drawn on the anterior and posterior surfaces of the uterus. An incision is made into both cavities, and a wedge is removed. Vasopressin may be injected along the line of the incision prior to removal of the wedge. The entire septum is removed to create one uterine cavity. The anterior and posterior surfaces are sutured together with 3–0 polyglactin suture (Fig. 19–7).

The modified Jones procedure is different from the traditional Jones procedure in that a smaller portion of the septum is removed by incising the septum medially to laterally. The Tompkins metroplasty divides the uterine septum and corpus in half. The lateral septal half is incised, and the incision is carried inferiorly until the endometrial cavity is reached. The Tompkins procedure conserves all myometrial tissue.

The Strassman procedure is particularly suited for two endometrial cavities with externally divided corpora such as a bicornuate or didelphys uterus. The procedure is performed by first dividing the rectoves-

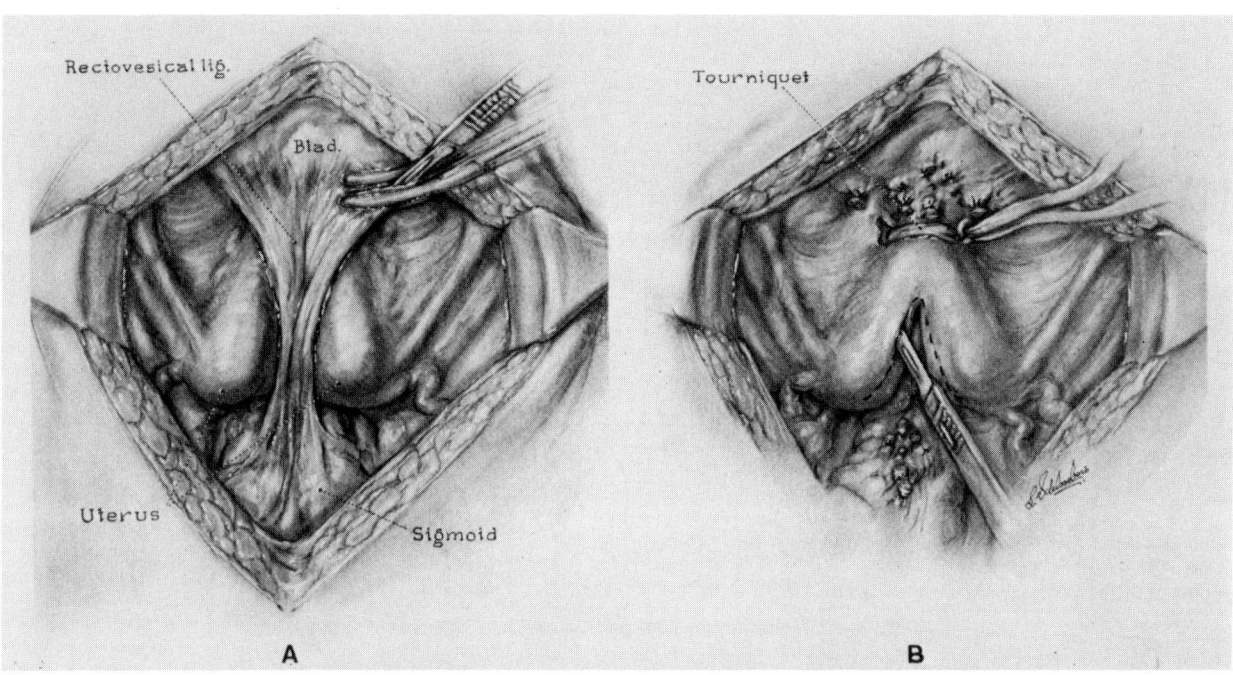
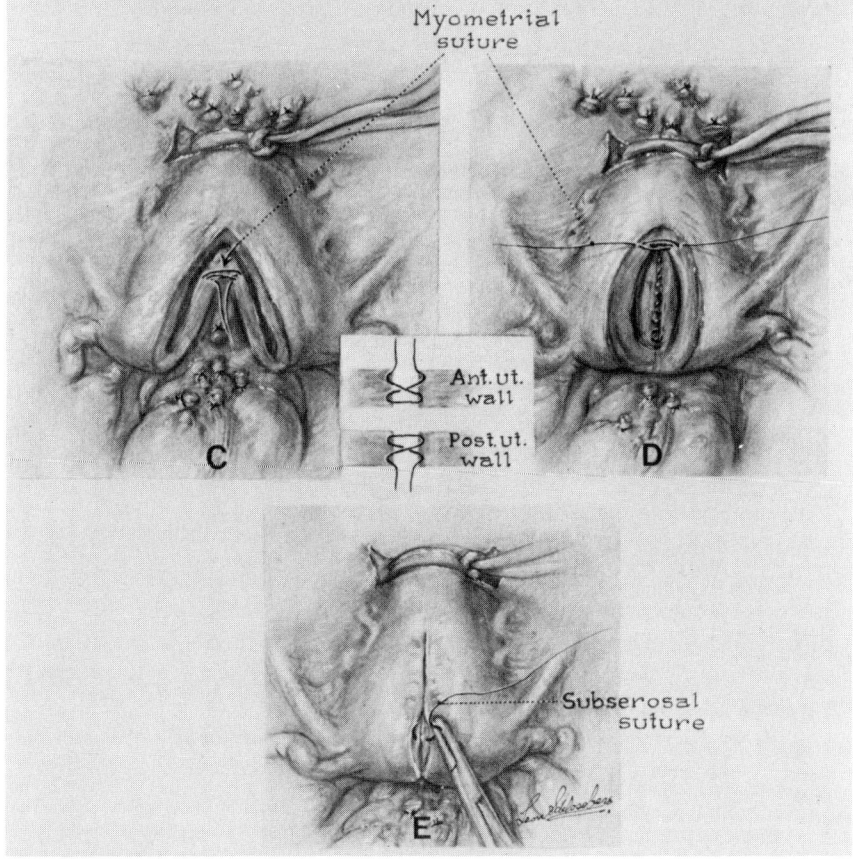

Figure 19–6
Strassman's metroplasty. A, If a rectovesical ligament is found, it should be removed. B, An incision is made on the medial side of each hemicorpus and carried deep enough to enter the uterine cavity. C and D, The myometrium is approximated using interrupted vertical figure-of-eight 3–0 polyglactin acid sutures. E, A continuous 5–0 polyglactin acid subserosal suture is used as a final layer. (From Mattingly R, Thompson J: TeLinde's Operative Gynecology, 6th ed. Philadelphia, JB Lippincott, 1985, pp 372–373.)

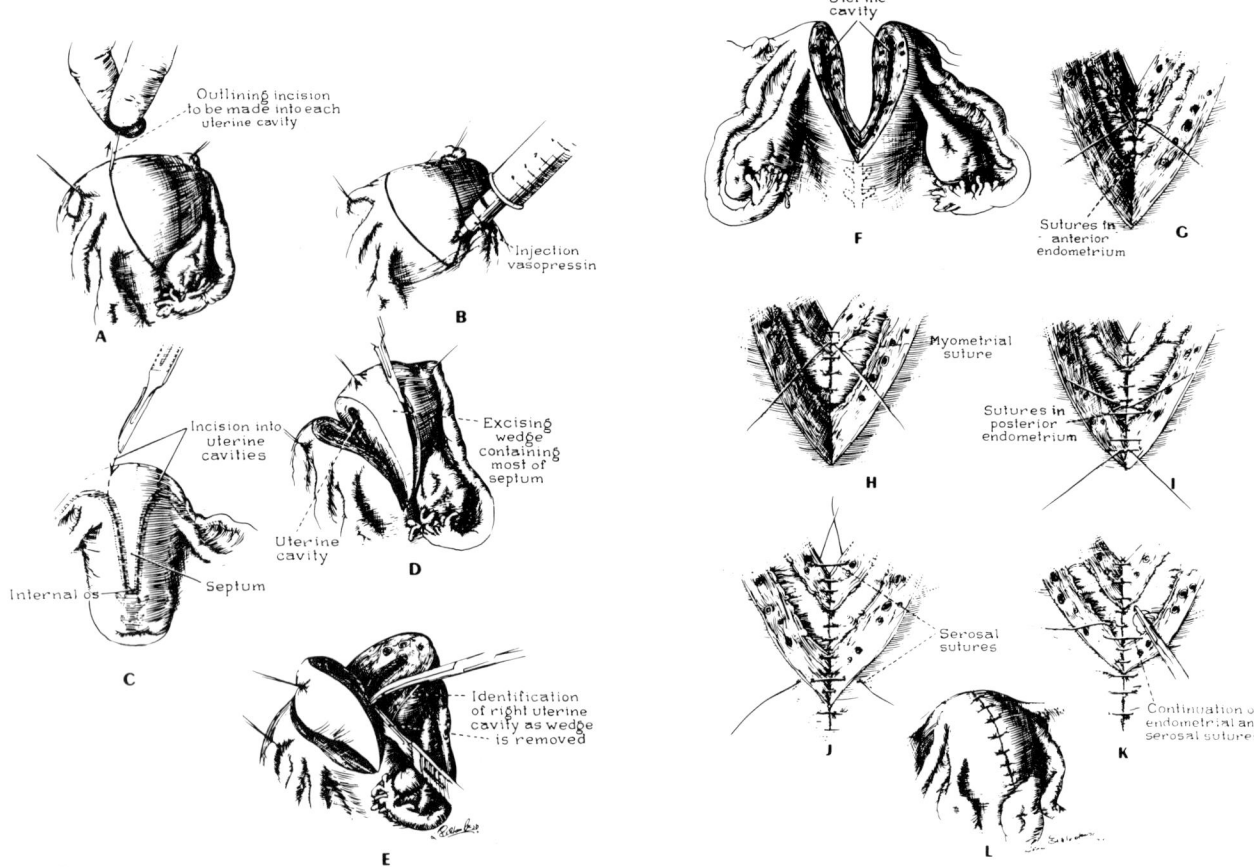

Figure 19–7
A to L, The Jones procedure. (From Jones H Jr: Reproductive impairment and the malformed uterus. In Wallach E, Kempers R (eds.): Modern Trends in Infertility and Conception Control, Vol. 2. Philadelphia, JB Lippincott (Harper Medical), 1982, pp. 282–293.)

ical ligament. Once the septum is identified, an incision is then made medially along the longitudinal axis to expose the uterine cavity. The uterine cavities are joined in a similar fashion to the Jones metroplasty.

Transcervical Hysteroscopic Metroplasty

The septate uterus is amenable to hysteroscopic metroplasty. The technique of hysteroscopic metroplasty was first proposed by Edstrom in 1974[63] but was not widely employed until distention media, illumination, and approved accessory instruments were developed.

The procedure is usually performed in an outpatient or ambulatory center under general anesthesia. It is recommended to perform a diagnostic laparoscopy with hysteroscopy to confirm one uterine corpus and to protect the bowel from the most common complication—uterine perforation. The two most common operative instruments include a wire loop urologic resectoscope with an 8-mm diameter and a semirigid or (7 Fr) rigid scissors used through a 21 Fr sheath.

The surgery should be scheduled in the first half of the menstrual cycle when the endometrium is thin prior to the build-up caused by prolonged estrogen stimulation. Some investigators have advocated the use of progestational agents to have the endometrial lining undergo atrophy. This is probably not necessary because the removal of the septum is not well correlated with hormonal changes within the uterine cavity.

Since the introduction of lasers into the gynecologic armamentarium of medical instruments, Daniel and coworkers have used a KTP/532 laser for transection of the uterine septum.[64] The KTP/532 laser cuts by vaporization, whereas the Nd:YAG laser cuts by excision. All safety precautions must be observed when utilizing these powerful lasers for intrauterine surgery. If the septum is complete with two cervices, a pediatric Foley catheter may be placed into one of the cervical ora to stop the transgression of the liquid distending media out the opposite cervical canal. The electrocautery is set at 30–40 watts of cutting power. Thin septa are usually cut or electrocoagulated in the mid-portion between the two halves. Larger septa require a zigzag approach, with the operator of the urologic resectoscope remembering that the objective of the procedure is to decrease the septal surface area. The most challenging part of the transcervical hysteroscopic metroplasty is knowing when the septum is completely resected and flush with the uterine fundus. The safest way to avoid uterine perforation and subsequent peritoneal or bowel injury is with the coexistence of a laparoscopy.

Postoperatively, prophylactic antibiotics, high levels of estrogen, and a pediatric Foley catheter or intrauterine devices have been suggested.[65] Essentially, all of these techniques have been discontinued. Postoperative infections are rare when the procedure is performed under sterile technique, the estrogen from the menstrual cycle appears to be adequate to regenerate endometrial growth, and synechia formation is rare within the uterine cavity. Two to three months after the procedure, a hysterosalpingogram should be repeated to confirm removal of the septum.

In contrast to the abdominal wedge resection, metroplasty performed by the transcervical hysteroscopic approach does decrease the total uterine volume. Postoperative evaluations have indicated that over 90% of the uterine septum has been removed during the procedure.[65] The results from hysteroscopic metroplasty are excellent. In a study by DeCherney and colleagues, 72 out of 103 patients underwent successful resection of a uterine septum.[72] A 86% pregnancy rate was observed after hysteroscopic metroplasty. In a literature review by Siegler and associates, 367 procedures were performed from 1974 to 1988, and 216 pregnancies were delivered at term with 23 spontaneous abortions and 8 premature deliveries[66] (Table 19–1).

The advantages of hysteroscopic metroplasty are numerous. It allows the removal of a septum to be performed on an outpatient basis without an abdominal incision and with minimal postoperative morbidity. There is little residual damage to the uterine cavity, and vaginal delivery is typical after these procedures. Thus, the appropriate procedure for patients with a uterine septum with poor reproductive history is a hysteroscopic metroplasty. The results are comparable with the transabdominal approach performed by the Tompkins procedure and should be performed only in those patients with primary infertility after a sophisticated evaluation has failed to identify other causes and empiric treatment has failed.

Endometrial Ablation

Women with abnormal uterine bleeding due to dysfunctional or associated pathology may have severe enough symptoms to require transfusions and be chronically anemic. Hormonal therapy and surgical curettage often control the majority of these problems, but occasionally therapy fails and until recently the only option was the removal of the uterus. The removal of the uterus may not be the best option for patients with serious medical illnesses or blood dyscrasias or who are poor surgical candidates. Considering that 1 in 1000 patients will die from the procedure and over 20% will have some associated morbidity, other options should be considered when treating these patients with refractory bleeding.[67]

Several methods have been developed to destroy the endometrial lining but the most successful approaches appear to be electrosurgery and the laser. Laser or electrocautery removal of the endometrium creates intrauterine adhesions with hypomenorrhea or amenorrhea. Preoperatively, the patient should understand that endometrial ablation is not a sterilization procedure and pregnancy can theoretically occur. Endometrial pathology should be ruled out with an office endometrial sampling, hysteroscopy, and hysterosalpingogram. Removal of submucous leiomyomas or polyps that are identified or even the occurrence of endometrial carcinoma will change the direction of the therapeutic approach. A thin endometrial lining will increase the success of the procedure. Medroxyprogesterone acetate, megestrol acetate, leuprolide acetate, or danazol may be used preoperatively to decrease the endometrial lining.

Laser endometrial ablation is performed with a powerful Nd:YAG laser causing photocoagulation by "cooking" the endometrium at just under 100° C. The endometrium passes through several stages until it actually is carbonized with 50–55 watts of power by a "touching" technique or with 20–30 watts using a "no-touch" technique. Using the Nd:YAG laser, Goldrath and colleagues treated 216 patients from 12 to 53 years of age with excessive uterine bleeding and found that 130 had leiomyomas, 30 had adenomyosis, and 16 had bleeding disorders; an overall 98% success rate was achieved.[68] Lomano compared the dragging versus the no-touch technique,[69] and Loffer described a box technique of endometrial ablation.[70] DeCherney and associates described the use of a modified urologic resectoscope for endometrial ablation in 21 patients with intractable bleeding who could not undergo a major operative procedure.[71] Eighteen patients who survived their primary illness were still found to be amenorrheic 6 months postoperatively. An easier method of endometrial ablation using electrocautery in place of the urologic wire loop employs a rollerball electrode. Both procedures appear to have a very high success rate with resolution of menstrual symptoms without the morbidity associated with hysterectomy. In a literature review by Valle and coworkers, a 94% success rate was achieved in 366 patients who underwent the endometrial ablation procedure.[70] A 4.9% complication rate was noted with uterine perforation or postoperative endometritis. The disadvantages of this procedure include the unknown long-term follow-up

Table 19-1

Results from Hysteroscopic Metroplasty

Author	Cases (No.)	Medium Used	Technique	IUD in Place	Estrogen/ Progestogen Treatment	Pregnancy			
						Term	Spontaneous Abortion	Premature	Undelivered
Edström	2	Hyskon	Rigid biopsy forceps	Yes	No	0	0	1 (19 wks)	0
Chervenak/Neuwirth	2	Hyskon	Scissors adjacent hysteroscope	Yes	Yes	1	0	0	0
Daly et al	25	Hyskon	Semirigid scissors	No	Yes	7	1	0	2
DeCherney et al	72	Hyskon	Resectoscope	No	No	58	4	0	0
Corson/Batzer	18	CO_2/Hyskon	Rigid scissors/ resectoscope	No	No	10	2	1	2
Fayez	19	Hyskon	Rigid scissors	Yes (Foley)	No	14	0	0	0
March/Israel	91	Hyskon	Flexible scissors	Yes	Yes	44	7	4	7
Valle/Sciarra	59	Hyskon/D5W	Flexible/rigid/ semirigid scissors	No	Yes	44	5	2	0
Daniell et al.	18	Saline	Laser KTP/argon	No	Yes	NA	0	NA	10
Perino et al.	61	CO_2/glycine	Semirigid scissors/ resectoscope	No	No	38	4	0	0
Totals	**367**					**216**	**23**	**8**	**21**

The outcome is unknown for 99 pregnancies.
NA, not available.
From Siegler A, et al.: Therapeutic Hysteroscopy: Indications and Techniques. St. Louis, CV Mosby, 1990, p. 79.

and side effects, possible damage to the surgeon's eyes, and combustion caused by the laser beam.

References

1. Castiglioni A: A History of Medicine, 2nd ed., tr. and ed. by EB Krumbhaar. New York, Alfred A Knopf, 1958.
2. Garrison FH: An Introduction to the History of Medicine, 4th ed. Philadelphia, WB Saunders Co., 1929.
3. Ramsey EM: Biology of the Uterus. Wynn 1989, p. 13.
4. Soranus: Gynecology, tr. by O Temkin. Baltimore, Johns Hopkins Press, 1956.
5. Mondino dei Luzzi: Anatomia Mundini, per Joannem Dryandrum, In officina Christiani Egenolph, Marburg, 1541.
6. Vesalius A: De Humani Corporis Fabrica, Basilae (facsimile, Brussels, 1964), 1543.
7. da Vinci L: Quaderni d'Anatomia. III. Organi della Generazione-Embrione, Dodici Fogli della Royal Library di Windsor, Casa Editrice Jacob Dyburad, Christiana, 1513.
8. Miller NF, Ludovici PP: On the origin and development of uterine fibroids. Am J Obstet Gynecol 1955; 70:720.
9. Townsend DE, Sparkes RS, Baluda MC, et al.: Unicellular histogenesis of uterine leiomyomas as determined by electrophoresis of glucose-6-phosphate dehydrogenase. Am J Obstet Gynecol 1970; 107:1168.
10. Spellacy WN, LeMaire WJ, Buhi WC, et al.: Plasma growth hormone and estradiol levels in women with uterine myomas. Obstet Gynecol 1972; 40:829.
11. Goodman AL: Progesterone therapy in uterine fibromyoma. J Clin Endocrinol Metab 1946; 6:402.
12. Farber M, Conrad S, Heinrichs WL, et al.: Estradiol binding by fibroid tumors and normal myometrium. Obstet Gynecol 1972; 40:479.
13. Gabb RG, Stone GM: Uptake and metabolism of tritiated oestradiol and oestrone by human endometrial and myometrial tissue in vitro. J Endocrinol Gr Britain 1974; 62:109.
14. Ylikorkala O, Kauppila A, Rajala T: Pituitary gonadotrophins and prolactin in patients with endometrial cancer, fibroids or ovarian tumors. Br J Obstet Gynaecol 1979; 86:901.
15. Reddy W, Rose LI: 4, 3-Ketosteroid 5-oxidoreductase in human uterine leiomyoma. Am J Obstet Gynecol 1979; 135:415.
16. Persaud V, Arjoon PD: Uterine leiomyoma: Incidence of degenerative change and a correlation of associated symptoms. Obstet Gynecol 1970; 35:432.
17. Sehgal N, Haskins AL: The mechanism of uterine bleeding in the presence of fibromyomas. Am J Surg 1960; 26:21.
18. Buttram V, Reiter R: Uterine leiomyomata: Etiology, symptomatology and management. Fertil Steril 1981; 36:433.
19. Berkeley AS, DeCherney AH, Polan ML: Abdominal myomectomy and subsequent fertility. Surg Gynecol Obstet 1983; 156:319.
20. Kelly N, Noble C: Gynecology and Abdominal Surgery. Philadelphia, WB Saunders Co., 1908.
21. Mayo W: Myomectomy. Surg Gynecol Obstet 1922; 34:548.
22. Bonney J: The technic and results of myomectomy. Lancet 1931; 220:171.
23. Rubin I: Progress in myomectomy. Am J Obstet Gynecol 1942; 44:196.
24. Babaknia A, Rock J, Jones H Jr: Pregnancy success following abdominal myomectomy for infertility. Fertil Steril 1978; 30:644.
25. Ranney B, Frederick I: The occasional need for myomectomy. Obstet Gynecol 1979; 53:437.
26. Rosenfeld DL: Abdominal myomectomy for otherwise unexplained infertility. Fertil Steril 1986; 46:328.
27. Starks GC: CO_2 laser myomectomy in an infertile population. J Reprod Med 1988; 33:184.
28. Gatti D, Falsetti L, Viana A, Gastaldi A: Uterine fibroma and sterility: Role of myomectomy. Acta Eur Fertil 1989; 20:11.
29. Brown JM, Malkasian GD, Symmonds RE: Abdominal myomectomy. Am J Obstet Gynecol 1967; 99:126.
30. Finn W, Muller P: Abdominal myomectomy: Special relevance to subsequent pregnancy and to the reappearance of fibromyomas of the uterus. Am J Obstet Gynecol 1950; 60:109.
31. Friedman AJ, Rein MS, Harrison-Atlas D, et al.: A randomized, placebo-controlled, double blind study evaluating leuprolide acetate depot treatment prior to myomectomy. Fertil Steril 1989; 52:728.
32. Neuwirth RS, Amin HK: Excision of submucous fibroids with hysteroscopic control. Am J Obstet Gynecol 1976; 131:95.
33. Neuwirth RS: A new technique for and additional experience with hysteroscopic resection of submucous fibroids. Am J Obstet Gynecol 1978; 131:91.
34. Hallez JP, Perino A: Endoscopic intrauterine resection: Principles and technique. Acta Eur Fertil 1988; 19:17.
35. Lin BL, Miyamoto N, Aoki R, et al.: Transcervical resection of submucous myoma. Acta Obstet Gynaecol Jpn 1986; 38:1647.
36. Brooks PG, Loffer FD, Serden SP: Resectoscopic removal of symptomatic intrauterine lesions. J Reprod Med 1989; 34:435.
37. Grainger DA, DeCherney AH: Hysteroscopic management of uterine bleeding. Baillieres Clin Obstet Gynecol 1989; 3:403.
38. Davids AM: Myomectomy in the relief of infertility and sterility and in pregnancy. Surg Clin North Am 1957; 37:563.
39. Golan D, Aharoni A, Gonen R, et al.: Early spontaneous rupture of the post myomectomy gravid uterus. Int J Gynaecol Obstet 1990; 31:167.
40. Jarcho J: Malformation of the uterus. Am J Surg 1946; 71:106.
41. Rock J, Jones H Jr: The clinical management of the double uterus. Fertil Steril 1979; 28:798.
42. Thompson DP, Lynn HB: Genital anomalies associated with solitary kidney. Mayo Clin Proc 1966; 41:538.
43. Green L, Harris R: Uterine anomalies: Frequency of diagnosis and associated obstetric complications. Obstet Gynecol 1976; 47:427.
44. Strassman P: Die operative Vereinigung eines doppelten Uterus. Zentrbl Gynaek 1907; 31:1322.
45. Jones HW, Seeger-Jones GE: Double uterus as an etiological factor in repeated abortion: Indications for surgical repair. Am J Obstet Gynecol 1953; 65:325.
46. Jones HW, Delfs E, Seeger-Jones GE: Reproductive difficulties in double uterus: The place of plastic reconstruction. Am J Obstet Gynecol 1956; 72:865.
47. Perino A, Catinella E, Comparetto G, et al.: Hysteroscopic metroplasty: The role of ultrasound in the diagnosis and monitoring of patients with uterine septa. Acta Eur Fertil 1987; 18:349.
48. Buttram V, Gibbons W: Müllerian anomalies: A proposed classification. Fertil Steril 1979; 32:40.
49. March CM, Israel R: Hysteroscopic management of recurrent abortion caused by septate uterus. Am J Obstet Gynecol 1987; 156:834.
50. Heinonen P, Saarikoski S, Pystynen P: Reproductive performance of women with uterine anomalies: An evaluation of 182 cases. Acta Obstet Gynecol Scand 1982; 61:157.
51. Jewelewicz R, Husami N: When uterine factors cause infertility. Cont Obstet Gynecol 1980; 16:95.
52. Capraro VJ, Chuang JT, Randall CL: Improved fetal salvage after metroplasty. Obstet Gynecol 1968; 31:97.
53. Jones HW Jr, Jones GES: Double uterus as an etiological factor of repeated abortion: Indication for surgical repair. Am J Obstet Gynecol 1976; 65:325.
54. Strassman EO: Operations for double uterus and endometrial atresia. Clin Obstet Gynecol 1961; 4:240.
55. McShane PM, Reilly RJ, Schiff I: Pregnancy outcomes following Tompkins metroplasty. Fertil Steril 1983; 40:190.
56. Rock JA, Murphy AA: Anatomic abnormalities. Clin Obstet Gynecol 1986; 29:886.
57. Mahgoub SE: Unification of a septate uterus: Mahgoub's operation. Int J Gynaecol Obstet 1979; 15:400.
58. Mizuno K, Koike K, Ando K, et al.: Significance of Jones-Jones operation on double uterus: Vascularity and dating of endometrium in uterine septum. Jpn J Fertil Steril 1978; 23:9.
59. O'Leary JL, O'Leary JA: Rudimentary horn pregnancy. Obstet Gynecol 1963; 22:371.
60. Musick J, Behrman S: Obstetric outcome before and after metroplasty in women with uterine anomalies. Obstet Gynecol 1978; 52:63.

61. Tompkins P: Comments on the bicornuate uterus and twinning. Surg Clin North Am 1962; 42:1049.
62. Jones HW: Reproductive impairment and the malformed uterus. Fertil Steril 1981; 36:137.
63. Edstrom K: Intrauterine surgical procedures during hysteroscopy. Endoscopy 1974; 6:175.
64. Daniell JF, Osher S, Miller W: Hysteroscopic resection of uterine septi with visible light laser energy. Colpos Gynecol Laser Surg 1987; 3:217.
65. DeCherney AH, Russell JB, Graebe RA, Polan ML: Resectoscopic management of müllerian fusion defects. Fertil Steril 1986; 45:728.
66. Siegler AM, Valle RF, Lindemann HJ, Mencaglia L: Therapeutic Hysteroscopy: Indications and Techniques. St. Louis, CV Mosby, 1990; p. 79.
67. Dicker RC, Greenspan JR, Strauss LT, et al.: Complications of abdominal and vaginal hysterectomy among women of the reproductive age in the United States. Am J Obstet Gynecol 1982; 144:841.
68. Goldrath MH: Hysteroscopic laser surgery. In Baggish MS (ed.): Basic and Advanced Laser Surgery in Gynecology. Norwalk, CT, Appleton-Century-Crofts, 1985, pp. 357–372.
69. Lomano JM: Dragging technique versus blanching technique for endometrial ablation with the Nd:YAG laser in the treatment of chronic menorrhagia. Am J Obstet Gynecol 1988; 159:152.
70. Loffer FD: Hysteroscopic endometrial ablation with Nd:YAG laser using a noncontact technique. Obstet Gynecol 1987; 69:679.
71. DeCherney AF, Diamond MP, Lavy G, et al.: Endometrial ablation for intractable uterine bleeding: Hysteroscopic resection. Obstet Gynecol 1987; 70:668.

Surgery for Malignant Tumors of the Uterine Corpus

20

Thomas W. Burke
Mitchell Morris

A variety of malignant tumors can arise from the fundal portion of the uterus. Most commonly, these are adenocarcinomas that originate from the glandular epithelium of the endometrium. Indeed, endometrial carcinoma is by far the most frequent cancer of the female genital tract, accounting for about one-half of all female pelvic tumors.[1] Well-differentiated and superficially invasive adenocarcinomas are seen in about two-thirds of patients. The excellent outcome associated with this clinical setting has led some investigators to underestimate the true impact of endometrial cancer.[2] Careful surgical and pathologic risk assessments published over the past 10–15 years have done much to further our ability to identify high- and low-risk patients. Much of this information has been incorporated into a surgical staging system for uterine cancer adopted by the International Federation of Obstetricians and Gynecologists (FIGO) in 1988.[3] Current approaches to therapy in patients with endometrial cancers are focusing on individualized treatment based upon a surgically determined estimate of risk for recurrence.

Sarcomas are the second major category of uterine cancer. These tumors arise from mesenchymal tissues of the uterine wall or lining and include leiomyosarcoma, endometrial stromal sarcoma, and rare forms derived from nonspecific supporting tissues like fibrous stroma and vessels. Malignant mixed müllerian tumors contain a mixture of sarcomatous and carcinomatous elements. Most commonly, these tumors are a mixture of endometrial adenocarcinoma and stromal sarcoma, but bizarre components such as chondrosarcoma or osteosarcoma can be seen. Surgical resection is the major therapeutic modality for uterine sarcomas.

Malignant tumors arising in other pelvic organs commonly involve the uterus when patients present with advanced local disease. Rarely, tumors arising in distant sites can metastasize to the uterine wall or lining. A general classification of uterine fundal cancers is outlined in Table 20–1.

ENDOMETRIAL ADENOCARCINOMA

Epidemiology

Two subgroups of patients with endometrial adenocarcinoma have been described. The first exhibits historical or lifestyle features that have been associated with prolonged, unopposed exposure to estrogens.[4–7] Estrogen exposure may be categorized as endogenous or exogenous. Women with early menarche, late menopause, anovulatory menstrual patterns, nulliparity, estrogen-secreting ovarian tumors, or obesity experience episodes of chronic endogenous estrogenic stimulation. Postmenopausal women using continuous estrogen therapy without progestational agents have similar chronic exogenous estro-

Table 20-1
Malignant Tumors of the Uterine Fundus

Epithelial Tumors
Endometrioid adenocarcinoma (Grades 1-3)
Papillary endometrioid adenocarcinoma
Papillary serous carcinoma
Clear cell carcinoma
Adenosquamous carcinoma
Mucinous adenocarcinoma

Mesenchymal Tumors
Endometrial stromal sarcoma
Leiomyosarcoma
Nonspecific mesenchymal sarcomas

Mixed Tumors
Adenosarcoma
Malignant mixed müllerian tumor

Tumors Originating at Another Site
Direct extension (cervix, ovary, colon)
Metastatic involvement

gen exposure. Because the normal response of the endometrial glands to estrogen is proliferation, it makes sense that long-term estrogen exposure can lead to overstimulation and ultimately neoplastic transformation.[8-12]

Patients who develop endometrial cancer in association with chronic estrogen exposure tend to develop well-differentiated and superficially invasive tumors. Often, the tumor arises in an area of atypical adenomatous hyperplasia, suggesting a continuum between this condition and early cancer. Despite the logic of this estrogen-stimulation hypothesis, it is important to remember that as many as half of patients with endometrial cancer have no risk factors that can be tied to chronic estrogen exposure. Diabetes mellitus, hypertension, high-fat diet, and home in an industrialized nation have also been implicated as increasing the risk of endometrial cancer.[4-7] A genetic predisposition to endometrial cancer can be identified in some women. Those with a strong family history of endometrial cancer and those with previous malignant tumors of the breast, colon, or ovary are at greater risk.[13] Cancer families in which endometrial cancer (often in association with breast or ovarian cancer) appears to be inherited as an autosomal dominant trait have also been described.[14]

The second subgroup of endometrial cancer patients are those whose tumors follow a much more aggressive clinical course. These women tend to be slightly older. Their tumors tend to be poorly differentiated or demonstrate some of the rarer cell types of endometrial carcinoma such as papillary serous,[15-17] clear cell,[18-20] papillary endometrioid,[21,22] or adenosquamous.[23-25] Deep myometrial invasion and extrauterine tumor spread are more common in this subgroup. The risk of tumor recurrence is high and survival is low when these women are compared with patients with well-differentiated tumors.

Clinical Presentation

Most patients with uterine fundal cancers are postmenopausal, and most present with vaginal bleeding. Fortunately, this symptom is generally recognized as abnormal by both the woman who has it and her physician. Prompt endometrial sampling will usually provide a diagnosis. This combination of prompt symptom recognition and early biopsy results in a large number of diagnoses when disease is clinically limited to the uterus. All large clinical reviews of endometrial carcinoma report that 70–80% of patients have clinical Stage I or II tumors at the time of diagnosis (Fig. 20–1). Less common presentations include pelvic pain, pelvic mass, bowel or bladder symptoms, ascites, or symptoms of extraabdominal metastases. These presentations are associated with advanced tumors that have been rapidly progressive or neglected.

Malignant cells can be shed through the cervix and occasionally are noted on routine Papanicolaou smears performed to screen for cervical cancer (Fig. 20–2). Although a number of women known to have uterine cancer will have abnormal cytologic smears, this method of diagnosis in the asymptomatic patient is rare.

Tumors that involve the cervix or have a large polypoid growth pattern may present as a cervical lesion readily visible on speculum examination. Polypoid tumors that extend down the cervical canal and on biopsy demonstrate histologic patterns typical of

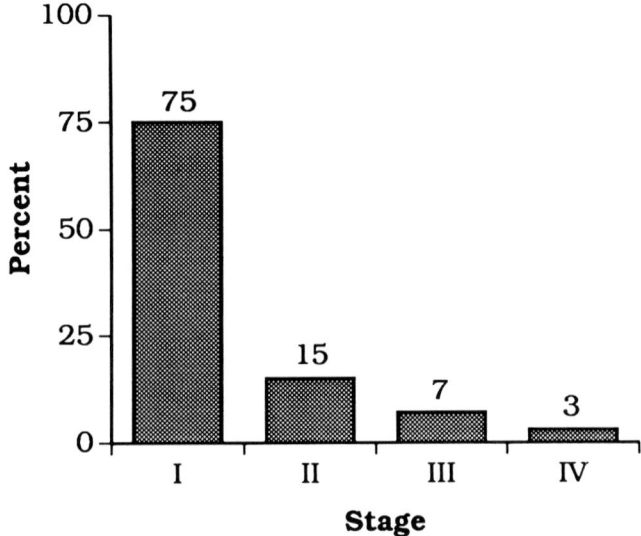

Figure 20-1
Most patients with endometrial cancer present with postmenopausal bleeding and are promptly diagnosed by endometrial biopsy. Diagnosis in clinical Stage I or II is common and probably accounts for the excellent overall prognosis for patients with this disease.

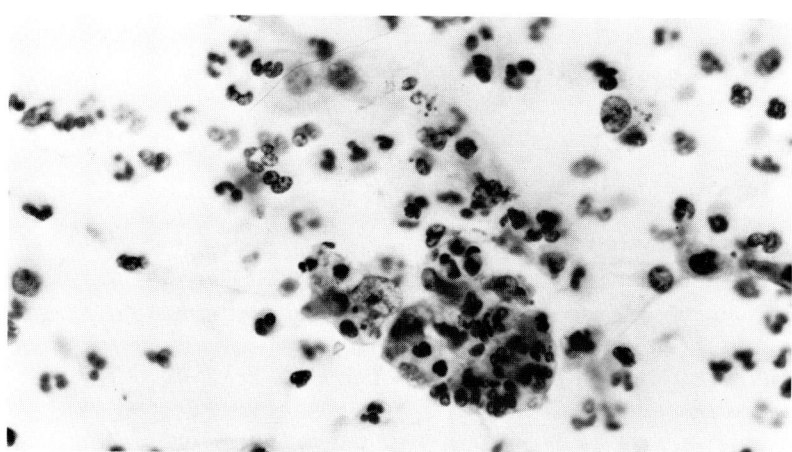

Figure 20–2
Small tumor fragments shed from the surface of endometrial carcinomas can be detected on cervical Papanicolaou smears. However, this method of diagnosis is uncommon in asymptomatic women. In this illustration, a malignant gland fragment is surrounded by inflammatory cells.

endometrial cancer do not usually present a diagnostic dilemma. This presentation is also common in patients with endometrial stromal sarcomas and malignant mixed müllerian tumors. The site of origin of endometrioid adenocarcinomas that grossly involve both the cervix and the uterine cavity can be difficult to determine because primary adenocarcinomas of the cervix occasionally demonstrate an endometrioid histologic appearance. The primary site of these "corpus et colli" tumors may be impossible to distinguish. An equally difficult diagnostic dilemma is encountered when papillary serous or endometrioid tumors involve the uterus and ovary. Tumors with these histologic patterns can arise as primary malignancies in either organ, and simultaneous primary tumors at both sites are not uncommon. Occasionally the organ of origin can be discerned on the basis of the relative degree of tumor involvement, but in patients with extensive, large-volume disease this may be impossible.

Mechanisms of Tumor Spread

Tumors arising in the uterine fundus exhibit a variety of mechanisms for disease spread (Fig. 20–3). Those that expand within the uterine cavity can invade the lower uterine segment and cervix. Direct extension from these sites will involve the upper vagina and paracervical and parametrial soft tissues. Tumors that burrow into the myometrium will ultimately reach the serosal surface, where they can directly extend into the adnexa or gain access to the peritoneal cavity. Viable tumor fragments that break free from the main tumor or traverse the fallopian tube may implant on any of the peritoneal surfaces. The lymphatic drainage of the uterus is complex and parallels the uterine, cervical, and ovarian vessels. Tumors that invade uterine lymphatics can, therefore, metastasize to the pelvic, para-aortic, or inguinal nodes. Para-aortic node metastases may occur high in the chain at the level of ovarian venous drainage into the vena cava or left renal vein. Unlike lymph node metastases in cervical cancer, which typically follow a predictable course of increasing levels of node involvement, para-aortic nodal spread in uterine cancer may occur in the absence of pelvic node involvement. Locally advanced tumors may obstruct regional lymphatic channels and cause retrograde lymphatic flow and metastasis. This mechanism may explain the relatively frequent finding of suburethral tumor nodules in patients with bulky tumors. If the tumor gains

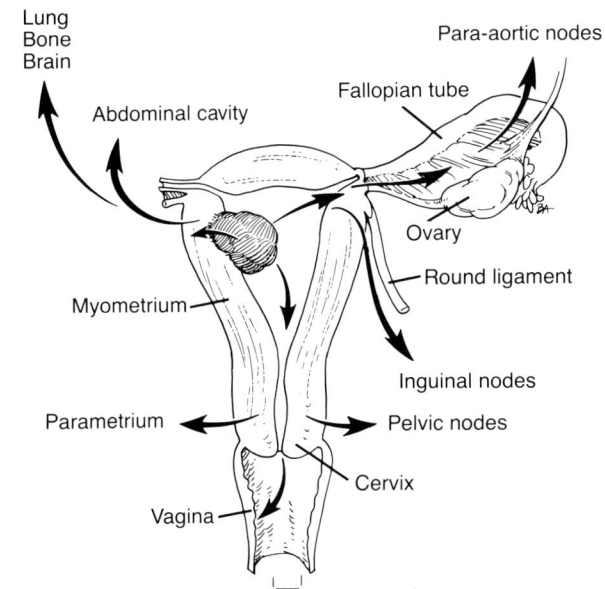

Figure 20–3
Uterine fundal tumors can spread by several mechanisms. Tumors that extend to the cervix can invade the upper vagina and parametrium by direct extension. Those that penetrate the myometrium have direct access to the adnexa, other pelvic organs, and the peritoneal cavity. Viable tumor cells may also reach the peritoneal cavity via the fallopian tube. Invasion of lymphatic channels can result in spread to the lower vagina or the pelvic, para-aortic, and inguinal lymph nodes. Hematogenous dissemination to the lung, brain, or bone can also occur. (Modified from Burke TW: Cancer Bull 1990; 42:78. Copyright, Medical Arts Publishing Foundation, Houston, Texas, 1990.)

access to vascular channels, hematogenous dissemination to any site can occur. Common locations include bone, brain, lung, and liver.

Diagnosis

The diagnosis of most uterine tumors can be easily established by endometrial biopsy. The classic approach of examination under anesthesia, uterine sounding, dilatation, and fractional curettage, although still useful, has largely been replaced by outpatient biopsy techniques.[26-28] A wide variety of flexible and rigid endometrial biopsy instruments are available. Most of these provide equivalent biopsy samples for histologic diagnosis. The authors begin by performing a routine visual inspection and bimanual pelvic examination. Polypoid tumors protruding through the cervical os are readily visible and can be easily biopsied using a cervical biopsy forceps. Bimanual examination provides information about the relative uterine size and position within the pelvis. Careful palpation of the cervix may be useful in determining whether the tumor has invaded the cervical stroma. An enlarged, firm, nodular cervix or lower uterine segment is strongly suggestive of tumor extension. Following antiseptic preparation of the cervix with an iodine solution, an endocervical curettage sample is obtained and submitted as a separate specimen. The uterine cavity is then sounded to confirm the depth and direction of the endometrial cavity. The endometrial biopsy instrument is then repeatedly inserted to the fundus and withdrawn while exerting pressure against the uterine wall. The authors obtain material by making at least one pass of the anterior, posterior, and each lateral uterine wall to ensure that the biopsy material contains tissue representative of the entire endometrial cavity. Specimens obtained from only one part of the uterus may miss a small exophytic tumor whose growth is limited to one segment of the uterine cavity, or they may provide only a small unrepresentative sample of a larger tumor (Fig. 20-4). The diagnostic accuracy of an appropriately obtained endometrial biopsy sample approaches that of a dilatation and curettage specimen.

Most patients tolerate outpatient biopsy with a minimum amount of cramping pain. Sedation or anesthesia is usually not required. Pre- and postbiopsy treatment with a nonsteroidal anti-inflammatory drug, such as ibuprofen, can minimize patient discomfort following biopsy. A small amount of vaginal bleeding is common for the first few days after biopsy.

In the authors' experience, 80% or more of patients with endometrial neoplasms can have their disease diagnosed in an outpatient setting. The re-

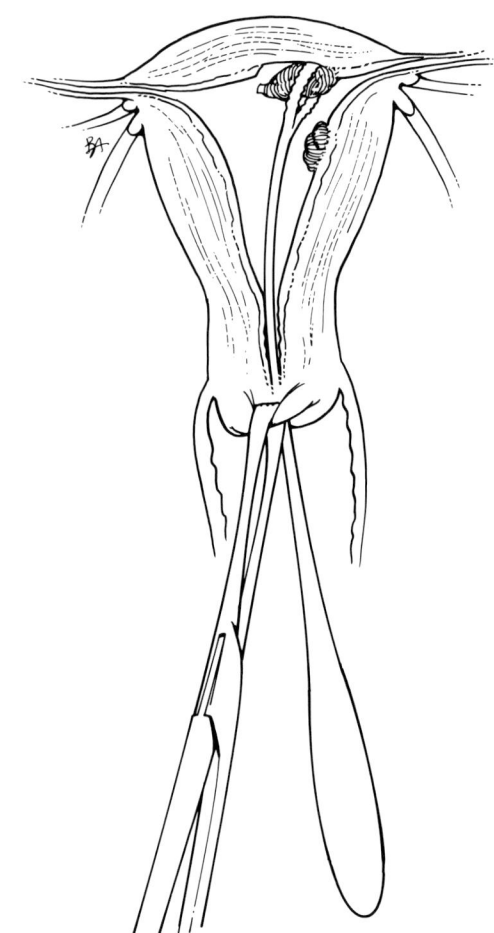

Figure 20-4
Many instruments provide excellent endometrial specimens for histologic diagnosis. Whatever sampling instrument is used, care must be taken to obtain tissue from all segments of the endometrium. Inadequate technique may miss tumors that involve only a small portion of the endometrium.

maining patients require operative biopsy by dilatation and curettage. Indications for operative evaluation include cervical stenosis that precludes access to the endometrial cavity, inconclusive or inadequate diagnosis from material obtained by outpatient biopsy, patient intolerance of outpatient biopsy, and patient anatomy or examination findings that are difficult to assess accurately without an examination under anesthesia.

Preoperative Assessment and Clinical Staging

Prior to the adoption of a surgical staging system by FIGO in 1988, endometrial cancer was a clinically staged disease. The criteria for assigning a clinical stage are summarized in Table 20-2. A pretherapy evaluation is used to clinically assess the extent of disease and to evaluate the anesthetic and operative risks for the patient. This evaluation should routinely

Table 20–2

Clinical Staging of Uterine Fundal Tumors*

Stage I	The tumor is limited to the uterine fundus
IA	The uterine cavity measures 8 cm or less
IB	The length of the uterine cavity is greater than 8 cm
Stage II	The tumor extends to the uterine cervix
Stage III	The tumor has spread to the adjacent pelvic structures
Stage IV	There is bulky pelvic disease or distant spread
IVA	Tumor invades the mucosa of the bladder or rectosigmoid
IVB	Distant metastases are present

*FIGO, 1971.

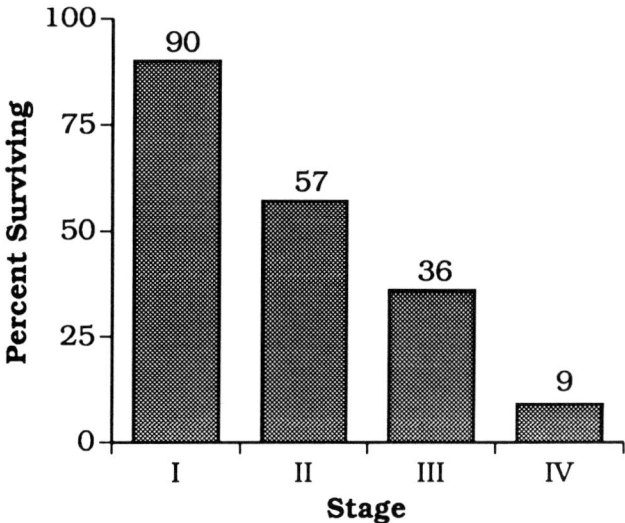

Figure 20–5
Probability of long-term (5-year) survival correlates well with clinical stage. Survival may be enhanced and treatment morbidity reduced with the institution of surgical staging. Precise knowledge of disease status will allow adjuvant or adjunctive therapy that is tailored to known tumor sites. Patients who are proved to be at low risk for treatment failure can be spared the morbidity of additional therapy.

include a careful physical examination, the diagnostic biopsies described previously, a chest radiograph, laboratory studies, and additional diagnostic studies as indicated by the clinical findings (Table 20–3). In most large series, clinical stage has proved to be a significant predictor of outcome.[29–34] Survival data by FIGO clinical stage that have been compiled from several publications are presented in Figure 20–5.

Patients with disease that appears limited to the uterus who are surgical candidates do not require an extensive metastatic evaluation. Definitive histopathologic information will be obtained at laparotomy in these cases. However, further diagnostic studies (Table 20–4) may be useful in patients with uncertain diagnosis, those with clinically advanced pelvic disease, and those who are not acceptable candidates for surgical exploration.

Magnetic resonance imaging (MRI), computed tomography (CT), and pelvic ultrasound (US) can be used to identify the area of greatest tumor volume within the uterus and may detect areas of extrauterine spread that are not appreciated clinically. Both pelvic MRI and US have been used to visualize the endometrial cavity and can often identify the exophytic tumor within the uterus, as well as provide an estimation of myometrial invasion.[35–39] The authors have been impressed that MRI provides good definition of tissue planes within the pelvis. It also provides a reasonably good image of structures in the retroperitoneal space, including the pelvic and para-aortic lymph nodes. In the authors' experience, MRI provides more detailed and reliable information about uterine and pelvic disease than CT. In most situations, pelvic US adds little additional information; therefore, the authors do not routinely use it. CT with contrast can, however, be used to provide a detailed examination of the liver, kidneys, ureters, spleen, and retroperitoneum. It is particularly valuable in identifying visceral metastases to the liver or spleen and hydronephrosis.

Noninvasive assessment of pelvic and para-aortic lymph nodes is difficult. Retroperitoneal adenopathy can be identified by MRI and CT. However, these modalities provide information about node size rather than node architecture. They can identify nodal metastases when the involved nodes are larger than 1.5–2.0 cm. Unfortunately, many nodal metas-

Table 20–3

Routine Pretreatment Evaluation in Early Disease

Detailed medical history
Complete physical examination
Endocervical and endometrial biopsy
Chest radiograph
Electrocardiogram
Complete blood count
Screening serum profile
Serum CA-125
Urinalysis and culture
Studies to assess specific organ systems

Table 20–4

Pretreatment Evaluation in Clinically Advanced Disease*

Cystoscopy
Proctosigmoidoscopy
Barium enema
Intravenous pyelogram
Computed tomography
Magnetic resonance imaging
Bipedal lymphangiography
Ultrasonography
Directed fine-needle aspiration biopsy

*Evaluation tailored to symptoms and clinical presentation.

tases in endometrial cancer are small and do not cause detectable enlargement. Lymphangiography provides detailed information about nodal size and architecture and seems to be better able to identify nodal metastases in the pelvic and para-aortic chains. However, this technique is not recommended in elderly, obese, or diabetic patients because of the risks of peripheral infection at the injection site or poor imaging once contrast has been injected. Pulmonary and renal complications of contrast injection are more frequent in older women. The authors have not been able to utilize this technique in endometrial cancer patients as successfully as they have in those with cervical cancer.

Directed fine-needle aspiration (FNA) cytology has substantially enhanced our ability to confirm questionable or suspicious findings on imaging studies without resorting to a major operative procedure. A skilled interventional radiologist and a trained cytopathologist can provide reliable diagnostic information from virtually any abdominal or pelvic site. Studies in gynecologic cancers have demonstrated a high degree of accuracy for FNA when positive or suspicious findings are reported.[40–44] Negative findings are slightly less accurate. FNA techniques are particularly valuable in assessing the uterine cancer patient who has an increased surgical risk and abnormal imaging findings. In this clinical setting, a positive FNA result may help to avoid laparotomy in a patient with extensive disease.

Cystoscopy, intravenous pyelography (IVP), proctosigmoidoscopy, and barium enema are obtained in patients with advanced pelvic disease or symptoms related to the urinary or lower gastrointestinal tracts. Cystoscopy and proctoscopy are mandatory for staging patients with bulky central tumors because assignment to Stage IVA requires biopsy confirmation of invasion of the bladder or rectal mucosa. IVP will identify occult ureteral obstruction, although comparable information can also be obtained from renal ultrasound or CT with intravenous contrast. Barium enema may identify a primary colorectal origin for the tumor and prevent misdiagnosis as cervical or uterine adenocarcinoma. Areas of invasion into bowel wall or luminal narrowing may be clearly demonstrated. The presence of diverticular disease or inflammatory disease of the large bowel may have an impact on the planning of surgery or pelvic irradiation. Upon completion of the pretherapy evaluation, patients can be assigned to one of the four clinical stage groups.

Most women with endometrial cancer are postmenopausal, about one-half are obese, and about two-thirds have significant medical problems that increase operative and anesthetic risks. The second goal of the pretreatment evaluation is to assess these risks for each patient. This evaluation should be directed toward the specific organ systems likely to be affected. An in-depth cardiac, pulmonary, or renal evaluation may be required to identify those patients who have unacceptable surgical risk or those who might benefit from invasive intraoperative monitoring and postoperative intensive care. The postoperative management of these high-risk patients can be greatly simplified if preoperative baseline function has been assessed and an aggressive management plan established by the surgeon, the anesthesiologist, and the intensive care specialist. Using current techniques, about 90% of patients with endometrial cancer can be surgically treated with reasonable safety. Patients who are judged to be unacceptable candidates for surgery, usually because of severe medical contraindication to anesthesia, should be clinically staged according to 1971 FIGO criteria. These patients may be successfully treated with radiotherapy alone. Two studies have reported 5-year survivals of 72% and 55%, respectively, in such patients.[45, 46] Both studies employed multiple brachytherapy applications, and both suggested that uterine packing with multiple sources (Heyman or Simon capsules) tended to give a superior result. It is interesting to note that the long-term survivals are so high, because patients treated with radiation alone were felt to be "too sick" for exploratory surgery. Several patients in the MD Anderson series successfully underwent hysterectomy when radiotherapy failed.

Histopathologic Prognostic Factors

During the 1970s and 1980s, several large retrospective and prospective series carefully examined a wide variety of potential prognostic features in patients with endometrial cancers.[47–50] The information evaluated came largely from patients whose tumors were limited to the uterus (clinical Stage I or II) and was based on a detailed histopathologic examination of the uterus and additional biopsy material obtained at laparotomy for hysterectomy. These studies demonstrated the inherent diagnostic deficiencies of the clinical staging system, including the following:

1. The length of the uterine cavity correlates poorly with tumor volume or prognosis and is commonly increased by benign conditions such as leiomyomas and adenomyosis.

2. Preoperative endocervical curettage is a poor predictor of tumor invasion of the cervix or lower uterine segment when compared with hysterectomy findings.

3. Tumor grade determined from endometrial curettage is not always reflective of tumor grade determined from the hysterectomy specimen.

4. Small metastases to the retroperitoneal lymph nodes and the peritoneal cavity are not clinically evaluable.

Table 20-5

Prognostic Factors in Endometrial Carcinoma

Uterine Factors
Cell type
Histologic grade
Depth of myometrial invasion
Cervix or lower uterine segment extension
Lymph–vascular space invasion
Extent of uterine cavity involvement

Extrauterine Factors
Lymph node involvement (pelvic, para-aortic, inguinal)
Adnexal spread
Vaginal metastases
Peritoneal spread (cytologic, macroscopic)
Adjacent organ invasion (bladder, rectosigmoid)

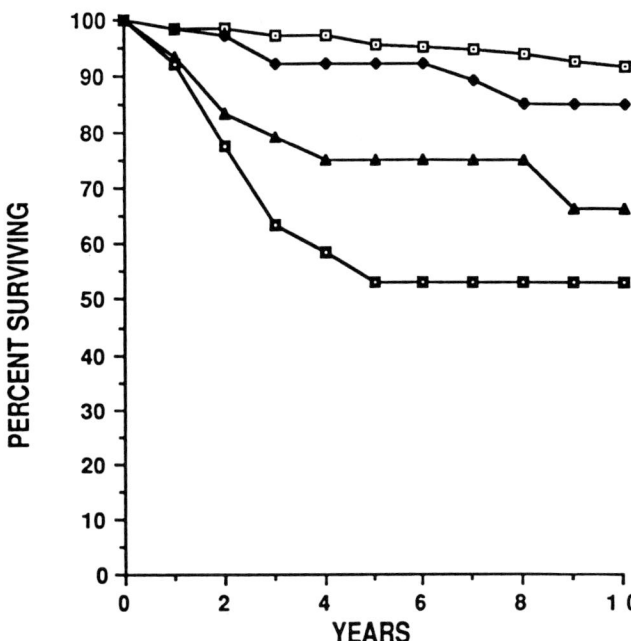

Figure 20–6
Tumor histology and grade are important prognostic factors in patients with early endometrial cancer. Grade 1 tumors rarely recur following hysterectomy, whereas treatment failure in Grade 3 or variant-histology tumors (papillary endometrioid, papillary serous, clear cell, adenosquamous) approaches 50%. Key: Open squares, Grade 1 (n = 287); closed diamonds, Grade 2 (n = 75); closed triangles, variant cell types (n = 31); closed squares, Grade 3 (n = 41). (Reprinted with permission from The American College of Obstetricians and Gynecologists [Obstetrics and Gynecology, 1990; 75:98].)

These histopathologic studies also served to identify and define a group of findings that were clearly tied to an increased risk of recurrence and a poor prognosis (Table 20–5). Major prognostic features include tumor grade and histologic findings (Fig. 20–6), depth of myometrial invasion, tumor invasion of the cervix, presence of lymph node metastases, and extrauterine spread within the pelvis or peritoneal cavity. Factors that have been associated with poor prognosis but are less clearly defined at present include tumor encroachment on the lower uterine segment, extent of tumor involvement in the uterine cavity,[51] presence of lymph-vascular space invasion,[52] and presence of malignant cells in peritoneal washings.[53-56]

Surgical staging studies focused attention on the one-third of early endometrial cancer patients who are at high risk for treatment failure. Based upon the information gained from these studies, FIGO adopted a surgical staging system for uterine fundal tumors (Table 20–6). This staging classification recognizes the prognostic importance of tumor grade, depth of myometrial invasion, cervical extension of tumor, peritoneal cytology, extrauterine spread, and bulky tumor volume. Although the staging criteria are well defined, the intended application of this system is not clearly stated.

Unanswered questions about staging of uterine cancer: What procedures constitute a staging operation? Which patients need a full staging operation? How should adjuvant or adjunctive treatments, particularly external irradiation, be administered relative to the staging procedure? Is there a proven benefit to surgical staging? Can it be assumed that the prognostic factors incorporated into the surgical staging scheme also apply to patients with uterine sarcomas?

The surgical staging system is readily applied to patients with uterine tumors that are clinically confined to the uterus. In this large group of patients, exploration for hysterectomy is usually an integral part of initial therapy. Staging procedures can then be performed at the time of hysterectomy. The authors have taken an approach to the surgical staging of endometrial cancer that combines a detailed as-

Table 20-6

Surgical Staging of Uterine Fundal Tumors*

Stage		Description
Stage I		The tumor is confined to the uterine fundus
	IA	Tumor is limited to the endometrium
	IB	Tumor invades less than one-half of the myometrial thickness
	IC	Tumor invades more than one-half of the myometrial thickness
Stage II		The tumor extends to the cervix
	IIA	Cervical extension is limited to the endocervical glands
	IIB	Tumor invades the cervical stroma
Stage III		There is regional tumor spread
	IIIA	Tumor has invaded the uterine serosa or adnexa, or there are positive peritoneal cytologic findings
	IIIB	Vaginal metastases are present
	IIIC	Tumor has spread to pelvic or para-aortic lymph nodes
Stage IV		There is bulky pelvic disease or distant spread
	IVA	Tumor invades the mucosa of the bladder or rectosigmoid
	IVB	Distant metastases are present

*FIGO, 1988.

sessment of uterine factors with a systematic sampling of the peritoneal cavity and retroperitoneal lymph nodes similar to that used in patients with early ovarian cancers. It is the authors' belief that there is a large number of early stage Grade 1 patients with very limited risk of extrauterine disease who do not require an extended staging procedure. The authors' scheme for surgical staging attempts to stratify patients into high- and low-risk subgroups based upon preoperative tumor histologic appearance and grade, coupled with intraoperative estimate of uterine risk factors. The approach employed is diagrammatically outlined in Figure 20–7. Using this method, the authors perform hysterectomy alone in about 60–70% of patients with tumors limited to the uterus; the remaining 30–40% of patients with identified risk factors are subjected to a more extensive staging operation. This surgical scheme is also designed to obtain a maximal amount of histopathologic and biochemical data, which may prove to be useful in future prognostic evaluations or treatment decisions.

Four groups of patients present problems: (1) patients who have serious medical conditions that make them poor surgical candidates, (2) patients who are acceptable candidates for surgery but who have medical conditions or obesity that makes them poor candidates for a more involved operation than hysterectomy, (3) patients with clinically advanced disease in whom hysterectomy may not be the most appropriate choice for initial therapy, and (4) patients with uterine sarcomas.

Patients who are not felt to be medical candidates for operation should be staged clinically (based upon 1971 FIGO criteria) and can be treated with nonsurgical modalities, such as radiotherapy and/or hormonal therapy. Because of significant physiologic impairment, many of these patients will not be candidates for aggressive cytotoxic therapy. Patients who present technical problems to staging laparotomy, particularly massive obesity, may be effectively treated by vaginal hysterectomy.[57-60] Many obese patients have low-grade, superficially invasive tumors that have developed in response to chronic estrogenic stimulation; hysterectomy alone should be curative for most. However, it is the authors' experience that vaginal hysterectomy in the massively obese patient can often be as challenging as abdominal hysterectomy. In patients who are felt to be suitable anesthetic risks, the authors prefer an abdominal approach regardless of patient size. This allows a careful abdominal exploration and cytologic assessment at the time of hysterectomy even if further staging procedures are not technically feasible.

Patients with clinically advanced pelvic tumors require an individualized treatment plan. Some surgeons have attempted initial surgical resection and tumor debulking in these cases so that disease volume and location can be clearly identified prior to institution of postoperative adjunctive therapy. The authors have typically initiated treatment with external-beam irradiation in many of these cases, followed by brachytherapy and surgical exploration for hysterectomy. The goal of this approach is to obtain palliative control of pelvic disease. Fortunately, patients with clinically advanced disease are rare. An approach that tailors treatment to the specific problems in a given patient is probably most appropriate. Initial treatment with external irradiation may reduce pelvic tumor volume and facilitate subsequent hysterectomy. Immediate exploration and attempted resection may be more appropriate in a patient with symptoms of early large bowel obstruction. No matter what treatment approach is employed in patients with clinically advanced tumors, prognosis is poor.

Most of the histopathologic features incorporated into the surgical staging scheme are based upon studies of patients with endometrial adenocarcinoma. It is not entirely clear that the same set of prognostic features can be extrapolated to patients with uterine sarcomas or malignant mixed müllerian tumors. Most investigators would agree that evidence of extrauterine disease carries a poor prog-

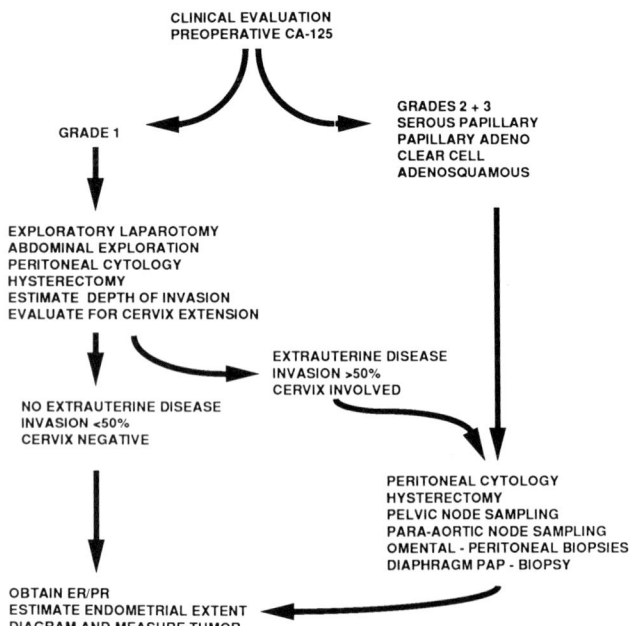

Figure 20–7
Selective approach to surgical staging. The authors' approach to surgical staging is to perform a complete staging procedure only in early disease patients with high-risk tumors. Patients with superficially invasive, Grade 1 tumors that do not involve the cervix are treated with hysterectomy alone. Patients with higher-risk histologic types and Grade 1 patients found to have poor prognostic factors at laparotomy undergo a full staging operation. This selective approach to surgical staging provides curative resection by hysterectomy while minimizing operative risks for the 60% of patients who have a negligible chance of tumor recurrence. ER, estrogen receptor; PR, progesterone receptor. (From Burke TW: Cancer Bull 1990; 42:80. Copyright, Medical Arts Publishing Foundation, Houston, Texas, 1990.)

nosis.[61] However, the significance of factors such as depth of invasion, extension to the cervix, and grade are less clear for nonepithelial tumors. Surgical evaluation of these patients is also hindered because the diagnosis is not established preoperatively in many cases. These patients would have to be returned to the operating room for a staging procedure, which the authors believe is, in general, unwarranted. When the diagnosis of sarcoma or malignant mixed müllerian tumor is known preoperatively, the authors perform a complete staging operation. This accomplishes the goal of obtaining a clear picture of disease extent and may provide useful information upon which to make decisions about the need for additional therapy.

Surgical Therapy for Primary Tumor

Extrafascial abdominal hysterectomy is the mainstay of therapy for endometrial carcinoma. Surgical removal of the uterus, without additional therapy, is curative for the majority of patients. The authors' approach is to open the abdomen through a generous midline vertical incision. Saline washings from the abdomen and pelvis are then obtained and sent as a single sample for cytologic examination. A careful abdominal examination that includes inspection and palpation of the intraperitoneal structures and retroperitoneal lymph node areas is then performed.

If there is no gross tumor outside of the uterus, the authors proceed with simple extrafascial hysterectomy and removal of the adnexa if they are still

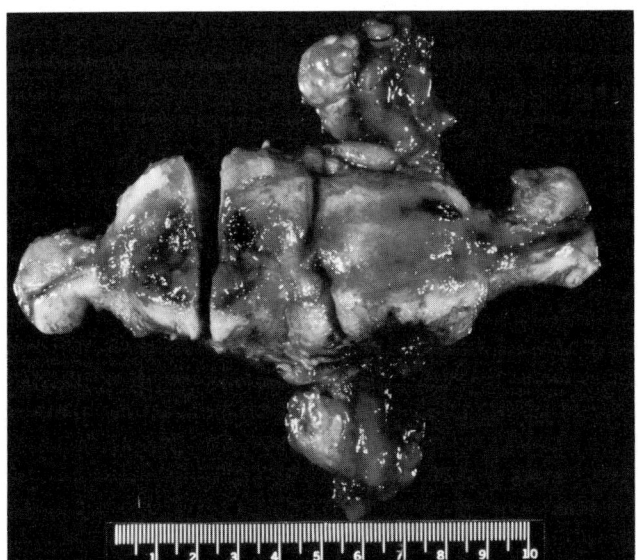

Figure 20–8
This photograph illustrates the technique for grossly estimating the depth of myometrial invasion intraoperatively. The uterus has been bisected, and a full-thickness segment of uterine wall has been excised at the center of the tumor.

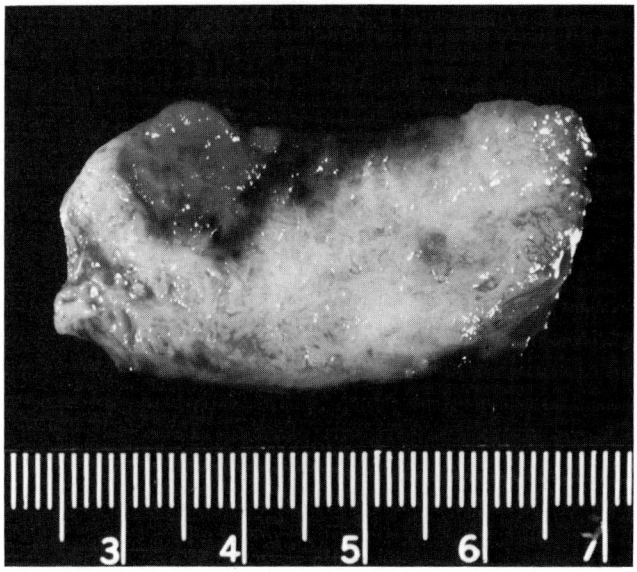

Figure 20–9
The excised segment from Figure 20–8 has an easily identified border between the invading tumor and adjacent myometrium. Intraoperative estimates of depth of invasion by visual inspection correlate with final histopathologic results in about 90% of cases.

present. No specific attempt is made to remove parametrial tissue or additional vaginal cuff unless there is clinically evident involvement of these areas by tumor. The uterus is sent directly to the pathology laboratory, where the specimen is opened. A gross visual estimation of the depth of invasion is made. This is done by bisecting the uterus using lateral incisions from the cervix to the fundus, as is shown in Figure 20–8. A full-thickness transverse segment of the uterine wall is removed at the level of the tumor. The cut surface of this segment is inspected, and an estimated depth of invasion is measured with a ruler (Fig. 20–9). This technique provides an accurate assessment of depth of myometrial invasion in about 90% of cases.[62] In situations in which the gross examination is equivocal or extensive benign disease such as leiomyomas or adenomyosis complicates it, frozen section estimate of depth of myometrial invasion may provide additional information. The authors also ask the pathologist to make a gross inspection for evidence of cervical or lower uterine segment extension and to estimate the extent of uterine cavity involvement by tumor (Fig. 20–10). Tumor samples for steroid hormone receptor analysis are obtained from the hysterectomy specimen by the pathologist in the frozen section laboratory.

The role of more radical types of hysterectomy is undefined. Some authors recommend using a classic type III radical hysterectomy for some patients with clinical Stage II endometrial cancer.[63] This recommendation must be modified to accommodate the new staging criteria. Patients with surgical Stage IIA disease may not be accurately diagnosed preoperatively.

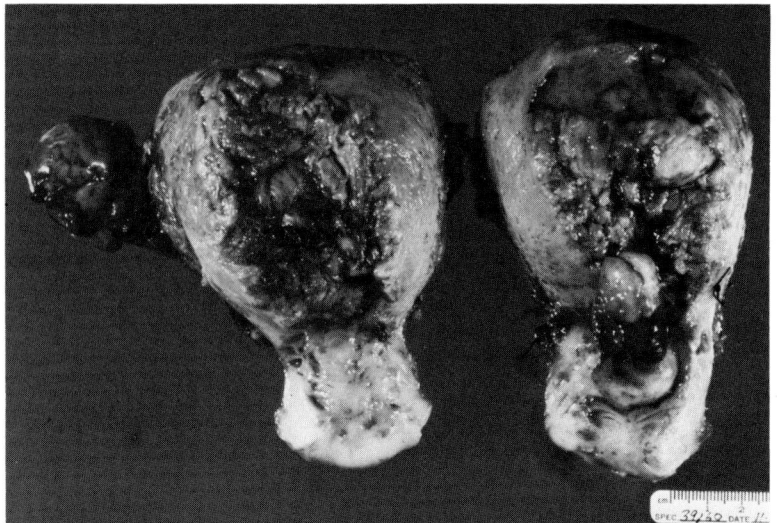

Figure 20–10
Tumor encroachment into the lower uterine segment and extensive involvement of the endometrial cavity have been associated with poor prognosis. The cancer in this illustration involves the entire endometrial surface and extends to the internal cervical os. Myometrial invasion can be grossly identified at the cut edge of the specimen.

Extrafascial hysterectomy will have already been performed when microscopic surface involvement of the cervix is detected. Planned radical hysterectomy is then limited to patients who might fall into the surgical Stage IIB category. Some of these patients have clinically detectable, firm, irregular cervical enlargement. They are at risk for extrauterine disease, particularly parametrial spread and pelvic lymph node metastases, and have a greater chance of pelvic recurrence. Radical hysterectomy may be a rational way to address these risks, although many investigators would prefer a combined surgical-radiotherapeutic approach in this setting.[64–68]

Occasionally, tumors that have penetrated the myometrium and extended into the medial parametria are unexpectedly encountered at laparotomy. Modified radical hysterectomy (type II) may be needed to provide complete resection of all gross disease in this setting. The technique for performing radical or modified radical hysterectomy in patients with uterine fundal tumors is identical to that described for the management of cervical cancers.

The role of tumor reductive surgery (or debulking) or exenterative resections in patients with advanced uterine cancer is controversial. Because these large, bulky tumors are rare, clinical experience with extensive resection is limited. Both epithelial and mesenchymal uterine cancers are relatively resistant to known chemotherapeutic agents. There is no current evidence to suggest that tumor reductive surgery will enhance the response to systemic postoperative chemotherapy. It seems reasonable to suggest that aggressive surgical resections should be reserved for patients likely to derive some palliative benefit from a more involved resection. Pelvic exenteration may provide complete surgical excision for the rare patient with Stage IVA disease. Because of the substantial morbidity and significant mortality associated with exenteration, these cases should be highly selective. Many patients with bulky central tumors will be found to have extrapelvic or retroperitoneal metastases, which would make curative ultraradical resection impossible.

Extended Staging Procedures

For patients with high-risk histopathologic features and a stable intraoperative course during initial hysterectomy, the authors proceed with an extended staging operation (Fig. 20–11). Cytologic specimens have already been obtained when the abdominal cavity was opened, the peritoneal cavity has been explored, and hysterectomy with adnexectomy has been completed. With the abdominal contents packed off into the upper abdomen, the authors first obtain random biopsy specimens of the pelvic peritoneum, bladder peritoneum, and sigmoid colon serosa. These specimens can be easily obtained by grasping the peritoneum with a long Allis clamp and elevating a small segment of tissue. Each sample is excised with fine scissors and forwarded for permanent section. Diffuse microscopic tumor implants may be detected on these specimens.

The authors then proceed with a selective pelvic lymph node sampling (Fig. 20–12). The retroperitoneal space is entered through a lateral peritoneal incision over the psoas muscle extending from the round ligament to the pelvic brim. Blunt dissection is used to open the pararectal space to visualize the pelvic vessels and mobilize the ureter medially. The authors arbitrarily divide the pelvic nodes into four regional groupings based upon their association with the pelvic arteries: (1) common iliac, (2) external iliac,

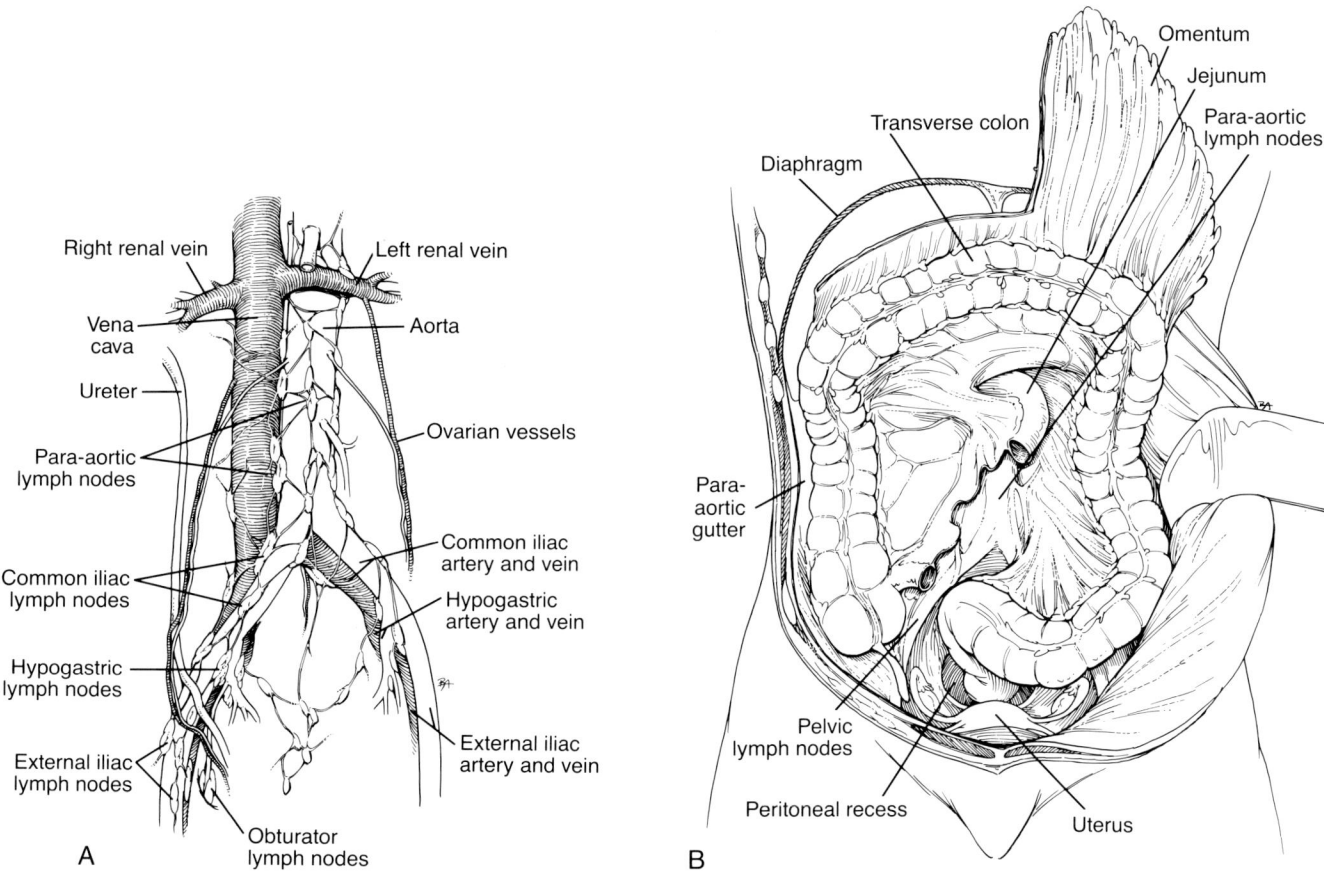

Figure 20–11
Extended surgical staging biopsy specimens should be systematically obtained. A, Lymphatic spread is evaluated by selective sampling of the pelvic and para-aortic lymph nodes. Para-aortic nodes should be biopsied at or near the level of the ovarian vessels. Pelvic node biopsy specimens are obtained from the common iliac, external iliac, hypogastric, and obturator nodal groups. Bilateral selective sampling provides a broad assessment of the lymphatic drainage pathways from the uterus. B, Intraperitoneal spread can be assessed with cytologic washings and biopsies of peritoneum, omentum, diaphragm, bowel serosa, and bowel mesentery. Additional specimens are taken from sites that look or feel abnormal.

(3) hypogastric, and (4) obturator. With the vessels exposed and the ureter retracted, the authors select one or two prominent nodes from each of the four groups for excisional biopsy. The lymph node is gently grasped with a Singley forceps and elevated away from the adjacent vessel. Dissecting scissors are used to separate adventitial tissue and to define the vascular supply to the node. The identified vessels are clipped with small hemoclips, and the node is excised. This sampling procedure is performed bilaterally and, because each node is visually identified, should provide a minimum of eight pelvic lymph nodes for histologic analysis. Closed suction drains are placed into the retroperitoneal space and brought out through separate lateral stab incisions.

If lymph nodes containing obvious tumor are encountered, the authors attempt to perform a formal pelvic lymphadenectomy that completely removes these positive nodes. They believe that postoperative external pelvic irradiation or chemotherapy may successfully sterilize small-volume nodal metastases but is unlikely to control gross nodal disease. Some investigators recommend that a complete bilateral pelvic lymphadenectomy be performed as part of the staging procedure.[69] They argue that selective nodal samplings are less accurate, that lymphadenectomy may provide a therapeutic benefit for patients with positive nodes, and that the morbidity of selective sampling and of lymphadenectomy is similar. The authors feel that a consistent and thorough approach to node sampling provides adequate prognostic information. Because postoperative external irradiation is often given to all patients with positive pelvic nodes regardless of the completeness of the nodal dissection, the more extensive dissection associated with pelvic lymphadenectomy provides no tangible benefit to the patient.

When the pelvic staging biopsies are completed, the abdominal packs and retractor are removed. Random peritoneal biopsy specimens from the par-

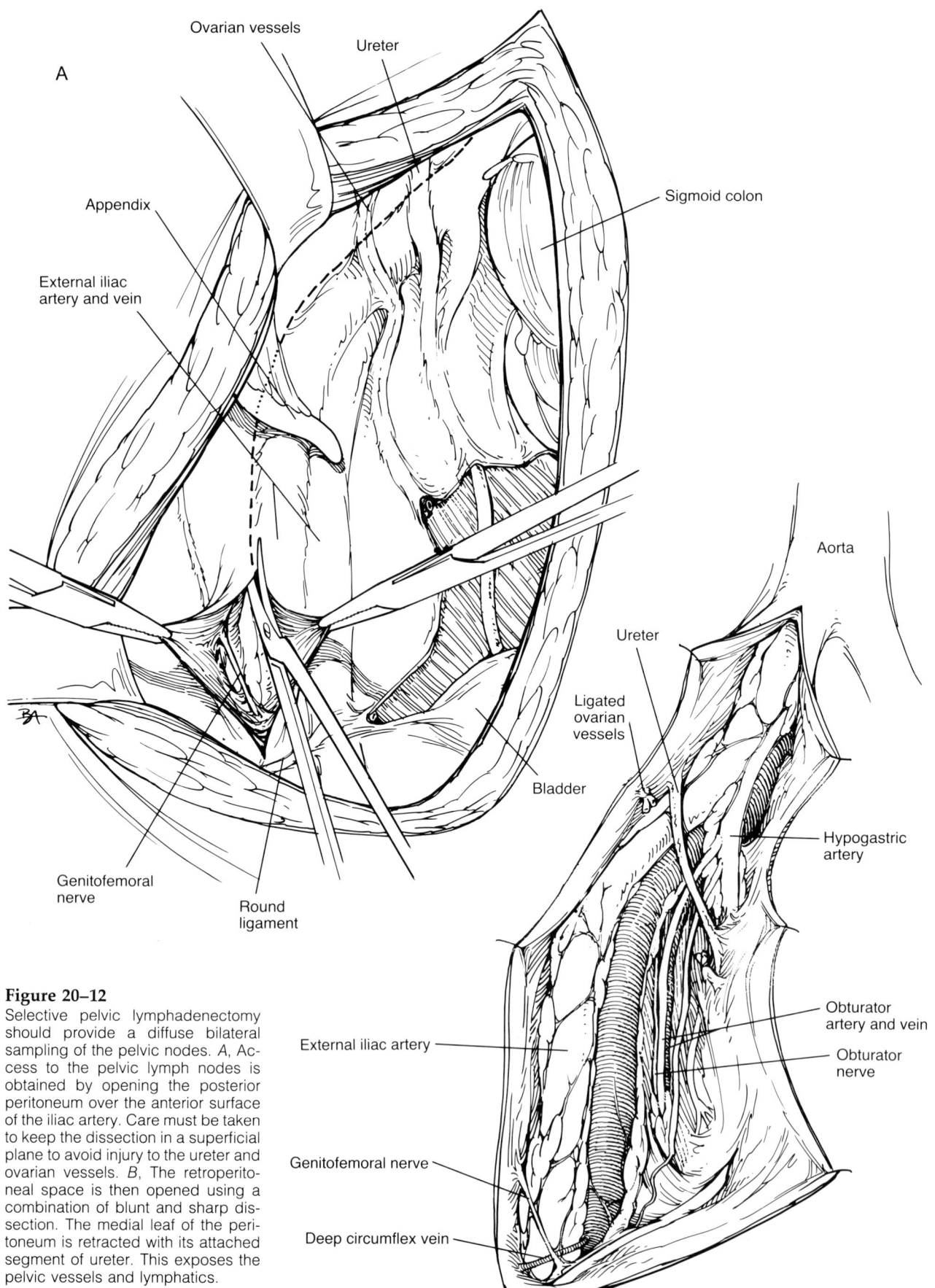

Figure 20–12
Selective pelvic lymphadenectomy should provide a diffuse bilateral sampling of the pelvic nodes. *A,* Access to the pelvic lymph nodes is obtained by opening the posterior peritoneum over the anterior surface of the iliac artery. Care must be taken to keep the dissection in a superficial plane to avoid injury to the ureter and ovarian vessels. *B,* The retroperitoneal space is then opened using a combination of blunt and sharp dissection. The medial leaf of the peritoneum is retracted with its attached segment of ureter. This exposes the pelvic vessels and lymphatics.

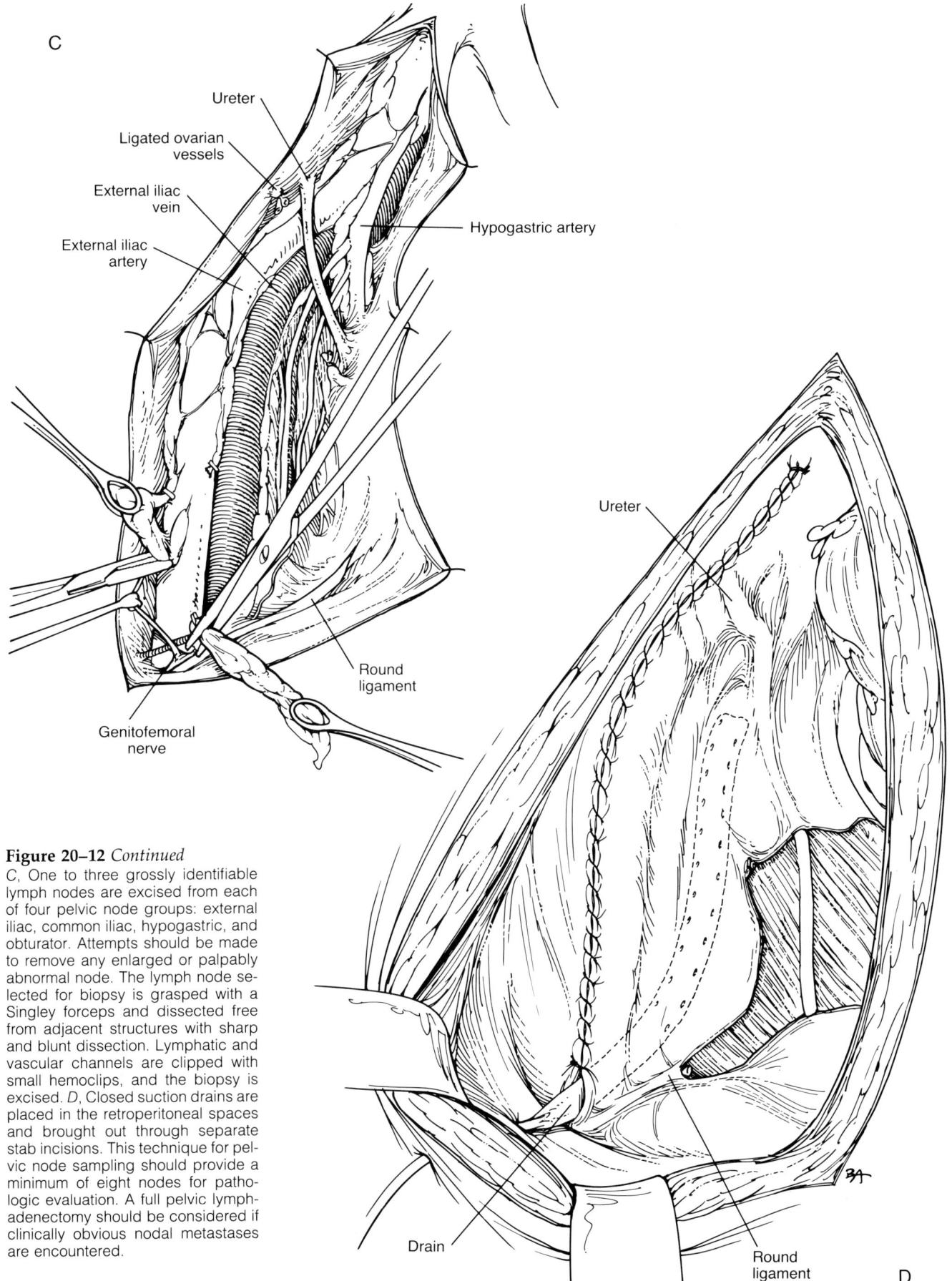

Figure 20–12 *Continued*
C, One to three grossly identifiable lymph nodes are excised from each of four pelvic node groups: external iliac, common iliac, hypogastric, and obturator. Attempts should be made to remove any enlarged or palpably abnormal node. The lymph node selected for biopsy is grasped with a Singley forceps and dissected free from adjacent structures with sharp and blunt dissection. Lymphatic and vascular channels are clipped with small hemoclips, and the biopsy is excised. *D*, Closed suction drains are placed in the retroperitoneal spaces and brought out through separate stab incisions. This technique for pelvic node sampling should provide a minimum of eight nodes for pathologic evaluation. A full pelvic lymphadenectomy should be considered if clinically obvious nodal metastases are encountered.

acolic gutters and the right diaphragmatic surface are taken by elevating the biopsy specimen with a long Allis clamp and excising it. A representative portion of the infracolic omentum is removed. The authors do not attempt to perform a complete omentectomy unless there is obvious tumor spread to the omentum. Serial application of the CO_2-powered ligating and dividing stapler (LDS, US Surgical) is a rapid and simple way to obtain this specimen. An alternative technique is to sequentially define, clamp, cut, and tie the omental vessels. Biopsy specimens of any other intraperitoneal abnormalities are then obtained. Sites to consider for additional biopsy include adhesions, palpable nodules or irregularities, capsular or parenchymal liver nodules, and abnormalities of the gastric or small bowel serosa.

Finally, the authors obtain right and left para-aortic lymph node biopsy specimens, as demonstrated in Figure 20–13. Access to the para-aortic lymph node chains can be obtained by extending the lateral peritoneal incisions up into the paracolic gutters or by opening the peritoneum directly over the aorta. Because uterine fundal tumors have access to lymphatics that parallel the ovarian vessels, metastases may be present in the para-aortic nodes even when pelvic nodes are negative. The authors attempt to obtain one to three nodes from both the right and left sides of the aorta at a level near the origin of the ovarian arteries.

Adequate exposure for the para-aortic node sampling usually requires an abdominal incision that extends slightly above the umbilicus. The authors' preference is to extend the lateral peritoneal incisions used for the pelvic node sampling up into the paracolic gutters. When the retroperitoneal space is developed with blunt dissection, the cecum and ascending colon or the descending colon can be shifted medially to expose the vena cava and aorta. Once the cecum has been mobilized, the right ureter and ovarian vessels are identified and retracted medially with a large curved retractor. A second curved retractor placed into the retroperitoneal space is used for superior retraction. Care should be taken to identify and mobilize the third portion of the duodenum superiorly and to limit tension placed on the retractors to avoid traction injury to the ovarian vessels. The major chain of right-sided lymph nodes usually lies on top of the inferior vena cava. These nodes can be elevated with a Singley forceps. Dissecting scissors are used to identify the plane of tissue anterior to the vena caval wall, and a 4–5 cm segment of the node chain is isolated. Small vessels

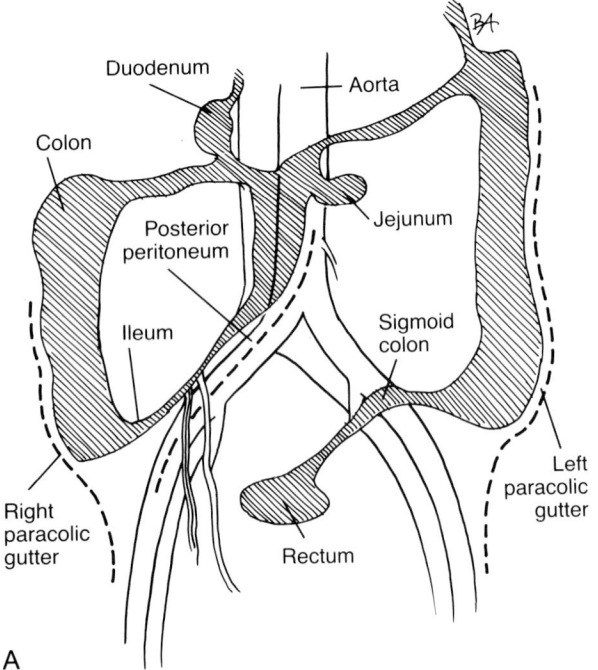
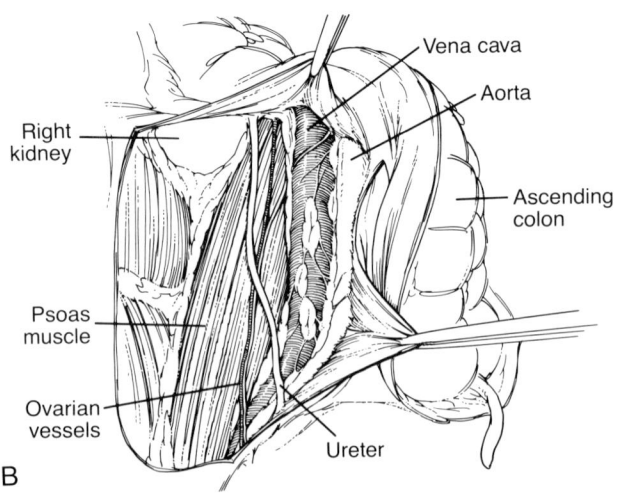

Figure 20–13
A, Retroperitoneal exposure of the vena cava and abdominal aorta can be obtained by vertically incising the peritoneum of the right and left paracolic gutter as outlined by the lateral markings. This is most easily accomplished by caudally extending the incisions made in the pelvic peritoneum created at the time of hysterectomy and pelvic node sampling. Medial mobilization of the large bowel and its mesentery provides access to the vena cava or aorta. An alternative approach is to open the posterior peritoneum along the anterior surface of the common iliac artery and lower aorta as indicated by the middle line. Dissection to the level of the arterial wall permits lateral mobilization of the more superficial structures and provides access to both the right and left para-aortic nodal chains. B, The cecum and ascending colon have been retracted medially to expose the vena cava. The ovarian vessels and right ureter are identified lying on the surface of the psoas muscle and can be protected with a large curved retractor. The duodenum is identified and mobilized superiorly.

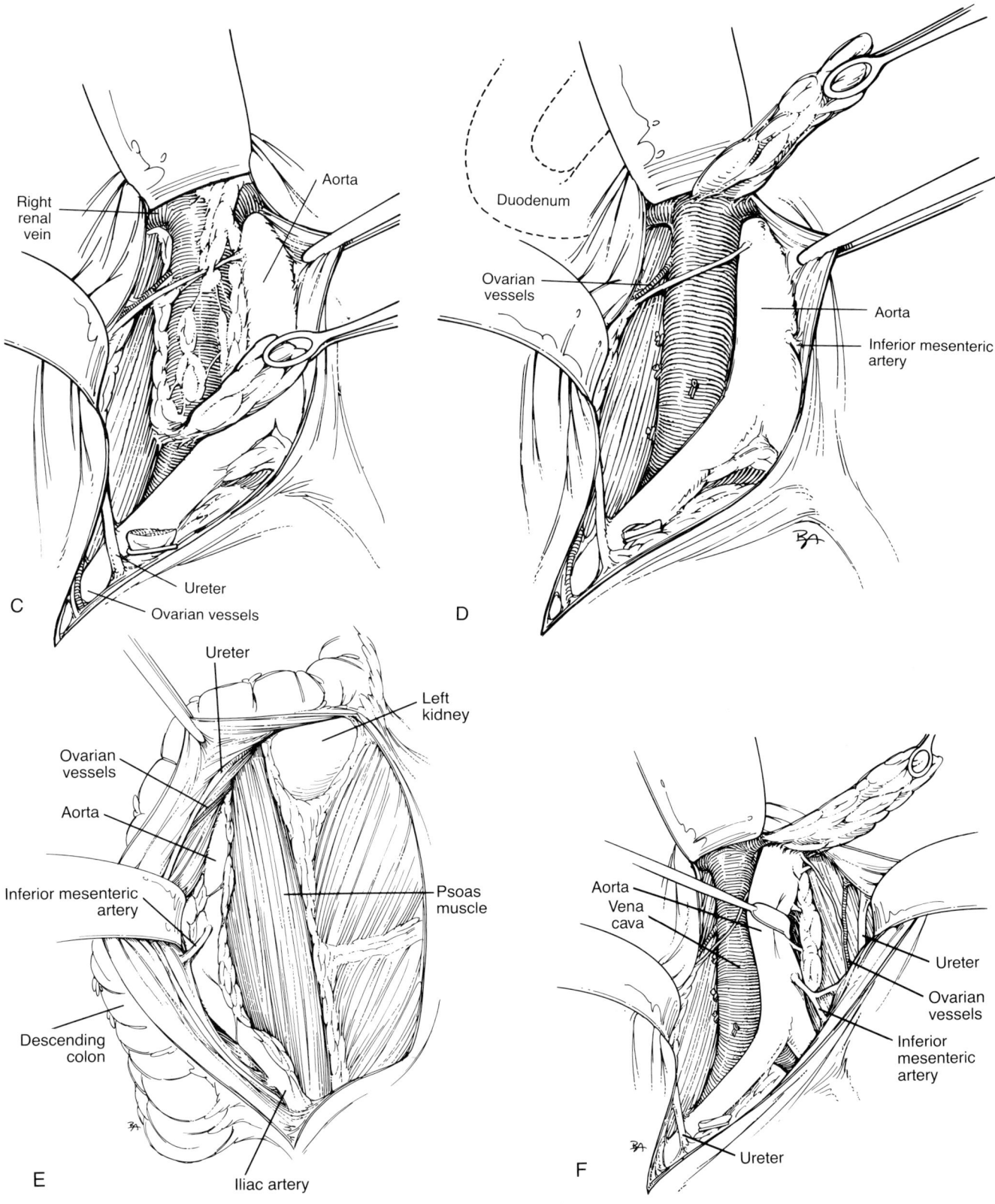

Figure 20–13 *Continued*
C and *D*, The nodal tissue lying on the anterior surface of the vena cava near the level of the right ovarian vein is dissected free and removed. Vascular and lymphatic channels are secured with hemoclips. *E*, The descending colon and its mesentery have been retracted medially to expose the abdominal aorta. The ureter and left ovarian vessels as well as the inferior mesenteric artery are identified and protected. *F*, The nodal chain on the left is located more posteriorly than on the right. As on the right, a 4–5 cm segment of nodal tissue is dissected free and excised. Care should be taken to avoid injury to the segmental lumbar vessels that lie just posterior to the para-aortic lymph nodes.

are clipped with hemoclips, as are the superior and inferior lymphatic trunks. The nodal biopsy specimen is then excised.

No major venous channels should be encountered below the level of the ovarian vein during the right-sided dissection. However, there is a fairly consistent small anterior vein entering the lower 3–4 cm of the vena cava, which can cause substantial bleeding if it is sheared off. An attempt should be made to identify and clip this vessel if present. Occasionally, small veins enter the vena cava from the psoas muscle laterally; therefore, care should be taken when freeing the lateral attachments of the node biopsy. The lumbar veins on the right generally enter the posterior aspect of the vena cava and are not encountered during dissection of the anterior node bundle. The authors usually close the peritoneal incision with a running 2-0 absorbable suture.

Sampling of the left-sided aortic nodal chain is performed in a similar manner. The peritoneal incision used for the pelvic node sampling is extended up into the left paracolic gutter. Using blunt dissection, the descending colon and upper sigmoid colon are mobilized medially. The large bowel, left ureter, and left ovarian vessels are retracted. Exposure on the left is often more difficult to obtain because the large bowel mesentery crosses the pelvic brim on this side. If the peritoneal incision is taken high up into the gutter, adequate mobilization of the bowel and lateral exposure to the aorta can usually be obtained. Superior or medial retraction must be performed carefully to avoid injury to the inferior mesenteric artery, which arises from the anterior aorta 8–10 cm above the bifurcation. The left-sided lymph node chains lie more posterior than those on the right. The authors again attempt to isolate a short segment of the nodal chain containing one to three obvious nodes at a level near the origin of the ovarian artery. Clips are used for hemostasis and to occlude lymphatic channels. Separation of the biopsy specimen from its posterior attachments should be done carefully because the lumbar arteries and veins often lie immediately behind the lymph nodes.

An alternative approach to the abdominal aorta is to open the peritoneum along the anterior surface of the common iliac artery and lower aorta, dissecting down to the level of the arterial wall. The retroperitoneal space can then be developed with sharp and gentle blunt dissection. Both ureters must be clearly identified and mobilized laterally during this dissection. The right and left sides of the aorta can then be exposed by lateral retraction and biopsy specimens obtained as described earlier. This approach generally provides excellent exposure to the lower aorta and vena cava but is less flexible than the lateral approach for obtaining exposure higher in the abdomen.

The management of clinically evident para-aortic nodal metastases is controversial. Some investigators would argue that patients with metastatic spread to these nodes have systemic disease and are already doomed to treatment failure. Difficult dissection of bulky lymph nodes may only expose the patient to the risks of major vascular injury. However, there are reports of a consistent proportion of patients whose only extrapelvic disease is in the para-aortic nodes, and some of these patients can be salvaged with extended-field irradiation.[70, 71] Because of the dose limitations of radiation therapy delivered to the para-aortic area, residual tumor volume may be important. The authors' approach to the patient whose only evidence of abdominal spread is clinically obvious para-aortic adenopathy is to make an estimate of the level of nodal involvement and the likelihood that all gross disease can be resected. Patients with positive nodes extending to the diaphragm or nodes densely encasing the major vessels are not likely to benefit from an aggressive attempt at resection. Patients with positive nodes confined to the lower or mid-portions of the abdomen that are not adherent to the vessel wall may be candidates for postoperative extended field therapy. The authors attempt resection of all gross disease in these cases. There would seem to be no advantage to difficult resection of grossly positive para-aortic lymph nodes in patients with other areas of obvious tumor outside the pelvis.

Tumor reductive or debulking surgery for uterine cancers is equally controversial. There is no current evidence to support the concept that surgical attempts to resect areas of gross disease within the abdominal cavity have an impact on postoperative therapeutic response or survival. Most patients with gross disease outside the uterus die of disease despite additional therapy. Unlike ovarian epithelial cancers, smaller volume residual endometrial cancer does not seem to be more responsive than larger disease to subsequent chemotherapy. Most probably, this is related to the lack of effective chemotherapeutic agents for advanced or recurrent endometrial cancer.

Tumor reduction may have a palliative benefit in selected patients. Resection of bulky omental metastases may be helpful in controlling ascites postoperatively. Total omentectomy should be considered in patients with widespread peritoneal disease and clinically significant ascites. Similarly, bowel resection to remove bulky disease in the pelvis or small bowel mesentery may prevent or delay postoperative bowel obstruction in some situations.

Risks of Surgical Staging

The general operative risks for extended surgical staging—infection, wound separation, atelectasis—are comparable with those of routine hysterectomy not associated with additional procedures.[72, 73] Complications specific to surgical staging procedures can be grouped into two categories: immediate perioperative complications and delayed complications. Vascular injuries during lymph node dissection have been reported in 2–5% of patients undergoing pelvic and para-aortic lymph node biopsies for staging.[72] Venous injuries are more common than arterial injuries because the normal anatomic relationship of thin-walled veins can be distorted by traction used to facilitate dissection. In addition, the variability in location, size, and number of branches of the major pelvic veins can make accurate identification more difficult. Blood loss from a major venous injury may be substantial before control of the bleeding site is obtained. Selective lymph node sampling also exposes the patient to a slightly higher risk of ureteral injury, although these injuries are uncommon. Operative injuries at other abdominal biopsy sites are rare; the tissue samples obtained are small and are obtained under direct vision.

The major delayed complications of surgical staging are related to postoperative adhesion formation involving the small bowel. Postoperative ileus and bowel obstruction occur more commonly after lengthy or extended surgical procedures. The incidence of severe small bowel injury following postoperative external irradiation rises substantially in patients who have had extensive transperitoneal procedures. Weiser and coworkers reported a fourfold increase in severe small bowel injuries for cervical cancer patients who had transperitoneal surgical staging prior to pelvic irradiation compared with patients who had extraperitoneal staging.[74] Because external-beam irradiation to the whole pelvis, extended fields, or whole abdomen is commonly employed as a postsurgical adjunct in uterine cancer, this is a significant concern. The authors believe that a risk-oriented approach to extended surgical staging as outlined previously will minimize the risks of postoperative irradiation bowel injury by reducing the number of patients who undergo a full staging operation.

Advantages of Surgical Staging

The major advantages of a surgical staging system for endometrial cancer are the accurate determination of disease extent and the elimination of the common errors introduced by clinical staging. Accurate determination of histologic grade and the presence of cervical extension are particularly difficult to evaluate on curettage specimens.[75] Discrepancy rates as high as 30% have been reported when the pathologic interpretation of curettage specimens and hysterectomy specimens have been compared.[76] Detection of small-volume extrauterine disease is virtually impossible using noninvasive clinical studies. The histopathologic risk factors that have been incorporated into the surgical staging system are generally recognized as being prognostically significant. Precise and reproducible evaluation of tumor histology, tumor grade, depth of myometrial invasion, cervix extension, and extrauterine disease should allow patients to be subgrouped into more comparable risk categories than is possible with clinical staging.

Surgical staging should make decisions about postoperative adjuvant or adjunctive therapy more uniform and logical. Different adjuvant approaches can be tailored to specific poor prognosis subgroups. For example, extended-field irradiation may be beneficial for a patient with positive para-aortic nodes, but not for one with omental metastases. An additional advantage of surgical staging is the reliable identification of a low-risk population that requires no additional therapy. Patients with early endometrial cancer who are surgically proved to have disease confined to the uterus may be spared the risks and morbidity of adjuvant treatment. Most of these women are cured by extrafascial hysterectomy alone. Finally, widespread application of surgical staging permits a detailed description of treatment results and allows more valid comparisons between institutions.

Disadvantages of Surgical Staging

There are some significant problems with surgical staging for uterine cancer. The staging system appears to be most applicable to patients with clinically limited disease who might benefit from a more detailed and complete assessment of disease and recurrence risk. Surgical staging is not likely to have a significant impact in patients with low-risk disease because their survival is already excellent. Subjecting these patients to the increased surgical risks of extended staging seems unwarranted. Conversely, patients at the other extreme who have advanced primary disease are uniformly refractory to currently available therapy. It is unlikely that information obtained at laparotomy will significantly alter therapy decisions or outcome for these patients. Fortunately, most patients with advanced disease have clinically detectable extrauterine tumor, which would preclude the need for surgical exploration.

Perhaps the largest issue related to extended surgical staging is proof that it influences outcome. It would be illogical to subject patients to the risks of additional surgical procedures unless there was a documented benefit to the performance of those procedures. Although risk assessment and stratification of prognostic groups are intellectually rewarding, a proven survival advantage must be shown for surgical staging efforts to continue. Ongoing critical evaluation of the impact of surgical staging on outcome is required.

Adjuvant and Adjunctive Therapy

A wide variety of adjuvant therapy options have been advocated for patients with endometrial cancer (Table 20–7). The fact that the options available are so numerous would suggest that no single approach has been clearly established as the most effective. The term "adjuvant therapy" should be applied to nonsurgical treatment given to patients who do not have extrauterine disease documented by surgical staging. Candidates for adjuvant therapy are those whose uterine specimens demonstrate deep myometrial invasion, cervical extension, or lymph–vascular space invasion. Patients with poor prognosis histologic subtypes or Grade 3 adenocarcinomas may also be candidates for adjuvant treatment. Treatment beyond hysterectomy is justified in these cases because of the documented risk for vaginal and pelvic recurrence as well as the potential for undetected disseminated disease. Extended surgical staging will identify a group of patients with proven small-volume disease outside the uterus. These patients will have known or suspected residual tumor following hysterectomy. Postoperative therapy in this setting is most appropriately termed "adjunctive." The options for adjuvant or adjunctive therapy can be grouped into three broad categories: radiotherapy, chemotherapy, and hormonal therapy. Combinations of these can also be considered.

Table 20–7

Adjuvant or Adjunctive Therapy Options

Radiotherapy
Preoperative
Tandem and ovoids
Whole-pelvis external beam

Postoperative
Vaginal ovoids or cylinder
Whole-pelvis external beam
Extended-field external beam
Whole-abdomen irradiation
Intraperitoneal isotopes (^{32}P)

Hormonal Therapy
Progestins
Medroxyprogesterone acetate (Provera)
Megestrol acetate (Megace)

Antiestrogens
Tamoxifen citrate (Nolvadex)

GnRH Antagonists
Leuprolide acetate (Lupron)

Chemotherapy
Doxorubicin
Cisplatin
Carboplatin
Doxorubicin-cyclophosphamide
Cisplatin-doxorubicin-cyclophosphamide

Critical examination of the available information regarding therapeutic additions to hysterectomy is exceedingly difficult. Most available studies are retrospective reviews. Although these studies contain large numbers of patients, the numbers of patients at significant risk of failure are relatively small. Most published data are based upon clinical staging, which has a known and significant error rate. Extrapolation of treatment results from clinically staged to surgically staged patients is complex, and interpretation of information derived from surgically staged patients is likely to be equally challenging because of the large number of significant prognostic factors. To further confuse the adjuvant therapy picture, Morrow and colleagues have presented data to suggest that each of the known prognostic features may be associated with a different relative risk of recurrence.[77] At present, decisions about types of adjuvant and adjunctive therapy are more a function of physician bias than proven therapeutic value. Current philosophies about adjuvant and adjunctive therapy are continuously evolving as new data become available. Surgical staging will undoubtedly cause further refinement of these concepts.

Radiotherapy

Radiotherapeutic options can be further subdivided into three groups: brachytherapy, external-beam therapy, and intraperitoneal isotopes. Both brachytherapy and external-beam therapy can be given either preoperatively or postoperatively. There are, therefore, many possible combinations of technique, dose, and timing for the delivery of adjuvant or adjunctive irradiation.

Brachytherapy can be delivered preoperatively with a standard tandem and ovoid apparatus such as that used in the routine radiotherapeutic treatment of cervical cancer. The authors routinely use this type of preoperative brachytherapy for patients with Grade 2 or 3 adenocarcinomas and variant histologic types when the tumor appears to be clinically confined to the uterus. The authors believe that these patients are at increased risk of vaginal apex recurrence and benefit from irradiation of the upper vagina. Compiled recurrence information from several large series demonstrates that the risk of vaginal apex failure can be reduced from 5–8% to 2–4% with upper vaginal irradiation.[78] The authors prefer to leave this system in place for a total of 72 hours and then proceed with hysterectomy and extended staging after 24 additional hours.[79] Rapid scheduling and completion of hysterectomy minimize the risk of infectious morbidity and do not significantly alter histopathologic assessment of the surgical specimens. In addition, both therapies can be delivered during a single hospitalization, although two anesthetizations are required.[80, 81]

An alternative approach, more commonly practiced, is to perform initial surgical exploration with hysterectomy and staging and then provide postoperative brachytherapy for those patients believed to be at risk for vaginal failure.[82, 83] This can be accomplished with either vaginal cuff ovoids or with a vaginal dome cylinder. Both techniques deliver acceptable doses to the vaginal surface. However, better depth penetration is achieved with the preoperative brachytherapy system because of the contribution of sources within the tandem.

For patients being treated solely with irradiation, there seems to be some advantage to brachytherapy techniques that use uterine packing of sources (such as Heyman's or Simon's capsules). Presumably, these approaches enhance dosimetry surrounding the uterine fundus and provide more complete coverage of the tumor than is provided by the linear arrangement of sources in a standard uterine tandem.[84] This advantage is not significant when hysterectomy is planned because the fundal portion of the tumor will be surgically removed. Techniques for brachytherapy application are described in another chapter of this text.

Preoperative external-beam irradiation has been utilized for high-risk patients in some centers.[85] Although whole-pelvis external irradiation is an integral part of treatment for patients with clinically advanced pelvic tumors, its use in an adjuvant setting has largely been abandoned in favor of more tailored postoperative therapy. Whole-pelvis therapy has been shown to sterilize nodal disease and to improve local and regional control for patients with extrauterine disease confined to the pelvis. Unfortunately, this improvement in local control has not been translated into improved survival. No significant survival advantage could be demonstrated in patients who received postoperative external pelvic irradiation in a large prospective randomized trial from the Norwegian Radium Hospital.[86, 87] Patients who were irradiated experienced failure outside the treatment field, suggesting that the real problem is systemic disease. Sites of treatment failure from two studies of patients with recurrent disease presented in Figure 20–14 demonstrate this problem.

Some limited success with extended-field and whole-abdomen irradiation has been reported in select subgroups of patients with small-volume para-aortic nodal or abdominal tumor.[90-92] These remain legitimate therapeutic options when the amount of residual extrauterine disease can be sterilized by radiation doses achievable with these techniques.

A few reports have described the use of intraperitoneal radioisotopes for patients with positive peritoneal cytologic findings or small-volume miliary peritoneal disease. If the information related to the use of intraperitoneal isotopes for minimal volume

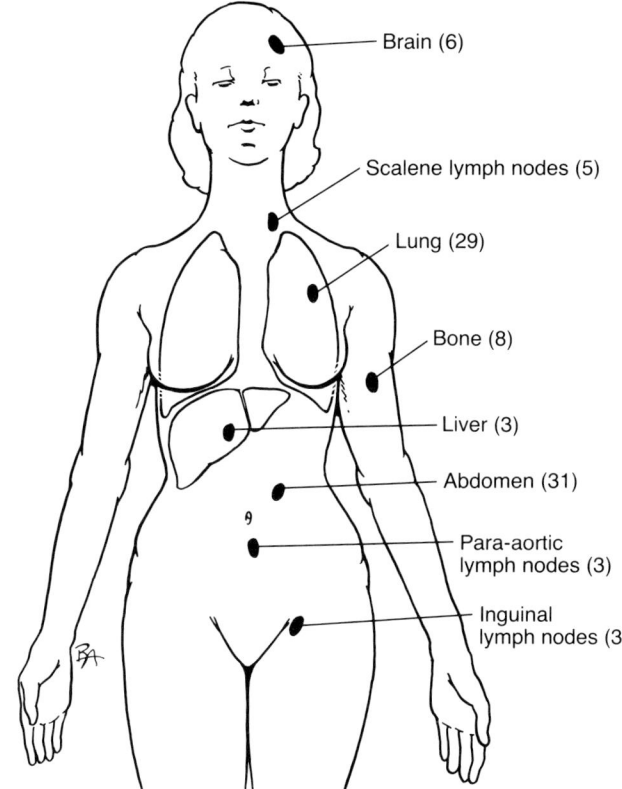

Figure 20–14
About 30–50% of endometrial cancer treatment failures occur outside the pelvis. Most of these recurrences are not amenable to local or regional therapy. Systemic hormonal or chemotherapy produces few cures in patients with recurrent disease. Data compiled from Burke et al., 1990 (ref. 34), and Burke et al., 1991 (ref. 103) (patient n = 74).

ovarian cancer can be extrapolated to the analogous situation in endometrial cancer, there may be a theoretical basis for this approach. A single intraperitoneal instillation of ^{32}P certainly presents less risk than a full course of whole-abdomen irradiation. Isotope therapy directed by monoclonal antibodies to endometrial tumors is a research concept that may provide the therapeutic advantage needed to make this technique more widely applicable.

UTERINE SARCOMAS

Surgery for Primary Disease

Patients with primary uterine sarcomas present several different clinical scenarios: (1) patients operated on for suspected benign gynecologic conditions, usually leiomyomas or dysfunctional bleeding, who postoperatively are found to have a malignant tumor; (2) patients with abnormal bleeding or a cervical mass who have preoperative biopsies documenting the presence of a sarcoma or mixed tumor; or (3) patients with advanced disease who present with extensive pelvic disease with or without clinically evident metastases.

Curative therapy for patients with uterine sarcomas can be directly correlated with resectability by hysterectomy.[93, 94] Patients whose tumors are confined to the uterus are appropriately treated by extrafascial hysterectomy. For smooth muscle tumors, the diagnosis is frequently not established preoperatively. Occasionally, intraoperative examination of the uterine specimen may provide a diagnosis of leiomyosarcoma, but this is uncommon unless extensive disease is encountered. Small tumors often have a gross appearance similar to that of benign leiomyomas, and frozen section analysis for prognostic features such as cytologic atypia and mitotic counts is difficult to perform. When the final pathology evaluation reveals the diagnosis of leiomyosarcoma, it is too late to perform staging biopsies; therefore, further treatment decisions must be based upon other criteria. Because smooth muscle tumors have a tendency for vascular and lymphatic spread, careful intraoperative assessment of these structures should be done when the diagnosis is known. Intraperitoneal surface spread is less common. The authors usually obtain a detailed radiographic assessment for metastatic disease preoperatively and proceed with lymph node sampling intraoperatively as described for the staging of endometrial adenocarcinomas.

The preoperative diagnosis of endometrial stromal sarcomas is more commonly possible because a significant portion of the tumor projects into the uterine cavity and is readily accessible to biopsy (Fig. 20–15). Tumors confined to the uterus are adequately resected by extrafascial hysterectomy. The authors routinely perform extended staging biopsies to assess potential subclinical spread and to accumulate additional data about these uncommon tumors. Both lymph-vascular and intraperitoneal spread patterns are common. The authors' staging approach is identical to that described previously for adenocarcinomas.

Malignant mixed müllerian tumors can also be diagnosed prior to surgery by endometrial biopsy. Occasionally, an erroneous preoperative diagnosis of endometrial adenocarcinoma is made if the epithelial component predominates in the biopsy specimen and obscures the sarcomatous element. When present, extrauterine metastases are often composed exclusively of the epithelial element while the sarcomatous component remains confined to the uterus. The authors approach these tumors surgically in the same way they treat high-risk endometrial adenocarcinomas.

Surgical resection of advanced uterine sarcomas is difficult and unlikely to be curative. Incomplete resection is associated with an exceedingly high failure rate and mortality, regardless of the volume of residual disease. There is no defined benefit to tumor reductive surgery. The surgical approach in patients with advanced disease must be tailored to the clinical situation. When feasible, resection of the bulk of the primary tumor by hysterectomy may help to provide pelvic control. Aggressive efforts to resect large-volume extrauterine disease should probably be avoided unless the goal of such resection is palliative. The exception to this caution is the rare case in which there is advanced or recurrent low-grade endometrial stromal sarcoma or smooth muscle tumor. The natural history of these lesions is long, and delayed pelvic or abdominal recurrences can often be controlled with repeated aggressive surgical resections.[95]

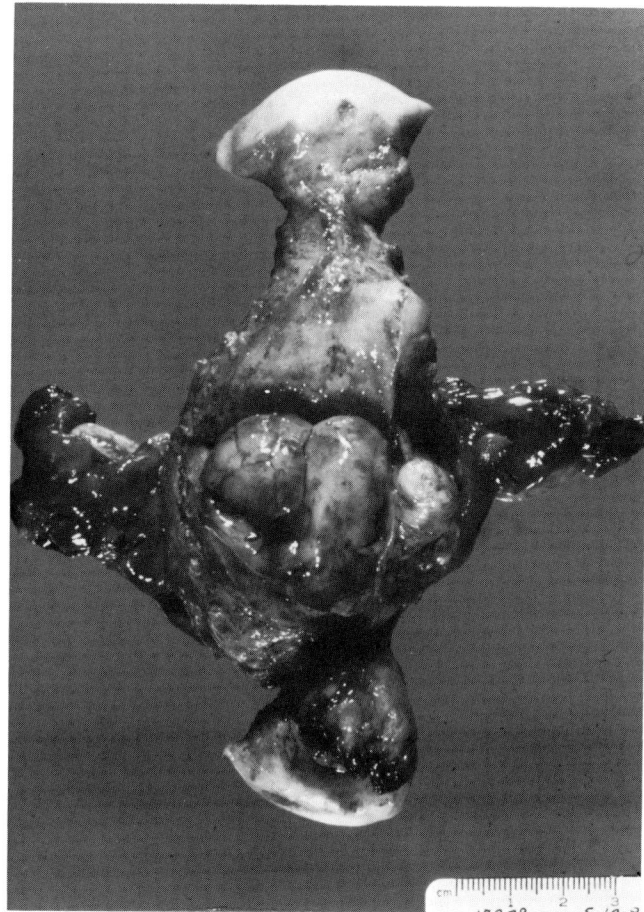

Figure 20–15
In contrast to the complex exophytic growth patterns of most endometrial adenocarcinomas, uterine sarcomas tend to grow as solid- or smooth-surfaced masses. This endometrial stromal sarcoma fills the fundal portion of the uterine cavity.

Surgery for Recurrent Adenocarcinoma and Sarcoma

Surgical therapy plays a limited role in the treatment of recurrent uterine cancer. As has been noted previously, most recurrent uterine cancers are relatively refractory to systemic therapy with hormonal or chemotherapeutic agents. Although responses can be achieved, long-term survival and cure are uncommon. Surgical approaches that do not provide complete resection of recurrent disease will not produce a cure. Most patients with uterine tumors who experience relapse present with disease that is technically unresectable. This group includes those with multiple sites of spread as well as those with a single recurrence at an unresectable site such as the pelvic sidewall, liver, or para-aortic lymph nodes.

Nevertheless, rare patients may derive curative benefit from ultraradical resections or resection combined with irradiation. Experience with pelvic exenteration for uterine cancer is limited.[96] Patients treated with exenteration include those with large, bulky tumors (Stage IVA) in whom curative resection is attempted as primary treatment. The success of this approach is limited by the age, body size, and medical status of the patient; and by the relative frequency of extrauterine disease, which defeats the goal of en bloc resection of disease. Patients who develop isolated vaginal apex recurrences following hysterectomy may also be candidates for curative resection by exenteration. If radiotherapy has not been previously used, it should be attempted prior to exenteration because some patients with recurrent disease can be cured with considerably lower morbidity.[97, 98] Vaginal apex failure presenting as an isolated area of recurrence is uncommon.[96] Because a significant proportion of patients will have other sites of spread discovered at exploration, the actual number of patients who go on to complete exenteration and subsequently remain disease-free is exceedingly small.[99]

Less radical surgical approaches, when combined with radiotherapy, may provide curative treatment of recurrence for some patients with isolated tumors. In these situations, gross tumor is surgically resected and the tumor bed is treated with external irradiation or implant therapy. Success with this combined approach has been described for patients with periurethral and some limited nodal recurrences. Long-term survival in these patients depends upon the absence of systemic disease and the ability to provide adequate dose to the site of disease.

Rare patients with uterine sarcomas who develop limited abdominal or pulmonary recurrences may benefit from surgical resection of their recurrence.[100, 101] Most of these patients have low-grade tumors with a long natural history.[102] Patients with high-grade lesions have a strong tendency for systemic dissemination and recurrence at multiple sites.

The range of palliative operations for patients with recurrent uterine cancers parallels that seen in patients with cervical or ovarian cancer. Laparotomy to relieve bowel obstruction or correct fistulas provides the most dramatic palliative benefit. A variety of possible surgical interventions are possible. The specific operation performed should be tailored to accomplish the immediate surgical goal in the most simple and direct manner. Complex palliative operations should be avoided if possible. Patient selection in this setting is critical. Patients subjected to a major palliative operation should have an acceptable functional status and a reasonable life expectancy. A patient who is not likely to outlive the time period needed for postoperative recovery should not be operated on. Percutaneous gastrostomy tube placement may be the least morbid approach to dealing with bowel obstruction in the patient with end-stage disease.

References

1. Boring CC, Squires TS, Tong T: Cancer statistics, 1991. Cancer 1991; 41:19.
2. Boronow RC: Endometrial cancer: Not a benign disease. Obstet Gynecol 1976; 47:630.
3. Creasman WT: New gynecologic cancer staging. Obstet Gynecol 1990; 75:287.
4. Wynder EL, Escher GC, Mantel N: An epidemiological investigation of cancer of the endometrium. Cancer 1966; 19:489.
5. MacMahon B: Risk factors for endometrial cancer. Gynecol Oncol 1974; 2:122.
6. Davies JL, Rosenshein NB, Antunes CMF, Stolley PD: A review of the risk factors for endometrial carcinoma. Obstet Gynecol Surv 1981; 36:107.
7. Parazzina F, La Vecchia C, Bocciolone L, Franceschi S: Review: The epidemiology of endometrial cancer. Gynecol Oncol 1991; 41:1.
8. Smith DC, Prentice R, Thompson DJ, Herrmann WL: Association of exogenous estrogen and endometrial carcinoma. N Engl J Med 1975; 293:1164.
9. Ziel HK, Finkle WD: Increased risk of endometrial carcinoma among users of conjugated estrogens. N Engl J Med 1975; 293:1167.
10. Gray LA, Christopherson WM, Hoover RN: Estrogens and endometrial cancer. Obstet Gynecol 1977; 49:385.
11. Antunes CMF, Stolley PD, Rosenshein NB, et al.: Endometrial cancer and estrogen use: Report of a large case-control study. N Engl J Med 1979; 300:9.
12. Ernster VL, Bush TL, Huggins GR, et al.: Benefits and risks of menopausal estrogen and/or progestin hormone use. Prev Med 1988; 17:201.
13. Lynch HT, Krush AJ, Larsen AL, Magnuson CW: Endometrial carcinoma: Multiple primary malignancies, constitutional factors and heredity. Am J Med Sci 1966; 252:381.
14. Lynch HT, Krush AJ, Thomas RJ, Lynch J: Cancer family syndrome. In Lynch HT (ed.): Cancer Genetics. Springfield, IL, Charles C Thomas, 1976, pp. 355–388.
15. Hendrickson M, Ross J, Eifel P, et al.: Uterine papillary serous carcinoma: A highly malignant form of endometrial adenocarcinoma. Am J Surg Pathol 1982; 6:93.
16. Jeffrey JF, Krepart GV, Lotocki RJ: Papillary serous adenocarcinoma of the endometrium. Obstet Gynecol 1986; 67:670.
17. Chambers JT, Merino M, Kohorn EI, et al.: Uterine serous papillary carcinoma. Obstet Gynecol 1987; 69:109.
18. Silverberg SG, De Giorgi LS: Clear cell carcinoma of the endometrium: Clinical, pathologic, and ultrasonic findings. Cancer 1973; 31:1127.
19. Kurman RJ, Scully RE: Clear cell carcinoma of the endometrium: An analysis of 21 cases. Cancer 1976; 37:872.

20. Christopherson WM, Alberhasky RC, Connelly PJ: Carcinoma of the endometrium. I. A clinicopathologic study of clear-cell carcinoma and secretory carcinoma. Cancer 1982; 49:1511.
21. Christopherson WM, Alberhasky RC, Connelly PJ: Carcinoma of the endometrium. II. Papillary adenocarcinoma: A clinical pathological study 46 cases. Am J Clin Pathol 1982; 77:534.
22. Sutton GP, Brill L, Michael H, et al.: Malignant papillary lesions of the endometrium. Gynecol Oncol 1987; 27:294.
23. Ng ABP, Reagan JW, Storasli JP, Wentz WB: Mixed adenosquamous carcinoma of the endometrium. Am J Clin Pathol 1973; 59:765.
24. Salazar OM, DePapp EW, Bonfiglio TA, et al.: Adenosquamous carcinoma of the endometrium: An entity with an inherent poor prognosis? Cancer 1977; 40:119.
25. Alberhasky RC, Connelly PJ, Christopherson WM: Carcinoma of the endometrium. IV. Mixed adenosquamous carcinoma: A clinical-pathological study of 68 cases with long-term follow-up. Am J Clin Pathol 1982; 77:655.
26. Greenwood SM, Wright DJ: Evaluation of the office endometrial biopsy in the detection of endometrial carcinoma and atypical hyperplasia. Cancer 1979; 43:1474.
27. Koss LG, Schreiber K, Moussouris H, Oberlander SG: Endometrial carcinoma and its precursors: Detection and screening. Clin Obstet Gynecol 1982; 25:44.
28. Grimes DA: Diagnostic office curettage—heresy no longer. Contemp Obstet Gynecol 1986; 28:96.
29. Malkasian GD: Carcinoma of the endometrium: Effect of stage and grade on survival. Cancer 1978; 41:996.
30. Malkasian GD, Annegers JF, Fountain KS: Carcinoma of the endometrium: Stage I. Am J Obstet Gynecol 1980; 136:872.
31. Connelly PJ, Alberhasky RC, Christopherson WM: Carcinoma of the endometrium. III. Analysis of 865 cases of adenocarcinoma and adenoacanthoma. Obstet Gynecol 1982; 59:569.
32. Hendrickson M, Ross J, Eifel P, et al.: Adenocarcinoma of the endometrium: Analysis of 256 cases with carcinoma limited to the uterine corpus. Gynecol Oncol 1982; 13:373.
33. Christopherson WM, Connelly PJ, Alberhasky RC: Carcinoma of the endometrium. V. An analysis of prognosticators in patients with favorable subtypes and stage I disease. Cancer 1983; 51:1705.
34. Burke TW, Heller PB, Woodward JE, et al.: Treatment failure in endometrial carcinoma. Obstet Gynecol 1990; 75:96.
35. Lehtovirta P, Cacciatore B, Wahlstrom T, Ylostalo P: Ultrasonic assessment of endometrial cancer invasion. JCU 1987; 15:519.
36. Gordon AN, Fleischer AC, Dudley BS, et al.: Preoperative assessment of myometrial invasion of endometrial adenocarcinoma by sonography (US) and magnetic resonance imaging (MRI). Gynecol Oncol 1989; 34:175.
37. Yazigi R, Cohen J, Munoz AK, Sandstad J: Magnetic resonance imaging determination of myometrial invasion in endometrial carcinoma. Gynecol Oncol 1989; 34:94.
38. Brown JJ, Thurnher S, Hricak H: MR imaging of the uterus: Low-signal-intensity abnormalities of the endometrium and endometrial cavity. Magn Reson Imag 1990; 8:309.
39. Harrill CD, Kopecky KK, Weaver SR, Sutton GP: Magnetic resonance imaging in the preoperative assessment of clinical stage I endometrial carcinoma. Comput Med Imaging Graph 1990; 14:191.
40. Nordqvist SRB, Sevin BU, Nadji M, et al.: Fine-needle aspiration cytology in gynecologic oncology. I. Diagnostic accuracy. Obstet Gynecol 1979; 54:719.
41. Sevin BU, Greening SE, Nadji M, et al.: Fine needle aspiration cytology in gynecologic oncology. I. Clinical aspects. Acta Cytol 1979; 23:277.
42. Flint A, Terhart K, Murad TM, Taylor PT: Confirmation of metastases by fine needle aspiration biopsy in patients with gynecologic malignancies. Gynecol Oncol 1982; 14:382.
43. Nash JD, Burke TW, Woodward JE, et al.: Diagnosis of recurrent gynecologic malignancy with fine needle aspiration cytology. Obstet Gynecol 1987; 71:333.
44. Layfield LJ, Heaps JM, Berek JS: Fine-needle aspiration cytology accuracy with palpable gynecologic neoplasms. Gynecol Oncol 1991; 40:70.
45. Landgren RC, Fletcher GH, Delclos L, Wharton JT: Irradiation of endometrial cancer in patients with medical contraindication to surgery or with unresectable lesions. AJR 1976; 126:148.
46. Andersen WA, Peters WA III, Fechner RE, et al.: Radiotherapeutic alternatives to standard management of adenocarcinoma of the endometrium. Gynecol Oncol 1983; 16:383.
47. Berman ML, Ballon SC, Lagasse LD, Watring WG: Prognosis and treatment of endometrial cancer. Am J Obstet Gynecol 1980; 136:679.
48. Boronow RC, Morrow CP, Creasman WT, et al.: Surgical staging in endometrial cancer: Clinical-pathologic findings of a prospective study. Obstet Gynecol 1984; 63:823.
49. DiSaia PJ, Creasman WT, Boronow RC, Blessing JA: Risk factors and recurrence patterns in stage I endometrial cancer. Am J Obstet Gynecol 1985; 151:1009.
50. Morrow CP, Creasman WT, Homesley H, et al.: Recurrence in endometrial carcinoma as a function of extended surgical staging data. In Morrow CP, Smart G (eds.): Gynaecological Oncology: Proceedings of the Second International Conference on Gynaecological Cancer. New York, Springer-Verlag, 1986, p. 147.
51. Schink JC, Lurain JR, Wallemark CB, Chmiel JS: Tumor size in endometrial cancer: A prognostic factor for lymph node metastasis. Obstet Gynecol 1987; 70:216.
52. Hanson MB, van Nagell JR Jr, Powell DE, et al.: The prognostic significance of lymph-vascular space invasion in stage I endometrial cancer. Cancer 1985; 55:1753.
53. Harouny VR, Sutton GP, Clark SA, et al.: The importance of peritoneal cytology in endometrial carcinoma. Obstet Gynecol 1988; 72:394.
54. Konski A, Poulter C, Keys H, et al.: Absence of prognostic significance, peritoneal dissemination and treatment advantage in endometrial cancer patients with positive peritoneal cytology. Int J Radiol Phys 1988; 14:49.
55. Lurain JR, Rumsey NK, Schink JC, et al.: Prognostic significance of positive peritoneal cytology in clinical stage I adenocarcinoma of the endometrium. Obstet Gynecol 1989; 74:175.
56. Turner DA, Gershenson DM, Atkinson N, et al.: The prognostic significance of peritoneal cytology for stage I endometrial cancer. Obstet Gynecol 1989; 74:775.
57. Pratt JH, Symmonds RE, Welch JS: Vaginal hysterectomy for carcinoma of the fundus. Am J Obstet Gynecol 1964; 88:1063.
58. Ingiulla W, Cosmi EV: Vaginal hysterectomy for the treatment of cancer of the corpus uteri. Am J Obstet Gynecol 1968; 100:541.
59. Peters WA III, Andersen WA, Thornton WN Jr, Morley GW: The selective use of vaginal hysterectomy in the management of adenocarcinoma of the endometrium. Am J Obstet Gynecol 1983; 146:285.
60. Bloss JD, Berman ML, Bloss LP, Buller RE: Use of vaginal hysterectomy for the management of stage I endometrial cancer in the medically compromised patient. Gynecol Oncol 1991; 40:74.
61. Peters WA III, Kumar NB, Fleming WP, Morley GW: Prognostic features of sarcomas and mixed tumors of the endometrium. Obstet Gynecol 1984; 63:550.
62. Doering DL, Barnhill DR, Weiser EB, et al.: Intraoperative evaluation of depth of myometrial invasion in stage I endometrial adenocarcinoma. Obstet Gynecol 1989; 74:930.
63. Rutledge F: The role of radical hysterectomy in adenocarcinoma of the endometrium. Gynecol Oncol 1974; 2:331.
64. Park RC, Patow WE, Petty WM, Zimmerman EA: Treatment of adenocarcinoma of the endometrium. Gynecol Oncol 1974; 2:60.
65. Hernandez W, Nolan JF, Morrow CP, Jernstrom PH: Stage II endometrial carcinoma: Two modalities of treatment. Am J Obstet Gynecol 1978; 131:171.
66. Kinsella TJ, Bloomer WD, Lavin PT, Knapp RC: Stage II endometrial carcinoma: 10-year follow-up of combined radiation and surgical treatment. Gynecol Oncol 1980; 10:290.
67. Onsrud M, Aalders J, Abeler V, Taylor P: Endometrial carcinoma with cervical involvement (stage II): Prognostic factors and value of combined radiological-surgical treatment. Gynecol Oncol 1982; 13:76.

68. Wallin TE, Malkasian GD, Gaffey TA, et al.: Stage II cancer of the endometrium: A pathologic and clinical study. Gynecol Oncol 1984; 18:1.
69. Orr JW, Orr P, Holloway RW: Surgical staging of corpus cancer: Perioperative morbidity (abstract). Proc Soc Gynecol Oncol 1991, p. 14.
70. Komaki R, Mattingly RF, Hoffman RG, et al.: Irradiation of paraaortic lymph node metastases from carcinoma of the cervix or endometrium. Radiology 1983; 147:245.
71. Potish RA, Twiggs LB, Adcock LL, et al.: Paraaortic lymph node radiotherapy in cancer of the uterine corpus. Obstet Gynecol 1985; 65:251.
72. Moore DH, Fowler WC Jr, Walton LA, Droegenmueller W: Morbidity of lymph node sampling in cancers of the uterine corpus and cervix. Obstet Gynecol 1989; 74:180.
73. Clarke-Pearson D, Cliby W, Soper J, et al.: Morbidity and mortality of selective lymphadenectomy in early stage endometrial cancer (abstract). Proc Soc Gynecol Oncol 1991, p. 14.
74. Weiser EB, Bundy BN, Hoskins WJ, et al.: Extraperitoneal versus transperitoneal selective paraaortic lymphadenectomy in the pretreatment surgical staging of advanced cervical carcinoma (a Gynecologic Oncology Group study). Gynecol Oncol 1989; 33:283.
75. Berman ML, Afridi MA, Kanbour AI, Ball HG: Risk factors and prognosis in stage II endometrial cancer. Gynecol Oncol 1982; 14:49.
76. Cowles TA, Magrina JF, Masterson BJ, Capen CV: Comparison of clinical and surgical staging in patients with endometrial carcinoma. Obstet Gynecol 1985; 66:413.
77. Morrow CP, Bundy BN, Kurman RJ, et al.: Relationship between surgical-pathological risk factors and outcome in clinical stage I and II carcinoma of the endometrium: A Gynecologic Oncology Group study. Gynecol Oncol 1991; 40:55.
78. Morrow CP, Townsend DE: Synopsis of Gynecologic Oncology. New York, Churchill Livingstone, 1987.
79. Delmore JE, Wharton JT, Hamberger AD, et al.: Preoperative radiotherapy for early endometrial carcinoma. Gynecol Oncol 1987; 28:34.
80. Underwood PB, Lutz MH, Kreutner A, et al.: Carcinoma of the endometrium: Radiation followed immediately by operation. Am J Obstet Gynecol 1977; 128:86.
81. Chambers JT, Kapp DS, Lawrence R, et al.: Immediate versus delayed hysterectomy for endometrial carcinoma: Surgical morbidity and hospital stay. Obstet Gynecol 1985; 65:245.
82. Chung CK, Stryker JA, Nahhas WA, Mortel R: The role of adjunctive radiotherapy for stage I endometrial carcinoma: Preoperative vs. postoperative irradiation. Int J Rad Oncol Biol Phys 1981; 7:1429.
83. Meerwaldt JH, Hoekstra CJM, van Putten WLJ, et al.: Endometrial adenocarcinoma, adjuvant radiotherapy tailored to prognostic factors. Int J Rad Biol Phys 1989; 18:299.
84. Wollin M, Kagan AR, Kwan DK: Radiation dose calculations in endometrial cancer treated with Heyman capsules or tandem. Gynecol Oncol 1982; 13:37.
85. Ritcher N, Lucas WE, Yon JL, Sanford FG: Preoperative whole pelvic external irradiation in stage I endometrial cancer. Cancer 1981; 48:58.
86. Onsrud M, Kolstad P, Normann T: Postoperative external pelvic irradiation in carcinoma of the corpus stage I: A controlled clinical trial. Gynecol Oncol 1976; 4:222.
87. Aalders J, Abeler V, Kolstad P, Onsrud M: Postoperative external irradiation and prognostic parameters in stage I endometrial carcinoma. Obstet Gynecol 1980; 56:419.
88. Potish RA, Twiggs LB, Adcock LL, Prem KA: Role of whole abdominal radiation therapy in the management of endometrial cancer; prognostic importance of factors indicating peritoneal metastases. Gynecol Oncol 1985; 21:80.
89. Greer BE, Hamberger AD: Treatment of intraperitoneal metastatic adenocarcinoma of the endometrium by the whole-abdomen moving-strip technique and pelvic boost irradiation. Gynecol Oncol 1983; 16:365.
90. Creasman WT, DiSaia PJ, Blessing J, et al.: Prognostic significance of peritoneal cytology in patients with endometrial cancer and preliminary data concerning therapy with intraperitoneal radiopharmaceuticals. Am J Obstet Gynecol 1981; 141:921.
91. Soper JT, Creasman WT, Pearson DL, et al.: Intraperitoneal chromic phosphate P 32 suspension therapy of malignant cytology in endometrial carcinoma. Am J Obstet Gynecol 1985; 153:191.
92. Heath R, Roseman J, Varia M, Walton L: Peritoneal fluid cytology in endometrial cancer: Its significance and the role of chromic phosphate therapy. Int J Rad Oncol Biol Phys 1988; 15:815.
93. Hannigan EV, Gomez LG: Uterine leiomyosarcoma: A review of prognostic clinical and pathological features. Am J Obstet Gynecol 1979; 134:557.
94. Larson B, Silfversward C, Nilsson B, Petterson F: Prognostic factors in uterine leiomyosarcoma. Acta Oncol 1990; 29:185.
95. Styron SL, Burke TW, Linville WK: Low-grade endometrial stromal sarcoma recurring over three decades. Gynecol Oncol 1989; 35:275.
96. Rutledge FN: Pelvic exenteration: An update of the University of Texas MD Anderson Hospital experience and review of the literature. In Rutledge FN, Freedman RS, Gershenson DM (eds.): Gynecologic Cancer: Diagnosis and Treatment Strategies. Austin, University of Texas Press, 1987, pp. 7–28.
97. Brown JM, Dockerty MB, Symmonds RE, Banner EA: Vaginal recurrence of endometrial carcinoma. Am J Obstet Gynecol 1968; 100:544.
98. Phillips GL, Prem KA, Adcock LL, Twiggs LB: Vaginal recurrence of adenocarcinoma of the endometrium. Gynecol Oncol 1982; 13:323.
99. Barber HRK, Brunschwig A: Treatment and results of recurrent cancer of corpus uteri in patients receiving anterior and total pelvic exenteration 1947–1963. Cancer 1968; 22:949.
100. McCormack PM, Martin M: The changing role of surgery for pulmonary metastases. Ann Thorac Surg 1979; 28:139.
101. Mountain CF, McMurtrey MJ, Hermes KE: Surgery for pulmonary metastasis: A 20-year experience. Ann Thorac Surg 1984; 38:323.
102. Gloor E, Schnyder P, Cikes M, et al.: Endolymphatic stromal myosis: Surgical and hormonal treatment of extensive abdominal recurrence 20 years after hysterectomy. Cancer 1982;50:1888.
103. Burke TW, Stringer CA, Morris M, et al.: Prospective treatment of advanced or recurrent endometrial carcinoma with cisplatin, doxorubicin, and cyclophosphamide. Gynecol Oncol 1991; 40:264.

Surgery of the Gastrointestinal Tract in Relation to Gynecology

21

Mitchell Morris
Thomas W. Burke

At first glance, a chapter on gastrointestinal procedures in a textbook of gynecologic surgery may seem out of place. However, the need for gastrointestinal surgery in patients with a gynecologic malignancy frequently arises. Gynecologic oncologists are often called on to perform many of the procedures described herein. The general obstetrician-gynecologist should also be familiar with these procedures. Although a generalist is usually not expected to perform intestinal surgery independently, knowledge of the disease process involved, of possible conservative options, and of the principles of pre- and postoperative evaluation is important in caring for these patients. The general surgeon who may serve as technician in these situations is often unfamiliar with the natural history of gynecologic cancer and of the particular problems experienced by this group of patients.

The procedures and techniques described herein all fall within the scope of the care required to treat women with gynecologic malignancies. They include surgical procedures for the primary treatment of pelvic cancer and the management of complications caused by therapy or disease progression.

Bowel resection in patients who have a gynecologic cancer is probably performed most often during the course of cytoreductive surgery for epithelial ovarian carcinoma, which often involves the sigmoid colon and terminal ileum. Achieving the therapeutic goal of minimal residual tumor following surgery often requires intestinal resection. Bowel resection is also a component of pelvic exenteration for advanced or recurrent pelvic cancers, as is the use of intestinal segments for reconstructive procedures. The latter procedures include sigmoid resection, low re-anastomosis, and formation of urinary conduits or continent pouches (the latter is discussed in Chapter 22).

Intestinal surgery may also be required in managing complications. Because many women with gynecologic cancer are primarily treated with radiation, radiation bowel injury to the terminal ileum or sigmoid colon is common. Intestinal dysfunction or obstruction secondary to progressive disease, postoperative obstruction, and fistula formation are other clinical entities frequently encountered in the woman with gynecologic malignancy.

ANATOMY REVIEW

Detailed knowledge of anatomy is a prerequisite to successful surgery. It is beyond the scope of this chapter to present a complete description of gastrointestinal anatomy. To serve as a reference, however, a brief review of some basic anatomic concepts, especially vascular supply, is in order.

The arterial supply to the stomach originates at the celiac trunk. The left gastric artery, which comes directly off the celiac artery, anastomoses with the right gastric branch of the hepatic artery (Fig. 21–1).

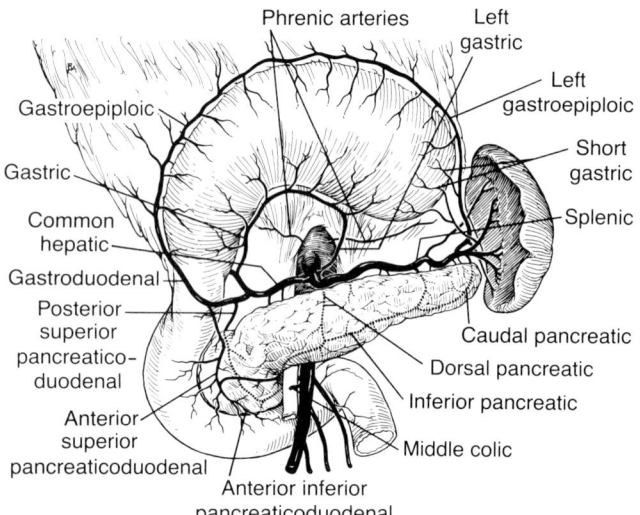

Figure 21–1
Arterial supply to the stomach, duodenum, and spleen. The stomach has been reflected superiorly with the posterior surface in view.

The gastroduodenal artery gives off an important branch known as the right gastroepiploic, which runs along the inferior greater curvature of the stomach and is a dominant blood supply to the greater omentum. The splenic artery, passing posterior to the stomach, gives rise to the short gastric arteries feeding the superior portion of the stomach and also to the left gastroepiploic artery. All of these vessels form a rich anastomotic plexus. The duodenum is also supplied from the celiac artery by means of the gastroduodenal artery, which gives rise to numerous branches.

The superior mesenteric artery arises from the anterior aspect of the aorta, immediately inferior to the celiac trunk (Fig. 21–2). This important vessel gives off numerous jejunal and ileal branches that feed the major portion of the small bowel. These anastomose to form arcades through which the vasa recta pass to the small intestine. The ileocolic artery is an important branch that supplies the terminal ileum and cecum. The right and middle colic arteries also arise from the superior mesenteric artery.

The inferior mesenteric artery arises more inferiorly on the aorta, below the level of the renal arteries (Fig. 21–3). Its major branches include the superior left colic artery and several sigmoid arteries (also known as inferior left colic arteries). The most inferior branch is known as the superior rectal artery. The lowermost part of the rectum is supplied by the middle and inferior rectal arteries, which are branches from the iliac vessels.

Venous drainage of the intestine is via the portal circulation. The exception to this is the veins of the most inferior portion of the rectum, which drain into the internal iliac veins.

PREOPERATIVE EVALUATION

Proper evaluation and preparation before performing intestinal surgery on a woman who has gynecologic

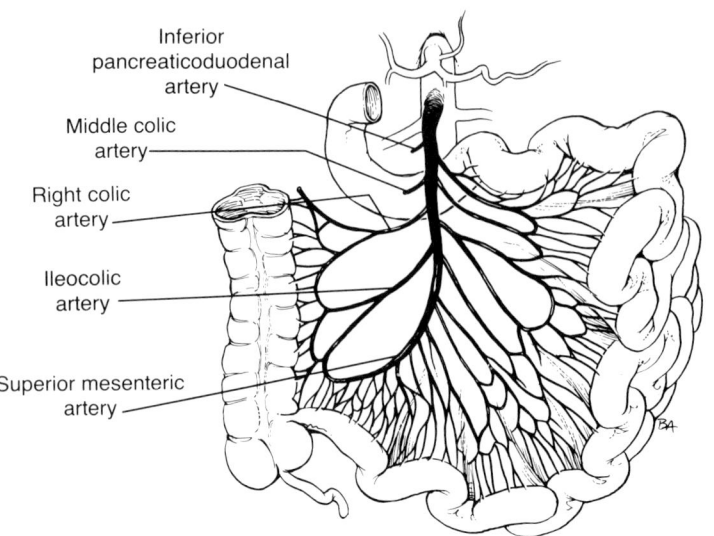

Figure 21–2
Distribution of the superior mesenteric artery.

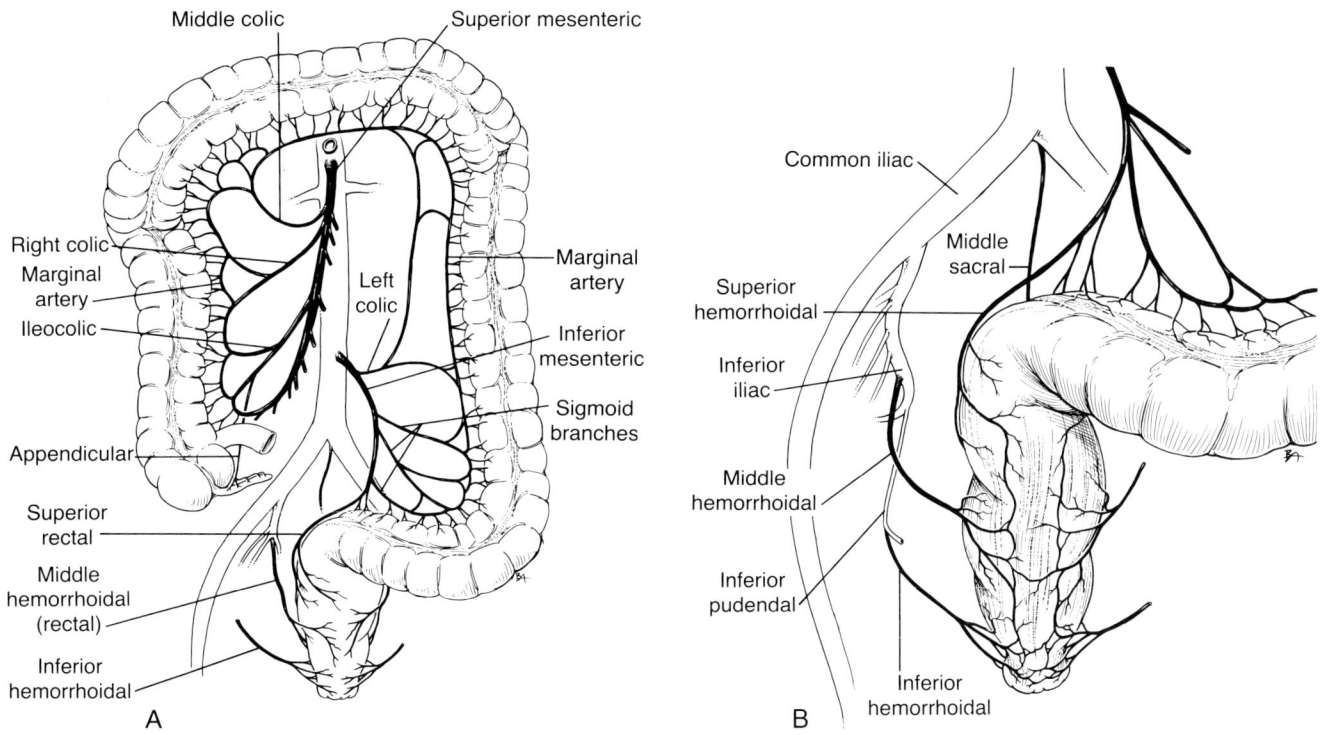

Figure 21–3
A, Arterial supply to the colon. *B*, The superior, middle, and inferior rectal arteries supply the sigmoid colon and rectum.

cancer are critically important. The preoperative testing selected should be determined by the patient's symptoms and findings on physical examination. Most patients who are scheduled for cytoreductive procedures should undergo either barium enema radiography (preferably double-contrast) or colonoscopy before coming to the operating room. This test can serve several evaluative purposes. It can identify narrowing or stricture of the sigmoid colon or of other colonic segments, which is often present in patients with ovarian cancer owing to involvement with the pelvic tumor. Occasionally, too, a patient believed preoperatively to have ovarian cancer will be found, after testing, to have diffuse disease secondary to colon carcinoma. Information regarding such a lesion would, of course, affect the preoperative evaluation and the operative approach. Radiographic evidence of intestinal involvement helps ensure that the patient has adequate bowel preparation prior to surgery, and that personnel are prepared for the eventuality of colon resection. Any patient who is suspected of having ovarian cancer and who has upper gastrointestinal symptoms should, in addition, undergo evaluation of the stomach and small intestine. Gastric carcinoma can occasionally present with ascites and a pelvic mass along with such symptoms as early satiety or nausea and vomiting. Evaluation with an upper gastrointestinal series or upper endoscopy can accurately identify these patients before they undergo exploratory surgery.

When a patient is considered a likely candidate for intestinal resection in the course of treatment for gynecologic malignancy, proper preoperative counseling is important. The patient should be informed of the possible need for small bowel or colonic resection; the implications of this surgery; and its possible effects on her lifestyle, including the possibility of fecal diversion through colostomy. Even when this eventuality is considered unlikely, the patient should know of it; performing suboptimal cytoreduction for fear of the patient's reaction to an unplanned colostomy would be a disservice to her. Most hospitals have an enterostomal therapist on staff who is available to meet with a patient and educate her about the possible need for fecal diversion. The role of the enterostomal therapist is discussed further in the section on stoma formation.

When the likelihood of intestinal resection is significant, proper preoperative bowel preparation is essential. The traditional 3-day bowel "prep" consists of a plethora of laxatives and cleansing enemas along with antibiotics, administered orally, intravenously, or by both routes (Table 21–1). Although this preparation cleanses the bowel effectively in preparation for surgery, its drawbacks include the prolonged administration time and the potential for fluid shift

Table 21-1

Traditional Three-Day Bowel Preparation

Day 1	Low-residue diet Bisacodyl, 1 capsule PO at 6 P.M.
Day 2	Continue low-residue diet Magnesium sulfate, 30 ml, 50% solution (15 g) PO at 10 A.M., 2 P.M., and 6 P.M. Saline enemas in evening until return is clear
Day 3	Clear liquid diet, supplemental IV fluids as needed Magnesium sulfate, in doses above, at 10 A.M. and 2 P.M. No enemas Neomycin, 1 g, and erythromycin base, 1 g PO at 1 P.M., 2 P.M., and 11 P.M.
Day 4	Cefoxitin, 2 g IV on call to OR Surgery

and electrolyte disturbance, which may be problematic in an elderly or sick patient.[1] Intravenous fluid replacement should start the day before surgery to avoid dehydration, and electrolyte levels must be monitored.

The 2–3 day regimen of bowel preparation has been largely supplanted by a 1-day procedure using polyethylene glycol mixed in an electrolyte solution. These products, when reconstituted in 4 liters of water, are administered orally over 3–4 hours. If patients are unable or unwilling to drink this large a volume, nasogastric tube administration should be considered. The osmotic activity of this solution results in little exchange of fluid or electrolytes across the mucosal membranes in the intestine and induces a prompt diarrhea. At the conclusion of the preparation, the rectal effluent should be nearly a clear liquid. Oral or intravenous antibiotics can be administered in conjunction with the fluid solution. Some clinicians prefer to add a stimulant such as bisacodyl (Dulcolax) at the conclusion of the administration to promote complete colonic evacuation of residual fluid. This whole-gut lavage regimen has been shown to reduce hospitalization time and produces results equivalent to those of the traditional 3-day preparation.[2] The standard bowel preparation regimen currently in use at The University of Texas MD Anderson Cancer Center is described in Table 21–2. The patient should begin intravenous hydration the evening before surgery; if she is to undergo a radical procedure, this is an opportune time to insert a central venous catheter.

Whether or not oral or intravenous antibiotics are helpful for a patient who is to undergo intestinal surgery remains somewhat controversial. Preoperative oral antibiotic preparations such as neomycin and erythromycin have been used for many years with good results.[3-5] Some clinicians, however, believe that intravenous antibiotics alone may provide as much protection as orally administered antibiotics.[6,7] Some use both oral and intravenous antibiotics with good results, although the oral preparations often have the disadvantage of causing abdominal discomfort. However, good evidence is contained in the literature that antibiotic prophylaxis of some sort is helpful for patients who undergo elective colonic resection.[6,8] Patients who have inadequate bowel preparation or have surgery on an unprepared colon should not receive a *prophylactic* regimen, but instead should be treated with a therapeutic course of antibiotics. A therapeutic course is also necessary when resection is performed in the presence of perforation, abscess, fecal spillage, or obstruction.

A number of different antibiotics are suitable for prophylaxis in conjunction with elective colon surgery. Broad-spectrum coverage is desirable, and most antibiotics that fall into that category provide good results. At MD Anderson, the authors have had success with cefoxitin and cefmetazole given as single agents, starting before surgery. There is no substitute, however, for good surgical technique. The formation of a secure anastomosis with a good vascular supply and a clean operative field are undoubtedly of overriding importance in preventing infection.

The benefit of prophylactic antibiotics in operations on the small intestine is less well defined. Small bowel contents are usually sterile or have a low bacterial count. However, for women with gynecologic malignancy, small bowel procedures are often combined with colonic resection. Exploratory surgery for obstruction or fistula frequently reveals bacterial overgrowth in the small intestine. For these reasons, this patient population should receive perioperative antibiotics.

The issue of preoperative nutritional assessment and administration of total parenteral nutrition (TPN) is addressed elsewhere. Because malnutrition is a known risk factor for poor healing and anastomotic breakdown,[9-11] 10–14 days of preoperative TPN should be considered when the clinical situation permits such a delay. Studies regarding the benefits of preoperative nutritional supplementation have been conducted with various results, but most suggest that morbidity is decreased following nutritional repletion.[12-15] It is clear, however, that administering

Table 21-2

Whole Gut Lavage Bowel Preparation

Day 1	GoLYTELY, 4 L PO over 4 h No enemas Bisacodyl, 2 capsules PO 1 h after lavage Neomycin, 1 g, and erythromycin base, 1 g PO at 1 P.M., 2 P.M., and 11 P.M. (PO antibiotics optional)
Day 2	Cefoxitin, 2 g IV on call to OR Surgery

TPN for a week or less does not result in a meaningful change in the patient's nutritional status, and unfortunately surgery for the gynecologic cancer patient often cannot be delayed for the time required to achieve significant benefit from TPN.

TECHNIQUES OF INTESTINAL SURGERY

Historical Perspective

The technique of intestinal resection has undergone a remarkable evolution, especially during the past 50 years. The first attempts at such surgery resulted in high mortality, with the greatest problems being the integrity of the anastomosis and infection. Rather than perform a resection, surgeons in the 1800s exteriorized the intestine to relieve obstruction. The first attempts at sutured anastomosis, credited to Travers,[16] were further advanced by Lembert,[17] whose name is still used to describe a common intestinal suture technique. A fascinating array of objects designed to be placed within the lumen of the intestine to approximate the severed ends was used as an alternative to sutures.[18] The most successful of these was the Murphy button, which served as an internal stent to hold the ends of the bowel together.[19] However, without the benefit of bowel preparation and antibiotics, resection remained a hazardous undertaking.

With the advent of modern antibiotics, colonic resection without fecal diversion was greatly advanced by Dixon,[20] and in the 1950s it became a reasonable surgical option. During these years, the principles of intestinal surgery were defined and expanded. Preoperative intestinal cleansing, meticulous hemostasis, and creation of a secure anastomosis without tension were recognized as key elements of successful bowel surgery.

During the years that the sutured bowel anastomosis was becoming the established method, the search for mechanical devices that could reliably coapt the resected ends of intestine was in progress. De Petz is credited with developing the first functional surgical stapler.[20a] However, it was at the Institute for Experimental Surgical Apparatus and Instruments in Moscow that the forebears of modern surgical staplers were invented.[21] Although ingenious in design, the Russian devices required that individual staples be manually loaded after each firing, which limited their acceptance. Nevertheless, their safety and effectiveness in operations such as low anterior-sigmoid resection were well documented.[22, 23] The importation of the Russian devices to the United States led to their radical redesign and improvement and to the introduction of new stapling concepts.

Staplers for intestinal procedures consist of the thoracoabdominal (TA), the gastrointestinal anastomosis (GIA), and the end-to-end anastomosis (EEA). The ligating and dividing stapler (LDS) is also a useful adjunct in bowel surgery.*

The advent of stapling devices has by no means eliminated the need for conventional suture techniques. Many surgeons prefer hand-sewn anastomoses to stapled ones, and in some situations the use of staples is not advisable. Surgeons must, therefore, retain familiarity with suture techniques. A valid criticism of the use of stapling devices in training programs is that students may be insufficiently exposed to techniques of hand sewing. Furthermore, most staplers are disposable devices that add significant cost to the surgery.

Several reports in the gynecologic literature have documented good results for stapled anastomoses.[24-27] In a retrospective comparison of staple and suture techniques, Delgado found that staple use decreased operative time, caused less contamination of the abdominal cavity, and provided a better blood supply to the anastomosis.[24] However, in a prospective randomized trial comparing suture technique to staples, Reiling and associates found no difference in operative time, length of hospital stay, or complication rate.[28] In a review of 812 operative procedures, Chassin and coworkers also found no difference in complication rate between staples and sutures.[29] Although this controversy will not be resolved anytime soon, suffice it to say that training programs should prepare surgeons in both techniques.

General Principles of Intestinal Anastomoses

Intestinal anastomoses may be performed by a variety of techniques, and the results are uniformly excellent if the operator adheres to the following principles:

1. Blood supply to both sides of the anastomosis must be adequate.
2. The anastomosis should be under no tension.
3. Hemostasis must be excellent.
4. The anastomotic ring should be complete and secure.

---

*TA, GIA, EEA, and LDS are trademarks of the United States Surgical Corporation. This organization has been largely responsible for the development of modern surgical staplers. Other companies market similar devices under a variety of trade names. Because there are no generic designations for surgical staplers, in this text the authors refer to them using the US Surgical Corporation nomenclature.

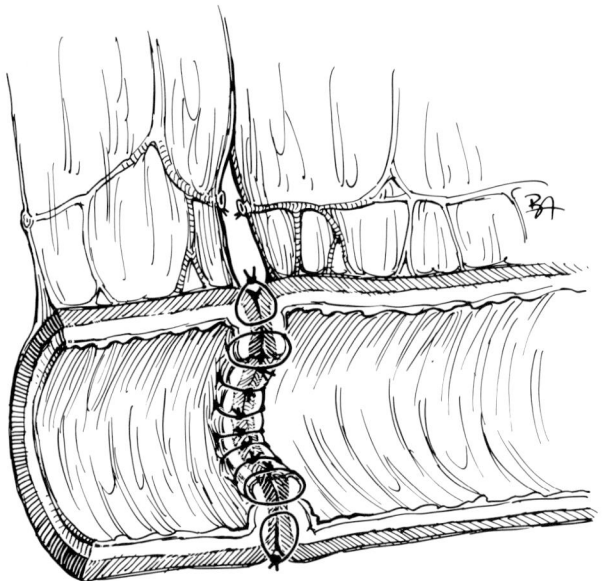

Figure 21–4
Two-layer inverting intestinal anastomosis.

5. The resultant lumen must be of sufficient caliber for the passage of intestinal contents.

If the surgeon follows these principles, the precise method of anastomosis, by suture or staple, probably has little effect on the eventual outcome.

Hand-Sewn Intestinal Anastomosis

The time-honored method for intestinal closure is the two-layered inverting anastomosis (Fig. 21–4). In this technique, a row of Lembert sutures is first placed on the posterior wall through the seromuscular layer using either 3-0 silk or a long-term absorbable suture such as Dexon or Vicryl, which serves equally well.* The inner mucosal layer is then sewn, starting at the back wall and ending anteriorly, using a 3-0 absorbable suture. The anastomosis is completed with Lembert sutures on the anterior wall.

Although this method provides a secure anastomosis, a two-layered closure is probably unnecessary. The additional inversion of the bowel wall results in luminal narrowing, and the second layer takes time to stitch and adds to the trauma of the tissues in the anastomosis.

An alternative method commonly used at MD Anderson is the single-layer inverting closure similar to that described by Gambee[30] (Fig. 21–5). Interrupted 3-0 sutures begin at the posterior wall, pass through the seromuscular layer, and pick up a small amount of mucosa. A single mattress suture is used to complete the closure of the lumen. Some surgeons advocate a single-layer running closure using a resorbable monofilament such as 3-0 Maxon for both small bowel and colonic anastomoses.[31] Whether such a technique is advisable in the authors' patient population remains to be determined.

Stapled Anastomoses

Intestinal closure using staples seems simple and straightforward to the novice, yet the surgeon must still be cognizant of the five principles elaborated earlier. Staplers for intestinal division and those for closure work on a similar principle. A staggered double row of fine wire staples is forced through the tissue until the ends strike an anvil that causes the staples to bend into a "B" figure (Fig. 21–6). The configuration of the B-staple is deliberately different from the shape of a staple used on paper. It provides secure approximation of the tissues without impairing capillary blood flow to the anastomotic site. Staples used to be constructed of stainless steel, but these have been largely replaced by staples made from titanium, a nonferrous substance that does not interfere with magnetic resonance imaging.

The GIA stapler (Fig. 21–7) places four rows of staples through the tissue while a center knife divides between them, leaving a double row of staples on each side. This instrument allows intestinal segments to be divided without spilling of their contents and is also used in anastomosis and reconstructive procedures. The GIA stapler comes in several lengths (55–90 mm) to accommodate different intestinal diameters. The staples, however, are all the same size. This instrument should not be used on extremely edematous bowel.

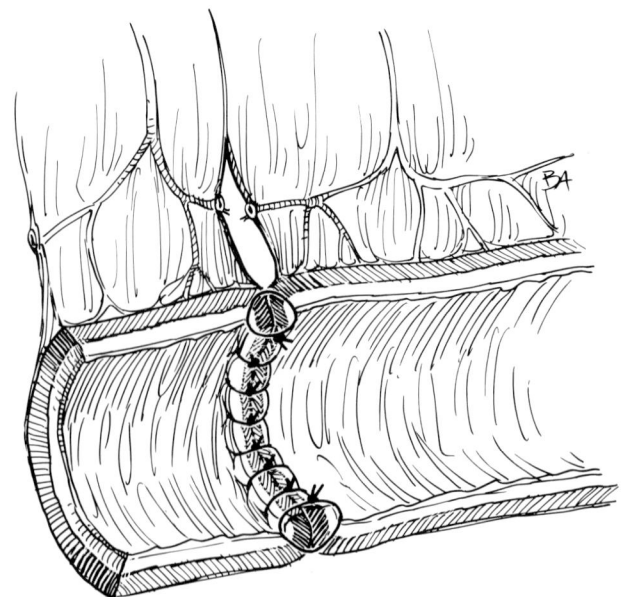

Figure 21–5
Single-layer inverting intestinal anastomosis.

---

*It is the authors' practice to use a long-term absorbable suture material and not silk for all intestinal procedures. In this chapter, unless otherwise specified, the material in use is Dexon or Vicryl.

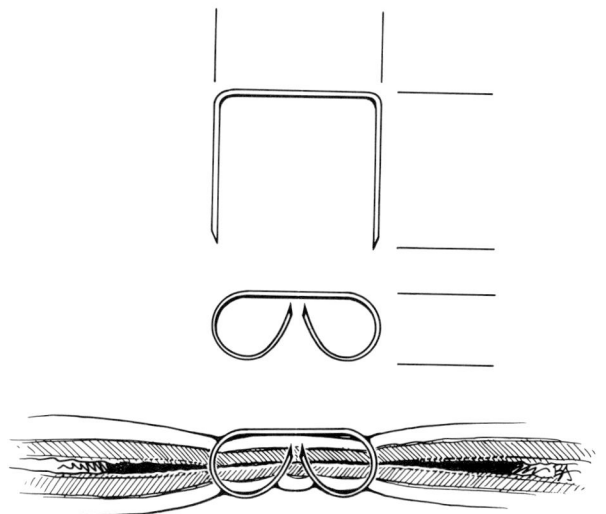

Figure 21–6
Wire staple is bent into a "B" figure, allowing for secure tissue approximation without compromise of blood supply.

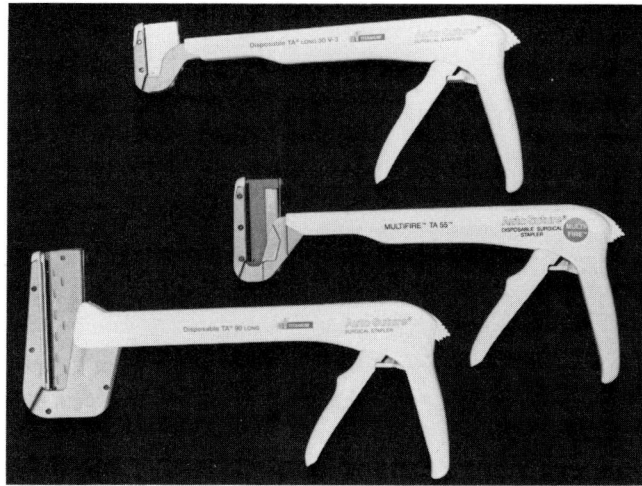

Figure 21–8
The TA stapler, shown here in three available sizes, places a double row of staples across an intestinal segment. (United States Surgical Corporation. All rights reserved.)

The TA family of staplers (Fig. 21–8) places a double row of staples and can be used to approximate tissue or as an adjunct to division. The devices come in three sizes (30, 55, and 90 mm) and have different size staples. The usual size of the staple used for small bowel or colon is 3.5 mm (blue cartridge); after firing, it has a height of 1.5 mm. The larger, 4.8 mm, staple (green cartridge) may be used for thicker tissues, such as stomach, but should be avoided for most anastomoses because inadequate tissue approximation may result. The TA-55 device also comes in a configuration that has a rotating and articulating head that allows for its use in the deep pelvis.

Even those surgeons who remain firmly committed to suture techniques find use for the EEA device (Fig. 21–9). Modeled after the Russian SPTU gun, the EEA places a circular double row of staples to form an inverting anastomosis while a circular knife within cuts out the excess inverted tissue. Although the EEA can be used to create anastomoses at any site and has also been used for colostomy formation,[32] its greatest utility is in low rectal re-anastomosis.

The LDS stapler (Fig. 21–10) is a disposable device powered by a CO_2 cartridge. It was designed to ligate and divide mesentery, although it may also be used on other tissues such as omentum. The operator must first use a small clamp to develop a pedicle, which is placed within the jaws of the LDS. As the device is fired, two staples ligate the pedicle while a center knife divides between them. The LDS can save time over traditional hand-tied pedicles, but it does have limitations. It is useful in thin patients, but in those with a thick mesentery the surgeon may have difficulty developing pedicles that fit within the jaws of the LDS.

PROCEDURES

The following is not meant to be an exhaustive listing of possible intestinal procedures, but rather descrip-

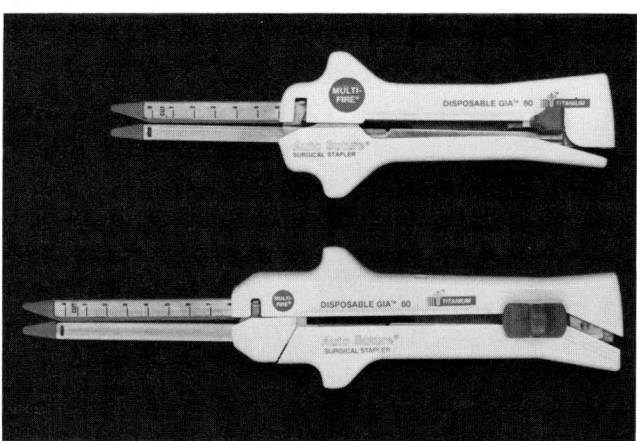

Figure 21–7
The GIA stapler is used to divide a segment of intestine. (United States Surgical Corporation. All rights reserved.)

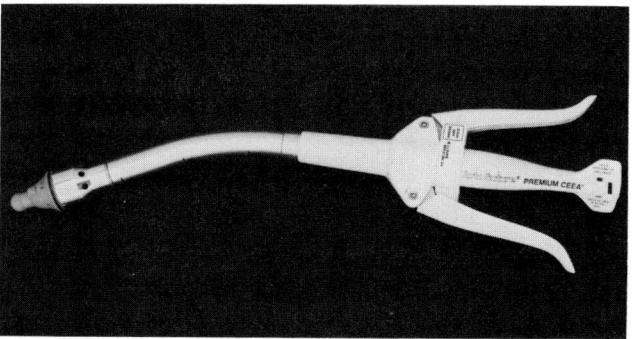

Figure 21–9
The EEA device is most useful for the creation of a low rectal anastomosis. (United States Surgical Corporation. All rights reserved.)

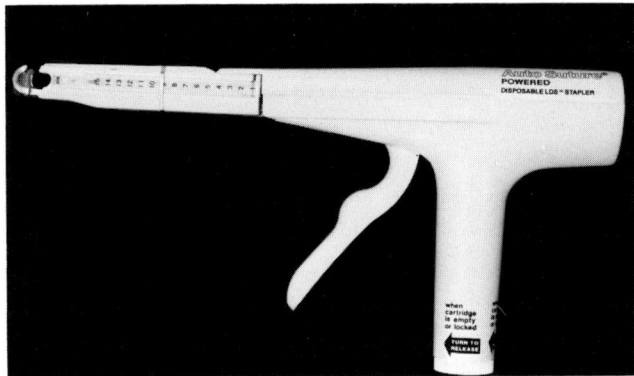

Figure 21-10
The LDS powered stapler. (United States Surgical Corporation. All rights reserved.)

tions of some of the operations performed most frequently in the course of surgery for gynecologic malignancy. The techniques described are those used at the authors' institution with good results.

Small Bowel Procedures

The resection of a portion of small intestine is often a procedure of last resort. Because maintaining intestinal length is of prime importance, all alternatives should be exhausted before resorting to resection. Intestinal involvement in a patient with ovarian cancer is usually located in the terminal ileum (Fig. 21-11). Because ovarian cancer is noninfiltrating by nature, the surgeon can often find a plane between the intestinal wall and the tumor and perform an adequate tumor resection without compromising the bowel. Using the ultrasonic surgical aspirator in cytoreductive surgery may allow more frequent intestinal salvage.[33, 34] In many instances, however, infiltration and destruction of the normal bowel require resection to achieve optimal cytoreduction. Other indications for small bowel resection include radiation injury, obstruction, and fistula, which will be discussed in more detail.

The surgeon should first identify which portion of small intestine must be excised, aiming always for minimal functional loss. The surgeon must find a segment free of tumor, because the presence of tumor at the anastomotic line results in poor healing. A knife or electrocautery is used to score the mesentery and delineate the segment to be excised (Fig. 21-12). Using either the LDS stapler or crushing clamps, the surgeon ligates and divides the mesentery. The intestine may then be divided by using a GIA stapler (Fig. 21-13). If a suture anastomosis is planned, division may be performed by GIA or by double-clamping with crushing clamps and dividing between them with a knife.

Open End-to-End Sutured Anastomosis

Once the diseased segment has been excised, rubber-shod clamps are placed on the proximal and distal bowel segments and clean laparotomy pads are placed around the site of proposed anastomosis to limit intestinal content spillage. Fat and mesentery are cleaned off the bowel for a distance of 5 mm from the anastomosis, and the staple line or crushed tissue should be trimmed off. The surgeon then brings the ends of the two bowel segments together, using single interrupted 3-0 Gambee sutures to approximate the posterior wall first (Fig. 21-14). The anterior wall is then approximated and the final mattress suture placed to form a completely inverted anastomosis. When the size of the proximal and distal lumina are disparate, a Cheatle cut (Fig. 21-15) can be made along the antimesenteric border to correct for this. To check the anastomosis' patency, the surgeon should inspect the suture line carefully and invaginate the distal bowel wall with a finger through the anastomotic ring. The mesenteric defect should then be closed.

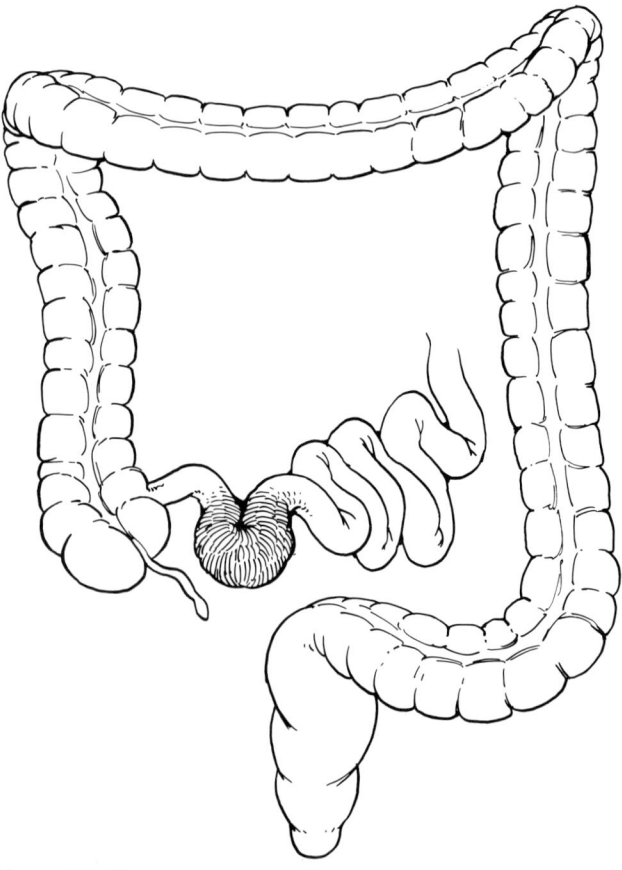

Figure 21-11
Ovarian cancer or radiation bowel injury often involves the terminal ileum.

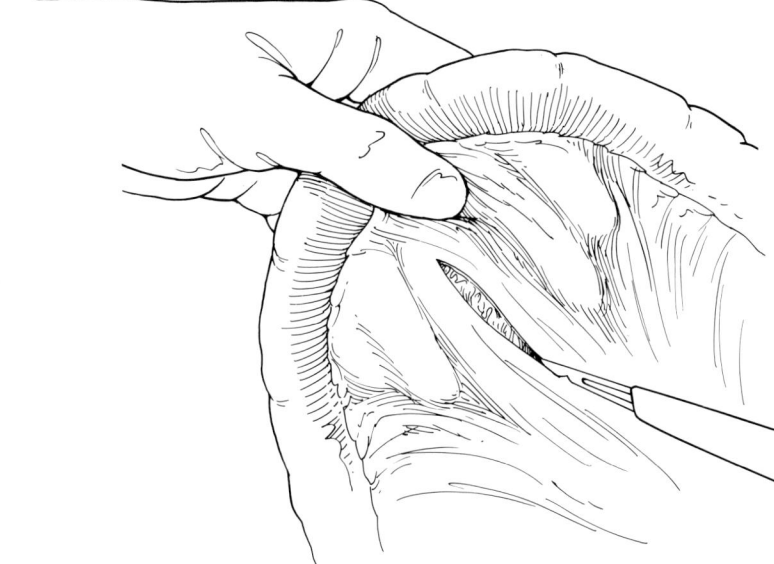

Figure 21–12
The mesentery is scored using a knife.

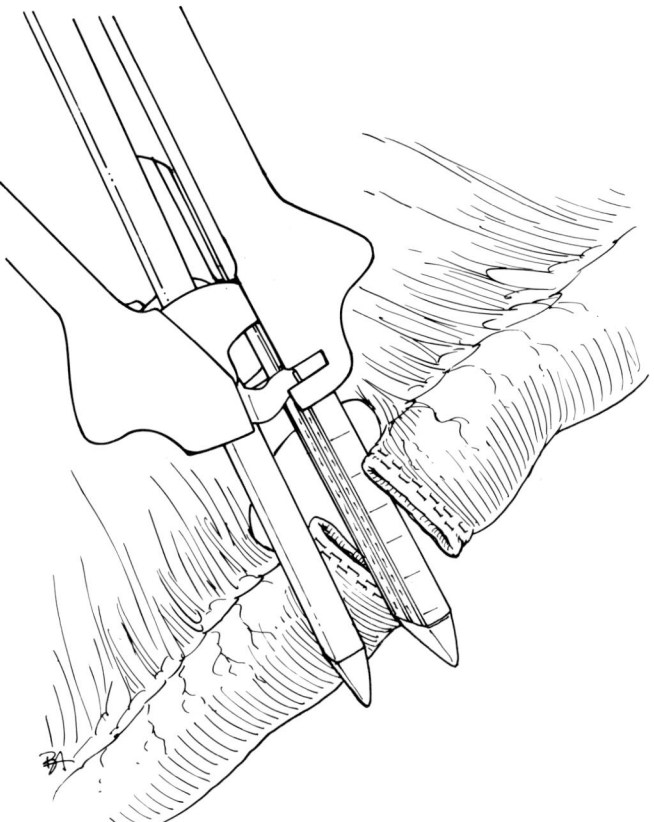

Figure 21–13
The GIA stapler is used to divide the small intestine, simultaneously sealing the proximal and distal limbs with a double row of staples.

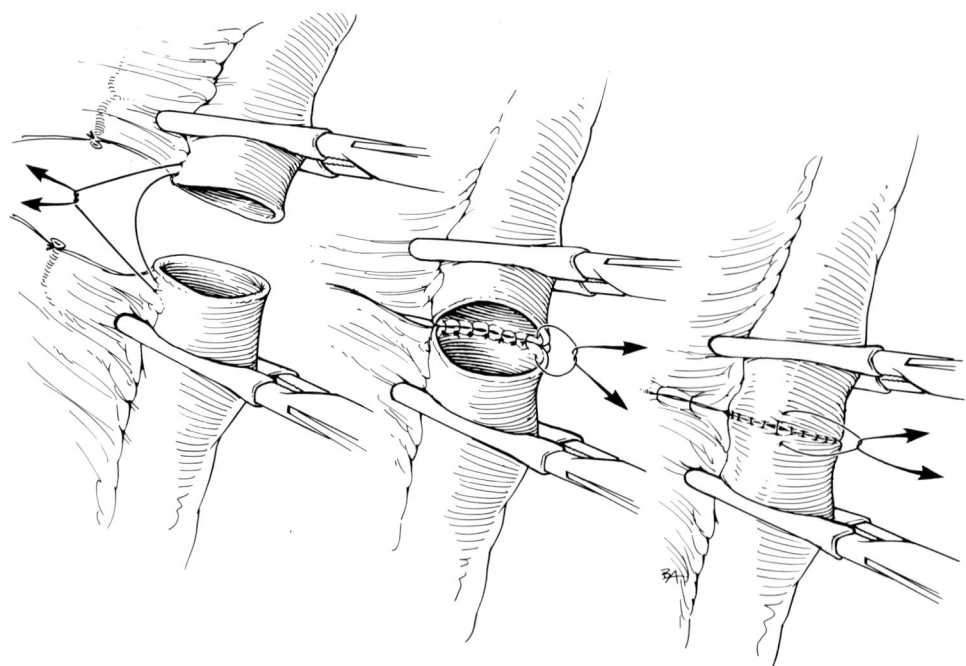

Figure 21–14
With rubber-shod clamps applied to prevent intestinal spillage, the intestinal segments are sewn together.

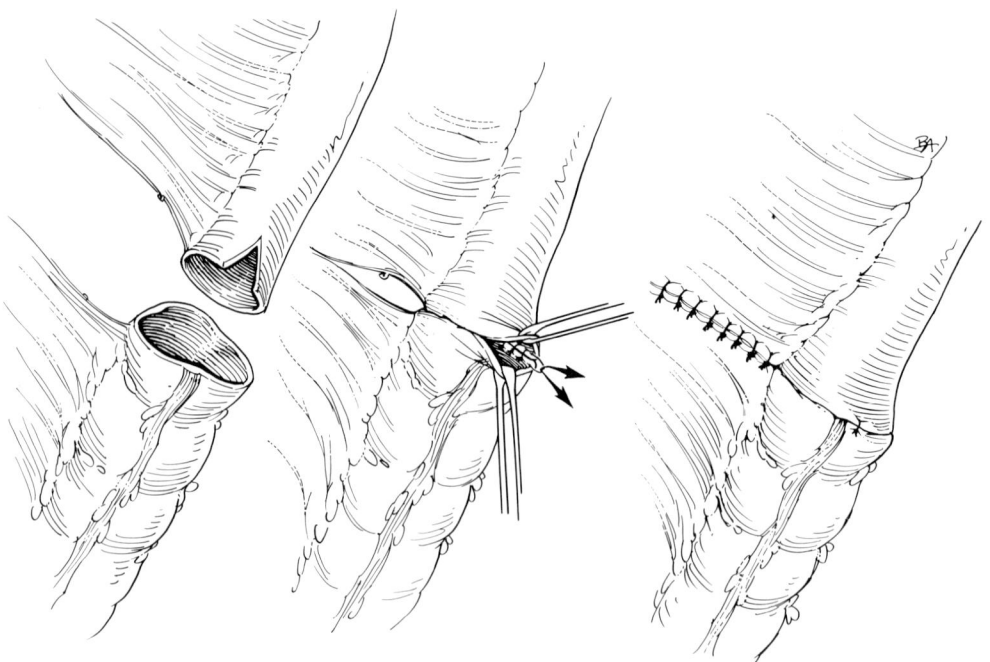

Figure 21–15
A Cheatle cut is used to allow for disparity in luminal size. The mesenteric defect is sewn closed.

Side-to-Side (Functional End-to-End) Stapled Anastomosis

The bowel proximal and distal to the excised segment should have been divided using a GIA stapler and rubber-shod clamps placed as described earlier. A small nipple of tissue is trimmed off the staple line on the antimesenteric surface of the two bowel ends, creating in each a defect just large enough to admit one jaw of the GIA stapler (Fig. 21–16). Placing 3-0 stay sutures often helps to guide the placement of the stapler. The GIA is then fired along the antimesenteric aspects of the bowel, thus creating an inverted union between the two segments. The remaining defect is closed using a TA-55 stapler, and the mesentery is reapproximated. The staple line should be carefully inspected to ensure that it is complete, and the adequacy of the lumen should be checked. Hemostasis must be ensured. Reinforcing sutures outside the staple line are not necessary; they would narrow the lumen and might devascularize the anastomosis.

Postoperative Care

After an intestinal anastomosis, adequate time for healing must be allowed before the patient can resume oral intake. This is perhaps most critical when the anastomosis is in the small bowel. Ileus typically lasts for 3–7 days after surgery, and the patient should receive nothing by mouth and remain on nasogastric suction during this time. Following some of the more radical procedures such as exenteration or extensive cytoreductive surgery, ileus frequently persists for 10–14 days. Because nasogastric tubes are so uncomfortable, it is the authors' practice to insert a gastrostomy tube at the time of surgery (see later discussion). When a prolonged ileus is expected, the authors begin TPN on the first day after surgery and continue until the patient has resumed adequate oral intake.

An alternative to TPN is to insert a tube jejunostomy at the time of surgery. An elemental feeding may then be started on the first postoperative day, even when a colonic or ileal anastomosis is present. Elemental diets are, for the most part, absorbed before they reach the ileum. Enteral feeding prevents brush border hypoplasia in the small bowel, which develops in patients receiving TPN for long periods of time, and may also allow a more rapid return to a regular diet. Gastric drainage is recommended with tube jejunostomy. Once the patient passes flatus or has a bowel movement, she may begin taking clear liquids and can advance to a regular diet as tolerated.

Patients whose terminal ileum is removed require chronic vitamin B_{12} replacement. The most common regimen involves monthly injections of 1000 μg.

Complications

When a patient has any intestinal anastomosis, the physician must be concerned about possible breakdown or leakage. The risk of these complications is particularly high for those patients whose wound healing is impaired to begin with—such patients as the malnourished, the previously irradiated, or ones with extensive malignancy. Anastomotic disruption usually produces signs of peritonitis and needs

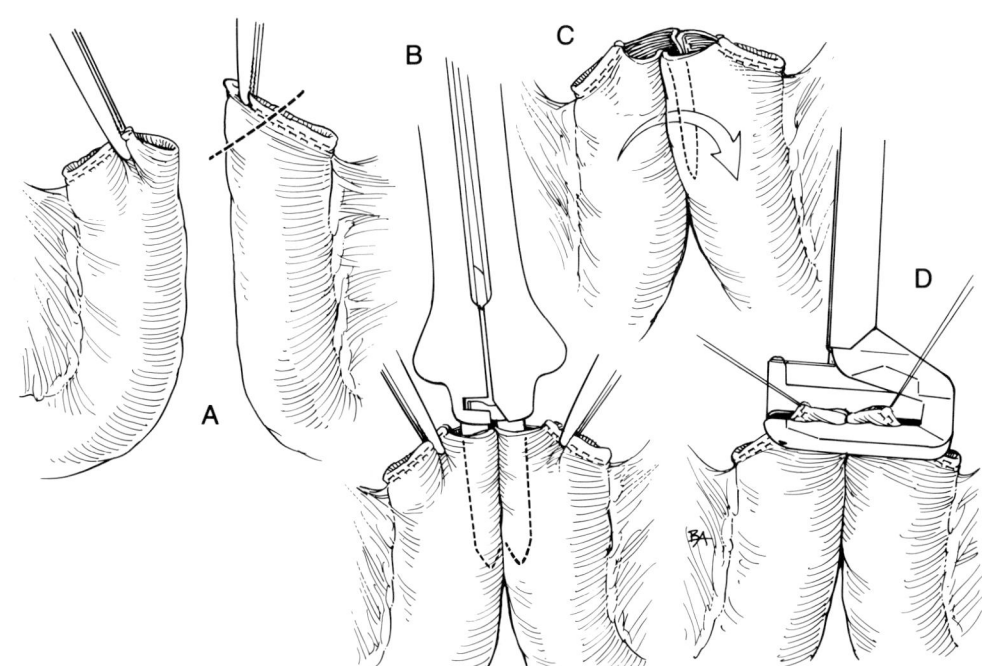

Figure 21–16
A, The two segments of small intestine are approximated by the antimesenteric aspect. A small nipple of tissue is trimmed off as shown. B, The jaws of the GIA stapler are placed, one in each intestinal segment. C, After the GIA is fired, the two segments are now connected with a lumen between. D, A TA stapler is used to seal the remaining defect.

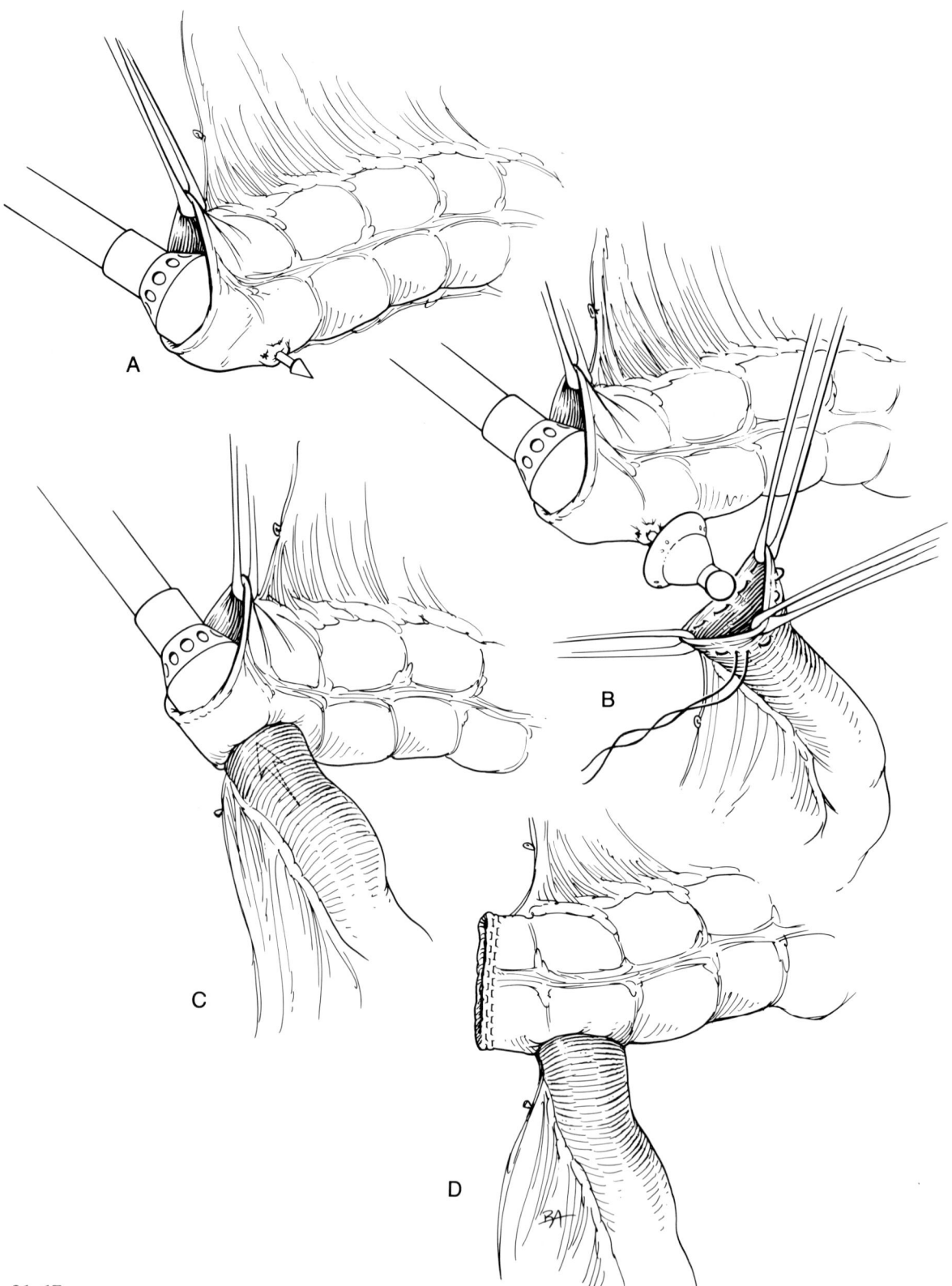

Figure 21–17
A, The trocar of the instrument is introduced through the open colonic end. B, The anvil is then placed on the EEA and inserted into the open lumen of the ileum. A pursestring suture has been placed around the lumen. C, The EEA is closed and fired. D, The colon is closed using a TA stapler.

prompt exploration and repair. In some patients, a leak walls itself off and presents more insidiously through fevers, an elevated white blood cell count, and persistent ileus. Radiographic studies with water-soluble contrast, ultrasound, or computed tomography can help in diagnosing this situation. Anastomotic leaks may also present with a fistula (see later).

Obstruction at the anastomotic site may be the result of poor technique, fibrosis, or impaired healing owing to poor blood supply. The management of obstruction is discussed in a later section.

Large Bowel Procedures

Ileocolectomy: End-to-Side Sutured Anastomosis

Ovarian cancer or radiation injury can extend to the ileocecal area, requiring resection of the terminal ileum and a portion of the ascending colon. After the bowel and mesentery have been separated, the bowel may be divided using a GIA or clamps.

In this procedure, the proximal end of the colon is oversewn if not previously stapled. An area along the antimesenteric border of the ascending colon is cleaned of fat along one of the taeniae coli. After taking the usual measures to limit spillage of intestinal contents, the surgeon then opens the distal ileum. An incision of sufficient size to accommodate the proximal ileum is made in the colonic wall along the taenia. The surgeon places a single row of inverting sutures to approximate the two ends, again starting with the posterior wall and moving to the anterior wall. After ensuring hemostasis, security of the suture line, and patency, the surgeon repairs the mesenteric defect.

Ileocolectomy: End-to-Side Stapled Anastomosis

The procedure begins with a pursestring suture placed in the terminal ileum (Fig. 21–17). The EEA instrument with its anvil removed is placed through the open transected end of the proximal colon, and the trocar is advanced through the antimesenteric border of the colon several centimeters from the transected end. The anvil is then placed in the open lumen of the distal ileum, and the pursestring suture is tied. The anvil is reset on the center rod of the EEA, the tissues are approximated, and the instrument is fired. The remaining defect in the proximal colon may be closed with a TA-55.

Partial Colectomy and Re-anastomosis

A severed colon can be reapproximated by one of three methods. One is via a hand-sewn, single-layer, end-to-end anastomosis, as described earlier. Second, a side-to-side stapled anastomosis can be performed using the GIA and TA instruments. A potential limitation to the latter technique, however, is limited mobility of the colon. When this is a problem, the solution may be an end-to-end anastomosis using the principle of triangulation (Fig. 21–18). Two stay sutures are placed so as to lay out the posterior wall of the anastomosis, and a TA-55 instrument is used to form an inverted staple line. A third stay suture is then placed in the mid-portion of the remaining open area. The TA-55 is then fired twice more to close the remaining two arms of the triangle in an everting fashion. The staple line is inspected and the lumen palpated.

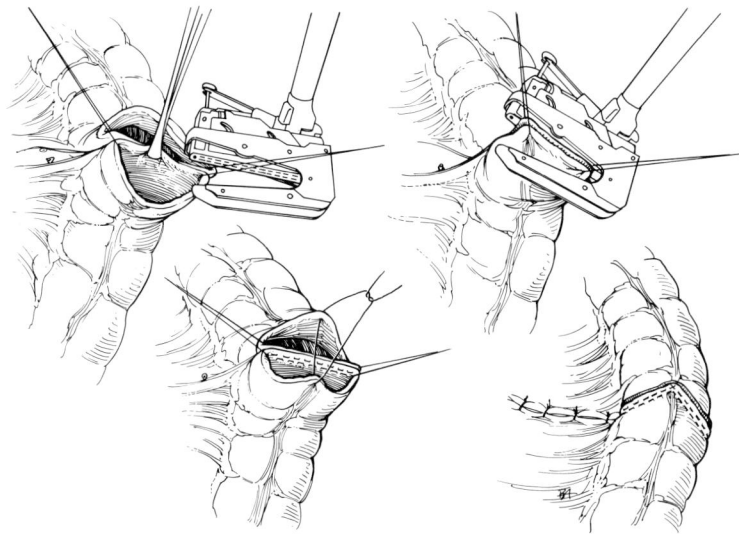

Figure 21–18
Anastomosis of the colon using the triangulation technique.

Sigmoid Colectomy

The removal of the sigmoid colon en bloc with the pelvic reproductive organs is often indicated in women undergoing cytoreductive surgery for ovarian cancer. It is also an integral part of pelvic exenteration, and it may be needed when patients have radiation-induced proctosigmoiditis. High resections of the sigmoid (where the distal line of resection is above the peritoneal reflection) are relatively straightforward. The anastomosis may be handled as described previously.

Low anterior resection refers to a distal line of resection below the peritoneal reflection. In some patients, the condition of the distal rectum is too poor to allow for re-anastomosis. For example, severe radiation injury, active infection secondary to perforation, or the presence of unresectable tumor contraindicates the re-establishment of intestinal continuity. In these situations, low anterior sigmoid resection should be followed by an end-descending colostomy and a Hartmann pouch (Fig. 21–19). Re-anastomosis is sometimes possible at a later date when, for example, infection has been treated and the tissues return to their normal state.

With proper bowel preparation, re-anastomosis following low anterior resection is frequently possible. Sigmoid resection should therefore be carried out with this possibility in mind. The procedure should be performed with the patient in the modified lithotomy position to allow the EEA device to be inserted through the anus.

The surgeon should first identify the proximal line of sigmoid resection and make sure that the tissue at this level is free of disease and mobility is adequate to effect re-anastomosis. To gain additional mobility, the surgeon may have to mobilize the descending colon and the splenic flexure.

A mesenteric defect is made directly below the bowel wall with a small clamp, and the colon is then divided using the GIA instrument. The mesentery is then scored and the line of resection planned. The superior rectal artery may be sacrificed without concern for the distal rectal stump, because the middle and inferior rectal arteries will provide an adequate blood supply. Care should be taken to identify the ureters to avoid damaging them inadvertently. As the mesenteric dissection proceeds inferiorly, the attachments to the presacral fascia are encountered. They should be sharply dissected until the avascular plane between the sacrum and rectum is reached. Care should be taken not to attempt blunt dissection near the sacral promontory, because this may result in brisk bleeding. Bleeding in this area may arise directly from the bone and is difficult to control. Using a gloved hand, the physician enters the avascular retrorectal space in the hollow of the sacrum. Blunt dissection here creates a characteristic sucking sound and may continue down to the pelvic floor. Depending on the level of the distal resection, the lateral rectal ligaments may need to be ligated and divided. When the distal margin of resection is reached, the rectum is skeletonized of fat and mesentery and a TA-55 Roticulator is placed across it

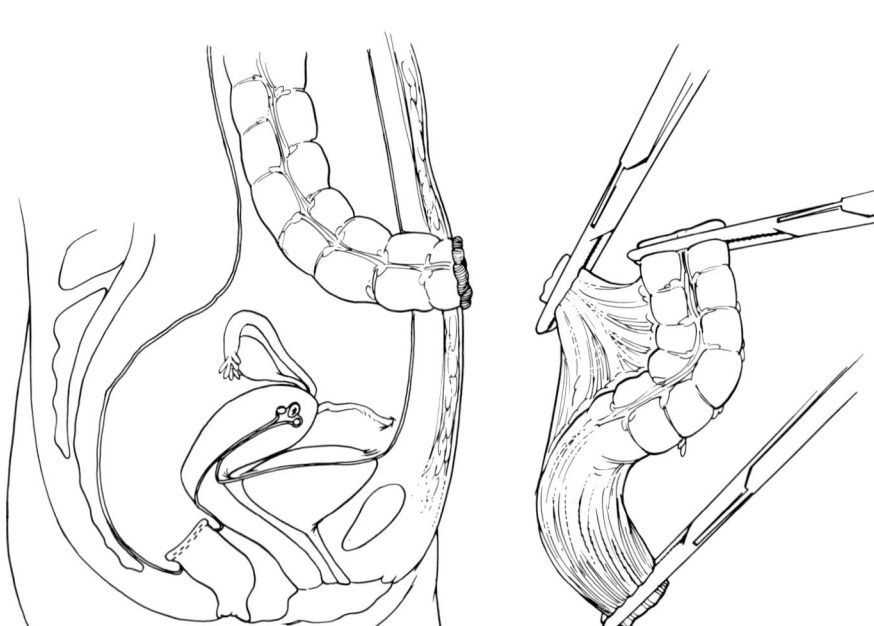

Figure 21–19
End-descending colostomy with Hartmann pouch.

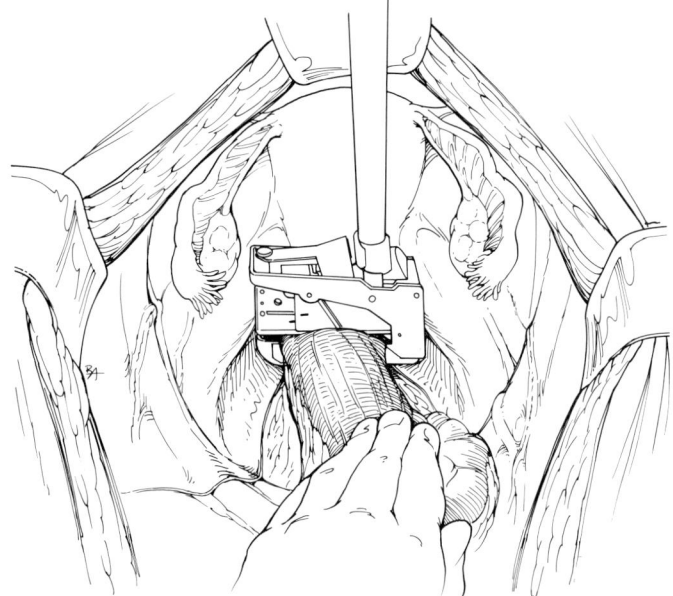

Figure 21-20
A TA instrument with a rotating and articulating head can be used to place a double row of staples in the pelvis.

(Fig. 21–20). The operator fires the instrument and excises the specimen with a knife, using the stapler edge as a cutting guide. If an en bloc dissection of the uterus and ovaries with the sigmoid is desired, the final transection of the sigmoid may take place from an anterior approach after the vagina has been transected.

After hemostasis has been achieved, preparation can be made for low re-anastomosis. To be sure that mobility is adequate to effect anastomosis without tension, the proximal sigmoid should be prepared first. The surgeon cleans fat and mesentery off the resected end for 10 mm and places a rubber-shod clamp proximally to limit spillage of intestinal contents. Using a pursestring clamp or the pursestring instrument (Fig. 21–21), the surgeon places a pursestring suture and trims the staple line above it. Care should be taken to leave only 2–4 mm bowel distal to the pursestring suture.

Anastomosis is best performed with the EEA instrument, which is available in several sizes (25, 28, and 31 mm); the largest should be used whenever

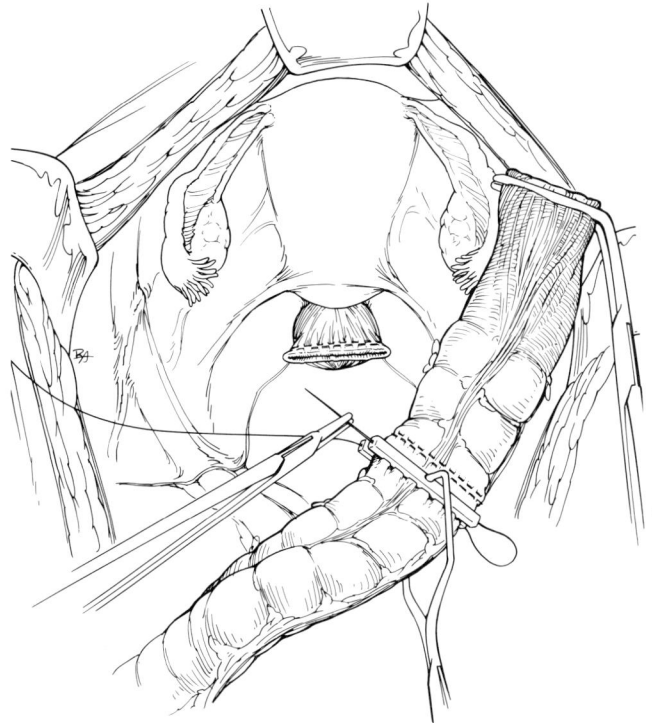

Figure 21-21
A pursestring clamp is used to assist in the placement of a pursestring suture.

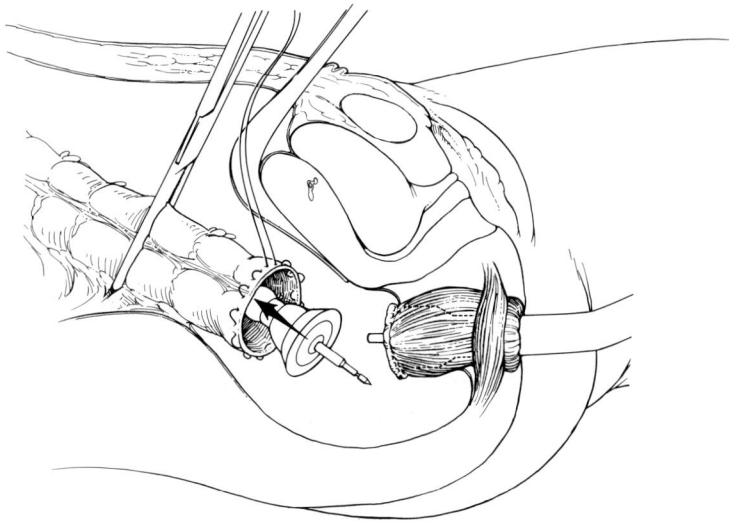

Figure 21–22
The EEA is placed through the anus by an assistant. The sharp trocar is advanced to puncture the staple line in the mid-portion. The anvil of the EEA is then placed in the proximal colon, and the pursestring suture is tied around the shaft.

possible. The surgeon assesses the proximal bowel to determine which size is appropriate, using metal "sizers" that determine the size without dilating the proximal lumen.

The surgeon now detaches the anvil from the EEA instrument, places it into the proximal sigmoid, and ties the pursestring suture (Fig. 21–22). An assistant gently inserts the EEA instrument, now fitted with the removable trocar in the center rod, into the anus and advances it to the staple line. The center rod is then advanced until the trocar has perforated the staple line (Fig. 21–23). The trocar is removed and the anvil reattached to the center rod. The EEA is closed by turning the wing nut to approximate the bowel ends. Care should be taken to ensure that the mesentery lines up and that no fat or other tissue is included within the staple line. The surgeon now places a seromuscular stay suture anteriorly through the anastomosis (Fig. 21–24), and the assistant fires the EEA instrument. The wing nut is then opened three full turns, and the EEA is removed by a gentle rocking motion. The surgeon should hold the stay suture during this maneuver to stabilize the anastomosis.

After removing the EEA instrument from the anus, the assistant should open the device to be sure that two complete rings of excised tissue ("donuts") lie within. If this is not the case, the anastomosis is incomplete at some point. The surgeon then has the choice of reinforcing the incomplete area with suture or repeating the entire maneuver.

If the integrity of the anastomosis is in question,

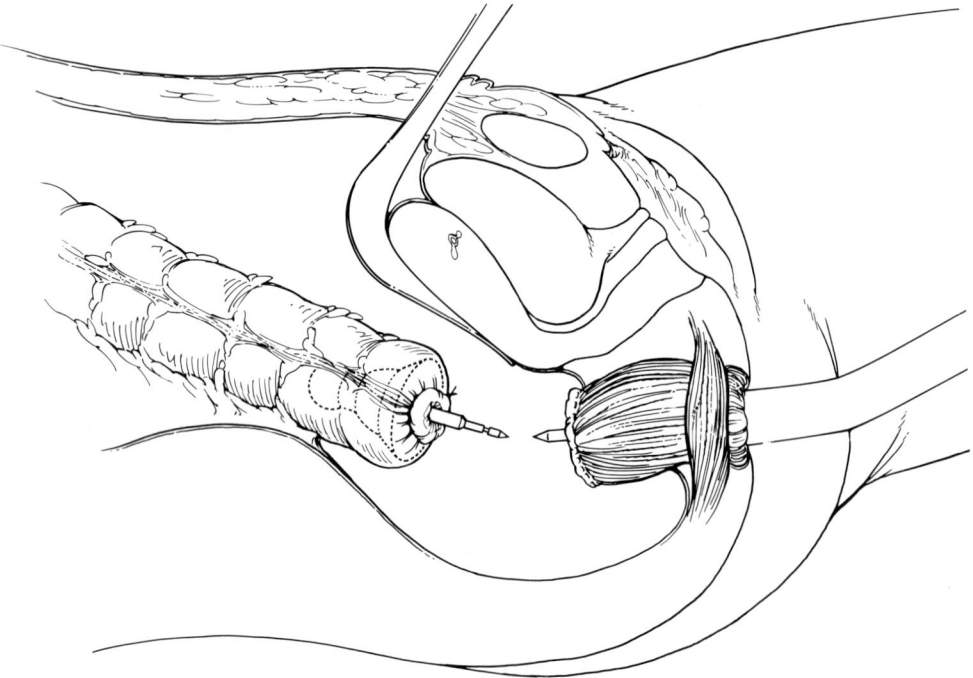

Figure 21–23
The center shaft of the anvil is then brought down and inserted into the center shaft of the EEA instrument.

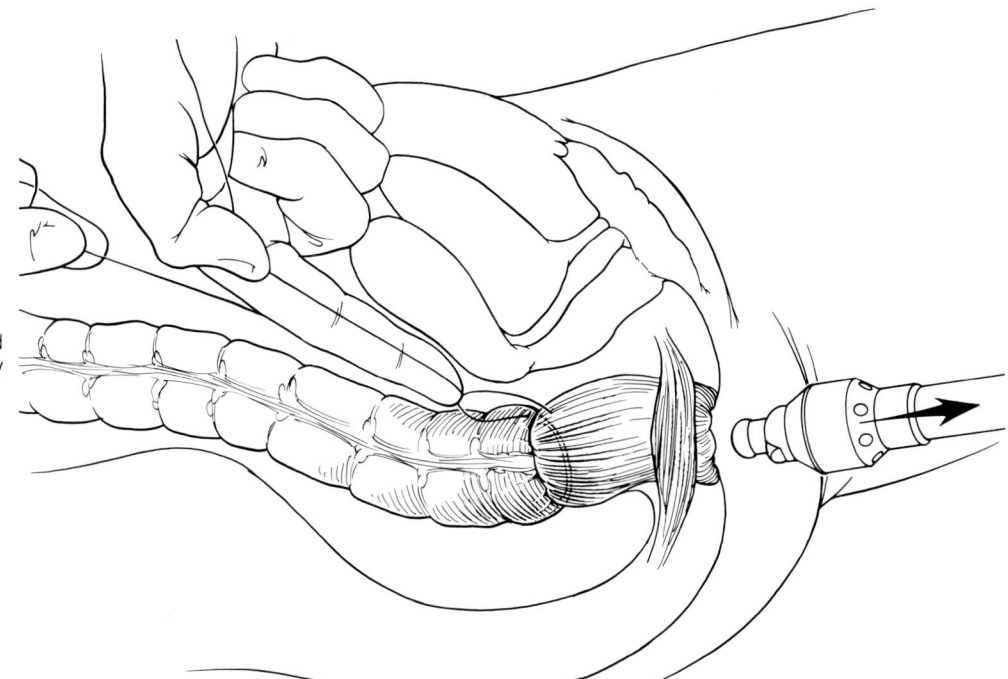

Figure 21–24
The instrument is closed and a stay suture placed anteriorly through the anastomosis.

the pelvis may be filled with saline and the rectum insufflated with air. If bubbles are seen, the surgeon has a problem! Some surgeons routinely inspect the anastomotic line through a flexible sigmoidoscope. The authors prefer to reserve this technique for patients whose anastomoses are suspect, because the sigmoidoscope is potentially traumatic.

Low anterior resection may also be carried out with a conventional suture technique. A single-layer open closure is satisfactory in most cases. Access to a deep or narrow pelvis, however, may be difficult, and therein lies the advantage of the EEA instrument. A caution: Staples should not be used when the tissue is very thick or too thin. In either setting, a sutured anastomosis should be performed or the patient should be given an end colostomy with a Hartmann pouch.

The minimal length of rectal stump that is required to maintain continence is controversial. In the course of radical resections, autonomic afferent nerve fibers are transected, which may contribute to incontinence in some patients. Theoretically, at least, continence should be possible if the internal and external anal sphincters have been preserved. Some patients experience difficulty with control at first, but it usually resolves over time. In the authors' experience, nearly all patients who have a rectal stump of 5 cm or more will be continent.

Postoperative Care

Patients who have undergone colonic resection with re-anastomosis may begin oral feeding after the passage of flatus. Progression from clear liquids to solid food should take place in the usual fashion. Nasogastric suction is probably not needed after low anterior resection alone. Most of the authors' patients, however, undergo other procedures in conjunction with the sigmoid resection, and prolonged ileus occurs frequently. The authors routinely either use nasogastric suction or place a gastrostomy tube at the time of surgery. Those patients in whom a prolonged ileus is anticipated should receive TPN as described previously.

Protective Colostomy

Whether or not to perform a protective transverse-loop colostomy at the time of low rectal re-anastomosis is a matter of individual preference. Dixon recommended a temporary diverting colostomy in all patients.[20] The rationale was to give time for the anastomosis to heal before allowing the passage of stool with the increased rectal pressures that result. Schrock and associates[11] reported no difference in the incidence of anastomotic leak when patients had a proximal diversion, and others have reported satisfactory results without colostomy.[35, 36] There are, however, some clear indications for a diverting colostomy, which are listed in Table 21–3. When a temporary colostomy has been created, closure may be performed 2–4 months later (see later). Before reversing the colostomy, however, the distal bowel segment should be evaluated by a contrast radiograph to ensure patency and an intact anastomosis. Narrowing of the anastomosis has been reported more frequently in patients who have undergone proximal diversion,[23] although this can usually be treated by noninvasive measures.

Table 21–3

Indications for Protective Loop Colostomy Following Low Rectal Re-anastomosis

Poor bowel preparation
Radiated bowel
Infection or perforation
Marginal blood supply or tension
Tumor near the anastomotic line

Complications

Anastomotic leak is perhaps the most serious complication of low rectal re-anastomosis. Its incidence varies widely in the literature, ranging from 15% to 69%.[10, 36] Those studies that find a high proportion of leaks may be biased by the method of detection. Most instances of a minor leak are clinically insignificant and would not be detected without radiographic screening. The true incidence of significant anastomotic disruption is probably in the range of 10–15%. Forming a diverting colostomy does not protect against leaks, but it does appear to reduce mortality should they occur.[10] Some of the factors that contribute to anastomotic breakdown are listed in Table 21–4.

Management of anastomotic breakdown is based on the clinical presentation. A minor disruption may be corrected with proximal diversion. If eventual repair is anticipated, a transverse-loop colostomy can provide a temporary diversion. Otherwise, the treatment of choice is a descending end colostomy with Hartmann pouch. When the anastomosis suffers a major breakdown and abscesses form, fecal diversion is still performed. However, the pelvic infection must be addressed by laparotomy and drainage. For those patients who are too ill to withstand a major procedure, loop colostomy and percutaneous drainage may be a satisfactory temporizing measure.

Anastomotic stricture is a complication seen more frequently in stapled closures. Mild stricture is fairly common during the initial months postoperatively and tends to improve with time. Severe stricture is less common. Mild to moderate stricture can be managed with a variety of dilatation techniques and only occasionally requires reoperation.

Stoma Formation

When a stoma may be part of a planned surgical procedure, the patient should be evaluated preoperatively as described earlier. The operating room is clearly not the best place in which to select the stoma site. The enterostomal therapist should perform a preoperative evaluation of the patient's abdomen and mark the best site for stoma placement after consultation with the surgeon. Once the patient is in the supine position in the operating room, stoma placement may inadvertently occur at a site where the patient wears her slacks or skirts or over a skinfold that is apparent only when she is sitting. These factors are taken into account by the enterostomal therapist, who examines the patient in the sitting and standing position as well as supine. The stoma should not be placed too close to the wound, ribs, or iliac crest. In general, there should be a 5-cm margin of smooth skin from the center of the stoma. The surgeon should specify what type of diversion is planned.

The enterostomal therapist plays a vital role in all aspects of care of the patient with a stoma. In addition to marking the patient for stomal placement, the therapist provides education and counseling in the preoperative setting to help prepare the patient to care for her stoma. Postoperatively, the educational process continues as the patient is taught how to manage her appliance. The enterostomal therapist will continue her relationship with the patient over time, assisting with changes in appliance needs, managing skin problems, and providing emotional support.

End-Colostomy

End-colostomy is the procedure of choice for patients who are not expected to undergo colostomy reversal in the future. It is most frequently created using the sigmoid or descending colon. The technique is the same for more proximal colon segments as well. To maintain the maximal absorptive capacity of the colon, the most distal segment possible should be chosen.

The surgeon should first be sure that the colon will reach the proposed stoma site without tension. Mobilizing the splenic or hepatic flexure may be necessary to achieve adequate mobility. When tension or technical difficulty prevents stomal placement at a satisfactory site, it is occasionally necessary to sacrifice an additional portion of colon.

The distal colon should be cleaned of fat and

Table 21–4

Factors Contributing to Anastomotic Leak Following Low Rectal Re-anastomosis

Poor blood supply
Tension
Infection or abscess
Hematoma
Incomplete anastomosis
Poor preparation and fecal spillage
Anastomosis <6 cm from the anal verge
Prior radiation therapy
Poor nutritional status or medical problems

mesentery for approximately 5–10 mm. When a patient is obese with large epiploicae, the surgeon should remove these structures to facilitate passage of the colon through the abdominal wall. The surgeon grasps the skin at the proposed stoma site with a Kocher clamp and excises a circular piece of skin of sufficient diameter to accommodate the colon. In obese patients, it is helpful to excise an additional plug of underlying fat down to the level of the fascia (Fig. 21–25). The surgeon incises the anterior rectus sheath in a cruciate fashion and the rectus muscle in a longitudinal fashion. It is desirable to have the colon pass through the rectus, which may help prevent stomal herniation. Last to be incised is the peritoneum. The resultant abdominal wall defect should be large enough to allow the colon to pass through easily without tension. The abdominal wall should now be carefully inspected for damage to the inferior epigastric vessels and hemostasis ensured. The distal colon is now brought through the defect, and the stoma may be matured. Most surgeons, however, prefer to close the abdomen first.

If the exterior colon contains a staple line, it should be trimmed off. The stoma is then sewn to the skin with interrupted fine absorbable sutures. For distal colonic stomas, it is not necessary to have the stoma protrude significantly above the level of the skin. The final step is to place a transparent bag over the stoma in anticipation of eventual function yet permitting observation during the postoperative period.

Stoma Formation with the EEA Instrument

The EEA instrument can be used to form a terminal colostomy, as described by Burke and colleagues.[32] The abdominal wall defect is created from below, leaving the skin intact: the peritoneum, rectus, and fat are incised to a level just below the skin, and the incision must allow adequate space for the colon to pass through. The physician fires the pursestring instrument just below the staple line on the distal colon and then trims off the staple line. The sizers are used to determine the proper size EEA instrument. The distal anvil with the anvil shaft attached is then placed within the lumen of the colon, and the pursestring suture is tied (Fig. 21–26). A small incision is then made in the skin, through which the anvil shaft is carefully introduced. After the surgeon has determined that the colon is not twisted and is free of tension, he or she joins the anvil shaft to the center rod of the EEA, closes the instrument, and fires it. Placing several seromuscular sutures to the peritoneum and posterior rectus sheath helps to support the stoma. The staples are left in place and do not seem to affect the stoma adversely; they are usually spontaneously extruded over time.

Ileostomy

The surgical technique is similar to that of an end-colostomy with an important exception. Because of the irritating nature of the small bowel effluent, an ileostomy should be elevated above the level of the skin to allow intestinal contents to flow more directly into the appliance, avoiding prolonged skin contact. The abdominal wall defect is prepared as described earlier, and the ileum brought through the defect so that 4 or 5 cm is protruding. The mesentery should be trimmed over this length (Fig. 21–27). The intestine is then everted by placing a 3-0 suture through the skin, taking a seromuscular bite at the level of the skin, and finally passing the suture through the intestinal edge. This maneuver "rosebuds" the intestine to form a nipple.

An alternative method of stoma formation that is especially useful for ileostomy is the Turnbull or J-loop stoma. In this procedure, a loop of ileum several centimeters from the distal stump is brought through the abdominal wall and allows for a rosebud stoma

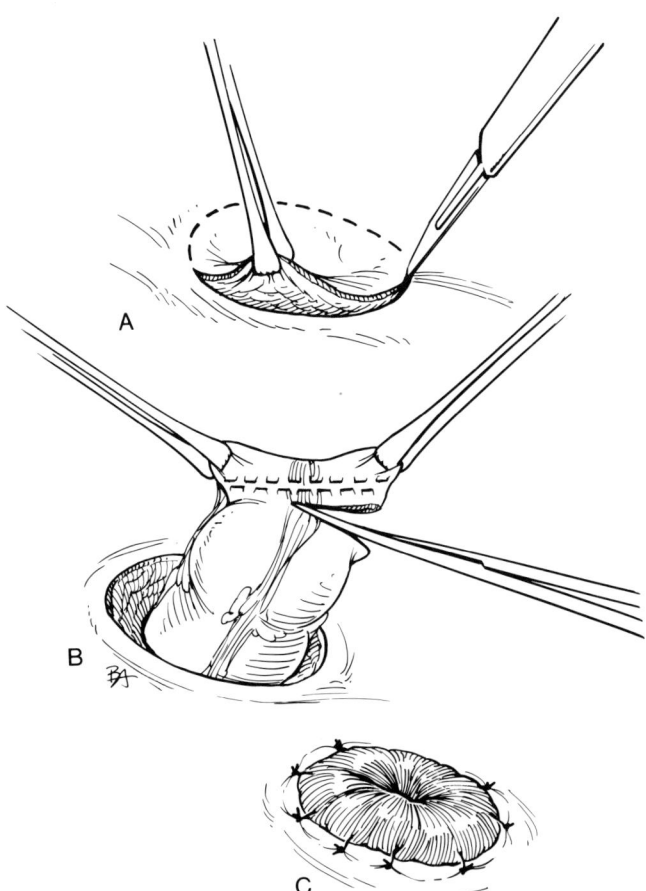

Figure 21–25
A, A circular plug of skin and underlying fat is excised. *B*, The colon is easily brought through the defect without tension. *C*, The stoma is matured and sewn to the skin with several interrupted sutures.

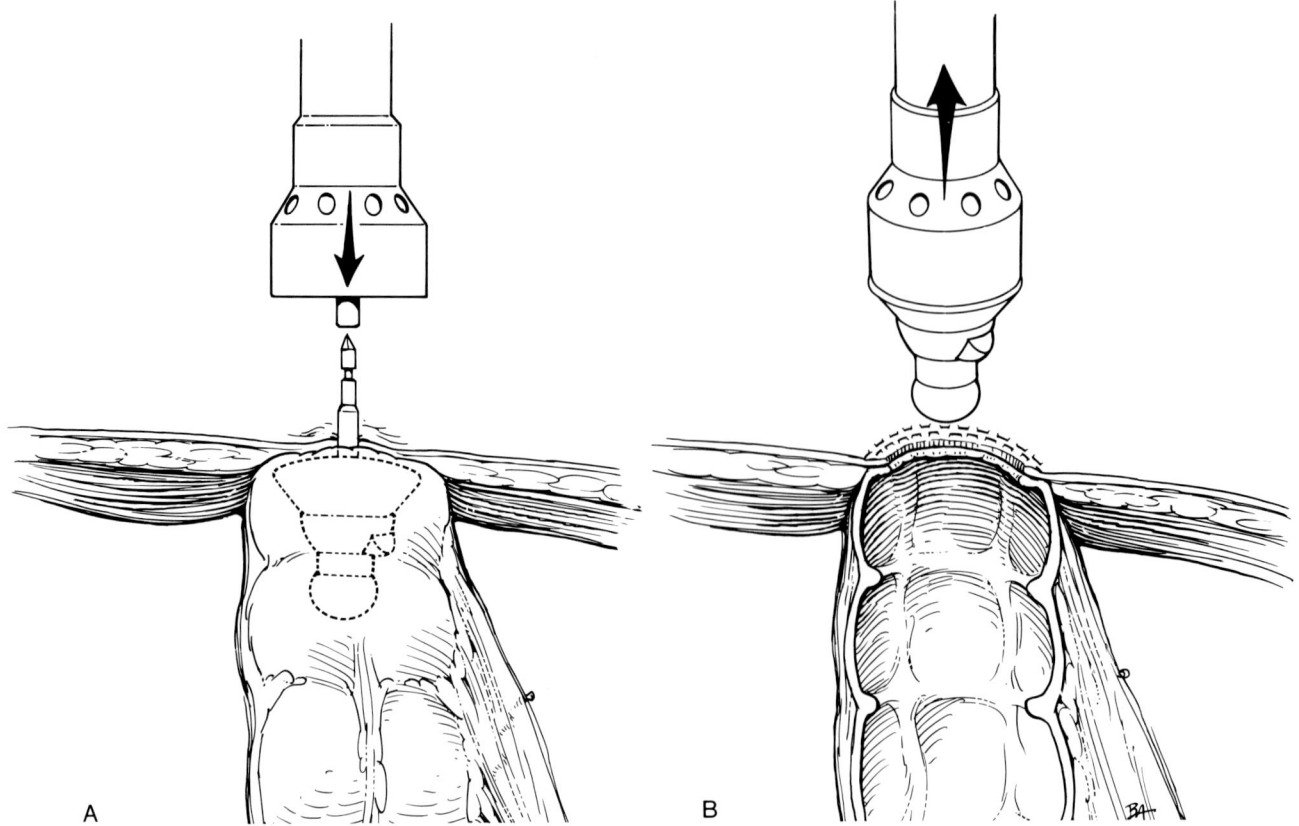

Figure 21–26
A, With the anvil in the colon, the trocar pierces the skin. The EEA device is then linked to the anvil via the center rod. B, After firing, the EEA instrument is removed, leaving a circular stoma flush with the skin. Additional support may be obtained by interrupted seromuscular sutures between the colon and interior abdominal wall.

with an excellent vascular supply. A J-loop colostomy is useful in obese patients with a thick abdominal wall or in cases in which there is some compromise of the vascular supply.

Management of an ileostomy can be a frustrating problem for the patient, surgeon, and enterostomal therapist. The approach to appliance selection and skin care should be initiated before significant skin breakdown has a chance to occur and should be pursued aggressively.

Mucous Fistula

When the distal segment of bowel is long or obstructed, the surgeon must provide a means for mucus and sloughed epithelium to escape; therefore, the surgeon forms a mucous fistula. The technique involved in creating a mucous fistula is similar to that of end-colostomy. The fistula should be placed far enough away from the active stoma so as not to interfere with appliance placement. A mucous fistula may be dressed with gauze and usually grows smaller over time. Because an appliance is not worn over this stoma, the surgeon has more latitude regarding its placement on the abdominal wall.

Loop Colostomy

When a temporary fecal diversion is desired, loop colostomy is the preferred procedure because closing the resultant stoma is relatively simple. It is indicated to protect a distal anastomosis, as a preliminary step to closing a rectovaginal fistula, or to bypass obstruction. When a patient with advanced pelvic malignancy—even a frail woman—has sigmoid obstruction, a loop colostomy can be formed swiftly. A loop colostomy usually uses the transverse colon, although the descending colon and proximal sigmoid occasionally have sufficient mobility. The same principles of stoma site selection elaborated earlier apply in this situation as well. When the colostomy is performed as part of a laparotomy, the abdominal wall defect is created as described previously, although it is often larger to accommodate the loop.

The surgeon creates a small mesenteric defect immediately below the bowel wall and passes a Penrose drain through it. Epiploic fat should be excised, because it may impair passage of the colon through the abdominal wall. The surgeon uses gentle traction on the Penrose drain while simultaneously feeding the colon up from below, delivers the colon

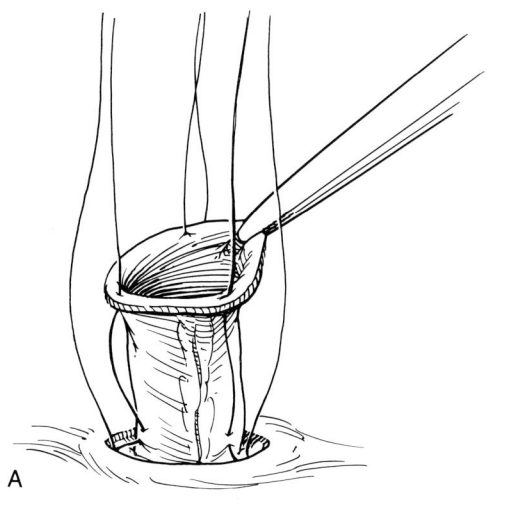

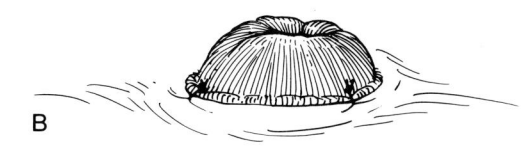

Figure 21–27
A and B, Ileostomy formation with elevated stoma.

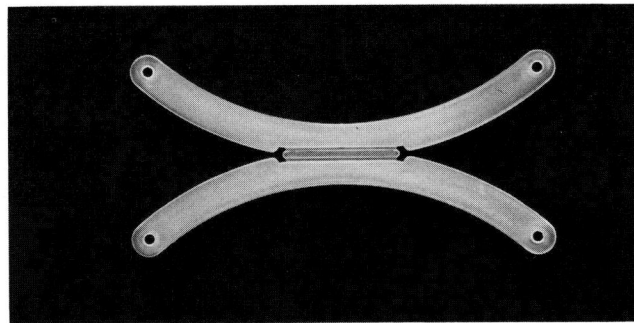

Figure 21–28
Hollister bridge.

through the abdominal wall defect, and closes the abdomen before maturing the stoma. In years past, some surgeons waited several days after surgery before maturing the stoma in the patient's room. The resultant flow of feces and blood in full view of the patient often led to suboptimal stomal formation, not to mention the negative impact on the patient's perception of her new stoma.

Support for the loop after Penrose drain removal was classically achieved with a glass rod. The rod was bulky and made appliance placement difficult. The authors prefer instead to use a Hollister bridge, which is effective and unobtrusive (Fig. 21–28). After sewing the bridge in place to the skin with 3-0 nylon, the surgeon matures the colostomy in a crescent fashion and sews the edges to the skin (Fig. 21–29).

Although some physicians express concern that fecal material may "spill over" to the distal limb of the loop, this rarely, if ever, happens in a well-constructed stoma. The opening of the loop colostomy serves as a mucous fistula. The bridge or rod may be removed in a week.

In some patients, a loop colostomy may be created to palliate a distal obstruction by making a small transverse incision at the proposed stoma site and bringing the transverse loop up through it. Preoperative abdominal films can help the physician assess the location of the transverse colon. Although this approach avoids a full laparotomy, the surgeon must exercise caution. Before operating, he or she must be sure that no other obstruction exists proximal to the transverse colon. In not fully exploring the abdomen, the surgeon risks the possibility of missing necrotic bowel or a perforation. The authors reserve this colostomy approach for patients who have end-stage malignancy and who may be too ill to withstand laparotomy.

A loop colostomy may be reversed by any number of techniques. The procedure carries a significant risk of infectious morbidity, although good bowel preparation and intravenous antibiotics can usually prevent this complication. Whole-gut lavage as described previously should be performed. Proximal irrigation of the distal limb should also be performed.

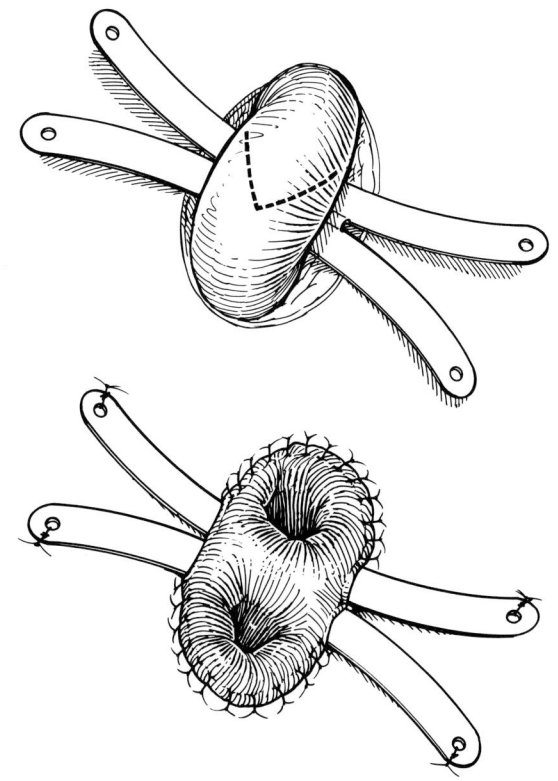

Figure 21–29
Loop colostomy is matured.

The reversal procedure begins with circumferential incision around the stoma, including several millimeters of skin (Fig. 21–30). The dissection then proceeds down through the abdominal wall to the level of the fascia. The colon is freed from the fascia, and the peritoneal cavity is opened. The skin and any scar tissue are then excised, leaving viable colon behind. The anterior bowel wall is then closed in a transverse fashion with a single layer of inverting sutures.

In some instances, the colon adjacent to the stoma is too edematous or the resultant lumen too narrow to permit this technique. In these situations, the colon near the stoma may be resected and re-anastomosis carried out as described earlier.

The colonic anastomosis is then replaced in the peritoneal cavity and the wound closed. Because of the high incidence of wound infection following this procedure, the authors leave the skin at the stomal site open and allow it to heal secondarily.

Stomal Complications

Acute stomal complications include hemorrhage and necrosis. The latter can be prevented by ensuring that the stomal segment is not under tension. A slightly bloody stomal edge without retraction at the conclusion of the procedure is a good sign. Stomal necrosis requires reoperation and revision. Significant bleeding at the stomal edge may be controlled with cautery, pressure, or suture ligation.

Given the inevitable spillage of intestinal contents during stoma formation, parastomal abscess is not an uncommon problem. In addition to antibiotics, management is surgical and usually requires relocating the stoma.

Long-term problems with stomas include stenosis and retraction, prolapse, and hernia formation. Immediate retraction may be prevented by mobilizing the intestine adequately before creating the stoma. Using sutures to fix the colon to the fascia also helps prevent retraction. Ostomy patients who gain weight are at risk for retraction and stenosis, regardless of the technique originally used. The enterostomal therapist can assist with mild cases by changing the appliance and giving support. For more severe cases, revision is required.

Peristomal hernia is a common late complication. Placing the stoma lateral to the rectus muscle may be a contributing factor. Hernias may be asymptomatic. If the patient becomes uncomfortable or the appliance becomes difficult to fit, repair is indicated. A small hernia may be directly repaired by taking down the stoma and repairing the defect. Relocating the stoma is another option, especially if the problem results from poor selection of the first site. Large defects are more difficult to fix and may require the insertion of synthetic material along with relocation of the stoma.

Prolapse of the stoma is not commonly seen. A mild prolapse can be dealt with by careful appliance selection. More severe cases require surgical repair.

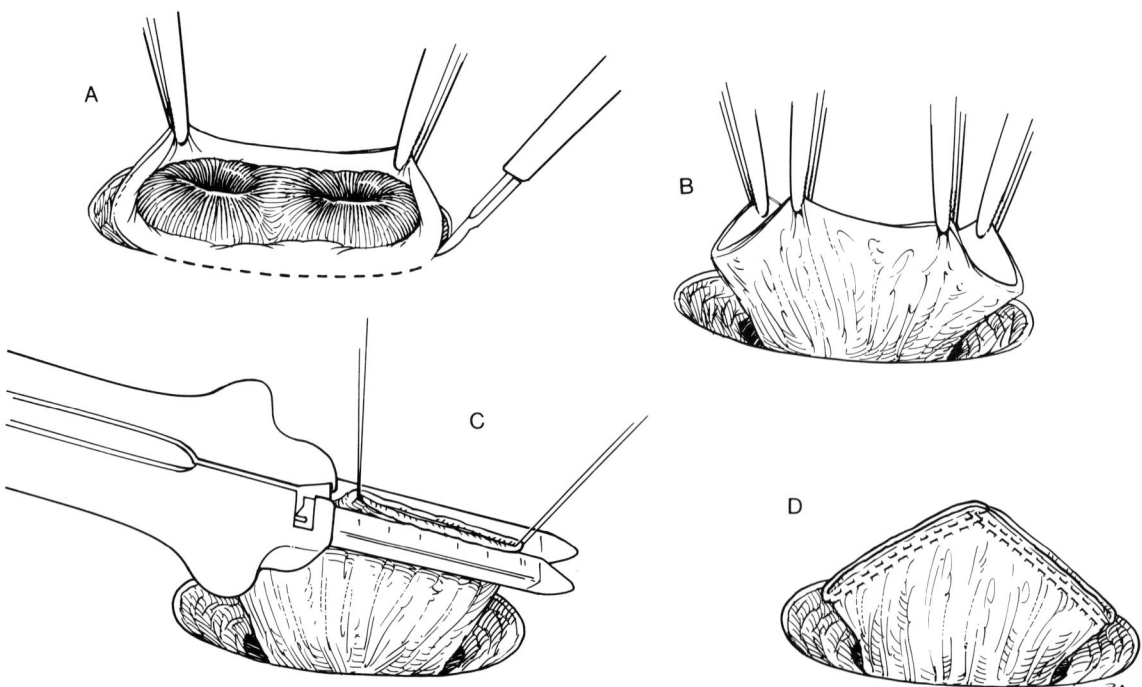

Figure 21–30
A, The stoma site and a few millimeters of surrounding skin are excised. *B*, The loop is mobilized from its fascial and peritoneal attachments. *C*, A GIA is used to seal each limb of the loop. *D*, Intestinal integrity is restored and the colon dropped into the peritoneal cavity.

Gastrostomy

As described earlier, a common indication for operative gastrostomy is the expectation of a prolonged ileus. The gastrostomy tube thus averts the discomfort of the nasogastric tube. The gastrostomy tube can also be used for tube feeding when required. The other major indication for gastrostomy in patients who have gynecologic cancer is to provide palliative relief of intestinal obstruction not amenable to operative correction. The most common setting involves a patient with end-stage ovarian cancer who has diffuse bowel dysfunction with multiple obstructed segments. Gastrostomy in this setting can provide tremendous relief.

A gastrostomy tube may be placed percutaneously under fluoroscopic guidance. In this procedure, a needle is inserted through the abdominal wall into the stomach and a guide wire is then placed through the needle. The needle is then removed and a succession of dilators inserted until the defect is large enough for a gastrostomy tube of the desired size to pass through. This technique is safe and requires only a local anesthetic.[37] In some centers, this procedure is most commonly performed with endoscopic guidance.

A gastrostomy tube may also be placed intraoperatively. The procedure employed most often at MD Anderson Cancer Center is a modification of the Stamm technique. The surgeon grasps the anterior wall of the stomach at its mid-point with a Babcock clamp. He or she loops a seromuscular pursestring suture of 0-0 or 2-0 chromic catgut around the clamp and places a second pursestring suture just beyond that. A spot on the anterior abdominal wall in the midclavicular line just below the lowermost rib is usually a good site for tube passage and should not interfere with any stomas that may be present. The surgeon makes a small skin incision, grabs a Malecot gastrostomy tube with a clamp, and brings it through the abdominal wall. Using a scalpel, the surgeon punches a full-thickness stab wound in the stomach wall in between the pursestring sutures. The gastrostomy tube is slipped through this wound and the pursestrings are tied, thereby inverting the gastric mucosa. The gastrostomy site on the stomach is then sewn to the posterior rectus sheath with several interrupted 0-0 chromic catgut sutures. Last, a nylon suture is used to fix the Malecot tube to the skin.

The nasogastric tube may be removed 24 hours after gastrostomy has been completed. The gastrostomy tube should not be placed on suction; gravity drainage will suffice. After gastrostomy tube removal, the resultant temporary fistula usually seals within 1–3 days.

RADIATION BOWEL INJURY

Caring for patients with radiation-induced bowel injury is an exercise in frustration. It requires a careful balancing act between medical management and surgical intervention. The patient who requires operative intervention presents a tremendous surgical challenge.

Radiation is employed for a number of gynecologic malignancies. It is the treatment of choice for the majority of women with cervical cancer and an important adjuvant therapy for those with endometrial malignancy. In addition, some centers still use whole-abdomen radiation to treat ovarian cancer. Patients who receive a total dose of more than 45 Gy to the pelvis or are treated with an extended field are particularly apt to experience toxicity. A brachytherapy device inserted close to the rectum or bladder may exceed the tolerance of these tissues. Other factors, such as prior abdominal surgery or a history of pelvic inflammatory disease, also increase the risk from pelvic radiation. Patients who have had prior abdominal or pelvic surgery frequently have intestinal adhesions to pelvic structures that may result in an excessive radiation dose to the bowel.

Sigmoid Injury

Portions of the gastrointestinal tract inevitably receive a significant radiation dose during pelvic radiotherapy.[38] The sigmoid colon is within the radiation field, and portions of the small intestine, usually the terminal ileum, often enter the pelvis as well. Given the intimate anatomic relationship of the sigmoid to the cervix, it is not difficult to imagine how a tandem and ovoid radiation system placed relatively posteriorly can result in a high dose of radiation to the sigmoid.

The acute effects of radiation on the sigmoid, described as proctosigmoiditis, include diarrhea, at times with passage of blood and mucus, and possibly tenesmus. These effects may begin after 1–2 weeks of external-beam therapy. This type of acute toxicity usually subsides shortly after external-beam treatment is concluded. A small proportion of patients, however, have chronic diarrhea, occasionally with significant bleeding and resultant microcytic anemia. The diagnosis of chronic proctosigmoiditis can be confirmed by flexible sigmoidoscopy. The mucosa is smooth and pale and has prominent friable blood vessels. There is no satisfactory treatment for chronic proctosigmoiditis. Patients who have this problem within the first few months after irradiation may be assured that frequently the disorder is self-limited. For some, however, proctosigmoiditis is a progressive illness. It has been suggested that treatment with hydrocortisone enemas may be of some value, although there is little objective evidence that significant improvement results. Chronic proctosigmoiditis can lead to a more serious condition of stricture or obstruction (Fig. 21–31).

Patients with a narrowed rectosigmoid often present with diarrhea alternating with constipation. Bloating, gaseousness, and crampy abdominal pain are common, frequently leading to anorexia and weight loss. The physician must be careful to distinguish between patients with this complication of radiation therapy and those who have recurrent disease.[39] The diagnosis can be confirmed by flexible sigmoidoscopy or barium contrast studies. The involved sigmoid can be narrowed for several centimeters, and the sigmoidoscopist may note that this portion of the colon is relatively fixed.

When the stricture is mild, patients can be treated with laxatives. Dilation of the narrowed segment, using balloons and other such devices, may be hazardous and may cause perforation if the tissue is significantly ischemic and fibrotic. Patients with a high-grade obstruction require surgical intervention. In selected patients, it may be possible to resect the narrowed area of colon and perform a re-anastomosis. In all such situations, however, it is important to perform a protective loop colostomy, because any anastomosis in irradiated bowel must be considered at high risk for impaired healing, leakage, or stricture. Unfortunately, in most cases this severe, the remaining sigmoid colon also has severe radiation change with ischemia, edema, and tethering of the mesentery. Patients with these problems are frequently left with a transverse or descending end-colostomy with a Hartmann pouch. The use of an irradiated portion of the colon to form the colostomy stoma can also be venturesome; stoma stenosis or retraction is always a possibility.

Chronic radiation injury to the sigmoid may also result in progressive ischemia leading to necrosis. Depending on the site of the greatest injury, necrosis of the intestinal wall can have several effects.[40] Injuries that occur above the peritoneal reflection can result in perforation. The diagnosis is easy when a chest x-ray shows fulminant peritonitis and free air under the diaphragm. In retrospect, these patients often have a history of progressive chronic crampy abdominal pain and bowel irregularity. Occasionally, the perforation presents subacutely, having been walled off with subsequent abscess formation. In this situation, patients may demonstrate fevers, a pelvic mass, and pelvic pain. At times, differentiating this disorder from recurrent cancer or pelvic inflammatory disease is difficult. When intestinal necrosis is a consideration, prompt surgical intervention is indicated, because the patient with a perforated sigmoid will soon develop sepsis.

Surgical management of sigmoid perforation can be especially difficult in the irradiated patient.[41] Re-establishing intestinal continuity is usually not possible. The necrotic segment should be resected and fecal diversion carried out. Simply performing a loop colostomy and placing a drain often result in repeated abscess formation. As a result of the intense local fibrosis and ischemia in the surrounding tissues that accompany these injuries, re-anastomosis at a later date is usually not possible, either. Whereas mortality from sigmoid perforation has been estimated to be as high as 50%, in recent years, thanks to broad-spectrum antibiotics and intensive care units, most patients with this serious injury survive.

When necrosis of the sigmoid colon occurs below the peritoneal reflection, patients may develop a rectovaginal fistula and present with flatus or stool per vagina. Whether the necrosis began primarily in the vagina or rectum is of academic interest only. Because fistulas are the result of recurrent tumor as often as of radiation injury, patients should be ex-

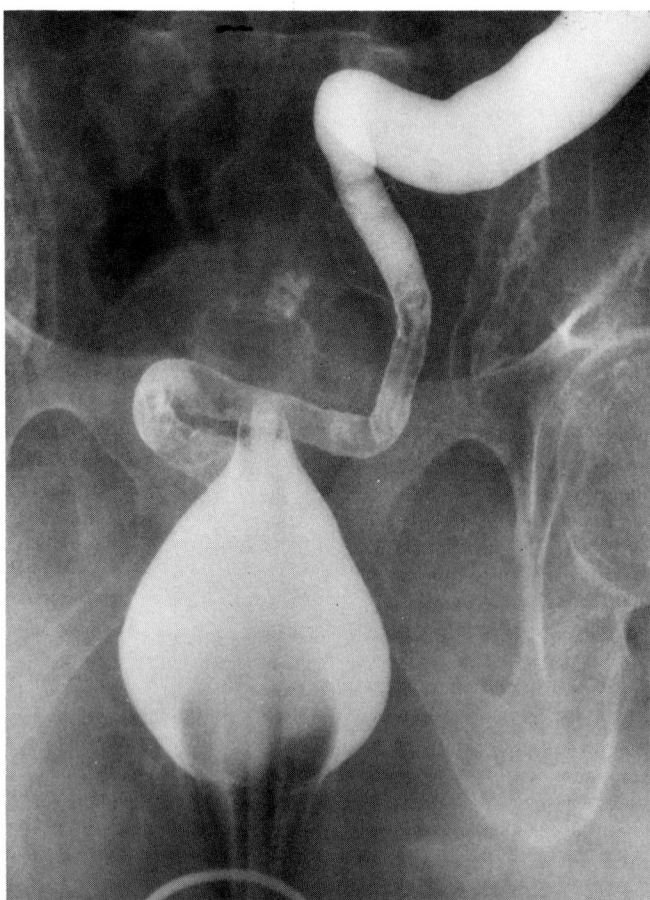

Figure 21–31
Barium enema radiograph showing stricture.

amined carefully and indicated biopsy specimens taken to exclude the possibility of recurrent disease. When the fistula is caused by radiation, primary healing is rare and repair is difficult at best. Initial treatment should include fecal diversion and observation. If recurrent disease is not evident and the area of necrosis does not spread, a resection of the involved area with a low re-anastomosis of the sigmoid to the anus can be effective in selected patients. Because their anastomosis is in the irradiated field, these patients need to maintain their diverting colostomy after this type of surgery. Should the repair be successful, the colostomy can subsequently be reversed. Even in the best of hands, however, the failure rate is high, and some patients also suffer from incontinence.

Small Bowel Injury

The acute reaction of the small intestine to irradiation is often manifested as diarrhea and abdominal cramping, sometimes with nausea and vomiting. These symptoms may arise within 1–2 weeks after external-beam therapy begins and are especially common when treatment is to extended fields. Fortunately, this is often a short-lived side effect that promptly disappears when radiation ceases. However, as with injury to the rectosigmoid, chronic injury can take years to develop. The section of small bowel that is most prone to injury is the terminal ileum, although other small bowel segments can be involved, especially in patients who have had prior abdominal surgery. Those patients who have extended-field or whole-abdomen irradiation are at particular risk for small bowel complications.

Patients whose chronic small bowel injury is secondary to irradiation have a progressive symptom complex that often starts with intermittent distention, nausea, weight loss, and diarrhea. The diarrhea is caused by rapid transit and malabsorption. Crampy abdominal pain is often a prominent feature. Often the severity of these symptoms can wax and wane over a period of months to years. Rarely, more severe injuries progress to focal stricture, obstruction, and, in the most severe cases, perforation.[42]

The diagnosis of small intestinal injury can be confirmed by radiologic studies. Results of the small bowel series (Fig. 21–32) have a characteristic appearance, including tethering and narrowing of the lumen. Plain abdominal films of patients who present with acute exacerbations often show multiple air-fluid levels or dilated intestinal loops. Initial treatment of these patients should include bowel rest, nasogastric decompression, and observation. The decision of whether to intervene operatively is often difficult. The surgeon who is experienced in treating

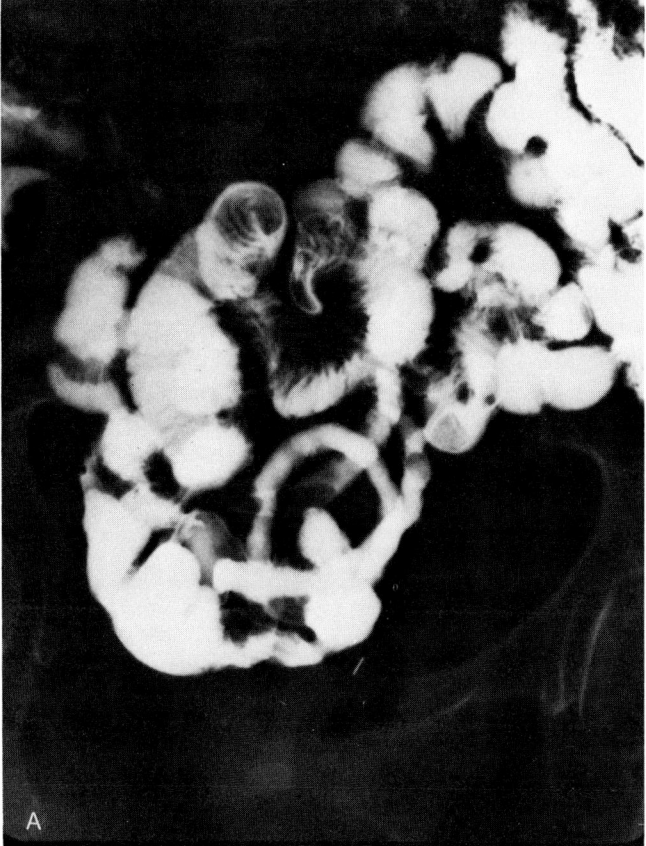

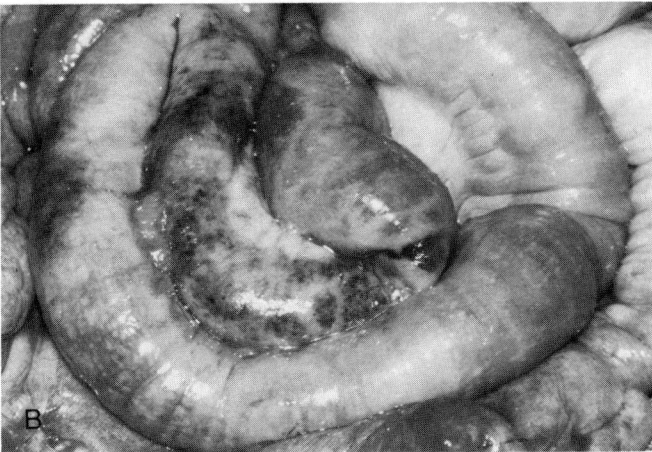

Figure 21–32
A, Barium contrast small bowel radiograph shows a narrowed and irregular small intestine. B, Findings at surgery include agglutinated loops of fibrotic small intestine.

the irradiated small intestine recognizes that the surgery is technically difficult and often results in other complications, such as inadvertent enterotomy, shortening of an already compromised intestine, and prolonged hospitalization, often with serious morbidity. Alternatively, the consequences of prolonged observation of a patient with a complete obstruction are perforation and death.

Patients whose symptoms are mild to moderate can often be treated expectantly with a low-residue diet and careful observation. Patients with more severe symptoms, especially repeated episodes of partial obstruction, deserve surgical intervention.[43] If a physician is debating whether or not surgery is indicated, it is probably best to go ahead and operate. In the authors' experience, they have never performed a laparotomy on a patient with radiation bowel injury without discovering significant abnormality.

The abdomen is best opened through a vertical midline incision. When patients have had pelvic radiation only, the authors often begin with an upper abdominal incision before approaching the pelvis. Extensive adhesive disease is the rule and, because irradiated intestine is injured easily, the surgeon must exercise patience while searching for the problem.

Sometimes it is possible to identify an isolated short necrotic segment or perforation surrounded by apparently normal small intestine. More often, however, the defect is diffuse and several areas show stricture. Although the goal of the surgeon should be to preserve as much intestinal length as possible, injured bowel should not be left in situ. If possible, the entire small bowel should be examined, because areas of injury may be discontinuous. This procedure also helps to exclude the presence of recurrent cancer, always a concern in this patient population.

The surgeon has a choice of either bypassing or resecting the diseased area. Bypass was considered to be the operative procedure of choice in the past,[40] because physicians believed that patients could not withstand the additional time and trauma associated with a definitive resection. The availability of TPN, modern antibiotics, and improved critical care skills render this opinion somewhat outdated. Nevertheless, some patients remain too ill to withstand a prolonged procedure or have such dense adhesions that a bypass remains the only viable option.

Intestinal bypass may be performed via a stapled technique (Fig. 21–33). Two areas of reasonably normal intestine both proximal and distal to the lesion should be identified. The surgeon makes a small defect in the antimesenteric border of each segment, only large enough to admit the jaws of the GIA instrument. He or she inserts the instrument and fires it, creating a communication between the two segments. The remaining defect is then closed using a TA-55 instrument. The resulting lumen restores intestinal continuity but does not isolate either limb of the obstructed segment, thereby preventing "blind loop" syndrome. Intestinal bypass may also be per-

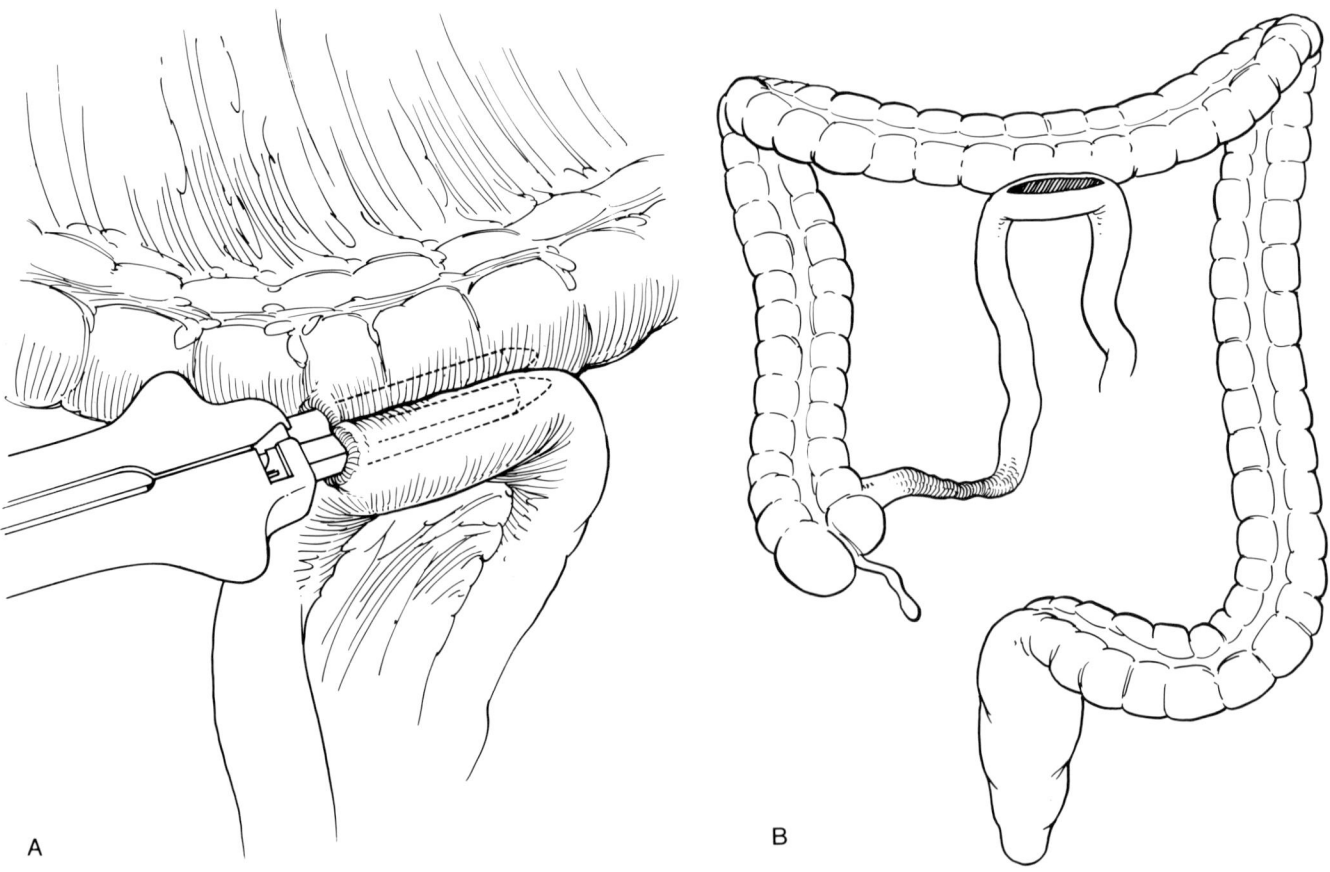

Figure 21–33
A, Side-to-side intestinal bypass may be performed with staplers. *B*, The areas of damaged ileum are now bypassed.

formed via a hand-sewn technique, which may be necessary when the bowel wall is extremely edematous.

It should be pointed out that a bypass procedure may also be indicated for women with obstruction who are not candidates for aggressive cytoreductive procedures because their ovarian cancer is too advanced. Many of these patients have diffuse intestinal involvement and may be better served by a diverting gastrostomy.

As stated earlier, the definitive procedure in treating severe radiation injury to the small intestine is resection and anastomosis. Every attempt should be made to exclude diseased bowel from the anastomosis. Unfortunately, subclinical injury may be present in bowel that appears grossly normal. For that reason, and because end-to-end anastomosis often has a narrow lumen that may be prone to further narrowing, the authors prefer to perform a side-to-side anastomosis (functional end-to-end) to ensure an adequate lumen. Although a stapled anastomosis as described previously has been shown to be safe in irradiated patients,[35] staples may be unwise when intestinal edema is significant; therefore, the hand-sewn technique should be considered the approach of choice.

When an anastomosis is performed on irradiated small intestine, the surgeons at MD Anderson routinely withhold oral feeding for at least 2 weeks postoperatively to allow adequate time for healing. During this interval, patients are supported with TPN. Those patients who present with preoperative evidence of nutritional depletion may benefit from 1–2 weeks of TPN prior to surgery if they are stable and the surgery is elective. Following surgery, patients often require a prolonged recovery period during which nutritional support and surveillance are critically important. Tube feeding may be necessary, because this group of patients often have absorptive impairment of the remaining bowel.

Intestinal-Sling Procedure

In an attempt to avoid intestinal complications associated with radiation therapy, some investigators have advocated using a synthetic sling to suspend the intestine out of the pelvis in advance of irradiation. Devereux and coworkers have reported on the use of the polyglycolic-acid (Dexon) mesh intestinal-sling procedure for patients undergoing pelvic irradiation for colorectal carcinoma.[44] A laparotomy is required to position the mesh, which enables the small intestine to be temporarily suspended out of the pelvic cavity (Fig. 21–34). Approximately 3 months after placement the mesh is resorbed, allowing the small bowel to return to its natural position

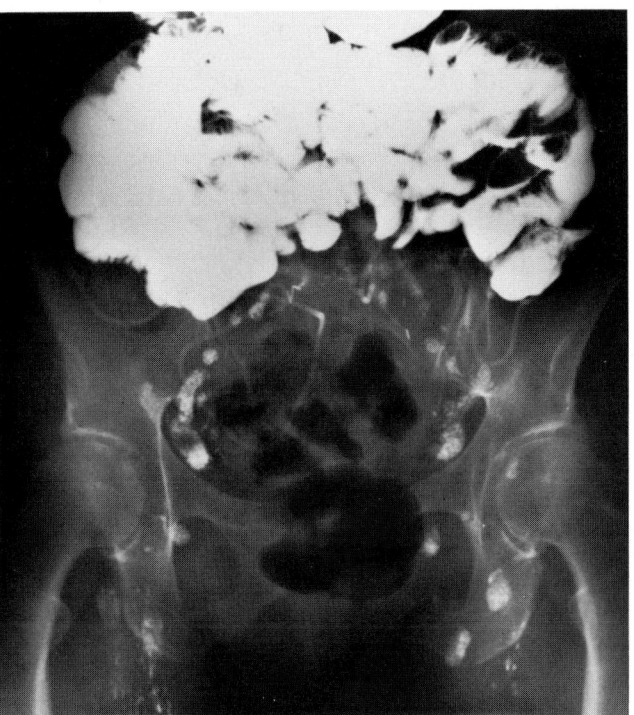

Figure 21–34
Barium contrast small bowel radiograph showing the small intestine suspended out of the pelvis by a Dexon mesh sling.

when radiation therapy is completed. The encouraging results in patients with colorectal cancer have yet to be duplicated in women who are undergoing irradiation for cervical cancer. The radiation field for cervical cancer does tend to extend more cephalad than that for rectal carcinoma, requiring that the mesh be placed higher and the intestine squeezed into a smaller volume.

Some surgeons have been reluctant to use the mesh based on early poor experience with another product (910-polyglactin).[45] Complications such as postoperative abscess and fistula formation have been reported.[46] Prolonged postoperative ileus and early satiety are common, although transient, problems in patients who have undergone the sling procedure. If a sling procedure is contemplated, patients must be carefully chosen; those who have had prior irradiation or infection are probably not good candidates for the insertion of a foreign body. Whether the Dexon intestinal-sling procedure will provide an advantage to patients receiving routine pelvic radiation remains to be determined. Certainly, the cost and effort involved in the surgery require that the benefit derived be significant. If a Dexon mesh is placed, the surgeon should be confident that extended-field radiation to the periaortic region is not in the treatment plan, because the mesh would fix the position of the small bowel, potentially leading to disastrous consequences. Prospective trials are needed to evaluate this new technology.

ENTERAL FISTULAS IN THE CANCER PATIENT

An enteral fistula is a devastating complication. The three most common causes of enteral fistulas are progressive cancer, complications of surgery, and radiation injury. Many times it is a combination of these causes that results in fistula formation.

The management of rectovaginal fistulas is discussed in detail in Chapter 12.

Enteral fistulas, which are classified and named according to the communications formed, include enterocutaneous fistulas, enterovaginal fistulas, and complex (involving more than one bowel segment) fistulas.

In many patients, the presentation of an enteral fistula is abrupt and its origin obvious. The passage of feculent material and flatus from the vagina in the presence of grossly visible tumor makes the diagnosis evident. In other patients, however, the onset is insidious. An enterocutaneous fistula may initially present as a low-grade fever and a reddened or indurated area on the abdominal wall. This may then progress to a small skin defect with drainage. At times, the cause of the drainage may not be clear; is it the result of an enteral fistula or of necrotic subcutaneous metastases or abscess? Diagnostic studies help to clarify the abnormality. Radiography of the small bowel or colon, using barium, is one method—or, if peritoneal spillage is a concern, a water-soluble contrast material may be used. A quick and simple test that the authors prefer, however, involves the oral administration of a vital dye such as brilliant green or blue. A charcoal slurry may also be used. The appearance of these substances as they move through the fistula tract confirms the diagnosis of an enteral fistula. Radiographic studies are still needed to rule out the presence of a complex fistula and to identify the area of intestine that is involved. However, when the dye study is negative, in a nonobstructed patient, an enteral fistula is probably not present.

Initial treatment of the patient with an enteral fistula is supportive. If recurrent disease is suspected, the physician should attempt to identify it and to determine its extent. When the fistula is enterocutaneous, an enterostomal therapist should be consulted and should attempt to fit an appliance to the patient's abdomen. Particularly when the fistula is in the proximal small bowel, the irritating and corrosive intestinal effluent can be a significant nursing problem.

Patients with an enteral fistula should not be fed orally and should begin receiving TPN. In the authors' experience, nearly half the fistulas—depending on their source—resolve spontaneously with this approach. However, when an enteral fistula is associated with tumor, this approach rarely provides a definitive result.

Surgical treatment of the enteral fistula should be undertaken only when the patient has been nutritionally repleted and conservative measures have failed. At laparotomy, it is best to identify the fistula site and to assess the type of repair required. In most cases, resection of the involved segment of bowel should be performed. The extent of resection is governed by the factor inciting fistula formation. When a fistula is secondary to a failed anastomosis or other surgical trauma, the resected portion may be locally limited. If recurrent cancer is uncovered, the resection must be sufficient so as not to incorporate metastatic deposits in the anastomosis. The surgeon should also be sure that obstruction is not impending in other bowel segments. Where it is, either a bypass procedure or a diverting gastrostomy may be indicated. If the bowel shows radiation injury, the anastomosis should incorporate grossly normal intestine. In all instances, the entire length of small intestine should be carefully examined. Diversion proximal to the anastomosis (ileostomy or colostomy) should be strongly considered, depending on the site of the fistula and the condition of the tissues. Proximal small bowel fistulas do not require diversion.

Postoperatively, patients should receive TPN until full bowel function returns.

INTESTINAL OBSTRUCTION

Obstruction of the intestinal tract in the woman with a gynecologic malignancy is a common problem. The most frequent causes include postoperative mechanical obstruction, tumor-related obstruction, and radiation bowel injury. The approach to these patients varies based on the cause of obstruction and the potential for resolution.

Diagnosis

The patient with acute mechanical small bowel obstruction is easy to recognize—abrupt onset of nausea and vomiting, a distended tympanitic abdomen, and abnormal bowel sounds allow for rapid diagnosis. However, patients with gynecologic cancer often present with a symptom complex reflecting progression of disease or complications of therapy. Management of complete or partial obstruction in this patient group should be based on knowledge of the underlying disease process involved and the severity of symptoms.

Women with carcinomatosis will often present with subacute obstruction with progressive symptoms. Based on physical examination alone, it may be difficult to distinguish distention secondary to tumor or ascites from dilated loops of bowel. The early satiety and nausea that accompany distention from ascites may also be a sign of impending obstruction due to progressive disease. Women with radiation bowel injury may progress to obstruction and, as described previously, may have mild symptoms that belie the severity of the underlying disease.

Because of these problems, clinicians are obligated to maintain a high degree of clinical suspicion when cancer patients present with abdominal complaints. Because the physical findings may be difficult to evaluate, the clinician must often make use of radiographic assessment techniques.

When partial or complete intestinal obstruction is suspected, the initial radiographic test should be an abdominal obstructive series. The finding of dilated intestinal loops and air-fluid levels will confirm the diagnosis. This test may also give some information regarding the site of obstruction based on whether gas is seen in the colon. Ascites or fecal impaction may also be seen. An upright chest radiograph will often be obtained with the obstructive series to search for free air under the diaphragm, an indication of intestinal perforation.

In some patients, especially those with diffuse abdominal tumor, the findings of the obstructive series may not be diagnostic. Some women may have what is best described as a tumor ileus—a dysfunctional intestine secondary to metastatic involvement of the bowel wall with aperistaltic areas and multiple sites of partial obstruction. Contrast studies may be used to further define the situation in this group of patients.

When the diagnosis of obstruction is unclear and in cases in which surgical intervention is contemplated, radiographic contrast studies may provide useful information. Barium enema and upper gastrointestinal series study can definitively localize the site of obstruction and exclude the presence of multiple obstructed sites. The authors are comfortable using barium contrast in patients with obstruction provided that there is no concern for peritoneal spillage. Barium from a small bowel series may be readily removed via nasogastric suction. Water-soluble contrast agents may also be used but do not provide the same degree of detail.

Management

The management of obstruction must be based on the reason for obstruction, the condition of the patient, and her life expectancy. The urgency of the situation is determined by the presence of impending strangulation or perforation. Initial management must include fluid and electrolyte correction and decompression. If the patient can be stabilized, diagnostic studies may be completed. When progressive ischemia or necrosis of the bowel is suspected, immediate operative intervention is indicated.

In patients with small bowel obstruction in the postoperative setting, observation with decompression should be considered. Obstruction may spontaneously resolve without surgery in a significant number of these patients. Whether or not to use a long intestinal tube, such as the Cantor tube or Miller-Abbott tube, remains controversial.[47, 48] It is likely that nasogastric decompression serves as well. Advocates of the long intestinal intubation point out that loose or filmy adhesions may be lysed by the passage of the tube through that segment. However, most of these patients have an adynamic ileus, making complete intubation of the small intestine difficult to achieve. For those patients with extensive adhesion, the long tube can help identify the course of the intestine intraoperatively.

In selecting this conservative approach, the surgeon must maintain vigilance for signs of a worsening condition. Frequent physical assessment, vital signs, repeat radiographic studies, and surveillance of the electrolytes and white blood cell counts are essential to this approach. Should there be signs of deterioration, prompt surgical intervention is indicated. Patients must also receive nutritional support through this period, usually with TPN.

When mechanical obstruction arises during a period more remote from surgery, operative intervention is almost always required. At laparotomy, the surgeon must decide whether the obstructed segment must be resected or if lysis of adhesions will suffice. "When in doubt, take it out" is good advice. An intestinal segment that has had a significant or prolonged interruption of blood supply may not recover and should be resected. Necrotic or perforated bowel should be removed. If the obstruction was due to extensive adhesions, consideration should be given to intraoperative long tube intubation because this may prevent subsequent kinking of the intestine in the postoperative period. Intraoperative decompression may also allow for a more secure abdominal closure.[49]

As noted earlier, when one is dealing with intestinal obstruction in previously irradiated patients, there is no such thing as being too careful. Though all surgeons are reluctant to operate on these patients, the changes in an obstructed segment are usually not reversible. These women may harbor necrotic or perforated intestine with only moderate symptomatology. Observation and nasogastric decompression of these patients should only be undertaken with caution.

The obstructed patient with advanced ovarian cancer presents a separate problem. Intestinal obstruction is a result of the natural progression of ovarian cancer and is probably the most common cause of death for these patients. Women who have untreated ovarian cancer have the potential to benefit from an aggressive approach with cytoreductive surgery and resection of involved intestinal segments. Patients who have progressive disease after first-line therapy usually do not benefit from an aggressive surgical approach, which carries significant morbidity and mortality.[50,51]

In the patient with obstruction secondary to recurrent ovarian cancer, the clinician must decide whether this is due to focal or diffuse tumor. Further treatment options, the functional status of the patient, and her potential life span must also be considered. A woman with a slow growing ovarian cancer with a focal obstruction may benefit from resection or bypass. Unfortunately, the more common situation is a malnourished patient with diffuse disease. She is probably best served by the placement of a percutaneous gastrostomy tube as described previously.

References

1. Davis GR, Morawski SG, Fordtran JS: Development of a lavage solution associated with minimal water and electrolyte absorption of secretion. Gastroenterology 1980; 78:991.
2. Soballe PW, Greif JM: Preoperative whole-gut lavage vs. traditional three-day bowel preparation in left colon surgery. Milit Med 1989; 154:198.
3. Clarke J, Condon R, et al.: Preoperative oral antibiotics reduce septic complications of colon operations: Results of prospective, randomized, double-blind clinical study. Ann Surg 1977; 186:251.
4. Condon RE, Bartlett JG, Greenlee H: Efficacy of oral and systemic antibiotic prophylaxis in colorectal operations. Arch Surg 1983; 118:496.
5. Nichols RL, Broido P, Condon RE: Effect of preoperative neomycin-erythromycin intestinal preparation on the incidence of infectious complications following colon surgery. Ann Surg 1973; 178:453.
6. Stellato TA, Danziger LH, Gordon N, et al.: Antibiotics in elective colon surgery. A randomized trial of oral, systemic, and oral/systemic antibiotics for prophylaxis. Am Surg 1990; 56:251.
7. Silva M, Cornick NA, Gorbach SL: Suppression of colonic microflora by cefoperazone and evaluation of the drug as potential prophylaxis in bowel surgery. Antimicrob Agents Chemother 1989; 33:835.
8. Herter F, Slanetz C Jr: Influence of antibiotic preparation of the bowel on complications after colon resection. Am J Surg 1967; 113:165.
9. Nazari S, Dionigi R, Comodi I, Campani M: Preoperative prediction and qualification of septic risk caused by malnutrition. Arch Surg 1982; 117:266.
10. Morgenstern L, Yamakawa T, Ben-Shoshan M, Lippman H: Anastomotic leakage after low colonic anastomosis. Am J Surg 1972; 123:104.
11. Schrock TR, Deveney CW, Dunphy JE: Factors contributing to leakage of colonic anastomoses. Ann Surg 1973; 177:513.
12. Bellantone R, Doglietto G, Bossola M, et al.: Preoperative parenteral nutrition of malnourished surgical patients. Acta Chir Scand 1988; 154:249.
13. Detsky AS, Jeejeebhoy KN: Cost-effectiveness of preoperative parenteral nutrition in patients undergoing major gastrointestinal surgery. Jpn J Parenter Enteral Nutr 1984; 8:632.
14. Leite JF, Antunes CF, Monteiro JC, Pereira BT: Value of nutritional parameters in the prediction of postoperative complications in elective gastrointestinal surgery. Br J Surg 1987; 74:426.
15. Smith RC, Hartemink R: Improvement of nutritional measures during preoperative parenteral nutrition in patients selected by the prognostic nutritional index: A randomized controlled trial. Jpn J Parenter Enteral Nutr 1988; 12:587.
16. Travers B: "An inquiry into the process of nature in repairing injuries of the intestine." 1812, Longmans, Green, and Co., London.
17. Lembert A: Memoire sur l'enterorrhaphie avec la description d'un procede nouveau pour pratiquer cette operation chirugicale. Rep Gen Anat Physio Path 1826; 2:100.
18. Fraser I: An historical perspective on mechanical aids in intestinal anastomosis. Surg Gynecol Obstet 1982; 155:566.
19. Murphy JB: Cholecysto-intestinal, gastro-intestinal and enterointestinal anastomosis, and approximation without sutures. Med Rec NY 1892; 42:665.
20. Dixon C: Anterior resection for carcinoma low in the sigmoid and the rectosigmoid. Surgery 1944; 15:367.
20a. De Petz A: Aseptic technic of stomach resections. Ann Surg 1927; 86:388.
21. Androsov PI: Experience in the application of the instrumental mechanical suture in surgery of the stomach and rectum. Acta Chir Scand 1970; 136:57.
22. Fain S, Patin C, Morgenstern L: Use of a mechanical suturing apparatus in low colorectal anastomosis. Arch Surg 1975; 110:1079.
23. Heald RJ, Leicester RJ: The low stapled anastomosis. Br J Surg 1981; 68:333.
24. Delgado G: The automatic staple versus the conventional gastrointestinal anastomosis in gynecological malignancies. Gynecol Oncol 1981; 12:302.
25. Harris WJ, Wheeless CRJ: Use of the end-to-end anastomosis stapling device in low colorectal anastomosis associated with radical gynecologic surgery. Gynecol Oncol 1986; 23:350.
26. Wheeless C: Avoidance of permanent colostomy in pelvic malignancy using the surgical stapler. Obstet Gynecol 1979; 54:501.
27. Wheeless C, Dorsey J: Use of the automatic surgical stapler for intestinal anastomosis associated with gynecologic malignancy: Review of 283 procedures. Gynecol Oncol 1981; 11:1.
28. Reiling R, Reiling W Jr, Bernie W, et al.: Prospective controlled study of gastrointestinal stapled anastomoses. Am J Surg 1980; 139:147.
29. Chassin J, Rifkind K, Sussman B, et al.: The stapled gastrointestinal tract anastomosis: Incidence of postoperative complications compared with the sutured anastomosis. Ann Surg 1978; 188:689.
30. Gambee LP, Garnjobst W: Ten years experience with a single-layer anastomosis in colon surgery. Am J Surg 1956; 92:222.
31. Max E, Sweeney WB, Bailey HR, et al: Results of 1,000 single-layer continuous polypropylene intestinal anastomoses. Am J Surg 1991; 162:461.
32. Burke TW, Weiser EB, Hoskins WJ, et al.: End colostomy using the end-to-end anastomosis (EEA) instrument. Obstet Gynecol 1987; 69:156.
33. Adelson MD, Baggish MS, Seifer DB, et al.: Cytoreduction of ovarian cancer with the Cavitron ultrasonic surgical aspirator. Obstet Gynecol 1988; 72:140.
34. Deppe G, Malviya VK, Malone, JMJ: Debulking surgery for ovarian cancer with the Cavitron Ultrasonic Surgical Aspirator (CUSA)—a preliminary report. Gynecol Oncol 1988; 31:223.
35. Berek JS, Hacker NF, Lagasse LD: Rectosigmoid colectomy and reanastomosis to facilitate resection of primary and recurrent gynecologic cancer. Obstet Gynecol 1984; 64:715.
36. Goligher J, Graham N, De Dombal F: Anastomotic dehiscence after anterior resection of rectum and sigmoid. Br J Surg 1970; 57:109.

37. Malone JMJ, Koonce T, Larson DM, et al.: Palliation of small bowel obstruction by percutaneous gastrostomy in patients with progressive ovarian carcinoma. Obstet Gynecol 1986; 68:431.
38. Chau PM, Fletcher GH, Rutledge FN, Dodd GD: Complications in high dose pelvic irradiation in female pelvic cancer. Am J Roent Radium Ther Nucl Med 1962; 87:22.
39. Schmitz RL, Chao JH, Bartolome JS: Intestinal injuries incidental to irradiation of carcinoma of the cervix of the uterus. Surg Gynecol Obstet 1974; 138:29.
40. Smith JP, Golden PE, Rutledge FN: The surgical management of intestinal injuries following irradiation for carcinoma of the cervix. In Cancer of the Uterus and Ovary. Chicago, Year Book Medical Publishers, 1966.
41. Allen-Mersh T, Wilson EJ, Hope-Stone HF, Mann CV: The management of late radiation induced rectal injury after treatment of carcinoma of the uterus. Surg Gynecol Obstet 1987; 164:521.
42. Morgenstern L, Thompson R, Friedman NB: The modern enigma of radiation enteropathy: Sequelae and solutions. Am J Surg 1977; 134:166.
43. van Nagell JR, Maruyama Y, Parker JC, Dalton WL: Small bowel injury following radiation therapy for cervical cancer. Am J Obstet Gynecol 1974; 118:163.
44. Devereux DF, Thompson D, Sandhaus L: Protection from radiation enteritis by an absorbable polyglycolic acid mesh sling. Surgery 1987; 101:123.
45. Soper JT, Clarde-Pearson DL, Creasman WT: Absorbable synthetic mesh (910-polyglactin) intestinal sling to reduce radiation induced small bowel injury in patients with pelvic malignancies. Gynecol Oncol 1988; 29:283.
46. Patsner B, Mann WJ, Chalas E, Orr JW: Intestinal complications associated with use of the Dexon mesh sling in gynecologic oncology patients. Gynecol Oncol 1990; 38:146.
47. Krebs H, Goplerud DR: The role of intestinal intubation in obstruction of the small intestine due to carcinoma of the ovary. Surg Gynecol Obstet 1984; 158:467.
48. Peetz DJ, Gamelli RL, Pilcher DB: Intestinal intubation in acute mechanical small bowel obstruction. Arch Surg 1982; 117:334.
49. Wickstrom P, Haglin JJ, Hitchcock CR: Intraoperative decompression of the obstructed small bowel. Surgery 1973; 73:212.
50. Krebs H, Goplerud DR: Mechanical intestinal obstruction in patients with gynecologic disease: A review of 368 patients. Am J Obstet Gynecol 1987; 157:577.
51. Morris M, Gershenson DM, Wharton JT: Secondary cytoreductive surgery in epithelial ovarian cancer: Nonresponders to first-line therapy. Gynecol Oncol 1989; 33:1.

Surgery of the Genitourinary Tract in Relation to Gynecology

22

Mitchell Morris
Thomas W. Burke

Because of the intimate relationship between the urinary tract and the pelvic reproductive organs, treatment of gynecologic malignancies must include certain urologic procedures. The realm of the gynecologist has traditionally extended to the treatment of certain urologic problems such as incontinence and fistulas. In the patient with cancer, though, the surgeon's skills are extended to include partial or complete resection of the collecting system, management of ureteral injury, treatment of radiation injury, and reconstructive procedures.

SURGICAL ANATOMY

As with surgery at any anatomic site, complete knowledge of regional anatomy is essential for success. Whereas the kidney and bladder are often represented in some detail in anatomy texts, the ureter is given brief mention. However, for the surgeon performing radical pelvic operations, the integrity of the ureters in a major concern. The importance of the ureters is reflected in the following discussion. Because this chapter deals with surgery of the ureters and bladder, the reader is referred to other sources for information on renal anatomy.

The Ureters

The ureters are paired muscular ducts that transport urine from the renal pelvis to the bladder (Fig. 22-1). Entirely retroperitoneal, in the female the ureters are 24–28 cm in length. The abdominal ureters start at the renal pelvis and run inferiorly along the anterior aspect of the psoas muscle. The gonadal vessels cross the ureters somewhere between the third and fifth lumbar vertebrae. The left abdominal ureter lies behind the mesentery of the descending colon and may be identified by medial reflection of the colon. Similarly, the right abdominal ureter is posterior to the cecum and ascending colon. The pelvic ureters start at the pelvic brim. Though their course may be somewhat variable, there are several points at which they may be reliably located. The right pelvic ureter will most often cross the external iliac artery just after it arises from the common iliac artery. The left pelvic ureter will cross the left common iliac artery just above its bifurcation. The ureters run inferior to the infundibulopelvic ligament and enter the medial leaf of the broad ligament. They then pass directly under the uterine arteries (hence the expression "water under the bridge"). At this point, the ureters are approximately 2 cm lateral to the uterine cervix. They then pass through the cardinal ligament and terminate in the trigone of the bladder.

The ureter can be tremendously distorted by altered pelvic anatomy. It may be greatly displaced either laterally or medially by pelvic masses, especially retroperitoneal tumors.

When locating the pelvic ureter, it is best to start by longitudinally dividing the pelvic peritoneum lat-

428 SURGERY OF THE GENITOURINARY TRACT IN RELATION TO GYNECOLOGY

is distorted by a pathologic process such as tumor, infection, or endometriosis, the ureter may be initially identified above the pelvic brim by dividing the peritoneum lateral to the colon and reflecting the

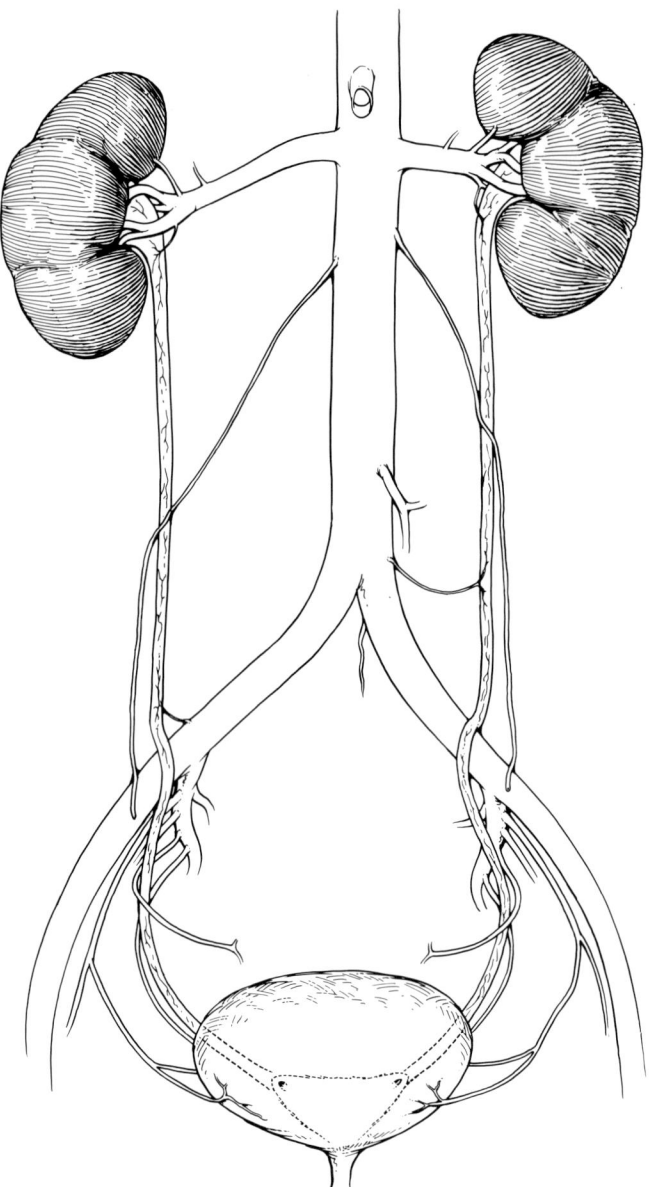

Figure 22–1
Anatomic relationships of the ureters. Note their passage under the uterine arteries.

eral to the infundibulopelvic ligament. Taking care not to injure the fragile venous plexus surrounding the gonadal artery, blunt dissection will part the loose and (usually) avascular areolar tissue within the broad ligament. The ureter will be posterior to the ovarian vessels and is readily identified by its white glistening appearance and peristaltic contractions. In some patients, especially those who are obese or who have undergone prior pelvic radiation therapy, the dissection may be guided by palpation. When rolled between the thumb and forefinger, the ureter has a characteristic feel and will "snap" like a rubber band. Once the ureter is located in this position, the remainder of the ureter can be easily traced cephalad or caudad. When the pelvic anatomy

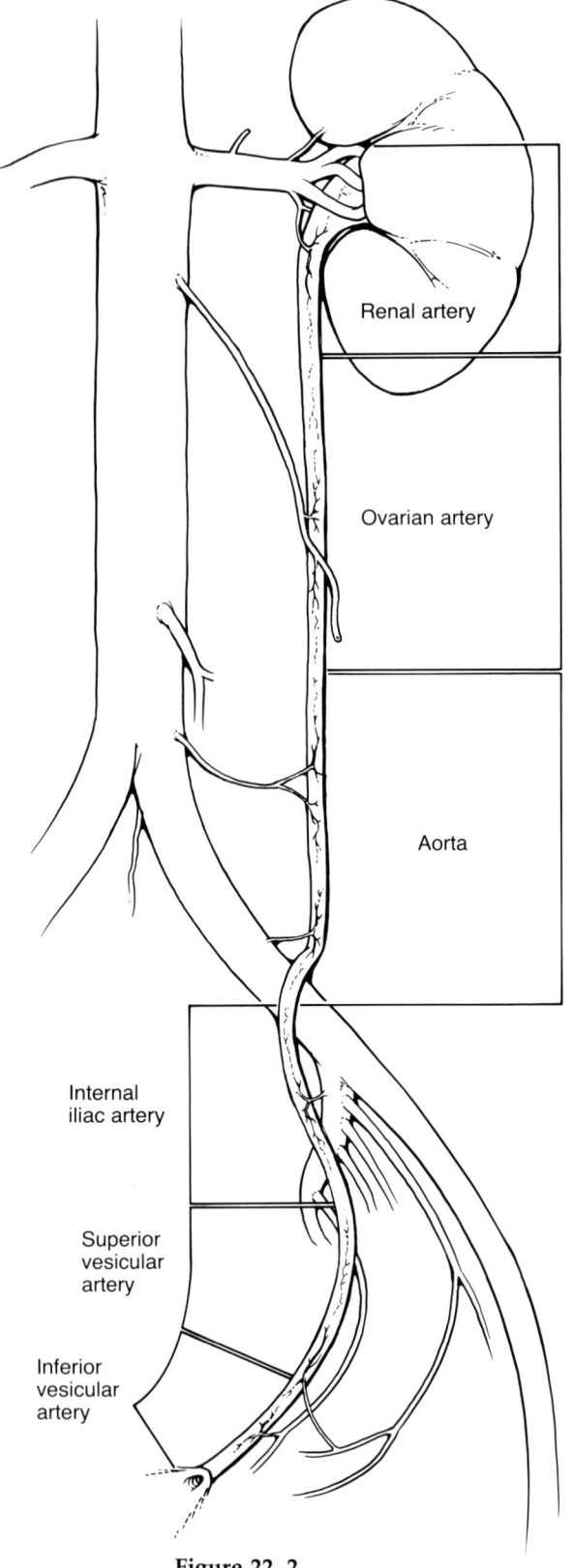

Figure 22–2
Ureteral blood supply.

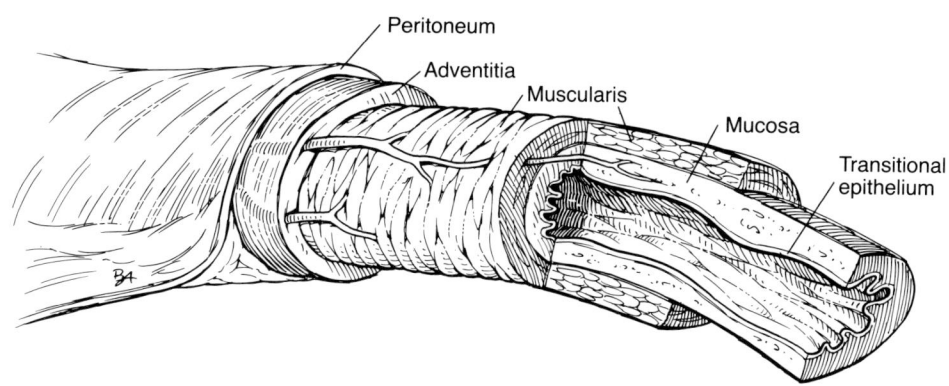

Figure 22–3
Layered view of the ureter. Care should be taken not to disturb the delicate vascular supply carried by the peritoneum and adventitia.

bowel medially. The ureter may then be traced down into the pelvis by direct visualization or palpation.

The surgeon should be alert for possible ureteral anomalies, most commonly duplication of the ureter. A double ureter may run from the renal pelvis down to the bladder or be fused at some point. Duplicated ureters tend to run in the same vascular sheath. Injury to a double ureter may occur when ligating the infundibulopelvic ligament, mistaking it for the ovarian vessels.

The blood supply of the ureter is variable (Fig. 22–2). The ureter may receive arterial branches from the renal artery; from the aorta; from the ovarian artery; from the common, internal, and external iliac vessels; and from the superior vesicular artery. These small unnamed arteries form a rich longitudinal anastomotic plexus that courses through the adventitial sheath of the ureter. During the course of pelvic surgery, some of these vessels may be sacrificed without causing harm to the ureter, provided that the adventitial sheath remains intact (Fig. 22–3).

Below the adventitia, the ureter is made up of an outer layer of circular smooth muscle fibers and an inner layer of longitudinal fibers. The innermost portion of the ureter is the transitional epithelium, which is in direct contact with urine.

The Bladder

The bladder is a retroperitoneal structure composed of three layers—serosa, muscularis, and mucosa. The muscular layer is itself arranged into three layers of crossing smooth muscle fibers, which results in efficient emptying. Like the ureter, the inner surface of the bladder is lined by transitional epithelium. The base of the bladder contains the trigone (Fig. 22–4), the inferior angle of which is formed by the internal urethral orifice. The superior border is formed by the

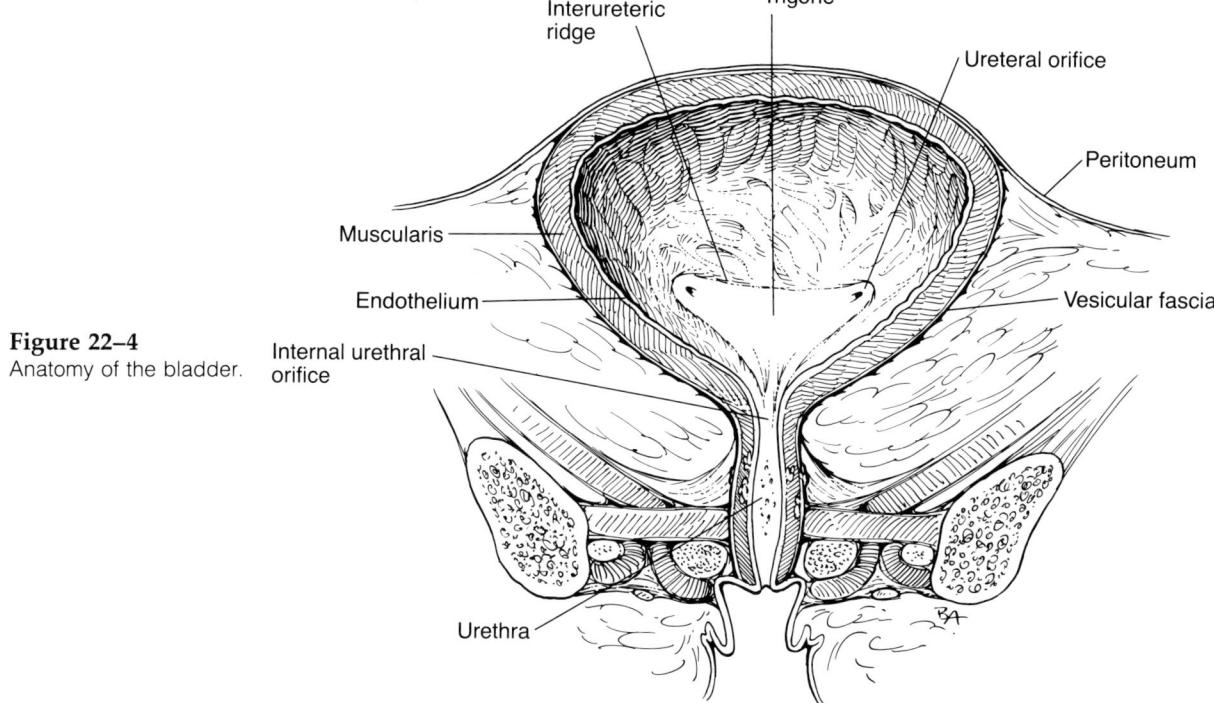

Figure 22–4
Anatomy of the bladder.

interureteric ridge, which connects the two ureteral orifices.

Blood is supplied to the bladder by the superior, middle, and inferior vesicular arteries. Also, it receives a rich collateral supply from the vaginal and pudendal arteries. Venous drainage is by a broad plexus of veins draining into the iliac veins.

INVOLVEMENT OF THE URINARY TRACT BY GYNECOLOGIC CANCERS

Involvement of the urinary tract by gynecologic tumors is common. The pattern and extent of involvement will depend on the type of cancer. Metastases to the kidney are a curiosity; however, extension to the ureters and bladder is common and may produce functional disturbance.

Cervical Cancer

Cervical cancers most often spread by direct extension and lymphatic dissemination and may affect the urinary tract either way. Because cervical cancers first spread to the immediate paracervical tissues, the bladder and lower ureters are at risk. Pretreatment evaluation of all but the most early cervical cancers requires intravenous pyelography (IVP) and cystoscopy. Ureteral obstruction is common in patients with large lesions. Occasionally, the first sign of advanced cervical cancer will be uremia resulting from bilateral ureteral obstruction.

In patients with hydroureter from cervical cancer, ureteral patency may be restored following administration of pelvic radiation therapy. When there has been direct extension of tumor to the bladder mucosa, "successful" radiation therapy will often leave the patient with a vesicovaginal fistula. In some cases, continence is preserved if the resolving tumor is replaced by fibrotic tissue.

Lymph nodal metastases may result in ureteral obstruction. Pelvic nodes may compress the pelvic ureter and cause obstruction, but they rarely directly infiltrate the ureter. Tumor-involved nodes can adhere to the ureter tightly, however, and attempts at surgical resection may devascularize the ureter. The upper ureter may be obstructed by enlarged paraaortic lymph nodes. This type of obstruction may be evident at primary presentation but is probably more common in patients with recurrent carcinoma.

Ovarian Cancer

Epithelial ovarian cancer primarily spreads by peritoneal dissemination. The peritoneum overlying the bladder is commonly involved with tumor, but this rarely causes any functional deficit. The tumor is rarely infiltrating, and if desired, the peritoneal covering of the bladder may be stripped. This removes the tumor but leaves the underlying musculature intact. When the cancer infiltrates further, a portion of the lower urinary tract may be resected.[1] Alternatively, an approach gaining in acceptance is use of the ultrasonic surgical aspirator, which can selectively remove tumor while leaving the vascular supply and muscular wall of the bladder intact.[2]

Epithelial lesions also spread through lymphatics but, when compared with lymph nodal metastases from cervical cancer, tend to displace rather than obstruct the ureter.

Malignant germ cell tumors and stromal tumors of the ovary may spread in a similar fashion, but they rarely directly involve the urinary tract.

Endometrial Cancer

Endometrial cancer involves the bladder and ureters less often than cervical cancer. Advanced lesions, however, may extend into much of the uterine cervix, and the cancer may then spread like a cervical cancer, with the potential to obstruct the ureter.

Endometrial cancers also spread by means of lymphatic channels but, similar to ovarian lesions, tend to displace rather than obstruct the ureters.

Sarcoma

Pelvic sarcomas have the potential for significant local destruction. In addition to spread by direct extension and through the lymphatics, sarcomas often metastasize through the bloodstream. The pelvic ureters are often involved with recurrent pelvic sarcoma. These lesions are often deeply infiltrative and destructive. If a therapeutic goal is resection of the tumor, resection of the involved portion of the urinary tract is often necessary.

Benign Conditions

The ureters and bladder are often involved by a host of benign lesions, which in terms of anatomic distortion may be as difficult to approach as pelvic malignancies. Advanced pelvic endometriosis can obstruct the ureter with an impenetrable sheath of inflammation and fibrosis, as can pelvic inflammatory disease. A variety of benign neoplasms may also displace or obstruct the ureter.

PREOPERATIVE EVALUATION OF THE URINARY TRACT

When significant pelvic pathology exists, some preoperative evaluation of the collecting system is indicated. The findings of such an evaluation may impact on the procedure performed and also document any pre-existent abnormality. The patient who is to undergo a routine exploration for an ovarian cyst or myomatous uterus or to undergo any other relatively straightforward procedure probably derives little benefit from a preoperative evaluation. Whenever a radical pelvic procedure is planned or the patient's anatomy is significantly distorted, information regarding the urinary tract is essential. Patients may include those with advanced pelvic cancer, candidates for radical hysterectomy, and those with urinary tract symptoms. Retroperitoneal dissections may be more difficult in patients with extensive endometriosis, pelvic infection, or multiple prior surgeries than in those with malignant disease; thus, the former may also benefit from evaluation.

The most common method of urinary tract evaluation remains IVP. This examination identifies the 2–5% of patients with congenital anomalies and determines the patency of their ureters. It is better to discover a nonfunctioning kidney before surgery than after, when there may be some question as to the timing and cause of the damage.

Many patients undergo computed tomography (CT) scans prior to surgery. When these are performed using intravenous contrast, the kidneys and ureters may be imaged with sufficient detail for most purposes. However, CT may not show as much anatomic detail of the ureters as will IVP.

There are several options for patients who cannot tolerate intravenous contrast. A nuclear renal scan may be used to visualize the kidneys and ureters; however, mild degrees of abnormality and duplication of the ureter are difficult to distinguish by this technique because it does not provide sufficient anatomic detail. Nevertheless, the renal scan gives more information than IVP about the function of the kidney, because flow of urine from each side may be quantified. The renal scan may also be used to evaluate relative blood flow to each kidney and can be used to estimate the glomerular filtration rate. This can be especially useful when planning a urinary conduit, as to be discussed.

Another option for patients with an allergy to the contrast material is the retrograde pyelogram. This procedure is performed through the cystoscope by inserting catheters into each ureteral orifice and threading them up to the renal pelvis. Injection of contrast through each catheter during fluoroscopy may provide the clinician with excellent anatomic detail without systemic exposure to the contrast.

Perhaps because of the popularity enjoyed by ultrasound examination in other areas of obstetrics and gynecology, many gynecologists initially evaluate the urinary tract by this modality. Although ultrasound can accurately determine the size and location of the kidneys and exclude the presence of hydroureter, it gives less information than the tests described previously.

Preoperative cystoscopy is probably not necessary for most patients. If bladder invasion is supected, cystoscopy is useful. Epithelial ovarian cancer rarely invades the bladder, even in cases of very extensive pelvic tumor. Cervical cancer, however, may involve the bladder by direct extension, and cystoscopy is part of the authors' routine evaluation prior to pelvic exenteration for recurrent cervical cancer.

URETERAL INJURY

All pelvic surgeons have caused inadvertent injury to the ureter at one time or another. Though avoidable in the majority of cases, intraoperative ureteral injury brings to mind the old adage, "Those who play with fire will eventually get burned." The gynecologist should be familiar with the types of ureteral injuries that may be induced and the factors contributing to injury and should know how to recognize ureteral injury. Even if repair is to be accomplished by a urologist, the gynecologist should be familiar with the operative approach.

Ureteral injuries most commonly occur during abdominal hysterectomy.[3–5] There are two times at which such injuries typically occur. As noted earlier the ureter passes remarkably close to the cervix. Improper placement of the clamp on the cardinal ligament or insufficient dissection of the bladder can lead to a crush injury or ligation of the ureter during hysterectomy. Similarly, even though the clamp may miss the ureter itself, a suture ligature may pass through the ureter, resulting in obstruction or fistula formation.

The other time during simple hysterectomy at which ureteral injury may occur is during the ligation of the infundibulopelvic ligament. This may be avoided by carefully identifying the ureter below the ovarian vessels by either palpation or, preferably, direct visualization prior to ligation.

Radical hysterectomy increases the likelihood of ureteral injury. Dissection of the lower half of the ureter risks devascularization of the ureteral wall and creates the potential for subsequent obstruction or fistula formation. During the early experience with radical hysterectomy, ureteral fistula or obstruction occurred in as many as 13% of cases.[6] Advances in the technique of radical hysterectomy have taken into account the potential for this problem, and surgeons are careful to minimize handling of and trauma to the ureter, thereby preserving blood supply as much as possible. Improvements in surgical technique along with modern antibiotics and the use of closed suction drainage in the pelvis have decreased the incidence of ureteral injury to between 1 and 3% in more recent series. In the patient with gynecologic disease, ureteral injury may also occur at the time of lymphadenectomy if the ureter has not been exposed adequately. The ureters are also vulnerable during para-aortic node dissection because they are often more medial than the surgeon expects. Injuries in this area are more difficult to correct.

A number of factors may contribute to ureteral injury. Certainly, the presence of pelvic malignancy increases the potential for such damage. Devascularization of the ureter during the course of cytoreductive surgery, especially for retroperitoneal tumors, is a known risk. Conditions such as endometriosis and pelvic inflammatory disease and previous pelvic radiation therapy also predispose the ureter to injury; all of these conditions make identification of the ureter more difficult and, at the same time, all the more important.

The most important factor predisposing the ureter to injury is the surgeon. During pelvic procedures, the operator should always be aware of the location of the ureters, preferably by direct visual identification early in the procedure. When confronted with pelvic bleeding, many surgeons will "stitch first and ask questions later." A more logical approach to hemorrhage, and one that avoids injury to other pelvic structures, is to isolate and skeletonize the damaged vessel and ligate it under direct vision. At the very least, an assistant may apply pressure to stop the bleeding while the surgeon verifies that the ureter is free and clear.

Recognition of Ureteral Injury

Even the most capable and exacting surgeon may injure a ureter at some time. The skillful surgeon will recognize the problem and take the appropriate intraoperative measures to correct the situation. Failure to detect the injury is a more serious error and has the potential to create a more serious problem.

Management of ureteral injury is based on the nature and location of the injury and on the timing of the diagnosis (intraoperative vs. postoperative). The ureter may be crushed, ligated, or divided; the extent of the injury will determine the need for repair.

The ureter also may be injured by factors other than surgical trauma. Occasionally, a ureter will become obstructed secondary to fibrosis or tumor. This is most common in women with cervical malignancies. The overwhelming majority of cases of ureteral obstruction in these patients are due to progressive cancer, and surgical repair is usually not an issue. Other malignancies, such as ovarian carcinoma, pelvic sarcomas, and lymph nodal metastases from tumors at a variety of primary sites, also may involve the ureter. It is unusual for the ureter to be invaded directly, but the adventitia is often involved. Stripping tumor off the ureter in this location may result in devascularization and subsequent injury. Also, a small number of patients develop severe retroperitoneal fibrosis secondary to radiation therapy and are candidates for surgical correction of the problem. Retroperitoneal fibrosis resulting from other causes, including drugs, chemicals, and idiopathic processes, may also result in ureteral obstruction.

When ureteral injury is suspected during the course of pelvic surgery, the surgeon may take a number of steps to ascertain the site and degree of the problem. At times, there is a clean transection of the ureter that is noticed immediately. A misapplied clamp or suture may also be recognized to have injured the ureter. In many cases, however, injury occurs by placing sutures into an obscured field to control bleeding or a clamp may be placed too close to the ureter. In these cases, the ureter should have been identified *before* the injury, not after.

Intraoperative Detection of Ureteral Injury

When ureteral injury is suspected, careful identification of the pelvic ureter is essential. The middle third of the ureter may be exposed by relatively simple dissection and then be inspected for injury. Crush injuries should be inspected carefully to determine the extent of devascularization. When the ureter is clamped along with a large bundle of tissue, the injury may be minor and the clamp simply removed. Similarly, a misplaced stitch may be removed. The surgeon then can decide whether to resect this area and effect anastomosis or to leave the crushed area in situ, perhaps with the addition of a stent. If the ureter appears to be intact and peristalsis can be seen through the area, the ureter may be left in place.

As soon as the need for a stent is even considered, the authors go ahead and place one. The stent is inserted to provide for drainage and to minimize the effects of edema or fibrosis on urinary flow. This may be especially important when the vascular supply is tenuous or the patient has previously received pelvic radiation. Ureteral stenting carries little morbidity and is easily carried out. For many of the authors' operative procedures, the patient is placed in the modified lithotomy position (Allen's stirrups). This has the added benefit of easily permitting concurrent intraoperative cystoscopy with stent placement. When cystoscopy is not possible or the patient is in the supine position, stents may be placed by opening the dome of the bladder and directly inserting them into the ureteral orifice. The authors prefer to use double-J catheters with multiple holes. They are simple to place, minimally reactive, and stay in place without suturing. Also, double-J stents can be removed through a cystoscope in the outpatient setting with minimal discomfort to the patient.

When an injury is suspected in the lower third of the ureter, evaluation may be more difficult because the ureter passes through the bladder. Dissection of this area may cause problems of its own.

When the anatomy cannot be fully exposed or a question of injury or ligation remains, there are several intraoperative maneuvers that should be considered. Intravenous injection of a vital dye such as indigo carmine can be helpful in identifying a ureteral leak, which will release blue dye into the operative field. When the urine passing from the Foley catheter turns blue, one is reassured that both ureters have not been ligated (of course, only one may be patent).

Intraoperative IVP may document ureteral patency; unfortunately, these studies do not provide great detail. Hydroureter will usually not be seen yet, and the passage of contrast, especially through the lower third of the ureter, may be difficult to document. Small amounts of extravasation from the ureter are also difficult to see.

As described previously, catheters may be passed into the ureter. Failure of the catheter to pass beyond a certain point can signal a site of obstruction. Palpation of the catheter may also assist the surgeon in identifying the ureter throughout its course.

Postoperative Detection of Ureteral Injury

Unrecognized ureteral injury will manifest as obstruction, abscess, fistula, or urinoma. In the case of an obstructed renal unit, many patients remain asymptomatic. The percentage who remain asymptomatic is unknown, because it is not known how many patients have silent death of a kidney following procedures such as hysterectomy. If the contralateral kidney is healthy, it will compensate for the loss and there may only be a transient increase in serum creatinine. If undiagnosed, the obstructed kidney will gradually lose its capacity for function over a period of several months, the end result being autonephrectomy. One can only hope that a patient will become symptomatic, so that appropriate diagnostic tests may be conducted. Symptoms may include unilateral flank pain, fever, or fistula formation. The patient who has had both ureters ligated does not present a diagnostic dilemma.

When ureteral obstruction is suspected, the ideal diagnostic study is IVP. The authors' second choice would be nuclear renal scan, for the reasons described earlier. Ultrasound is good at identifying hydroureter but has difficulty locating the exact point of obstruction. Additionally, the ureter may not have had time to dilate immediately after surgery. Cystoscopy with stent placement attempted under fluoroscopic control may also be diagnostic.

After gynecologic surgery, the most common site for a ureteral fistula is through the vagina. The appearance of profuse watery vaginal discharge will be suggestive of a urinary fistula. Intravenous administration of a vital dye may be helpful in showing that this fluid is, in fact, urine. Another reliable test is to analyze the fluid for urea nitrogen and creatinine. If the vaginal fluid is urine, the levels of urea nitrogen and creatinine will be several times higher than the levels in the patient's serum.

Instillation of methylene blue by means of a Foley catheter after insertion of a vaginal tampon can help in differentiating between vesicovaginal and ureterovaginal fistulas. In the case of a bladder defect, the tampon should stain blue. Unless ureteral reflux is significant, a patient with a ureterovaginal fistula will not show blue on the tampon.

Patients who have had complete transection of the ureter will present with a urinoma. This may manifest in a relatively benign manner with accumulation of "ascites." In most cases, however, the patient will develop abdominal pain, fever, and ileus. An abscess is often suspected in these situations. An IVP may document extravasation of urine or urine may be obtained on aspiration, thus specifying the diagnosis of urinoma.

When ureteral injury is identified in the postoperative setting, operative intervention is usually indicated. Patients with obstructions should be explored. In some cases, cutting a ligature may relieve the blockage. In other cases, a more complex repair will be indicated (see later discussion). If a patient is too ill to undergo surgery, percutaneous nephrostomy may suffice until definitive repair can be undertaken. Patients in whom urine is being extravasated into the abdomen should also be explored and repairs made. If surgery is not possible, percutaneous nephrostomy may temporarily relieve the situation. The continued presence of urine in the abdomen will lead to inflammation and fibrosis, making any subsequent repair more difficult.

Patients with a ureterovaginal fistula may be approached in a more conservative manner. In some cases the ureter may be stented, either retrograde through a cystoscope or antegrade by means of percutaneous nephrostomy. If stenting can be accomplished, many patients will have spontaneous resolution of the fistula provided that there is no infection and that a reasonable nutritional status can be maintained.[4] In patients with malignancy or prior pelvic irradiation, spontaneous healing is less frequent and surgical repair is required.

Surgical Repair of Ureteral Injuries

The method of ureteral repair depends on the location and extent of the injury. When the injury is minor, such as inadvertent ligature or the application of a crushing clamp, it may be managed by stenting the ureter and draining the surrounding area. The stent may be removed after 1 week and then IVP performed to ensure that stricture has not developed.

When the ureter has been partially transected, the surgeon must decide whether to repair the injury or resect the involved segment. When the cut is clean and there appears to be an adequate blood supply to the segment, the defect may be closed in a transverse fashion using 4-0 or 5-0 interrupted absorbable suture. The authors prefer to stent these repairs and drain the operative bed.

If the injury has resulted in the loss of a portion of the ureter, a more involved repair must be undertaken.

Ureteroureterostomy

When an injury such as complete transection or a severe crush injury occurs in the middle portion of the ureter, it is often possible to effect an end-to-end anastomosis. The damaged section must be excised, leaving the ureteral ends to be used in the anastomosis with a satisfactory blood supply. If the transected end of the ureter does not bleed freely, the viability of that segment is in question. If length is a problem, the ureter may be mobilized in several ways. When only a short segment has been excised, freeing the ureter from its peritoneal attachments will create a few centimeters of additional length. Great care must be taken, however, not to strip the ureteral blood supply during this maneuver. Additional length may also be obtained by mobilization of the kidney. The most common method to ensure a tension-free anastomosis is by a psoas hitch (see later).

The principles of ureteral anastomosis are similar to those of intestinal anastomosis: (1) the blood supply to both sides of the anastomosis must be adequate; (2) there should be no tension on the anastomosis; (3) the anastomosis should be watertight; and (4) the anastomotic site must be drained.

Ureteroureterostomy should be performed using a fine absorbable suture. The authors prefer to use 4-0 or 5-0 chromic catgut for ureteral repairs. In a modification of the technique originally reported by Hamm and coworkers,[7] the ureteral ends should be spatulated to prevent stricture (Fig. 22–5). Between 6 and 10 interrupted sutures are sufficient to effect the closure. The authors prefer to perform the anastomosis over a ureteral stent (Fig. 22–6), although there is no clear evidence that the use of stents is necessary. Some surgeons mobilize the greater omentum and place it over the anastomotic site in the belief that this brings in an additional blood supply to the ureter.[8] Although this practice is not harmful, the authors doubt that a significant new blood supply results.

Drainage of the site is important. The presence of free urine around the anastomotic site often results in stricture, fibrosis, and possibly infection. If the drain has minimal output, the authors remove it several days after the surgery. Depending on the clinical situation, the ureteral stent is left in place for 1–4 weeks. Patients with impaired healing capability because of cancer, prior radiation therapy, poor nutritional status, or questionable blood supply may benefit from a longer period of stenting.

Ureteroneocystostomy

Injuries to the ureter close to the bladder are best repaired by direct ureteral reimplantation, because

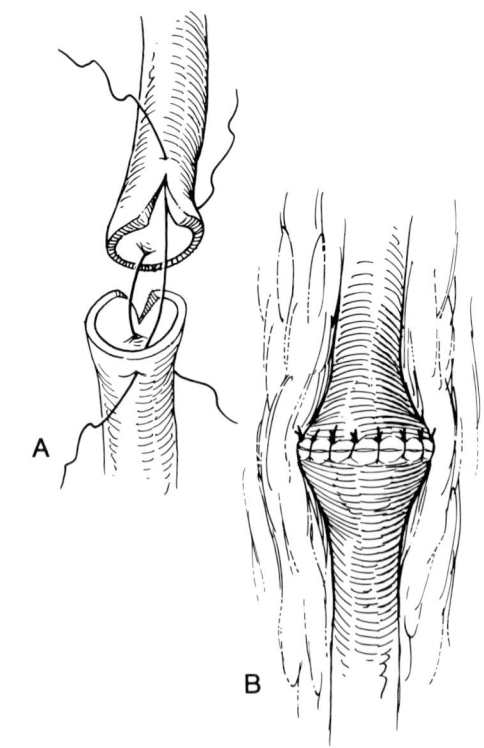

Figure 22–5
A, The ureteral ends are spatulated to provide a greater anastomotic diameter. *B*, Fine sutures are used to complete the anastomosis.

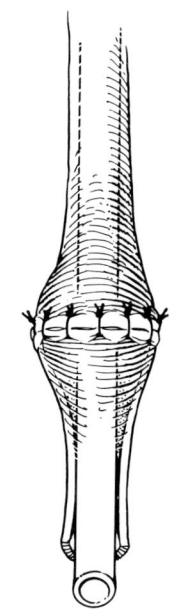

Figure 22–6
Ureteral anastomosis may be performed over a ureteral stent.

ureteroureterostomy is usually not feasible in the deep pelvis. The principles of repair elaborated previously must be followed. The damaged section of ureter is excised and the distal segment ligated using nonresorbable suture. Some mobilization of the bladder is usually required to achieve a tension-free anastomosis. The authors prefer an open bladder technique (Fig. 22–7), although an extravesical procedure may also be used.[9]

The dome of the bladder should be opened and a curved clamp used to create a submucosal tunnel for several centimeters. Submucosal passage of the ureter is used to prevent reflux. In the adult, mild reflux at the ureterovesical junction is probably of little consequence. The authors do not recommend more elaborate procedures such as the creation of a nipple valve.[10] At the end of the tunnel, a passage is created through the muscularis and serosa; the ureter is then pulled through the tunnel and the end spatulated. Using fine interrupted sutures, the ureter is sewn to the inner bladder wall. Care should be taken to ensure that the ureter is not twisted as it passes through the tunnel. The bladder is then closed. Stenting of this type of repair is optional.

Although the rate of complications from this procedure is low, all patients should undergo evaluation of the collecting system 4–6 weeks after ureteroneocystostomy, preferably by IVP. A small percentage will develop stricture or a fistula.

When significant hydroureter is present, a tunneled anastomosis is not appropriate. In these cases, a direct anastomosis to the bladder may be performed by excising a button of bladder wall and, using a single layer of interrupted sutures, performing and end-anastomosis like that used in ureteroileoneocystostomy (see later discussion).

Psoas Hitch

The most significant problem faced by the surgeon during repair of ureteral injury is insufficient ureteral length. Although more drastic solutions to this problem exist, the psoas hitch is a relatively straightforward procedure that carries little morbidity and that can add several centimeters of reach to a damaged ureter. According to Ehrlich and colleagues,[11] the psoas bladder hitch was first described in 1896 by Witzel but was largely ignored until 1969, when Turner-Warwick and Worth described 23 patients in whom ureteral implantation was successfully effected above the iliac vessels.[12]

The bladder should be mobilized by first incising the overlying peritoneum and partially developing the space of Retzius. Opening the paravesical spaces on each side will result in additional mobility. These maneuvers alone will often allow the bladder to be transfixed to the psoas muscle; in some cases, however, it may be necessary to take down the contralateral vesical pedicle to achieve sufficient mobility. The dome of the bladder is then opened, and the sites of psoas attachment and ureteral implantation are identified. The authors prefer to create the submucosal tunnel prior to psoas attachment using the technique described previously. Once the tunnel has been prepared, the bladder is transfixed to the psoas muscle using several 0-0 or 2-0 nonabsorbable interrupted sutures (Fig. 22–8). Care should be taken to avoid the genitofemoral nerve. After the bladder and psoas muscle are attached, the ureter is brought through the submucosal tunnel and sewn in place and the bladder is closed. The surgeon must ensure that neither the ureter nor the bladder is subject to significant tension. Despite the significant deformaton of the bladder that results from this procedure, most patients are able to void normally.[11, 12]

Boari Flap

An alternative to the psoas hitch procedure, the Boari flap may give the additional length needed to effect reimplantation. Like the psoas hitch, the Boari flap has been around for some time, being first described by Boari in 1894, according to Ehrlich and colleagues.[11] Although the procedure gained greater early acceptance than the psoas hitch, concerns regarding its technical complexities and postoperative complications have kept the Boari flap an infrequently performed operation.[12]

The Boari flap is made by creating a tapered flap from the posterior wall of the bladder (Fig. 22–9). The ureter is then implanted into the end of the flap

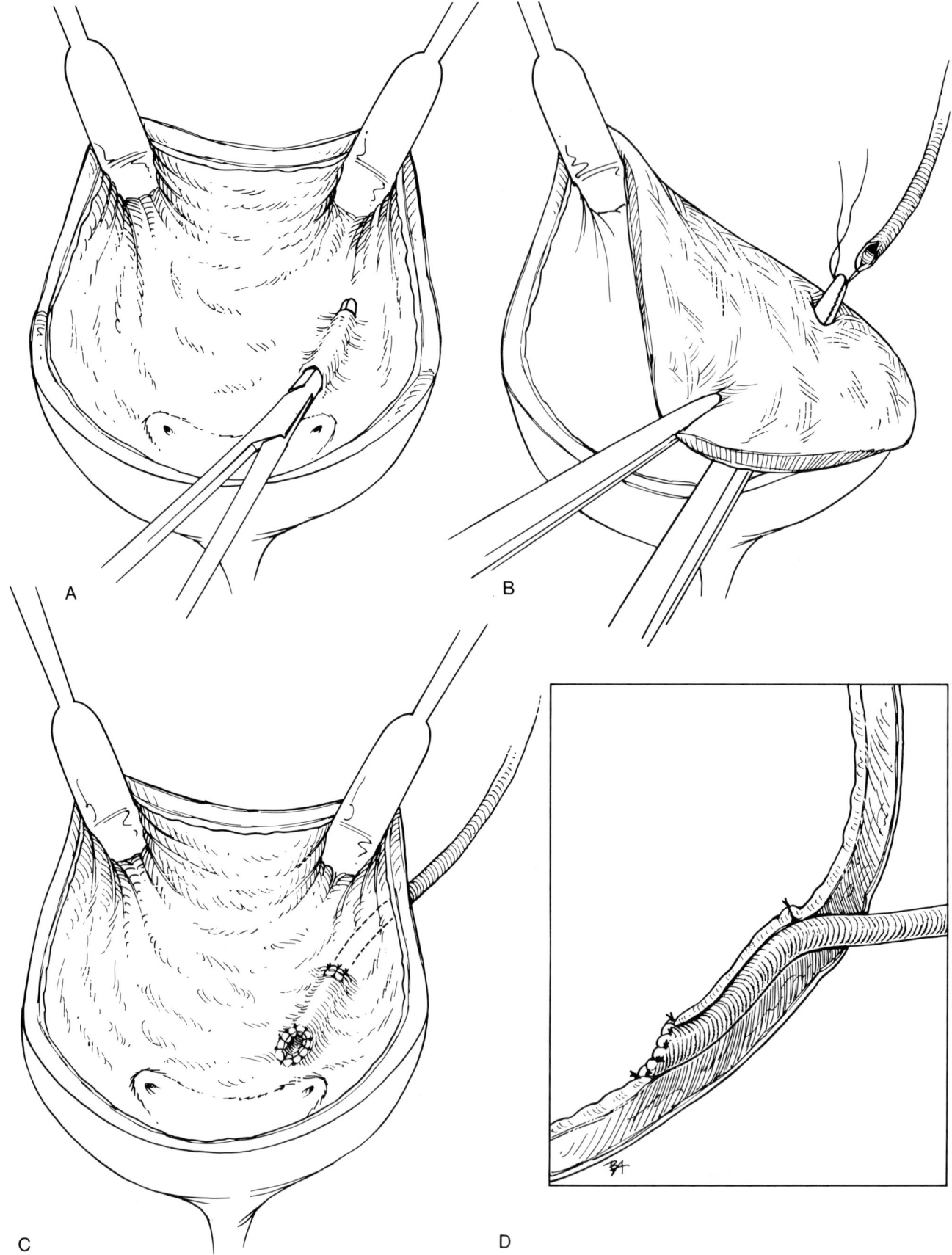

Figure 22-7
Ureteral reimplantation. *A*, A submucosal tunnel is created above the ureteral orifice. *B*, The spatulated ureter is brought through the bladder wall and drawn through the tunnel. *C*, The ureter is sewn in place with fine interrupted sutures. *D*, Cross-section showing the passage of the ureter through the bladder wall.

SURGERY OF THE GENITOURINARY TRACT IN RELATION TO GYNECOLOGY 437

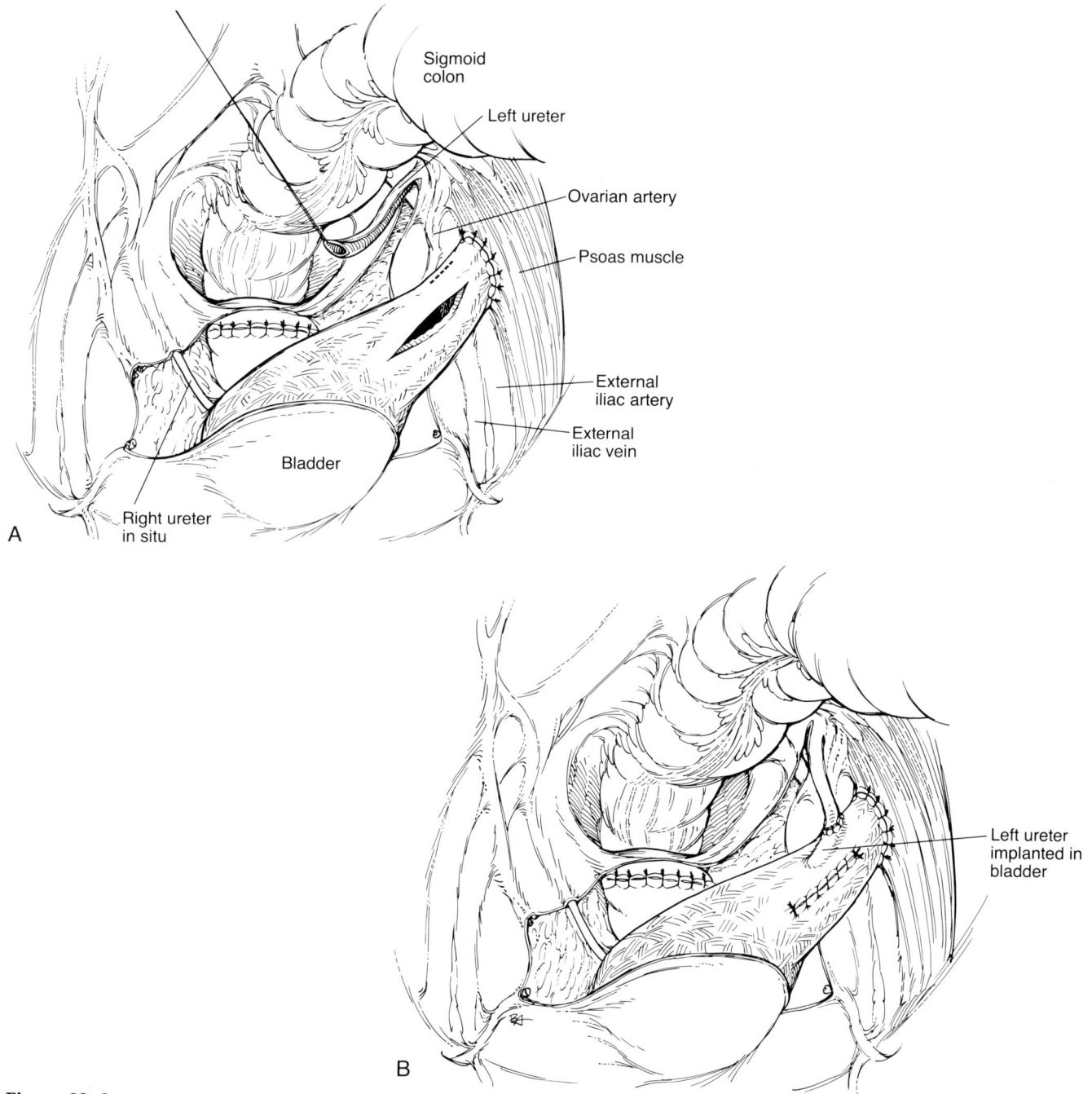

Figure 22–8
Psoas hitch. *A*, The bladder has been sewn to the psoas tendon. The dotted line indicates the site of ureteral reimplantation. *B*, The ureter has been reimplanted through a submucosal tunnel and the remaining bladder defect closed.

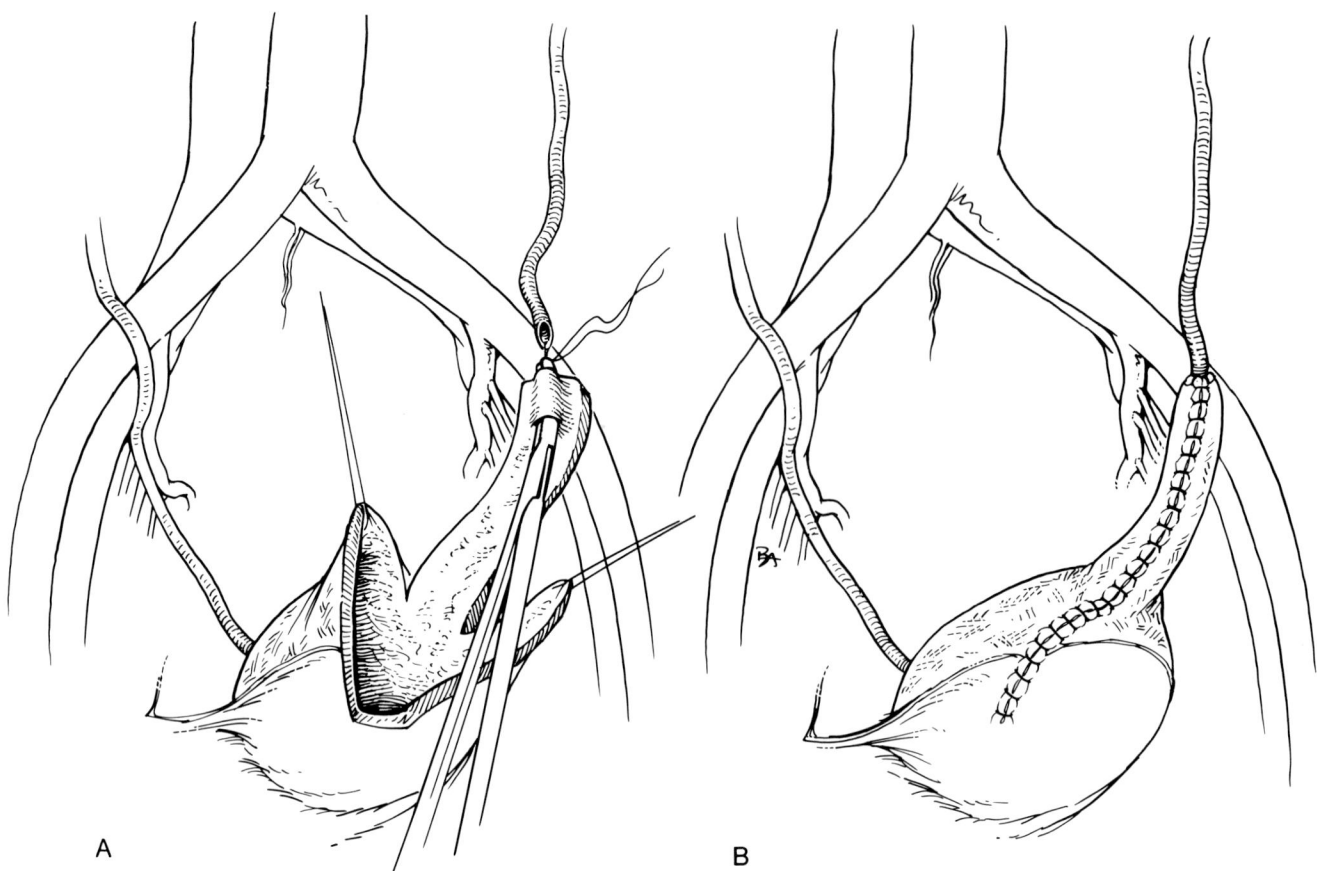

Figure 22-9
Boari flaps. *A*, A tongue of bladder is excised to reach the ureter, which is reimplanted. *B*, The bladder is closed.

and the bladder and flap closed using 3-0 absorbable suture. A Boari flap may be used with a higher pelvic injury than the psoas hitch. Complications may include stricture, fistula formation, or injury to the contralateral ureter.

Ureteroileoneocystostomy

Extensive injury to the ureter, especially in the middle or upper thirds, cannot be mended using the procedures described previously. In such instances, ureteroileoneocystostomy or transureteroureterostomy (described later) is called for. In the former procedure, a bridge between the ureter and bladder is constructed using an isolated segment of intestine, usually the terminal ileum.

According to Moore and coworkers,[13] the first human ureteral repair using a segment of ileum was performed by Shoemaker in 1906. Since then, numerous clinical reports have documented the usefulness and safety of the procedure.[13-16] Segments of colon have also been used for this type of repair,[17] but the middle to proximal ileum remains the most often used intestinal segment. The advantages of ileum for use in this type of repair include its excellent blood supply, peristaltic action, and wide mobility.

This procedure can replace the entire ureter, running the ileum from the renal pelvis to the bladder. Most often, however, the intestine is substituted for the inferior half of the ureter (Fig. 22-10).

Ureteroileoneocystostomy is performed similar to an ileal conduit, except the stoma end is attached to the bladder instead of the skin. The damaged ureteral segment is excised and the distal stump ligated with nonabsorbable suture. The end of the ureter to be placed into the ileal loop must have a good blood supply, and the cut end should bleed freely. In patients who have undergone prior pelvic irradiation, the ureter should be transected at or above the pelvic brim. The ileal segment should then be prepared. The authors prefer to use a portion at least 15 to 20 cm from the ileocecal valve. In previously irradiated patients, a segment free of obvious radiation injury should be used. The authors add 3-5 cm to their estimation of the length from the ureter to the bladder, because the intestine will contract somewhat and both anastomotic sites should be tension-free. The ileal loop is then isolated and its mesentery mobilized. Intestinal continuity is then restored anterior to the isolated segment (see Chapter 21).

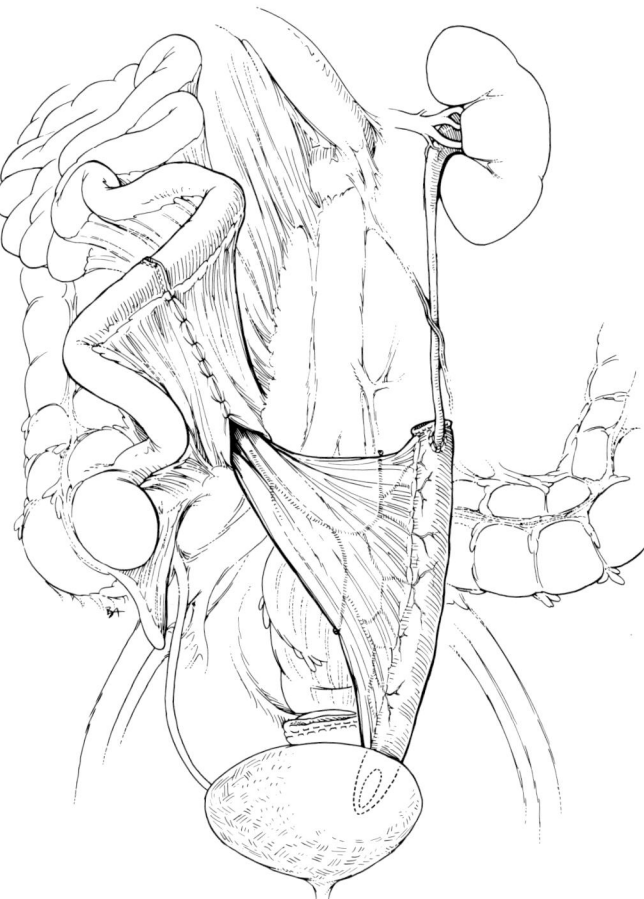

Figure 22–10
Ureteroileoneocystostomy.

Long-term results from this operation are good,[14, 18] but the authors recommend periodic surveillance with IVP. Complications include stricture or fistula formation at the ureteroileal anastomosis, repeated upper tract infection, and stone formation. Significant renal damage, however, is unusual.[18]

Transureteroureterostomy

Like the ileal segment substitution procedure, transureteroureterostomy is useful when the middle third of the ureter is damaged. However, viability of the procedure is dependent upon a normal contralateral ureter and a reasonably normal upper ureter on the involved side. Transureteroureterostomy is simpler to perform than ureteroileoneocystostomy, although both operations have their devotees. In this operation, the remaining portion of a damaged ureter is brought across to create an anastomosis with the contralateral normal ureter (Fig. 22–11).

Like the other procedure described, transureteroureterostomy is not new. According to Udall and associates,[19] the procedure was envisioned by Boari and Casati in 1894. However, it took until 1935 for Higgins to describe its first use in a human.[20] Since then, a number of reports have documented the good results that may be obtained with this procedure.[19, 21–23]

The nonviable portion of the damaged ureter must be excised with the distal stump tied off. Once again, irradiated ureter should not be included in the anastomosis. The damaged ureter should be mobilized only to the extent necessary to reach the ureter on the other side without tension. To preserve the

A small defect is then made in the mesentery of the colon; the ileal segment is carefully passed through so that it may lie in the retroperitoneal position. Care should be taken to avoid twisting the mesentery of the loop. The proximal end should remain stapled or be sewn closed. The distal end, which will be attached to the bladder, is opened and any residual stool or mucus irrigated away. The surgeon should be sure to place the segment in an isoperistaltic fashion. A small defect is then made in the proximal end of the intestine, and, using fine absorbable sutures, a mucosa-to-mucosa everting anastomosis is sewn between the ureter and bowel. The authors prefer to stent this anastomosis, but it is not essential.

A circular button of mucosa is then excised from the bladder wall, as close as possible to the trigone. An anastomosis between the distal end of the loop and the bladder is then hand-sewn using resorbable suture. The technique used is essentially that for an end-to-side anastomosis, described in Chapter 21. The pelvis is drained and a Foley catheter left in place for 1 week. If a ureteral stent is used, it may be removed by means of cystoscopy shortly thereafter.

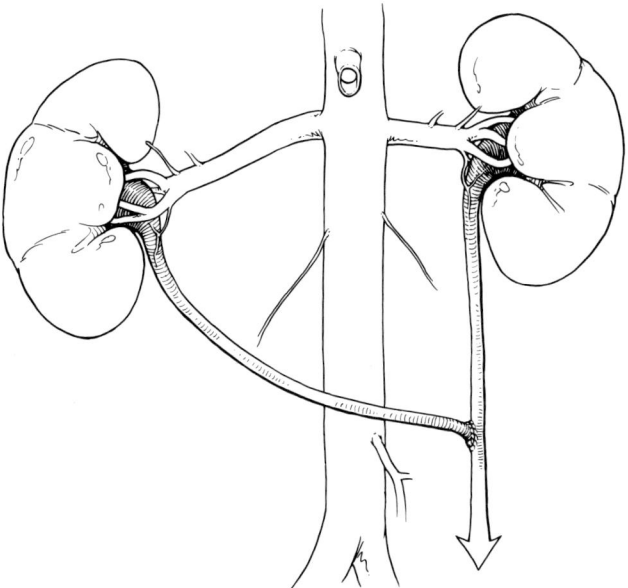

Figure 22–11
Transureteroureterostomy.

blood supply as well as possible, the ureter should not be dissected away from its retroperitoneal tissue. It has been suggested that the infundibulopelvic ligament be brought along with the ureter to provide an additional blood supply.[21] After it is mobilized, the ureter is passed through the retroperitoneal space anterior to the great vessels until it reaches the contralateral ureter. Care should be taken not to run the ureter under the inferior mesenteric artery, which may result in stricture. The operator must also be sure that the donor ureter is not twisted or kinked during this maneuver. The recipient ureter should not be mobilized toward the midline when the damaged ureter is too short, because this may result in angulation; in such cases, the patients are best served by ureteroileoneocystostomy.

The site for anastomosis should be on the medial wall of the recipient ureter. At the recipient site, a longitudinal ureterotomy of approximately 15 mm should be made, corresponding to the spatulated end of the donor ureter. The anastomosis should be hand-sewn using fine absorbable sutures placed close enough to each other to ensure a watertight closure.

The authors prefer to stent these repairs with a double-J multi-holed catheter. The stent should travel from the bladder through the recipient ureter, cross into the donor ureter, and end in the renal pelvis of the donor unit. The anastomotic site should also be drained.

Considering the nature of this procedure, complications are surprisingly infrequent.[21–23] Reflux and infection are not usually a problem, provided that the ureterovesical junction on the recipient side is normal. The recipient ureter has no problem accommodating the additional flow. Problems arise when the blood supply to the distal donor ureter is inadequate or when the surgical technique is faulty.

BLADDER INJURY

Injury to the urinary bladder is infrequent, even during radical oncologic surgery. If promptly recognized, most repairs of such injuries are quite simple and straightforward.

Bladder injury most often occurs during abdominal hysterectomy when the bladder is dissected from its cervical attachments. Injury is more likely to occur when normal anatomy is distorted by tumor, endometriosis, infection, or multiple prior surgeries. Most injuries occur when the surgeon fails to stay within the proper tissue plane and inadvertently enters the bladder.

When opening the bladder flap during the course of hysterectomy, blunt dissection should be avoided. The authors prefer sharp dissection, which allows continued visualization of the avascular plane between the bladder and the cervix. Although blunt dissection works well in most cases, it is when the anatomy is distorted that the technique can run into problems. Meticulous sharp dissection permits the surgeon to stay within the proper tissue plane.

When the surgical plane between the bladder and cervix is totally obscured, it may be helpful to open the dome of the bladder to help guide the dissection. In some instances of extensive tumor infiltration of the anterior cul-de-sac, this may be the only way to safely perform hysterectomy. In some cases of ovarian cancer, a portion of the bladder must be resected to achieve minimal residual tumor volume.

Intraoperative Detection

In patients with distorted pelvic anatomy, often the first sign of bladder injury is direct visualization of the Foley catheter. Small bladder defects, however, may be difficult to document. An intravenous vital dye such as indigo carmine can sometimes demonstrate a hole in the bladder. A more direct method involves instilling saline with methylene blue into the bladder through the Foley catheter. Blue liquid in the pelvis signals the presence of a bladder defect rather than a ureteral injury. Some surgeons prefer to fill the bladder with sterile milk, which they claim is easier to see spilling from the bladder.

Intraoperative cystoscopy can also be used to evaluate the bladder but may have difficulty finding a small defect. The authors prefer to use the cystoscope to verify the site of a small injury and, in particular, to ensure that the trigone is secure.

Postoperative Detection

If a bladder defect is not found during surgery, patients will present either with a fistula, usually vesicovaginal, or with a urinoma. When what is believed to be urine drains from the vagina, the diagnostic work-up is the same as that described in the section on ureteral injury. Initial management of a postoperative vesicovaginal fistula is Foley catheterization or suprapubic drainage, because many smaller fistulas will spontaneously resolve if there is a good blood supply, no infection, and no tumor. Surgical repair is indicated in cases that do not resolve, as discussed in Chapter 12.

Intra-abdominal spillage is of more immediate concern. If the pelvic peritoneum has been closed over the defect, urinoma may present as a pelvic mass and mimic a hematoma or abscess. Eventual fistulization is likely in these cases. A cystogram or IVP may assist in the diagnosis. In urinoma, immediate laparotomy and repair are usually indicated, although vaginal drainage and delayed repair may be more beneficial to some patients.

In some cases, urine spillage will fill the peritoneal cavity. Patients may present with signs of severe peritoneal reaction, but some present only with what appears to be ascites. The diagnosis can be made following IVP or cystogram, which will document contrast material in the peritoneal cavity. This situation cannot be managed conservatively, and immediate laparotomy is indicated.

Bladder Repair

Repair of the bladder injury is based on its location. Cystotomy in the dome of the bladder can be repaired using any number of techniques with excellent results. The authors prefer to use a two-layer inverting closure with 3-0 chromic catgut (Fig. 22–12). The use of suture materials that have a slower resorption time, such as those made from polyglycolic acid, is unnecessary and may predispose the patient to stone formation.

Following cystotomy repair, the authors prefer to rest the bladder for 5–7 days by either Foley catheterization or suprapubic drainage. Draining the pelvis is probably not necessary. Complications rarely follow this procedure, and nearly all patients can expect complete recovery.

Injury to the trigone is another matter. Simple closure of a laceration in the trigone can interfere with the function of the bladder and will not correct an undetected ureteral injury. When the bladder is lacerated near the trigone, the integrity of each ureter must be proved before *and after* repair. This can be done in two ways. The dome of the bladder may be opened (if it is not already) and repair of the trigone carried out with the ureters under direct visualization. Ureteral catheters can be placed to ensure that the ureters are not strictured or severely angulated. If the repair comes close to the ureteral orifice, a ureteral catheter will also ensure that the ureter will not become obstructed secondary to postoperative edema.

If the patient has been placed in a modified lithotomy position for the procedure, repair may be performed abdominally while an assistant observes through the cystoscope. Ureteral catheters may also be placed at that time.

Repair of a trigone laceration should take place with complete exposure of the defect and good hemostasis. This may entail additional dissection of the bladder base, which carries further potential for ureteral injury. Trigone laceration repair should be performed only by those thoroughly familiar with the anatomy of the region.

When the injury involves the ureteral orifice, the repair is more complex. In most cases, the pelvic ureter should be transected where it enters the bladder and reimplantation performed as described previously.

When infection is absent and hemostasis good, the great majority of patients recover from bladder laceration with no functional deficit. For injuries of the trigone, an IVP should be obtained after removal of stents and drains.

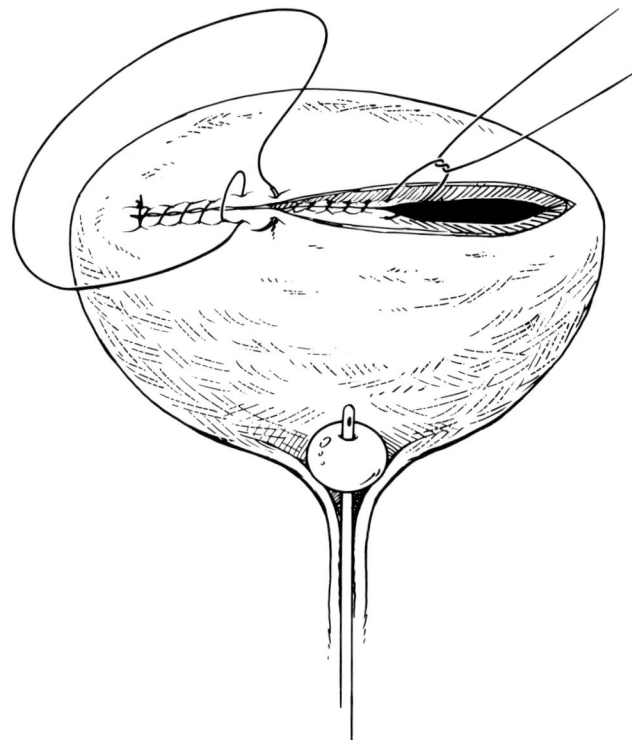

Figure 22–12
Two-layer inverting closure of the bladder.

URINARY DIVERSION

In women who have undergone cystectomy or who have a nonfunctional bladder, urinary diversion continues to present a challenge to pelvic surgeons. In the patient with gynecologic cancer, complete urinary diversion is necessary after pelvic exenteration. Diversion is also needed in patients who have severe radiation-induced injury to the bladder (see later). Despite great advances in urinary diversion in the past few decades, no single method is ideal. Surgeons must be familiar with the various procedures and tailor their approach to each patient.

Nephrostomy

Percutaneous nephrostomy tube placement is a relatively simple technique that has been mastered by interventional radiologists. Guided by fluoroscopy and ultrasound, a needle is used to locate the renal pelvis. A guide wire is passed through the needle, and the catheter is then inserted into the renal pelvis over the wire. This approach is useful for diversion of an obstructed kidney. If the ureter is not obstructed, significant amounts of urine will continue to pass down that channel.

Nephrostomy is a safe procedure and has been associated with few acute complications.[24, 25] Injury to the renal vessels may result in hematoma formation.[26] If the kidney is infected, significant bacteremia may occur during the procedure, creating the potential for sepsis. Nephrostomy is most useful for temporary diversion of an obstructed renal unit prior to definitive repair. Long-term complications include chronic pyelonephritis, which occurs in nearly all patients. The tube itself becomes encrusted and eventually obstructed. In most patients, the tubes must be changed every 3 months. After several months, many patients experience leakage of urine around the tubes and the tubes sometimes fall out (usually, it seems, at 3 A.M.). Therefore, nephrostomy should be considered a temporary method at best.

Cutaneous Ureterostomy

The technique of cutaneous ureterostomy involves bringing the end of the ureter up to the skin surface. Cutaneous ureterostomy is mentioned only to condemn it, because the associated morbidity precludes its practice in modern medicine.

Stomal problems are common. Ureters at the skin level will often undergo stenosis or retraction. Most patients suffer from skin irritation around the ureterostomy, and it is difficult to fit an appliance to the stomal site. Chronic infection is also a significant problem. The poor outcomes achieved by cutaneous ureterostomy led to the development of the operations described in the following sections.

Ureterosigmoidostomy

According to Blandy,[27] ureterosigmoidostomy was first conceived by Simon in 1852. In this procedure, the ureters are directly implanted into the sigmoid colon, where urine is then mixed into the fecal stream (Fig. 22–13). Continence is maintained (theoretically, at least) by the anal sphincter. It is also possible to direct the ureters into the colon in a patient with an end-sigmoid colostomy following a procedure such as pelvic exenteration. As one might imagine, the main problem with this procedure is ascending infection. This was partially addressed by Coffey in 1921,[28] when he described an antireflux valve created through a tunneled anastomosis. Ureterosigmoidostomy became the standard method of urinary diversion during the first half of the twentieth century, and many surgeons documented what they considered to be satisfactory results.[29–31]

The problem of ascending infection has never been solved satisfactorily, and many patients suffer from repeated bouts of pyelonephritis. The intact colon also has significant absorptive capacity, and

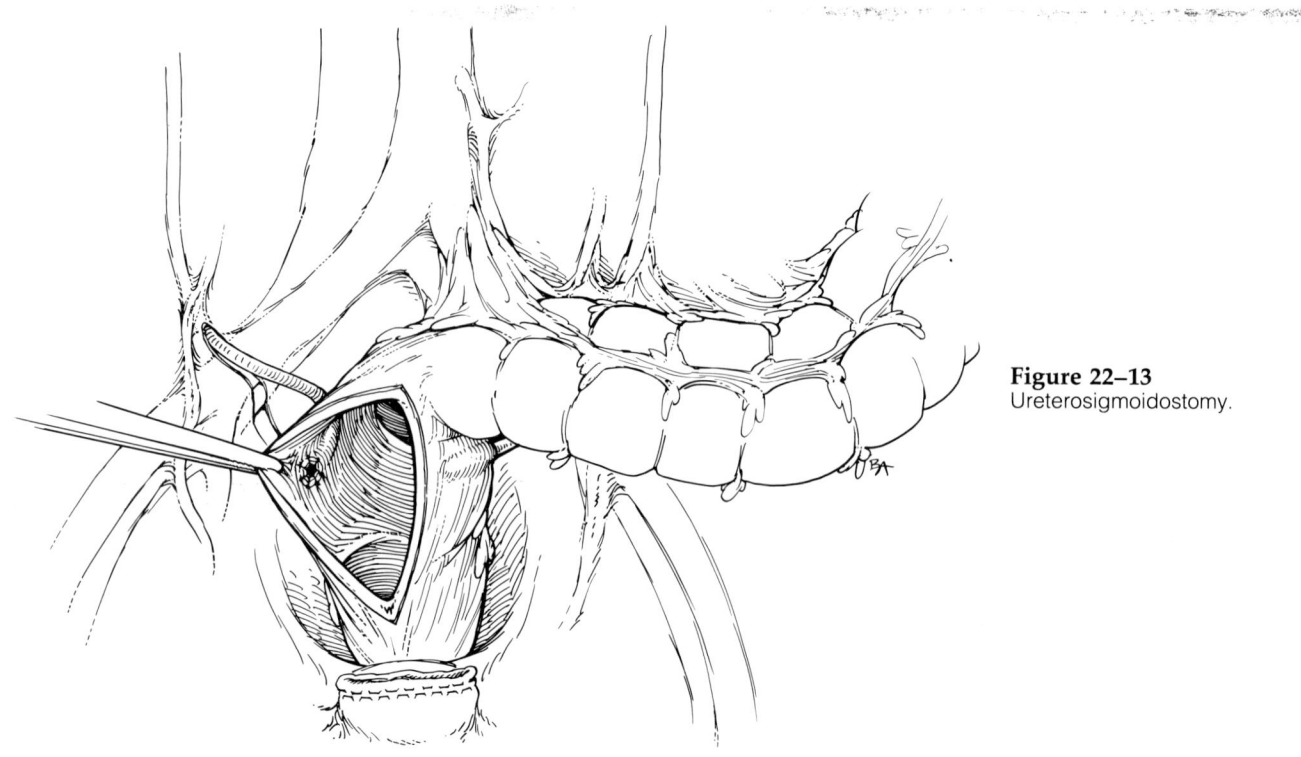

Figure 22–13
Ureterosigmoidostomy.

most patients have some degree of electrolyte disturbance, most notably hyperchloremic acidosis.[31] Incontinence is also a problem for many patients, especially at night.

In an attempt to decrease the problem of infection, some patients have undergone a descending colostomy in which the ureters are plugged into a sigmoid pouch. This decreased the incidence of infection, because the fecal stream was diverted. However, the patients were required to have an external stoma, and the incontinence problem was not solved.

Brunschwig used ureterosigmoidostomy during his early experience with pelvic exenteration with unsatisfactory results.[32] The reader can appreciate, then, the tremendous advance that urinary conduits and reservoirs represent.

Urinary Conduit

The need for diversion following pelvic exenteration and the development of a satisfactory external appliance led Eugene Bricker to develop the ileal conduit in 1950.[33] The procedure became the standard technique of urinary diversion for the next 40 years. At MD Anderson, the most common indication for ileal conduit has been reconstruction following pelvic exenteration, though some patients have undergone creation of a conduit for severe radiation injury or for palliation of disease recurrence.[34] Although the procedure may be performed for a number of other reasons in patients with gynecologic conditions, the following discussion is based on experience with patients undergoing pelvic exenteration.

Preoperative Preparation

Prior to undertaking conduit diversion, the patient should undergo extensive counseling regarding the procedure and the changes it will bring to the patient's lifestyle. Both the surgeon and an enterostomal therapist should be involved in this process. The stomal therapist has an especially important role in the preoperative assessment of the abdomen. To achieve proper placement of the stoma, the abdominal wall should be inspected with the patient standing, sitting, and supine and the skinfolds noted carefully. The level at which the patient wears her slacks and skirts must also be taken into account. If possible, the stomal therapist should mark more than one site on the abdominal wall suitable for stomal placement so that the surgeon has some latitude to deal with intraoperative factors such as the length and mobility of the intestinal segment and the thickness of the abdominal wall. Proper placement of a urinary stoma is perhaps of greater importance than placement of a colostomy, because even a minor skinfold can cause a very significant leak of urine. The discomfort and embarrassment of such a problem often result in a house-bound patient and psychosocial as well as physical pathology.

Preoperative evaluation must also include assessment of the kidneys and ureters. The function of the kidneys should be checked prior to surgery. Especially in patients with recurrent cervical cancer, it is not uncommon to have some degree of hydroureter. If the obstruction is relatively acute, the kidney should be capable of nearly full function following diversion.[34] However, if the renal unit has been obstructed for a prolonged period, it is doubtful that significant function can be regained. Preoperative IVP assesses the function of an obstructed side and also reveals ureteral anomalies.

When there is some doubt regarding the potential of an obstructed kidney, a nuclear renal scan may give more functional information than IVP. Using a renal scan, a percentage of the total glomerular filtration rate may be assigned to each kidney. A kidney that is "dead" will be identified by this test, thereby letting the surgeon avoid its inclusion in a conduit. In general, if a kidney carries out at least 15–20% of the total glomerular filtration, it should be preserved and included in the conduit; when the functional capacity is less than this, the deficient side should probably not be included.

Prior to surgery, the patients should undergo a complete mechanical and antibiotic bowel preparation, as outlined in Chapter 21. If there is evidence of pyelonephritis, a full course of antibiotic therapy is also indicated.

Technique of Ileal Conduit

In the case of pelvic exenteration, the extirpative phase of the procedure should be completed before the urinary diversion. In most cases, the ureters have been transected at the pelvic brim. To include a portion of irradiated ureter within the anastomosis is hazardous because of the potential for anastomotic breakdown.

The procedure is illustrated in Figure 22–14. The terminal ileum should be carefully inspected for radiation damage, and if significant injury is found, another intestinal segment should be used. If the ileum is not satisfactory, the ideal choice would be a colonic segment. The use of jejunum should be avoided, because it creates a greater chance of long-term electrolyte disturbance.[35] If the ileum is in good condition, the authors prefer to use a segment approximately 20 cm long, with the distal line of resection about 15 cm from the ileocecal valve.

The ileal segment should be isolated and intestinal continuity restored by either a stapled or a hand-sewn technique, as described in Chapter 21. The use

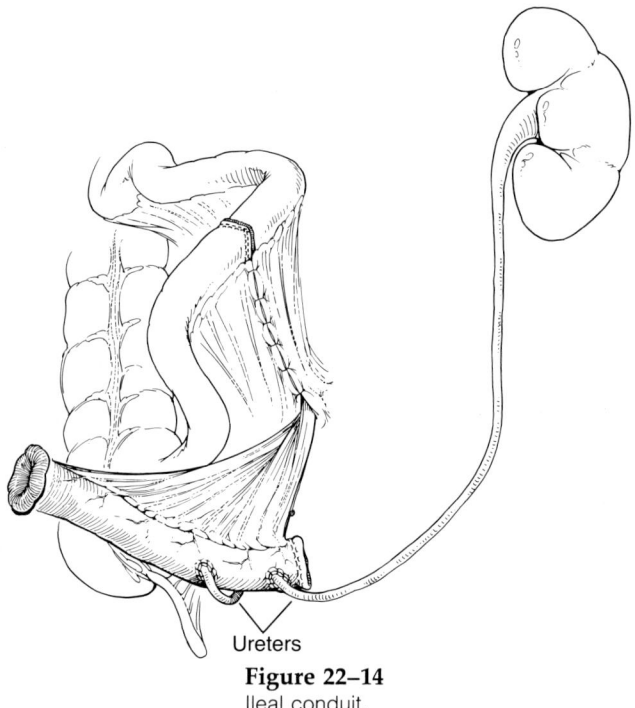

Figure 22–14
Ileal conduit.

of staples in conduit formation has been the source of some controversy, though a number of surgeons report good results.[36, 37] Some have expressed concern regarding the use of staples that may remain in the butt end of the conduit and thus have the potential to form stones.[38] The authors have found that using a GIA stapler, with its everting closure of the butt end, is satisfactory and have not seen stone formation. After healing, there should be no exposed staple within the lumen of the conduit. The authors restore intestinal continuity by means of a stapled side-to-side anastomosis.

When dividing the mesentery, one should take care not to devascularize the conduit while trying to achieve maximum mobility. The mesenteric defect in the remaining bowel should then be closed anterior to the conduit. The stomal end of the conduit is then opened after ensuring that the flow of urine will be in the direction of peristalsis. Any residual intestinal contents should be irrigated away.

Attention is then turned to the ureters, which should be mobilized as much as needed to reach the butt end of the conduit without tension or sharp angulation. Keeping in mind that dissection can decrease the vascular supply to the ureter, excessive mobilization should be avoided. Every effort should be made to preserve the periureteral adventitia. The distal end of the ureter should be trimmed and an adequate blood supply ensured. Further handling of this area should be kept to a minimum.

A small transmural defect is then made in the conduit wall near the butt end and a Silastic catheter pulled through. This stent is fixed in place with a single 4-0 chromic catgut suture. The ureter is then threaded on the catheter, and ureteroconduit anastomosis is completed using the mucosa-to-mucosa anastomotic technique described by Bricker.[39] This procedure is repeated with the other ureter. The stomal end of the conduit is then carefully brought through the abdominal wall, and a "rosebud" stoma is created as described in Chapter 21. Much attention has been given to the technique of ureteral anastomosis and a number of variations described.[40–42] However, there is little evidence that the more involved techniques improve on Bricker's direct method.

Postoperative nutritional support is of great importance in these patients. Because nearly all patients with gynecologic cancer will have received prior radiation therapy, the small bowel anastomosis has a higher than average risk of breakdown or obstruction. The authors routinely support patients by total parenteral nutrition and give them no oral feedings for at least 2 weeks following surgery to give the bowel anastomosis time to heal.

The ureteral stents will be spontaneously extruded 10–14 days after surgery, when the chromic suture dissolves. The temptation to pull on the stents should be avoided. The ureteral stents have several functions. They ensure that urine will pass from each kidney in the immediate postoperative period. That each kidney is making urine can also be verified when the stents are in place. Though stenting is routinely used in the larger clinical series,[34, 43] the operation can be successfully completed without it.[44] In a comparison of the results of stented versus nonstented anastomoses, Beddoe and coworkers[45] found that those patients who were stented had significantly fewer complications. Though a nonrandomized review, this report is important because all but one of the patients were previously irradiated, a recognized risk factor not often taken into account in the urologic literature.

Colon Conduits

As experience with ileal conduits increased, the shortcomings of the procedure became apparent and it was recognized that certain patients were not good candidates for the operation. A major disadvantage to the use of ileum in a conduit is the resulting small bowel anastomosis. This is of particular concern in previously irradiated patients.[34, 46, 47] The other concern has been the long-term deterioration of the kidneys observed in patients with ileal diversions,[48, 49] owing in most part to chronic infection. As a result, interest in colonic segments for use in the urinary conduit increased.

The sigmoid conduit was first described in 1967 by Mogg.[50] Since then, numerous reports have

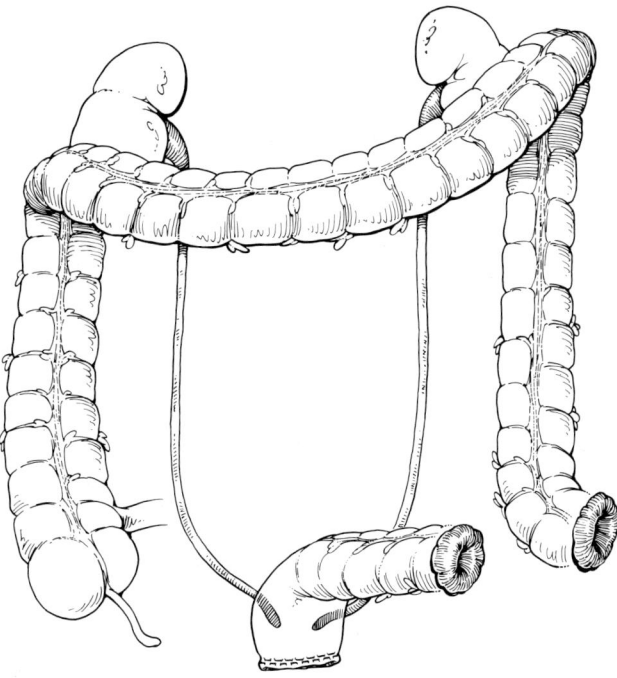

Figure 22–15
Sigmoid conduit.

documented the safety and feasibility of the procedure.[40, 44, 51–53] The sigmoid conduit has been successful in patients with gynecologic cancers in the course of pelvic exenteration.[34, 54]

The main advantage to the sigmoid conduit is the avoidance of an intestinal anastomosis (Fig. 22–15). Most patients who undergo pelvic exenteration will also have a colostomy; therefore, the use of 15–20 cm of sigmoid colon is of little consequence. The segment to be used for the conduit is divided from the descending colon, which is made into an end-colostomy. It is often necessary to mobilize the splenic flexure to achieve a tension-free colostomy. The remainder of the procedure is carried out in a fashion similar to that for an ileal conduit. For those surgeons who are fond of an antireflux anastomosis, a tunneled technique is more easily carried out with the colon.[40, 52]

There are some disadvantages to the sigmoid diversion, especially in women who have had prior pelvic irradiation, which of course always includes the sigmoid colon. If there is significant radiation-induced change or if the patient is obese, mobility of the sigmoid mesentery may be limited. Even when mobility is ideal, it is difficult to place the stoma above the umbilicus. Especially in elderly patients, the upper abdomen may be the only site for satisfactory appliance placement. It has been suggested that stomal complications are more frequent with the sigmoid loop.[34] Finally, in long-term follow-up, the results are nearly identical to those obtained using ileal diversion.[55]

The use of the transverse colon overcomes some of these disadvantages (Fig. 22–16). The procedure was first reported by Schmidt and colleagues,[46] and good results have since been reported by others, even for patients with gynecologic cancers.[43–47] The authors use the segment of transverse colon supplied by the middle colic artery. Because of the redundancy of the transverse colon, the portion for the conduit can be removed easily. Colocolostomy is easily accomplished, and although this is a bowel anastomosis, it is outside the radiated field and heals well with few complications. The transverse colon conduit is highly mobile, and the stoma may be placed nearly anywhere on the abdominal wall. There are few stomal complications, and the ureterocolonic anastomosis has a better chance of healing in an intestinal segment that has never been irradiated. Because radiation therapy inevitably affects the terminal ileum and sigmoid colon, the transverse colon conduit has been the urinary diversion of choice at MD Anderson for the past 10 years.

Complications of Urinary Conduits

Early reports noted that early and late complication rates in urinary diversion were as high as 50% each.[56–58] More recent reports give a much lower complication rate; this may be attributed to improve-

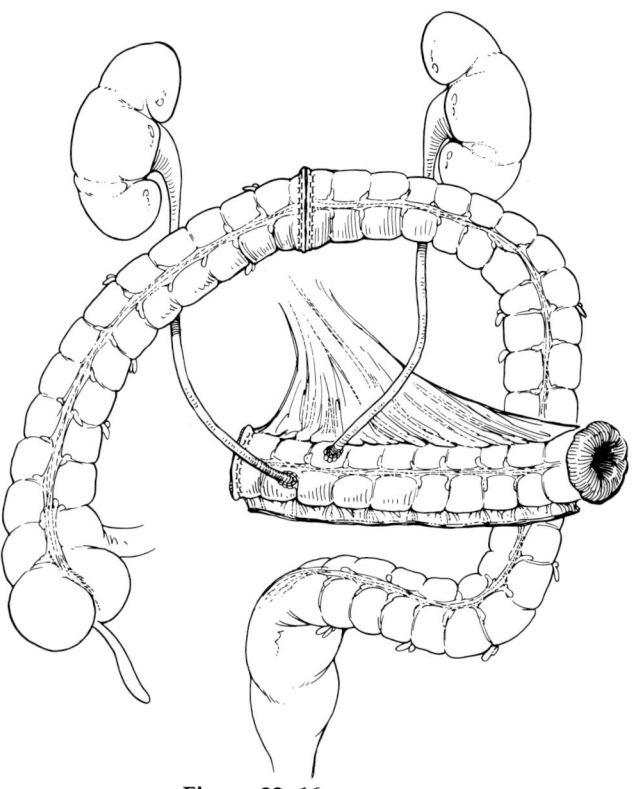

Figure 22–16
Transverse colon conduit.

ments in postoperative care, especially nutritional support.[34, 59]

Infections. Despite the use of perioperative prophylactic antibiotics, many women develop urinary tract infections before leaving the hospital. Long-term chronic infections have always been a major problem. There are no accurate statistics regarding the true incidence of chronic pyelonephritis in these patients. The appliance is always colonized, and accurate cultures of the upper tract are difficult to obtain. To some degree, at least, infection is due to stasis, and intestinal segments used to construct conduits should be no longer than necessary. Partial obstruction at the ureteroconduit anastomosis may also contribute to infection. When patients present with repeated episodes of upper urinary tract infection, they may benefit from chronic antibiotic prophylaxis.

Obstruction. In a series of patients treated at MD Anderson, the incidence of obstruction at the ureteroconduit anastomosis was 8%.[34] Although many cases occur during the perioperative period, some may have a gradual onset and occur years later. The authors recommend annual examination with an IVP or renal scan for all their conduit patients. Factors contributing to obstruction include poor surgical technique, prior irradiation, infection, and malnutrition.

Initial management of these obstructions is percutaneous nephrostomy. A renal scan should be performed when a long-standing obstruction is suspected, because the kidney may have no residual function to save. When the obstruction is partial, it may be possible to pass a stent through this area. This may be done in a retrograde fashion (through the conduit by means of a cystoscope or pediatric sigmoidoscope) or an antegrade fashion (through a percutaneous nephrostomy under fluoroscopic guidance). Stent placement is a temporary measure only. These tubes frequently become blocked and increase the risk of infection. Most patients should undergo conduit revision as the definitive procedure.

Anastomotic Leaks. Anastomotic leaks are an infrequent complication but one that requires prompt intervention. If too ill for surgery, these patients may be stented and the site of leakage drained. Conduit revision should be performed.

Stomal Complications. Stomal complications of urinary conduits are similar to those outlined in Chapter 21. Urinary stomas are particularly prone to stenosis. The resulting increase in back pressure on the urinary tract increases the risks of infection. Stomal revision should be performed when stenosis is significant. It is normal for the stoma of a colon conduit to shrink somewhat, but it should always admit the tip of a finger. The risk of stomal complications may be increased by the use of irradiated bowel.

Electrolyte Imbalance. Changes in the absorptive capacity of the intestine can adversely affect the serum electrolyte balance. This effect is most pronounced when using the more proximal segments, with hypochloremic acidosis the result.[35] These changes are often transient because the absorptive surface area of the conduit decreases over time.[60, 61] Electrolyte disturbances are rare in colon conduits.

Continent Diversions in Women

The urinary conduit was a major advance in reconstructive surgery, but it requires the patient to constantly wear an external appliance. It was felt that the ideal bladder substitute would provide a continence mechanism of some sort. It has been well established that women who undergo a urinary conduit procedure suffer from poor body image and have difficulty with sexual adjustment. Many fear leakage and odor and avoid social situations. In comparison, patients who undergo continent diversions benefit from an overall improvement in the quality of life.[62–65] These patients report improvements in sex life and body image, and 97% would undergo reoperation to revise a reservoir rather than revert to wearing an appliance. The development of a continent urinary diversion was a major advance in urologic surgery.

About the same time that Bricker[39] developed the ileal conduit, Gilchrist and associates[66] described a continent diversion using a pouch constructed from the cecum and terminal ileum. Though the patient still had a stoma, it was designed to be continent, a mechanism predicated on a competent ileocecal valve. At regular intervals, the patient would insert a catheter through the stoma to drain the cecal reservoir at a socially acceptable time. The procedure was not widely used because of its complexity and concerns about continence and reflux in this high-pressure reservoir.

In 1969, Nils Kock made a major advance toward developing a functionally continent diversion with his description of a reservoir constructed from detubularized bowel.[67] To decrease the pressures created by the peristaltic actions of the intestine, Kock split the intestine along the antimesenteric border and folded the split intestine twice. Once sewn together, the discordant contractions of the resulting pouch canceled each other out, thus producing a low-pressure reservoir. Borrowing the concept of an intussuscepted nipple valve from Basso[68] and from Smith and Hinman,[69] the Kock pouch was developed for continent urinary diversion (Fig. 22–17).[70–72] The nipple valves provide continence and prevent reflux, and the detubularized pouch serves as a low-pressure reservoir.

The procedure does have some drawbacks. Creation of the nipple valves is complex, and a surgeon must perform a number of these procedures before becoming proficient. Creating the Kock pouch is also a lengthy procedure, adding about 3 hours to the time needed for a standard urinary diversion. When one considers performing both this procedure and a pelvic exenteration, the added time is an important factor for both the patient and the surgeon.

The Kock procedure also requires the sacrifice of a significant length of small intestine, which may be difficult to spare in the previously irradiated patient. The Kock pouch also has a significant incidence of valve failure necessitating reoperation.[73, 74] As experience with the procedure has increased, the complication rate has decreased;[75, 76] nevertheless, the complexity of the procedure impedes its widespread acceptance.

The concept of the cecal reservoir in which continence is achieved by the ileocecal valve continued to attract attention.[77–79] Unpredictable continence mechanisms, ureteral reflux, and a high-pressure reservoir remained major problems. In 1987, Rowland and coworkers[80] described the Indiana continent urinary reservoir. In this procedure, the cecum was transformed into a low-pressure reservoir by using a patch of ileum to form a nontubular bowel segment (Fig. 22–18). Continence was provided by the ileocecal valve augmented by a plication of the ileal lumen.

The Indiana pouch was modified by Bejany and Politano (Fig. 22–19).[81] A portion of intestine from the terminal ileum 20 cm from the ileocecal valve through to the mid-portion of the transverse colon is isolated. The proximal ileum is anastomosed to the transverse colon to restore intestinal continuity, and an appendectomy is performed. The colonic segment is then opened along its antimesenteric border through its entire length. It is folded over in half, and the back wall is sewn or stapled closed. The authors prefer to use a single layer of running 3-0 absorbable suture for this closure. The two ureters are brought through the posterior wall of the pouch and sewn in place using fine sutures. The anterior wall of the pouch is then closed. The terminal ileum segment becomes the stoma. Using the GIA stapler, the ileum is tapered to improve the continence mechanism. Finally, three silk pursestring sutures are placed at the base of the ileocecal valve. The detubularized colon pouch exerts low pressure, which results in minimal reflux into the ureters. The ileal segment exerts high pressure, which maintains continence. The patient catheterizes herself using a rubber catheter as required.

This Indiana pouch has proved successful in patients with recurrent cervical cancer who undergo pelvic exenteration.[82] This procedure is more simple to learn than creation of the Kock pouch and takes less time to perform.

The long-term consequences of continent diversion remain to be studied. It is hoped that compli-

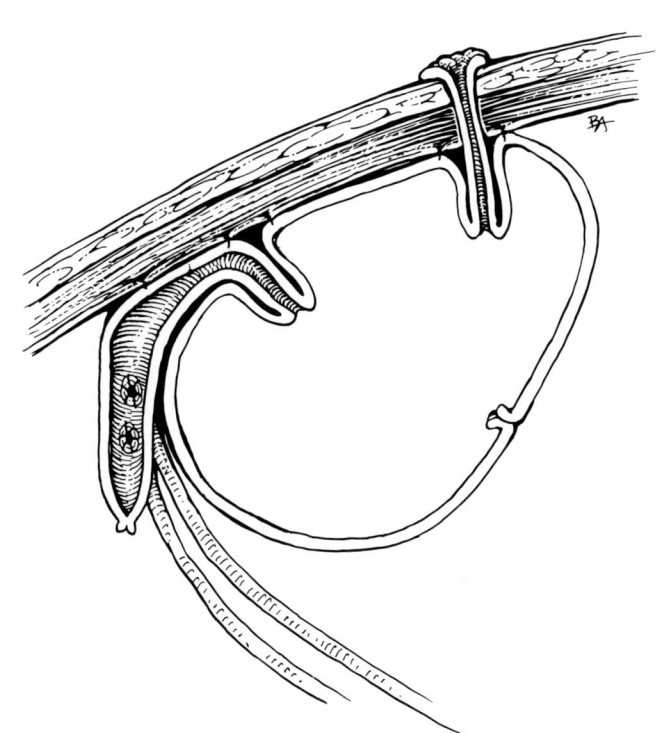

Figure 22–17
Kock pouch.

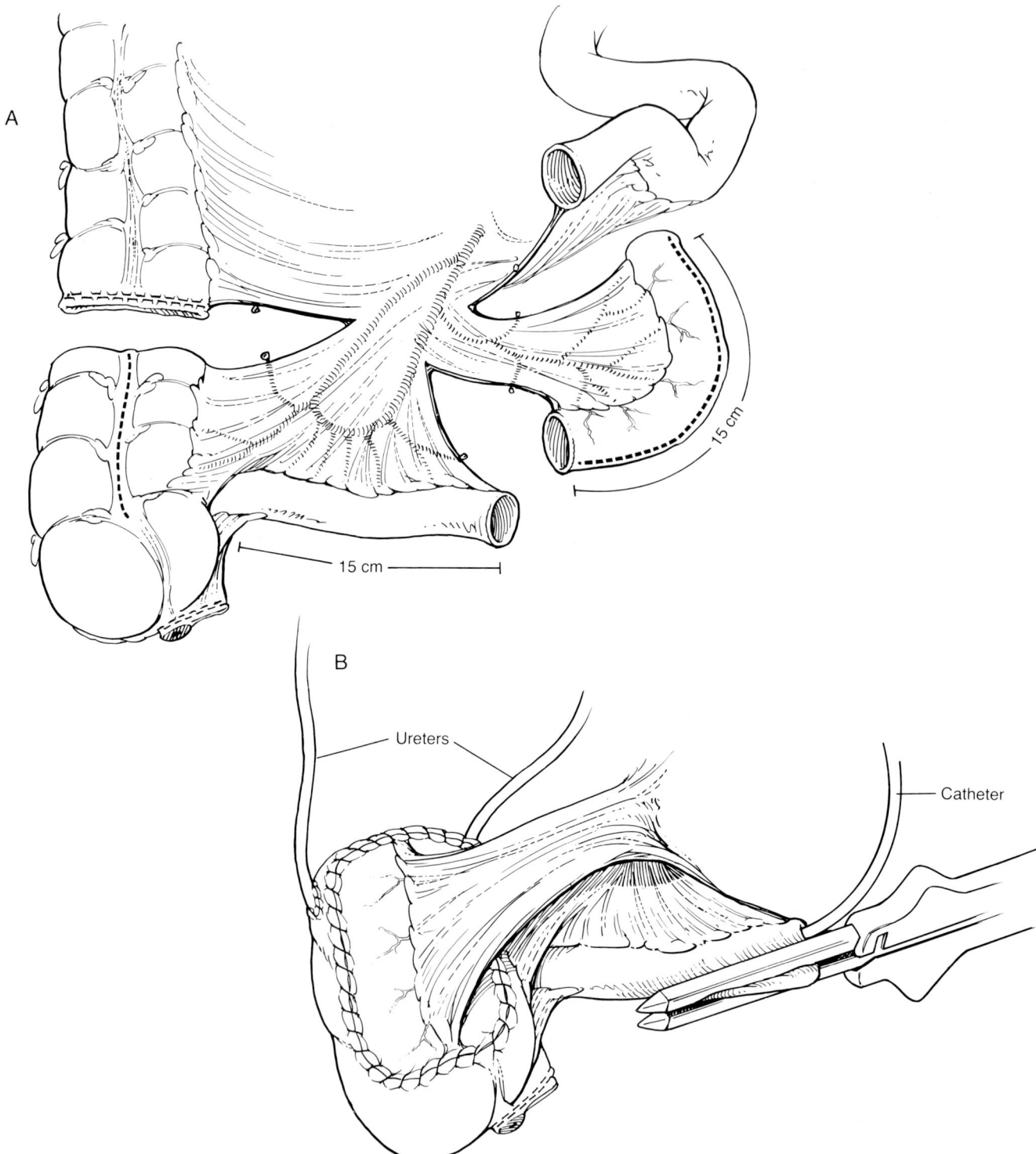

Figure 22–18
Ileocecal reservoir. *A,* The cecum and terminal ileum are isolated. A separate length of ileum is also isolated. *B,* The separate ileum is opened and placed as a "patch" on the cecum. The ureters have been implanted in the cecum.

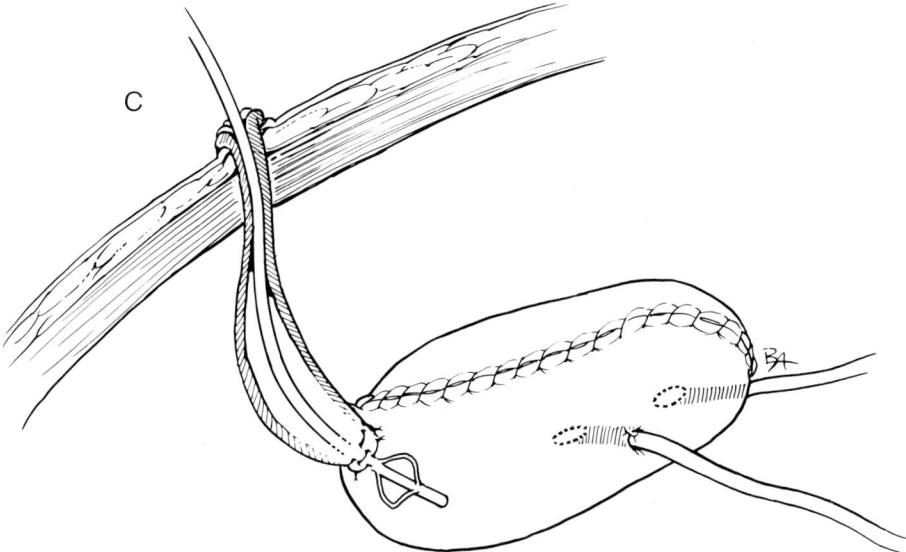

Figure 22–18 *Continued*
C, The ileal end is brought to the skin surface as a continent stoma.

cations of urinary conduits, such as renal deterioration, may be avoided by the use of continent procedures.

Many patients gain an undeniable improvement in quality of life with a continent diversion. The use of the procedure should be tailored to the needs of the patient. The authors have found that some women prefer an appliance to intermittent catheterization and that some are unable to catheterize themselves. This group is clearly in the minority, however, and it is expected that the use of continent urinary diversions will continue to increase.

UROLOGIC COMPLICATIONS OF RADIATION THERAPY

Irradiation of the pelvis is common in the treatment of gynecologic cancer. Though effects on the intestine are of most concern, the bladder and lower ureters receive a major dose of radiation. The gynecologist should be familiar with the acute and chronic effects of radiation on the urinary tract and the approaches to treatment.

During external-beam radiation therapy to the pelvis, patients will sometimes note urinary frequency. In the majority, this is a short-lived side effect that rapidly resolves upon completion of therapy. A small percentage of patients, however, may develop chronic problems.[83] Some women develop a contracted fibrotic bladder, leading to frequent urination and in some cases incontinence. Hemorrhagic cystitis is sometimes present; for some patients, this may be an incidental microscopic finding, although occasional severe exacerbations with gross hematuria may occur. When the bleeding is significant enough to cause clot formation in the bladder, emergency intervention is indicated.

Hemorrhagic cystitis due to radiation therapy presents a challenging treatment situation.[84] Cystoscopy should be carried out with clot evacuation. If the bladder can be appropriately visualized, a search for recurrent disease or other lesions should be made, with indicated biopsies performed. Often, the operator will see an edematous bladder with prominent friable bleeding vessels. Following clot evacuation, patients may benefit from continuous inpatient irrigation of the bladder using a three-way Foley catheter. A variety of solutions have been proposed for the irrigant; those most commonly used include one-quarter-strength acetic acid and potassium permanganate (1:10,000), both of which act as mild oxidizing agents to stop the bleeding. There are those that suggest that simple saline irrigation may be just as effective. Extreme care should be taken that blood clots do not obstruct the outflow tract of the catheter during irrigation; continued influx of fluid in this circumstance may lead to bladder perforation. When the urine has cleared, the irrigation may be discontinued.

Those patients with hemorrhagic cystitis who do not respond to irrigation may be treated using a variety of techniques, all of which have varied success. Occasionally, electrocoagulation of bleeding vessels under cystoscopic visualization can be helpful. Tamponade of the bladder using the Helmstein balloon technique is also effective when performed by experienced hands.[85] As a measure of last resort, instillation of formalin into the bladder can be performed.[86] Because of the severe pain associated with this procedure, it must be performed when the patient is under general anesthesia. It is also usually recommended that Fogarty catheters be inserted into

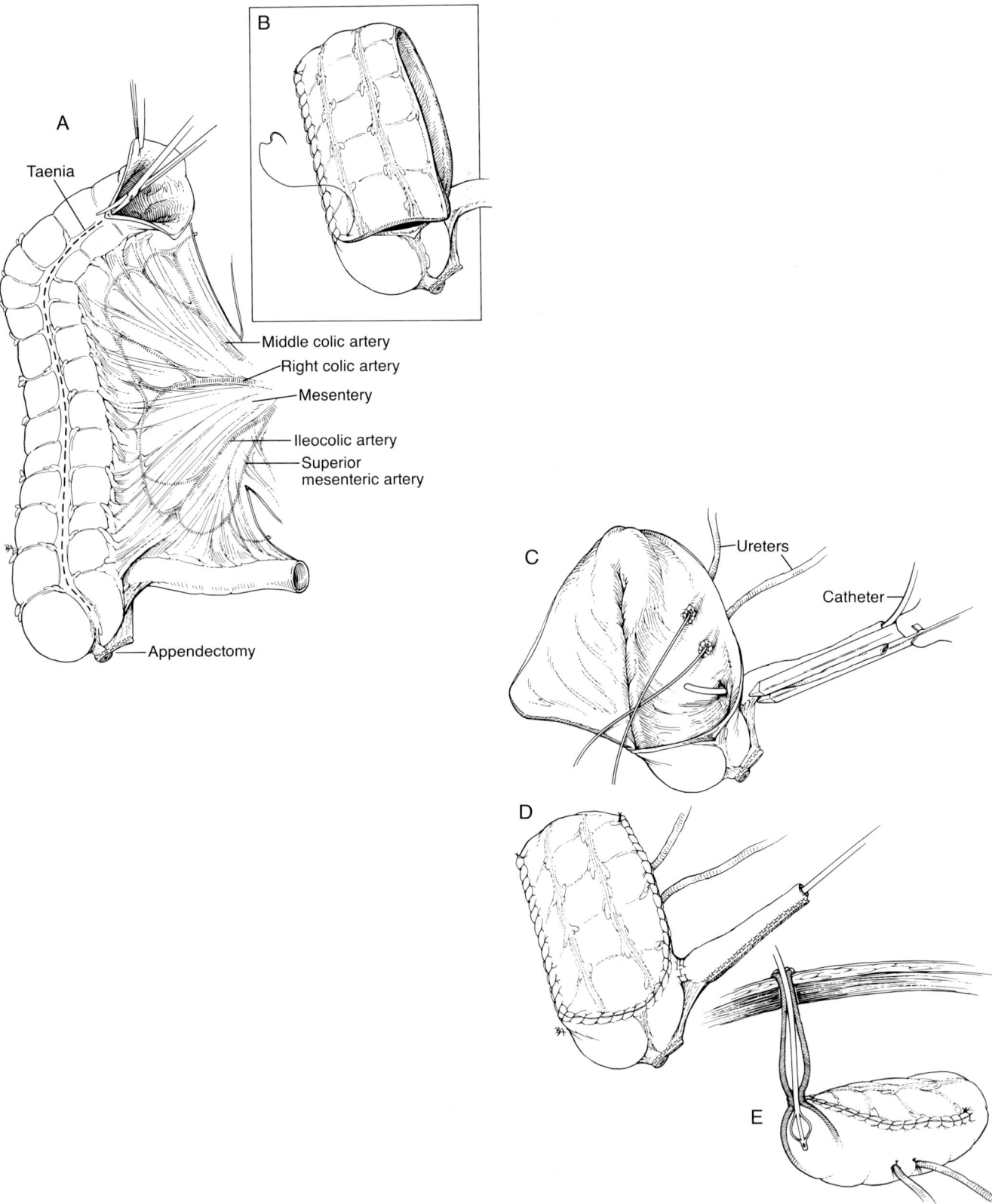

Figure 22–19
Indiana pouch. *A*, The terminal ileum and ascending colon are isolated. The colon is opened along its entire antimesenteric border. Appendectomy is performed. *B*, The colon is folded over to create a detubularized reservoir. The posterior wall is closed. *C*, The ureters are brought through the posterior wall of the colon and sutured in place. A GIA stapler is used to taper the ileum over a catheter. *D*, The closure of the colon is completed. Three silk pursestring sutures are placed at the ileocecal valve to ensure continence. *E*, The ileal end is brought to the skin, and a drain is left in place during the postoperative period. Thereafter, intermittent catheterization is performed.

the ureteral orifices to prevent reflux of the formalin.[87] Reflux of formalin into the renal pelvis can result in papillary necrosis and renal failure. Also, one must be extremely cautious about the pressure under which the formalin is injected, because bladder rupture and death have resulted from this treatment. Although formalin instillation often stops the bleeding, the resultant scarred and contracted bladder is frequently nonfunctional. Those patients who have persistent bleeding may ultimately require cystectomy with urinary diversion.

More severe cases of bladder injury due to radiation can result in focal necrosis. Depending on the site of necrosis, this may result in perforation of the bladder and subsequent peritonitis. Most often, necrosis occurs at the interface between the bladder and the vaginal vault, resulting in the formation of a vesicovaginal fistula. As with rectovaginal fistulas, these defects may be difficult to repair. Initial treatment should include drainage through a Foley catheter and local care to the perineum to prevent skin breakdown. Indicated biopsies should be performed to eliminate the possibility of recurrent disease. Unfortunately, most radiation-induced vesicovaginal fistulas do not heal spontaneously. Surgical repair can be performed by swinging a flap of healthy tissue into the area, such as the bulbocavernosus flap or an omental pedicle graft. In many patients, especially those with larger fistulas, repair cannot be effected and surgical urinary diversion is required.

As noted in the section dealing with ureteral injury, ureteral obstruction following pelvic radiation therapy most often connotes recurrent cancer. There are some cases, however, in which the obstruction is due to radiation fibrosis. This is a diagnosis of exclusion, and the patient should undergo the appropriate diagnostic studies and biopsy procedures to dismiss the possibility of recurrent tumor. Initial management of ureteral obstruction from radiation fibrosis depends on the function remaining in the occluded renal unit. In women with a long-standing obstruction, salvage of significant function is not likely. Relief of an occlusion of 3 months' duration or less may allow the affected kidney to have nearly complete recovery. A nuclear renal scan may be helpful in determining the relative function of the obstructed side.

Initial management is the insertion of a ureteral catheter by means of cystoscopy. Not surprisingly, the attempt is often unsuccessful, in which case percutaneous nephrostomy should be performed. Occasionally, antegrade insertion of a ureteral catheter is then successful. Although such catheters may be left in place for months at a time, problems such as repeated infection and obstruction make definitive repair desirable. At best difficult and often impossible, ureteral repair in the previously irradiated patient should be attempted only by surgeons who have experience with this challenging situation.

References

1. Berek JS, Hacker NF, Lagasse MD, Leuchter RS: Lower urinary tract resection as part of cytoreductive surgery for ovarian cancer. Gynecol Oncol 1982; 13:87.
2. Adelson MD, Baggish MS, Seifer DB, et al.: Cytoreduction of ovarian cancer with the Cavitron ultrasonic surgical aspirator. Obstet Gynecol 1988; 72:140.
3. Fry DE, Milholen L, Harbrecht PJ: Iatrogenic ureteral injury. Arch Surg 1983; 118:454.
4. Gangai MP, Agee RE, Spence CR: Surgical injury to ureter. Urology 1976; 8:22.
5. Guerriero W: Ureteral injury. Urol Clin North Am 1989; 16:237.
6. Green TH, Meigs JV, Ulfelder H, Curtin RR: Urologic complications of radical Wertheim hysterectomy: Incidence, etiology, management, and prevention. Obstet Gynecol 1962; 20:293.
7. Hamm F, Weinberg S, Waterhouse R: End-to-end ureteral anastomosis: A simple original technique. J Urol 1962; 87:43.
8. Turner-Warwick R: The use of the omental pedicle graft in urinary tract reconstruction. J Urol 1976; 116:341.
9. Pearse HD, Barry JM, Fuchs EF: Intraoperative consultation for the ureter. Urol Clin North Am 1985; 12:423.
10. Grey D, Flynn P, Goodwin W: Experimental methods of ureteroneocystostomy: Experiences with the ureteral intussusception to produce a nipple or valve. J Urol 1957; 77:154.
11. Ehrlich RM, Melman A, Skinner DG: The use of vesico-psoas hitch in urologic surgery. J Urol 1978; 119:322.
12. Turner-Warwick R, Worth PHL: The psoas bladder-hitch procedure for the replacement of the lower third of the ureter. Br J Urol 1969; 41:701.
13. Moore E, Weber R, Woodward E, et al.: Isolated ileal loops for ureteral repair. Surg Gynecol Obstet 1956; 102:87.
14. Boxer RJ, Fritzsche P, Skinner D, et al.: Replacement of the ureter by small intestine: Clinical application and results of the ileal ureter in 89 patients. J Urol 1979; 121:728.
15. Creevy C: Misadvantages following replacement of ureters with ileum. Surgery 1964; 58:497.
16. Prout G Jr, Stuart W, Witus W: Utilization of ileal segments to substitute for extensive ureteral loss. J Urol 1963; 90:541.
17. Struthers N, Scott R: Reconstruction of the upper ureter with colon. J Urol 1974; 112:179.
18. Fritzsche P, Skinner D, Craven J, et al.: Long-term radiographic changes of the kidney following the ileal ureter operation. J Urol 1975; 114:843.
19. Udall DA, Hodges CV, Pearse HM, Burns AB: Transureteroureterostomy: A neglected procedure. J Urol 1973; 109:817.
20. Higgins C: Transuretero-ureteral anastomosis: Report of a clinical case. J Urol 1934; 34:349.
21. Hendren W, Hensle T: Transureteroureterostomy: Experience with 75 cases. J Urol 1980; 123:826.
22. Hodges C, Barry J, Fuchs E, et al.: Transureteroureterostomy: 25-year experience with 100 patients. J Urol 1980; 123:834.
23. Ehrlich R, Skinner D: Complications of transureteroureterostomy. J Urol 1975; 113:467.
24. Chapman ME, Reid JH: Use of percutaneous nephrostomy in malignant ureteric obstruction. Br J Radiol 1991; 64:318.
25. Cochran ST, Barbaric ZL, Lee JJ, Kashfian P: Percutaneous nephrostomy tube placement: An outpatient procedure? Radiology 1991; 179:843.
26. Cronan JJ: Contemporary concepts in imaging urinary tract obstruction. Radiol Clin North Am 1991; 29:527.
27. Blandy J: The feasibility of preparing an ideal substitute for the urinary bladder. Ann R Coll Surg Engl 1964; 35:287.
28. Coffey R: Transplantation of the ureters into the large intestine in the absence of a functioning urinary bladder. Surg Gynecol Obstet 1921; 32:383.
29. Cordonnier J: Ureterosigmoid anastomosis. J Urol 1950; 63:276.
30. Jacobs A: A review of long-term results of uretero-colic anastomosis. Br J Urol 1967; 39:670.

31. Zincke H, Segura J: Ureterosigmoidostomy: Critical review of 173 cases. J Urol 1975; 113:324.
32. Brunschwig A: Complete excision of pelvic viscera for advanced carcinoma. Cancer 1948; 1:177.
33. Bricker EM: Bladder substitution after pelvic evisceration. Surg Clin North Am 1950; 30:1511.
34. Hancock KC, Copeland LJ, Gershenson DM, et al.: Urinary conduits in gynecologic oncology. Obstet Gynecol 1986; 67:680.
35. Klein E, Montie J, Montague D, et al.: Jejunal conduit urinary diversion. J Urol 1986; 135:244.
36. Delgado G: Use of the automatic stapler in urinary conduit diversions and pelvic exenterations. Gynecol Oncol 1980; 10:93.
37. Heney NM, Dretler SP, Hensle TW, Kerr WS Jr: Autosuturing device in intestinal urinary conduits. Urology 1978; 12:650.
38. Bergman SM, Sears HF, Javadpour N: Complication with mechanical stapling device in creation of ileoconduit. Urology 1978; 12:71.
39. Bricker E: The technic of ileal segment bladder substitution. Prog Gynecol 1964; 3:695.
40. Scardino PT, Bagley DH, Javadpour N, Ketcham AS: Sigmoid conduit urinary diversion. Urology 1975; 6:167.
41. Månsson W, Colleen S, Stigsson L: Four methods of ureterointestinal anastomosis in urinary conduit diversion. Scand J Urol Nephrol 1979; 13:191.
42. Lockhart J, Bejany D: Antireflux ureteroileal reimplantation: An alternative for urinary diversion. J Urol 1987; 137:867.
43. Orr JW, Shingleton HM, Hatch KD, et al.: Urinary diversion in patients undergoing pelvic exenteration. Am J Obstet Gynecol 1982; 142:883.
44. Lindenauer S, Cerny J, Morley G: Ureterosigmoid conduit urinary diversion. Surgery 1974; 75:705.
45. Beddoe AM, Boyce JG, Remy JC, et al.: Stented versus nonstented transverse colon conduits: A comparative report. Gynecol Oncol 1987; 27:305.
46. Schmidt J, Hawtrey C, Buchsbaum H: Transverse colon conduit: A preferred method of urinary diversion for radiation-treated pelvic malignancies. J Urol 1975; 113:308.
47. Loening S, Navarre R, Narayana A, Culp D: Transverse colon conduit urinary diversion. J Urol 1982; 127:37.
48. Orr J, Shand E, Watters D, Kirkland I: Ileal conduit urinary diversion in children. An assessment of the long-term results. Br J Urol 1981; 53:424.
49. Pitts WR Jr, Muecke E: A 20-year experience with ileal conduits: The fate of the kidneys. J Urol 1979; 122:154.
50. Mogg R: Urinary diversion using the colonic conduit. Br J Urol 1967; 39:687.
51. Mogg R, Syme R: The results of urinary diversion using the colonic conduit. Br J Urol 1969; 49:434.
52. Althausen A, Hagen-Cook K, Hendren W III: Non-refluxing colon conduit: Experience with 70 cases. J Urol 1978; 120:35.
53. Gonzales ET Jr, Baum NH, Friedman A, Carlton CE: Sigmoid conduit: Review and description of technique. Urology 1977; 10:579.
54. Morley G, Lindenauer S: Pelvic exenterative therapy for gynecologic malignancy: An analysis of 70 cases. Cancer 1976; 38:581.
55. Elder D, Moisey C, Rees R: A long-term follow-up of the colonic conduit operation in children. Br J Urol 1979; 51:462.
56. Cordonnier JJ, Nicolai CH: An evaluation of the use of an isolated segment of ileum as a means of urinary diversion. J Urol 1960; 83:834.
57. Schmidt J, Hawtrey C, Flocks R, Culp D: Complications, results and problems of ileal conduit diversions. J Urol 1973; 109:210.
58. Wrigley JV, Prem KA, Fraley EE: Pelvic exenteration: Complications of urinary diversion. J Urol 1976; 116:428.
59. Fallon B, Loening S, Hawtrey CE, et al.: Urologic complications of pelvic exenteration for gynecologic malignancy. J Urol 1979; 122:158.
60. Philipson B, Kock N, Jagenburg R, et al.: Functional and structural studies of ileal reservoirs used for continent urostomy and ileostomy. Gut 1983; 24:392.
61. Philipson B, Nilsson L, Norlen L, et al.: Mucosal adaptation in ileum after long time-exposure to urine: A study in patients with continent urostomy. In Robinson JWL, Dowling RH, Riecken EO (eds.): Mechanisms of Intestinal Adaptation. Proceedings of the Second International Conference on Intestinal Adaptation (Falk Symposium 30). Titisee, Germany, Lancaster MTM Press, 1981, pp. 613–620.
62. Boyd SD, Feinberg SM, Skinner DG, et al.: Quality of life survey of urinary diversion patients: Comparison of ileal conduits versus continent Kock ileal reservoirs. J Urol 1987; 138:1386.
63. Gerber A: Improved quality of life following a Kock continent ileostomy. West J Med 1980; 133:95.
64. McLeod R, Fazio V: Quality of life with the continent ileostomy. World J Surg 1984; 8:90.
65. Nilsson L, Kock N, Kylberg F, et al.: Sexual adjustment in ileostomy patients before and after conversion to continent ileostomy. Dis Colon Rectum 1981; 24:287.
66. Gilchrist R, Merricks J, Hamlin H, Rieger I: Construction of a substitute bladder and urethra. Surg Gynecol Obstet 1950; 90:752.
67. Kock N: Intra-abdominal "reservoir" in patients with permanent ileostomy. Arch Surg 1969; 99:223.
68. Basso D: The efficacy and applicability of an intussuscepted conical valve in preventing regurgitation and leakage of intestinal contents. Ann Surg 1951; 133:477.
69. Smith G, Hinman F Jr: The intussuscepted ileal cystostomy. J Urol 1955; 73:261.
70. Madigan M: Aspects of treatment: The continent ileostomy and the isolated ileal bladder. Ann R Coll Surg Engl 1976; 58:62.
71. Leisinger H, Sauberli H, Schauwecker H, Mayor G: Continent ileal bladder: First clinical experience. Eur Urol 1976; 2:8.
72. Kock N, Nilsson A, Norlen L, et al.: Urinary diversion via a continent ileum reservoir. Scand J Urol Nephrol Suppl 1978; 49:23.
73. Kock N, Nilsson L, et al.: Urinary diversion via a continent ileal reservoir: Clinical results in 12 patients. J Urol 1982; 128:469.
74. Montie J, MacGregor P, Fazio V, Lavery I: Continent ileal urinary reservoir (Kock pouch). Urol Clin North Am 1986; 13:251.
75. Skinner DG, Boyd SD, Lieskovsky G: Clinical experience with the Kock continent ileal reservoir for urinary diversion. J Urol 1984; 132:1101.
76. Skinner D, Lieskovsky G, Boyd S: Technique of creation of a continent internal ileal reservoir (Kock pouch) for urinary diversion. Urol Clin North Am 1984; 11:741.
77. Webster GD, Bertram RA: Continent catheterizable urinary diversion using the ileocecal segment with stapled intussusception of the ileocecal valve. J Urol 1986; 135:465.
78. Sullivan H, Gilchrist R, Merricks J: Ileocecal substitute bladder: Long-term follow-up. J Urol 1973; 109:43.
79. Benchekroun A: Continent caecal bladder. Eur Urol 1977; 3:248.
80. Rowland R, Mitchell M, Bihrle R, et al.: Indiana continent urinary reservoir. J Urol 1987; 137:1136.
81. Bejany D, Politano V: Stapled and nonstapled tapered distal ileum for construction of a continent colonic urinary reservoir. J Urol 1988; 140:491.
82. Penalver MA, Bejany DE, Averette HE, et al.: Continent urinary diversion in gynecologic oncology. Gynecol Oncol 1989; 343:274.
83. van Nagell JR, Parker JC, Maruyama Y, et al.: Bladder or rectal injury following radiotherapy for cervical cancer. Am J Obstet Gynecol 1974; 119:727.
84. McGuire EJ, Weiss RM, Schiff M, Lytton B: Hemorrhagic radiation cystitis treatment. Urology 1974; 3:204.
85. Schiff M, McGuire EJ: Experience with the use of an intravesical hydrostatic pressure balloon. Surg Gynecol Obstet 1980; 150:322.
86. Behnam K, Patil UB, Mariano E: Intravesical instillation of formalin for hemorrhagic cystitis secondary to radiation for gynecologic malignancies. Gynecol Oncol 1983; 16:31.
87. Bright JF, Tosi SE, Crichlow RW, Selikowitz SM: Prevention of vesicoureteral reflux with Fogarty catheters during formalin therapy. J Urol 1977; 118:950.

Tubal Surgery: Isthmic Tube

23

Lamia Haj-Hassan
Gad Lavy

FUNCTIONAL ANATOMY AND PHYSIOLOGY

The isthmic tube begins at the uterotubal junction (UTJ) and extends laterally for 2–3 cm to the ampullary-isthmic junction (AIJ). This portion of the fallopian tube has unique anatomy, physiology, and function. Surgical therapy of conditions affecting the isthmic tube must take these special characteristics into consideration, and an attempt should be made to preserve its functional anatomy. In this chapter, the unique features of the isthmic tube are discussed, its pathology reviewed, and surgical therapy of conditions affecting the isthmic tube are examined along these guidelines.

Function of the Isthmic Tube

The fallopian tube exhibits complex physiologic functions in gamete transport and maintenance, in supporting fertilization, and in preimplantation embryo development. The passage of the gametes to the ampulla, the site of fertilization, is dependent upon tubal motility,[1] as is the retention of the fertilized ovum in the ampullary portion prior to its release into the endometrial cavity. The isthmic tube, with its highly developed musculature and nerve supply, is an active participant in these processes.

Isthmic Musculature and Its Regulation

The typical appearance of the isthmic tube is that of thick muscle surrounding a narrow lumen. At the UTJ, three muscle layers can be identified: an inner longitudinal, a middle circular, and an outer layer in which fibers run in both directions (Fig. 23–1). The inner layer disappears in the middle of the isthmus, whereas the circular muscle layer increases in thickness from the ampulla to the interstitial portion. The thickness of the muscle layer in this region (1.3 mm) by far exceeds the luminal diameter (0.2 mm).

Tubal contractility is under neural and hormonal control.[2-4] In general, estrogens are believed to increase while progestogens decrease tubal contractile activity. This effect is even more pronounced in the isthmic tube, owing to its abundant musculature and dense adrenergic innervation. This hormonal effect may explain the retention of the embryo in the ampulla during the early luteal phase, when the estrogen-progesterone (E/P) ratio is high, whereas the dominant progestational environment present in the mid-late luteal phase causes relaxation of the isthmic and the interstitial portions, thus allowing the embryo to complete its journey into the endometrial cavity.

Innervation

The pattern of innervation of the isthmic tube is complex and involves the sympathetic and parasympathetic systems. Many surgical procedures interrupt this intricate network. The implications of this disruption on tubal function are not clear. It appears, however, that tubal function is at least partially preserved in these instances, as evidenced by the success of many of these surgical procedures.[5]

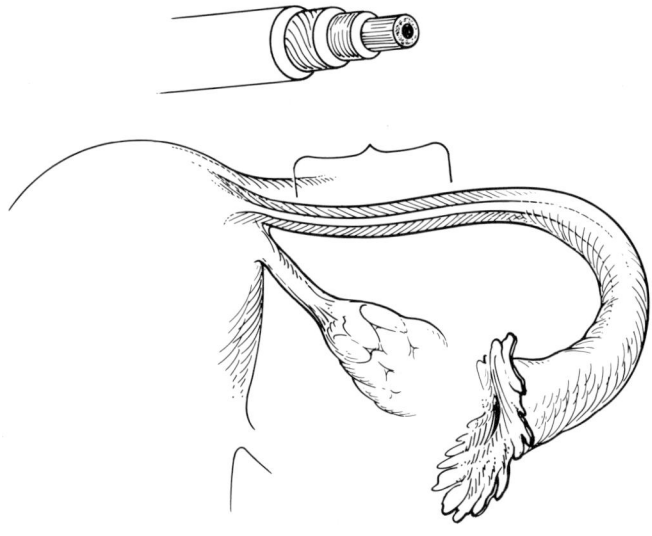

Figure 23–1
Isthmic musculature.

The sympathetic innervation of the tube is derived from the hypogastric nerves. The postsynaptic fibers are nonvascular and are located mainly in the circular smooth muscle layer, where high concentrations of catecholamines have been demonstrated. The density of intrinsic adrenergic innervation is the highest in the area of the isthmus, and the isthmic musculature functions as a sympathetically innervated sphincter.

The interaction between the neural and hormonal systems in this area is evidenced by the sensitivity of the isthmic sympathetic fibers to steroid hormones,[6] and by the modulation by these hormones of tubal smooth muscle response to norepinephrine. The high concentration of norepinephrine in the isthmus in the luteal and ovulatory phases of the cycle suggests that the sympathetic system is involved in the "tubal locking" mechanism, the mechanism by which the fertilized egg is retained in the fallopian tube prior to being released into the uterine cavity.

The parasympathetic innervation is derived from the vagus nerve and the pelvic plexus; its functional significance, however, remains to be elucidated.

The Isthmic Epithelium

The isthmic endosalpinx consists of ciliated and secretory cells (Fig. 23–2). Both cell types demonstrate functional and morphologic changes in response to the changing levels of ovarian steroid hormones and to the E/P ratio.[7] The estrogen-dominated follicular phase is characterized by an increase in the size and activity of the secretory cells and by the maturation of the ciliary cells, both peaking at ovulation. In the progesterone-dominated luteal phase, the secretory cells produce thick mucus and the cilia undergo degenerative changes.

The ciliary beat frequency varies in the different phases of the ovarian cycle, and within different regions of the tube. In the preovulatory phase, the cilia beat in the direction of the ovary; in the luteal phase, the direction is reversed.[8]

SURGICAL THERAPY OF PATHOLOGIC CONDITIONS OF THE ISTHMIC TUBE

The unique physiology and anatomy of the isthmus determine the disease processes that affect this area and at the same time dictate a unique therapeutic approach. The surgical approach to isthmic pathology is tailored to accommodate the narrow lumen and the thick musculature, and thus differs from therapy for distal tubal disease. Despite proper selection of surgery and meticulous technique, it is likely that surgery will be unable to completely restore physiology and function. Tubal surgery is therefore generally followed by tubal dysfunction. This is due in part to prior irreversible tubal damage following inflammation or tubal occlusion, or a result of the surgery itself. Normal anatomy is difficult to restore even with the use of magnification. This is especially true for the proper alignment of the mucosal folds during tubal anastomosis. Peritubal adhesions are common sequelae after surgery, restricting motility of the tube and disrupting function. Partial denervation of the tube usually accompanies tubal surgery, but it does not seem that disruption of the rich adrenergic isthmic innervation causes significant impairment of tubal function.[5]

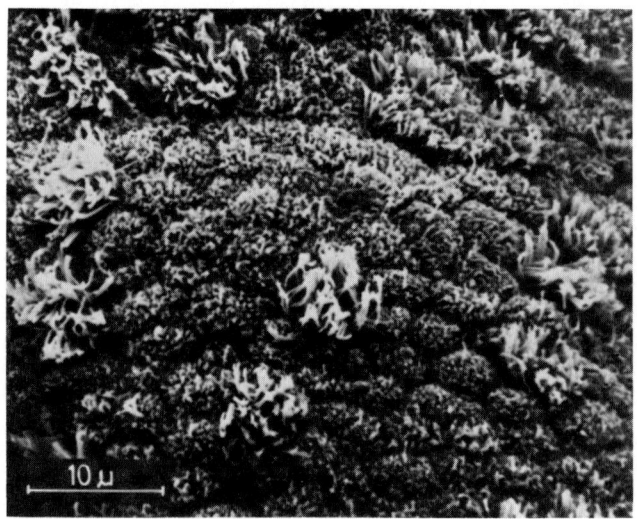

Figure 23–2
Isthmic epithelium.

The principles used for isthmic surgery do not differ from those employed in other parts of the tube or the female pelvis. Microsurgical technique emphasizes gentle tissue handling, meticulous hemostasis, and the use of fine, nonreactive suture material and is recommended in all gynecologic surgical procedures performed in women of reproductive age wishing to preserve their reproductive potential.

The use of magnification aids in restoration of functional tubal anatomy. However, there is no clear advantage of using surgical loupes as compared with the operating microscope.

The surgical approach (laparoscopy vs. laparotomy) should be tailored to the individual patient. Improvements in equipment now allow for many of the surgical procedures that previously required laparotomy to be performed laparoscopically. Linear salpingostomy, partial salpingectomy, segmental resection, and total salpingectomy can all be performed laparoscopically. Tubal anastomosis still requires laparotomy.

The following represent common disease conditions that affect the isthmic tube and the surgical approach to these conditions.

Salpingitis Isthmica Nodosa (SIN)

SIN (adenomyosalpingitis, endosalpingitis, diverticulosis of the fallopian tube, endosalpingoblastosis, epitheliomyosis) is a pathologic diagnosis first described in 1887 by Chiari.[9, 10] One hundred years later, controversy still exists regarding the etiology, pathogenesis, and clinical significance of this condition.

SIN is a disease of the fourth and fifth decades. The weight of evidence regarding its etiology supports a primary noninflammatory process similar to adenomyosis uteri and diverticulosis of other organs. The condition affects almost exclusively the highly muscular and densely innervated isthmic tube and may be a late morphologic expression of chronic tubal spasm. Infection may be present as a primary or secondary phenomenon.[10]

The incidence of SIN was 0.6%, 2.8%, and 50% in a control population, a group of patients with an ectopic pregnancy, and an infertile population, respectively.[10] Freakly and colleagues reported the disease to be more common in blacks than in whites,[11] whereas Homm and associates reported it to be present in almost 46% of specimens associated with isthmic ectopic pregnancy.[12] The characteristic features of SIN are multiple collections of irregular alveolar spaces in the myosalpinx lined by tubal epithelium. These spaces are continuous and indistinguishable from the tubal epithelium. The myosalpinx is frequently hypertrophic or hyperplastic (Fig.

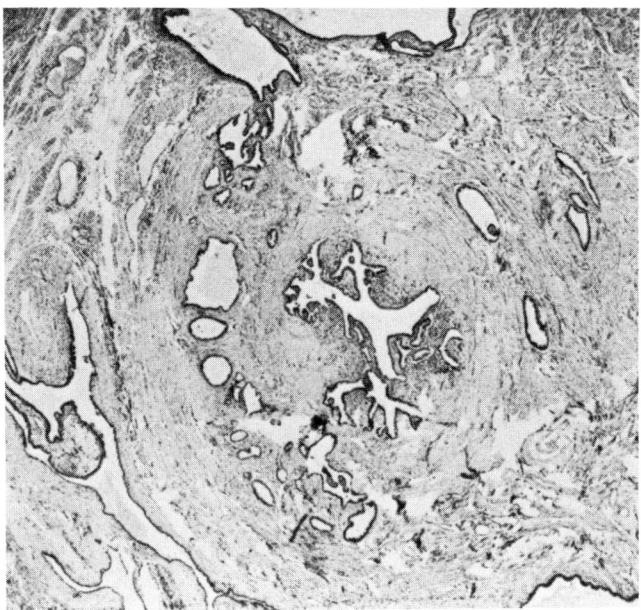

Figure 23–3
Salpingitis isthmica nodosa.

23–3). These lesions can be differentiated from endometriosis of the tube by the presence of normal appearing tubal columnar epithelium and the absence of endometrial stroma.

Radiographically, SIN presents as bilateral honeycomb stippled lesions affecting the proximal portions of the tubes.

Clinical Significance of SIN

SIN is associated with ectopic pregnancy and infertility. The incidence of SIN in a group of isthmic ectopic pregnancies was 45.9%.[12] SIN was also associated with an increased risk of recurrent ectopic pregnancy.

Infertility, however, is the most common clinical association of SIN.[11] The incidence of SIN was reported to be 50% in a small group of infertile patients.[10] Among infertile patients, hydrosalpinx and tubal obstruction were more common in the presence of SIN. The establishment of a causal relationship between SIN and infertility in cases in which no hydrosalpinx or obstruction is present is less clear and much more difficult.

Treatment of SIN

Management of SIN relies on accurate diagnosis and determination of the extent of tubal involvement. Observation or medical therapy with danazol (Danocrine) is of questionable merit and is reserved for mild conditions and where tubal patency has been established and when an endoscopic examination reveals only mild isthmic nodularity. In all other cases, surgical therapy is the treatment of choice. During surgery, a special effort should be made to ensure that the surgical margins are free of disease, because surgical failures and recurrences usually represent residual disease from the time of the initial surgery. In some cases, extensive resection may be necessary to remove all diseased tube. The optimal management for isthmic ectopic pregnancy associated with SIN is resection of the involved segment and microsurgical anastomosis. Again, extensive resection may be necessary to remove all diseased tube. Tubotubal, tubocornual, and tubal reimplantation are then performed on the disease-free margins.[13] Owing to the bilateral nature of the disease, the contralateral tube should be examined carefully at the time of surgery. Because a preoperative hysterosalpingogram (HSG) is usually not available in these cases, it should be obtained postoperatively in order to check for residual disease in the ipsilateral tube and for the presence of unrecognized disease in the contralateral tube.

Pelvic Inflammatory Disease (PID)

Pelvic infection resulting in distortion of tubal anatomy and impairment of its functional integrity is a major and ever increasing cause of female infertility. The degree of destruction following an acute episode of PID depends on the severity of infection, the nature of the organisms involved, the number of recurrences, and the antibiotic therapy used. Sequelae of pelvic infections include tubal epithelial damage, peritubal and intratubal adhesions, and tubal occlusion.

Endosalpingeal damage is common following an acute episode of PID. Vasquez and colleagues have shown a reduction in ciliary number and an impairment of ciliary function following an acute infection and demonstrated the process of deciliation that accompanies the development of hydrosalpinx.[38] In the rabbit tube, instillation of *Escherichia coli* endotoxin was associated with severe ciliary damage and changes on the surfaces of secretory cells.[14] The pattern of injury and regeneration in response to *E. coli* was almost identical to that caused by its endotoxin alone and differed from the patterns seen from experimental endosalpingeal damage caused by introduction of *Neisseria gonorrhoeae* and *Chlamydia trachomatis*.[15] A more extensive involvement of the tube is seen with tuberculosis, in which the various tubal layers are involved.

Tubal function following an episode of PID may also be impaired as a result of peritubal adhesions restricting tubal motility and affecting the ovum pickup mechanism. Intratubal adhesions can interfere with the safe passage of the ovum or zygote and give rise to infertility or ectopic pregnancy. The isthmic tube, with its narrow lumen, is most prone to inflammatory occlusions.

The success of the surgical management of the aftermath of pelvic infection is dependent on the extent of irreversible damage that has already occurred. Although tubal occlusion can be surgically corrected in most cases, tubal function postoperatively is dependent on the extent of epithelial damage that has been sustained. Review of the results of surgical correction of tubal disease illustrates this point quite clearly. Tubal anastomosis involving the isthmic tube is more successful in patients whose occlusion was the result of surgical sterilization than in those who suffer a postinfective obstruction.[16] Similarly, tubal occlusion resulting from peritubal disease and not involving the endosalpinx, such as that following an episode of acute appendicitis, is associated with a higher success rate.

Endometriosis

Endometriosis affects the fallopian tube by serosal implants and peritubal adhesions. Direct involvement of the tubal wall is uncommon. When present, the serosal implants can show varying degrees of extension into the muscularis and may lead to complete or incomplete tubal occlusion, depending on the segment involved and on the severity of the disease. Endometriosis may also affect tubal function by increased prostaglandin (PG) production. $PGF_{2\alpha}$ and PGE_2 were found to be elevated in peritoneal fluid of infertile women with endometriosis. Disturbances of tubal function may lead to failure of ovum pickup or rapid transfer of a fertilized egg and infertility.[17] The isthmic tube is no more prone than other tubal segments to become involved in endometriosis. The general principles that apply to the treatment of endometriosis elsewhere should be utilized in this situation. Expectant management, medical therapy, and conservative surgery should be considered in an infertile patient with endometriosis. Isthmic occlusion resulting from endometriosis can be treated medically with standard regimens of Danocrine or gonadotropin-releasing hormone agonists. The effect of this form of therapy should be assessed following 4–6 months of treatment by HSG to determine tubal patency. Persistent obstruction can be treated surgically by segmental resection and tubal anastomosis.

Ectopic Pregnancy (EP)

Tubal ectopic pregnancy accounts for 95–98% of all cases of extrauterine pregnancy. Isthmic EP contributes to 5–15% of all tubal pregnancies.[18] Structural abnormalities of the fallopian tube have long been recognized as the most common etiologic factors for EP. On the other hand, an abnormal hormonal milieu is thought to provide an explanation for the increased risk of EP associated with certain conditions such as infertility, induction of ovulation, and use of certain contraceptive techniques.

The ability to make the diagnosis earlier and more accurately has altered the therapeutic approach to EP. Whereas in the past, tubal rupture and life-threatening intraperitoneal bleeding were common occurrences, developments in diagnostic techniques allow the diagnosis to be made in most cases prior to tubal rupture. Thus, the emphasis of surgery has shifted towards a conservative approach, one that allows the individual to retain the involved tube and her reproductive potential. Radical surgery (salpingectomy) is currently reserved for patients who are not interested in preserving their reproductive potential and who have had multiple prior EPs, and for those with a badly damaged tube as a result of rupture. Following salpingectomy, the incidence of intrauterine pregnancy is 36.5% and the incidence of recurrent EP is 15.4%.[19] These figures do not differ significantly from those found following conservative surgery. This observation paved the way for conservative surgery, that in which the involved tube is retained, to become the "gold standard" of therapy for EP.

Crucial to the selection of the proper therapeutic approach is the understanding of the pathophysiology of this disease, and assessment of the extent of damage to tubal anatomy at the time of diagnosis. The evolution of the management of tubal EP has occurred through recognition of peculiarities in implantation of the ectopic trophoblast in different areas of the fallopian tube. It appears that the anatomic characteristics of isthmic ectopics differ from those of ampullary ectopics in the extent of invasion into the muscularis and resultant muscular destruction (Fig. 23–4). Whereas ampullary ectopics appear to remain intraluminal and produce relatively little mucosal and muscular destruction, isthmic pregnancy invades earlier and causes significant damage. Pauerstein and coworkers reported on a group of patients with EP in whom 67% of the ampullary EPs were found in an intraluminal position.[20] In another study of seven isthmic EPs, three were extraluminal, two were mixed extra- and intraluminal, and one was entirely intraluminal.[21] Prominent muscular and mucosal destruction was seen in the first two groups. The narrow lumen and the lack of decidual formation in the mucosa seem to predispose the patient to early trophoblastic invasion into the tubal wall. In the same study, 56% of the ampullary EPs were entirely intraluminal and in the majority the muscularis was

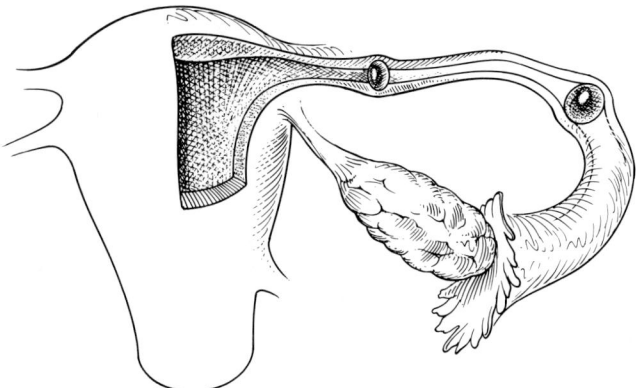

Figure 23–4
Anatomic location of isthmic and ampullary ectopic pregnancy.

preserved. It appears that isthmic and ampullary pregnancies differ in the location of the developing pregnancy in relation to the tubal lumen, which in turn determines the extent of tubal damage and thus the surgical procedure most appropriate for these two types of EP.

In isthmic EP, linear salpingostomy is often complicated by tubal occlusion. This may be due to the extensive muscular destruction found in these cases. A segmental resection with primary or secondary anastomosis appears to be the procedure of choice. In a review of 12 cases of intact isthmic EP, two patients had a salpingectomy, four had a linear salpingostomy, and six underwent segmental resection with delayed microsurgical anastomosis. None of the patients who had linear salpingostomy conceived, and in three tubal occlusion was demonstrated by HSG. Four of the six patients who were managed by segmental resection conceived (three intrauterine, one EP in the preserved tube). An HSG was performed in only three of the six patients, because three conceived before HSG could be performed; the tubes were patent in all three women in whom HSG was done.[18] Stangel and Reyniak reported postoperative tubal patency in all 11 patients managed by segmental resection and immediate anastomosis.[22] Support for segmental resection in patients with an isthmic EP is provided by other investigators.[22–25] Anastomosis of the tube can be performed immediately[22, 24] or at a later date.[18, 23] The extent of destruction in unruptured ampullary EP is more limited, and linear salpingostomy proves to be the treatment of choice in these cases.

Laparoscopic salpingostomy has been described for both isthmic and ampullary pregnancies. A study by Pouly and associates reported on 81 ampullary EPs treated with laparoscopic linear salpingostomy. Sixty two per cent of those attempting conception achieved an intrauterine pregnancy. The intrauterine pregnancy rate in 22 patients with isthmic EP who were treated in a similar fashion by linear salpingostomy was 54.5%.[26] The apparent discrepancy between the results of this study—that is, the better results obtained by linear salpingostomy in patients with isthmic pregnancy—may be attributed to the laparoscopic technique or to patient selection. DeCherney and associates reported a 50% incidence of intrauterine pregnancy in a group of 18 patients with no recurrent EPs.[27] Bruhat and coworkers reported on 25 patients undergoing laparoscopic linear salpingostomy. The incidence of intrauterine pregnancy was 72%, and that of recurrent EP was 12%.[28]

Segmental resection in cases of isthmic EP is combined by some authorities with an immediate tubal anastomosis,[22, 24] whereas others prefer to delay the definitive surgery to a later date when the edema and other tissue changes associated with pregnancy have subsided.[18, 23] In cases in which the anastomosis is delayed, both the proximal and the distal end are ligated using nonabsorbable suture. The anastomosis is performed 3–6 months later. If the contralateral tube is patent, the patient should be advised of the theoretical risk of an EP in the blind distal segment.

Medical therapy of tubal pregnancy is being explored. Systemic administration of methotrexate (MTX)[29, 30] and local injection by laparoscopy or transvaginal ultrasound guidance of MTX,[31] PG,[32, 33] or potassium chloride[34] have been associated with resolution of EP without surgery. The patency rates following these procedures also appear to be high.[29–34] Further work is needed to enable one to comment on the efficacy of these procedures in isthmic versus ampullary pregnancies.

SURGERY FOR ISTHMIC TUBAL PREGNANCY

Linear Salpingostomy for Isthmic Ectopic Pregnancy

Linear salpingostomy has become the standard therapy of ampullary EP and is being practiced for isthmic EP when performed laparoscopically. Meticulous microsurgical technique is applied whether the procedure is performed by laparotomy or laparoscopically. The use of diluted vasopressin (Pitressin) injected into the antimesenteric aspect of the tube reduces blood loss and simplifies the procedure. A small linear incision 1.0–1.5 cm in length is made on the antimesenteric side of the fallopian tube immediately over the EP using the CO_2 laser, electrocautery, or scissors (Fig. 23–5A). This will be followed by extrusion of the products of conception (Fig. 23–5B). Débridement of the base of implantation site should be avoided to minimize bleeding and tissue damage. The incision is closed or left to heal by secondary intention. Disappearance of serum human chorionic gonadotropin (hCG) is the rule following this approach.

The same procedure can be performed laparoscopically in patients who are hemodynamically stable. A standard double- or triple-puncture laparoscopic technique is employed. The antimesenteric border of the tube is injected with a dilute solution of Pitressin, and a small incision is made in the area immediately over the EP. The tissue will usually

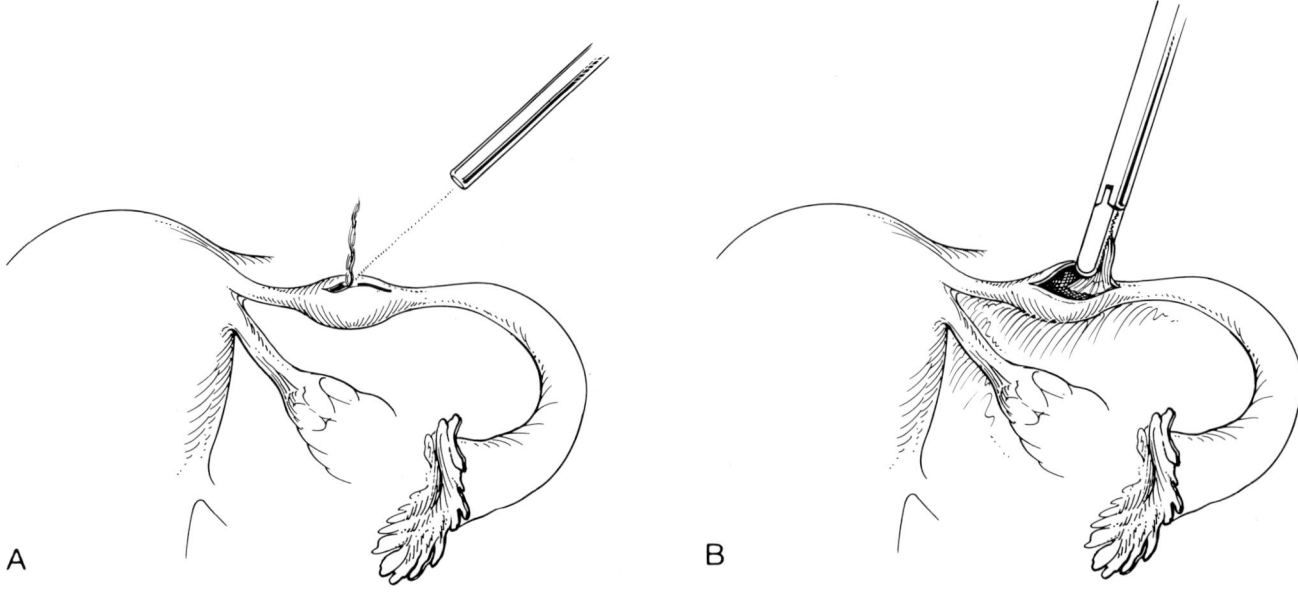

Figure 23–5
A and B, Linear salpingostomy for isthmic ectopic pregnancy.

extrude spontaneously or can be removed utilizing spoon forceps.

Segmental Resection with Immediate or Delayed Anastomosis

Segmental resection is performed by elevation of the maximum bulge of the swelling and excision of the involved tubal segment. Tubal anastomosis can be delayed or performed immediately if the conditions are favorable (Fig. 23–6). In cases in which anastomosis is delayed, both the proximal and the distal ends are ligated using nonabsorbable suture. The anastomosis is performed 3–6 months later. In all instances, standard microsurgical technique is utilized; gentle tissue handling, meticulous hemostasis, and constant irrigation minimize tissue damage and postoperative adhesions. Prophylactic antibiotics and intraperitoneal Hyskon solution may also assist in prevention of postoperative adhesions.

TUBAL ANASTOMOSIS

Tubal anastomosis is performed to relieve an obstruction resulting from prior tubal sterilization, segmental resection, or PID.

An end-to-end anastomosis is performed between the distal and proximal tubal segments. The anastomosis can thus be intramural-isthmic, intramural-ampullary, isthmic-isthmic, isthmic-ampullary, ampullary-ampullary, or ampullary-infundibular, depending on the involved segments. The surgical technique should align the mucosal folds to the best degree possible and compensate for the disparity in luminal size, if any, between the proximal and distal segment.

Despite the achievement of patency, the degree to which tubal function has been restored following prolonged tubal occlusion and tubal anastomosis is variable. Tubal patency as assessed by HSG and laparoscopy alone gives no guarantee to the functional integrity of the repaired tube. Tubal function can be estimated only indirectly by examining the incidence of pregnancy following the procedure, the incidence of EP, and the interval from surgery to conception.

Many factors are thought to play a role in affecting the outcome in tubal microsurgery. The site of anastomosis, the technique used, the underlying tubal pathology, the presence of pelvic disease, the length of the tube after repair, and the presence of functional fimbriae all seem to be important in the final outcome. An inverse relation between the length of the tube and the interval between surgery and conception has also been observed. When tubal length was more than 6 cm, most pregnancies occurred within the first five cycles. When the tube length was less than 4 cm, that interval reached a mean of 19 months. The role of tubal length was noticed in another group of 25 women who had tubal sterilization by different techniques following microsurgical re-anastomosis. Intrauterine pregnancy was found to be directly related to tubal length.[35] When the length was less than 3 cm, no pregnancy occurred; when the length was greater than 4 cm, all patients had normal intrauterine pregnancy. Seven patients had a tubal length of 3–4 cm; only three of these women had normal intrauterine pregnancy. Ampullary length had little or no effect on the chance of pregnancy, as long as the 1-cm ampulla remained.

Isthmic-isthmic and isthmic-cornual anastomoses carry the highest rate of successful outcome. Technically, the presence of proximal and distal tubal segments of equal size and the thick muscularis facilitate the alignment of the tubal segments, thus increasing the likelihood of tubal patency and normal tubal function. The incidence of intrauterine pregnancy within 1 year was found to be 74% in such types of anastomosis and was the highest compared with other forms of anastomosis (Table 23–1).[36]

Tubal anastomoses involving the isthmic tube are technically easier, owing to the thick muscularis. As with tubal anastomoses elsewhere, the occluded ends of the tube are excised. Straight scissors or CO_2 laser is used to minimize damage to healthy tissue. Hemostasis is achieved by pinpoint coagulation and mild compression. Mucosal bleeders are not coagu-

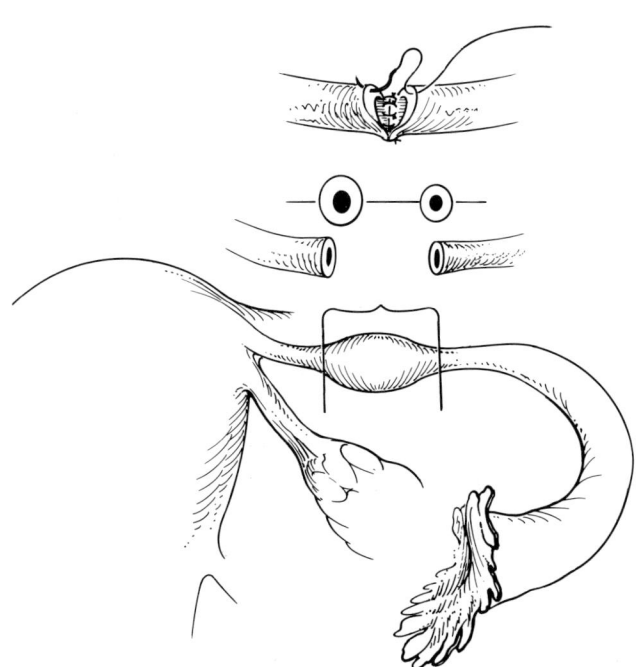

Figure 23–6
Resection and anastomosis for isthmic ectopic pregnancy.

Table 23–1

Success Rate of the Various Types of Anastomosis

Type of Anastomosis	No. of Patients in Each Group	Success Rate (%)
Isthmic-isthmic Isthmic-cornual	62	74
Uterine, intramural, cornual-ampullary	16	56
Isthmic-ampullary Ampullary-ampullary	55	69

All patients had two tubes anastomosed. In each group, the same type of anastomosis was performed on both sides. Success rate was defined as the percentage of intrauterine pregnancy within 1 year of the surgical procedure.

Modified from te Velde ER, et al.: Factors influencing success or failure after reversal of sterilization: A multivariate approach. Fertil Steril 54:274, 1990. Reproduced with permission of the publisher, The American Fertility Society.

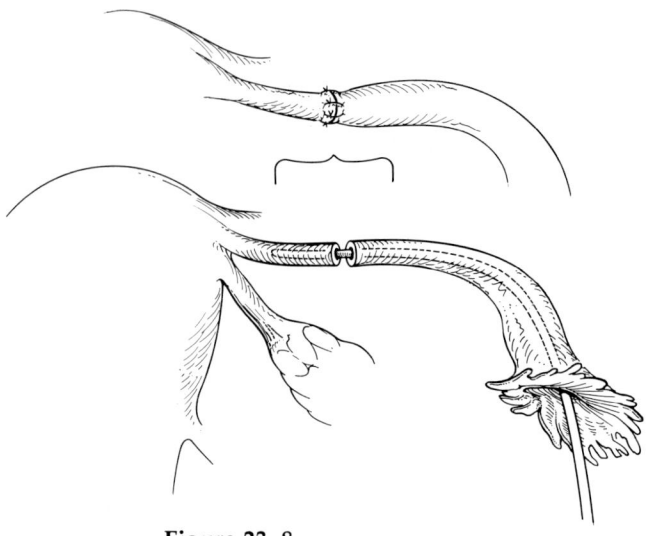

Figure 23–8
Isthmic-ampullary anastomosis.

lated, if possible, to avoid mucosal damage. An attempt is made, particularly in anastomosis of the isthmic tube, to avoid the mucosa, for fear of stenosis and postoperative occlusion. This technique should also be modified depending on the existence of a disparity between the proximal and distal segments.

In cases in which no luminal disparity exists between the proximal and distal segments, such as isthmic-isthmic anastomosis, a two-layer closure is performed. The muscularis is sutured circumferentially with three or four interrupted sutures, using 8–0 Vicryl, and knots are kept distal to the mucosa. When suturing the isthmic muscularis, only the inner one-third or one-half of the muscularis is included in the suture in order to avoid stenosis. The serosa is sutured with continuous sutures using 8–0 Vicryl (Fig. 23–7).

When luminal disparity exists, as is the case in isthmic-ampullary anastomoses, the surgical technique should attempt to decrease this disparity. The ampullary opening is created over a blunt probe to match the isthmic opening. In addition, the isthmic lumen can be enlarged by incising the proximal tube at an angle. The serosa is incised in a similar fashion to match the other segment.

Anastomosis is performed as previously described (Fig. 23–8).

ISTHMIC-CORNUAL ANASTOMOSIS

Isthmic-cornual anastomosis is performed if a small portion of the interstitial tube is occluded. A knife is used to core out the obstructed segment, thus creating a crater around the intramural tube. The isthmic portion is approximated to the intramural part, and anastomosis is performed in two layers as previously described, using high magnification. Diluted Pitressin may be used to decrease bleeding and facilitate the surgical procedure.

TUBAL STERILIZATION AND ITS REVERSAL

The various forms of tubal sterilization are some of the most common gynecologic procedures. The high demand for reversal of tubal sterilization should be taken into account in counseling patients as to the type of sterilization to be performed. The factors

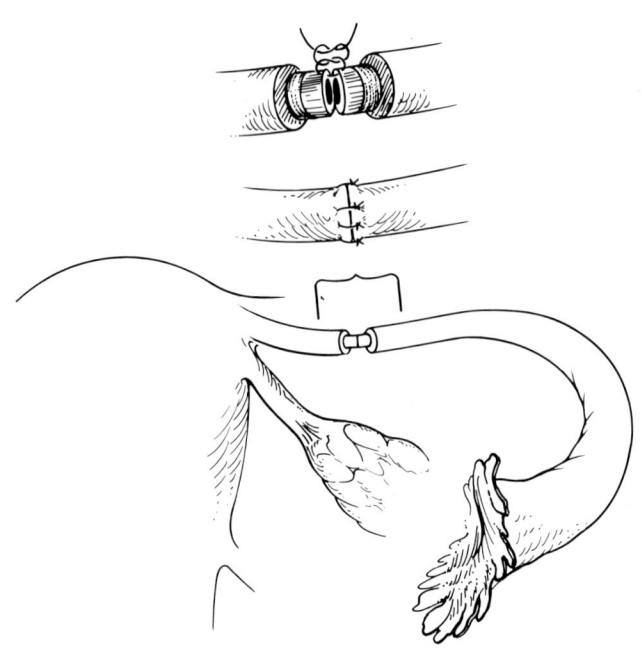

Figure 23–7
Isthmic-isthmic anastomosis.

determining the success of sterilization reversal are similar to those discussed for tubal anastomosis. Success may be correlated with (1) the extent of tubal destruction as a result of the sterilization, (2) the isthmus being the site of sterilization, (3) the presence of functioning fimbriae, and (4) a short interval from sterilization to repair.

The success of reversal is highest following sterilization procedures that destroy only a limited portion of tube. Thus, reversal of Hulka clip sterilization has the highest rate of success. This is followed by Falope ring, modified Pomeroy, Irving, Uchida, and last, by electrocoagulation. Sterilization by unipolar coagulation carries the poorest prognosis, owing to extensive tissue damage.[37]

The success of reversal is also related to the interval from sterilization to attempted repair. Vasquez and coworkers demonstrated the effects of prolonged tubal occlusion such as deciliation, flattening of the mucosal folds, and presence of mucosal polyps.[38]

Finally, the site of sterilization also affects the outcome of the reversal procedure: isthmic sterilization carries the highest rate of successful reversal. As mentioned earlier in the discussion of tubal anastomosis, isthmic-isthmic and isthmic-cornual anastomoses carry the highest rate of success. Thus sterilization procedures that preserve the isthmic portion are most likely to be reversible.

The overall success of microsurgical reversal following a variety of sterilization procedures was assessed in 118 patients. Sixty-five per cent conceived, and the mean surgery-conception interval was 10.2 months.[39]

The breakdown of success by sterilization procedure is presented in Table 23–2.[37, 40, 41]

The principles of tubal anastomosis described previously apply to reversal of tubal sterilization.

DIAGNOSTIC PROCEDURES

Laparoscopy and HSG are the "gold standard" in diagnosis of tubal disease. Peritubal as well as tubal occlusion can be diagnosed by one or both of these techniques. Direct inspection of tubal mucosa by endoscopy has shed new light on tubal pathology and its therapy.

The procedure of tubal endoscopy (salpingoscopy) can be performed hysteroscopically in the evaluation of the UTJ and proximal intramural portions, or in a retrograde fashion through the distal tubal ostium for evaluation of the distal tube. A transcervical approach to tubal endoscopy allowing visualization of the entire tube has been reported.[42] The technique of salpingoscopy has diagnostic and therapeutic applications. The properties of normal tubal mucosa, its folds, and vascularity can readily be evaluated. Nonobstructive tubal diseases, such as mild adhesions and mucosal scars impairing tubal function, can be diagnosed. Minor adhesions and other lesions such as polyps can be removed. The procedure is thought to have a prognostic value in predicting reproductive success. Cornier and colleagues reported a good correlation between the endoscopic result and postoperative patency and pregnancy rates following tubal repair.[43]

Investigation of the UTJ and the proximal portion of the intramural tube is performed with the aid of a CO_2 hysteroscope. The UTJ, the endosalpinx, mucosal folds, and mucosal vascularity can readily be evaluated. The endosalpinx in this area is usually smooth with minimal vascularity. Periosteal adhesions causing proximal tubal obstruction have been seen hysteroscopically.

Exploration of the distal tube and the ampullary-isthmic junction (AIJ) is performed in a retrograde fashion by cannulating the fimbrial end of the tube

Table 23–2

Tubal Anastomosis for Reversal of Sterilization: Outcome by Procedure

Author	Year	Method	Patients	Pregnant	%	Ectopic	%
Rock et al.[37]	1982	Caut uni: unipolar cautery	48	25	52	4	8.3
		Pomeroy: Pomeroy's tubal ligation	31	22	71	1	3.2
		Falope ring: Falope ring sterilization	22	18	82	0	0
		Irving: Irving's tubal ligation	6	4	66	0	0
Seiler[40]	1983	Caut uni: unipolar cautery	22	15	67	2	9.0
		Pomeroy: Pomeroy's tubal ligation	40	25	62	0	0
		Falope ring: Falope ring sterilization	6	3	50	0	0
		Irving: Irving's tubal ligation	4	3	75	0	0
Total		Pomeroy: Pomeroy's tubal ligation	71	47	66	1	1.4
		Caut uni: unipolar cautery	70	40	57	6	8.5
		Falope ring: Falope ring sterilization	28	21	75	0	0
		Irving: Irving's tubal ligation	10	7	70	0	0

From Lavy G, et al.: Ectopic pregnancy: Its relationship to tubal reconstructive surgery. Fertil Steril 47(4):543–556, 1987. Reproduced with permission of the publisher, The American Fertility Society.

during laparoscopy or laparotomy. The endoscope is visually guided through the ampulla during perfusion with saline solution under low pressure. The procedure allows the exploration of the distal tube to the AIJ. The normal ampullary mucosa is pinkish and shows parallel folds around its entire circumference. A variety of intratubal nonobstructive lesions have been identified, such as adhesions, epithelial scarring, and intraluminal debris. Cornier and associates have reported on the good correlation between HSG and endoscopic findings. No patient with abnormal HSG had normal endoscopy.[43] The therapeutic use of tubal endoscopy is being explored while the technology that will permit smaller fibers and surgical instruments that can be passed through an operating channel is being developed.

Kerin and coworkers reported on the correlation between transvaginal salpingoscopic findings, hysterosalpingography, and laparoscopy in 47 patients. In 74% of the cases, the salpingoscopic finding of an intraluminal defect correlated with an abnormal HSG or laparoscopic findings. In 12 of the 47 patients, an abnormal HSG or laparoscopy was associated with a normal salpingoscopy.[42]

In other studies, salpingoscopy was found to be a better predictor of reproductive outcome than laparoscopy.

SUMMARY

The isthmic tube has unique anatomic and physiologic characteristics. Some disease processes affect the isthmic tube exclusively, whereas others present a unique pathologic appearance when involving this part of the tube. Understanding of isthmic tube physiology and pathology is instrumental in the planning and execution of proper surgical therapy.

References

1. Hafez ESE: Transport of spermatozoa in the female reproductive tract. Am J Obstet Gynecol 1973; 115:703.
2. Lindblom B, Wilhelmsson L, Wikland M, et al.: Prostaglandins and oviductal function. Acta Obstet Gynecol Scand 1983; 113:43.
3. Caschetto S, Lindblom B, Wiqvist N, et al.: Prostaglandins and the contractile function of the human oviductal ampulla. Gynecol Obstet Invest 1979; 10:212.
4. Lindblom B, Ljung B, Hamberger L: Adrenergic and novel nonadrenergic neuronal mechanisms in the control of smooth muscle activity in the human oviduct. Acta Physiol Scand 1979; 106:215.
5. Winston RML, McLure M, Browne JC: Pregnancy following autograft transplantation of the fallopian tube and ovary in the rabbit. Lancet 1974; 2:294.
6. Owman C, Alm P, Sjoberg NO: Pelvic automomic ganglia: Structure, transmitters, function and steroid influence. In Elfin LG (ed.): Autonomic Ganglia. New York, John Wiley & Sons, 1983, p. 125.
7. Jansen RPS: Endocrine responses in the fallopian tube. Endocr Rev 1984; 5:525.
8. Critoph FN, Dennis KJ: Ciliary activity in the human oviduct. Br J Obstet Gynaecol 1977; 84:216.
9. Ansari AH, Bondell SP, Squires HR: Salpingitis isthmica nodosa. In Siegler AM (ed.): The Fallopian Tube: Basic Studies and Clinical Contributions. Mount Kisco, NY, Futura Publishing, 1986, p. 225.
10. Louis HH: Salpingitis isthmica nodosa in female infertility and ectopic tubal pregnancy. Fertil Steril 1978; 29:164.
11. Freakly G, Norman WJ, Ennis JT, et al.: Diverticulosis of the fallopian tubes. Clin Radiol 1974; 25:535.
12. Homm RJ, Holtz G, Garvin AJ: Isthmic ectopic pregnancy and salpingitis isthmica nodosa. Fertil Steril 1987; 48:756.
13. Ansari AH, Bondell SP, Squires HR: Salpingitis isthmica nodosa. In Siegler AM (ed.): The Fallopian Tube: Basic Studies and Clinical Contributions. Mount Kisco, NY, Futura Publishing, 1986, p. 227.
14. Laufer N, Sekeles E, Cohen R, et al.: The effects of E. coli endotoxin on the tubal mucosa of the rabbit. A scanning electron microscopic study. Path Res Pract 1980; 170:202.
15. Draper DL, Donegan EA, James JF, et al.: In vitro modeling of acute salpingitis caused by N. gonorrhoeae. Am J Obstet Gynecol 1980; 138:996.
16. Lavy G, Diamond MP, DeCherney AH: Pregnancy following tubocornual anastomosis. Fertil Steril 1986; 46:21.
17. Badawy SZA, Cuenca V, Marshall L, et al.: Cellular components in the peritoneal fluid in patients with and without endometriosis. Fertil Steril 1984; 42:704.
18. DeCherney AH, Boyers SP: Isthmic ectopic pregnancy: Segmental resection as the treatment of choice. Fertil Steril 1985; 44:307.
19. Oesiner G, Tarlatzis BC: Radical surgery for extrauterine pregnancy. In DeCherney AH (ed.): Ectopic Pregnancy. Rockville, MD, Aspen Publishers, 1986, p. 127.
20. Pauerstein CJ, Croxatto HB, Eddy CA, et al.: Anatomy and pathology of tubal pregnancy. Obstet Gynecol 1986; 67:301.
21. Senterman M, Jibodh R, Tulandi T: Histopathologic study of ampullary and isthmic tubal ectopic pregnancy. Am J Obstet Gynecol 1988; 159:939.
22. Stangel JJ, Reyniak JV: Conservative techniques for the management of tubal pregnancies. In Reyniak JV, Lauersen NH (eds.): Principles of Microsurgical Techniques in Infertility. New York, Plenum Publishers, 1982, p. 207.
23. Gomel V: Conservative surgical treatment of tubal pregnancy. In Gomel V (ed.): Microsurgery in Female Infertility. Boston, Little, Brown, 1983, p. 253.
24. Stangel JJ, Gomel V: Techniques in conservative surgery for tubal gestation. Clin Obstet Gynecol 1980; 23:1221.
25. Siegler AM, Wang CF, Westoff C: Management of unruptured tubal pregnancy. Obstet Gynecol Surv 1981; 35:599.
26. Pouly JL, Manhes H, Mage G, et al.: Conservative laparoscopic treatment of 321 ectopic pregnancies. Fertil Steril 1986; 46:1093.
27. DeCherney AH, Romero R, Naftolin F: Surgical management of unruptured ectopic pregnancy. Fertil Steril 1981; 35:21.
28. Bruhat MA, Manhes H, Mage G, Pouly JL: Treatment of ectopic pregnancy by means of laparoscopy. Fertil Steril 1980; 33:411.
29. Stovall TG, Ling FW, Buster JE: Reproductive performance after methotrexate treatment of ectopic pregnancy. Am J Obstet Gynecol 1990; 162:1620.
30. Sauer MV, Gorrill MJ, Rodi IA, et al.: Non-surgical management of unruptured ectopic pregnancy: An extended clinical trial. Fertil Steril 1987; 48:752.
31. Feichtinger W, Kemeta P: Conservative treatment of ectopic pregnancy by transvaginal aspiration under sonographic control and methotrexate injection. Lancet 1987; 1:381.
32. Lang PF, Weiss PA, Mayer HO, et al.: Conservative treatment of ectopic pregnancy with local injection of hyperosmolar glucose solution or prostaglandin-F_2 alpha: A prospective randomized study. Lancet 1990; 336:78.
33. Lindblom B, Hahlin M, Källfelt B, Hamberger L: Local prostaglandin F_2-α injection for termination of ectopic pregnancy. Lancet 1987; 1:776.

34. Timor-Tritsch I, Baxi L, Peisner DB: Transvaginal salpingocentesis: A new technique for treating ectopic pregnancy. Am J Obstet Gynecol 1989; 160(2):459.
35. Silber SJ, Cohen R: Microsurgical reversal of female sterilization: The role of tubal length. Fertil Steril 1980; 33:598.
36. te Velde ER, Boer ME, Looman CWN, Habbema JDF: Factors influencing success or failure after reversal of sterilization: A multivariate approach. Fertil Steril 1990; 54:270.
37. Rock JA, Bergquist CA, Zacur HA, et al.: Tubal anastomosis following unipolar cautery. Fertil Steril 1982; 37:613.
38. Vasquez G, Winston RML, Boeckx W, Brosens I: Tubal lesions subsequent to sterilization and their relation to fertility after attempts at reversal. Am J Obstet Gynecol 1980; 138:86.
39. Gomel V: Microsurgical reversal of female sterilization. Fertil Steril 1980; 33:587.
40. Seiler JC: Factors influencing the outcome of microsurgical tubal ligation reversal. Am J Obstet Gynecol 1983; 146:292.
41. Lavy G, Diamond MP, DeCherney AH: Ectopic pregnancy: Its relation to tubal reconstructive surgery. Fertil Steril 1987; 47:543.
42. Kerin J, Daykhovsky L, Segalowitz J, et al.: Falloposcopy: A microendoscopic technique for visual exploration of the human fallopian tube from the uterotubal ostium to the fimbria using a transvaginal approach. Fertil Steril 1990; 54:390.
43. Cornier E, Feintuch MJ, Corccora L: Fibrotuboscopie ampullaire. J Gynecol Obstet Biol Reprod 1984; 1:4.

Tubal Surgery: Distal Fallopian Tube

24

Eli Reshef
Joseph S. Sanfilippo

The earliest suggestion of the presence of uterine tubes is found in Hindu medical writings as early as 800 B.C.[1] In 1543, the famous anatomist Vesalius mentioned the tube but failed to recognize its uterine origin in his book *De humani corporis fabrica*.[2] His pupil, Gabriel Fallopius, however, provided the first anatomically accurate description of the uterine tube, published in *Observations Anatomicae* in 1561.[2] The fallopian tube was subsequently named in his honor.

Tubal surgery was first reported in modern times by Schroeder,[3] who in 1884 performed five tubal operations, one of which involved tubal resection. A summary of historic milestones in distal tubal surgery is presented in Table 24–1. Results of distal tubal surgery in the first half of this century were disappointing. In a survey presented to members of the Chicago Gynecologic Society in 1936, Greenhill[7] reported a cumulative rate of 4.4% live births out of more than 800 procedures. As knowledge of tubal function and pathology expanded in the second half of this century, along with improvement in surgical techniques, the live birth rate has improved to 20–30% following distal tubal surgery. This improvement is largely attributed to the application of meticulous surgical techniques, primarily microsurgical.

In the late 1940s, prosthetic devices made of nylon and, subsequently, of silicone were introduced by Mulligan and colleagues[8] to maintain tubal patency following surgical repair. Other devices followed (Fig. 24–1).[14,15] Tubal surgery under magnification was introduced to gynecology by Swolin in 1967.[11] As improved technical expertise in tubal microsurgery accrued, outcome equal or superior to conventional "macroscopic" tubal surgery with or without

Table 24–1

Historic Milestones

Year	Author	Contribution
1561	Fallopius[2]	First anatomically correct description of the uterine tube
1884	Schroeder[3]	First description of tubal surgery (five cases, one salpingostomy)
1889	Skutsch[4]	First used the term *salpingostomy*
1891	Martin[5]	First postoperative pregnancy in 24 cases of distal tubal surgery (aborted)
1932	Holden and Sovak[6]	Described cuff salpingostomy (two methods)
1937	Greenhill[7]	Survey showing poor live birth rate following tubal surgery (4.4% out of 818 cases)
1953	Mulligan et al[8]	Silicone prosthesis (Mulligan hood)
1956	Greenhill[9]	Report of 15% live birth rate among 2000 patients following distal salpingostomy
1959	Walz[10]	First salpingostomy under magnification
1967	Swolin[11]	Microsalpingostomy
1974	Semm[12]	First laparoscopic salpingostomy
1988	American Fertility Society[13]	Classification of tubal occlusion and adnexal adhesions

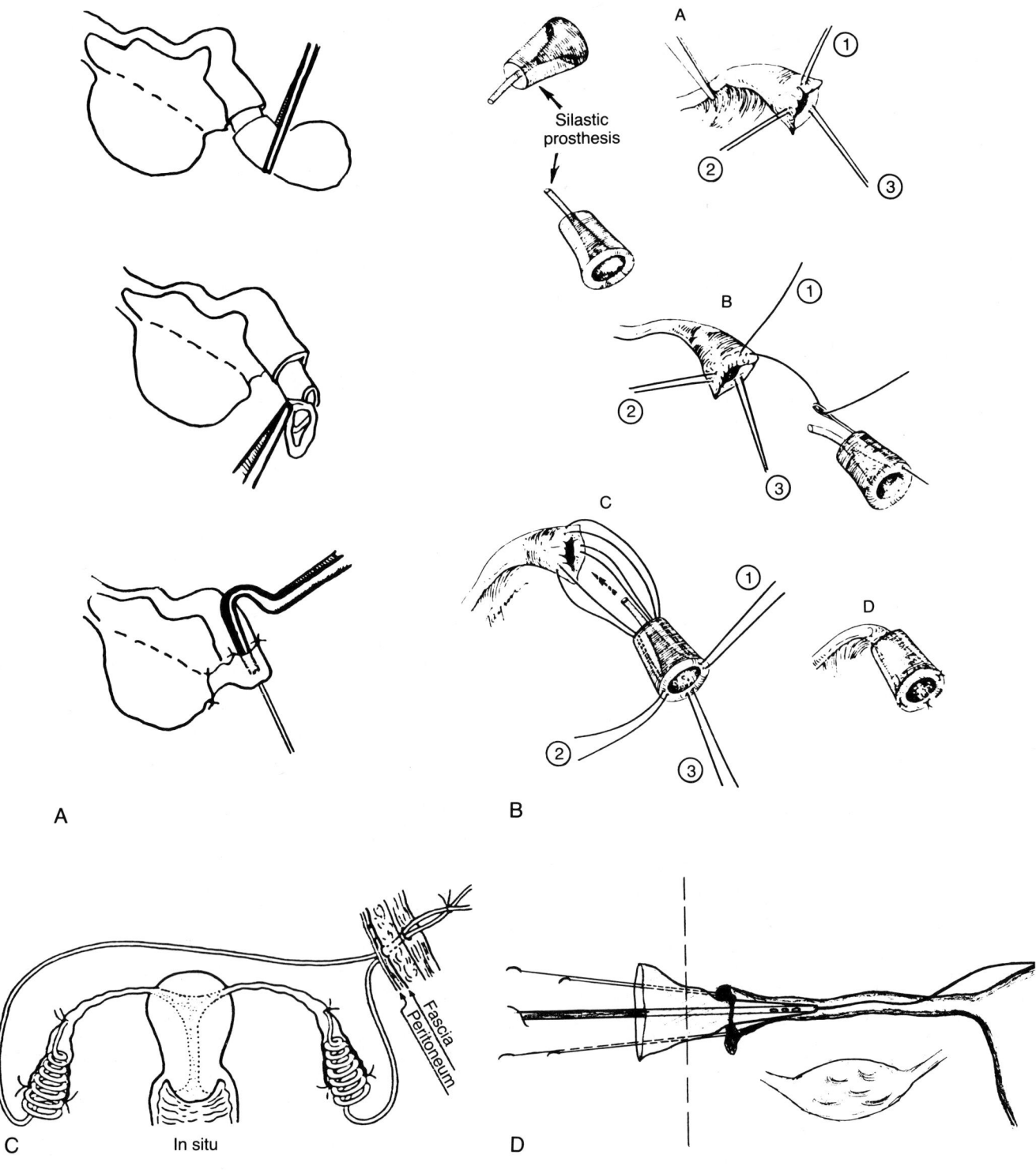

Figure 24–1
Historical milestones in distal tubal surgery. *A*, Bonney cuff salpingostomy, used by Holden and Sovak in 1932.[6] (From Palmer R: Discussion on modern methods of salpingostomy. Proc R Soc Med 1960; 53:357.) *B*, Silastic Mulligan hood. (From Mulligan WJ: Int J Fertil 1966; 11:424.) *C*, Roland prosthesis. (Reprinted with permission from The American College of Obstetricians and Gynecologists [Obstetrics and Gynecology, 1970; 36:359].) *D*, Cognat hood. (Courtesy of Marvin A. Yussman, M.D., Professor of Obstetrics and Gynecology, University of Louisville, School of Medicine.)

prosthetic devices resulted, and thus, the cornerstone of reparative distal tubal surgery was established. The popularity of prosthetic devices rapidly declined. As the extent of tubal disease was classified into prognostic categories (as noted subsequently), it became apparent that the inferior live birth rate following surgery for severe distal tubal damage should be weighed against modern assisted reproductive technologies such as in vitro fertilization (IVF), which in experienced hands may yield more than 15% live births per cycle.[16]

TUBE: PATHOPHYSIOLOGY

Normal Function

The fallopian tube is a dynamic structure with complex gross and intrinsic motion designed to capture and transport the ovum toward the uterus. In addition, it facilitates sperm transport in the opposite direction. The fimbria ovarica, a bridge of collagen and smooth muscle connecting the fimbriated end of the tube to its ovary, exhibits maximum activity at ovulation and probably aids in ovum pickup. At ovulation, the fimbriated end of the tube sweeps over the ovarian surface and captures the ovum.[17] In the ampullary portion of the tube, approximately 65% of the mucosal epithelial cells are ciliated, and the remainder are secretory cells (Fig. 24–2A).[18] The cilia at this segment beat toward the uterus approximately seven times per minute.[19] The egg is swept into the fimbria primarily by ciliary action.

The success of capture is inversely related to the degree of fimbrial deciliation.[20] Ciliary motion is probably more responsible for ovum transport than is gross tubal motion, although the normal or nearly normal fertility rate in immotile cilia syndrome challenges this notion. Intraluminal secretion volume and thickness increase in the periovulatory period, perhaps masking ciliary activity toward the uterus to allow sperm transport into the distal tube near the ovary.[21] Luminal secretions then clear, allowing prouterine ciliary motion to predominate.[20]

Pathology

Pelvic inflammatory disease (PID) is the most common etiology of tubal damage and can be deleterious to tubal function through several mechanisms. Gross tubal motion may be impaired by pelvic adhesions,

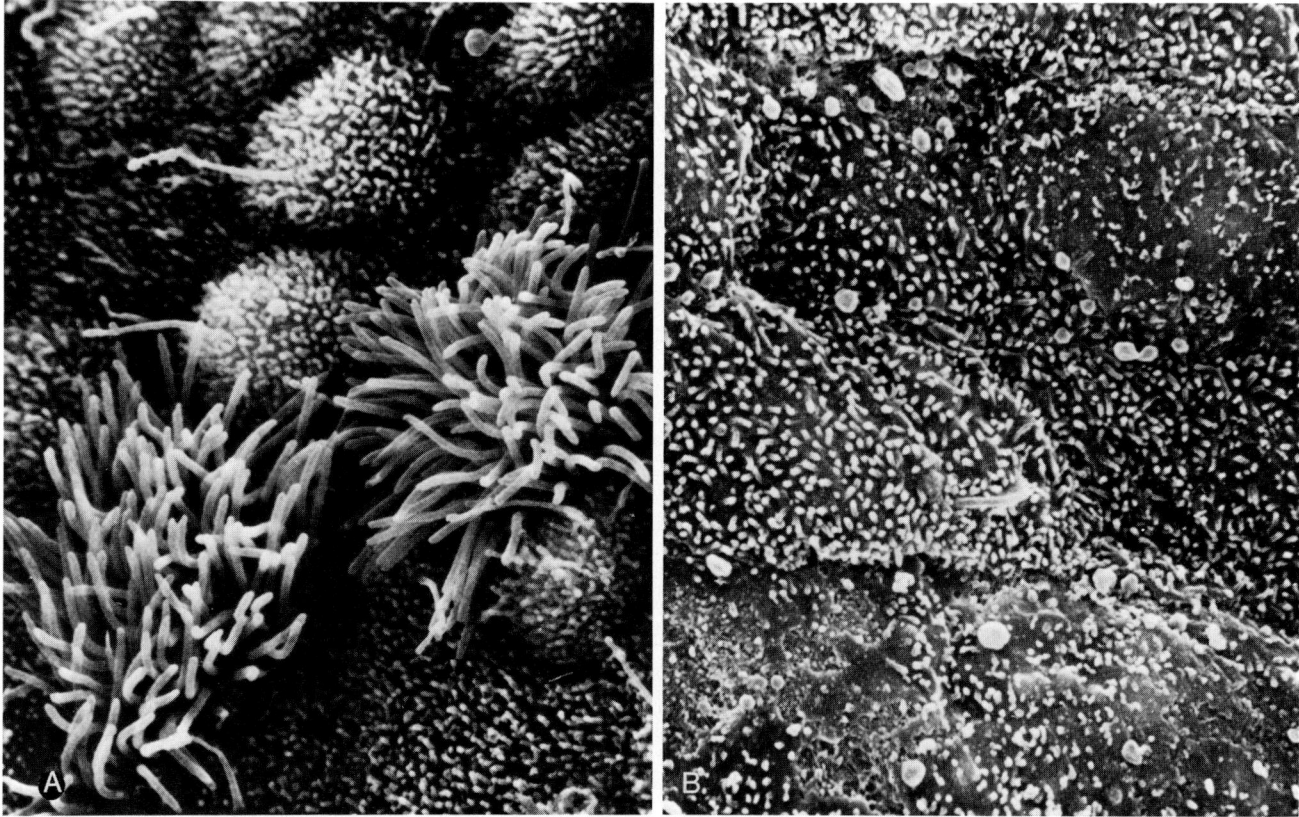

Figure 24–2
Scanning electron microscopy images of the ampullary portion of human fallopian tubes. *A*, Healthy ampullary mucosa. Note both ciliated and secretory cells (magnification 5000×). *B*, Ampullary mucosa of a hydrosalpinx. Note the marked absence of cilia (one seen at the center) (magnification 5000×). (Courtesy of Marvin A. Yussman, M.D., Professor of Obstetrics and Gynecology, University of Louisville, School of Medicine.)

thus preventing ovum pickup. The latter can also be prevented by adhesive bands that block the distal tube. Ovum extrusion can be disrupted by extensive periovarian adhesions. Intrinsic tubal damage is yet another mechanism by which PID can impair fertility. Destruction of the cilia may also prevent ovum transport (Fig. 24–2B). Fimbrial agglutination and phimosis, as well as partial or complete distal occlusion secondary to thickened visceral peritoneum, are the sequelae of chronic inflammation.

The white lines often noted at the distal end of a hydrosalpinx represent demarcation of peritoneal fusion. Complete distal occlusion will result in increased internal tubal pressure, a consequence of impaired egress of tubal secretions. The myosalpinx then thickens, and eventually the tubal wall weakens and becomes dilated (hydrosalpinx) with fibrous tissue replacing smooth muscle. Increased internal pressure will result in attenuation and eventual complete destruction of mucosal folds and cilia (Fig. 24–3). Hydrosalpinx (sactosalpinx in European literature) is usually a consequence of infectious salpingitis and is often associated with intrinsic tubal disease. Two histopathologic types have been characterized: hydrosalpinx simplex (h. simplex) and hydrosalpinx follicularis (h. follicularis). H. simplex has a single lumen, whereas h. follicularis has multiple luminal compartments as a result of septae formed by fusion of mucosal plicae. The latter is often associated with tubal wall thickening, which is due to chronic interstitial tubal disease (Fig. 24–3).

The degree of deciliation correlates positively with the severity of distal tubal disease by radiographic criteria and negatively with pregnancy rates following surgical repair.[22] A decrease in cytosolic estrogen and progesterone receptors has also been demonstrated.[23] Exogenous estrogen administration may reverse some cilial damage and promote regeneration.[24] Most studies of experimental hydrosalpinx investigated the sequelae of mechanical obstruction of the tube without infection. In rabbits and primates, the progressive loss of mucosal plicae was duplicated by ligating the oviducts. The effect on cilia was variable, with some studies showing preservation of ciliary activity and morphology as well as normal ovum transport[25, 26] and others demonstrating deciliation and decreased capillary volume and number.[27, 28]

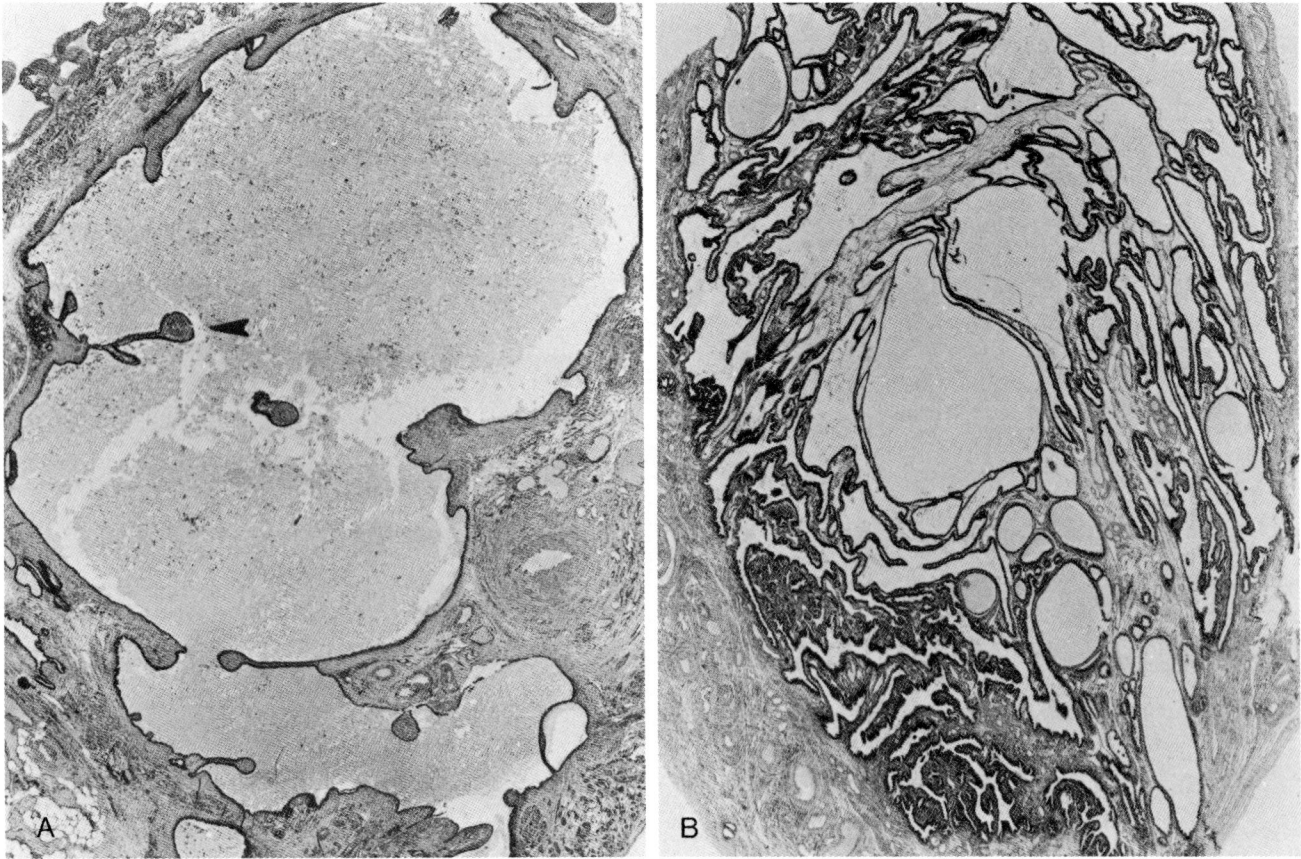

Figure 24–3
Light microscopy of hydrosalpinx. A, Hydrosalpinx simplex. Note the absence of mucosal folds (one intact fold marked by arrowhead) and the presence of a thin-walled enlarged lumen. B, Hydrosalpinx follicularis. (From Woodruff JD, Pauerstein CJ: The Fallopian Tube. Baltimore, Williams & Wilkins, 1969, p. 1.)

In the past, *Neisseria gonorrhoeae* was considered the major etiologic factor in the pathogenesis of salpingitis. However, *Chlamydia trachomatis* is now implicated as the primary agent as manifested by the identification of high antichlamydial IgG titer in greater than 60% of patients with acute salpingitis.[29] Cervical inoculation with chlamydia results in ascending infection with subsequent endometritis and salpingitis.[20] Proximal ligation of the oviducts appears to prevent such infection.[20] Primary inoculation of the fallopian tubes results in salpingitis.[30] Chlamydial salpingitis results in progressive deciliation and endothelial damage. Lymphocytic infiltration suggests a lymphocyte-mediated cytotoxic process. Repeat chlamydial infection may be the key for the evolution of a hydrosalpinx. Chlamydial infection may indeed be silent and associated with progressive tubal damage.[31]

N. gonorrhoeae has been isolated in 5–65% of patients with acute PID.[20] It is thought to disseminate via the lymphatics and endometrium, and primarily affects epithelial secretory cells. *Mycoplasma* and *Ureaplasma urealyticum*, in general, account for a small percentage of salpingitis cases and may actually cause primary endomyometritis. Anaerobes are thought to be secondary invaders in salpingitis and are frequently isolated from tubo-ovarian complexes during the acute phase. Detrimental effects of coliform organisms, especially gram-negative bacteria, are thought, in part, to be due to direct action of the endotoxin on tubal epithelium.[32]

CLASSIFICATION OF DISTAL TUBAL DISEASE

In 1966, Shirodkar[33] emphasized the importance of considering various factors that affect severity of tubal disease when judging the results of salpingostomy. He and other gynecologists recognized that the extent of tubal damage was of paramount importance in determining the postoperative outcome. Although specific data were not given by Shirodkar, he proposed a classification based on five factors: (1) the size of the hydrosalpinx (less than or greater than thumb size); (2) the consistency of peritubal adhesions (flimsy or firm); (3) the condition of the tubal wall (normal; pale and overstretched; or soft, hard, or nodular); (4) the status of the fimbria (normal, few buds, or absent); and (5) the condition of the ciliary epithelium after biopsy (good, fair, or poor).

Through the years, several classifications of distal tubal disease have been proposed. One of the most popular has been that of Rock and coworkers from 1978[34] that is based on preoperative hysterosalpingography (HSG) as well as on intraoperative findings. Tubal disease is classified as mild, moderate, or severe on the basis of the size of the hydrosalpinx, the extent and consistency of tubal adhesions, the status of the fimbria, and the mucosal pattern of the tubal lumen on HSG. In 1983, Boer-Meisel and associates[35] proposed a numeric classification based on intraoperative findings regarding the diameter of the hydrosalpinx, extent and consistency of pelvic adhesions, gross appearance of the mucosa, and tubal wall thickness. Both research groups presented data supporting an inverse relationship between the extent of distal tubal disease and the rate of live births per patient.[34, 35]

In 1986, Mage and colleagues[36] proposed a classification based on HSG and laparoscopic findings, rather than on actual intraoperative observations at laparotomy. This classification is based on the extent and consistency of tubo-ovarian adhesions, as well as on information regarding tubal patency, hysterographic appearance of the tubal mucosa, and the appearance of the tubal wall at laparoscopy. The most commonly accepted classification of distal tubal disease is that of the American Fertility Society (Fig. 24–4).[16] This numeric classification utilizes intraoperative laparotomy findings based on the assertion that although laparoscopy and HSG may be effective in diagnosing cases at both extremes of tubal disease, certain factors can only be assessed after appropriate exposure or palpation. These include the extent of tubal wall rigidity and thickness and the status of the mucosal folds at the neostomy site. The utility of salpingoscopy in determining prognosis preoperatively is yet unproved, although preliminary studies show good correlation between salpingoscopic and histologic findings.[37] The development of flexible hysteroscopic salpingoscopy may prove useful for preoperative evaluation of distal tubal disease.[38]

PREOPERATIVE EVALUATION

The selection of patients best suited for distal tubal surgery is of utmost importance because there is an inverse relationship between the severity of tubal disease and the conception rate. Definitions of types of surgical procedures are conveyed in Table 24–2. Assisted reproductive techniques such as IVF should be considered alternatively in patients with moderate or severe tubal damage. An operative endoscopic (pelviscopic) approach may be an appropriate alternative. Therefore, thorough preoperative evaluation and discussion with patients are required in order to optimize the therapeutic alternatives. The surgeon's experience clearly influences success rates.[40, 41] Absolute contraindications to distal tubal surgery are shown in Table 24–3.

A thorough infertility evaluation should be conducted prior to attempting tubal repair. Potential

Patient's Name _____ Date _____ Chart # _____
Age _____ G _____ P _____ Sp Ab _____ VTP _____ Ectopic _____ Infertile Yes _____ No _____
Other Significant History (i.e. surgery, infection, etc) _____

HSG _____ Sonography _____ Photography _____ Laparoscopy _____ Laparotomy _____

		<3 cm	3-5 cm	>5 cm
Distal ampullary diameter				
	L	1	4	6
	R	1	4	6
Tubal wall thickness		Normal/Thin	Moderately Thickened or Edematous	Thick & Rigid
	L	1	4	6
	R	1	4	6
Mucosal folds at neostomy site		Normal/ >75% Preserved	35% to 75% Preserved	<35% Preserved Adherent Mucosal Fold
	L	1	4	6
	R	1	4	6
Extent of adhesions		None/Minimal/Mild	Moderate	Extensive
	L	1	3	6
	R	1	3	6
Type of adhesions		None/Filmy	Moderately Dense (or Vascular)	Dense
	L	1	2	4
	R	1	2	4

Prognostic Classification for Terminal Salpingostomy (Salpingoneostomy)

	LEFT		RIGHT
A. Mild	_____	1-3	_____
B. Moderate	_____	9-10	_____
C. Severe	_____	>10	_____

Treatment (Surgical Procedures):
Salpingostomy   L   R
   A. Terminal   _____   _____
   B. Ampullary   _____   _____

Other: _____

Prognosis for Conception & Subsequent Viable Infant*

_____ Excellent (> 75%)
_____ Good   (50 - 75%)
_____ Fair   (25% - 50%)
_____ Poor   (< 25%)

*Physician's judgment based upon adnexa with least amount of pathology.

Recommended Followup Treatment: _____

Additional Findings: _____

DRAWING
L   R

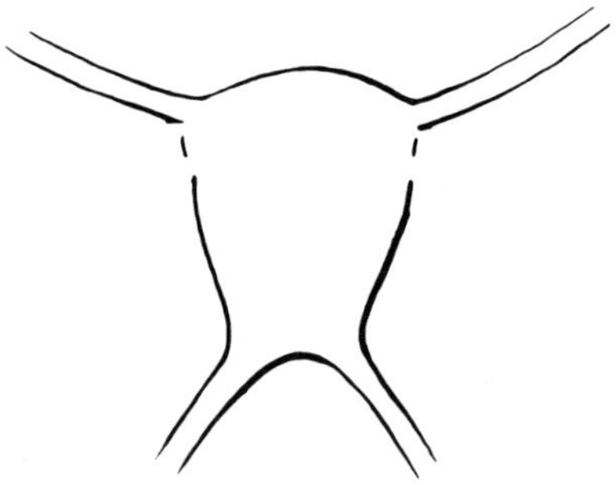

For additional supply write to:
The American Fertility Society
2140 11th Avenue, South
Suite 200
Birmingham, Alabama 35205

Property of
The American Fertility Society

Figure 24-4
The American Fertility Society classification of distal tubal occlusion. (From Fertil Steril 49(6):948, 1988. Reproduced with permission of the publisher, The American Fertility Society.)

Table 24–2
Definitions of Tubal Surgery

Salpingostomy (salpingoneostomy): surgical creation of a new tubal ostium
  a. Terminal
  b. Ampullary
  c. Isthmic
  d. Combination: different type anastomosis on right and left tubes

Fimbrioplasty: reconstruction of existent fimbria
  a. By deagglutination and dilatation
  b. With serosal incision (for completely occluded tube)
  c. Combination: different type fimbrioplasty on right and left tubes

Lysis of periadnexal adhesions (salpingo-ovariolysis): classified according to the adnexa with least pathology
  a. Minimal: 1 cm of tube or ovary involved
  b. Moderate: partially surround tube or ovary
  c. Severe: encapsulating peritubal or periovarian adhesions

Classification by the International Federation of Fertility and Sterility (IFFS) at the Ninth and Tenth World Congress of Fertility and Sterility, 1977 and 1980.
Adapted from Gomel V: Classification of operations for tubal and peritoneal factors causing infertility. Clin Obstet Gynecol 1980; 23:1259.

Table 24–3
Absolute Contraindications to Distal Tubal Surgery

Active pelvic infection
Genital tuberculosis
Serious medical or psychologic contraindications to pregnancy
Absence of ampullary segment of fallopian tube
Absence of sufficient ovarian surface

---

infertility factors, such as ovulatory dysfunction, male factors, and cervical abnormality, should be excluded. The extent of intrinsic tubal disease as well as intracavitary uterine architecture are evaluated by HSG. The HSG, particularly when using water-soluble contrast, can suggest the presence or absence of distal tubal rugae, an important prognostic factor (Fig. 24–5). The presence or absence of tubal occlusion as well as the size of the hydrosalpinx (another important prognostic factor) can also be identified on HSG.

Diagnostic laparoscopy may serve as an important adjunct to the assessment of the severity of tubal disease. The extent and consistency of adhesions can only be determined reliably by direct vision (Fig. 24–6). This can well be coordinated with immediate surgical repair of the tube and lysis of adhesions. Other prognostic factors such as tubal wall texture and status of the fimbria can often be examined via laparoscopy.

Although laparoscopic distal tubal surgery has gained popularity with the increased acceptance of pelviscopic surgery, data specifically addressing the choice and efficacy of laparoscopic salpingostomy versus laparotomy with microsurgical salpingostomy are scant. Table 24–4 summarizes the results of laparoscopic salpingostomy from the literature. It shows that pregnancy rates using the laparoscopic approach are comparable with microscopic salpingostomy (Table 24–5). Until more data are available, one should consider the endoscopic approach, which involves less operative morbidity and discomfort and is more cost-effective, in the presence of moderate or severe distal tubal disease, or if IVF is not a feasible alternative.

Several authors recommend that distal tubal surgery be performed during the follicular phase of the cycle to take advantage of the "anabolic regenerative interval" of the cycle and to reduce bleeding that may be more prominent during the luteal phase.[62]

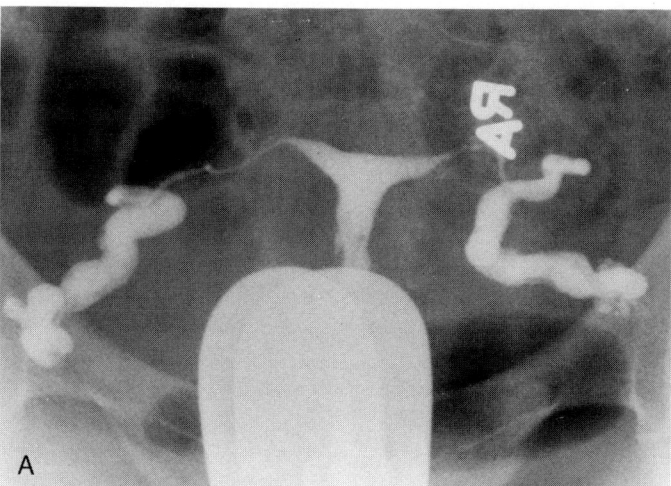
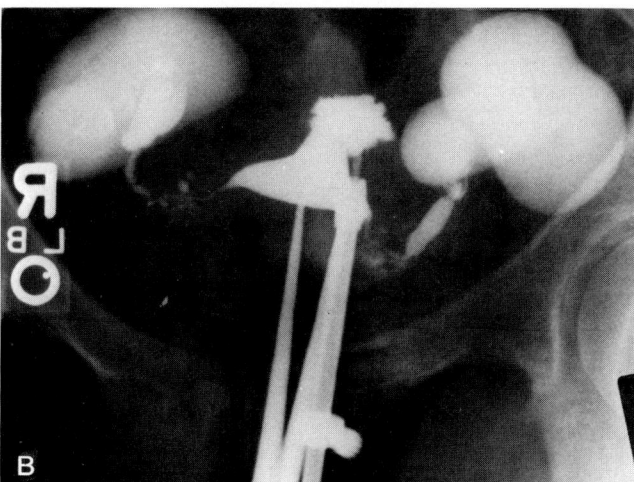

Figure 24–5
Hysterosalpingograms of two patients with bilateral distal tubal disease (water-soluble contrast medium). *A*, Bilateral small hydrosalpinges. Note the lack of spill bilaterally as well as the suggestion of mucosal rugae bilaterally. *B*, Bilateral large hydrosalpinges with occlusion. The presence of salpingitis isthmica nodosa is suggested by the radiographic appearance of the proximal isthmic segments.

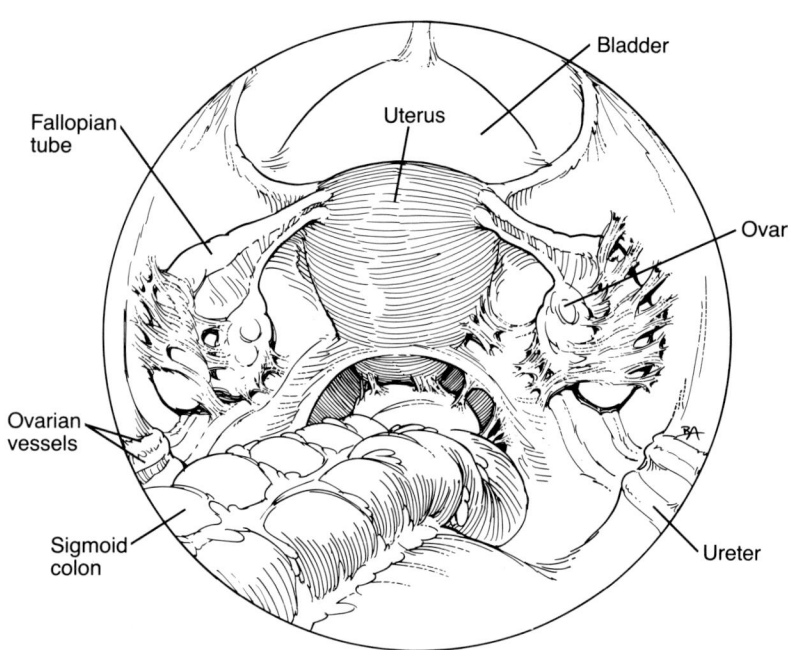

Figure 24–6
Illustration of a laparoscopic view of pelvic adhesions and distal tubal disease. Note tubo-ovarian adhesions as well as bilateral hydrosalpinges.

Table 24–4

Endoscopic Salpingostomy

Reference	Year	Patients	Pregnancy Rate (%)	Term (%)	Ectopic (%)	Aborted (%)	Comments
Gomel[42]	1977	9	44	—	0	—	No laser
Mettler et al[43]	1979	38	26	—	—	—	No laser
Fayez[44]	1983	19	10	0	10	—	No laser
Daniell and Herbert[45]	1984	21	24	19	5	—	Laser
Mage et al[46]	1990	87	33	—	—	—	Laser/pelvisc.

Table 24–5

Microsurgical Salpingostomy

Reference	Year	Patients	Pregnancy Rate (%)	Term (%)	Ectopic (%)	Aborted (%)
Swolin[47]	1975	33	45	—	18	—
Marik[48]	1977	52	23	—	2	—
Winston[49]	1980	241	18	—	10	—
Gomel[50]	1980	72	31	—	10	—
DeCherney and Kase[51]	1981	54	44	26	17	—
Larsson[52]	1982	54	39	31	0	7
Verhoeven et al[40]	1983	167	—	17	2	4
Tulandi and Vilos[53]	1985	30	23	20	3	—
Luber et al[54]	1986	17	35	18	18	0
Boer-Meisel et al[35]	1986	108	46	22	18	6
Kitchin et al[55]	1986	103	39	25	13	13
Russell et al[56]	1986	68	—	42	17	—
Carey and Brown[57]	1987	65	28	18	9	—
Williams and Griffin[58]	1988	62	21	—	16	—
Laatikainen et al[59]	1988	93	13	—	13	8
Jacobs et al[60]	1988	71	47	32	11	12
Wu and Minassian[61]	1989	36	25	—	—	—

One should consider the possibility of an early gestation and perform a pregnancy test if the surgery is performed in the luteal phase of the cycle. There are no studies that demonstrate an advantage to operating on the distal tube at any particular phase of the menstrual cycle. Patients should be apprised of the possibility of a unilateral salpingectomy or salpingo-oophorectomy if that adnexa is deemed irreparable and pelvic pain is a dominant complaint.

TUBAL SURGERY: LAPAROTOMY

Instruments and Accessories

For fimbrioplasty or salpingostomy under magnification, microsurgical instruments similar to those used in tubal reanastomosis are required. Table 24–6 lists recommended surgical instruments and "magnification instruments" for these procedures. For intraoperative chromopertubation, several devices may be useful. A simple and inexpensive one is a pediatric 8 Fr Foley catheter (Fig. 24–7), which is inserted through the cervix preoperatively under direct vision and then inflated with 3-ml fluid. It is connected to an intravenous extension line and a syringe filled with indigo carmine or methylene blue, which can be operated by the surgeon during the procedure. Any commercially available transcervical cannula for hydrotubation can also be used. Transfundal injection of dye after occlusion of the lower uterine segment with a Buxton or Shirodkar clamp is now used infrequently owing to obstruction of the surgical field by the clamp and the availability of the less traumatic alternatives previously discussed.

Table 24–6

Instruments and Equipment for Microsurgical Salpingostomy

Operating microscope
Operating loupes*
Bipolar coagulation unit
Bipolar microforceps
Unipolar coagulation unit
Unipolar needle microelectrode
Self-retaining retractor (e.g., Kirschner's)
Irrigator (Gomel's or a 20-ml syringe with 23–25-gauge clipped needle)
Heparinized lactated Ringer's solution (1-L IV bag)
Suction tips (small and regular)
Dissecting rods (glass or Teflon; quartz if laser is used)
Microscissors
Iris scissors
Microneedle carrier
Ring microforceps*
Platform microforceps
Toothed microforceps (2)
Smooth microforceps (2)
Nonabsorbable or delayed-absorption 8–0 sutures with tapered needle
Pediatric 8–10 Fr foley catheter
Indigo carmine (30-ml syringe or IV bag)

*Optional.

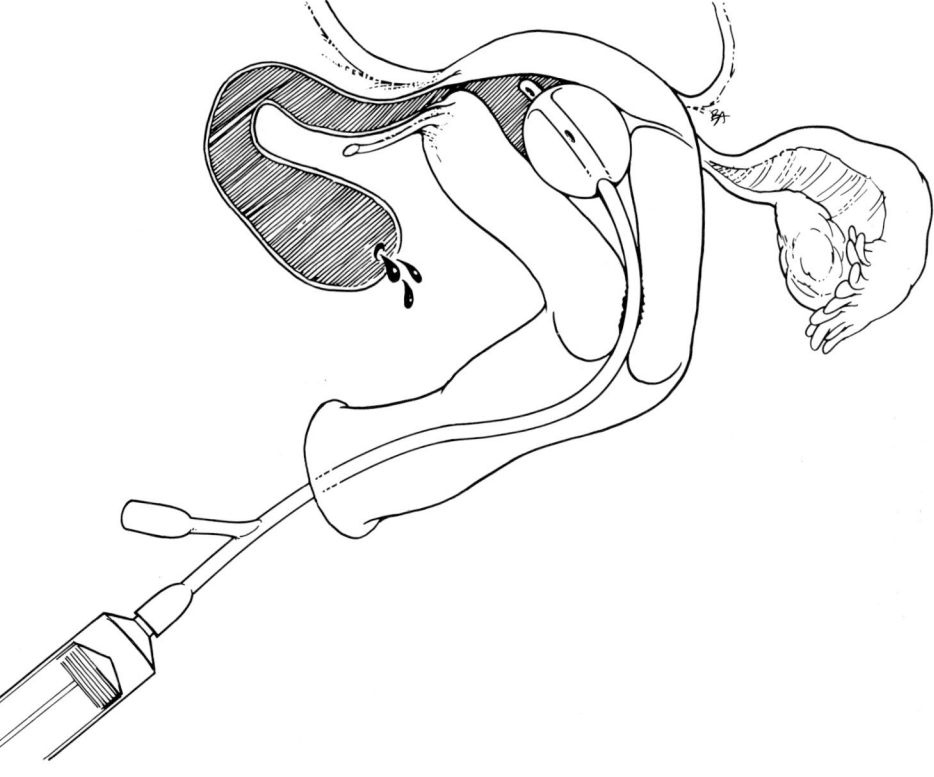

Figure 24–7
Chromopertubation. A size 8–10 Fr pediatric Foley catheter is inserted by direct visualization into the cervix prior to draping the patient. It is connected via an extension tubing to a 20- or 30-ml syringe containing blue dye.

Abdominal Incision and Exposure

The incision must provide room for adequate adhesiolysis and freeing of the adnexa. Care must be taken to provide hemostasis and avoid leakage of blood into the peritoneal cavity. The wound edges should be protected with lint-free moistened laparotomy pads prior to insertion of the retractor. A self-retaining retractor, such as a Kirschner, is excellent for four-way retraction (Fig. 24–8).

Moistened laparotomy pads or pads in plastic bags are suitable for displacement of the bowel to enhance exposure. The former are easier to handle but may cause abrasive injury to peritoneal surfaces if not handled carefully. The latter are slippery and therefore more difficult to handle but may cause less peritoneal trauma. If adhesions are present, they should be lysed initially before lap pad placement to provide maximum mobilization of the involved adnexa. Following adhesiolysis, the uterus and adnexa to be repaired are elevated to the level of the abdominal incision by packing the cul-de-sac as well as the lateral and anterior spaces with moistened laps (see Fig. 24–8). The contralateral adnexa should not be exposed to prevent trauma through drying.

All peritoneal surfaces should be irrigated periodically with warm isotonic irrigation solution such as lactated Ringer's solution. Addition of heparin to the irrigation solution offers no further benefits.[63] A syringe with a 23–25-gauge needle with a clipped tip can serve as an irrigation device. Alternatively, an irrigator devised by Gomel and Swolin,[64] which is connected to an intravenous set and turned on or off by the operator, can be used.

Adhesiolysis

The basic principles of reproductive surgery must be followed to minimize tissue trauma with resultant adhesion formation. Tissue should be handled with care. Peritoneal surfaces should be grasped with fine-toothed forceps whenever possible. Blotting action with surgical laps, as well as handling the adnexa with gloved hands, is discouraged. Elevation of the fallopian tube should be performed with Babcock

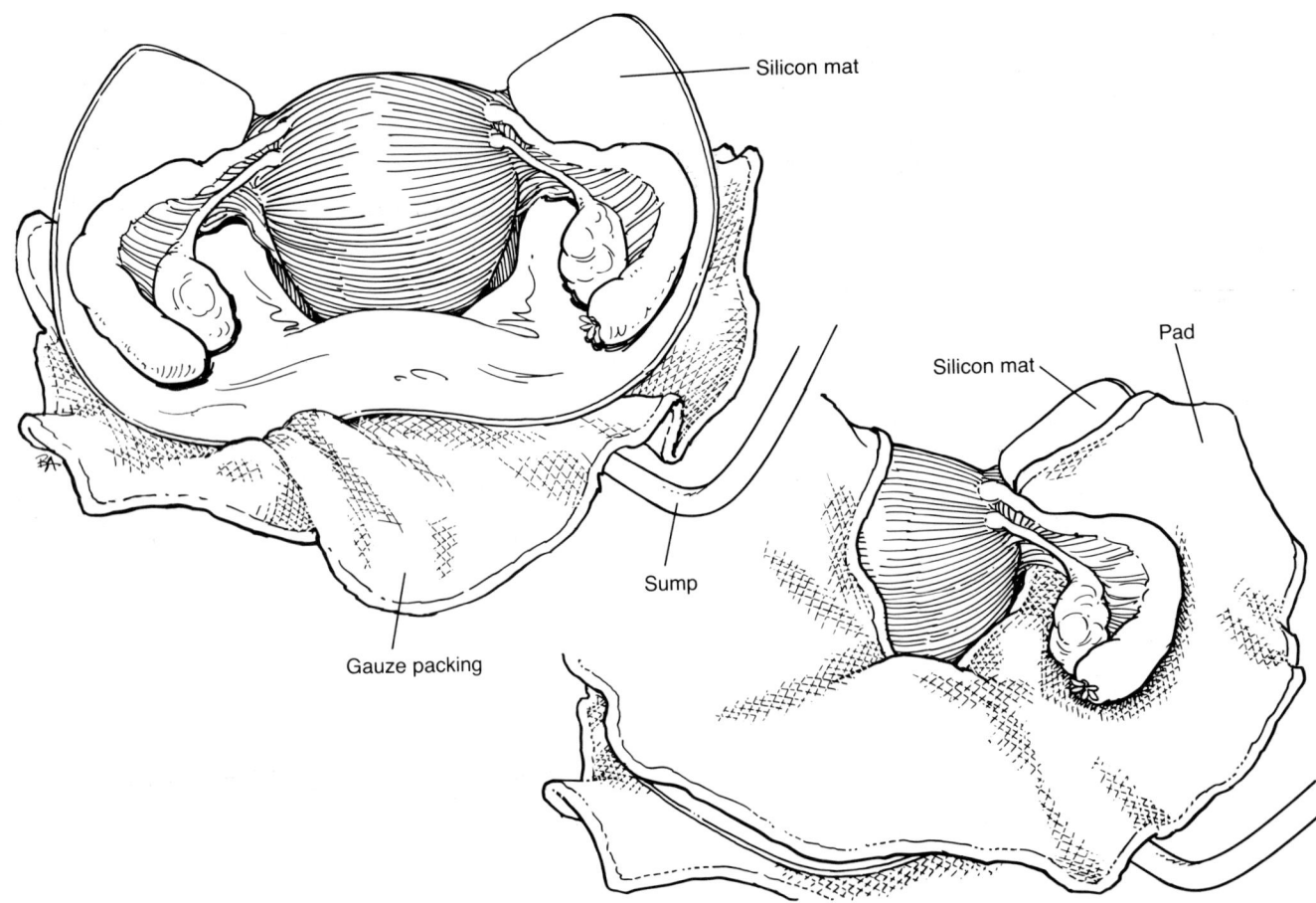

Figure 24–8
Retraction and packing during microsalpingostomy. Only one adnexa is exposed at a time to avoid drying or trauma to the contralateral adnexa. The abdominal incision edges are protected with moist sponges. A Kirschner retractor is excellent for four-way retraction. Packing is accomplished by using moist, lint-free laparotomy sponges or sponges in plastic bags. Alternatively, a silicone mat may be used.

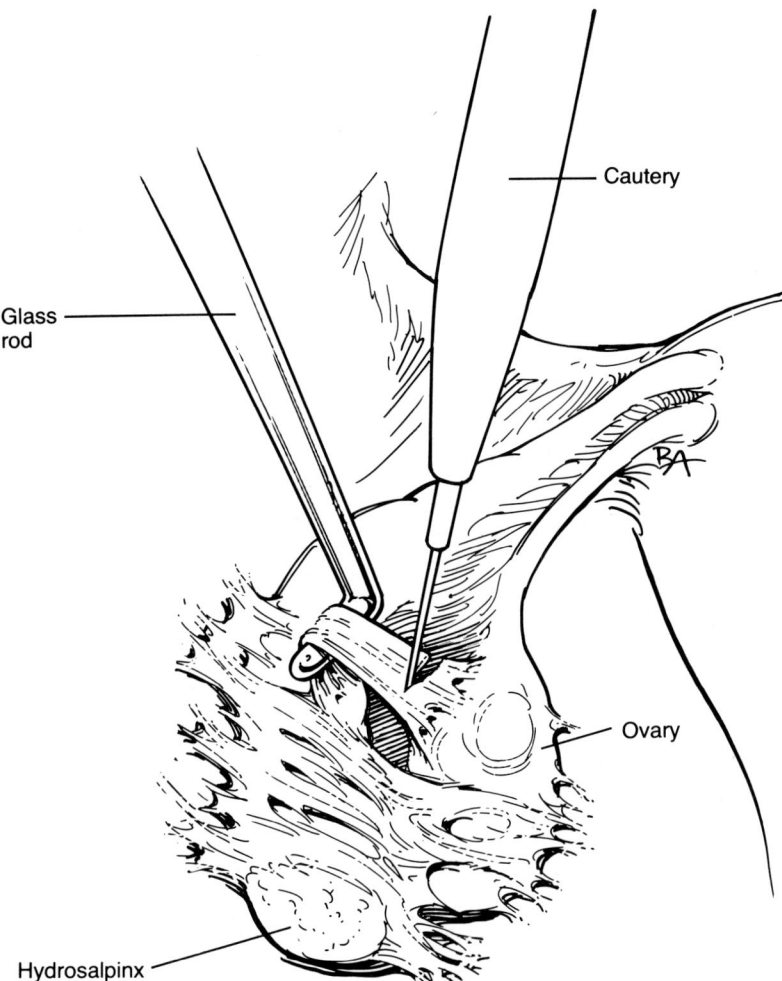

Figure 24–9
Lysis of adnexal adhesions (ovariolysis and salpingolysis). A glass, quartz, or Teflon-coated rod is inserted behind the adhesion. The adhesive band is severed in both attachments and then removed in its entirety using a fine-needle microelectrode, a hand-held laser, or fine scissors.

forceps or special cylindric tube forceps. Whenever electrocautery or laser are used, the tissue should be irrigated in order to reduce lateral thermal damage. One must avoid denuding peritoneal surfaces as much as possible. If this is inevitable, a graft taken from the parietal peritoneum at the abdominal incision site or a synthetic fabric should be considered. The use of omental graft in this instance is discouraged because it may promote adhesion formation. Agents that inhibit peritoneal inflammatory responses (e.g., steroids or methylxanthine derivatives) have also been suggested.

Lysis of adhesions is performed with a unipolar needle cautery device or with the hand-held laser. For locations deep in the pelvis, a long, insulated cautery needle is used. Lysis of pelvic adhesions that do not intimately involve the tube can be performed without magnification. Ovariolysis, and especially salpingolysis, often requires magnification in order to reduce potential damage to the adnexal surface. A glass or Teflon-coated rod is used as a backstop to avoid damage to tissue below the adhesion, provide local traction, and expose demarcation lines (Fig. 24–9). If electrocautery is used, a blended current is recommended to provide slight coagulating action to the cutting current. Large vessels within adhesions are coagulated and then divided. If possible, adhesions should be excised by lysing both attachments.

Salpingostomy (Salpingoneostomy)

Terminal salpingostomy is the procedure of choice for establishing tubal patency. Ampullary and especially isthmic salpingostomy for tubal occlusion have been virtually abandoned because of poor pregnancy rates following these procedures. The distal end of the tube is inspected—orientation is of great importance because the tube may be convoluted and its distal end buried in adhesions. The anatomic relationship between the ampulla and the ovary must be restored. The fimbria ovarica must first be identified (Fig. 24–10). One should avoid opening the ampullary or isthmic segments of the tube erroneously or incising through the fimbria ovarica. The latter should be reconstructed whenever possible.

Under magnification, an avascular central dimple is identified, along with several "suture" lines ra-

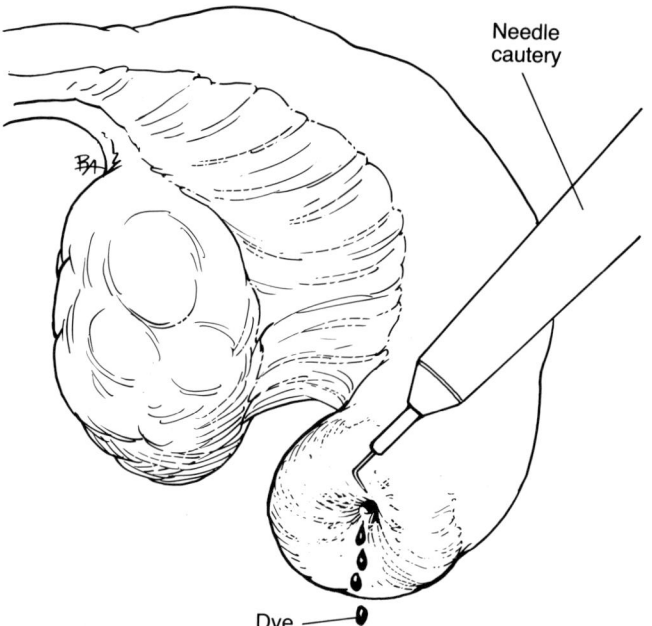

Figure 24–10
Salpingostomy. The fallopian tube has been freed from all adhesions and its orientation to the adjacent ovary established. The fimbria ovarica is identified. The tube is distended with blue dye. A central avascular dimple is seen, along with radial avascular lines of peritoneal closure. These are the sites of salpingostomy incisions. The vascular pattern should be discerned prior to incising the distal tube. The central dimple is entered with needle microelectrode or laser. Dye is seen escaping from the distal end of the tube.

diating peripherally (Fig. 24–10). The tube is then distended with diluted methylene blue or indigo carmine and entered at the central dimple with microcautery until dye escapes (Fig. 24–10). The opening is then enlarged by inserting a glass rod or a dropper, and radial incisions are made with a needle unipolar cautery device or hand-held laser along the avascular lines on the mucosal surface (Fig. 24–11A). One should avoid cutting through viable fimbria, ampullary mucosal folds, or blood vessels. Bleeding is controlled with a microbipolar device under magnification coupled with irrigation. Three to five radial incisions are usually made, resulting in distal tubal flaps (Fig. 24–11B). Interrupted sutures (8–0 polyglactic acid or nylon on a tapered needle) are then used to evert each flap (Fig. 24–11C and D).

One technique previously reported recommends placing these sutures at the least prominent portion of the flap and approximating the mucosa to the adjacent seromuscular portion of the ampulla in such a manner that the fimbriated ends remain free and the cuff so formed is not large (Fig. 24–11C).[64] This is designed to maintain a stable, open ostium without devitalizing the leaflet by impairing venous drainage. The reconstructed ostium should be positioned so that it is capable of moving over maximum ovarian surface. Other surgeons prefer to approximate the serosa or mucosa of the most distal edge of the flaps to the ampullary serosa, creating a somewhat larger cuff (Fig. 24–11D). Intratubal adhesions and fimbrial bridges are separated with needle microcautery against a glass rod with a fine tip. Resection of "redundant" fimbrial tissue is discouraged. Dye is then injected to confirm patency, and the tube is irrigated to remove clots and debris.

If the CO_2 laser is used, eversion of the newly created distal flaps can be performed by using the defocused beam on the ampullary serosa as described by Bruhat and Mage (Fig. 24–11E).[65] Tissue contraction at that site will result in eversion. It is unclear whether this technique produces results comparable with eversion by sutures, and the extent of tissue devitalization is yet unknown.

Fimbrioplasty

The reconstruction of existent fimbria involves a range of procedures, including separation of agglutinated fimbria; opening a partially occluded tube; releasing constricting bands of adhesions that cause partial occlusion; or dilating ampullary constriction (phimosis). The microsurgical approach to fimbrioplasty is similar to distal salpingostomy. Agglutinated fimbria may be separated by unipolar needle cautery or laser with an appropriate fine-tipped, nonconductive glass or quartz rod. Care must be taken not to grasp the fimbria, which can easily be traumatized and bleed. Avascular planes are identified and incised under magnification. A constricting peritoneal band should be carefully incised parallel to the long axis of the tube over a rod that is inserted through the patent ostium (Fig. 24–12). The fimbria may then be everted by using fine sutures or the Bruhat technique. If an area of constriction at the fimbriated end is encountered, gentle dilatation with fine mosquito forceps can be attempted.

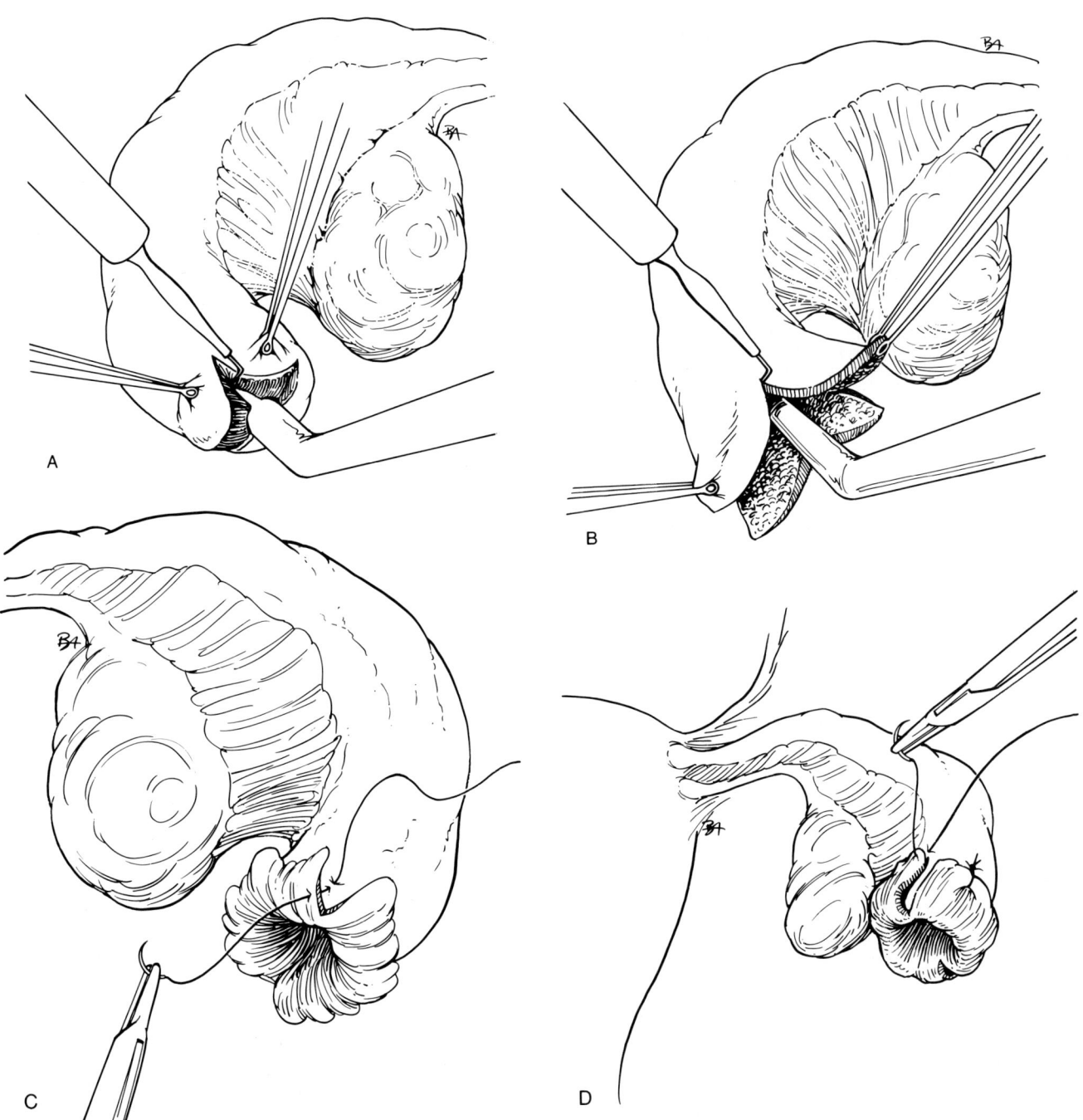

Figure 24–11
A, Salpingostomy. Radial incisions are made with needle microelectrode or laser in the avascular peritoneal lines of demarcation after inserting a glass rod through the neostomy site. This rod serves as a backstop and helps the surgeon to incise in a direction parallel to the long axis of the tube. Three to five radial incisions are usually made.
B, Salpingostomy. The newly formed distal tubal leaflets are incised further on the mucosal side to identify and avoid blood vessels. Traction is provided by holding the distal tube at the serosal surface by atraumatic forceps. Hemostasis is provided by microbipolar cautery under constant irrigation.
C, Salpingostomy. Eversion of the distal flaps is performed by suturing the mucosa to the adjacent serosal surface so that the fimbriated ends remain free and the cuff so formed is not very large. An 8–0 nylon or polyglactic acid suture on a tapered needle is used.
D, Salpingostomy. Another technique for eversion involves suturing the most distal portion of each leaflet to the ampullary serosa. The cuff so formed is usually larger but the fimbriated ends are not free.

Illustration continued on following page

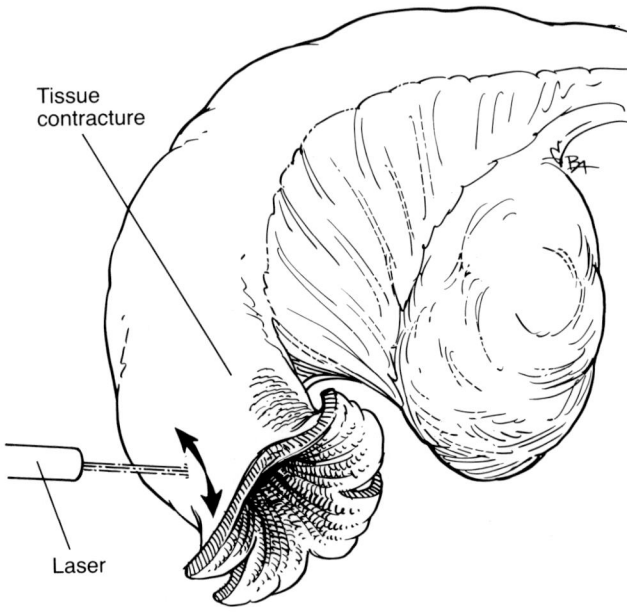

Figure 24–11 *Continued*
E, Salpingostomy. Eversion of the newly opened tube by the Bruhat maneuver with the CO_2 laser or needle microelectrode. The defocused laser beam is aimed at the distal serosal surface and is moved back and forth parallel to the long axis of the tube until tissue contracture causes eversion of the distal flap.

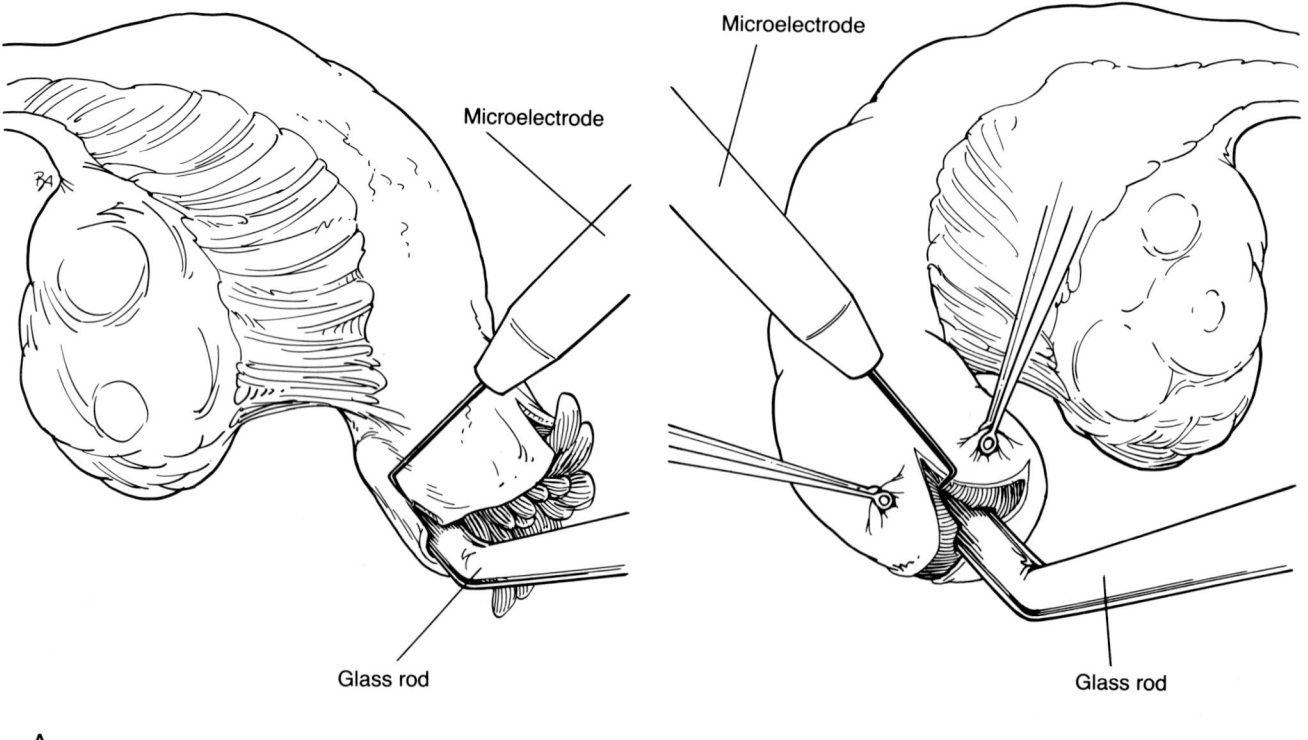

Figure 24–12
A and *B*, Fimbrioplasty. A glass rod is inserted through the pre-existing opening in the tube, and the serosa is incised with needle microelectrode or with the laser beam. A tuft of fimbria is seen, but the majority of the fimbria is buried underneath peritoneal covering and is exposed and everted in a manner similar to salpingostomy. An 8–0 nylon or polyglactic acid suture is used.

Abdominal Closure

The pelvis should be meticulously inspected for remaining adhesions or peritoneal damage and irrigated. The cut edge of the peritoneum should be everted to reduce the contact of raw surfaces with abdominal contents. Opinions vary regarding agents that aid in postoperative adhesion prevention; these are discussed in Chapter 8.

ENDOSCOPIC CORRECTION OF DISTAL TUBAL DISEASE

A list of instruments for laparoscopic salpingostomy, fimbrioplasty, and lysis of adhesions is shown in Table 24–7. The CO_2, KTP, and argon lasers have been shown to be useful in laparoscopic salpingostomy, fimbrioplasty, and salpingo-ovariolysis. Table 24–8 presents results of laser salpingostomy. The laser offers the theoretical advantage of superior hemostasis over laparoscopic incision with scissors. Conversely, one may use fine unipolar needle cautery during salpingostomy for lysis of adhesions, achieving a similar degree of hemostasis and resulting in limited thermal tissue damage.

Exposure is of primary importance during endoscopic tuboplasty. A steep Trendelenburg position is often mandatory, and well-padded shoulder braces may be helpful in preventing patient motion. Two or three punctures are required in addition to the umbilical incision. Ideally, the main operative (manipulating) instruments should be placed in the opposite lower abdominal quadrant to the involved adnexa to achieve maximum instrument mobility, and the atraumatic grasping instrument should be placed on the side of the involved adnexa. The grasping and manipulating instruments should be placed as far from each other as possible to avoid touching and restriction of motion.

The adnexa should be mobilized by lysis of adhesions, and the orientation of the tube as well as the location of the fimbria ovarica should be determined. The distal end of the tube must be free following lysis of adhesions to allow optimum tubal repair.

Table 24–7

Instruments and Equipment for Laparoscopic Salpingostomy

CO_2 insufflator (high flow)
Suction-irrigation unit
Bipolar cautery unit
Bipolar atraumatic forceps (Kleppinger's)
Unipolar needle cautery (with suction-irrigation*)
Laparoscope (operating or diagnostic, 10 mm)
Trocar and sleeve (10 mm)
Camera and video system
Veress needle
Second puncture trocar and sleeve (3 sets, 5 mm)
Atraumatic grasping forceps (3)
Hook scissors
Microscissors (with unipolar cautery attachment*)
Uterine manipulator
Endocoagulator*
Endosuture*

*Optional.

The tube should be distended by transcervical chromopertubation prior to creating the distal salpingoneostomy. This will facilitate visualization of the lines of peritoneal closure as well as demonstrate the moment of establishment of patency. After puncture of the hydrosalpinx and establishment of patency either by laser or by fine-needle cautery (Fig. 24–13A), the tube is grasped with atraumatic forceps and its distal end placed under gentle traction. Radial salpingostomy incisions are then made on the avascular demarcation lines in a manner similar to that described previously with tuboplasty procedures during laparotomy (Fig. 24–13B).

The newly created stoma is now everted as suggested by Bruhat (see Fig. 24–12C).[65] An endocoagulator or laser can be used to accomplish this task. If the CO_2 or KTP lasers are used, they are aimed in a defocused mode at a low power setting at the ampullary serosa 0.5–1.0 cm proximal to the newly formed distal tubal flaps. Short application will result in tissue contraction in that region and subsequent eversion with a "flowering effect." Irrigation should be used intermittently in order to minimize thermal tissue damage during this maneuver. Suturing the stoma has also been advocated,[66] as well as the use of absorbable clips.[67]

Table 24–8

Laser Salpingostomy (Laparotomy)

Reference	Year	Patients	Pregnancy Rate (%)	Term (%)	Ectopic (%)	Aborted (%)
Kelly and Robert[82]	1983	28	11	7	4	—
Tulandi and Vilos[53]	1985	37	41	24	5	—
Daniell et al.[83]	1986	48	21	19	2	—
Mage et al[36]	1986	76	26	—	9	—

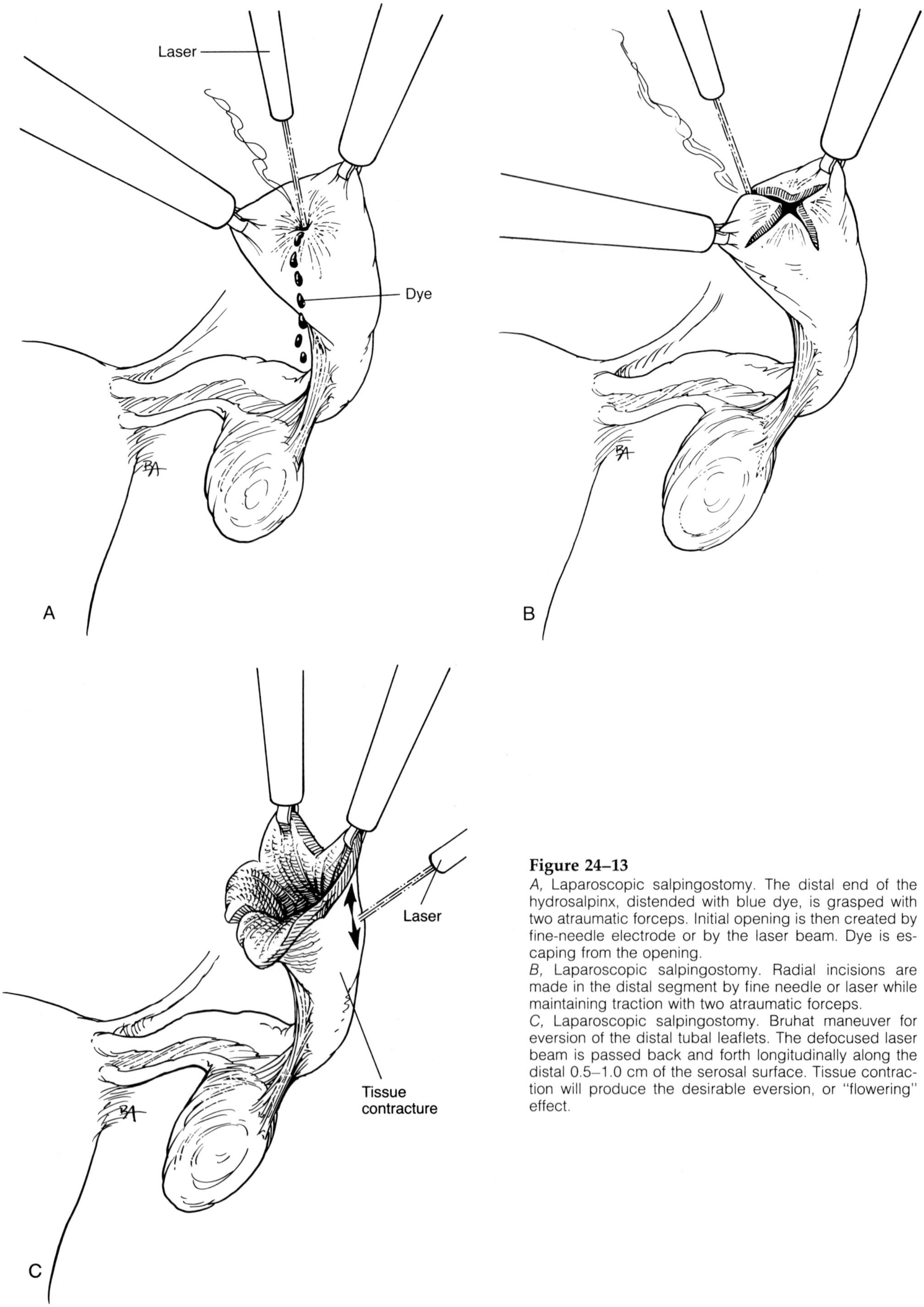

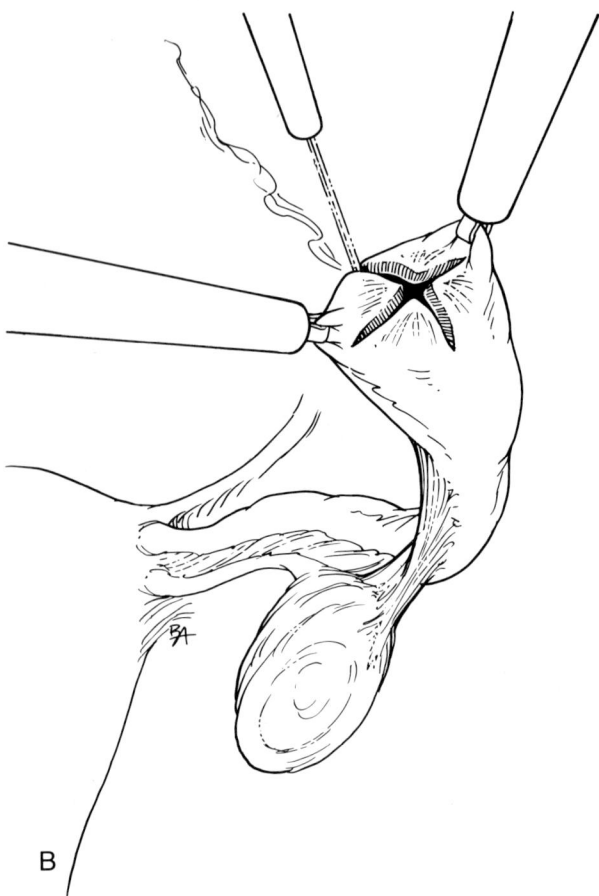

Figure 24–13

A, Laparoscopic salpingostomy. The distal end of the hydrosalpinx, distended with blue dye, is grasped with two atraumatic forceps. Initial opening is then created by fine-needle electrode or by the laser beam. Dye is escaping from the opening.
B, Laparoscopic salpingostomy. Radial incisions are made in the distal segment by fine needle or laser while maintaining traction with two atraumatic forceps.
C, Laparoscopic salpingostomy. Bruhat maneuver for eversion of the distal tubal leaflets. The defocused laser beam is passed back and forth longitudinally along the distal 0.5–1.0 cm of the serosal surface. Tissue contraction will produce the desirable eversion, or "flowering" effect.

Copious irrigation with normal saline or lactated Ringer's solution should be undertaken during the procedure to remove clots or char as well as to identify bleeding spots. A laparoscopic suction-irrigation device is recommended for that purpose and also aids in smoke evacuation during laser application. Postoperative instillation of 500–1000 ml of lactated Ringer's or 100 ml of dextran 70 32% (Hyskon, Pharmacia, Piscataway, NJ) has been recommended to prevent adhesion formation. Possible complications from the use of Hyskon are discussed in Chapter 26. Broad-spectrum prophylactic antibiotics should be administered preoperatively and continued for 24 hours postoperatively.

POSTOPERATIVE CARE

Postoperative broad-spectrum antibiotic administration should be continued for 24 hours. Attempts at conception should be delayed for one or two cycles. There is no evidence that postponing conception for longer periods enhances future fertility.[56] The patient should be apprised that approximately 60% of pregnancies following salpingostomy will occur beyond 1 year postoperatively and that the majority of pregnancies will occur within 3 years following the procedure.[62] This may represent the relatively long interval required for ciliogenesis and regeneration of the tubal mucosa.[56] The patient should be informed about the increased rate of ectopic pregnancies following tuboplasty, as discussed subsequently, and that any menstrual irregularity or suspicion of pregnancy should be brought promptly to the physician's attention.

Discussion of the postoperative use of agents to prevent adhesion formation is presented in Chapter 8. Second-look laparoscopy has been advocated in order to lyse newly formed adhesions and dilate or reconstruct a reoccluded distal tube.[68] The timing and utility of this procedure remain controversial, but the majority of studies favoring the second-look prefer 8 days to 6 weeks following laparoscopic or open microsurgical salpingostomy.[69] An HSG, performed 3 months following the procedure, may also aid in gauging the success of surgery. Repeat tuboplasty often produces poor results in terms of live births[20] but should be considered along with IVF when counseling the patient.

DISTAL TUBAL SURGERY: ASSESSMENT OF RESULTS

Distal tubal surgery results have improved significantly since Greenhill's discouraging survey in 1936,[7] which found only a 4.4% live birth rate following salpingostomy. Comparison between conventional and microsurgical salpingostomy is made difficult by the lack of consistency of reporting results, the length of postoperative follow-up period, and the poor distinction between "microsurgery" and "macrosurgery." A number of surgeons use microsurgical instruments and techniques without magnification. As shown in Table 24–9, the results of conventional salpingostomy have generally improved to approximately 20% live births per patient but reached a plateau in the 1970s. Although microsurgical distal tubal repair has produced slight improvement in overall results (20–25% live births per patient), the rate of ectopic pregnancies has also increased from 5% to approximately 10% (see Table 24–5).

Salpingostomy with prosthetic devices has not improved term pregnancy rates and has added complexity to the procedure (Table 24–10).[20] The use of the CO_2 laser for distal tubal surgery has not resulted in improved outcome and places a burden on the cost factor. The experience with endoscopic salpingostomy is limited (see Table 24–4). This less invasive method, which has the advantage of reducing postoperative recovery time and patient discomfort, needs to be carefully evaluated. Preliminary results are comparable to distal tubal surgery by laparotomy. The reader, however, should view these results with caution in light of the very small number of published reports.

The clinician must be able to clearly communicate his or her personal statistics of success and failure regarding tubal surgery. Previously published data regarding results of distal tubal surgery are presented in Table 24–11. The American Fertility Society classification of adnexal adhesions is presented in Figure 24–14. Clearly, surgical success depends on the condition of the tubes prior to or at the time of surgery. Mild distal tubal disease in general has a term pregnancy rate of 50–80%, whereas the rate for patients with moderate tubal disease is 16–25%. Correction of severe tubal disease generally results in less than 15% live births (per patient). Overall each category has a similar rate of ectopic pregnancy.

Preoperatively, the physician must also discuss alternatives to tubal surgery, including assisted reproductive technology and adoption. The In-vitro Fertilization–Embryo Transfer (IVF-ET) Registry of the American Fertility Society has reported an overall live birth rate per stimulation cycle of 12% in the United States in 1988.[9] Some clinics consistently achieve a higher rate of 20–30% live births per stimulation cycle. Most IVF procedures are performed transvaginally with significantly less operative morbidity compared with surgical repair of the tube by laparotomy. It appears reasonable, then, to consider

Table 24-9

Salpingostomy Without Magnification (Laparotomy)

Reference	Year	Patients	Pregnancy Rate (%)	Term (%)	Ectopic (%)	Aborted (%)
Siegler and Hellman[69]	1956	891	21	15	2	3
Palmer[70]	1960	396	34	13	6	15
Hanton et al[71]	1964	32	19	3	3	13
Arronet et al[72]	1969	85	27	—	2	—
Siegler[73]	1969	27	7	7	—	—
Jessen[74]	1971	25	52	44	8	0
Grant[75]	1971	217	22	15	2	4
Lamb and Muscovitz[76]	1972	37	24	11	8	5
Horne et al[77]	1973	52	38	29	—	—
Cognat and Rochet[78]	1977	118	24	20	—	—
Rock et al[34]	1978	87	28	18	6	—
Trimbos-Kemper et al[79]	1985	68	—	28	12	—
		95	—	25	25	—

Table 24-10

Salpingostomy with Prosthetic Devices (Laparotomy)

Reference	Year	Patients	Pregnancy Rate (%)	Term (%)	Ectopic (%)	Aborted (%)	Comments
Mulligan	1966	21	19	9	9	0	Polyethylene
	1966	45	36	20	9	7	Silastic hood
Garcia	1968	25	—	28	8	—	Silastic hood
Young	1970	18	17	17	0	0	Hood
Roland	1972	44	23	25	—	—	Spiral stent
Lamb and Muscovitz[76]	1972	35	20	9	9	3	Hood, splint
Rock et al[34]	1978	18	—	17	6	—	Hood, splint
DeCherney and Kase[51]	1981	9	22	22	0	0	Silastic hood
Wallach	1983	24	33	21	8	4	Silastic hood

Table 24-11

Surgical Results Based on Degree of Tubal Disease

Reference	Year	Patients	Pregnancy Rate (%)*	Term (%)			Ectopic (%)			Aborted (%)		
				I	II	III	I	II	III	I	II	III
Rock et al[34]	1978	87	28	80	17	5	6	13	0	—	—	—
Mage et al[36]	1986	76	26	58	25	0	8	12	0	—	—	—
Donnez and Casanas-Roux[22]	1986	83	39	48	25	22	0	6	12	—	—	—
Boer-Meisel et al[35]	1986	108	46	59	16	3	4	27	16	18	5	0
Winston[80]	1990	184	†	37	19	15	—	—	—	—	—	—
Schlaff et al[81]	1990	95	26	60	17	13	10	14	4	—	—	—

*Total number of pregnancies.
†Total number of pregnancies could not be calculated as Winston did not report the number of ectopic pregnancies in his study.

Patient's Name _____ Date _____ Chart # _____

Age ____ G ____ P ____ Sp Ab ____ VTP ____ Ectopic ____ Infertile Yes ____ No ____

Other Significant History (i.e. surgery, infection, etc.) _____

HSG _____ Sonography _____ Photography _____ Laparoscopy _____ Laparotomy _____

EXAMPLES

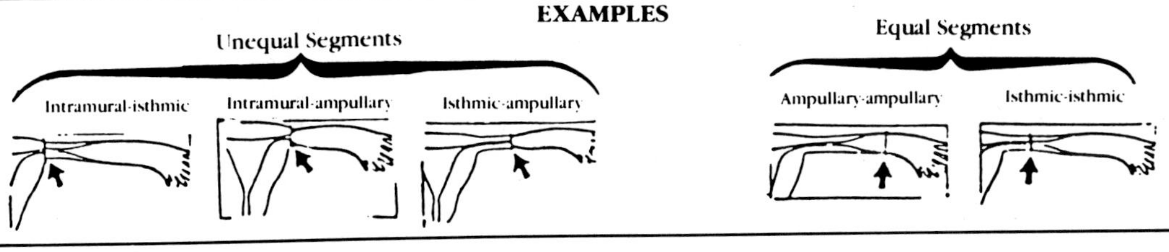

Unequal Segments: Intramural-isthmic | Intramural-ampullary | Isthmic-ampullary

Equal Segments: Ampullary-ampullary | Isthmic-isthmic

Segmental length (cm)   AFTER REPAIR   **Additional Findings:** _____
(Extramural)   Proximal   Distal

Right ____ ____
Left ____ ____

Treatment (Surgical Procedures):

ANASTOMOSIS	Right	Left
IM-IS		
IM-AM		
IS-IS		
IS-AM		
AM-AM		

Other: _____

DRAWING

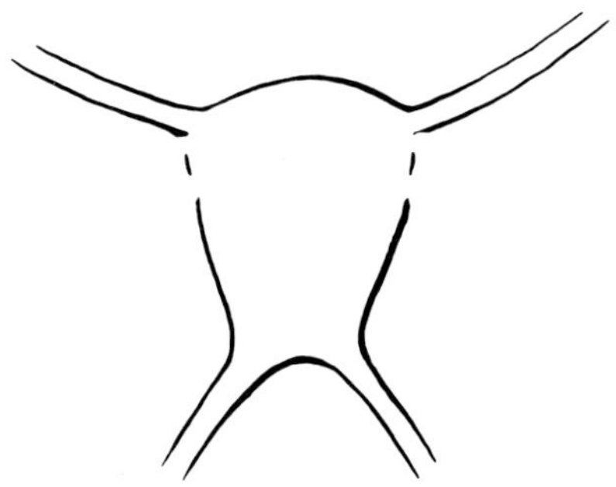

L   R

Prognosis for Conception & Subsequent Viable Infant*

____ Excellent (> 75%)
____ Good (50-75%)
____ Fair (25%-50%)
____ Poor (< 25%)

*Physician's judgment based upon adnexa with least amount of pathology.

Recommended Followup Treatment: _____

For additional supply write to:
The American Fertility Society
2140 11th Avenue, South
Suite 200
Birmingham, Alabama 35205

Property of
The American Fertility Society

Figure 24–14
The American Fertility Society classification of adnexal adhesions. (From Fertil Steril 49(6):945, 1988. Reproduced with permission of the publisher, The American Fertility Society.)

IVF-ET as the primary therapeutic procedure in patients with severe tubal disease and perhaps even for those with moderate tubal disease because the success of assisted reproductive technology may equal or exceed that of tubal repair in these circumstances.

In summary, if the fallopian tubes are moderately or severely diseased, one should consider the surgeon's expertise and his or her results following microscopic or endoscopic tuboplastic procedures; the availability and rate of success of assisted reproductive technology; the cost factors; and above all, the potential surgical risks to the patient.

References

1. Woodruff JD, Pauerstein CJ: The Fallopian Tube. Baltimore, Williams & Wilkins, 1969, p. 1.
2. Siegler AM: The Fallopian Tube. New York, Futura Publishing, 1986, p. 359.
3. Schroeder C: Die Excision von Ovariun Tumoren mit Erhaltung des Ovariun. Zentralb Gynakol 1884; 8:716.
4. Skutsch F: Beitrag zur Operativen Therapie der Tubenerkrankungen. Zentralb Gynakol 1889; 13:565.
5. Martin A: Über Tuben und Ovarialresektion. Zentralb Gynakol 1891; 15:515.
6. Holden FC, Sovak FW: Reconstruction of the oviducts: An improved technic with reported cases. Am J Obstet Gynecol 1932; 24:684.
7. Greenhill JP: Evaluation of salpingostomy and tubal implantation for treatment of sterility. Am J Obstet Gynecol 1937; 33:39.
8. Mulligan WJ, Rock J, Easterday CL: Use of polyethylene in tuboplasty. Fertil Steril 1953; 4:428.
9. Greenhill JP: Present status of plastic operations on the fallopian tubes. Am J Obstet Gynecol 1956; 72:516.
10. Walz W: Fertilitats Operationen mit Hilfe eines Operationenmikroskopes. Geburtshilf Gynakol 1959; 153:49.
11. Swolin K: 50 Fertilitats Operationen I. Literatur und Metodik. Acta Obstet Gynecol Scand 1967; 46:234.
12. Semm K: History. In Sanfilippo JS, Levine RL (eds.): Operative Gynecologic Endoscopy. New York, Springer-Verlag, 1989, pp. 1–15.
13. The American Fertility Society classification of adnexal adhesions, distal tubal occlusion, tubal occlusion secondary to tubal ligation, tubal pregnancies, müllerian anomalies and intrauterine adhesions. Fertil Steril 1988; 49:944.
14. Roland M: Spiral Teflon splint for tuboplasty involving fimbria. Obstet Gynecol 1970; 36:359.
15. Cognat M: Presentation d'une prosthese-drain destinee a la chirurgic tubulaire pour sterilite. Bull Fed Soc Gynecol Obstet Fr 1971; 23:4.
16. In vitro fertilization–embryo transfer in the United States: 1988 results from the IVF-ET Registry. Fertil Steril 1960; 53:13.
17. Blandau RJ: Observing ovulation and egg transport. In Daniel JC (ed.): Methods in Mammalian Embryology. San Francisco, WH Freeman, 1971, p. 1.
18. Vasquez G, Winston RML, Beockx W, et al.: The epithelium of human hydrosalpinges: A light optical and scanning electron microscopic study. Br J Obstet Gynaecol 1983; 90:764.
19. Critoph FN, Dennis KJ: Ciliary activity in the human oviduct. Br J Obstet Gynaecol 1977; 84:216.
20. Bateman BG, Nunley WC, Kitchin JD: Surgical management of distal tubal obstruction—are we making progress? Fertil Steril 1987; 48:523.
21. Jansen RPS: Cyclic changes in the human fallopian tube isthmus and their functional importance. Am J Obstet Gynecol 1980; 136:292.
22. Donnez J, Casanas-Roux F: Prognostic factors of fimbrial microsurgery. Fertil Steril 1986; 46:200.
23. Devoto L, Pino AM, Heras JL, et al: Estradiol and progesterone nuclear and cytosol receptors of hydrosalpinx. Fertil Steril 1984; 42:594.
24. Yussman MA: Unpublished data.
25. Halbert SA, Patton DL: Hydrosalpinx: Effect of oviductal dilatation on egg transport. Fertil Steril 1981; 35:69.
26. Patton DL, Halbert SA: Mechanically induced hydrosalpinx: Long term oviductal dilatation does not impair ciliary transport function. Fertil Steril 1981; 36:808.
27. Vemer HM, Boeckx WD, Vasquez G, Brosens IA: Experimental hydrosalpinx and salpingostomy in rabbits. Eur J Obstet Gynecol Reprod Biol 1984; 18:95.
28. Donnez J, Cuprasse J, Casanas-Roux F, et al.: Morphologic study of mechanically induced hydrosalpinges in rabbits. Acta Eur Fertil 1985; 16:257.
29. Treharne JD, Ripa KT, Mardh PA, et al.: Antibodies to Chlamydia trachomatis in acute salpingitis. Br J Vener Dis 1979; 55:26.
30. Patton DL, Halbert SA, Kuo C-C, et al.: Host response to primary Chlamydia trachomatis infection of the fallopian tubes in pig-tailed monkeys. Fertil Steril 1983; 40:829.
31. Patton DL, Moore DE, Spadon LR, et al.: A comparison of the fallopian tube's response to overt and silent salpingitis. Obstet Gynecol 1989; 73:622.
32. Laufer N, Sekeles E, Cohen R, et al.: The effects of E. coli endotoxin on the tubal mucosa of the rabbit. A scanning electron microscopic study. Path Res Pract 1980; 179:202.
33. Shirodkar VN: Factors influencing the results of salpingostomy. Int J Fertil 1966; 1:361.
34. Rock JA, Katayama KP, Martin EJ, et al.: Factors influencing the success of salpingostomy techniques for distal fimbrial obstruction. Obstet Gynecol 1978; 52:591.
35. Boer-Meisel MF, te Velde ER, Habbema JDF, Kardaun JWPF: Predicting the pregnancy outcome in patients treated for hydrosalpinx: A prospective study. Fertil Steril 1986; 45:23.
36. Mage G, Pouly JL, de Joliniere JB, et al.: A preoperative classification to predict the intrauterine and ectopic pregnancy rates after distal tubal microsurgery. Fertil Steril 1986; 46:807.
37. Hershlag AJ, Seifer DB, Carcangiu ML, et al.: Salpingostomy: Clinical, light microscopic and electron microscopic correlations (abstract). Forty-sixth Annual Meeting of the American Fertility Society, Washington, 1990.
38. Kerin J, Daykhovsky L, Grundfest W, Surrey E: Falloposcopy: A microendoscopic transvaginal technique for diagnosing and treating endotubal disease incorporating guide wire cannulation and direct balloon tuboplasty. J Reprod Med 1990; 35:606.
39. Gomel V: Classification of operations for tubal and peritoneal factors causing infertility. Clin Obstet Gynecol 1980; 23:1259.
40. Verhoeven HC, Berry H, Frantzen C, Schlosser HW: Surgical treatment for distal tubal occlusion. J Reprod Med 1983; 28:293.
41. Procea C, Mastrianni L: Microsurgery for treatment of adnexal disease. Fertil Steril 1980; 34:413.
42. Gomel V: Salpingostomy by laparoscopy. J Reprod Med 1977; 18:265.
43. Mettler L, Giesel H, Semm K: Treatment of female infertility due to tubal obstruction by operative laparoscopy. Fertil Steril 1979; 32:384.
44. Fayez JA: An assessment of the role of operative laparoscopy in tuboplasty. Fertil Steril 1983; 39:476.
45. Daniell JF, Herbert CM: Laparoscopic salpingostomy utilizing the CO_2 laser. Fertil Steril 1984; 41:558.
46. Mage G, Canis M, Pouly JL, et al.: Laparoscopic distal tuboplasty, results and comparison with microsurgery (abstract). Forty-sixth Annual Meeting of the American Fertility Society, Washington, 1990.
47. Swolin K: Electromicrosurgery and salpingostomy: Long-term results. Am J Obstet Gynecol 1975; 121:418.
48. Marik JJ: Microsurgical repair of hydrosalpinx. In Philips JM (ed.): Microsurgery in Gynecology. St. Louis, CBP, 1977, pp. 126–134.
49. Winston RML: Microsurgery of the fallopian tube: From fantasy to reality. Fertil Steril 1980; 34:521.
50. Gomel V: Clinical results of infertility microsurgery. In Crosig-

nani PG, Rubin BL (eds.): Microsurgery in Female Infertility. London, Academic Press, 1980, p. 77.
51. DeCherney AH, Kase N: A comparison of treatment for bilateral fimbrial occlusion. Fertil Steril 1981; 35:162.
52. Larsson B: Late results of salpingostomy combined with salpingolysis and ovariolysis by electromicroscopy in 54 women. Fertil Steril 1982; 37:156.
53. Tulandi T, Vilos GA: A comparison between laser surgery and electrosurgery for bilateral hydrosalpinx: A 2-year follow-up. Fertil Steril 1985; 44:846.
54. Luber K, Beeson CC, Kennedy JF, et al.: Results of microsurgical treatment of tubal infertility and early second-look laparoscopy in the post–pelvic inflammatory disease patient: Implications for in vitro fertilization. Am J Obstet Gynecol 1986; 154:1264.
55. Kitchin JD, Nunley WC, Bateman BG: Surgical management of distal tubal occlusion. Am J Obstet Gynecol 1986; 155:524.
56. Russell JB, DeCherney AH, Laufer N, et al.: Neosalpingostomy: Comparison at 24- and 72-month follow-up time shows increased pregnancy rate. Fertil Steril 1986; 45:296.
57. Carey M, Brown S: Infertility surgery for pelvic inflammatory disease: Success rates after salpingolysis and salpingostomy. Am J Obstet Gynecol 1987; 156:296.
58. Williams KM, Griffin WT: Distal tuboplasty: Is it appropriate? South Med J 1988; 81:872.
59. Laatikainen TJ, Tenhunen AK, Venesma PK, Apter DL: Factors influencing the success of microsurgery for distal tubal occlusion. Arch Gynecol Obstet 1988; 243:101.
60. Jacobs LA, Thie J, Patton PE, Williams TJ: Primary microsurgery for postinflammatory tubal infertility. Fertil Steril 1988; 50:855.
61. Wu CH, Minassian SS: Assessment of infertility surgery by a pelvic scoring system. Int J Fertil 1989; 34:56.
62. Garcia CR, Aller J: Surgical approach to tubal disease. Clin Obstet Gynecol 1974; 17:102.
63. Jansen RPS: Failure of peritoneal irrigation with heparin during pelvic operations upon young women to reduce adhesions. Surg Gynecol Obstet 1988; 166:154.
64. Gomel V, Swolin K: Salpingostomy: Microsurgical technique and results. Clin Obstet Gynecol 1980; 23:1243.
65. Bruhat M, Mage G: Use of the CO_2 laser in neosalpingostomy. In Kaplan I (ed.): Proceedings of the Third International Congress for Laser Surgery. Tel Aviv, Jerusalem, Academic Press, 1979, p. 271.
66. Semm K: Operative Manual for Endoscopic Abdominal Surgery. Chicago, Year Book Medical Publishers, 1987, p. 168.
67. Leventhal JM: Tubal reconstructive surgery. In Sanfilippo JS, Levine RL (eds.): Operative Gynecologic Endoscopy. New York, Springer-Verlag, 1989, p. 143.
68. Tulandi T: Reconstructive tubal surgery by laparoscopy. Obstet Gynecol Surv 1987; 42:193.
69. Siegler AM, Hellman LM: Tubal plastic surgery: Report of a survey. Fertil Steril 1956; 7:170.
70. Palmer R: Discussion on modern methods of salpingostomy. Proc R Soc Med 1960; 53:357.
71. Hanton EM, Pratt JH, Banner EA: Tubal plastic surgery at the Mayo Clinic. Am J Obstet Gynecol 1964; 89:934.
72. Arronet GH, Eduljee SY, O'Brien JR: A nine-year survey of fallopian tube dysfunction in human infertility: A diagnosis and therapy. Fertil Steril 1969; 20:903.
73. Siegler AM: Salpingoplasty: Classification and report of 115 operations. Obstet Gynecol 1969; 34:339.
74. Jessen H: Forty-five operations for sterility. Acta Obstet Gynecol Scand 1971; 50:105.
75. Grant A: Infertility surgery of the oviduct. Fertil Steril 1971; 22:496.
76. Lamb EJ, Muscovitz W: Tuboplasty for infertility. Int J Fertil 1972; 17:53.
77. Horne HW, Clyman M, Debrovner C, et al.: The prevention of postoperative pelvic adhesions following conservative operative treatment for human infertility. Int J Fertil 1973; 18:109.
78. Cognat M, Rochet Y: Notre experience de la salpingoplastie. J Fr Gynecol Obstet Biol Reprod 1977; 6:839.
79. Trimbos-Kemper TCM, Trimbos JB, Van Hall EV: Adhesion formation after tubal surgery: Results of the eighth day laparoscopy in 188 patients. Fertil Steril 1985; 43:395.
80. Winston RML: Additional aspects of tubal surgery: The British perspective. In Seibel M (ed.): Infertility: A Comprehensive Text. Norwalk, CT, Appleton & Lange, 1990, pp. 417–432.
81. Schlaff WD, Damewood MD, Rock JA: Treatment of distal tubal obstruction: Prognostic factors and impact of surgical technique (abstract 226). Society of Gynecologic Investigations Annual Meeting, St. Louis, 1990.
82. Kelly RW, Robert DK: CO_2 laser laparoscopy: A potential alternative to danazol in the treatment of stage I and II endometriosis. J Reprod Med 1983; 28:638.
83. Daniell JF, Miller W, Tosh R: Initial evaluation of the use of the potassium-titanyl-phosphate (KTP/532) laser in gynecologic laparoscopy. Fertil Steril 1986; 46(3):373.

Surgery for Ectopic Pregnancy

25

Steven J. Ory

The diagnosis and management of ectopic pregnancy have undergone substantial change during the past two decades. A sharp increase in prevalence, improved diagnostic modalities, broader therapeutic options, and a greater appreciation of the natural course of ectopic pregnancy have contributed to these changes.

The Arabian writer Albucasis is credited with first describing ectopic pregnancy in A.D. 963. It was considered to be almost a universally fatal event for the subsequent 900 years. The management of ectopic pregnancy was revolutionized by Lawson Tait, who reported the successful treatment of four women in England who survived following salpingectomy. This rapidly became the treatment of choice and was practiced almost without exception until the 1950s, when Stomme provided the first description of successful conservative surgery.

EPIDEMIOLOGY

The incidence of ectopic pregnancy has increased over fivefold since 1970; 17,800 ectopic pregnancies were reported to the United States Centers for Disease Control (CDC) in 1970 and over 88,000 were described in 1987, the last year the CDC published data.[1] This increase has occurred throughout all regions of the United States and was most dramatic for women over 30 and for nonwhite women. Similar increases in the incidence of ectopic pregnancy have been reported to occur in Czechoslovakia, England, Wales, Scotland, Finland, and Sweden.[2]

During the same time interval, the relative and absolute mortality rates of ectopic pregnancy have declined. In 1987, 30 women in the United States died of ruptured ectopic pregnancy, producing a mortality rate of 0.034%. Despite this encouraging development, ectopic pregnancy is still considered to be a major cause of maternal mortality in the United States and is currently the most common cause of death during the first half of pregnancy. The risk of death is greater in black and in unmarried women. Also, interstitial and abdominal pregnancies confer a fivefold greater risk of being fatal.[3]

PATHOPHYSIOLOGY

Several potential mechanisms may account for the occurrence of tubal ectopic pregnancy. Previous tubal damage from infection or surgical trauma is the most commonly cited predisposing factor. Such abnormalities in the fallopian tube might result in altered embryo transport arising from damaged or absent cilia; intraluminal synechia, which could trap the embryo and impede migration into the uterus; or adhesions on the tubal serosa, which could impair peristaltic motion. In fact, histologic evidence of previous pelvic inflammatory disease is present only in 30–50% of cases, suggesting that other factors play a role.[4,5]

Transmigration of the oocyte from one ovary to the contralateral fallopian tube has been suggested as a potential source of delay of ovum or embryo migration with resultant tubal nidation. The presence of a corpus luteum on the opposite side from the tubal pregnancy has been reported to occur in 24–33% of cases.[4] However, there is no difference in the site of implantation whether the corpus luteum is ipsilateral or contralateral to the implantation site, suggesting that the additional delay that occurs with transmigration does not produce an obvious difference in location of implantation within the tube.[6] Also, patients treated with salpingo-oophorectomy have a subsequent ectopic pregnancy rate comparable with those treated with salpingectomy alone. These data do not support the notion that transmigration is a predisposing cause of ectopic pregnancy.

Salpingitis isthmica nodosa has also been associated with ectopic pregnancy. This uncommon inflammatory condition of the tubal isthmus may produce partial or complete obstruction of the fallopian tube, impeding passage of the embryo. Curiously, many ectopic pregnancies in patients with salpingitis isthmica nodosa occur in the ampullary portion of the tube, presumably secondary to alterations in tubal transport.

Pauerstein has proposed two additional explanations for the pathophysiology of ectopic pregnancy.[5] In some cases, the oviduct may be unsuccessful in picking up the ovum and the egg may be released into the cul-de-sac, where fertilization occurs. This could occur following ovulation from either ovary, and both oviducts would be equally accessible to the embryo. If fertilization and blastocyst development began in this environment, ultimate pickup of the embryo could be delayed and tubal implantation might result from the larger cell mass becoming obstructed in the tubal ampulla prior to entering the isthmus, or the stimulus for nidation could be initiated before the embryo reached the uterine cavity.

Alternatively, ovulation, ovum pickup, and fertilization could occur normally, but with tenuous attachment within the tube. The ovum or embryo could be dropped into the cul-de-sac, to be retrieved by either tube later. This would result in a delay of embryo transfer, and implantation could occur prematurely.

Previous tubal surgery is associated with increased risk of ectopic pregnancy because of preexisting tubal disease or resultant iatrogenic tubal injury. Patients undergoing conservative surgery of tubal pregnancy incur a 12–15% risk of future ectopic pregnancies. Ectopic pregnancy rates as high as 50% have been reported in women conceiving following tubal sterilization by laparoscopic fulguration.[7] In contrast, microsurgical tubal re-anastomosis after tubal ligation is associated with only a 4% risk of ectopic pregnancy, presumably owing to minimal tubal damage.

Several authors have noted an association between high serum estradiol levels and an increased risk of ectopic pregnancy. This has been described in women receiving high doses of estrogen post ovulation to prevent pregnancy, following human menopausal gonadotropin therapy, and with clomiphene citrate therapy.[8–10] Tubal motility and cilia activity are altered by elevated estradiol and progesterone levels.

Abnormal embryonic development has been suggested as a potential contributing factor as well. Genetic abnormalities per se do not appear to be a cause of ectopic pregnancy; ectopic gestations are not more likely to have abnormal karyotypes, and there is no increased familial incidence.[11]

The fallopian tube was the site of 97.7% of ectopic pregnancies in one large series; 1.4% of ectopics were abdominal, and less than 1% were ovarian or cervical.[4] The tubal ampulla is the most common implantation site in the tube (81%). Implantation in the isthmus occurs in 12% of cases, the fimbria in 5%, and the interstitium in 1%.

Heterotopic or combined pregnancies were previously reported to occur in 1 in 30,000 tubal pregnancies. This calculated incidence, reported in 1948, represented the product of the incidence of ectopic pregnancy and dizygotic twinning. The incidence of ectopic pregnancy has increased dramatically in the last 45 years, and dizygotic twinning is more common as a result of the availability of ovulation induction agents. The current estimate of heterotopic pregnancy ranges from 1 in 3899 to 1 in 15,000.[12]

Currently, there is some controversy regarding the mode of dissemination of trophoblasts after implantation within the tube. Historically, intraluminal spread had been suspected. Budowick and colleagues suggested that the trophoblast invades the lamina propria shortly after attachment and then spreads through the muscularis in both a longitudinal and circumferential manner early in the course of disease.[13] Hemorrhage is extraluminal until tubal rupture occurs or there is extrusion from the fimbriated end. However, Pauerstein and coworkers, in a similar pathologic review, reported that early invasion of the lamina propria and dissection through the muscularis occur in only a third of ectopic gestations.[5] Dissemination of trophoblasts through the muscularis layer may account for the occurrence of persistent ectopic pregnancy following conservative surgery.

CLINICAL PRESENTATION

Ectopic pregnancy may present in two clinically distinct forms. The classic presentation of ectopic pregnancy includes the triad of abnormal vaginal bleeding, pelvic pain, and an adnexal mass. Greater than 95% of patients experience abdominal or pelvic pain, and 75% of cases are associated with amenorrhea or abnormal vaginal bleeding.[14] The possibility of ectopic pregnancy should be considered in all women with lower abdominal pain and a positive pregnancy test. Syncope, shoulder pain, and the urge to defecate are reported by 10–15% of patients, and 5–10% will pass a decidual cast, which is often mistaken for products of conception. An adnexal mass can be palpated in 30–50% of patients. The differential diagnosis includes pelvic inflammatory disease, adnexal torsion, degeneration of a uterine leiomyoma, threatened or incomplete abortion, ruptured corpus luteum, endometriosis, appendicitis, and gastrointestinal disorders.

The second type of presentation is now more common but is more insidious. These patients are usually diagnosed earlier, often prior to developing symptoms. Increasingly, patients who are at increased risk for ectopic pregnancy because of a history of previous ectopic pregnancy, tubal surgery, or pelvic infection are followed prospectively with laboratory tests and ultrasound from the time that pregnancy is confirmed. The diagnosis can usually be established early, and more therapeutic options are available to this group of patients.

DIAGNOSIS

Physical findings associated with ectopic pregnancy are highly variable. Many patients with early ectopic pregnancies have no demonstrable findings. Assessment of vital signs is helpful in the initial evaluation. Many young, healthy individuals can tolerate a large reduction of intravascular volume without exhibiting signs of cardiovascular collapse. Tachycardia and orthostatic changes may represent the first clue. Hypovolemia must be distinguished from sepsis as a cause of shock. Some patients with intra-abdominal hemorrhage will have temperature elevations that may represent a nonspecific response to peritoneal irritation provoked by blood.

Deep tenderness with or without rebound may be present on abdominal examination. The tenderness is usually localized to the lower abdomen, but with greater amounts of abdominal bleeding it may be generalized. With massive intra-abdominal bleeding, the abdomen may be distended and the umbilicus may become blue (Cullen's sign).

On vaginal examination, nonspecific signs of pregnancy, including vaginal and cervical cyanosis, may be present. Cervical motion tenderness may be present, and the posterior cervix may be particularly tender as a result of its proximity to blood. A tender, enlarged adnexal mass can be palpated in 30–50% of cases. The uterus may be enlarged to 8 weeks' size. Irregularities over the cornua may suggest the presence of an interstitial pregnancy.

One-quarter of patients will have hematocrits of less than 30% following tubal rupture. About one-half of the patients have an associated leukocytosis, which is usually in the 10,000–15,000/mm^3 range.

Quantitative Human Chorionic Gonadotropin Testing

The development of sensitive serum radioimmunoassays for the detection of human chorionic gonadotropin (hCG) has been a major advance in the diagnosis of ectopic pregnancy. In contrast to previous urinary hCG tests, which were positive in ectopic pregnancies in 50% of cases, currently available radioimmunoassays (RIA), enzyme-linked immunoabsorbant assays (ELISA), and immunoradiometric assays (IRMA) detect the presence of hCG in over 99% of ectopic pregnancies.[15] Moreover, the hCG levels are reflective of the status of the pregnancy; hCG concentrations are roughly correlated to the amount of trophoblastic mass present, which, in turn, is indicative of the length of gestation. Normal intrauterine pregnancies are associated with a characteristic doubling time of the hCG concentration of 1.98 days.[16] This observation has been helpful in identifying abnormal pregnancies. hCG increases of less than 66% within 48 hours are predictive of ectopic pregnancies or intrauterine pregnancies destined to abort in 87% of cases. Fifteen per cent of normal pregnancies may be associated with abnormal doubling times. Obtaining serial hCG levels has been helpful in following pregnant patients in whom the site of implantation has not been determined. One prospective study has challenged the accuracy of following doubling times in early asymptomatic patients, but most investigators have found it to be reliable.[17]

Elimination of hCG has been studied following term pregnancy and therapeutic abortion.[18] There appear to be two phases—the major elimination has a half-life of 5–9 hours, and the second, longer phase has a 22–32 hour half-life. Similar rates of excretion have been described following salpingectomy and conservative surgery for ectopic pregnancy.[19]

Progesterone

Several authors have found a single serum progesterone determination within the first 6 weeks of gestation to be predictive of the viability of the pregnancy.[20-22] Serum progesterone values greater than 15 ng/ml are more often associated with normal intrauterine pregnancy, and those below 15 ng/ml are more commonly associated with ectopic pregnancies and spontaneous abortions. Neither serum progesterone determinations nor suboptimal hCG doubling times distinguish ectopic pregnancy from spontaneous abortion.

Ultrasound

Ultrasound has been an integral part of the evaluation of ectopic pregnancy for over 15 years. Transabdominal ultrasound (TAUS) has been primarily used to exclude the presence of an intrauterine pregnancy in clinically suspicious circumstances. Ectopic pregnancy is associated with intrauterine "pseudogestational sacs" in 10–20% of cases.[23] These can be distinguished from genuine gestational sacs by the absence of a second ring around the fluid collection. In 1981, Kadar and associates defined a discriminatory zone as a range of serum hCG concentrations (6000–6500 mIU/ml, IRP [see later]) above which a normal intrauterine gestational sac can be visualized in 94% of cases and below which an intrauterine sac is usually not visible.[24] The absence of a gestational sac when hCG levels exceed the discriminatory zone is indicative of ectopic pregnancy in 86% of cases. These investigators were unable to consistently locate the site of implantation when hCG levels were less than 6000 mIU/ml.

Although the discriminatory zone is a useful diagnostic aid, diagnosis is usually not possible until 6 weeks' gestation with TAUS. Moreover, only 25–40% of ectopic pregnancies are associated with hCG concentrations greater than 6000 mIU/ml at the time of the initial presentation.[25]

Transvaginal ultrasonography (TVUS) has offered improved resolution and the opportunity to make the diagnosis earlier. The determination of the discriminatory zone is dependent upon the quality of ultrasound resolution, the sensitivity of the hCG assay, and the reference standard with which it is calibrated. These factors produce significant variation at lower hCG levels, and specific discriminatory zones vary depending upon the particular equipment and assay used at each institution.

Currently, there are two reference standards for hCG—the Second International Standard (Second IS) and the International Reference Preparation (IRP).[26] The Second IS, which was paradoxically the first reference standard developed, was made available as a bioassay for hCG in 1964. The material is heterogeneous, containing various amounts of alpha and beta subunits in addition to containing approximately 20% intact hCG molecule. The IRP was introduced as an hCG standard in 1974. It consists of a highly purified hCG material (CR 119) and contains

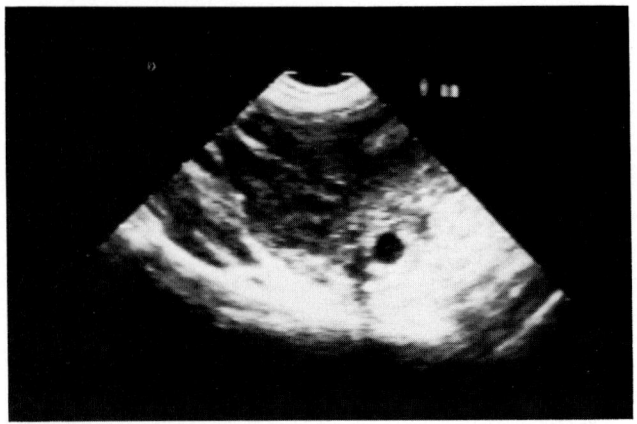

Figure 25–1
Pelvic ultrasound showing gestational sac within the fallopian tube.

insignificant amounts of the hCG subunits. There are separate IRP reference standards for the alpha and beta subunits. The IRP is the preferred reference standard, but references to the Second IS and erroneous references to the IRP are in the literature.

It is possible to detect an intrauterine gestational sac with TVUS when the hCG concentrations are approximately 1400 mIU/ml (IRP) utilizing a 5.0- or 7.5-MHz transducer.[27] A gestational sac can be detected at 35 days' gestation, or 1 week earlier than with TAUS. An ectopic gestational sac can occasionally be identified using TVUS (Fig. 25–1).

In addition to locating the site of the gestational sac, ultrasound provides other valuable information. The presence of a complex adnexal mass is predictive of ectopic pregnancy in 83% of cases, and an ectopic pregnancy will be found in 94% of cases if free peritoneal fluid is present with the mass.[28]

Serial hCG determinations and ultrasound have reduced the need to perform culdocentesis, because the presence of fluid in the cul-de-sac can frequently be confirmed with ultrasound. However, a culdocentesis is very effective in detecting ectopic pregnancy. A positive culdocentesis (>5 ml of nonclotting blood) in association with a positive serum pregnancy test is indicative of ectopic pregnancy in 99% of cases.[29] A positive culdocentesis is found in 62% of unruptured ectopic pregnancies; 45% of patients with positive test results have no peritoneal signs at initial evaluation. Currently, the principal role for culdocentesis is to determine whether immediate surgery is indicated in patients with otherwise equivocal findings.

Dilatation and Curettage

Dilatation and curettage (D & C) may be helpful in the evaluation of patients with possible incomplete abortion in which the gestational age is greater than 5 weeks and sonographic evidence of an intrauterine gestation is absent. Histologic examination of the curettings can be performed by frozen section, and laparoscopy should be performed if no chorionic villi are identified. Occasionally, chorionic villi can be identified grossly by floating the tissue in saline. A variety of types of endometrial histology may be associated with ectopic pregnancy, including proliferative endometrium, secretory endometrium, decidua, and Arias-Stella reaction. None of these findings are diagnostic of ectopic pregnancy.

Laparoscopy

The definitive diagnosis of ectopic pregnancy is usually made at laparoscopy, although it is now occasionally possible to establish the diagnosis with ultrasound alone if an ectopic gestational sac can be visualized. The false-negative and false-positive rates for laparoscopy are 2–5%.[30]

THERAPY

Patients with suspected ectopic pregnancy should be evaluated as expeditiously as possible. Those with evidence of intra-abdominal hemorrhage with obvious tubal rupture and with significant pelvic pain require immediate surgery. If the diagnosis is less obvious, ultrasound, serial hCG determinations, and serum progesterone levels may be useful. In addition to the greater diagnostic options, there are more therapeutic alternatives available to patients being followed prospectively, because they tend to have earlier, less symptomatic ectopic pregnancies. Prior to surgery, all reasonable therapeutic options and the risks and benefits of each should be reviewed with the patient. An in-depth knowledge of the patient's fertility desires, previous tubal surgery, and concerns about future ectopic pregnancy should be established before surgery. Conservative surgical procedures generally confer improved subsequent fertility potential but may be associated with an increased risk of recurrent ectopic pregnancy (15–30%) and persistent ectopic pregnancy (5%). The general risks of abdominal surgery and unique risk of laparoscopy should be reviewed, as well.

Continued observation, systemic methotrexate, and salpingocentesis have been reported to be successful alternatives to conventional surgery. Many tubal pregnancies resolve by spontaneous tubal abortion without obvious clinical sequelae if surgery is not performed. Evolving and complete spontaneous tubal abortions are often noted at surgery. Tubal abortion is usually presaged by declining hCG levels.

Several studies have confirmed the safety and reliability of expectant management of patients with early ectopic pregnancies with falling hCG concentrations.[31-33] This approach should be limited to the infrequent, asymptomatic patient in whom ectopic pregnancy is suspected, but not confirmed. In general, patients with initial hCG levels below 1000 mIU/ml have the most rapid and uneventful clinical courses.[25]

Several series have confirmed the safety and efficacy of systemic methotrexate for the treatment of ectopic pregnancy.[34-40] Regimens utilizing intramuscular or intravenous methotrexate (1 mg/kg/day every other day for four doses, with administration of leucovorin on alternating days) are successful in 95% of cases. Treatment has generally been well tolerated, and side effects are mild. Variations in the regimen, including outpatient administration, shorter courses of therapy, and administration without laparoscopic confirmation, have also been successful.[38-39] The preliminary evaluation of subsequent fertility has been encouraging as well.[40] Clinical response is less complicated and more rapid with hCG levels below 5000 mIU/ml. However, most patients still require laparoscopy for diagnosis, and methotrexate treatment offers no distinct advantage if definitive treatment can be accomplished at laparoscopy.

Injection of methotrexate, potassium chloride, prostaglandin $F_{2\alpha}$, or hypertonic glucose into the gestational sac at the time of laparoscopy or by TVUS-directed needle guide is termed salpingocentesis. The latter technique may offer the patient the opportunity to avoid a general anesthetic and hospitalization. Although the technique has been successful in small series, clinical efficacy is not established and concerns regarding local tissue effects of methotrexate and potassium chloride have not been resolved.[41-43] At this time, salpingocentesis is investigative.

Surgery

Laparoscopy is performed initially except when the patient is in obvious shock or there are contraindications to laparoscopy. In all cases, the necessary instruments for laparotomy should be available in the room at the initiation of the procedure. Laparoscopic treatment of ectopic pregnancy has become the procedure of choice in many locales and offers the advantage to the patient of shorter hospitalization and the opportunity to return to work earlier. Safety and efficacy appear to be comparable with procedures performed at laparotomy. Laparoscopic treatment requires additional equipment and surgical training but should be offered if appropriately trained personnel are available. All conservative surgical procedures except re-anastomosis after segmental excision can be accomplished through the laparoscope.

The choice of procedure depends on several factors. Salpingectomy should be performed on patients with obvious tubal rupture, uncontrolled hemorrhage, or no desire for additional pregnancies. In addition, salpingectomy should be considered for patients who have already had two ectopic pregnancies in an affected tube and for those unwilling to accept a future increased risk of repeat ectopic pregnancy. However, they should be aware that they have a comparable risk of future ectopic pregnancy in the contralateral tube. In patients wishing to preserve their fertility potential, the choice of procedures will also be influenced by the site of the ectopic pregnancy within the tube, the size of the ectopic pregnancy, the condition of the contralateral tube, prior history of infertility or previous ectopic pregnancies, and the relative availability of in vitro fertilization.

Tubal Surgery

Subsequent fertility following treatment of tubal pregnancy is significantly improved if microsurgical principles are employed. Although magnification is not essential, gentle tissue handling, copious irrigation, meticulous hemostasis, and use of fine, nonreactive suture material are important. The majority of tubal pregnancies occur in the ampullary portion of the fallopian tube, and linear salpingostomy is the procedure of choice (Fig. 25–2). The tube is grasped

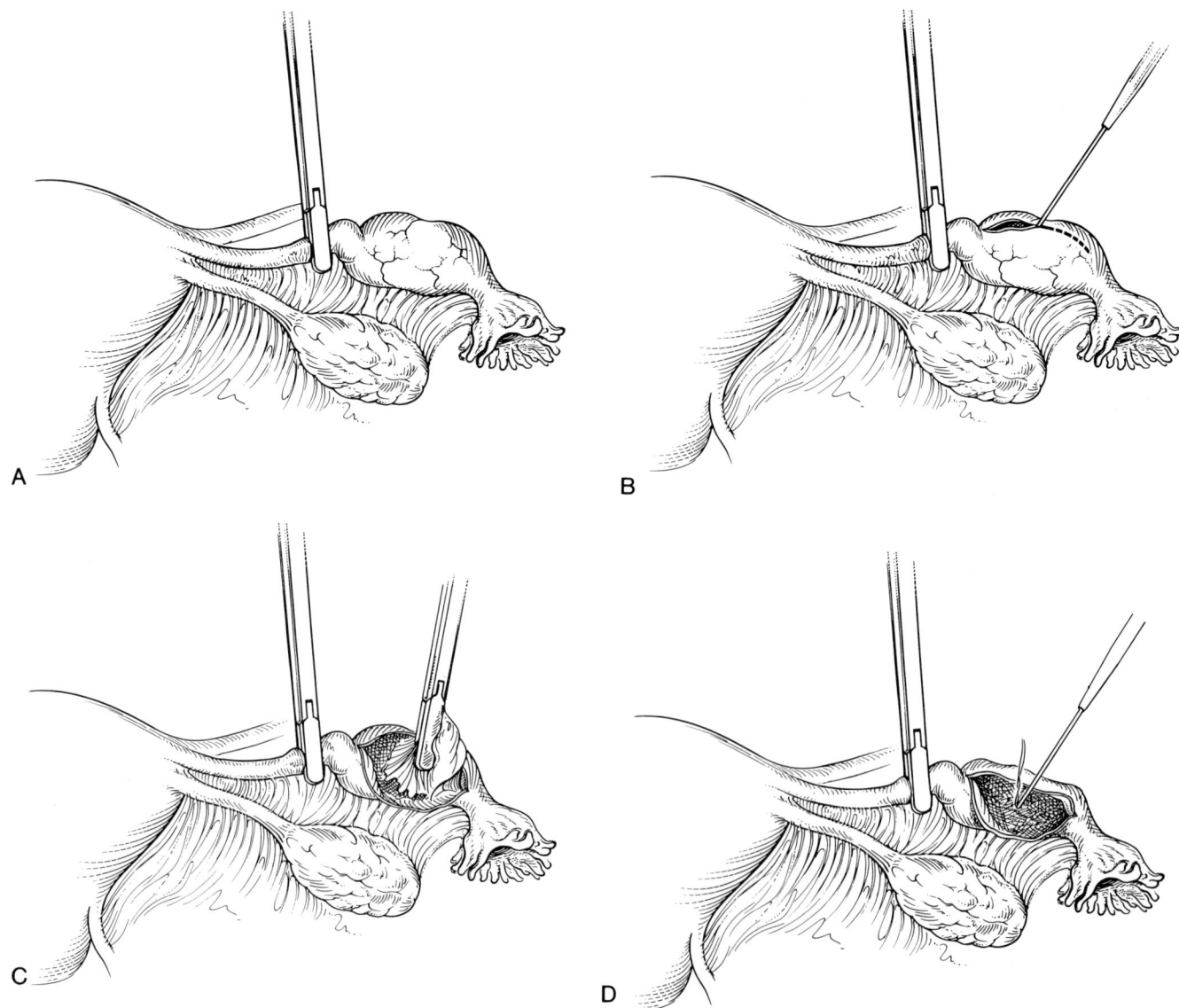

Figure 25–2
Linear salpingostomy. *A*, An unruptured ampullary ectopic pregnancy is identified, and the tube is grasped proximally. *B*, The tube is incised with microcautery over the most distended portion of the antimesenteric surface. *C*, The tissue is atraumatically removed from the tubal lumen. *D*, Hemostasis is achieved with microcautery.

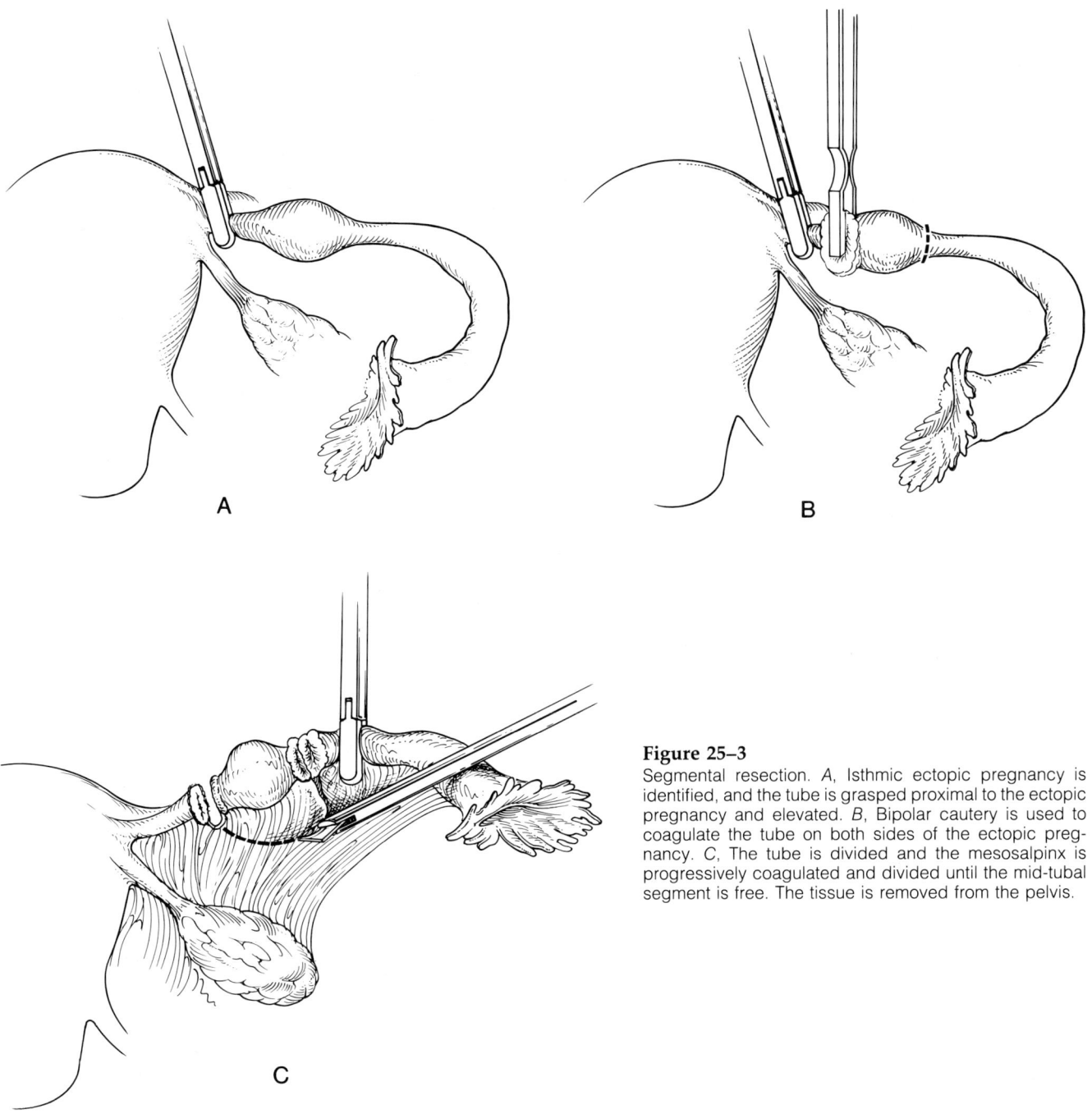

Figure 25–3
Segmental resection. *A*, Isthmic ectopic pregnancy is identified, and the tube is grasped proximal to the ectopic pregnancy and elevated. *B*, Bipolar cautery is used to coagulate the tube on both sides of the ectopic pregnancy. *C*, The tube is divided and the mesosalpinx is progressively coagulated and divided until the mid-tubal segment is free. The tissue is removed from the pelvis.

proximally, and a small incision is made over the antimesenteric surface of the tube at the point of maximum distention of the ectopic pregnancy. This can be accomplished at laparotomy with a scalpel or microelectrode or at laparoscopy with microelectrode, laser, or scissors. The products of gestation are grasped and gently extruded from the tube. Bleeding occurs at the serosal edges and at the implantation site and can usually be controlled with electrocautery. In more difficult circumstances, compression of the underlying mesosalpinx, placing a suture in the mesosalpinx, or injection of vasopressin (Pitressin) may be helpful. Following salpingos-

tomy and achieving hemostasis, the opening is left to close by secondary intention. Alternatively, some authors have recommended salpingotomy in which the tubal defect is closed with fine (5-0 to 7-0), interrupted, nonreactive suture material. Although there is currently no compelling evidence that salpingostomy yields better results than salpingotomy, salpingostomy is virtually always used during laparoscopy because of the difficulty in placing sutures. Also, the sutures employed with salpingotomy may provide more tissue ischemia and be associated with additional adhesion formation.[44]

Fimbrial expression has also been used for treat-

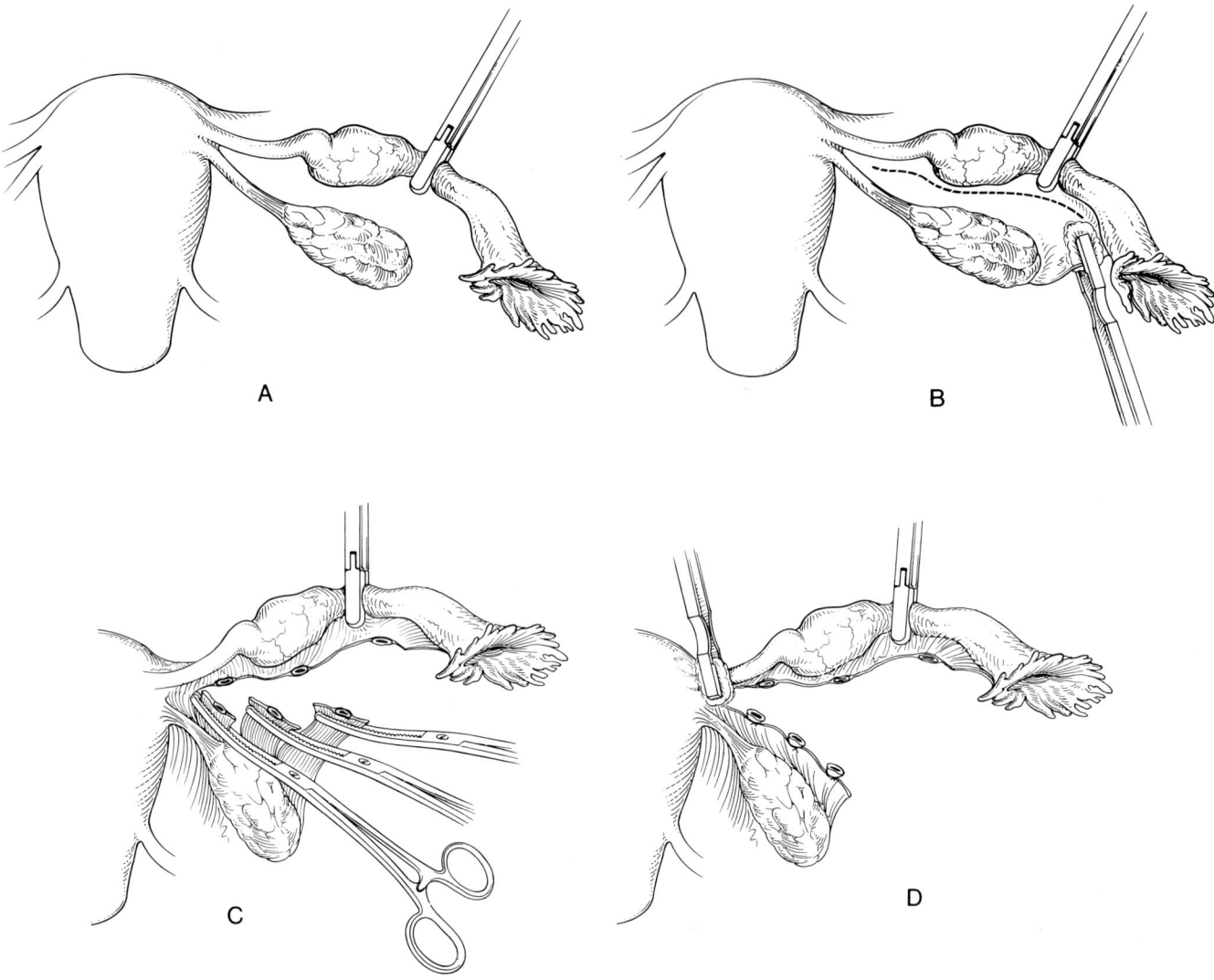

Figure 25–4
Salpingectomy. *A,* Tubal pregnancy is identified; the tube is grasped immediately distal to the ectopic pregnancy and is elevated. *B,* Beginning at the distal end of the tube, the mesosalpinx is divided using bipolar cautery to coagulate and scissors to cut progressive pedicles at laparoscopy or (*C*) Kelly clamps to clamp, ligate, and cut the pedicles until the length of the mesosalpinx has been divided. *D,* The tube is then removed by coagulating with bipolar cautery and dividing the tissue with scissors (laparoscopy) or

ment of ampullary ectopic pregnancy. The products of conception are extruded from the fimbriated end of the tube by squeezing the tube proximally. This technique results in greater tissue trauma and potentially more dissection of the trophoblastic tissue through the adventitia. Fimbrial expression has been associated with a higher incidence of persistent trophoblastic tissue and recurrent ectopic pregnancy.[45] It should not be used except in instances in which partial tubal abortion has occurred and tissue is already protruding from the tubal ostium. In this circumstance, forceps can be used to gently tease the tissue away from the fimbria. Encouraging reproductive potential has been described in this situation.

Although some authors have reported successful utilization of linear salpingostomy with isthmic tubal pregnancy, the tubal lumen is more likely to be significantly damaged and the risk of subsequent fertility impairment and tubal occlusion is greater. For this reason, segmental excision is preferred for most isthmic ectopic pregnancies. Laparoscopically, this can be performed by using bipolar cautery to coagulate the tube immediately proximal and distal to the ectopic pregnancy (Fig. 25–3). The tissue can then be excised with scissors and removed. Additional cauterization of the mesosalpinx may be necessary for hemostasis. At laparotomy, the same procedure is usually performed by clamping, cutting, and ligating the pedicles surrounding the tubal pregnancy.

Anastomosis of the tubal segments can be accomplished as either a primary or a secondary procedure. It is generally preferable not to attempt primary anastomosis, because the tissues are usually edema-

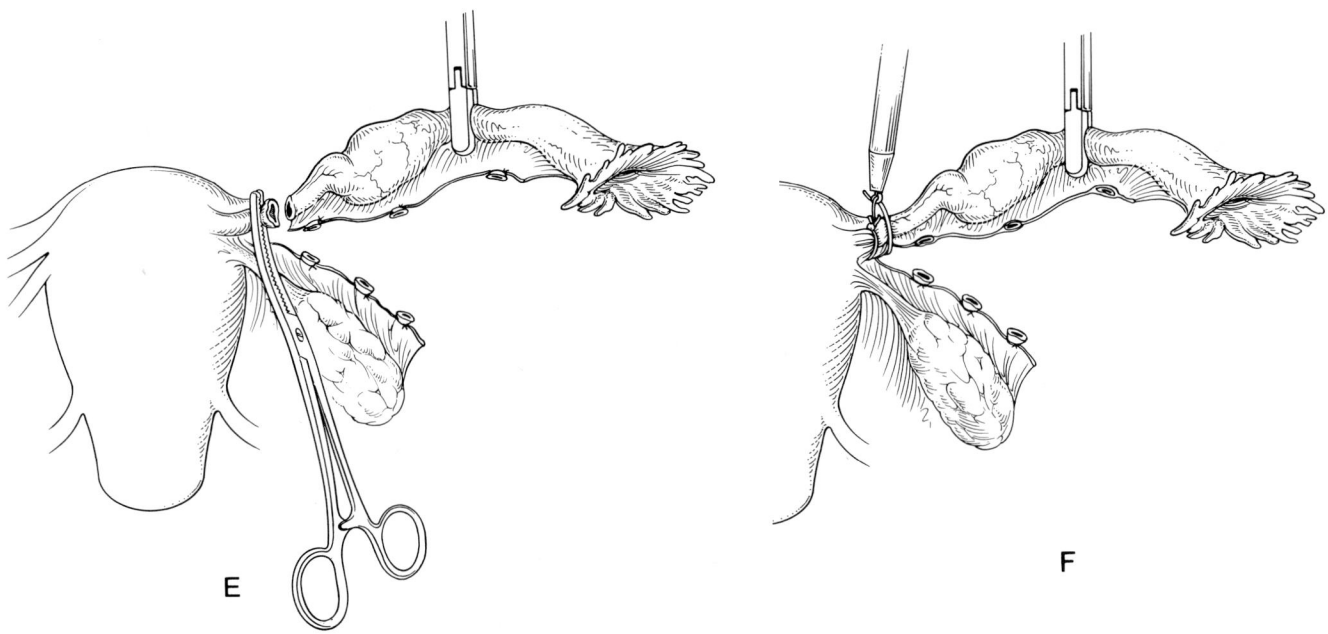

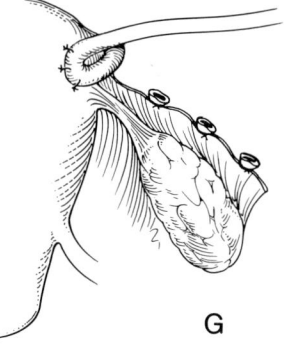

Figure 25–4 *Continued*
(*E*) placing a Kelly clamp across the tube at the uterine surface and ligating and dividing the tissue (laparotomy). *F*, Alternatively, an Endoloop suture can be placed over the tube in the final portion of the mesosalpinx. *G*, The round ligament can be pulled over the cornual surface and secured with 2-0 Vicryl to cover the raw defect. This cannot be easily accomplished at laparoscopy.

tous and friable and subsequent tissue reaction may compromise the results. Primary anastomosis cannot be performed at laparoscopy. However, some investigators have reported excellent results with primary anastomosis at laparotomy. Repeat ectopic pregnancy has occurred in the isolated distal segment.

Salpingectomy should be performed in patients who are not interested in subsequent fertility or have tubal rupture or uncontrolled bleeding. It can be easily accomplished at laparoscopy by grasping and elevating the fallopian tube with a forceps and progressively coagulating and dividing the mesosalpinx with bipolar cautery and scissors, respectively (Fig. 25–4). The tube can then be removed at the site of its uterine attachment. Tubal closure may be secured with sutures placed through the laparoscope or with bipolar coagulation.

The same procedure can be performed at laparotomy by clamping, cutting, and ligating the mesosalpinx. The site of excision may then be covered by either the round ligament or broad ligament to minimize risk of recannulation of the tubal cornu and to prevent adhesion formation over the cornual surface.

Previously, cornual resection or excision of the distal portion of the interstitial fallopian tube was recommended at the time of salpingectomy in the hopes of preventing subsequent interstitial pregnancy.[46] However, later studies showed that these procedure are ineffective in eliminating the risk of interstitial pregnancy.[47] Furthermore, they may serve to weaken the uterus in subsequent intrauterine pregnancies and disrupt myometrial blood flow.

Earlier authors also recommended that oophorectomy be performed at the time of salpingectomy for ectopic pregnancy to ensure that subsequent ovulation occurred on the same side as the remaining fallopian tube.[48] Although there is a mixed consensus regarding the effect of this procedure on subsequent fertility, the practice can no longer be supported with the availability of in vitro fertilization (IVF). IVF is the only means by which some patients can conceive following ectopic pregnancy, and the loss of an ovary adversely affects their fertility potential.

Laparoscopy

If a laparoscopic procedure is planned, a technique utilizing three punctures or two punctures with an operating laparoscope should be employed. The two ancillary trocars should be in suprapubic sites approximately 5 cm lateral to the midline. Contraindications to laparoscopic treatment include inability to adequately visualize the pelvis, inability to mobilize the affected tube, and uncontrolled hemorrhage. Previously, some clinicians recommended that laparoscopic treatment not be attempted if the ectopic pregnancy was greater than 4 cm in diameter. However, with the availability of morcellators and other instruments for removing tissue, size alone need not be a contraindication to laparoscopic management. Necessary equipment includes unipolar and bipolar cautery, a variety of grasping forceps, laparoscopic scissors, and a means of removing the tissue. The tube may be incised with laser, unipolar electrocautery with a microtip, or scissors. A dilute Pitressin solution (4 units/20 ml saline) can be injected into the tubal serosa for hemostasis. If salpingectomy or segmental excision is planned, bipolar cautery or appropriate laparoscopic suture such as Endoloops (pre-tied suture) should be available for hemostasis. The availability of a video system with camera is essential for appropriate assistance.

Interstitial Pregnancy

Pregnancy in the tubal interstitium poses unique therapeutic challenges. Interstitial pregnancy usually does not produce symptoms until approximately 12 weeks' gestation or later. The advanced gestational development, proximity to large uterine vessels, and usual pre-existing uterine distention make management particularly hazardous. Hysterectomy may be necessary for advanced, ruptured interstitial pregnancies. Conservative options include wedge resection of the involved region, systemic methotrexate, and salpingocentesis, all of which have been successfully employed.[41, 49] Salpingocentesis may be the least deleterious to future fertility. If wedge resection is performed, injection of a dilute Pitressin solution and placement of sutures under the area to be resected are helpful in reducing blood loss. Cesarean section in subsequent pregnancies may be advisable to reduce the risk of uterine rupture.

Ovarian Pregnancy

Ovarian pregnancy may be treated by oophorectomy, salpingo-oophorectomy, wedge resection, or cystectomy. The patient's clinical status, the size of the involved ovary, and the amount of surrounding tissue destruction and reaction determine which procedure is most appropriate. All of these procedures may be performed through the laparoscope or at laparotomy.

Cervical Pregnancy

Cervical pregnancy, like interstitial pregnancy, is associated with risk of profuse hemorrhage and significant mortality. Hysterectomy has been recommended as the treatment of choice in the past, but success with conservative measures, including cervical amputation, hypogastric artery ligation, ligation of cervical branches of the uterine arteries with curettage, transabdominal evacuation of the trophoblast, and systemic methotrexate, has been reported. Fertility potential is usually poor with all modalities.

Abdominal Pregnancy

Primary abdominal pregnancies often undergo spontaneous abortion resulting in hemoperitoneum, which usually precipitates diagnosis and management. This usually occurs in the first trimester. At surgery, a small eroded bleeding area may be identified with chorionic villi present at the base. Abdominal pregnancies may occur throughout the abdomen but are most often encountered in the pelvis. They can usually be managed with excisional biopsy and interrupted sutures to achieve hemostasis. A laparoscopic approach may be possible in selected cases. Advanced abdominal pregnancies are less common and should be managed by prompt delivery of the fetus at laparotomy and resection of the placenta if it appears that the blood supply can be effectively controlled. If the implantation site is extensive and large vessels are involved, removal may not be possible. In this instance, the cord should be ligated and the placenta left in place. Treatment should not be delayed to await fetal viability.[50] Hemorrhage and fetal loss as a result of abruptio placentae are common, and there is a high incidence of significant malformation generally attributed to the oligohydramnios noted in surviving infants. Methotrexate treatment of abdominal pregnancy has been associated with several deaths and should not be considered.[51]

Rh FACTOR

All Rh-negative unsensitized women should receive 50 µg of Rh immunoglobulin following an ectopic gestation of less than 12 weeks' duration and 300 µg if it has advanced beyond 12 weeks. Unfortunately, the majority of Rh-negative women in the United States do not receive Rh$_o$(D) immunoglobulin following ectopic pregnancy because prior Rh screening is inconsistently performed. The risk of sensitization increases with the duration of gestation and may be as high as 9% at 3 months' gestation.[52]

PERSISTENT ECTOPIC PREGNANCY

Persistent ectopic pregnancy, the continued proliferation of trophoblast after conservative surgical treatment of tubal pregnancy, is a unique complication of conservative surgery that was initially described by Kelly and colleagues in 1979.[53] It is common for hCG levels to be detectable for 6 weeks or longer following salpingectomy or conservative surgery for ectopic pregnancy. Continued hCG production is indicative of remaining trophoblastic tissue but is not a clinical concern unless the tissue begins to proliferate. This latter event is consistently depicted by an increase in hCG levels. Patients with increasing hCG levels following conservative surgery for ectopic pregnancy may present anew with symptoms of ectopic pregnancy and are at further risk for tubal rupture. Approximately 5% of patients undergoing conservative surgical treatment will experience persistent ectopic pregnancy, and this risk may be higher following laparoscopic treatment.[54] Patients undergoing conservative surgical procedures for tubal pregnancy should have weekly hCG determinations until nonpregnant results are attained.

Treatment options for persistent ectopic pregnancy include repeat conservative surgical procedure, salpingectomy, or systemic methotrexate therapy. Many persistent ectopic pregnancies are associated with trophoblastic dissection through the muscularis layer. The inability to see this tissue at the time of the initial surgery may again be a limiting factor if a second conservative procedure is being considered. Salpingectomy is effective but adversely affects future fertility potential. Systemic methotrexate therapy is effective and well tolerated, although no large series have yet confirmed this. At present, it seems to be the best choice for patients with persistent ectopic pregnancy.

FERTILITY FOLLOWING ECTOPIC PREGNANCY

With the great strides made in the diagnosis and management of ectopic pregnancy, the major remaining challenge is preservation of fertility potential. Many patients are infertile prior to their ectopic pregnancy, but others become infertile after treatment. Reviews of fertility potential following salpingectomy before 1970 cited a 30% chance of having a live-born child.[45, 55] Intrauterine pregnancy rates of 50–70% were reported with conservative microsurgical procedures during the 1970s and 1980s. These limited series were responsible for the rapid adoption of conservative surgical techniques in women desiring additional children. However, comparison of fertility potential following conservative surgery to salpingectomy has been confounded by several variables. As noted previously, there has been a dramatic increase in the incidence of ectopic pregnancy during the past 20 years, which is in part a consequence of improved diagnosis and earlier intervention. Studies have demonstrated that fertility potential following salpingectomy has significantly improved, and intrauterine pregnancy rates of 50–70% have also been reported.[56, 57, 59] These results must be interpreted with caution. There is an absence of appropriate prospective controlled studies comparing results of the two modalities. Women have a higher risk of spontaneous abortion following treatment of ectopic pregnancy. Most studies have looked at intrauterine pregnancy rates rather than live-birth rates, and live-birth rates may be substantially lower than the intrauterine pregnancy rates.

Several studies have failed to notice a difference in fertility outcome between patients who have been treated conservatively and radically (Table 25–1).[56,]

Table 25–1

Studies of Fertility Following Ectopic Pregnancy: Conservative Versus Radical

Author	Follow-up (yr)	Patients		Overall (%)		IUP (%)		Live Birth (%)		Ectopic (%)		Factors Associated with Infertility
		Con	Rad	Con	Rad	Con	Rad	Con	Rad	Con	Rad	
Sherman et al., 1982[56]	11.2	65	159			83.0	72.0			6.4	5.8	A, B, C, D
Nagamani et al., 1984[57]	3–13		71		62		52.0				12.6	B, D
Toumivaara and Kauppila, 1988[58]	1–11	86	237	80	82					14.0	13.0	B
Querleu and Boutteville, 1989[59]	2	141	332			58.5	52.0			22.9*	4.4	A
Makinen et al., 1989[60]	4–8	42	68					69	63	29.0*	15.0	D, E
Langer et al., 1990[61]	3–15	118				70.3		63.5		12.7		B

*Significant difference.
Con, Conservative surgery; Rad, Radical surgery; A, Previous infertility; B, Pelvic adhesions; C, Tubal rupture; D, Advanced age; E, Non-IUD user.

[59, 62] Most of these studies have failed to adequately stratify for other factors that affect subsequent fertility, including the presence of pelvic adhesions, status of the contralateral tube, occurrence of tubal rupture, age of patients, and, most importantly, a history of infertility prior to the ectopic pregnancy. Definitive data are not available, but overall, conservative surgery does appear to offer improved fertility potential over salpingectomy. This is most obvious in patients who have a single remaining tube.

However, some of these same studies describe a significantly higher risk of repeat ectopic pregnancy than when salpingectomy is performed.[59, 60] These findings are in contrast to earlier studies that suggested that there was no difference in risk of repeat ectopic pregnancy for patients treated with conservative versus radical surgery. Risk of recurrent ectopic pregnancy may be as high as 30%.

References

1. Ectopic pregnancy—United States, 1987. MMWR 1990; 39(24):401.
2. Westrom L, Bengtsson LPH, Mardh PA: Incidence, trends, and risks of ectopic pregnancy in a population of women. Br Med J 1981; 282:15.
3. Dorfman SF, Grimes DA, Cates W Jr, et al.: Ectopic pregnancy, United States: Clinical aspects, 1979 to 1980. Obstet Gynecol 1984; 64:386.
4. Breen JL: A 21-year survey of 654 ectopic pregnancies. Am J Obstet Gynecol 1970; 106:1004.
5. Pauerstein CJ, Croxatto HB, Eddy CA, et al.: Anatomy and pathology of tubal pregnancy. Obstet Gynecol 1986; 67:301.
6. Saito M, Koyama T, Yaoi Y, et al.: Site of ovulation and ectopic pregnancy. Acta Obstet Gynecol Scand 1975; 54:227.
7. McCausland A: High rate of ectopic pregnancy following laparoscopic tubal coagulation failures. Am J Obstet Gynecol 1980; 136:97.
8. Morris JM, Van Wagenen G: Interception: The use of postovulatory estrogen to prevent implantation. Am J Obstet Gynecol 1973; 115:101.
9. McBain JC, Evans JH, Pepperell RJ, et al.: An unexpectedly high rate of ectopic pregnancy following the induction of ovulation with human pituitary and chorionic gonadotropin. Br J Obstet Gynaecol 1980; 87:5.
10. Gemzell CA: Experience with the induction of ovulation. J Reprod Med 1978; 21(Suppl.):205.
11. Elias S, LeBeau M, Simpson JL, et al.: Chromosome analysis of ectopic human conceptuses. Am J Obstet Gynecol 1981; 141:698.
12. Bello G, Schonholz D, Mosirpur J, et al.: Combined pregnancy: The Mount Sinai experience. Obstet Gynecol Surv 1986; 41:603.
13. Budowick M, Johnson TRB, Genardy R, et al.: The histopathology of the developing tubal ectopic pregnancy. Fertil Steril 1980; 34:169.
14. Weckstein LN: Current perspectives on ectopic pregnancy. Obstet Gynecol Surv 1985; 40:259.
15. Schwartz RD, DiPietro DL: Beta hCG as a diagnostic aid for suspected ectopic pregnancy. Obstet Gynecol 1980; 56:197.
16. Kadar N, Caldwell B, Romero R: A method of screening for ectopic pregnancy and its indications. Obstet Gynecol 1981; 58:162.
17. Shepherd RW, Patton PE, Novy MJ, Burry KA: Serial beta hCG measurements in the early detection of ectopic pregnancy. Obstet Gynecol 1990; 75:417.
18. Midgley A, Jaffe P: Regulation of human gonadotropin II. Disappearance of human chorionic gonadotropin following delivery. J Clin Endocrinol 1968; 28:1712.
19. Kamrava M, Taymor M, Berger M, et al.: Disappearances of human chorionic gonadotrophin following removal of ectopic pregnancy. Obstet Gynecol 1983; 62:486.
20. Milwidsky A, Adoni A, Segal S, Palti Z: Chorionic gonadotropin and progesterone levels in ectopic pregnancy. Obstet Gynecol 1977; 50:145.
21. Matthew CP, Coulson PB, Wild RA: Serum progesterone levels as an aid in the diagnosis of ectopic pregnancy. Obstet Gynecol 1986; 68:390.
22. Buck RH, Joubert SM, Worman RJ: Serum progesterone in the diagnosis of ectopic pregnancy: A valuable diagnostic test? Fertil Steril 1988; 50:752.
23. Romero R: The diagnosis of ectopic pregnancy. In DeCherney AH (ed.): Ectopic Pregnancy. Rockville, MD, Aspen Publishers, 1986, pp. 15–33.
24. Kadar N, DeVore G, Romero R: Discriminatory hCG zone: Its use in the sonographic evaluation for ectopic pregnancy. Obstet Gynecol 1981; 58:156.
25. Leach RE, Ory SJ: Modern management of ectopic pregnancy. J Reprod Med 1989; 34:324.
26. Bangham DR, Storring PL: Standardization of human chorionic gonadotropin, hCG subunits, and pregnancy test. Lancet 1982; 1:390.
27. Fossum G, Davajan V, Kletzky O: Early detection of pregnancy with transvaginal ultrasound. Fertil Steril 1988; 49:788.
28. Romero R, Kadar N, Castro D, et al.: The value of adnexal sonographic findings in the diagnosis of ectopic pregnancy. Am J Obstet Gynecol 1988; 158:52.
29. Romero R, Copel J, Kadar N, et al.: Value of culdocentesis in the diagnosis of ectopic pregnancy. Obstet Gynecol 1985; 65:519.
30. Samuellson S, Sjovall A: Laparoscopy in suspected ectopic pregnancy. Acta Obstet Gynecol Scand 1972; 51:31.
31. Garcia A, Aubert J, Sama J, Josimovich J: Expectant management of presumed ectopic pregnancies. Fertil Steril 1987; 48:395.
32. Mashiach S, Carp H, Serr D: Nonoperative management of ectopic pregnancy: A preliminary report. J Reprod Med 1982; 27:127.
33. Dericks T, Scholz C, Tauber H: Spontaneous recovery of ectopic pregnancy: A preliminary report. Eur J Obstet Gynecol Reprod Biol 1987; 25:181.
34. Ory SJ, Villanueva AL, Sand PK, Tamura RK: Conservative treatment of ectopic pregnancy with methotrexate. Am J Obstet Gynecol 1986; 154:1299.
35. Goldstein DP: Treatment of unruptured ectopic pregnancy with methotrexate with folinic acid rescue (MTX-FA). Presented at the Thirty-Fourth Annual Clinical Meeting of the American College of Obstetricians and Gynecologists, New Orleans, May 1986.
36. Sauer M, Gorrill M, Rodi I, et al.: Nonsurgical management of unruptured ectopic pregnancy: An extended clinical trial. Fertil Steril 1987; 48:752.
37. Ichinoe K, Wake N, Shinkai N, et al.: Nonsurgical therapy to preserve oviduct function in patients with tubal pregnancies. Am J Gynecol 1987; 156:484.
38. Stovall TG, Ling FW, Buster JE: Outpatient chemotherapy of unruptured ectopic pregnancy. Fertil Steril 1989; 51:435.
39. Stovall TG, Ling FW, Carson SA, Buster JE: Nonsurgical diagnosis and treatment of tubal pregnancy. Fertil Steril 1990; 54:537.
40. Stovall TG, Ling FW, Buster JE: Reproductive performance after methotrexate treatment of ectopic pregnancy. Am J Obsstet Gynecol 1990; 162:1620.
41. Robertson DE, Smith W, Moye MA, et al.: Reduction of ectopic pregnancy by injection under ultrasound control. Lancet 1987; 1(8539):974.
42. Lindblom B, Hahlin M, Kallfelt B, Hamberger L: Local prostaglandin F2 alpha injection for termination of ectopic pregnancy. Lancet 1987; 1:776.
43. Feichtinger W, Kemeter P: Conservative treatment of ectopic pregnancy by transvaginal aspiration under sonographic control and injection of methotrexate injection. Lancet 1987; 1:381.
44. McComb P, Gomel V: Linear ampullary salpingotomy heals better by secondary versus primary closure. Fertil Steril 1984; 41:454.

45. Timonen S, Nieminen U: Tubal pregnancy, choice of operative method of treatment. Acta Obstet Gynecol Scand 1967; 46:327.
46. Malkasian GD, Hunter JS, Remine WH: Pregnancy in the tubal interstitium and tubal remnants. Am J Obstet Gynecol 1959; 77:1301.
47. Kalchman GG, Meltzer RM: Interstitital pregnancy following homolateral salpingectomy. Am J Obstet Gynecol 1966; 96:1139.
48. Jeffcoate TNA: Salpingectomy or salpingo-oophorectomy. Br J Obstet Gynaecol 1955; 135:74.
49. Tanaka T, Hayashi H, Kutsuzawa T, et al.: Treatment of interstitial ectopic pregnancy with methotrexate: Report of a successful case. Fertil Steril 1982; 37:851.
50. Fredericks CM, Holtz G: Nontubal ectopic pregnancy. In Fredericks CM, Paulson JD, Holtz G (eds.): Ectopic Pregnancy: Pathophysiology and Clinical Management. New York, Hemisphere Publishing, 1989, p. 193.
51. Hreschchyshyn MM, Naples JD Jr, Randall CL: Amethopterin in abdominal pregnancy. Am J Obstet Gynecol 1965; 93:286.
52. Grimes DA, Geary FH Jr, Hatcher RA: Rh immunoglobulin utilization after ectopic pregnancy. Am J Obstet Gynecol 1981; 140:246.
53. Kelly RW, Martin SA, Strickler RC: Delayed hemorrhage in conservative surgery for ectopic pregnancy. Am J Obstet Gynecol 1979; 133:225.
54. DiMarchi J, Kosasa T, Kobara T, Hale R: Persistent ectopic pregnancy. Obstet Gynecol 1987; 70:555.
55. Schenker J, Eyal Z, Polishuk W: Fertility after tubal surgery. Surg Gynecol Obstet 1972; 135:74.
56. Sherman D, Langer R, Sadovsky G, et al.: Improved fertility following ectopic pregnancy. Fertil Steril 1982; 37:497.
57. Nagamani M, London S, Amand P: Factors influencing fertility after ectopic pregnancy. Am J Obstet Gynecol 1984; 149:533.
58. Tuomivaara L, Kauppila A: Radical or conservative surgery for ectopic pregnancy? A follow-up study of fertility of 323 patients. Fertil Steril 1988; 50:580.
59. Querleu D, Boutteville C: Fertility after ectopic pregnancy (letter). Fertil Steril 1989; 51(6):1069.
60. Makinen JI, Salmi TA, Nikkanen VPJ: Encouraging rates of fertility after ectopic pregnancy. Int J Fertil 1989; 34(1):46.
61. Langer R, Raziel A, Ron-El R, et al.: Reproductive outcome after conservative surgery for unruptured tubal pregnancy: A 15-year experience. Fertil Steril 1990; 53:227.
62. Thorburn J, Philipson M, Lindblom B: Fertility after ectopic pregnancy in relation to background factors and surgical treatment. Fertil Steril 1988; 49:595.

Gynecologic Endoscopy: Laparoscopy, Falloposcopy, and Hysteroscopy

26

Randle S. Corfman

In recent years, gynecologic endoscopy has progressed from chiefly a diagnostic procedure to a method by which surgical therapy can be rendered. The gynecologic surgeon has awaited development of technology that would permit transition from the traditional approaches to gynecologic pathologies to endoscopic techniques. Viewed by many with skepticism, much of the mystique of operative endoscopy has been replaced with the realization that endoscopic approaches to gynecologic pathologies can often afford the patient many benefits.[1]

The basic maneuvers required for gynecologic surgery are well established, as described elsewhere in this text. Adaptations of these maneuvers are required with an endoscopic technique.[2, 3] These adaptations must be safely and effectively rendered in order for this approach to be efficacious. Given that an endoscopic approach is merely a variation of *access*, the endoscopic gynecologic surgeon must realize that basic techniques used by the surgeon at laparotomy and at laparoscopy are the same.

This chapter addresses laparoscopy, falloposcopy, and hysteroscopy separately, even though it is recognized that the basic surgical maneuvers are similar. Basic surgical maneuvers, drawn from the very foundations of surgery, are reviewed in order to create a working environment for the endoscopic surgeon.

LAPAROSCOPY

Basic Equipment

Several basic equipment items are considered to be absolutely necessary for performing operative laparoscopic procedures. Appropriately assembled, these items will provide the endoscopic surgeon with appropriate visualization of the abdominal and pelvic contents, permitting effective and safe application of gynecologic surgical principles.

The *laparoscope* can be configured in a variety of optical designs as well as physical variations, as demonstrated in Figure 26–1. The straight laparoscope, long the mainstay of laparoscopy, continues to provide the most clear view of pelvic structures. In order to accommodate an operative channel, the head of the laparoscope must be either offset at 45 degrees from the longitudinal axis of the laparoscope or placed parallel to the main shaft of the laparoscope. These offset configurations significantly decrease visibility in low-light settings. The straight, nonoperative laparoscope is used most frequently for diagnostic maneuvers as well as for maneuvers that do not require the use of an operative channel.

The optics of the laparoscope can also vary, ranging from 0 degrees to 30 degrees. With a 0-degree

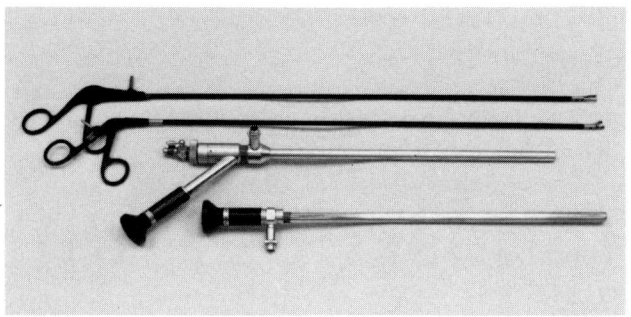

Figure 26–1
The straight laparoscope (*bottom*) and operating 45-degree offset laparoscope (*top*) with instruments designed for the operating laparoscope.

optical system, a straight-ahead view is obtained, whereas the 30-degree laparoscope provides visualization of structures to the side of the laparoscope. The endoscopic surgeon will soon become aware of the utility of having each of these available on the operating table.

The *illumination* of the abdominal and pelvic structures is gained by a variety of cold-light sources. Although halogen sources were often used for laparoscopic surgery, the xenon sources have virtually replaced the halogen elements by virtue of their splendid illumination. In addition, many light sources have capabilities for generating a flash that can be used with photodocumentation using a single lens reflex camera.

The light cables that connect the laparoscope to the light source must be carefully handled in order to ensure that breakage of the fibers within the cables does not occur. It should also be recognized that the fiberoptics can generate considerable heat, providing potential for heating of surgical drapes directly in front of the fiberoptics. As a safety measure, the light source should not be switched on until the laparoscope is ready to be inserted into the abdominal cavity.

The chip *video camera* may be the single most important contribution to the development of endoscopic approaches to gynecologic surgery. These cameras have replaced early, heavy cameras, providing a lightweight system that can be either directly attached to the laparoscope or attached to the laparoscope via a beam-splitter, as shown in Figure 26–2. The direct coupling type requires less illumination than the beam-splitting configuration. A disadvantage of the direct coupler is that direct visualization through the laparoscope cannot be made without removing the camera from the laparoscope. Even though significant advances have been made with the camera systems, it is this author's opinion that there are times when tissue planes are most clearly identified using direct visualization through the laparoscope. The television *monitors* are placed at a variety of positions around the operating room. By judicious placement of the monitors, the surgeon as well as the assistants can easily visualize what is taking place in the abdomen.

Documentation of the procedure can be easily attained either by video recording of the procedure or by still photography methods. Advantages of the video documentation include a permanent record of the procedure, which can be either provided to other physicians for future care of the patient or saved by the surgeon for his or her own records. A major disadvantage of this approach is that storage of these tapes becomes difficult. A single lens reflex camera can also be adapted to the laparoscope. When used with the flash generating light sources, a detailed image can be obtained. Unfortunately, application of the single lens reflex camera to the laparoscope can be cumbersome, making routine use of this modality tenuous.

The need for appropriate distention of the peritoneal cavity is obvious when one considers that the peritoneal cavity is a potential space. *Insufflation* can be achieved by placing the Veress needle into the abdominal cavity and taking steps to ensure that the insufflation will not occur in the preperitoneal space, in a vascular structure, or in other abdominal organs. A variety of gases can be employed, although carbon dioxide is one used by most endoscopic surgeons. Carbon dioxide is readily absorbed, and any residual gas will be cleared from the abdominal cavity over several hours. This frequently leads to referred shoulder pain, and the patient should be made aware of this adverse effect. The high-flow insufflator has replaced the conventional insufflator, permitting rapid placement of gas into the peritoneal cavity. This replacement is necessary as a result of the loss of distention gas during an operative procedure. Most high-flow insufflators currently permit the surgeon to specify the desired intra-abdominal pressure, and flow rates ranging from 3 to 6 liters/minute can be employed to maintain this pressure.

Potential complications of insufflation include

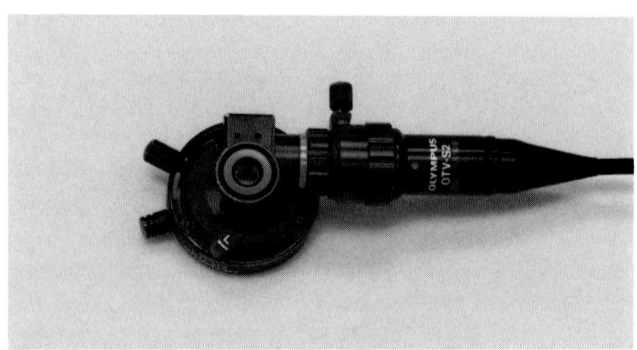

Figure 26–2
A lightweight chip video camera, of the beam-splitting type, provides clear color images.

overdistention leading to a decreased venous return to the heart and increased ventilatory pressures. If the Veress needle is inserted into a vascular structure, gas embolism can occur with disastrous results. Preperitoneal insufflation can also occur, particularly in the obese patient. A variety of techniques exist for ensuring that these complications do not occur.

Availability of a *high-power-density energy source* is absolutely necessary. An electrocautery power source should always be present in the room and ready for use. This would require placement of a grounding pad on the patient prior to draping, and the system should be turned on, ready for use. Many endoscopic surgeons find it advantageous to have access to laser technology, and these laser units should be in position and ready for use prior to the operative endoscopy.

A variety of *suction-irrigation systems* are available, providing capability to rapidly evacuate smoke plume, fluid (blood), or solid gel (clots) from the abdomen. It is necessary to be able to rapidly deliver irrigation fluids to a specific location, and this can be achieved by simply using the hanging intravenous fluid bag. Several commercial irrigation systems are available for each application. A suction device can be connected to wall suction or to a smoke treatment and filtering system. Selection of a suction-irrigation probe that permits dual function with minimal changing of hand position is preferable. This will permit the surgeon to quickly and efficiently change from irrigation to suction, greatly increasing his or her ability to maintain the adequate visualization of pelvic structures.

When large blood clots must be evacuated from the abdominal cavity, a chest tube can be modified for use, connecting it to the suction tubing with an adapter. The tube can then be introduced through a 10-mm port into the abdominal cavity, and a ringed forceps used to control the application of suction force. Very large clots can be evacuated easily using this technique.

Many of the items just described should be assembled on a portable cart for rapid, dependable access. This will permit portability between operating rooms.

LAPAROSCOPIC INSTRUMENTATION AND BASIC MANEUVERS

Unlike laparotomy, with instruments that have stood the test of time (e.g., Mayo scissors, Kelly clamps, etc.), laparoscopy instruments are evolving quickly in an attempt to meet the needs of the endoscopic surgeon. When faced with the large variety of instruments that can be used in endoscopic procedures, the endoscopic surgeon is often impressed by the lack of uniform designation for a given instrument. What follows is a grouping of instruments that correlate with the basic surgical maneuvers for which they were designed or adapted. With this grouping, provision is made for a convenient method of operative table organization, further improving efficiency and minimizing some of the frustrations that can face both the surgeon and endoscopic surgery team.

Manipulation Instruments and Maneuvers

The objective of the manipulation instrument is to aid in obtaining visualization of abdominal or pelvic structures and to establish adequate traction-countertraction forces in order to facilitate dissection. The *blunt probe* is the preferred instrument for intraabdominal manipulations. The blunt probe is devoid of sharp edges and is relatively atraumatic. The endoscopic surgeon should avoid vigorous manipulations, which can render the pelvic tissues edematous, hemorrhagic, and damaged.

A great deal of torque can be generated using the laparoscopic instruments, and the surgeon should be aware that the lever arm that exists when using instruments through a laparoscopic port can contribute significantly to the pressures that are sustained by the tissue. Furthermore, the surgeon should avoid the use of instruments as alternatives to the blunt probes. The potential for laceration increases when instruments that are other than round and smooth are utilized. Finally, a "fingertip" approach should be used, thereby facilitating gentle manipulation of pelvic and abdominal structures.

Grasping forceps are available in two general types, each with various grasping mechanisms (Fig. 26–3). A scissor type grasper is configured so that active force is required to approximate the jaws of the instruments. Self-retaining graspers require an active force to open the jaws. When force is relieved, the jaws grasp the tissue in question so that no active force is necessary for maintenance of the tissue within the grasp of the instrument. In general, scissor type graspers are used whenever many relatively quick, repetitive movements are required. Self-retaining graspers are used when it is anticipated that the tissue will be held for relatively long periods of time. Despite the exponential growth in the number of laparoscopic instruments that are available, the "alligator" and biopsy forceps remain the most useful. It may be no accident that many of the instruments that the endoscopic surgeon finds most useful are those that have existed for several years.

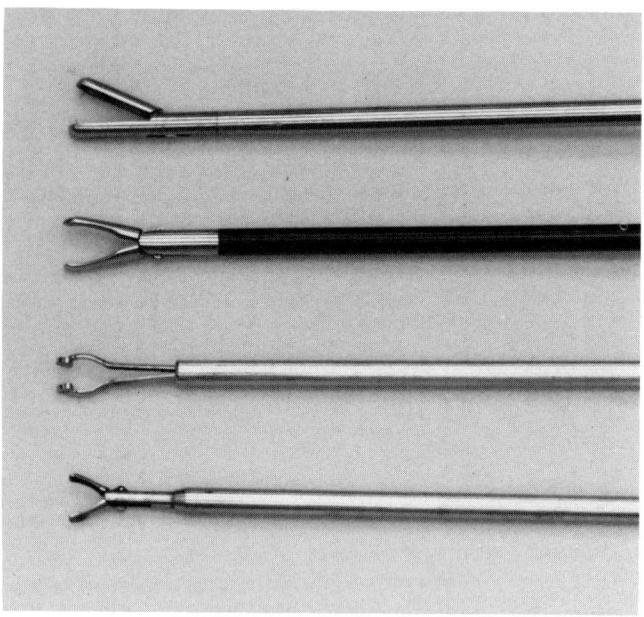

Figure 26–3
Grasping forceps include (*top to bottom*) spoonbill biopsy forceps, atraumatic (alligator) forceps, self-retaining tissue forceps, and self-retaining atraumatic grasping forceps.

Incising Instruments

Incision of tissue is one of the most basic maneuvers used by the surgeon. In order to gain incision, the chosen modality must use a force to provide the incision effect. The force of the scalpel is gained from the surgeon's hand, whereas the force of the electrocautery or laser modalities uses the flow of electrons or photons, respectively. As one moves from a purely cutting modality, such as a scalpel, a "field effect" must be reckoned with, as well as the sequelae that may result from this field effect.

Sharp incision is the ultimate in a modality that generates no field effect. However, the lack of field effect contributes to hemorrhage from the incised tissues. The *scalpel* can be used endoscopically, attached to the end of a probe that can be inserted through a 5-mm sheath. *Scissors* can also be employed, which achieve incision by crushing of tissue between two sharpened jaws. With proper sharpening, the crushing effect is minimized. A variety of scissors are available for endoscopic use, including the hook, peritoneum, and microdissecting scissors, shown in Figure 26–4. The hook scissors are designed so that the tips of the scissor jaws approximate before the more proximal portions of the jaws, thereby entrapping the tissue to be incised. The advantage of the scalpel and the scissors is that minimal field effect results if the instruments are properly sharpened. Again, the disadvantage of these modalities is the lack of any inherent hemostatic properties.

Field Effect–Producing Incising Instruments

The incising effect of the high-power-density energy systems is created using energy either in the form of electrons (electrocautery) or photons (laser). Simply put, as electrons or photons impinge upon the tissue, energy is absorbed by intracellular components, leading to tissue heating and destruction. The degree of peripheral heating is determined in part by the vascularity of the tissue, because the blood and lymphatic vessels contribute to dissipation of heat.

The heating around the periphery of the vaporized or desiccated tissue has both advantages and disadvantages. The advantage of incising with these modalities is that there is a sealing of vessels and lymphatics that occurs with application of the energy, resulting in hemostasis. However, this field effect can be disadvantageous, owing to the ischemia and zone of thermal necrosis that occurs.

If energy delivered to tissues is pulsed, there is less average heating of the tissue, thereby permitting a significant contribution to dissipation of heat by the vascular or lymphatic channels. Super- and ultra-pulsing are variations that permit low average powers while achieving very high peak powers. Currently, lasers are the only high-energy modalities to employ pulsing of the energy.[4,5]

The power density of the energy delivered to a issue determines the zone of ischemia and necrosis. The power density is approximated by the equation:

$$Pd = \frac{W \times 100}{sd^2}$$

where Pd is the power density in watts/cm^2, W is the power in watts, and sd is the spot diameter in

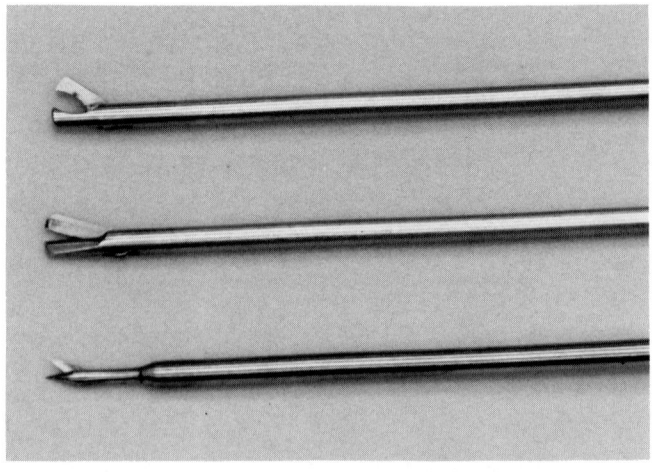

Figure 26–4
Laparoscopic scissors include (*top to bottom*) hook scissors, peritoneum scissors, and microdissecting scissors.

millimeters. This approximation is thought to apply to both laser and electrocautery energies.

The usefulness of this equation has been demonstrated for the carbon dioxide laser, revealing that the field effect, or zone of thermal damage, is related inversely to the power density.[6] For the carbon dioxide laser, a power density of greater than 2500 watts/cm^2 must be maintained for the pulsed waveforms, whereas a power density of greater than 5000 watts/cm^2 must be maintained for continuous waveforms in order to minimize the zone of thermal damage. If the power density is allowed to go below these values, the field effect rapidly increases. When incising tissue that appears to have the propensity toward hemorrhage, lower power densities may be employed in order to increase the field effect, enhancing the hemostatic properties of the energy. On the other hand, when working in areas where minimal field effect is desired, such as the fallopian tube, power densities greater than those mentioned earlier should be maintained.

Lasers that are amenable to laparoscopic use include the carbon dioxide laser, the argon laser, the neodymium:yttrium-aluminum-garnet (Nd:YAG) laser, and the KTP-532 laser. Each of these have their own unique properties, including differences in color dependency, wavelength, beam-scattering effect, and depth of penetration. Several excellent texts exist that address the use of lasers in operative gynecologic surgery.[5, 6]

The needle-tip and microtip electrocautery devices (Fig. 26–5) have been adapted for endoscopic use, permitting very high power densities to be attained. Use of these significantly decreases the cost for a high-power-density energy system.

Regardless of which energy source is chosen, achieving optimal incision depends on proper tissue positioning and attaining appropriate traction-countertraction forces.

INSTRUMENTS FOR APPROXIMATING TISSUE

Approximation of tissue is used for a variety of indications, including achievement of hemostasis, pedicle procurement, and restoration of anatomic relationships. In general, the trend in gynecologic surgery is toward less suturing, owing to a variety of studies revealing that sutures predispose the patient to adhesion formation. Although easily placed at laparotomy, laparoscopic suturing is time consuming and requires significant training before the surgeon is proficient with this approach. Two major categories of suturing include the intra-abdominal and the extracorporeal knotting techniques.

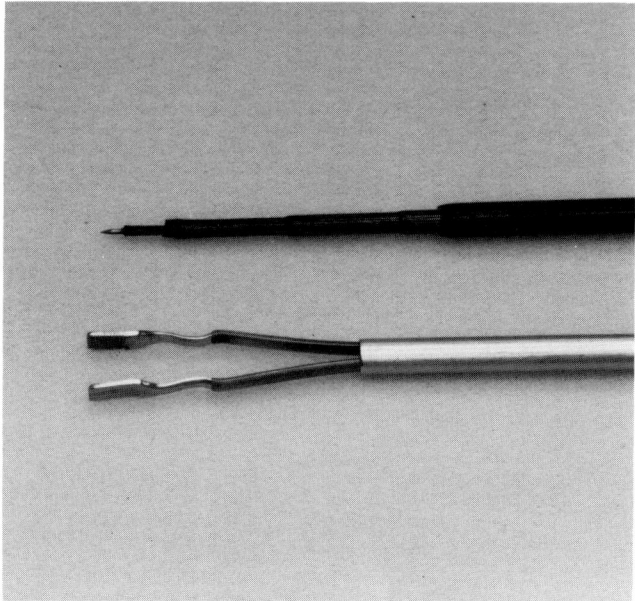

Figure 26–5
Laparoscopic electrocautery instruments include (*top to bottom*) the needle-tip unipolar electrocautery and the bipolar coagulation forceps.

Laparoscopic Suturing and Intra-abdominal Knotting Techniques

Approximation of tissues is achieved using laparoscopic placement of sutures.[7] The needle is grasped with laparoscopic needle holders (Fig. 26–6), and the suture is placed. A variety of sutures can be chosen, and either a straight or a "ski" needle can be used. The knot is then tied using either an instrument tie within the abdominal cavity or a modification of a fisherman's knot,[8] shown in Figure 26–7. Tying an instrument knot endoscopically is tedious and time consuming; a modified fisherman's knot is much more easily tied intracorporeally than an instrument knot.

Sutures can be placed and the knot tied outside the abdomen, or extracorporeally. Following laparoscopic placement of the sutures, the needle is withdrawn via the same port through which it was introduced into the abdominal cavity, and the knot is applied. Two commonly used knots include the Roeder knot and the Duncan knot (Fig. 26–8). Following the tying of the knot, the knot is introduced into the abdomen and positioned using a laparoscopic knot applicator. It should be noted that the slipping strength of the knot is significantly improved with the addition of a half-hitch, as shown in Figure 26–9.

Another variation of extracorporeal knotting can be achieved using a series of half-hitches, each of which is pushed into the abdominal cavity using a

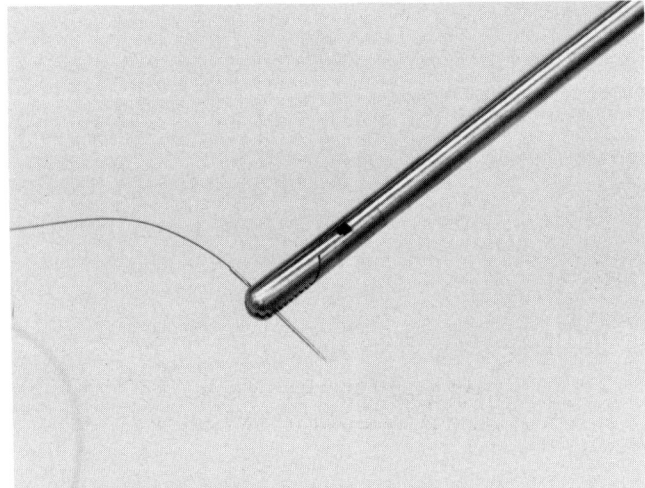

Figure 26-6
Laparoscopic needle holder grasping needle.

specialized knot applicator. Using this approach, simple and secure knots can be placed without the need for tying the more sophisticated but difficult Roeder and Duncan knots.

Pretied loops are commercially available and are easily placed into the abdominal cavity. The tissue to be sutured is pulled through the loop within the abdominal cavity, and the loop is closed and the knot secured. Previously available in chromic and plain catgut sutures, the pretied loops are now available in a variety of suture materials. Alternatively, the surgeon can tie his or her own Roeder or Duncan knot, creating a loop that can easily be placed into the abdominal cavity. This permits variations in the type of suture and the diameter of suture to be used.

Laparoscopic Stapling Devices

With the entry of endoscopic surgery into general surgical use, a variety of stapling devices and clip applicators have become available to the endoscopic gynecologic surgeon. One such device delivers a titanium clip that can be placed for tissue approximation. It should be kept in mind, however, that these clips are permanent and may preclude future application of techniques such as magnetic resonance imaging or diathermy.

A variety of stapling devices have been introduced that function in similar fashion to those used for performing bowel resections at laparotomy. Following application of the stapling device, a series of

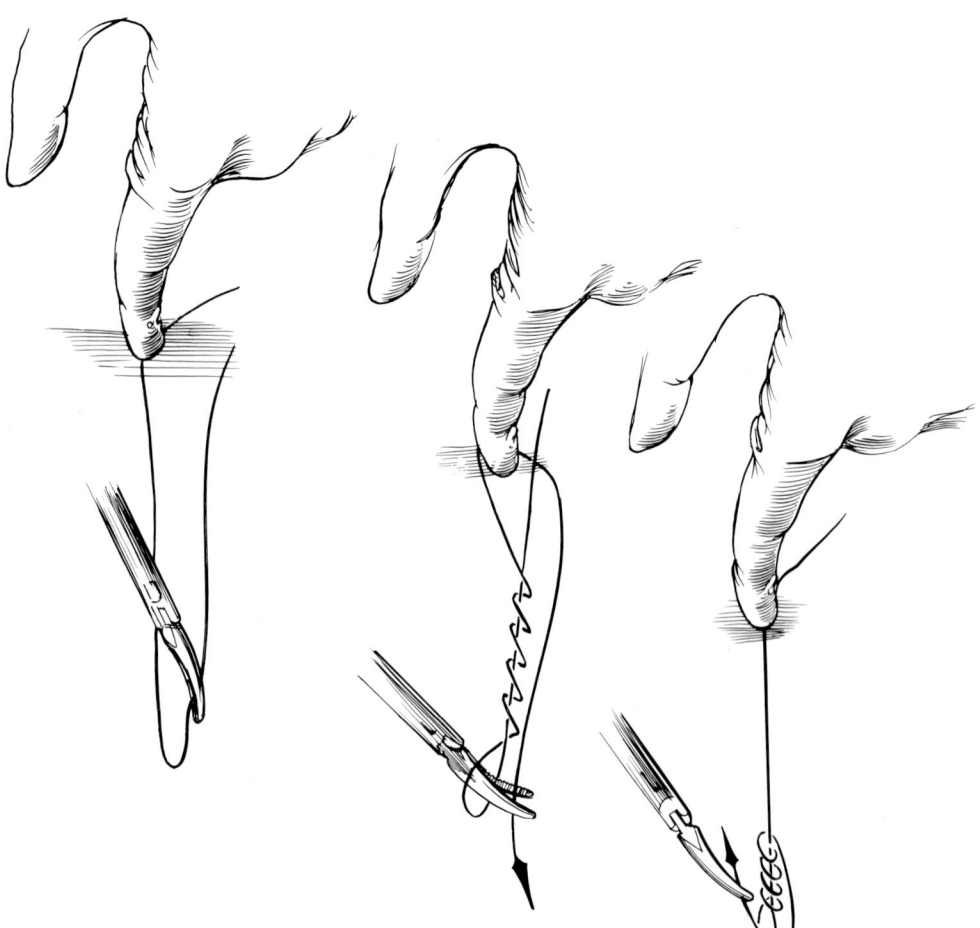

Figure 26-7
Modified fisherman's knot for intracorporeal knotting (see ref. 8).

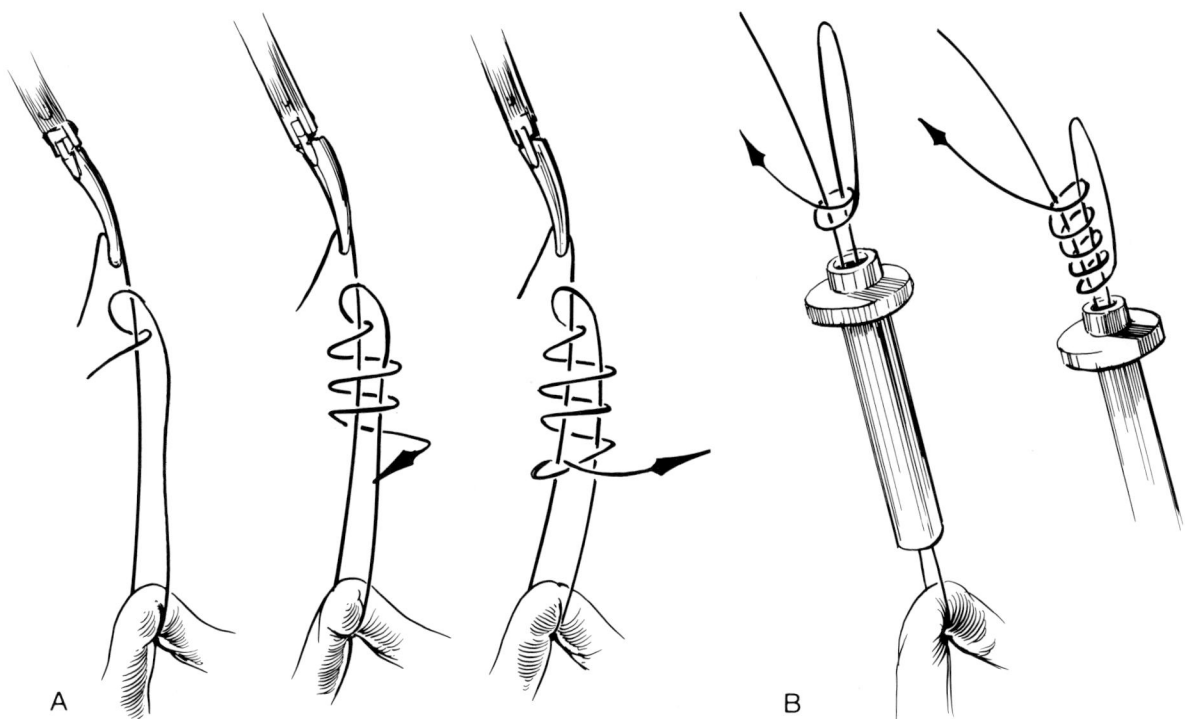

Figure 26–8
The Roeder (*left*) and Duncan (*right*) knots are useful extracorporeal knots.

staples are left in place, as well as a clean incision. These stapling devices are potentially useful for adnexectomy, laparoscopic-assisted vaginal hysterectomy, and appendectomy.

Tissue Removal Instrumentation

Often the endoscopic surgeon is faced with tissue inside the abdomen that is too large to pass through the 5-mm diameter accessory sheaths. Several methods can be used to remove this tissue.

If the surgeon has placed a 10-mm port through the umbilicus, the operative channel of the laparoscope can be used, placing grasping forceps through the operative channel in order to grasp the tissue. With one smooth motion, the grasped forceps, along with the laparoscope, is withdrawn from the abdominal cavity while the assistant maintains the trumpet valve of the 10-mm port in the open position. This method obviates the need for placement of a second 10-mm operative port at another location.

Another option includes placement of a 10-mm port at one of the suprapubic accessory sites. A variety of 10-mm diameter instruments (Fig. 26–10) can then be placed into the abdominal cavity, including scissors, biopsy forceps, claw forceps, and a morcellating instrument. These instruments permit fragmentation of tissue prior to removal, greatly enhancing the ability to remove tissue from the abdominal cavity. It is important to recognize, however, that spring retainers have been designed into the instrument to preclude inadvertent opening of the jaws within the abdominal cavity. This is particularly important with the 10-mm instruments. The instruments should neither be placed into nor withdrawn from the abdominal cavity except under direct visualization. This will preclude inadvertent injury to the abdominal structures.

In the instance that a 5-mm port must be removed and a larger port placed, a set of dilators can be used

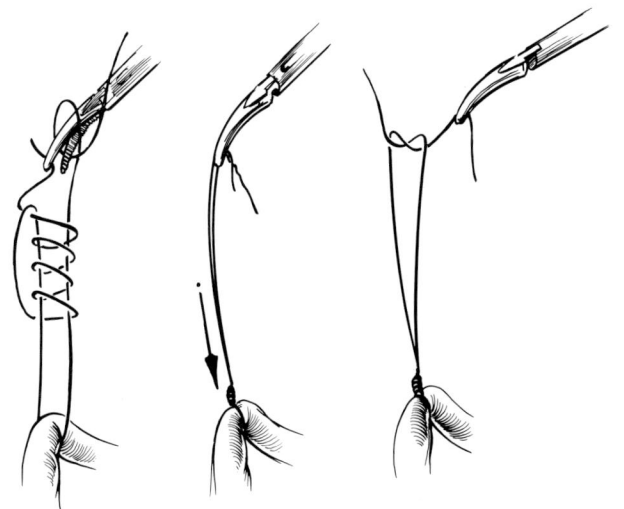

Figure 26–9
Addition of a half-hitch to either the Roeder or the Duncan knot significantly improves the slipping strength of the knot.

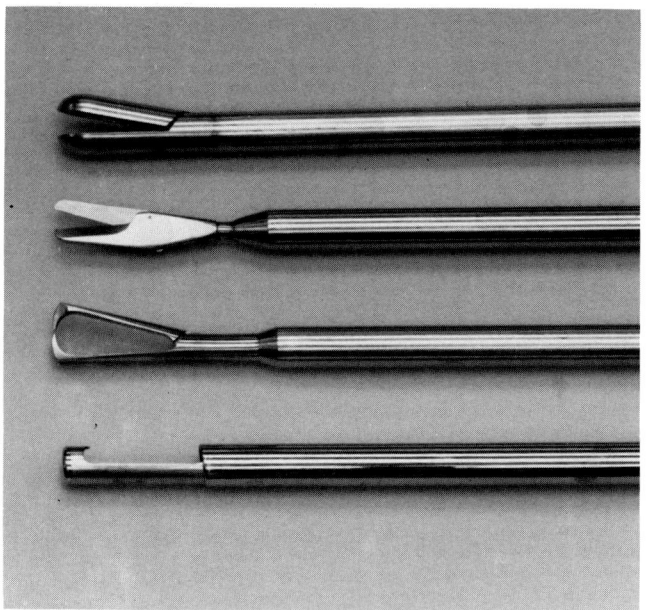

Figure 26–10
The larger (10-mm diameter) instruments include (*top to bottom*) spoonbill biopsy forceps, scissors, claw grasping forceps, and tissue morcellator.

to dilate the incision to the desired diameter. Alternatively, a 10-mm trocar and sheath can be initially placed into the abdominal cavity via a suprapubic accessory site, and an adapter used to downsize from the larger 10-mm or 12-mm diameter to the diameter of the 5-mm instruments.

The final option includes provision of a larger incision via the anterior abdominal wall or cul-de-sac for tissue removal. This technique is particularly useful for removal of large tissues. A posterior culdotomy can also be performed laparoscopically using a laser for incision.

Ablation Instrumentation

Ablative methods achieve the desired tissue result utilizing field effects. Ablation can be obtained with the bipolar coagulation forceps, needle-tip electrocautery, and laser. Each modality is useful, but limitations should be kept in mind for each.

The bipolar coagulation forceps (see Fig. 26–5), owing to the very low power density, has a large field effect. When desiccation is achieved, it is unlikely to yield postoperative adhesions, but damage to adjacent structures must be anticipated and proper application of the forceps made. The needle and microtip electrocautery devices are unipolar modalities and have the potential for arcing. Field effects with unipolar devices can be considerable, inducing damage peripheral to the application site.

The laser energy forms are also popular for ablation. In general, vessels of the diameter of greater than 0.5 mm cannot be sealed adequately with laser modalities. Pulsed, super-pulsed, and ultra-pulsed waveforms are less likely to provide hemostasis, owing to the extremely high peak power densities that can be achieved. It is recognized that the pigment-dependent lasers, including the Nd:YAG, argon, and KTP-532 lasers, are more likely to coagulate and ablate colored lesions preferentially.

It is very important to have rapid access to ablative methods, particularly for hemostasis needs. For example, the bipolar coagulation forceps must be on the table with a grounding plate on the patient, ready for immediate use in the case that immediate hemostasis must be made. In addition, a thorough knowledge of the location of adjacent vital structures (e.g., the ureters) must be exercised.

Trocars and Sheaths

A variety of trocars and sheaths can be used, providing a port of access to the peritoneal cavity. These come in a variety of sizes ranging from 3 mm through 12 mm and greater.

The 10-mm diameter sheaths are most frequently used for positioning the laparoscope and for tissue removal. On the other hand, the 3-mm and 5-mm diameter sheaths are frequently used for placement of laparoscopic instruments and for manipulations of the pelvic and abdominal contents. Adapters are currently available that permit downsizing from a 10-mm to smaller diameters, precluding the loss of an adequate pneumoperitoneum. There are two types of valves available for preserving the pneumoperitoneum. The *ball valve* type is useful, but it must be recognized that it is difficult to remove tissue through this valve, owing to entrapment of the tissue by the ball valve as it closes. The *trumpet valve* type permits the surgeon to keep the valve open for tissue removal.

With the larger diameter trocars and sheaths, the surgeon must keep in mind that herniation or occult entrapment of bowel or omentum can occur with removal of the sheaths. These adverse outcomes can be minimized using two maneuvers. First, insertion of a blunt probe into the sheath prior to removal prevents the withdrawal of abdominal contents through the incision. Second, reapproximation of the fascia occasionally must be achieved by suturing. Special care must be taken to prevent inadvertent bowel damage with suture placement.

HYSTEROSCOPY

Until the last decade, the hysteroscope has been an instrument in search of a use.[9] Faced with chiefly a diagnostic tool, the hysteroscopist had only scissors and biopsy forceps for operative procedures until the resectoscope and the fiberoptic lasers could be adapted for hysteroscopic use.

In order to perform hysteroscopy, distention of the potential space within the endometrial cavity must be safely attained, permitting visualization of structures therein. This discussion centers around fluid distention media and basic maneuvers that can be safely performed at hysteroscopy.

Distention Media

In order to gain expansion of the potential space within the endometrial cavity, a variety of agents have been safely used, including high-molecular-weight dextran (Hyskon, Pharmacia), Ringer's lactate solution, sorbitol, and glycine. The ideal medium would possess properties that include nontoxicity, immiscibility with blood for excellent clarity, ease of delivery into the intrauterine cavity, and low cost. Unfortunately, none of the currently available media possess all of these properties.

Hyskon provides excellent visualization as a result of its immiscibility with blood. Its high viscosity allows slow egress from the endometrial cavity, providing excellent distention. It is nonionic, permitting its use with the electrocautery-powered resectoscope. Major drawbacks to its use include potential for anaphylactic reactions that manifest as disseminated intravascular coagulation and adult respiratory distress syndrome. These reactions are not limited to cases in which large volumes of Hyskon are used, although they can be minimized by keeping the total volume of Hyskon used to less than 500 ml. It should be recognized that fluid overload can also occur in the patient, because 1 ml of absorbed Hyskon pulls 3 ml of fluid into the intravascular space. Other deficiencies of Hyskon include the tendency for the Hyskon to caramelize when it is sufficiently heated, forming a coating around the wire loop of the resectoscope or rollerball electrode. It is quite sticky and tends to gum up the instruments, making cleaning difficult. The viscosity of the solution, although providing excellent clarity, makes delivery to the uterine cavity difficult, requiring either a strong-armed assistant or a special pump. Despite these disadvantages, Hyskon remains the preferred distention medium of many hysteroscopic surgeons.

Lactated Ringer's solution, sorbitol, and glycine are also frequently used. With the development of the continuous flow hysteroscope, the surgeon is able to gain excellent visibility with these media, despite the ease with which blood mixes with each of these fluids. Advantages of these media include ease of delivery, lack of anaphylactic reactions, and low cost. Disadvantages include the miscibility with blood, which leads to decreased visibility, and the potential for fluid overload. In addition, absorption of sorbitol and glycine solutions can lead to dilutional hyponatremia, a very serious sequela. These potential problems require fastidious accounting of the fluids that have been used. If more than 2000 ml of fluid is unaccounted for, the procedure is terminated. Serum electrolytes are monitored if greater than 1200 ml of sorbitol or glycine is used. Patients with significant medical problems, including heart disease, pulmonary disease, or renal disease, should be carefully monitored.

Regardless of which distention medium is selected, it should be recognized that when large quantities of distention media are used, significant hypothermia can result. It is preferable for the anesthesiologist to be particularly aware of the complications that can occur with distention media in hysteroscopy so that prompt recognition of an adverse effect can be made.

Hysteroscopes

Two major components of the hysteroscope include the optical system and the delivery system. The *optics* of the hysteroscope determine the angle of view that is provided to the surgeon, with this angle ranging from 0 degrees (straight ahead) to 30 degrees (from the longitudinal axis). These choices permit selection of a view that maximizes visualization of the working elements of the hysteroscope.

The *delivery system* that is chosen can include a diagnostic hysteroscope without an operative channel or a hysteroscope with an operative channel, as shown in Figure 26–11. When the latter is chosen, a variety of attachments can be placed into the endometrial cavity, including flexible or rigid operative instruments.

Biopsy and Tissue Removal Instruments

Biopsy and tissue removal instruments permit directed biopsy as well as removal of tissue or foreign objects from the endometrial cavity. For smaller biopsies or for those in the uterine cornu, the flexible biopsy forceps can be introduced via the working channel of the hysteroscope into the uterine cavity (Fig. 26–12). Foreign objects such as intrauterine devices or retained bone from an induced or spontaneous abortion are more easily removed with the rigid forceps.

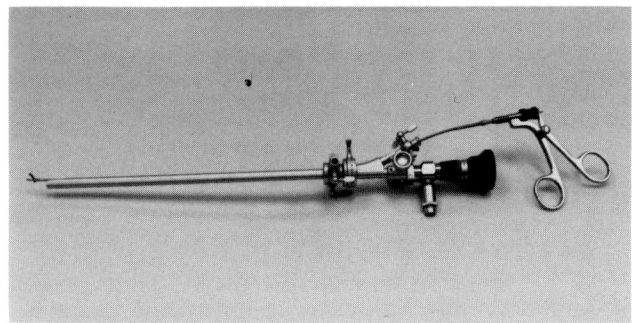

Figure 26-11
Operating hysteroscope with flexible scissors in position.

Incision Instruments

Tissues can be incised or excised with either hysteroscopic scissors or fiberoptic lasers. Scissors have been designed with either a flexible shaft or a rigid design. The fiberoptic lasers that are used most commonly in the endometrial cavity include the Nd:YAG and argon lasers, each of which can be used for incision. In addition, the wire loop resectoscope is also used for incision or excision, particularly for treating the septate uterus or submucous leiomyomas.

Ablation and Coagulation Instruments

Either the wire loop resectoscope or the fiberoptic laser can be used to ablate tissue within the endometrial cavity. Used for years by the urologist, the resectoscope has been adapted as an instrument for incision or ablation within the uterus. Any of the nonionic distention media can be used with the resectoscope, including Hyskon, glycine, and sorbitol. As previously mentioned, the advent of the continuous flow hysteroscope has permitted greater use of the less viscous media. Regardless of the medium chosen, bubble production with application of current is frequently a problem, requiring the surgeon to occasionally rid the cavity of bubbles.

The wire loop resectoscope can be used for a variety of applications, including incision, excision, and ablation. The rollerball electrode, an adaptation of the wire loop resectoscope, has been used extensively as an ablative instrument. Incorporation of the conductive metal ball onto the wire loop adds a degree of safety to the instrument by reducing, but not eliminating, the potential for uterine perforation.

The Nd:YAG laser has also been used for ablative therapy. It can be applied with either a "no-touch" or a contact technique. The flexibility of the fiberoptic lasers permits ablation of remote areas within the uterus, particularly the uterine cornu.

A combination of these techniques has been used effectively for endometrial ablations by employing electrocautery for treatment of the larger surface areas within the endometrial cavity and the Nd:YAG laser for treatment of the cornu.

FALLOPOSCOPY

The final endoscopic frontier facing the gynecologist is the lumen of the fallopian tube.[10] Adequate visualization of this space has been slow in coming, owing to the need for technologies that would permit tiny endoscopes to be passed into the fallopian tube, which has a diameter of 200 μ at the uterotubal junction. The bias that the interstitial portion of the fallopian tube is most commonly tortuous in course has also had to be overcome.

The distal portion of the fallopian tube has been assessed primarily via a laparoscopic approach. With this technique, a "salpingoscope" was placed through the ampullary portion of the fallopian tube and images obtained.[11] Hysteroscopic cannulation had to await the demonstration that a transcervical access to the tube could be effectively and safely used.[12] Kerin and colleagues[13] coined the term "falloposcopy," demonstrating for the first time that a fiberoptic device could be directed hysteroscopically into the proximal fallopian tube, providing the first endoscopic views of the tube's entire length.

These new techniques may permit a diagnostic approach to the fallopian tube, permitting triage of

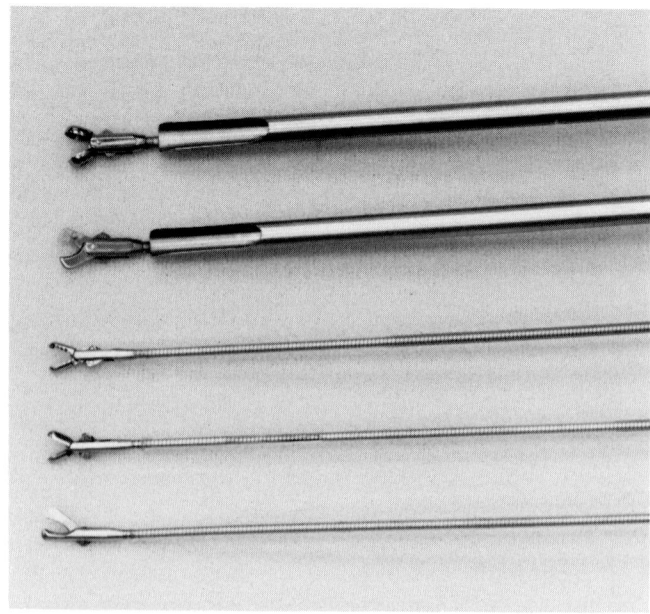

Figure 26-12
Hysteroscopic instruments include (*top to bottom*) rigid biopsy forceps, rigid scissors, flexible grasping forceps, flexible biopsy forceps, and flexible scissors.

the subfertile woman. As an example, patients with unexplained infertility could be examined prior to undergoing the assisted reproductive technologies in order to determine the health of the fallopian tube. The falloposcope could also be used in patients with hydrosalpinx and distal tubal obstruction prior to a surgical approach to evaluate the health of the tubal mucosa.

Therapeutic modalities must also be developed that can be delivered with the falloposcope. Perhaps adhesiolysis can be performed in treating intratubal synechiae. Interest also exists in the development of the ability to deposit gametes or pre-embryos into the fallopian tube via a transcervical approach, in conjunction with the assisted reproductive technologies.

Before the falloposcope can be widely used clinically, prospective studies must be performed to determine the clinical significance of falloposcopic findings. Development of delivery systems that permit atraumatic access to the fallopian tube is desirable.

OPERATIVE ENDOSCOPIC GYNECOLOGIC SURGICAL PROCEDURES

Having described each of the maneuvers that is possible using the laparoscope, hysteroscope, and falloposcope, the similarities between the endoscopic approach and the laparoscopic approach are obvious. Truly, the endoscopic gynecologic surgeon is limited only by his or her expertise in performing certain maneuvers and determining what can and cannot be performed endoscopically. Tables 26–1 and 26–2 list gynecologic procedures that have been effectively performed endoscopically.

It should also be emphasized that the efficacy of many of these procedures performed endoscopically

Table 26–1

Partial Listing of Laparoscopic Gynecologic Procedures

> Adhesiolysis
> Appendectomy
> Laparoscopic-assisted hysterectomy
> Myomectomy
> Neosalpingostomy
> Oocyte retrieval
> Oophorectomy
> Ovarian cystectomy
> Ovarian wedge resection
> Salpingectomy for ectopic pregnancy
> Salpingo-oophorectomy
> Salpingostomy for ectopic pregnancy
> Transection of uterosacral ligaments
> Uterine suspension
> Vaporization-excision of endometriosis

Table 26–2

Partial Listing of Hysteroscopic Procedures

> Cannulation of proximal fallopian tube
> Directed biopsy
> Endometrial ablation
> Excision of endometrial polyps
> Excision of submucous fibroids
> Removal of foreign body
> Resection-incision of uterine septum
> Resection of endometrial synechiae (Asherman's syndrome)

has yet to be proved. This is perhaps best summarized by Alan H. DeCherney, MD, who said, "The days of show and tell are over," in commenting on the widespread application of gynecologic procedures at endoscopy.[14] It is important that clinical trials be performed to demonstrate that these techniques can be safely and effectively performed. The endoscopic gynecologic surgeon must be aware that just because we can perform a procedure endoscopically does not mean that we should.

ACQUISITION AND DEVELOPMENT OF ENDOSCOPIC SURGICAL SKILLS

Having discussed the basic surgical maneuvers that can be performed endoscopically, it becomes obvious that application of these skills can be made only after a firm working knowledge of pelvic and abdominal anatomy is realized. It is only after this knowledge is obtained that a safe and effective transition to an endoscopic approach can be made. It would be desirable to integrate endoscopic surgical training into residency training programs so that at completion of the training program, the basic surgical maneuvers can be comfortably and safely applied at laparotomy and endoscopy. Of course, this mandates that the faculty must be able to provide necessary direction to the resident physician in obtaining these skills.

For physicians who have completed residency training prior to the general availability of operative endoscopic gynecologic surgery, it is necessary to gain some postgraduate training for development of the these skills. Attendance at several postgraduate hands-on courses should be made in order to gain familiarity with endoscopic techniques and instrumentation.

It should be recognized that, owing greatly to the relative youth of this approach, a wide variety of techniques are available to the endoscopic surgeon. Many of these techniques have limited clinical application and should be considered in a stage of evolution. By attending several workshops, the endoscopic surgeon will be able to more effectively ascertain the usefulness of a variety of techniques to his or her practice.

Many of medicine's greatest surgeons have expanded their skills by observing experienced surgeons performing procedures. Often a visiting surgeon could directly assist the master, further promoting a rich experience. Unfortunately, these possibilities have been virtually eliminated in modern medicine, owing chiefly to today's medicolegal environment. Observing surgery is still possible, however, permitting the preceptee to see the extracorporeal movements and techniques that contribute significantly to the success or failure of a given procedure. These preceptorships will greatly enhance the experiences gained in postgraduate didactic courses.

Procurement of a training device that simulates a laparoscopic perspective is also desirable. Such devices can be used with the video system in order to gain the ability to operate using the video monitor for imaging. The trainers permit the surgeon to hone skills, making the transition from the three-dimensional perspective available by laparotomy to the two-dimensionality of the endoscopic approach.

Having gained the skills necessary for endoscopic surgery, it is important to maintain proficiency. The general aviation community has emphasized the fact that an instrument aviator's competence decreases significantly more quickly than his or her confidence levels. This creates a dangerous situation, both for the instrument aviator and the endoscopic surgeon.

Finally, it should be recognized that operative endoscopy is not for every gynecologic surgeon. The physician must weigh the need to perform the endoscopic surgery against the time commitment that must be sacrificed in order to gain the necessary skills. This honest assessment will undoubtedly permit specialization opportunities and further contribute to quality medical care for our patients.

References

1. DeCherney AH: The leader of the band is tired. Fertil Steril 1985; 44:299.
2. Semm K: Operative Manual For Endoscopic Abdominal Surgery. Chicago, Year Book Medical Publishers, 1987.
3. Sanfilippo JS, Levine RL: Operative Gynecologic Endoscopy. New York, Springer-Verlag, 1989.
4. Taylor MV, Martin DC, Poston WM, et al.: Effect of power density and carbonization on residual tissue coagulation using the continuous wave carbon dioxide laser. Colpos Gynecol Laser Surg 1986; 2:169.
5. Keye WR: Laser Surgery in Gynecology and Obstetrics, 2nd ed. Chicago, Year Book Medical Publishers, 1990.
6. McLaughlin DS: Lasers in Gynecology. Philadelphia, JB Lippincott, 1991.
7. Marrero MA, Corfman RS: Laparoscopic use of sutures. Clin Obstet Gynecol 1991; 34:387.
8. Thompson RG, Reich H: Intraabdominal laparoscopic suturing: A new technique. Forty-Sixth Annual Meeting, American Fertility Society, Washington, 1990.
9. Corfman RS: Indications for hysteroscopy. Obstet Gynecol Clin North Am 1988; 15:41.
10. Corfman RS: Falloposcopy: Frontiers realized . . . a fantastic voyage revisited. Fertil Steril 1990; 54:574.
11. Nezhat F, Winer WK, Nezhat C: Fimbrioscopy and salpingoscopy in patients with minimal to moderate pelvic endometriosis. Obstet Gynecol 1990; 75:15.
12. Confino E, DeCherney A, Corfman R, et al.: Transcervical balloon tuboplasty: A multicenter study. JAMA 1990; 264:2079.
13. Kerin J, Daykhovsky L, Segalowitz J, et al.: Falloposcopy: A microendoscopic technique for visual exploration of the human fallopian tube from the uterotubal ostium to the fimbria using a transvaginal approach. Fertil Steril 1990; 54:390.
14. DeCherney AH: Personal communication.

Adnexal Surgery

27

Ann Jeanette Davis

OVARIAN CYSTECTOMY

Indications

Ovarian cystectomy, removal of a cystic structure from the ovary, is performed for a variety of pathologic conditions. In contrast to oophorectomy, it allows the patient to retain her fertility potential.

Functional Ovarian Cysts

During each successive menstrual cycle, a group of follicles is recruited to begin the maturation process. The dominant, or ovulatory, follicle reaches a size of an approximately 2-cm cyst at the expense of the other, degenerating follicles. The cellular residue surrounding the dominant follicle becomes the corpus luteum. Thecal lutea represent the cellular components of nonovulatory follicles or the residue from all the follicles in an anovulatory patient.

Physiologic cysts may represent follicular cysts, ovulatory cysts, corpus luteum cysts, or thecal luteum cysts. Cysts larger than 3–4 cm of these same structures are called functional ovarian cysts. Physiologic cysts are fluid collections representing the normal physiologic stimulation of the ovary by gonadotropin. Functional cysts are non-neoplastic enlargements of physiologic cysts.

The treatment of cystic adnexal masses must depend on the age of the patient and size of the mass. Spanos, in a classic study of 286 reproductive age women with cystic adnexal masses, treated patients with an estrogen-progestin combination for 6 weeks.[1] All patients in whom the mass did not resolve with treatment were surgically explored. Every patient explored had a pathologic condition, which included endometriosis, benign teratomas, parovarian cysts, and malignancies. All patients with functional cysts had regression of the cyst during the 6-week treatment cycle and avoided operative intervention. Most of the malignant neoplasms were in the 8–10 cm size group.

A prudent approach in the reproductive age woman with a cystic mass 7 cm or less in size is to place the patient on an estrogen-progestin combination for 6 weeks. Although Steinkampf and colleagues have shown that estrogen-progestin therapy does not hasten the resolution of functional cysts,[2] the combination may help prevent any large new cystic structures from forming. Surgical exploration is performed on any patient with an unresolving mass. Radiographic flat plates of the abdomen to rule out calcifications are also helpful. Tumor markers should be considered.

The rare functional cyst that does not resolve in a 6-week treatment cycle can be removed by ovarian cystectomy. Differentiating a functional cyst from some dermoids or mucinous cystadenomas by initial gross inspection can be difficult.

Benign Ovarian Teratoma

The most common ovarian neoplasm in young women is the benign ovarian teratoma, sometimes referred to as a dermoid cyst. This germ cell tumor of the ovary arises from all the germ cell layers.

Dermoids often contain sebaceous material, hair, cartilage, and teeth.

On examination, dermoids will usually present as mobile adnexal masses that may have a cystic or solid feel. Vague lower quadrant pain or ovarian torsion is another common presentation. Dermoids may be very mobile and present as a mass anterior to the bladder.

Ultrasonographic studies have shown that dermoids do not always have the typical appearance of an echogenic focus within a predominately cystic mass. Approximately 25% of dermoids will appear predominately solid on ultrasound.[3]

Diagnosis of a benign teratoma can be aided by a flat plate of the abdomen. Approximately 40% of dermoids will have radiologic calcifications compatible with teeth.

Cystectomy, with preservation of the ovary, is the treatment of choice. Even very small amounts of ovarian tissue can be reconstructed into a functional ovary.

Benign teratomas are bilateral in approximately 15% of cases. The opposite ovary should be palpated carefully. Doss and coworkers reviewed 213 cases of benign teratoma.[4] They concluded that covert bilaterality was not common, and that if the opposite ovary was normal in appearance and to palpation it should not be routinely bivalved or biopsied. Routine biopsy of the opposite ovary could lead to periovarian adhesive disease.

Endometrioma

Cystectomy may be appropriate for patients with an endometrioma (see also Laparoscopy). Except for very small endometriomas, medical therapy is of little help. These patients require experienced microsurgical techniques if they are seeking future fertility.

Surgical Procedure

The initial ovarian incision is made carefully through the outermost tissue layer with a fresh, sharp blade (Fig. 27–1A). The area adjacent to the tube and the

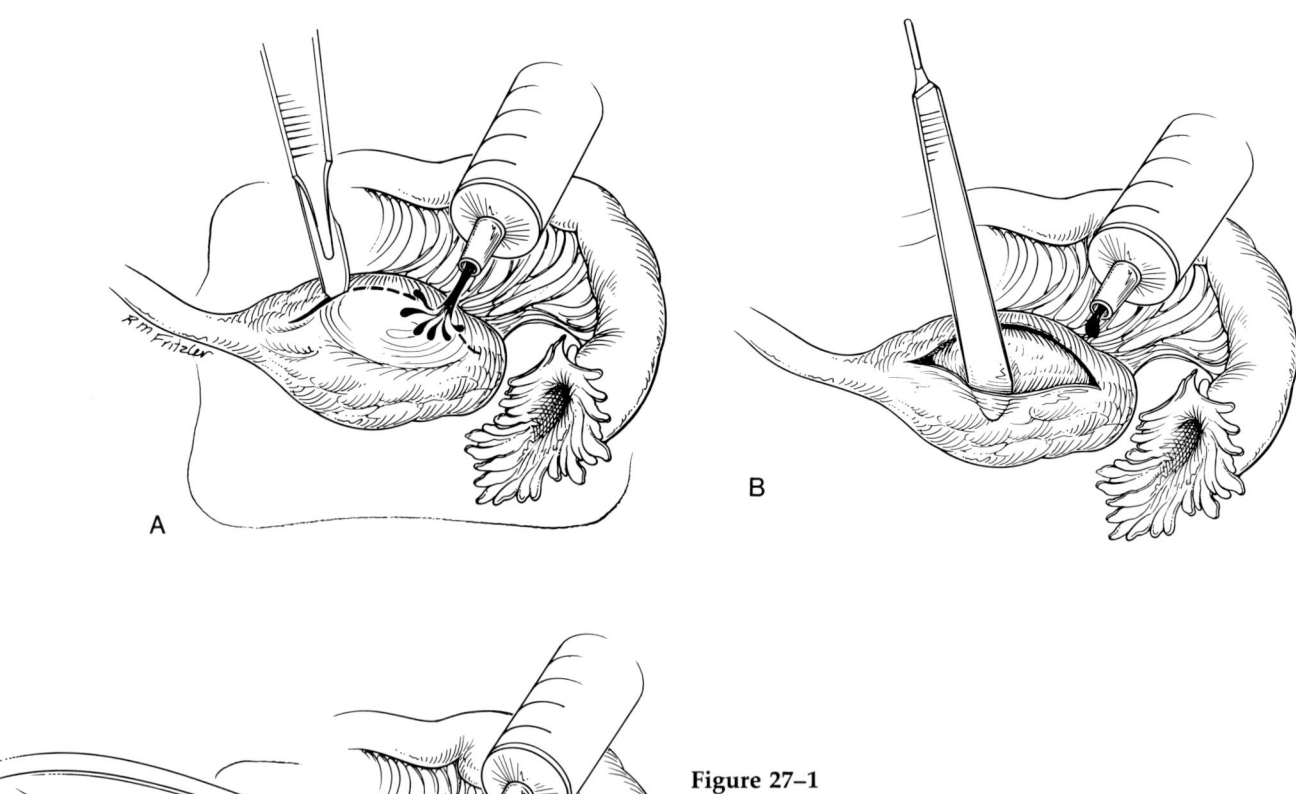

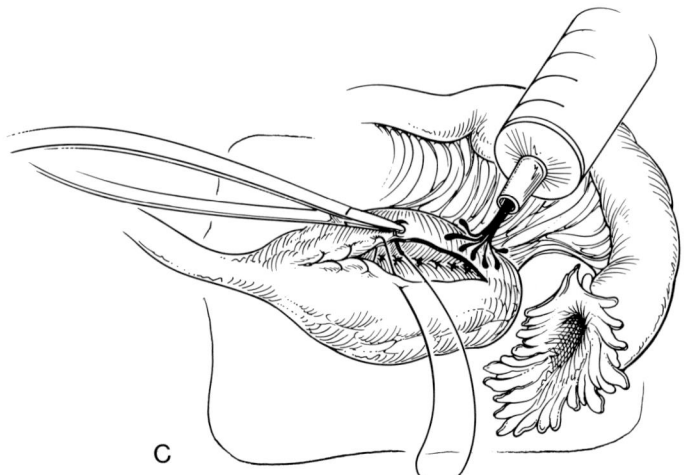

Figure 27–1
A, An incision is made through the outermost tissue layer, with the ovary elevated on a silicone mat. Constant irrigation keeps the operative field damp. B, A scalpel blade is used to dissect between the cyst wall and the ovary. C, Microsurgical technique is used to close the ovary. Deep interrupted sutures have been placed. The ovarian surface is closed with a baseball stitch. A continuous suture is directed from the inside of the defect to the outside.

fimbria ovarica are avoided. The ovary may be placed on a silicone mat to avoid unnecessary manual handling, which may predispose the patient to adhesive disease. Constant irrigation with a Ringer lactate heparin solution (5000 units heparin to 1 liter) is an excellent method to keep the operative field moist. Microsurgical techniques should be employed. The fimbriae are to be placed in a position that will not crush them or impinge on their blood supply.

Grasping the ovarian cortex should be avoided if at all possible. If it is necessary to directly grasp the tissue, atraumatic forceps such as Singley's or DeBakey's forceps is ideal. A "pool" suction device is less traumatic to the peritoneum than a standard suction device and may result in decreased postoperative adhesions.

After the initial incision is made, the cystic structure, such as a dermoid, can be shelled out of the ovary. The blunt end of a scalpel can be placed between the epithelial lining of the cyst and the ovarian tissue (Fig. 27–1B). An attempt is made to deliver the cyst intact without rupture. If incidental rupture occurs, a Kelly clamp can often be placed across the defect. Care should be taken to avoid spilling the contents into the abdominal cavity, because the cyst may contain substances capable of causing a chemical peritonitis.

The base of the cyst may require sharp dissection or incision with Metzenbaum's scissors or electrocautery to free the cyst from the ovarian stroma. The residual ovarian tissue may require trimming so that closure can be best performed.

Closure of the ovary should be performed with microsurgical techniques to lessen the chance of postoperative adhesive disease. Deep sutures are placed, using fine absorbable suture (5–0 or 6–0) in an interrupted fashion. The ovarian surface can be closed with the "baseball technique" (Fig. 27–1C). A fine absorbable suture is used, and each stitch is directed from the inside of the incision towards the outside. The "baseball technique" prevents cortical surface exposure of suture material by pulling ovarian cortex from one side over the previous suture. This decreases the risk of periovarian adhesions.

Small hemostatic ovarian defects may be allowed to heal by secondary intention. Preliminary data by some investigators appear to indicate that this healing process actually lessens the chance of periovarian adhesions.

Modified oxidized regenerated cellulose (TC7, brand name INTERCEED) has been shown to significantly reduce the incidence of adhesion formation and also to reduce the severity of adhesions.[5] This sheet of cellulose is applied over the ovarian defect and dampened with saline or Ringer's lactate.

Laparoscopy

Physicians skilled in multiple-puncture surgical laparoscopy may elect to perform an ovarian cystectomy through the laparoscope. Advantages of a laparoscopic technique include decreased recovery time and a probable decrease in the incidence of postoperative adhesive disease. Oxidized regenerated cellulose can also be applied via the laparoscope.[6]

Removal of any benign ovarian mass may be appropriate. Endometriomas are commonly treated laparoscopically because they are relatively easy to diagnose and differentiate from malignant conditions.[7] Treatment may include stripping, cauterization, or laser ablation of the cyst wall. The comparative efficacies of these various modalities remain unclear.

Dermoids may also be removed laparoscopically. However, controlled studies comparing cystectomy at laparotomy versus laparoscopy and future fertility have yet to be performed. Nezhat and associates reported a retrospective series of nine cases of laparoscopic dermoid cyst removal.[8] Four patients had second-look laparoscopies. One patient had periovarian adhesion, and the pelvis appeared normal in the other three. In three cases, the cysts were removed intact through a colpotomy incision.

The laparoscopic approach should be investigated in prospective controlled studies to determine its efficacy with the conventional approach.[9] Laparoscopic removal of dermoids usually requires rupture.[8] The sebaceous material of a dermoid may lead to peritoneal irritation. Laparotomy has a potential for the formation of peritubal adhesions. Some surgeons elect to perform laparoscopic dermoid cystectomies only in women who do not wish to retain fertility.

Future studies will provide needed data regarding the appropriate operative procedure (laparoscopy vs. laparotomy) for patients with adnexal disease. Currently, surgeons must base their decisions on less than ideal data. The ultimate goal is to select the operative procedure that will maintain or enhance fertility (if that is desired) and provide optimal therapy for adnexal masses that could have malignant potential. Although malignant potential in young women is very low, spillage of a malignant cyst may complicate staging and possibly lead to peritoneal seeding of malignant cells.

Surgeons must be aware that laparoscopic surgery is often more difficult than laparotomy. Laparoscopic equipment is often not "user friendly" to the novice laparoscopic surgeon. The surgeon's selection of appropriate laparoscopic cases will usually broaden with more laparoscopic experience. Good operative judgment is essential. Converting a laparoscopic case to a laparotomy may be very appropriate. Patients must be carefully counseled and prepared preoperatively regarding this possibility.

The surgical techniques for laparoscopic cystectomy are discussed thoroughly elsewhere in this text.

OOPHOROPEXY

Oophoropexy (ovariopexy) may be performed in an attempt to shield the ovary from radiation or to fix the ovary in a position where it is less likely to experience torsion.

Ovarian Torsion

The majority of cases of ovarian torsion occur in patients with a predisposing mass such as an ovarian teratoma or a large functional cyst of the ovary. These masses create mechanical factors that predispose the heavy ovary to twisting.

Torsion of a normal ovary, however, occurs more frequently than is generally appreciated. One out of four oophorectomies performed in a series of 88 children was the result of torsion and necrosis of a normal ovary.[10]

Diagnosis

In the past, the majority of patients with ovarian torsion were taken to the operating room with the preoperative diagnosis of appendicitis. This has been changing as surgeons more commonly use ultrasound in the preoperative evaluation of the patient with possible appendicitis. The normal appendix is usually not visible on ultrasound, in contrast to an inflamed appendix, which is typically visible. Use of ultrasonography has a sensitivity of approximately 75% in the diagnosis of appendicitis.[11] Unsuspected pelvic masses, typical of ovarian torsion, may be found during this evaluation, resulting in the preoperative diagnosis of ovarian torsion.

The clinical differentiation between appendicitis and ovarian torsion can be difficult. Both can present with lower abdominal pain, peritonitis, and leukocytosis. Torsion more frequently involves the right adnexa than the left, further complicating the diagnosis.[12] This phenomenon is probably due to the mass effect of the sigmoid, which lessens the chance of the left adnexa twisting.

There are, however, clinical differences between appendicitis and torsion. Appendicitis tends to be more gradual in its onset, in contrast to the very acute pain of torsion. Emesis often accompanies the onset of the pain in torsion, whereas it is a later symptom in appendicitis.

Ultrasonography should be part of the routine evaluation of the patient with suspected torsion. Quick preoperative diagnosis may allow salvage of an ovary. Oophorectomy is required if the ovary has had enough time to reach the stage of necrosis. Patients with ovarian torsion of most durations will have an echogenic mass on ultrasound whether or not they had a predisposing mass. Torsion of the adnexa apparently disrupts lymphatic and venous flow, which can result in ovarian enlargement secondary to edema.[13] Edema can be considered a stage in the process of torsion. If untwisting does not occur, the ovary will become necrotic and unsalvageable. If an echogenic adnexal mass is found on ultrasound, the patient can be immediately taken to the operating room and the ovary potentially saved.

Treatment

Clearly necrotic adnexa that are the result of torsion should be excised without untwisting the pedicle. The ureter must be identified to confirm that it is not included in the torsed pedicle.

The surgical treatment of torsion without necrosis remains controversial. Doppler ultrasound may be useful in determining whether the ovary has any vascular flow. However, untwisting the torsed pedicle has the potential of releasing thrombi.

No matter what decision an individual surgeon makes, many other questions arise. If torsion occurred once, what will prevent it from recurring? If one ovary is lost to torsion, should something be done to the contralateral ovary to prevent it from the same fate?[14] If oophoropexy is performed, how effective is it? There are no clear-cut answers to these questions.

Surgical Procedure

Various methods of oophoropexy have been performed. Elkins and Stock have proposed using permanent suture and securing the ovary to the pelvic sidewall[15] (Fig. 27–2).

In the patient with massive ovarian edema, wedge resection will confirm a diagnosis by frozen section and reduce ovarian size to allow for proper fixation.[16, 17]

An alternative method of oophoropexy is to shorten the supportive ligamentous support of the ovary, teetering it on a shorter pedicle, which would be less likely to twist. The ovarian ligament is folded into pleats and secured with permanent suture (Fig. 27–3). This method has the theoretical advantage of avoiding suturing ovarian tissue, which could contribute to adhesion formation.

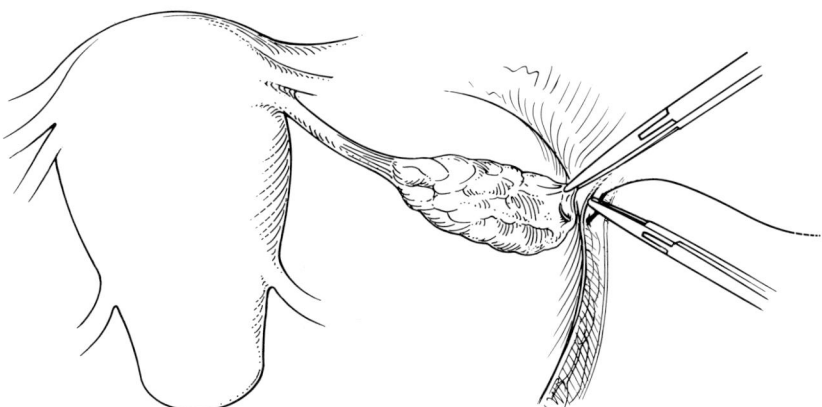

Figure 27–2
Permanent suture is used to pex the ovary to the peritoneum of the pelvic sidewall.

STERILIZATION (EXCLUDING LAPAROSCOPY)

Indications

Sterilization is the most common contraceptive method in the United States today. Most females are sterilized by laparoscopic techniques (see Chapters 23 and 26). Postpartum sterilization can be accomplished via a small infraumbilical incision. Mini-laparotomy may be used for sterilization in nonpuerperal patients who cannot tolerate laparoscopic procedures because of concurrent medical problems. Mini-laparotomies are also utilized by surgeons who are not comfortable with laparoscopic surgery.

Preoperative Evaluation

Patients requesting sterilization deserve careful counseling. Studies have shown that women less than 25 years of age are more likely to request reversal, as compared with women over age 30. This finding is independent of parity. Many women who have reversal procedures made their initial decision to be sterilized as a result of interpersonal stress and not primarily in regard to fertility. A history of unreliable contraception, such as pregnancies during oral contraceptive use, is more likely to be seen in patients who later request sterilization reversal procedures, as compared with their satisfied counterparts.[18]

Physicians must counsel patients regarding sterilization failure rates. Failure rates from sterilization via mini-laparotomy are equivalent to those of similar laparoscopic techniques. Failures can be reduced by approximately one-third by avoiding the so-called luteal phase pregnancy. Sterilization should be performed during the early proliferative phase to prevent these factitious failures. Simultaneous dilatation and curettage at the time of sterilization are not indicated. Curettage provides no guarantee of interrupting all pregnancies and increases the morbidity of the sterilization procedure.[19]

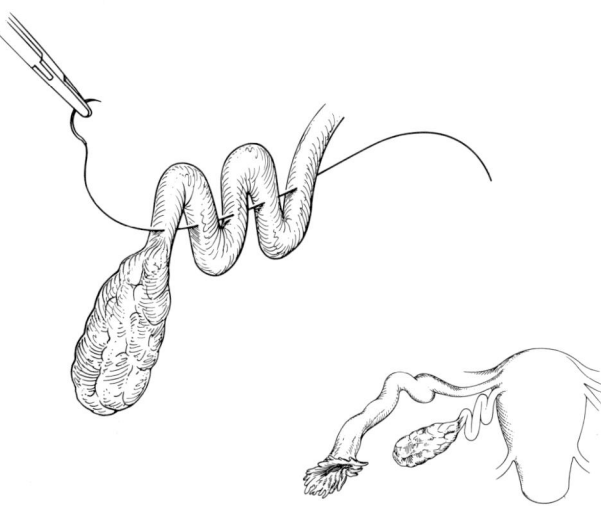

Figure 27–3
The ovarian ligament is folded "accordion style," tethering the ovary on a shortened pedicle, which is less likely to twist. A permanent suture is placed through the multiple folds.

Surgical Procedure

Mini-Laparotomy

A small suprapubic incision, approximately 3 cm in size, is made transversely several centimeters above the symphysis pubis. A manipulating device, such as a Cohen cannula, has been previously inserted in the uterus. The peritoneum is entered, and the uterus is pushed into an anteverted position. Clips, rings, coagulation (see discussion of laparoscopic sterilization in Chapter 23), or the Pomeroy technique (see later discussion) can be used to occlude the tubes. Other techniques such as the Irving and the Kroener procedures are infrequently used in the United States today (Figs. 27–4 and 27–5). The Kroener technique (Fig. 27–5) may be appropriate in patients with extensive adhesive disease in whom the mid-portion of the tube is not accessible. The suture ligatures must be placed proximal to all the fimbrial tissue to avoid sterilization failure. Chromic catgut suture, which may predispose the patient to tuboperitoneal fistulas, should be avoided.

Postpartum Sterilization

This procedure should be performed prior to significant uterine involution. A small (2-cm), infraumbilical, slightly curved incision is made. The fasciae and peritoneum are individually identified and entered. Small retractors pull forcibly toward the side that is to be ligated. The uterus can often be moved by external transabdominal pressure. Babcock's forceps are used to grasp the tube as soon as it is visualized. The fimbriae should be positively identified by "walking" the Babcock forceps toward the distal end of the tube (Fig. 27–6A).

The most common method of postpartum sterilization is the Pomeroy technique (Fig. 27–6B). The Babcock forceps grasp the ampullar portion of the tube. A loop of tissue is ligated with plain suture and held with a hemostat. It is prudent to remove as little of the tubal ampulla as possible to facilitate possible future re-anastomosis techniques. A second suture ligature is applied just proximal to the first. The tip of a small scissors can be used to perforate the mesosalpinx (Fig. 27–6C). The loop of tubal tissue is then excised (Fig. 27–6D).

Most failures following the Pomeroy method are the result of fistula formation. The use of plain catgut apparently reduces this risk, as compared with chromic suture.[20]

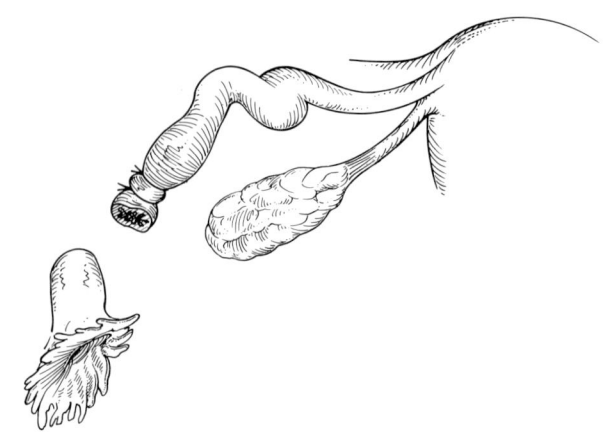

Figure 27–5
The Kroener fimbriectomy is accomplished by excising the fimbriated end of the tube. Two suture ligatures are placed at the distal end of the tube. Catgut suture should not be used.

OOPHORECTOMY

Indications

Oophorectomy may be indicated for a wide variety of pathologic conditions, including ovarian malignancies, endometriosis, and tubal ovarian abscesses that have not been responsive to antibiotic treatment.

Prophylactic oophorectomy at the time of hysterectomy remains controversial.[21] Many gynecologists offer prophylactic oophorectomy to women over the age of 40 who are undergoing pelvic operations for other indications. Advantages include potential prevention of ovarian cancer. Approximately 1 in 100 women will die of ovarian cancer. Unfortunately, most women are diagnosed with Stage III disease, because early detection is difficult. Given this alarming data, many patients will choose to have their ovaries removed when they are close to the menopausal years. The incidence of reoperation on residual ovaries, which ranges between 0.9 and 5.1%,[22,23] is yet another justification for prophylactic oophorectomy in women over 40 years of age.

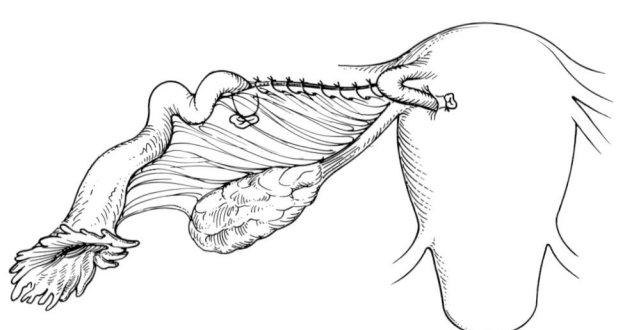

Figure 27–4
The Irving procedure buries the proximal tube into the myometrium. The distal end of the tube is placed into the broad ligament. Interrupted sutures are placed across the mesosalpinx.

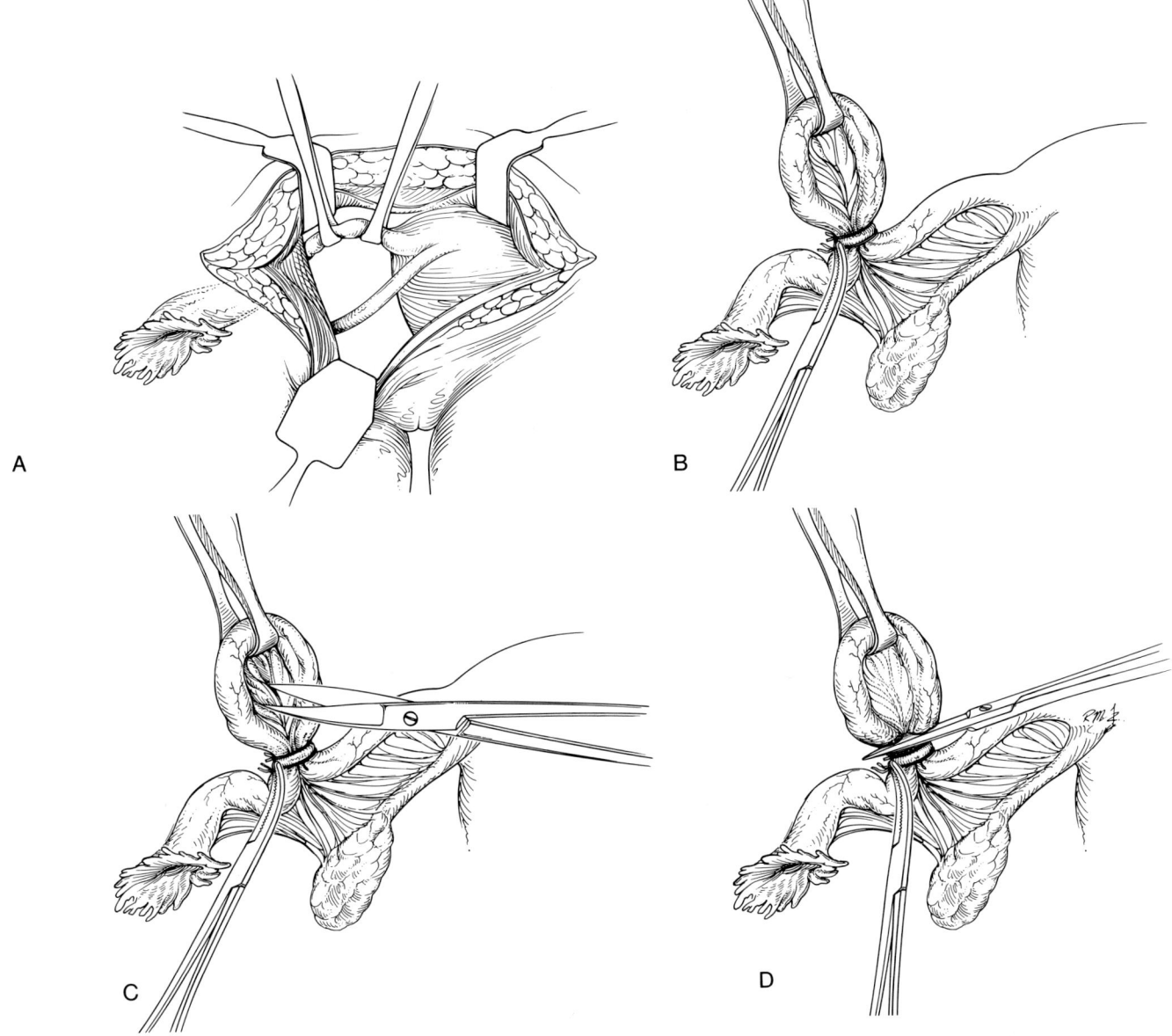

Figure 27-6
A, The Pomeroy technique utilizes an infraumbilical elliptical incision. Successive Babcock forceps are used to "walk" to the fimbriated ends of the tube. *B*, A nucha of tissue is formed in the midportion of the tube and doubly ligated with plain suture. *C*, Metzenbaum scissors create a window in the mesosalpinx. *D*, Metzenbaum scissors excise the anterior portion of the tubal nucha.

Surgical Procedure

The abdomen is entered with either a transverse or an abdominal incision, depending on the patient and the expected pathology. The infundibulopelvic ligament is isolated and the ureter identified. A finger can bluntly dissect the leaflets of the broad ligament anterior to the ureter. The infundibulopelvic ligament is triply clamped and incised, leaving an adequate pedicle. This pedicle is doubly ligated to ensure hemostasis of the ovarian artery.

If the adnexa are to be removed separately from the uterus, a similar pedicle is made, encompassing the tube and ovarian ligament (Fig. 27–7). Double clamps are placed, and an adequate pedicle is created.

In most cases requiring an oophorectomy, the tube is also removed. In the rare young patient, for whom reproductive potential is a consideration, it is possible to salvage the tube for use in assisted reproductive techniques. If the tube is to be saved, multiple pedicles are made between the ovary and the tube. Microsurgical technique and fine absorbable suture must be employed to decrease tubal adhesions. Assisted reproductive techniques such as gamete intrafallopian transfer (GIFT) require normal fallopian tubes.

Laparoscopy

Surgeons skilled in multiple-puncture laparoscopy may elect to use this technique to perform oophorectomies. Proper patient selection and good technical laparoscopic skills are essential. The surgical techniques are discussed elsewhere in this text.

WEDGE BIOPSY

Indications

Wedge biopsy is indicated in some cases of malignancy to evaluate the contralateral ovary if preservation is being considered. Use of wedge biopsy has declined in recent years. Gynecologists now appreciate that the procedure may produce adhesions, which could contribute to infertility. The use of the wedge biopsy in polycystic ovarian disease is largely outdated. Thus, the wedge procedure is reserved only for specific indications.

Surgical Procedure

A wedgelike incision is made in the ovary, taking care to avoid the fimbria ovarica and the infundibu-

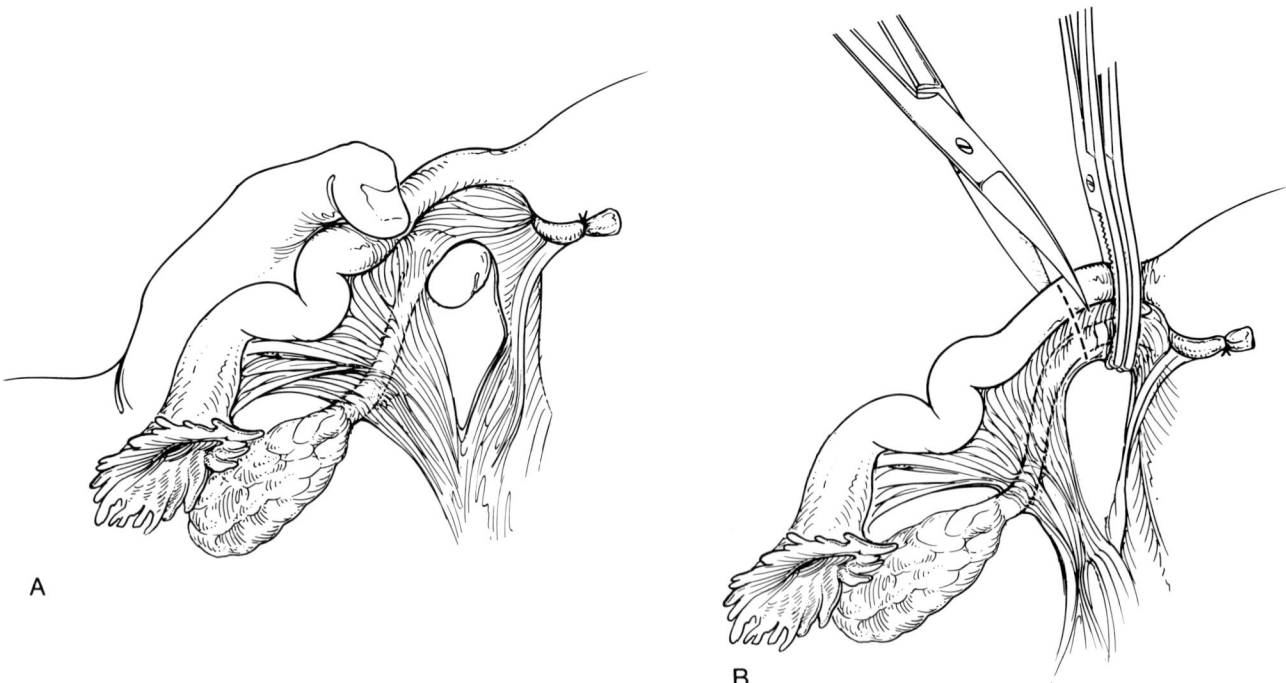

Figure 27–7
A, The infundibulopelvic ligament has previously been triply clamped superior to the ureter. The broad ligament is bluntly perforated with the surgeon's finger. *B*, In situations in which the adnexa is to be removed separate from the uterus, the tube and suspensory ligament of the ovary are doubly clamped and cut. The remaining peritoneal tissue is sharply or bluntly dissected near the ovary. Distal dissection may result in ureter injury.

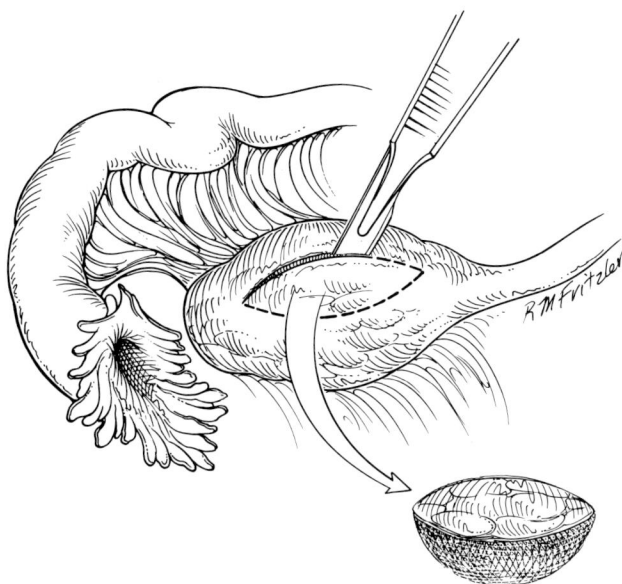

Figure 27–8
Wedge biopsy. A wedged incision is made into the ovarian tissue, avoiding the areas near the infundibulopelvic ligament and fimbria ovarica.

lopelvic ligament (Fig. 27–8). Microsurgical technique is employed. The ovary is best placed on a silicone mat. Handling of the cortex is avoided as much as is possible. The wedge is sent for frozen section.

Closure of the ovary is accomplished as detailed in the section on ovarian cystectomy.

References

1. Spanos WJ: Preoperative hormonal therapy of cystic adnexal masses. Am J Obstet Gynecol 1973; 116:551.
2. Steinkampf MP, Hammond KR, Blackwell RE: Hormonal treatment of functional ovarian cysts: A randomized, prospective study. Fertil Steril 1990; 54:775.
3. Laing FC, Van Dalsem F, Marks WM, et al.: Dermoid cysts of the ovary: Their ultrasonographic appearance. Obstet Gynecol 1981; 57:99.
4. Doss N, Forney JP, Vellios F, et al.: Covert bilaterality of mature ovarian teratomas. Obstet Gynecol 1977; 50(6):651.
5. INTERCEED (TC7) Barrier Adhesion Study Group: Prevention of postsurgical adhesions by INTERCEED (TC7), an absorbable adhesion barrier: A prospective randomized multicenter clinical study. Fertil Steril 1989; 51:933.
6. Diamond MP, Cunningham T, Linsky CB, et al.: Laparoscopic application of INTERCEED (TC7) in the pig. J Gynecol Surg 1989; 5:145.
7. Vercellini P, Vendola N, Bocciolone L, et al.: Reliability of the visual diagnosis of ovarian endometriosis. Fertil Steril 1991; 56:1198.
8. Nezhat C, Winter WK, Nezhat F: Laparoscopic removal of dermoid cysts. Obstet Gynecol 1989; 73:278.
9. Serafini P, Kerin J, Marrs R: Management of unexpected ovarian dermoid cyst during laparoscopy for oocyte pick-up. Fertil Steril 1987; 48:146.
10. Bower R, Adkins J: Surgical ovarian lesions in children. Am Surg 1981; 47:474.
11. Puylaert J, Rutger P, Lalisang R, et al.: A prospective study of ultrasonography in the diagnosis of appendicitis. N Engl J Med 1987; 317:666.
12. James D, Barber H, Graber E: Torsion of normal uterine adnexa in children. Obstet Gynecol 1970; 35:226.
13. Kleiner GJ, Solomon L, Greston WM, Lev-Gur M: Wedge resection in massive edema of the ovary. Am J Obstet Gynecol 1978; 132:107.
14. Davis AJ, Feins NM: Subsequent asynchronous torsion of normal adnexa in children. J Pediatr Surg 1990; 25:687.
15. Elkins T, Stock R: Recurrent massive edema of the ovary. South Med J 1982; 75:478.
16. Lupovitch A, Shanoski S: Massive edema of the ovary. Am J Obstet Gynecol 1974; 118:291.
17. Kalstone C, Jaffe R, Abell M: Massive edema of the ovary simulating fibroma. Obstet Gynecol 1969; 34:564.
18. Ballou J, Bryson J: The doing and undoing of surgical sterilization: A psychosocial profile of the tubal reimplantation patient. Psychiatry 1983; 46:161.
19. Grubb GS, Peterson HB: Luteal phase pregnancy and tubal sterilization. Obstet Gynecol 1985; 66:784.
20. Soderstrom RM: Sterilization failures and their causes. Am J Obstet Gynecol 1985; 152:395.
21. American College of Obstetricians and Gynecologists: Technical bulletin, No. 11, December 1987.
22. Ranney B, Abu-Ghazeleh S: The future function and fortune of ovarian tissue which is retained in vivo during hysterectomy. Am J Obstet Gynecol 1977; 128(6):626.
23. Grogan RH, Duncan CJ: Ovarian salvage in routine abdominal hysterectomy. Am J Obstet Gynecol 1955; 70(6):1277.

Surgery for Ovarian Cancer

28

David M. Gershenson
J. Taylor Wharton

Ovarian cancer, one of the most challenging diseases facing gynecologic oncologists, is currently the second most common malignancy of the female genital tract in the United States. According to the American Cancer Society, there were an estimated 21,000 new cases of ovarian cancer and 13,000 deaths from the disease in the United States in 1992.[1]

Surgery remains the cornerstone in the management of ovarian cancer. This chapter reviews current practices in surgical management, including primary surgery, secondary procedures, second-look laparotomy, and surgery for complications of ovarian cancer and its therapy. Although many of the concepts and principles apply equally to all three broad categories of ovarian cancer—epithelial, germ cell, and sex cord–stromal—whenever indicated, distinctions are discussed.

The material presented is based on the authors' personal experience at The University of Texas MD Anderson Cancer Center (UTMDACC) and a review of the literature. A comprehensive discussion of postoperative management is beyond the scope of this chapter, although reference is made when appropriate.

PRIMARY SURGERY

For a patient suspected of having ovarian cancer, primary surgery accomplishes the following goals:

1. Confirmation of the diagnosis of ovarian cancer

2. Precise determination of extent of disease—that is, surgical staging

3. Maximum cytoreductive surgery in patients with advanced disease

Preoperative Assessment and Preparation

Careful patient selection and preoperative evaluation are an important part of the surgical management of ovarian cancer. Current minimal studies for assessment of a patient with a possible or definite mass palpable on pelvic examination include a pelvic sonogram (by either the abdominal or the transvaginal approach) and a battery of serum tumor marker determinations. For patients younger than 45 years, recommended serum tumor marker screening includes CA-125, carcinoembryonic antigen, alpha-fetoprotein, and human chorionic gonadotropin. For older patients, only the first two are indicated. If results of these studies suggest a functional ovarian cyst, conservative management may be indicated. Such clinical management may vary from observation to percutaneous cyst aspiration to diagnostic laparoscopy, depending on several factors, including duration of the condition and characteristics of the cyst—size, consistency, presence and thickness of septae, and so forth. On the other hand, if findings suggest the possibility of a malignancy (e.g., elevated levels of tumor markers, sonographic characteristics com-

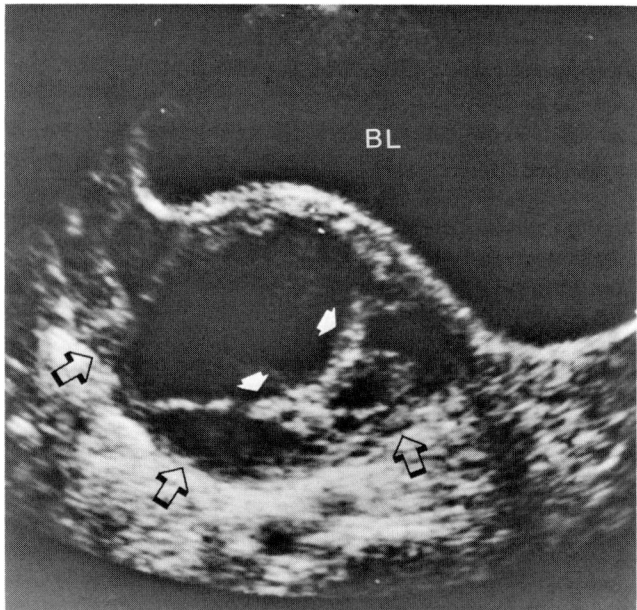

Figure 28–1
Longitudinal sonogram showing a 12-cm preponderantly cystic mass *(open arrows)* containing thick septations *(closed arrows)* representing a serous carcinoma of the ovary in a 57-year-old woman with ascites and pleural effusion. BL, bladder.

patible with malignancy) (Fig. 28–1), operative intervention is generally indicated. If, after careful evaluation, the physician recommends laparoscopy as an initial procedure, it is critical to ensure that expert frozen section analysis is available and that the surgeon and patient are prepared to proceed immediately to laparotomy if indicated. The report of Maiman and colleagues has emphasized the potential problems associated with the laparoscopic management of an ovarian mass subsequently found to be malignant.[2]

For a patient for whom surgery is indicated, the preoperative work-up should also include a chest radiograph. Chest radiography is useful for detecting the presence of pleural effusions or, rarely, pulmonary metastases. A barium enema study is valuable in some patients with a pelvic mass. This test, sometimes in conjunction with proctosigmoidoscopy, will help eliminate the possibility of such conditions as diverticular disease, cancer of the colon, inflammatory bowel disease, or involvement of the rectosigmoid colon by ovarian cancer (Fig. 28–2). It may be unnecessary for young patients or those with smaller, freely mobile masses.

Optional preoperative studies include intravenous pyelography, computed tomography (CT) or magnetic resonance imaging (MRI) of the abdomen and pelvis, upper gastrointestinal tract series, and bipedal lymphangiography. If CT is performed, intravenous pyelography is redundant. Neither CT nor MRI is reliable in detecting intraperitoneal disease smaller than 1–2 cm in diameter. However, both are superior to surgical exploration in the detection of parenchymal hepatic metastases (a rare initial finding).

Although CT or MRI will demonstrate enlarged retroperitoneal lymph nodes, if present, these modalities will not delineate the architecture of normal size nodes. Bipedal lymphangiography may be used to identify lymph node involvement, but it has not been used routinely.

Only if there is a strong suspicion of a nongynecologic primary cancer or hepatic metastases from ovarian cancer do the authors routinely obtain a preoperative CT or MRI study. Also, only if the patient has upper gastrointestinal tract symptomatology or a primary gastric cancer is suspected will they recommend endoscopy and upper gastrointestinal tract series.

Once the decision to proceed with surgery is made, the patient and her family are carefully counseled about the procedure, the indications, the possible complications, and the postoperative expectations.

In most, but not all, patients, a mechanical bowel preparation is indicated preoperatively because of the potential for intestinal surgery. Patients for whom intestinal resection is more likely include those with obvious advanced disease, those with a fixed pelvic mass, and those with obvious colonic involvement

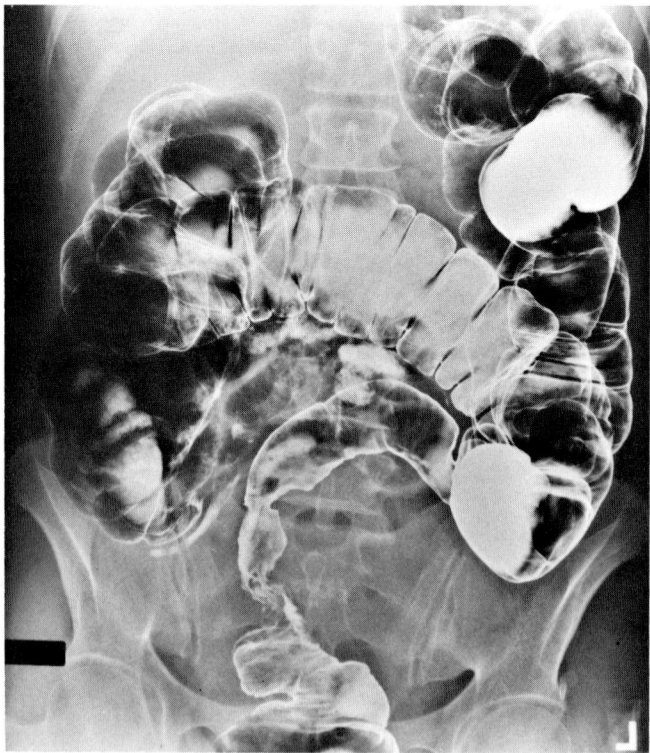

Figure 28–2
Preoperative air contrast barium enema showing constriction of the rectosigmoid colon related to tumor involvement from ovarian cancer.

or compromise found by barium enema study. The authors' standard bowel preparation at UTMDACC consists of a 1-day regimen of 3–4 liters of GoLYTELY (polyethylene glycol 3350 and electrolytes). Prophylactic antibiotics are also administered perioperatively. Some type of prophylaxis against thromboembolic phenomena—either subcutaneous heparin or a pneumatic compression device—is also recommended.

A central venous line is inserted preoperatively via either the subclavian or the antecubital route; this catheter can be used for hemodynamic monitoring in the perioperative period, for delivery of total parenteral nutrition postoperatively, or for subsequent chemotherapy administration.

Of course, an important component of preoperative preparation is assessment of the patient's general medical condition. Past history, medications, allergies, and previous medical problems should be carefully reviewed. Cardiopulmonary status is evaluated, especially in elderly patients or those with a pertinent medical history. If massive pleural effusions exist, preoperative thoracentesis may be indicated to allow for better pulmonary expansion. Occasionally, even insertion of a thoracostomy tube is prudent. Likewise, for patients with massive ascites causing excessive pain or pulmonary compromise, preoperative paracentesis may be indicated. In general, routine preoperative paracentesis is not recommended because of the risk of tumor implantation in the site and the small risk of intestinal puncture and contamination from bowel flora or bleeding.

Although initial surgery is the obvious choice for patients suspected of having an ovarian malignancy, there are exceptions. Patients who are poor surgical candidates because of massive reaccumulating effusions or severe medical problems may be best served by treatment with initial chemotherapy for two or three cycles prior to surgical intervention, performed after effusions have resolved or the medical condition has improved. In such cases, a presumptive diagnosis of ovarian cancer should be supported by a cytologic examination of the effusion or sample obtained by fine-needle aspiration. A decision to depart from standard management is often difficult and should be carefully made on an individual basis. The surgeon's previous experience is an important factor. Also, of course, the options and risks need to be thoroughly discussed with the patient and her family.

Surgical Staging

Stage of disease is determined by the extent of tumor at the time of initial diagnosis. The staging classification for ovarian cancer is a surgicopathologic system, last modified by the International Federation of Gynecology and Obstetrics (FIGO) in 1985[3] (Table 28–1).

Stage distribution varies, depending on the type of ovarian malignancy (Table 28–2). In addition, there is some variation from one study to another, especially with regard to sex cord–stromal tumors. As noted, epithelial tumors are most often diagnosed after spread to the upper abdomen and beyond, whereas sex cord–stromal tumors are rarely metastatic at diagnosis; germ cell tumors have intermediate metastatic potential, but the majority of these patients are still diagnosed with early-stage disease. Several studies have demonstrated a significant impact of FIGO stage on survival. Among the largest are the compiled series of Tobias and Griffiths and McGarrity and coworkers[4, 5] (Table 28–3).

The implication of the subdivisions of Stage I is that tumor rupture, surface excrescences, and the presence of ascites (Stage IC) are each unfavorable prognostic factors. It seems logical to theorize that penetration of the ovarian capsule will invariably lead to dissemination of tumor cells throughout the peritoneal cavity. Studies at the Mayo Clinic have indicated that these factors are associated with a worse prognosis than is Stage IA disease.[6] However, a number of studies have failed to show an adverse effect of tumor rupture or ascites on survival in patients with Stage I disease.[7–9] The findings of at least some of these studies are undoubtedly confounded by inadequate staging information and the effect of histologic grade. Dembo and associates reported that, for patients with Stage I epithelial ovarian cancer, histologic grade was the most powerful predictor of relapse.[10] In this large series, cyst rupture, capsular penetration, tumor size, histologic subtype, and bilaterality had no influence on survival.

The gynecologic literature is replete with inadequate staging information. Several reports (Table 28–4) have documented occult metastases in patients with apparent Stage I or II disease.[11–18] The problem of inadequate staging in ovarian cancer is illustrated by the collaborative study of Young and associates, in which 100 patients with apparent early disease (Stages IA–IIB) underwent a variety of restaging procedures upon referral to one of the member institutions.[18] Thirty-one patients were found to have more advanced disease than originally thought, and 23 of the 31 patients (74%) actually had Stage III disease. In 61% of patients found to have a more advanced disease stage, procedures other than a second laparotomy—that is, laparoscopy or lymphangiography—confirmed this evidence.

McGowan and associates reported that only 54% of 291 patients with ovarian cancer received proper staging procedures.[19] The most common examina-

Table 28–1

FIGO Staging for Primary Carcinoma of the Ovary

Stage	Description
I	Growth limited to the ovaries.
IA	Growth limited to one ovary; no ascites. No tumor on the external surface; capsule intact.
IB	Growth limited to both ovaries; no ascites. No tumor on the external surfaces; capsule intact.
IC	Tumor either Stage IA or IB but with tumor on surfaces of one or both ovaries; or with capsule ruptured; or with ascites present containing malignant cells or with positive peritoneal washings.
II	Growth involving one or both ovaries with pelvic extension.
IIA	Extension and/or metastases to the uterus and/or tubes.
IIB	Extension to other pelvic tissues.
IIC	Tumor either Stage IIA or IIB, but with tumor on surface of one or both ovaries; or with capsule(s) ruptured; or with ascites present containing malignant cells or with positive peritoneal washings.
III	Tumor involving one or both ovaries with peritoneal implants outside the pelvis and/or positive retroperitoneal or inguinal nodes. Superficial liver metastasis equals Stage III. Tumor is limited to the true pelvis but with histologically proven malignant extension to small bowel or omentum.
IIIA	Tumor grossly limited to the true pelvis with negative nodes but with histologically confirmed microscopic seeding of abdominal peritoneal surfaces.
IIIB	Tumor of one or both ovaries with histologically confirmed implants of abdominal peritoneal surfaces none exceeding 2 cm in diameter. Nodes are negative.
IIIC	Abdominal implants greater than 2 cm in diameter and/or positive retroperitoneal or inguinal nodes.
IV	Growth involving one or both ovaries, with distant metastases. If pleural effusion is present, there must be positive cytology to allot a case to Stage IV. Parenchymal liver metastasis equals Stage IV.

tions or procedures missed in incompletely evaluated cases included visualization and palpation of the undersurfaces of the diaphragm, biopsy of the pelvic peritoneum, observation and/or cytologic sampling of peritoneal fluid, and omental biopsy. Moreover, the completeness of the staging procedures varied, depending on the type of specialist performing the procedure: gynecologic oncologists, 97%; obstetrician-gynecologists, 53%; and general surgeons, 35%.

In a multicenter trial from the Netherlands, Trimbos and colleagues reported that surgical staging after one or two laparotomies was complete in only 53% of 86 patients.[20] The most frequently omitted staging steps were biopsy of the paracolic gutter, biopsy of the pelvic peritoneum, and sampling of the retroperitoneal lymph nodes. These investigators attributed the incompleteness of the staging procedures either to increased risk or difficulty of the procedure or to lack of knowledge of the sites at risk for metastases.

A major dilemma facing gynecologic oncologists is the referral of a patient with apparent Stage I epithelial carcinoma of the ovary who has had an incomplete staging procedure. We are in the midst of an evolution in which we are attempting to strictly define a subset of patients with early epithelial ovarian cancer who require no adjuvant therapy; inadequate staging information obviously escalates the difficulty in making a decision about the need for postoperative therapy in such patients. In addition to the study by Young and associates, other reports have addressed the rationale for a second laparotomy for patients referred after an initial incomplete surgical staging.[18, 21, 22]

An estimated three-fourths of patients referred to UTMDACC after having had primary surgery elsewhere for an apparent early-stage ovarian cancer have inadequate staging information. The authors make an effort to avoid repeat staging laparotomy whenever possible. For instance, if the probability of extraovarian disease is quite small based on known factors, if the patient requires adjuvant therapy regardless of any additional information, or if the

Table 28–2

Approximate Stage Distribution by Category of Ovarian Malignancy

	Percentage of Ovarian Malignancies*		
Stage	Epithelial	Germ Cell	Sex Cord–Stromal
I	15–25	50–70	85–100
II	15–20	5–15	0–5
III	40–50	25–35	0–10
IV	10–20	2–5	0–2

*Ranges reflect variation among reported series.

Table 28–3

Five-Year Survival Rates by Stage

	McGarrity et al.[5]		Tobias and Griffiths[4]	
Stage	No. of Patients	Five-Year Survival (%)	No. of Patients	Five-Year Survival (%)
IA	940	69.7	528	65
IB	227	63.9	130	52
IC	157	50.3	80	52
IIA	251	51.8	40	60
IIB	672	42.4	205	38
III	2074	13.3	539	5
IV	933	4.1	101	3

Table 28-4

Sites of Metastases in Patients with Apparent Stage I or II Epithelial Ovarian Cancer

	No. Patients with Metastasis at Site/Total No. Patients with Site Sampled				
Study	Peritoneal Cytology	Omentum	Diaphragm	Pelvic Nodes	Para-aortic Nodes
Knapp and Friedman, 1974		1/21		0/9	5/26
Musumeci et al., 1977				2/61	2/61
Creasman and Rutledge, 1971	1/10				
Keettel et al., 1974	16/44				
Rosenoff et al., 1975			7/16		
Piver et al., 1978	8/31	0/5	1/31		0/5
Chen and Lee, 1983				2/21	4/21
Young et al., 1983		6/57	2/58	1/11	6/52
Total	**25/85 (29.4%)**	**7/83 (8.4%)**	**10/105 (9.5%)**	**5/102 (4.9%)**	**17/165 (10.3%)**

findings of repeat laparotomy will not change the clinical management, no restaging laparotomy is recommended.

The emphasis on surgical staging has heightened our awareness of retroperitoneal nodal involvement associated with epithelial ovarian cancer. In 1974, Knapp and Friedman reported finding aortic nodal involvement with tumor in 19% of 26 patients with apparent Stage I ovarian cancer.[11] Since then, other studies have shown nodal involvement in over 50% of patients with epithelial ovarian cancer.[17,23,24]

Proper staging procedures should consist of the following:

1. Although a transverse abdominal incision is cosmetically superior, a vertical midline incision is preferable to provide adequate exposure for appropriate staging biopsies or resection of metastatic disease in the upper abdomen.

2. Ascites, if present, should be evacuated and submitted for cytologic analysis. If no peritoneal fluid is noted, cytologic washings of the pelvis, bilateral paracolic gutters, and subdiaphragmatic areas should be performed prior to manipulation of the intraperitoneal contents. Cytologic washings are obtained by instilling approximately 50–100 ml of normal saline into each area.

3. The entire peritoneal cavity and its structures should be carefully inspected and palpated in a systematic manner. The authors generally prefer to begin with the subphrenic spaces and move caudad, toward the pelvis. In particular, the subdiaphragmatic areas, hepatic capsule, omentum, colon, all peritoneal surfaces, the entire retroperitoneum, and small intestinal serosa and mesentery should be checked. If any suspicious areas are noted, they should be excised or sampled. During this process, one should be vigilant for non-gynecologic primary cancers.

4. The primary ovarian tumor and pelvis should be examined. Both ovaries should be carefully assessed for size, presence of obvious tumor involvement, capsular rupture, external excrescences, and adherence to surrounding structures. If the surgical findings are strongly suggestive of a benign ovarian mass in a young patient desirous of future childbearing, ovarian cystectomy may be indicated. Otherwise, a unilateral salpingo-oophorectomy should be performed and the specimen submitted for frozen section examination. If bilateral ovarian masses are present, the more suspicious side should be dealt with initially. If frozen section analysis reveals a malignant epithelial tumor, standard surgical therapy consists of hysterectomy and bilateral salpingo-oophorectomy. Exceptions to this rule—that is, conservative surgery—are discussed in the next section.

5. If disease seems to be limited—that is, confined to the ovary or localized to the pelvis—random staging biopsies of structures at risk should be performed. These sites include the omentum (either omentectomy or generous biopsy specimens from multiple areas) and the peritoneal surfaces of the following sites: bilateral paracolic gutters, cul-de-sac, lateral pelvic walls, vesicouterine reflection, and subdiaphragmatic areas. Any adhesions should be generously sampled. Some surgeons, including the authors, prefer cytologic analysis by saline lavage rather than scraping or biopsy of clinically normal subdiaphragmatic surfaces. Others prefer scraping the subdiaphragmatic surfaces with a wooden spatula or tongue depressor and making a cytologic smear. Still others perform biopsies using laparoscopic equipment. However, the advantage of one technique over another remains unclear and will require further study. In addition, no definitive studies demonstrate that total omentectomy or even infracolic omentectomy is more beneficial in terms of diagnostic accuracy or survival than generous sampling of the omentum in a patient without gross omental tumor.

6. If gross metastatic disease is present, it should be excised if feasible or at least sampled to document disease extent. The concept of cytoreductive surgery

and supporting evidence are discussed in a later section.

7. As noted earlier, the retroperitoneum has historically been the area of greatest neglect. The para-aortic and bilateral pelvic lymph node–bearing areas should be carefully palpated. Any suspicious nodes should be excised or sampled. If no suspicious nodes are detected, the authors generously sample these areas. There is no evidence at present that a complete para-aortic and/or pelvic lymphadenectomy is advantageous.

Conservative Surgery

Although the majority of ovarian malignancies occur in older women, for whom bilateral salpingo-oophorectomy and hysterectomy are standard treatment, a significant subset of patients are young and can be managed more conservatively. Conservative management is used in this discussion to denote surgery that preserves reproductive potential without compromising curability. With some exceptions, such a strategy may be applicable for women younger than 40 years old who wish to bear children.

When contemplating surgery on a young patient with a suspected ovarian malignancy, it is important to discuss with her all possible operative findings and procedures and the long-term implications of the various options. If the patient is a child, the parents need to clearly understand this information. Comprehensive preoperative counseling can be thwarted by any of a number of circumstances: the chaos that sometimes surrounds an emergency operation for acute abdominal pain; the surgeon's denial of the possibility of malignancy; or the surgeon's lack of understanding of the biology of the variants of ovarian cancer that may afflict young patients.

In most instances, young patients have their initial surgery performed outside major university hospitals or cancer centers. Common errors in surgical management include inadequate staging and unnecessary bilateral adnexectomy. In addition, some patients are mismanaged because of an error in the pathologic diagnosis of a rare ovarian neoplasm.

The ideal candidate for conservative surgical management is a young patient who has Stage IA disease. If, on initial inspection, the suspected cancer is confined to one ovary, unilateral salpingo-oophorectomy is appropriate. If the mass is thought to be benign, ovarian cystectomy may be preferable. The specimen should be sent for frozen section examination. If malignancy is diagnosed, appropriate staging biopsies should be performed, as discussed previously. If the contralateral ovary appears to be normal, the authors recommend that it be left undisturbed to avoid potential infertility caused by peritoneal adhesions or ovarian failure.

One should not rely too heavily on frozen section examination in making the decision to perform a hysterectomy and bilateral salpingo-oophorectomy. If the histologic diagnosis is in question, it is always preferable to wait for permanent section results for a young patient even if this requires a repeat laparotomy.

General criteria for conservative surgical management are listed in Table 28–5. Although strict criteria usually exclude patients whose tumors are bilateral, adherent, nonencapsulated, or ruptured and patients with ascites or positive cytologic washings, evidence suggests that such criteria can be liberalized, especially if adjuvant chemotherapy is used. There may be other exceptions to these guidelines, as to be discussed.

The advent of in vitro fertilization technology should also have an impact on intraoperative management. Convention has dictated that if a bilateral salpingo-oophorectomy is necessary, a hysterectomy should also be performed. However, current technology for donor oocyte transfer and hormonal support allows a woman without ovaries to sustain a normal intrauterine pregnancy. Similarly, if the uterus and one ovary are resected because of tumor involvement, current techniques allow retrieval of oocytes from the patient's remaining ovary, in vitro fertilization with sperm from her male partner, and implantation of the embryo into a surrogate's uterus. Therefore, traditional guidelines concerning surgical management of ovarian cancer may no longer be applicable in selected young patients.

Approximately 50–70% of malignant germ cell tumors are Stage I. As noted, except for dysgerminoma, in which the incidence of bilaterality is 10–15%, bilateral ovarian tumors are exceedingly rare. Such a finding almost always signifies advanced disease with metastatic spread from one ovary to the other or a mixed germ cell tumor with a dysgerminoma component. Benign cystic teratoma is associated with malignant germ cell tumors in 5–10% of

Table 28–5

Criteria for Conservative Surgical Management of Ovarian Cancer Patients

Young patient desirous of future childbearing
Patient and family consent and agreement to close follow-up
No evidence of dysgenetic gonads
Specific situations
    Any unilateral malignant germ cell tumor
    Any unilateral stromal tumor
    Any unilateral borderline tumor
    Stage IA invasive epithelial tumor

cases and may occur in one or both ovaries. Therefore, unilateral salpingo-oophorectomy, preserving the contralateral ovary and uterus, combined with surgical staging can be performed in most patients with these neoplasms, even many with advanced-stage disease. If the contralateral ovary is enlarged, most likely it represents a benign cystic teratoma that can be managed with an ovarian cystectomy only. With the exception of Stage IA pure dysgerminoma or Stage IA, Grade 1 immature teratoma, these patients require postoperative chemotherapy.

Most sex cord–stromal tumors are confined to the ovary. Stage I accounts for over 50% (in some series as high as 100%) of granulosa cell tumors. More than 90% of Sertoli-Leydig cell tumors are Stage IA. Bilaterality occurs in less than 5% of cases with either tumor type. Therefore, optimal surgical management of most patients with stromal tumors consists of unilateral adnexectomy combined with appropriate surgical staging. Because 5–15% of patients with granulosa cell tumors will develop endometrial cancer or hyperplasia, endometrial curettage should also be performed in any young patient whose uterus is preserved. For patients with metastatic disease or for selected patients with Stage I disease (e.g., poorly differentiated Sertoli-Leydig cell tumor or granulosa cell tumor with rupture), postoperative therapy may be indicated.

Approximately 10–15% of all ovarian neoplasms are of the borderline or low malignant potential classification. Although they were first described more than 60 years ago, only in the last few years have we begun to fully appreciate their biologic behavior. Approximately 33–60% of serous borderline tumors are limited to one ovary.[25] Extraovarian spread is noted in 16–18% of cases.[26] Approximately 80–90% of mucinous borderline tumors are confined to one ovary.[26] Both endometrioid and clear cell borderline tumors are almost always Stage I, and the vast majority are unilateral. For young patients with borderline tumors seemingly confined to one ovary, appropriate surgical management includes unilateral salpingo-oophorectomy with surgical staging. The use of ovarian cystectomy instead of unilateral adnexectomy has also been reported,[27, 28] although some patients treated in this manner will require repeat surgery for a recurrence of tumor in the same or opposite ovary. If bilateral borderline tumors are present, portions of one or both ovaries may be preserved with ovarian cystectomy, if feasible. Whatever the surgical approach, reported 5-year survival rates for patients with Stage I borderline tumors treated with surgery alone are 90% or better.[25, 26]

For patients with borderline tumors and peritoneal implants, the optimal management remains controversial. However, surgical excision is the mainstay of treatment. Even in the face of metastatic disease, a normal contralateral ovary may be preserved in young patients. However, the incidence of bilateral tumors is approximately 75% in patients with advanced-stage serous tumors.[29]

Invasive epithelial tumors account for approximately 70% of all ovarian malignancies. Despite the low overall survival rate associated with these tumors, selected young patients with Stage I disease can be treated conservatively. The major factors in addition to stage that influence the selection process are histologic grade and bilaterality. Serous tumors are bilateral in about 50% of cases. The incidence of bilaterality for mucinous tumors varies widely in reported series from as low as 5% to as high as 50% but probably is no greater than 10–20%. Approximately 30–50% of endometrioid and clear cell cancers are bilateral.

Within the Stage I category, histologic grade is the most powerful predictor of outcome.[10] Patients with well-differentiated or Grade 1 tumors have an excellent prognosis, with a 5-year survival rate of over 90%. On the other hand, the 5-year survival rates for patients with Grade 2 or 3 tumors are approximately 75–80% and 50–60%, respectively. If the tumor appears to be limited to one ovary, unilateral adnexectomy and surgical staging are appropriate for young patients. Surgery alone appears to be adequate treatment for patients with Stage I, Grade 1 disease.[10, 30] For patients with Grade 3 tumors, most experts recommend postoperative chemotherapy. The decision concerning Grade 2 tumors is more difficult, although the authors view them as having a biologic behavior more similar to that of Grade 3 tumors than that of Grade 1 tumors and, therefore, recommend postoperative chemotherapy.

Therefore, young patients with well-staged Stage I invasive epithelial tumors can be surgically managed with unilateral adnexectomy if only one ovary contains tumor. If postoperative therapy is deemed appropriate, a brief interval of chemotherapy will not disturb reproductive potential in the majority of patients.

Primary Cytoreductive Surgery

Cytoreductive or debulking surgery refers to a surgical procedure for which the goal is to reduce the amount of tumor as much as possible in a patient with metastatic ovarian cancer. Early studies suggested a relationship between the completeness of the surgery or the amount of residual tumor and survival.[26, 31, 32] Griffiths, in a landmark paper, demonstrated an inverse relationship between residual tumor diameter and survival; patients having residual disease less than 1.5 cm in diameter had a significantly improved survival compared with patients with bulky residual disease.[33] More recent reports subsequently confirmed these findings[34-36] (Table 28-6). As the philosophy about cytoreductive surgery has evolved over the last two decades, "optimal debulking" has come to denote minimal residual disease no greater than 1.5-2.0 cm in diameter; "suboptimal debulking" denotes bulky residual disease greater than 2.0 cm in diameter.

Cytoreductive surgery, of course, must be considered not in a vacuum but rather in the context of responsiveness of residual tumor to postoperative therapies. Both radiotherapy[33] and chemotherapy trials[37-39] have shown a higher response rate in patients with minimal residual disease. These observations are supported by basic studies that suggest that larger tumor masses have poorly perfused anoxic areas that are not accessible to cytotoxic agents. Furthermore, larger tumors may have a greater proportion of cells in the resting phase. These nonproliferating cells may be less sensitive to cytotoxic agents. Skipper espoused the "fractional cell kill hypothesis," stating that the ability of chemotherapeutic agents to eradicate cancer cells depends on both the dose of drug and the number of cells present.[40,41] A given dose of drug kills a constant fraction of cells with each exposure. However, certain factors such as cell repair mechanisms, tumor heterogeneity, the fraction of cells in G_0 phase, and the development of drug resistance serve to counteract this process. Goldie and Coldman[42] have shown that tumor cells have an intrinsic spontaneous mutation rate; larger tumors that go untreated for an extended period theoretically have a greater probability of containing cell populations resistant to anticancer agents. Therefore, even though patients with advanced ovarian cancer may undergo optimal debulking, the small residual tumor masses may still contain drug-resistant cells that preclude ultimate cure.

Several reports[34-36,43,44] have described the accomplishment of optimal cytoreductive surgery in a high percentage of patients, as high as 98% of those operated on by gynecologic oncologists.[44] The morbidity and mortality associated with cytoreductive surgery have also been analyzed.[36,43-46] These studies generally reflect an operative mortality rate of less than 2%, a mean operating time of 3-5 hours, and a mean blood loss of approximately 500-1500 ml. There is a wide range of postoperative complications, the most common of which are infection, hemorrhage (at times requiring re-exploration), prolonged ileus, and cardiopulmonary problems. The primary question concerning the efficacy of primary cytoreductive surgery is whether improved survival is related more to the biology of the tumor or to the skill and aggressiveness of the surgeon. In other words, are those tumors that can be debulked optimally also tumors that are less invasive, less infiltrative, and more indolent? Available studies do not suggest that this is the case.[34-36] All of these studies demonstrated that patients who required extensive surgery to achieve minimal residual disease and those who had minimal disease at the outset had similar survival rates. Unfortunately, there are no randomized studies to resolve important issues in this area. Moreover, prospects for such studies are not good because of several factors, including deeply established biases, the multiplicity of associated prognostic factors, and the highly individualized nature of each procedure. In the meantime, the efficacy of cytoreductive surgery remains controversial. Better information will ultimately be required to define its role.

In general, gynecologic oncologists are somewhat less than enthusiastic about the impact of aggressive cytoreductive surgery on survival because there has been little if any discernible improvement, despite the procedure's widespread application during the last decade. Perhaps this detectable reticence simply reflects a better appreciation of the virulence of ovarian cancer, the limitation of surgical debulking, and the recognition that the true hope for a dramatic improvement in cure rates for patients with advanced disease can only be realized through a systemic approach.

Exploration

The patient is placed in either the supine or semilithotomy or ski position, depending on the likeli-

Table 28-6

Survival by Residual Disease Following Cytoreduction

Study	No. of Patients	Optimal Cytoreduction Achieved	Median Survival (mo)	
			Optimal Cytoreduction	*Suboptimal Cytoreduction*
Griffiths[33]	102	72	28.6	11.0
Wharton and Herson[35]*	104	43	27.6	15.3
Hacker et al.[36]	47	66	22.0	6.0

*Not all patients operated on at authors' institution.
Modified from Hacker N, et al.: Ovarian cancer: More on cytoreduction. Contemp OB/Gyn 1983(November); 22:68.

hood of a rectosigmoid resection. A vertical midline incision is employed and extended cephalad as much as necessary. On entering the abdomen, the initial steps as outlined earlier under surgical staging are followed. After evacuation of ascites, if present, and inspection and palpation, the size of the primary tumors(s) and size and extent of metastatic deposits should be noted.

During this initial phase of the operation, the surgeon must make an assessment of the feasibility of cytoreductive surgery. In a typical patient with advanced disease, the omentum may be totally replaced by tumor and the pelvis may be filled with tumor, making it difficult or impossible for the surgeon to distinguish normal pelvic structures. Findings that may initially dissuade the surgeon from proceeding with aggressive tumor resection include extensive parenchymal hepatic involvement, massive diaphragmatic involvement, extensive infiltration of the small intestinal mesentery, and bulky nodal disease high in the para-aortic chain. On the other hand, even if minimal residual disease cannot be achieved, debulking of omental and pelvic masses may relieve production of ascites, reduce pressure on adjacent organs, and allow the patient increased comfort at least temporarily. Moreover, intestinal resection may still be indicated for relief of impending or true obstruction.

Omentectomy

If the omentum is largely or completely replaced by tumor, it is the authors' preference to perform an omentectomy prior to focusing on the pelvis. If the omental tumor is adherent to the parietal peritoneum of the anterior abdominal wall, the pelvic structures, or loops of small intestine, it should be dissected from these structures. Once the omentum is mobilized and lifted cephalad, a dissection plane is developed between it and the serosa of the transverse colon, extending the dissection laterally in both directions (Fig. 28–3). If the supracolic omentum is heavily involved with tumor and densely adherent to the transverse colon, it may also be necessary to establish a plane between the greater curvature of the stomach and the omentum by ligating the right and left gastroepiploic arteries and the individual gastric branches (Fig. 28–4). Occasionally, omental tumor may also involve the spleen or splenic hilum, necessitating splenectomy (see later discussion).

Resection of Pelvic Tumor

If there are any adhesions of small intestine or cecum to the pelvic structures, they should be lysed. A self-retaining retractor may then be inserted and the bowel packed for adequate exposure. If normal pelvic

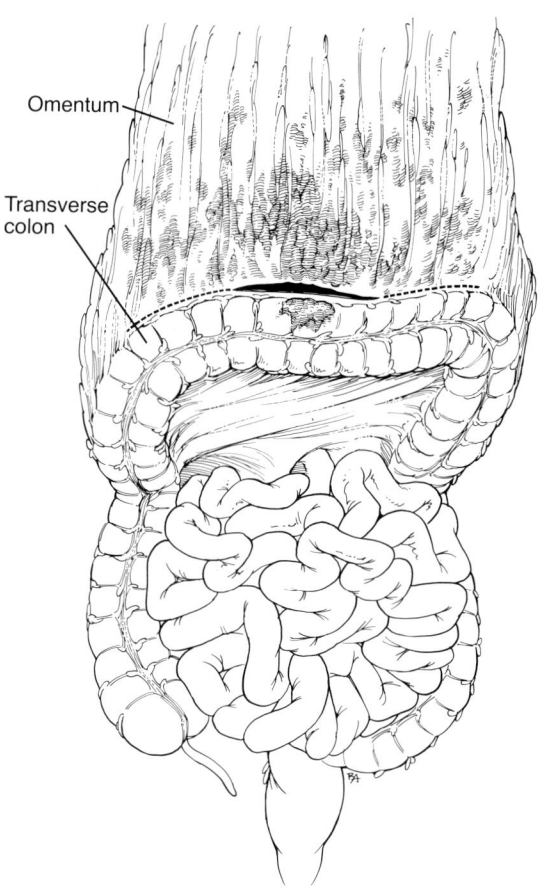

Figure 28–3
Omentectomy. Avascular dissection plane between omentum with tumor and transverse colon.

spaces and planes are obliterated by tumor, the retroperitoneal approach is preferred. The lateral pelvic peritoneum is incised, and the incision is carried cephalad and caudad (Fig. 28–5). As part of this maneuver, the round ligament is identified and ligated as well. The retroperitoneal space is thus entered and the structures—ureter, iliac vessels, and ovarian vessels—identified by using both sharp and blunt dissection (Fig. 28–6). A suction tip is a very nice instrument for dissecting areolar tissue planes if used properly. Next, the ovarian vessels are ligated. The identical procedure is performed on the opposite side of the pelvis, and the tumor mass(es) is mobilized medially.

If the ureters are densely adherent to the pelvic tumor, the surgeon may need to dissect them free, in some instances along the entire length of the pelvic portion of the ureter to the ureterovesical junction. In addition, the surgeon must establish a dissection plane between the sigmoid colon and the uterus and ovaries. This portion of the procedure may take considerable effort if this plane is obliterated by tumor. On the other hand, if the surgeon determines that such dissection is not feasible or that the wall of the colon is heavily infiltrated with tumor,

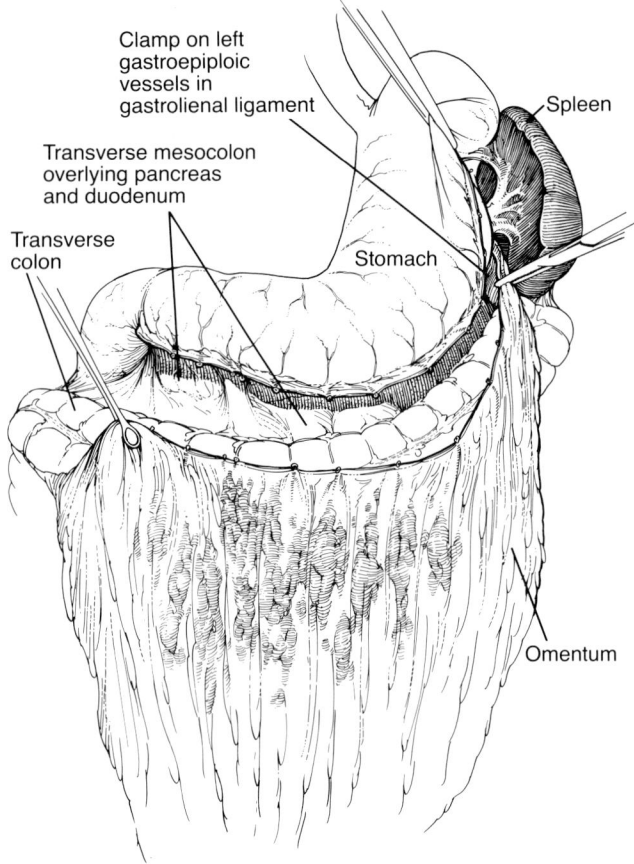

Figure 28–4
Omentectomy. Dissection of omentum with tumor from stomach with ligation of gastric branches.

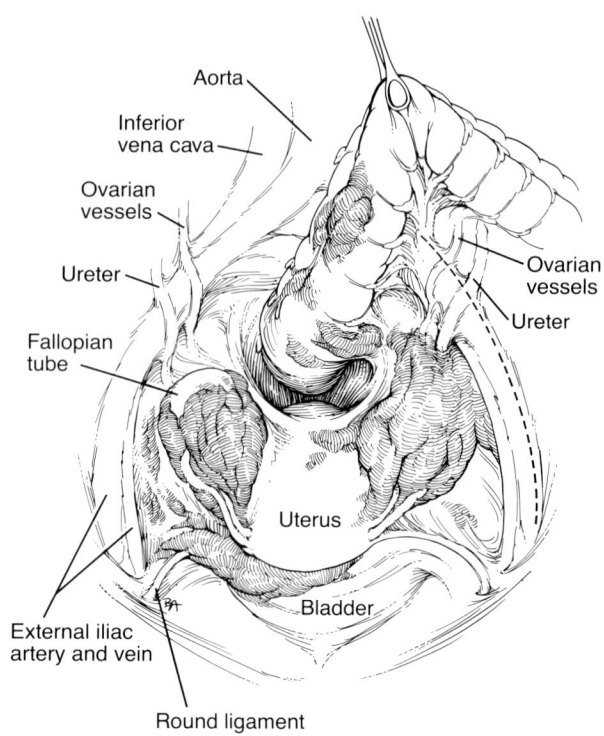

Figure 28–5
Pelvic dissection. Incision made in left lateral pelvic peritoneum to gain exposure to retroperitoneal space for identification of iliac vessels and ureter.

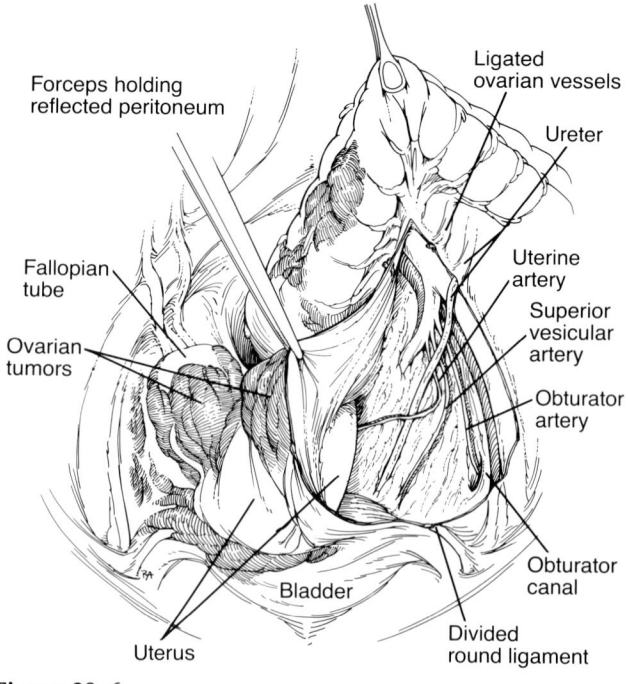

Figure 28–6
Pelvic dissection. Mobilization of ovarian tumor medially, with identification of iliac vessels and ureter.

resection of the rectosigmoid colon may be indicated (see later discussion). Resection of the pelvic portion of the colon allows the surgeon access to the avascular retrorectal space. The uterus is dissected from the bladder as well. It is extremely rare for ovarian cancer to involve the bladder mucosa at the time of primary surgery, but the vesicouterine peritoneum may be heavily infiltrated. In such cases, resection of this area may be necessary, occasionally in conjunction with a partial cystectomy (see later). Hysterectomy is then performed, the vagina is entered, and the mass is removed en bloc. In some instances, it may be necessary to ligate the uterine vessels at their origin rather than near the uterus if tumor is extensive in this area. Also, subtotal hysterectomy may be advisable if there is extensive unresectable tumor in the cul-de-sac.

Resection of Rectosigmoid Colon

As noted, a rectosigmoid resection may be performed in some patients during primary debulking, as it has been in approximately 10% of patients at UTMDACC (Fig. 28–7). The decision to perform this procedure depends on several factors, including the presence or absence of rectosigmoid obstruction, the amount of tumor infiltration of the lower colon and its contiguity with the ovarian tumor(s), and the probability that such a procedure will render the patient "opti-

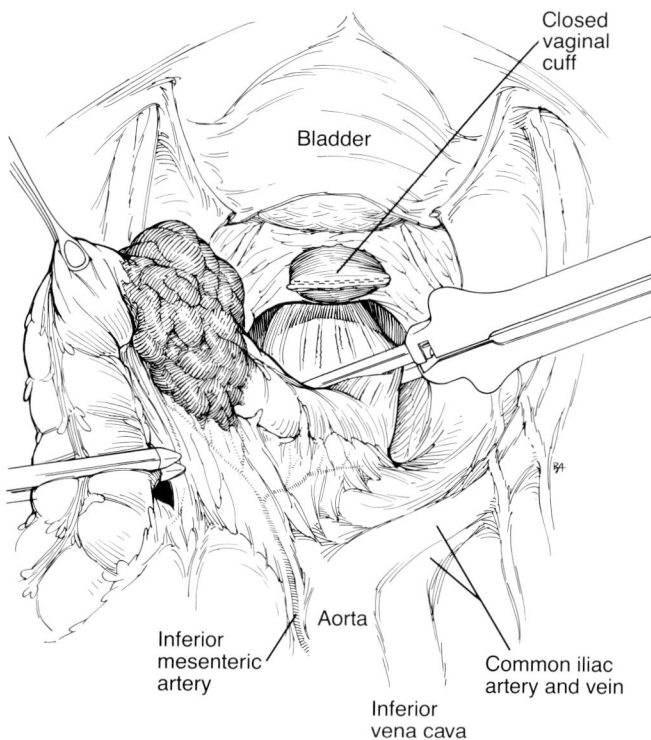

Figure 28–7
Resection of rectosigmoid colon involved with ovarian cancer. The uterus and bilateral ovarian tumors have already been removed. After mobilization and ligation of mesenteric vessels, transection is performed using GIA stapling devices (or roticulating stapler for distal transection) and remainder of mesentery is ligated. Usually, re-anastomosis using EEA stapler or suture technique can be accomplished.

mally debulked." Occasionally, a patient will limit the surgeon's intraoperative decision making ability by refusing to consent to possible colostomy. In the authors' experience, resection of the rectosigmoid colon can almost always be accomplished with consequent minimal residual disease in the pelvis; the limiting factor in achieving optimal cytoreduction, however, may be unresectable bulky residual tumor in the upper abdomen or retroperitoneum. In such cases, palliative resection in the absence of obstruction is not recommended. If a rectosigmoid colon resection is performed, in most cases the colon can be re-anastomosed using either a suture technique or the end-to-end anastomosis (EEA) stapler (see Chapter 21). For patients who undergo a re-anastomosis, a protective transverse loop colostomy may be indicated for those who have received pelvic radiotherapy, those with unprepared colon, or those whose anastomosis is judged to be suboptimal. Occasionally, a colostomy with a Hartmann pouch is necessary.

In 1984, Berek and colleagues reported their experience with 35 patients who underwent a rectosigmoid resection for ovarian cancer, 22 during primary debulking and 13 at secondary debulking.[47] Twenty-four patients underwent a re-anastomosis, and 11 had a colostomy without re-anastomosis. Seventy-five per cent of patients who underwent a re-anastomosis did not require a protective colostomy. Optimal cytoreduction (residual tumor < 1.5 cm in diameter) was accomplished in 94% of patients undergoing primary surgery and in 57% undergoing secondary surgery. Although major morbidity occurred in seven patients (20%), it was temporary in all except one, who developed an anastomotic stricture. There were no postoperative anastomotic leaks or pelvic abscesses.

In one report, Soper and associates described 40 women who underwent rectosigmoid colon resection during cytoreductive surgery, 21 (53%) as part of a primary procedure and 19 (47%) as part of a secondary procedure.[48] Residual disease was less than 1 cm in 54% of patients. A permanent colostomy was avoided in 78% of patients. Twenty-five per cent of patients experienced major morbidity, including one patient who developed an anastomotic dehiscence and pelvic abscess requiring a colostomy. One patient (3%) died in the immediate postoperative period. Despite aggressive surgical resection and postoperative therapy, the median survival for the entire group was only 14.5 months.

Small Intestinal Resection

Although the small intestine is a common site of metastasis, both to the serosa and the mesentery, extensive tumor involvement is an uncommon finding at primary surgery. If the small intestine is extensively involved with tumor, it is usually in the terminal ileum. Occasionally, small intestinal obstruction, either partial or complete, is present at diagnosis. As noted earlier, complete surgical staging includes careful examination of the entire length of the small intestine from the ligament of Treitz to the cecum. If, on exploration, loops of small intestine are adherent to the pelvic tumor, to omental tumor, or to other loops of intestine, these adhesions should be lysed. Indications for small intestinal resection include obstruction or impending obstruction by tumor and a nonobstructing extensive lesion of the small intestine for which resection would result in minimal residual disease.

The technique for small intestinal resection is discussed in Chapter 21. If the lesion involves the very terminal portion of the ileum, an ileocolectomy with resection of the cecum and portion of ascending colon adjacent to the small intestine may be necessary. Care should be taken to avoid the presence of tumor at the points of re-anastomosis. The re-anastomosis may be performed using either the suture or the stapling technique.

In the authors' experience, small intestinal resection is indicated in approximately 5–10% of primary operations for ovarian cancer. In other reported series, small intestinal resection has been performed in 2–8% of patients at primary surgery.[36, 43, 44]

Resection of the Urinary Tract

Indications for ureteral resection or partial cystectomy are uncommon during cytoreductive surgery. If ureteral obstruction is noted preoperatively, it is almost always a result of ureteral compression rather than tumor infiltration. Although adherence of the ureter(s) to masses of ovarian cancer is not an unusual finding, the surgeon can almost always separate the ureter from the tumor using sharp dissection. If the distal ureter is resected as part of cytoreductive surgery, it can usually be reimplanted into the bladder (see Chapter 22). More commonly, the ureter may be injured during the course of debulking surgery. Depending on the site of injury, a primary re-anastomosis, transureteroureterostomy, or ureteroneocystostomy may be indicated (see Chapter 22). In a report by Berek and associates, 16 of 848 patients (2%) underwent partial ureteral resection.[49] Five patients had transureteroureterostomy, two had re-anastomosis, and four had urinary diversion. Twelve of the operations were part of primary cytoreductive surgery, and four were part of secondary surgery. Nine of these 16 patients had evidence of ureteral obstruction on preoperative intravenous pyelograms.

On the other hand, tumor involvement of the peritoneum overlying the urinary bladder is not an uncommon finding during primary cytoreductive surgery. Occasionally, a partial cystectomy may be necessary to achieve optimal cytoreduction. In the series of Berek and colleagues, eight patients had a partial cystectomy for advanced ovarian cancer.[49] Reconstruction necessitated ureteral reimplantation in two patients and an ileal conduit in one patient. If a partial cystotomy is indicated, the authors prefer a simple closure with two layers of chromic catgut suture—the inner layer as a continuous running suture and the outer layer as interrupted sutures.

In the authors' experience, it is exceedingly rare to find involvement of the bladder mucosa with ovarian cancer at initial diagnosis. Such patients usually complain of hematuria in association with obvious massive disease. The definitive diagnosis can easily be made by preoperative cystoscopy.

Splenectomy

Splenectomy is occasionally indicated during primary cytoreductive surgery. Various series report the incidence of splenectomy during primary cytoreductive surgery in 5–11% of cases of advanced ovarian cancer.[50–52] In addition, the indications for splenectomy and the procedure itself have been described in case

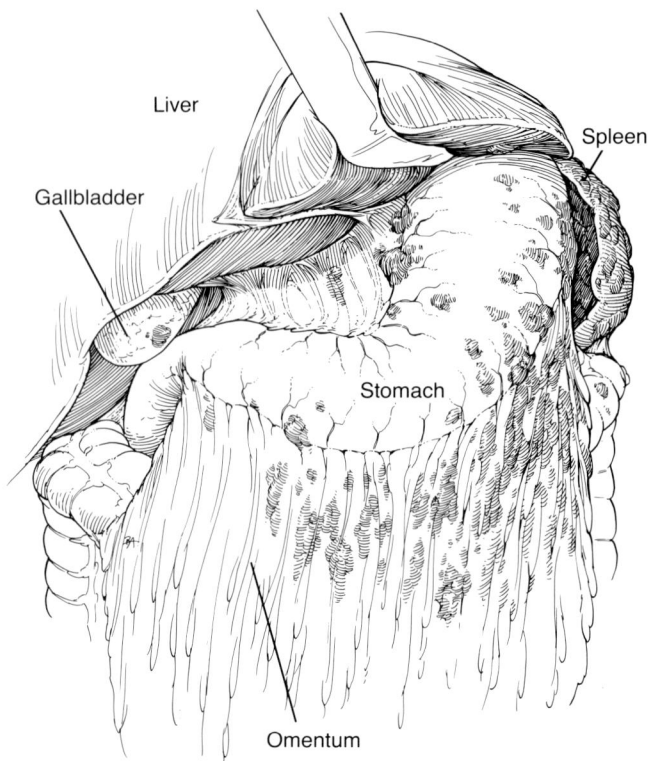

Figure 28–8
Involvement of splenic capsule and hilum with ovarian cancer.

reports.[53, 54] Most commonly, the hilum of the spleen is involved with ovarian cancer in association with extensive omental involvement (Fig. 28–8). Rarely, isolated splenic capsular involvement or even splenic parenchymal involvement may be found. In addition to tumor debulking, splenectomy may also be indicated during cytoreductive surgery because of a traction injury with avulsion of the splenic capsule during omentectomy or mobilization of the splenic flexure of the colon in association with descending colostomy or re-anastomosis after rectosigmoid colon resection. If a splenic capsular avulsion injury does occur in the absence of tumor involvement, splenorrhaphy may be indicated before resorting to splenectomy.

In the series of Sonnendecker and coworkers, five patients underwent splenectomy because of metastatic disease involving the spleen; one had parenchymal involvement, and one patient required splenectomy for capsular avulsion injury.[52] In a review of the UTMDACC Gynecology Service experience with splenectomy, Morris and associates reported on 23 patients for whom the procedure was performed as part of cytoreductive surgery for advanced ovarian cancer.[55] Splenectomy was planned preoperatively in only three of these patients. Seven patients had parenchymal involvement by tumor, eleven had capsular disease, and five had no pathologic involvement by tumor.

The methods of performing splenectomy during

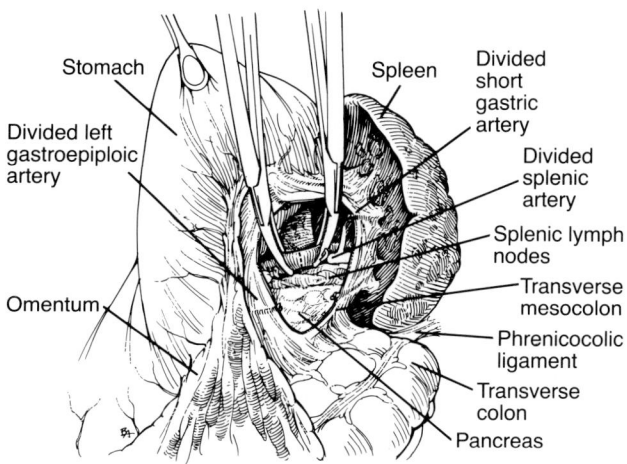

Figure 28–9
Splenectomy. Transection of splenic artery and vein along the superior border of the pancreas after access is gained to lesser sac with transection of gastrosplenic ligament.

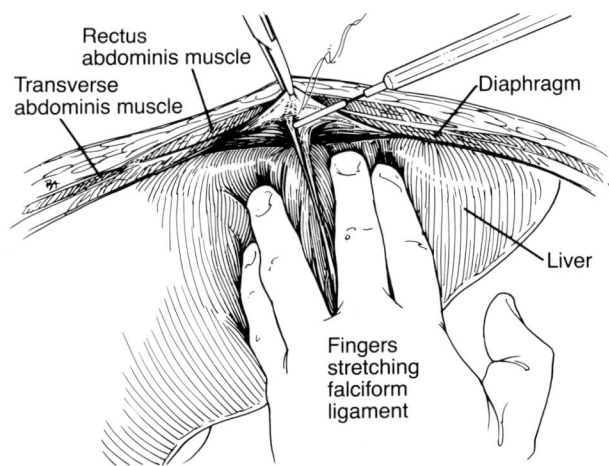

Figure 28–10
Gaining access to subdiaphragmatic tumor implants by transection of falciform ligament with cautery and mobilization of liver.

cytoreductive surgery may vary depending on the circumstances. Under controlled conditions (no uncontrolled hemorrhage), the surgeon may prefer to incise the gastrosplenic ligament, gain access to the lesser sac, and identify and ligate the splenic vessels as they run along the superior border of the pancreas (Fig. 28–9). The spleen can then be mobilized by transecting its attachments to the colon, the left kidney, and the diaphragm. If hemorrhage is occurring or if access to the lesser sac is limited by the distribution of tumor, the surgeon may prefer to first mobilize the spleen by dividing its peritoneal attachments while compressing the splenic vessels and then ligate the splenic vessels employing a posterior approach. In this technique, the spleen is rotated anteriorly and medially.

Complications associated with splenectomy include hemorrhage, infection, thromboembolic phenomena, left-sided atelectasis or pneumonia, injury to the tail of the pancreas (with resultant pancreatic pseudocyst), and injury to the stomach (with resultant gastric fistula). Because of the risk of severe infection following splenectomy, the patient should receive perioperative antibiotic coverage and postoperatively should be vaccinated with polyvalent pneumococcal vaccine. The authors also prefer to insert a drain in the splenic bed postoperatively to diagnose early postoperative hemorrhage and to reduce the infection rate.

Resection of Diaphragmatic Tumor

Several reports have described experience with resection of diaphragmatic metastatic deposits in patients with advanced ovarian cancer.[56–59] To gain access to the diaphragmatic surfaces, the abdominal incision is extended to just below the xiphoid process and the liver is mobilized by transecting the entire falciform ligament (Fig. 28–10) and the coronary and triangular ligaments. After it is adequately exposed, the diaphragmatic tumor may be resected by stripping the peritoneum from the diaphragmatic muscle using sharp dissection with either Metzenbaum's scissors or electrocautery (Fig. 28–11). Alternative techniques of debulking in this area are discussed in a later section. If the pleural cavity is entered, the anesthesiologist should be notified. Defects in the diaphragm may be closed with interrupted sutures. If a large defect cannot be closed primarily or can be closed only under tension, the defect may be closed using synthetic material such as Marlex mesh or Dexon mesh. If the pleural cavity is entered, a thoracostomy tube should be placed.

Possible complications associated with resection of diaphragmatic tumor include pneumothorax; hemorrhage; infection; and injury to such structures as the lung, the vena cava, or the phrenic nerves.

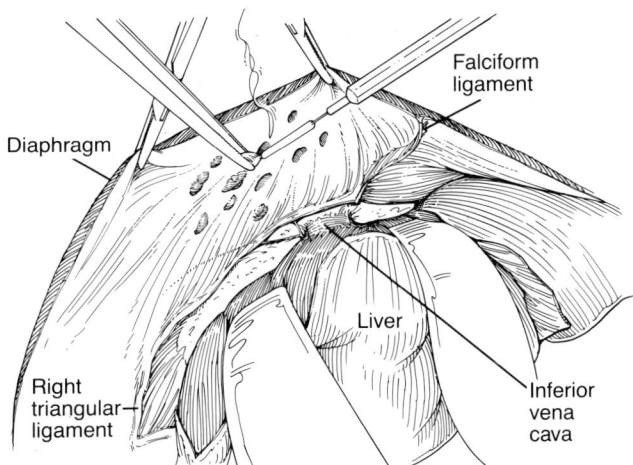

Figure 28–11
Ablation of subdiaphragmatic tumor implants with cautery after mobilization of liver. Sharp dissection or the Cavitron Ultrasonic Surgical Aspirator (CUSA) may also be used for the same purpose.

Whether aggressive resection of diaphragmatic metastases with associated potential complications is justified is unclear. Montz and associates reported that 13 of 14 patients with diaphragmatic tumor could be optimally debulked.[57] The size of resected specimens ranged from 12 × 7 cm to 17 × 11 cm. Kapnick and coworkers found that tumors that penetrated the entire thickness of the diaphragm to involve the pleura were 5.0 cm or greater in diameter.[59] Patients with tumors that penetrated the diaphragm had a median survival time of 8 months compared with a median survival time of 26 months for those patients without full-thickness diaphragmatic penetration by the tumor. Therefore, the assessment of the benefit of this procedure must await further studies.

Resection of Retroperitoneal Lymph Nodes

The benefit of radical resection of extensive retroperitoneal lymph node metastases also remains unclear. In the reports of Wu and colleagues and Burghardt and associates, the role of pelvic and para-aortic lymphadenectomy at initial surgery for ovarian cancer is discussed, but there is no particular discussion of debulking of grossly enlarged retroperitoneal nodes.[23, 24] For patients with malignant germ cell tumors, especially dysgerminoma, the advantages of debulking metastatic retroperitoneal nodes are even less apparent, because these tumors are generally much more sensitive to chemotherapy than are other ovarian tumors.

Until further information becomes available, it is probably reasonable to consider debulking enlarged retroperitoneal nodes if peritoneal metastases can be optimally cytoreduced, if there is no fixation to blood vessels, and if the surgeon believes that the procedure can be successfully accomplished without undue risk. Newer techniques for such debulking are discussed in the next section.

New Techniques for Cytoreductive Surgery

In the last few years, several reports described innovative techniques of debulking—the argon beam coagulator, the Cavitron Ultrasonic Surgical Aspirator (CUSA), and various types of laser therapy.

The argon beam coagulator is a new electrosurgical device that conducts current to tissue in a beam of inert argon gas. Brand and Pearlman reported the use of the argon beam coagulator for debulking in seven patients with advanced ovarian cancer.[60] Areas treated using the device included the diaphragm, stomach, duodenum, small intestine, colon, liver capsule, peritoneum, bladder and ureters, vaginal apex and parametrium, iliac vessels, and abdominal wall. Four of the patients had no gross residual tumor, and three had residual masses of no greater than 2–3 mm in diameter.

There have been several reports of the use of the CUSA for cytoreductive surgery.[61–65] The CUSA combines tissue fragmentation, irrigation, and aspiration while dissecting tumor from blood vessels without injuring them (Fig. 28–12). Adelson and colleagues described cytoreduction of tumors to less than 0.5 cm in 9 of 10 patients.[61] The authors particularly noted that intestinal resections were avoided because of the use of the CUSA. Deppe and coworkers reported on 11 patients who underwent optimal debulking using the CUSA.[62] In other reports, the same authors have described the utility of the CUSA in debulking diaphragmatic metastases[63, 64] and retroperitoneal lymph nodes.[65] In the latter report, the authors were able to optimally resect extensive para-aortic and pelvic lymph node masses in five of six patients with advanced ovarian cancer. Two patients sustained lacerations of the inferior vena cava during the procedure.

Use of the neodymium-yttrium-aluminum-garnet (Nd:YAG) laser for the resection of intra-abdominal tumors has been reported.[66] Other reports of laser therapy for metastatic deposits of ovarian cancer will undoubtedly follow during the next few years.

The benefit of any of these new techniques for cytoreductive surgery remains unproved. Further studies will be necessary to elucidate their proper role.

SECONDARY SURGERY

Second-Look Laparotomy

Second-look laparotomy for evaluation of disease status following treatment for cancer of the colon was initially proposed by Wangensteen and associates in 1948.[67] Since 1960, second-look laparotomy has been employed extensively in the management of ovarian cancer at UTMDACC. The procedure has gained popularity over the last two decades as more ovarian cancer patients have been treated with chemotherapy and fewer have received radiotherapy. Within the last 5 years or so, however, there has been increasing skepticism about the benefits of this procedure.

Definition

Interpretation of reports of experience with second-look laparotomy has been complicated by the fact that no standard definition of the procedure exists. Most experts agree that the term "second-look laparotomy" should be restricted to a laparotomy performed on a patient with no clinical evidence of persistent tumor for the purpose of determining disease status after a planned interval of treatment with chemotherapy. The term should not be applied

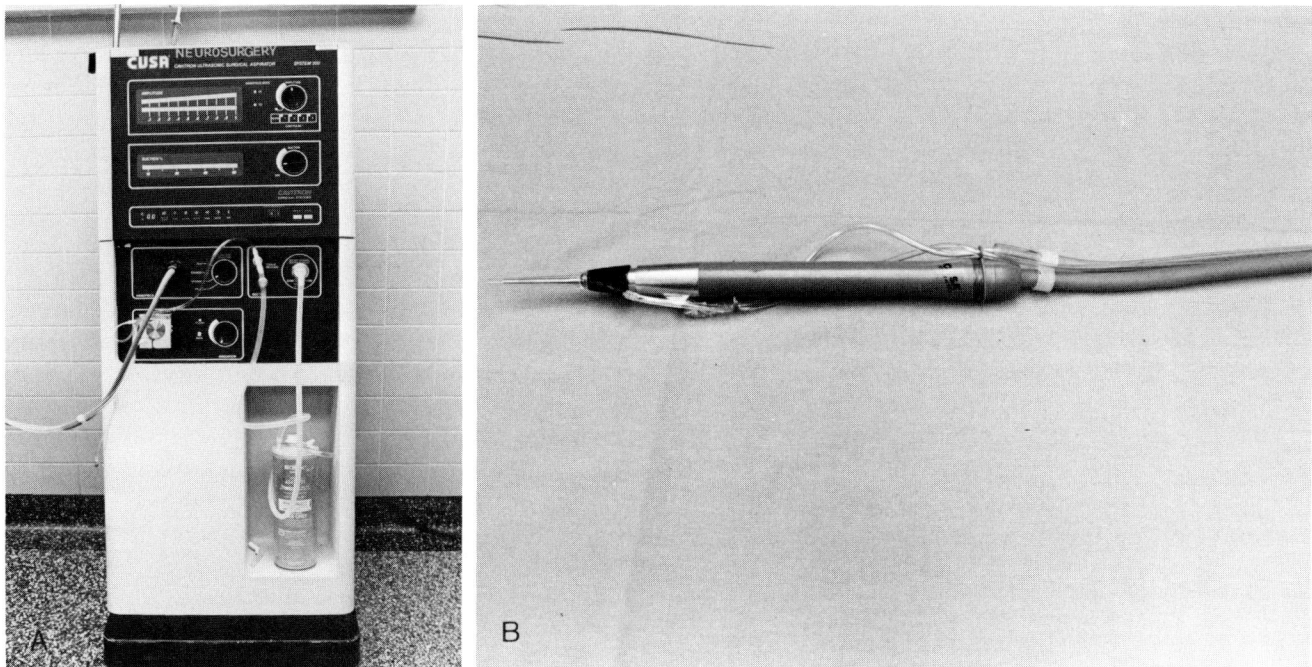

Figure 28–12
A, Cavitron Ultrasonic Surgical Aspirator (CUSA) console. *B*, Handpiece of CUSA.

to a surgical procedure performed in patients with clinical evidence of persistent or progressive disease for the primary purpose of debulking or treatment of complications. With current treatment regimens, at least 50–60% of patients with advanced ovarian cancer are candidates for second-look laparotomy.

Preoperative Assessment and Technique

Standard preoperative assessment of ovarian cancer patients at completion of the planned interval of chemotherapy includes physical examination, determination of serum tumor marker levels, and CT of the abdomen and pelvis. If these studies clearly document persistent ovarian cancer, then, with rare exceptions, second-look laparotomy is not performed. The operative technique of second-look laparotomy has been well described. It is essentially identical to a staging laparotomy, as discussed previously. An adequate vertical midline abdominal incision is made. Upon entering the abdomen, cytologic washings from the pelvis, bilateral paracolic gutters, and subdiaphragmatic areas are obtained, and the entire contents of the peritoneal cavity are inspected and palpated. If obvious macroscopic tumor is present, the procedure is usually limited. However, the extent of disease should be carefully determined, and a few biopsies should be taken for documentation of persistent disease (frozen section as well as permanent section). If no obvious macroscopic disease is noted, random biopsy specimens are routinely taken from the peritoneal surfaces, including the cul-de-sac, vesicouterine reflection, bilateral pelvic walls, bilateral paracolic gutters, and surfaces of the diaphragm. Omental biopsies and biopsies of the retroperitoneal lymph nodes are also performed. In the process of performing these biopsies, lysis of adhesions is not uncommon. Sites of previously documented tumor and adhesions should be carefully evaluated and generously sampled. An adequate procedure consists of a minimum of 20–30 biopsy specimens (Fig. 28–13).

Complications

Second-look laparotomy is a major operative procedure, although it is a very safe one. The average duration of the operation is 2 hours, and the usual hospital stay is 7 days. Operative mortality is a rarity. Operative morbidity is low, and most complications are minor. The most common complications include wound infection and prolonged ileus. Other reported complications include urinary tract infection, small intestinal obstruction, pneumothorax, intestinal injury, hemorrhage, pneumonia, and thromboembolic phenomena.[68–73]

Results

Findings at second-look laparotomy are classified as negative (grossly and pathologically negative), microscopically positive (grossly negative, pathologically positive), and macroscopically positive (grossly and pathologically positive). The clinical variables most

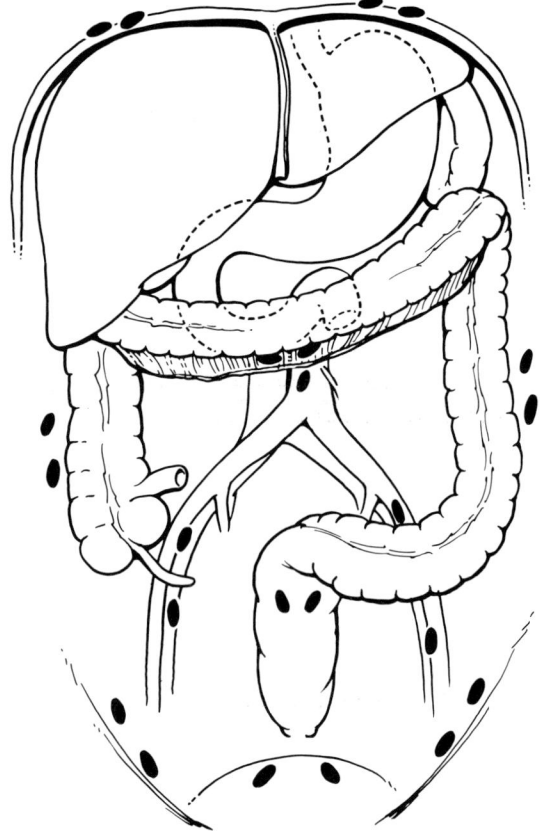

Figure 28–13
Random biopsy sites of peritoneum, residual omentum, and retroperitoneal nodes in standard second-look procedure.

Findings in approximately 50% of patients with advanced ovarian cancer (and a smaller percentage of those with early-stage disease) will be macroscopically positive at second-look laparotomy. Such patients, with the exception of those with low-grade tumors, have a very poor prognosis; more than 80% will eventually develop progressive disease and die. With rare exceptions, they are candidates for experimental therapies. The issue of cytoreductive surgery in this setting is discussed in a following section.

Approximately 20% of patients with advanced ovarian cancer who undergo second-look laparotomy will have microscopically positive findings. In 1985, Copeland and associates reported the experience at UTMDACC with 50 patients with advanced ovarian cancer who had microscopically positive findings.[80] The 2-year and 5-year actuarial survival rates of these patients were 81% and 70%, respectively—not statistically different from those achieved in patients with negative second-look findings.[81] However, most of the patients with microscopic disease received chemotherapy after second-look surgery, whereas those with negative findings did not. Moreover, the microscopic disease group contained a higher percentage of patients with low-grade tumors. After these studies were reported, a detailed pathologic analysis of the microscopic disease group revealed that in several cases, benign müllerian rests were misinterpreted as representing persistent tumor.[82] Another updated analysis of these patients revealed that when Grade 1 and borderline tumors were excluded, 58% of microscopic disease patients had recurrences.[83] Treatment approaches currently under study for microscopically positive disease include abdominopelvic radiotherapy, intraperitoneal chemotherapy, and radioisotope therapy.

Negative second-look laparotomy findings are noted in approximately 30% of patients with advanced ovarian cancer undergoing this procedure. At UTMDACC, the authors initially found a recurrence rate of 24% in 85 patients with advanced ovarian cancer who had negative second-look results.[81] An updated analysis revealed a recurrence rate of 44% in patients with Grades 2 and 3 disease.[83] Studies from other large centers have noted similar

consistently associated with findings at second-look laparotomy and survival afterward are histologic grade, amount of residual disease, and FIGO stage.[69–72, 74–79] Patients with low-grade tumors, minimal residual disease, and early-stage disease have a greater probability of having negative findings at second-look laparotomy than do those with high-grade tumors, bulky residual disease, or advanced-stage disease (Table 28–7). Other variables found to correlate with second-look findings and subsequent survival in some of these studies are histologic type, type of chemotherapy, amount of disease found at the initial surgery, age, performance status, and peritoneal cytology status.

Table 28–7

Per Cent Negative Findings at Second-Look Laparotomy

By Stage (1034 Patients)		By Histologic Grade (556 Patients)		By Residual Disease at Initial Surgery (753 Patients)	
Stage	% Negative	Grade	% Negative	Amount of Residual Disease	% Negative
I	80	1	61	None	77
II	68	2	50	Optimal*	45
III, IV	33	3	41	Suboptimal*	25

*Definition varies in original reports.
Modified from Rubin SC: The value of second-look laparotomy in ovarian cancer. Oncology 1987(October); 1:45. S Karger AG, Basel.

recurrence rates.[72, 75, 76, 84-87] The recurrence rates of 30–50% in patients with negative second-look findings after treatment for advanced ovarian cancer have prompted initiation of clinical trials evaluating a variety of therapies to follow negative second-look laparotomy. These treatments include external radiotherapy, intraperitoneal chemotherapy, and radioisotope therapy. It will probably be another 5 years, however, before results of prospective trials become available.

There is limited information in the literature regarding second-look laparotomy in patients with malignant germ cell tumors and virtually no meaningful information about patients with sex cord–stromal tumors. In a review of the experience with second-look laparotomy in patients with malignant germ cell tumors at UTMDACC, findings were negative in 52 of 53 such patients.[88] One patient with negative findings subsequently experienced a relapse and died. Thirteen patients had biopsy-proven evidence of mature teratoma—so-called chemotherapeutic retroconversion—at second-look laparotomy; treatment was discontinued in all patients, and none has developed a recurrence. It currently seems appropriate to limit the use of second-look laparotomy in this patient population as much as possible. For those patients with initially detectable levels of serum tumor markers, especially those with early-stage disease, the procedure is not recommended. Some patients with advanced disease, particularly those with initially undetectable serum tumor markers, continue to undergo second-look laparotomy. Nevertheless, as better therapies are developed and refined, the procedure will inevitably become obsolete except in unusual situations.

Alternatives

A number of alternatives to second-look laparotomy have been investigated. Laparoscopy has been evaluated as a substitute. With the availability of improved equipment, we may witness a revitalization of interest in this procedure for cancer patients. Approximately 30–50% of patients with ovarian cancer undergoing laparoscopy after chemotherapy will have positive findings,[89-92] thus avoiding the need for laparotomy. However, second-look laparoscopy is associated with several potential problems:

1. Several areas, including the bowel mesentery, the retroperitoneum, and areas obscured by adhesions are not accessible with this procedure.
2. If both laparoscopy and laparotomy are performed, total operating time may be significantly longer.
3. Ten to twenty per cent of patients develop complications, including hematomas and intestinal perforation.

The complication rate with the "open" laparoscopy technique is probably lower. With this technique, the surgeon makes a small incision through the abdominal wall layers into the peritoneal cavity and then inserts the scope. A pursestring suture is placed around the incision to avoid rapid escape of carbon dioxide, resulting in the loss of the pneumoperitoneum. Such a maneuver is generally associated with a lower incidence of intestinal perforation. If second-look laparoscopy is employed, it should be recognized that the false-negative rate is approximately 35%. Therefore, a negative laparoscopy should be followed by laparotomy.

CT has also been evaluated as a substitute for second-look laparotomy, but available information confirms the fact that tumor implants smaller than 2 cm in diameter are not reliably imaged.[93-99] Therefore, a negative CT scan does not obviate the need for second-look laparotomy. However, a positive study may avoid second-look laparotomy in approximately 20% of patients. Positive CT studies should always be confirmed with fine-needle aspiration. Whether MRI will prove to be superior to CT in defining persistent ovarian cancer remains unknown, although preliminary experience suggests that it will not.

The obvious substitute for second-look laparotomy is a reliable serum tumor marker. A negative CA-125 level at completion of chemotherapy, however, does not reliably predict lack of persistent disease. Second-look laparotomy has been negative in only 40–50% of patients with normal CA-125 levels.[100-102] Therefore, a negative CA-125 level is not a substitute for second-look laparotomy. Patsner and associates[102] reported that size of residual disease at second-look laparotomy did not correlate well with the serum level of CA-125. A positive CA-125 level, however, reliably predicts disease persistence and avoids a surgical procedure. Eventually, a battery of serum tumor markers or a more reliable single marker will most probably replace second-look laparotomy.

Therefore, despite its shortcomings, second-look laparotomy remains the most reliable method for detection of persistent cancer. Theoretically, negative findings allow the clinician to stop potentially toxic therapy, and positive findings prevent premature cessation of therapy. On the other hand, for one of several reasons (most commonly patient refusal or physician preference), many patients do not undergo the procedure. Currently, the most widespread alternative to second-look laparotomy is simply discontinuation of chemotherapy after a fixed interval (usually six to nine cycles) for a patient with no clinical evidence of disease.

Perspective

The benefits of second-look laparotomy have been seriously questioned in published articles and editorials.[103–106] There is general consensus that the findings at second-look laparotomy are of prognostic value; patients with macroscopic tumor have a worse survival rate than do those with either microscopic tumor or negative findings. Critics state, however, that although second-look laparotomy is superior to other methods of detecting residual ovarian cancer, the procedure still does not accurately predict the presence or absence of disease. The high recurrence rate after negative second-look laparotomy has essentially eliminated our ability to identify a subgroup of patients for whom therapy can be safely discontinued.

Another major criticism of second-look laparotomy is the lack of evidence that the procedure or the therapeutic decisions made based on the findings enhance survival. No prospective randomized clinical trials have compared patients who undergo second-look laparotomy with those who do not. The greatest impediment to improvement in survival for patients undergoing the procedure is the lack of success of salvage therapies. Few patients with persistent disease found at second-look laparotomy are cured of their disease with second-line therapy. Although there has been a flurry of enthusiasm for such modalities as external radiotherapy and intraperitoneal chemotherapy for patients with minimal persistent tumor, results with the former have been generally quite disappointing, and the benefits of the latter are being questioned increasingly despite reports of responses and prolonged survival.

Proponents of second-look laparotomy claim that resection of residual tumor in this setting improves survival. The issue of debulking at second-look laparotomy is very controversial; it is discussed in the following section. Until randomized clinical trials demonstrate a survival benefit of salvage therapies for patients with negative, microscopic, or macroscopic findings at second-look laparotomy, a cloud will remain over this procedure. Such trials are currently being conducted for patients with negative or microscopically positive findings. To the authors' knowledge, no randomized trials are assigning patients with no clinical evidence of disease after completion of chemotherapy to undergo surgery or not. Such a study might be quite difficult to execute in the present environment. In the meantime, it seems very reasonable to recommend that second-look laparotomy be performed only in a research setting until further information becomes available. For patients with Stage I epithelial ovarian cancer and those with malignant germ cell tumors, it is very difficult to justify second-look laparotomy because of the high probability of truly negative findings.

Secondary Cytoreductive Surgery

The term "secondary cytoreductive surgery" has no universal definition. It may denote cytoreductive surgery performed in one of several different settings:

1. In patients who are partial responders or nonresponders to primary chemotherapy
2. In patients who have developed recurrent disease after receiving primary therapy and who experience a prolonged disease-free interval off therapy (>6 months)
3. In patients who are referred to a gynecologic oncologist after a primary laparotomy resulting in inadequate debulking, usually biopsy alone
4. In patients who have persistent macroscopic tumor at second-look laparotomy

Tumors in these subgroups of ovarian cancer patients may have very different natural histories, principally defined by whether they are "platinum resistant" or "platinum sensitive." For example, patients whose tumor progresses during first-line chemotherapy, whether progression is noted clinically or at second-look laparotomy, are by definition "platinum resistant," whereas patients who have not yet received chemotherapy or are partial responders to chemotherapy, the response noted clinically or at second-look surgery, or who have developed recurrent disease after a prolonged interval off therapy may well be "platinum sensitive." These subgroups may thus have very different survival rates based on their responsiveness to second-line chemotherapy after secondary cytoreductive surgery. Therefore, it is extremely important for studies designed to assess the impact of these various secondary procedures on survival rates to carefully define their study populations. Because of the lack of prospective randomized studies in this area, it is difficult, if not impossible, to draw any firm conclusions about the influence of secondary debulking in these settings.

Secondary Cytoreductive Surgery for Nonresponders or Partial Responders to Primary Chemotherapy

Very little information is available about the possible benefits of secondary surgery for patients who have no or partial response to primary chemotherapy. Morris and associates reported the experience at UTMDACC with 33 ovarian cancer patients who had progressive or stable disease and who subsequently underwent an attempt at secondary cytoreductive surgery.[107] The tumors of 55% of the patients were cytoreduced to a residual diameter of 2 cm or less. Sixty-six per cent of the patients required intestinal resection during the procedure. Operative morbidity occurred in 24% of patients, mostly in those who underwent bowel resection. The overall median survival after secondary surgery was 9.4 months. For patients with residual tumor smaller than 1 cm, median survival after secondary surgery was 19.5

months, compared with 8.3 months for patients with residual tumor of 1 cm or more ($P < .004$). Patients with an interval between primary cytoreductive effort and secondary surgery of less than 12 months survived a median of 7.3 months, compared with an 18.3-month median survival for patients with an interval of 12 months or more ($P < .004$). The authors concluded that there is no definite evidence that secondary cytoreductive surgery is of significant benefit in most patients with ovarian cancer that is progressive or stable during chemotherapy. This issue can be resolved only by a prospective randomized study, the outcome of which would be significantly influenced by the effectiveness of postoperative second-line therapy.

Secondary Cytoreductive Surgery for Recurrent Disease

Equally scant information is available about the impact of secondary cytoreductive surgery for recurrent disease. Morris and colleagues reported the authors' experience at UTMDACC with 30 patients who underwent secondary debulking for recurrent ovarian cancer.[108] All had been initially treated with primary cytoreductive surgery and chemotherapy and had a period of clinical remission of at least 6 months thereafter. In 17 patients (57%), residual tumor was smaller than 2 cm. There were no postoperative deaths, but 40% of patients suffered postoperative morbidity, mostly prolonged ileus. The overall median survival after secondary surgery was 16.3 months. The interval between the primary and secondary cytoreductive surgeries and the amount of residual disease after the secondary procedure had no effect on survival. Morris and associates concluded that, although secondary cytoreductive surgery for recurrent ovarian cancer is technically feasible, in the absence of an effective second-line systemic therapy, its value is limited. Again, the true value of debulking surgery for recurrent ovarian cancer can be assessed only by a prospective randomized study.

Secondary Attempt at Cytoreductive Surgery After Suboptimal Debulking

The authors first became interested in secondary cytoreductive surgery after suboptimal debulking in the late 1970s when faced with the problem of how to treat a patient referred to their institution after undergoing only a laparotomy and biopsy because of presumed tumor unresectability. The authors reasoned that, on one hand, immediate re-exploration might incur the wrath of the referring physician, further compromise an already debilitated patient, and ultimately accomplish no greater cytoreduction;

it would also further delay initiation of chemotherapy. On the other hand, chemotherapy before an "interval debulking" might violate time-honored principles of therapy and potentially compromise curability.

The authors reported their experience with neoadjuvant chemotherapy and interval debulking using a matched-control design.[109] Twenty-two patients who were referred to their institution after laparotomy and biopsy alone received two to four cycles of cisplatin-based chemotherapy and then underwent interval debulking surgery; planned management consisted of six more chemotherapy cycles and second-look laparotomy. Two control groups were matched with the study group according to FIGO stage, histologic type and grade (2 or 3), and patient age plus or minus 5 years. The first control group (22 patients) had greater than 2 cm residual disease after initial surgery; their planned treatment was a minimum of six cycles of chemotherapy plus second-look laparotomy. The second control group (18 patients) had been referred after initial laparotomy and biopsy only; their disease was immediately re-explored and debulked; subsequent planned treatment was a minimum of six cycles of chemotherapy plus second-look laparotomy. Optimal cytoreduction to less than 2 cm was achieved for 77% of the interval debulking group versus 39% of the immediate re-exploration group ($P = .02$). There was also a suggestion that the operative morbidity was lower in the interval debulking group. However, median survival times for the three groups were not different. Within the interval debulking group, patients who were optimally debulked survived significantly longer than did those who were not (18.1 vs. 7.5 months) ($P = .02$).

Other investigators have similarly studied various aspects of cytoreductive surgery in this setting. In 1972, Griffiths and associates reported their experience with nine patients who received neoadjuvant chemotherapy with doxorubicin and cyclophosphamide before undergoing a definitive attempt at debulking.[110] In each instance, the referring surgeon had performed a laparotomy and staged the tumor but judged it to be unresectable. In seven of the nine (78%), the investigators were able to debulk the tumor to less than 1 cm. Median survival time for these 9 patients at the time of the report was over 6 months, considerably less than the median survival time of over 18 months for 15 patients who, during the same period, underwent primary debulking surgery and postoperative chemotherapy.

Wils and colleagues described a similar strategy employed in a Dutch cooperative group study.[111] Their study involved 88 previously untreated patients with advanced epithelial ovarian cancer whom they treated with the combination of cisplatin, doxorubicin, and cyclophosphamide. Optimal debulking (residual tumor not larger than 1.5 cm) at primary surgery could not be accomplished in 50 of the 88 patients but was achieved in 38. Comparison of the two groups showed a negative second-look rate of only 20% for those suboptimally debulked versus 70% for those with optimal surgical results; the respective actuarial survival rates at 3 years were 25% versus 60%. However, a select subgroup of these patients had a much more favorable prognosis. In 17 who were evaluable, response to a median of three cycles of chemotherapy made secondary optimal debulking surgery possible. These patients had a negative second-look rate of 29% and an actuarial 3-year survival rate of 50%, which approached the rate of the patients whose initial cytoreductive attempt was successful.

Neijt and coworkers, as part of a multicenter prospective randomized trial comparing the combination of cisplatin, hexamethylmelamine, doxorubicin, and cyclophosphamide with the cisplatin-cyclophosphamide regimen, described 47 patients who underwent neoadjuvant chemotherapy and interval debulking.[112] In 63% of these patients, the resultant residual disease was smaller than 1 cm. Unfortunately, their survival time was no better than that of patients whose interval debulking was unsuccessful. Furthermore, patients whose tumors measured less than 1 cm before chemotherapy survived significantly longer than those whose tumors were debulked to less than 1 cm at the interval procedure.

In 1989, Lawton and colleagues reported on 28 patients with bulky residual disease following an initial suboptimal debulking procedure.[113] After three cycles of cisplatin-based chemotherapy, tumors in 89% of these patients could be optimally debulked to less than 2 cm. Morbidity was minimal. In a subsequent study, the same group randomized 68 patients whose residual disease was greater than 2 cm after a primary debulking attempt to receive either chemotherapy alone or chemotherapy combined with interval debulking surgery that was performed after one to three cycles of chemotherapy.[114] Twenty-eight patients actually underwent the interval surgery, which optimally debulked the tumors of 18 (64%). The survival times of this group were not significantly different from those of patients with bulky residual disease treated with chemotherapy alone.

Based on the findings of most of the preceding reports, it appears that an interval debulking procedure after neoadjuvant cisplatin-based chemotherapy is feasible and may result in optimal cytoreduction for the majority of patients. The morbidity of the procedure is acceptable, possibly more so than after immediate re-exploration. With currently available therapy, however, the prognosis of patients with bulky disease following primary surgery remains uniformly poor, regardless of subsequent surgical intervention.

Secondary Cytoreductive Surgery at Second-Look Laparotomy

The issue of cytoreductive surgery at second-look laparotomy is very controversial and its value unproved. No prospective randomized trials exist to resolve this controversy. In the study of Raju and associates, complete resection of all macroscopic disease at second-look laparotomy in 9 patients seemed to confer no survival benefit when compared with survival of 29 patients with macroscopic residual disease after second-look surgery.[115] Other authors have questioned the value of secondary cytoreduction at second-look laparotomy.[71, 116] On the other hand, several authors have suggested a survival benefit associated with tumor resection at second-look laparotomy.[68, 117-121] In the study of Hoskins and coworkers, the 5-year survival rate of patients found to have microscopic disease at second-look laparotomy was 62%, similar to that of patients whose disease was rendered microscopic by tumor resection—51% ($P = .55$).[121] Especially in these retrospective studies, it is extremely difficult to evaluate the influence of all prognostic factors. As with all studies on the subject of cytoreductive surgery, it is virtually impossible to distinguish the effects of secondary tumor resection from the influence of the inherent tumor characteristics. Noninfiltrating tumors may be easier to resect but may also be inherently more indolent. In addition, survival after secondary debulking at second-look laparotomy is intimately linked to the effectiveness of postoperative therapy.

MISCELLANEOUS SURGICAL PROCEDURES

Management of Intestinal Obstruction

Approximately 25% of ovarian cancer patients will develop intestinal obstruction in the terminal phase of their illness. One of the major dilemmas facing the gynecologic oncologist is whether to operate on a patient with refractory ovarian cancer and an intestinal obstruction. Although current information provides some guidelines, the decisions concerning the wisdom of surgical intervention and intraoperative management are based more on the art of the discipline and the experience of the surgeon than on scientific criteria.

Signs and symptoms of intestinal obstruction resulting from ovarian cancer include nausea and vomiting, abdominal cramping, abdominal distention, and progressive constipation. In patients who have only partial obstruction, these complaints and findings may be episodic and more subtle. Plain films of the abdomen may support the diagnosis. Dilatation of the small intestine and air-fluid levels suggest involvement of the small bowel. Dilatation of the colon may characterize large bowel obstruction. In patients with early partial obstruction, the radiographic findings may be nonspecific.

The authors recommend a barium enema study for essentially all patients with suspected intestinal obstruction, unless a colon perforation is suggested by the plain films. This study will confirm colon obstruction for those with this condition or rule it out for a patient with a small bowel obstruction. The radiologist needs to be especially cautious when a colon obstruction is suspected; only a limited study may be prudent. Although recommended by some investigators, the authors have not found small bowel studies to be very helpful in the management of patients with overt obstruction. For patients with subtle findings suggestive of partial obstruction, a small bowel series may be indicated.

Although intestinal obstruction in patients with ovarian cancer may be caused by adhesions, progressive tumor is usually the inciting factor. Of course, if the patient has received abdominopelvic radiotherapy, this cause should also be considered. In the authors' experience and that of others, however, most cases of intestinal obstruction in ovarian cancer patients who have received prior radiotherapy are related primarily to tumor progression.

The site(s) of the obstruction may be solitary or multiple. In 5–10% of patients, there is simultaneous obstruction of the small and large bowel. Colon obstruction in the area of the sigmoid portion usually occurs from growth of pelvic tumor and resultant extrinsic compression, although occasionally there may be obstruction of more proximal segments. Small bowel obstruction is usually the result of adherence of loops of bowel by mesenteric or serosal tumor implants.

Once the appropriate evaluation is completed and the diagnosis of intestinal obstruction is made, the gynecologist must outline a plan of management. Many factors influence this decision, including age, the nutritional status and general condition of the patient, the amount of tumor present, the presence or absence of ascites, the options for postoperative salvage therapy, the attitude of the physician, and the wishes of the patient and her family. The decision of whether to operate or manage the patient nonoperatively is also colored by the fact that surgery for patients with refractory ovarian cancer is associated with significant morbidity and mortality, the obstruction cannot be relieved in almost 20% of those undergoing surgery, and the postoperative survival is disappointingly brief.[122–127] In reported series, the serious complication rate has ranged from 28% to 49%[122, 124] and the operative mortality rate is in the range of 12–16%.[122, 123, 126] The median survival rate for patients who have undergone surgery is in the range of 3–5 months.[123, 124, 126]

Although some investigators have used projected survival (usually > 2 months) as a parameter to decide on type of management, such an indicator is too unpredictable. Krebs and Goplerud devised a scoring system for selection of patients for surgery, which included patient age, nutritional status, amount of palpable tumor, presence of ascites, previous chemotherapy, and previous radiotherapy.[123] Outcome seemed to correlate with the prognostic score. Clarke-Pearson and coworkers later confirmed the influence of disease status, ascites, and nutritional status.[125]

For initial management of a patient with small bowel obstruction, the authors prefer the insertion of a nasogastric tube rather than a long tube (Cantor, Miller-Abbott, or Dennis) for intestinal decompression. After extensive experience with both, the authors have found no advantage from the latter. Furthermore, long tubes are associated with considerably greater discomfort. Long intestinal tubes seem to have the greatest success rate in patients with postoperative adhesions but are fairly ineffective in relieving obstruction resulting from cancer. In the study of Krebs and Goplerud, only 10% of patients had their obstruction relieved by tube decompression.[128] In patients for whom no surgery is planned, the authors have extensively utilized the technique of percutaneous gastrostomy since 1984[129] (Fig. 28–14). This procedure has resulted in excellent palliation for terminal-stage ovarian cancer patients, avoiding the discomfort of the nasogastric tube and allowing the patient to be easily cared for at home in most cases. With such a device, the patient may even continue to eat some, although, of course, the nutritional benefit is essentially nil.

If a patient is judged to be a suitable candidate for surgical intervention, optimal preoperative preparation is desirable. For patients with complete colonic obstruction or perforation of the small or large intestine, a surgical emergency exists unless the patient is in such poor condition that such an intervention is not feasible. In emergency cases, the patient should be stabilized with intravenous fluids and antibiotics prior to surgery. For patients with a small intestinal obstruction, emergency surgery is rarely indicated. It is preferable to optimize the patient's condition with nasogastric tube decompression and rehydration. In addition, a barium enema is usually indicated. If the patient is malnourished, intravenous hyperalimentation may be indicated preoperatively. Ample information suggests that hyperalimentation will place the patient in an anabolic state and will reduce the incidence of postoperative morbidity. Its effect on long-term survival is, however, unclear.

Colonic obstruction is usually treated by performing a colostomy. The selection of the site of colostomy depends on the area of obstruction. Most commonly,

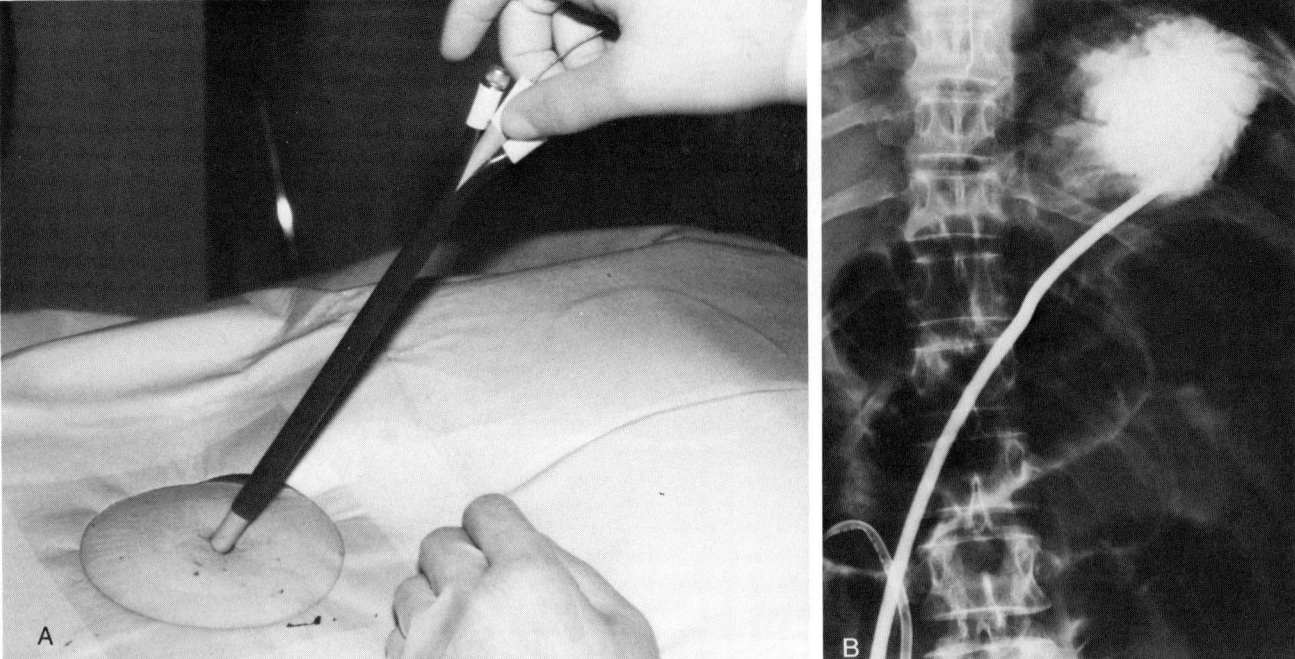

Figure 28–14
A, Percutaneous gastrostomy. 26 Fr peel-away sheath and dilator inserted over a guide wire prior to passage of Malecot catheter. *B*, Malecot catheter in stomach with contrast injected. Dilated loops of small intestine due to intestinal obstruction are noted.

a transverse loop colostomy is indicated in the presence of a sigmoid colon obstruction. For small bowel obstruction, a number of options are available, depending on the operative findings. Most commonly, there are multiple sites of obstruction in the terminal ileum, in which case an ileoascending colon bypass or ileotransverse colon bypass is preferable. In such situations, it is usually both unwise and inappropriate to attempt resection and re-anastomosis. If, on the other hand, there is an isolated area of obstruction, a resection and re-anastomosis may be indicated. The anastomosis may be either hand-sewn using a two-layer technique or approximated with surgical staplers. The authors generally prefer the latter because of the time-saving aspect. Not infrequently, there may be extensive tumor with multiple areas of obstruction, making both bypass and resection impossible. In such a situation, a tube gastrostomy is indicated, if possible. Procedures such as these are among the most demanding because of the meticulous, often tedious dissection required. Enterotomies are not uncommon and should be repaired as soon as they are identified. Complications of small intestinal procedures include wound infection, intraperitoneal abscess, sepsis, pneumonia, and enterocutaneous fistula. The details of these operative procedures mentioned are found in Chapter 21.

Intraperitoneal Therapy

Because of advances in technology and the availability of newer chemotherapeutic agents active against ovarian cancer, interest in the use of intraperitoneal chemotherapy has revived over the past decade. At the time of this writing, several ongoing randomized clinical trials are comparing intraperitoneal with intravenous chemotherapy as first-line postoperative treatment in patients with advanced epithelial ovarian cancer. In addition, several phase II studies of intraperitoneal chemotherapy have demonstrated activity in patients with persistent minimal residual tumor discovered at second-look laparotomy. Unfortunately, this approach has been prematurely embraced by community-based physicians. There is currently increasing skepticism about its possible efficacy. Nevertheless, the intraperitoneal route for administration of chemotherapy, immunotherapy, and monoclonal antibody therapy will undoubtedly continue to be used over the next few years.

The most popular intraperitoneal delivery system is the port-A-Cath, a completely implantable device. The catheter is inserted into the peritoneal cavity and the port is placed in the subcutaneous tissue, usually over the lower costal margin in the midclavicular line. Complications associated with the port-A-Cath include outflow or inflow obstruction and infection—either abdominal wall cellulitis or abscess or peritonitis.[130, 131]

References

1. American Cancer Society: Cancer Facts & Figures—1992: Ovarian Cancer. New York, American Cancer Society, 1992.
2. Maiman M, Seltzer V, Boyce J: Laparoscopic excision of

ovarian neoplasms subsequently found to be malignant. Obstet Gynecol 1991; 77:563.
3. Gynecol Oncol 1986; 25:383.
4. Tobias JS, Griffiths CT: Management of ovarian carcinoma: Current concepts and future prospects. N Engl J Med 1976; 15:818.
5. McGarrity KA, Pettersson F, Ulfelder H (eds.): Annual Report on the Results of Treatment of Gynecologic Cancer, Vol. 8. Statement of Results Obtained in 1973 to 1975 Inclusive. Stockholm, Radiumhemmet, 1982.
6. Malkasian GD Jr, Melton LJ III, O'Brien PC, et al.: Prognostic significance of histologic classification and grading of epithelial malignancies of the ovary. Am J Obstet Gynecol 1984; 149:274.
7. Hart WR, Norris HJ: Borderline and malignant mucinous tumors of the ovary: Histologic criteria and clinical behavior. Cancer 1973; 31:1031.
8. Smith JP, Day TG: Review of ovarian cancer at The University of Texas System Cancer Center, MD Anderson Hospital and Tumor Institute. Am J Obstet Gynecol 1979; 135:984.
9. Sigurdsson K, Alm P, Gullberg B: Prognostic factors in malignant epithelial ovarian tumors. Gynecol Oncol, 1983; 15:370.
10. Dembo AJ, Davy D, Stenwig AE, et al.: Prognostic factors in patients with stage I epithelial ovarian cancer. Obstet Gynecol 1990; 75:263.
11. Knapp RC, Friedman EA: Aortic lymph node metastases in early ovarian cancer. Am J Obstet Gynecol 1974; 119:1013.
12. Musumeci R, Banfi A, Bolis G: Lymphangiography in patients with ovarian epithelial cancer. Cancer 1977; 40:1444.
13. Creasman WT, Rutledge F: The prognostic value of peritoneal cytology in gynecologic malignant disease. Am J Obstet Gynecol 1971; 110:773.
14. Keettel WX, Pixley EE, Buschbaum HJ: Experience with peritoneal cytology in the management of gynecologic malignancies. Am J Obstet Gynecol 1974; 120:174.
15. Rosenoff SH, Young RC, Anderson T, et al.: Peritoneoscopy: A valuable staging tool in ovarian carcinoma. Ann Intern Med 1975; 83:37.
16. Piver MS, Barlow JJ, Lele SB: Incidence of subclinical metastasis in stage I and II ovarian carcinoma. Obstet Gynecol 1978; 52:100.
17. Chen SS, Lee L: Incidence of para-aortic and pelvic lymph node metastases in epithelial carcinoma of the ovary. Gynecol Oncol 1983; 16:95.
18. Young RC, Decker DG, Wharton JT, et al.: Staging laparotomy in early ovarian cancer. JAMA 1983; 250:3072.
19. McGowan L, Lesher LP, Norris HJ, et al.: Misstaging of ovarian cancer. Obstet Gynecol 1985; 65:568.
20. Trimbos JB, Schueler JA, vanLent M, et al.: Reasons for incomplete surgical staging in early ovarian cancer. Gynecol Oncol 1990; 37:374.
21. Greer BE, Rutledge FN, Gallager HS: Staging or restaging laparotomy in early-stage epithelial cancer of the ovary. Clin Obstet Gynecol 1980; 23:293.
22. Helewa ME, Krepart GV, Lotocki R: Staging laparotomy in early epithelial ovarian carcinoma. Am J Obstet Gynecol 1986; 154:282.
23. Wu P-C, Qu J-Y, Lang J-H, et al.: Lymph node metastasis of ovarian cancer: A preliminary survey of 74 cases of lymphadenectomy. Am J Obstet Gynecol 1986; 155:1103.
24. Burghardt E, Pickel H, Lahousen M, Stettner H: Pelvic lymphadenectomy in operative treatment of ovarian cancer. Am J Obstet Gynecol 1986; 155:15.
25. Russel P: The pathological assessment of ovarian neoplasms. I. Introduction to the common "epithelial" tumors and analysis of benign "epithelial" tumors. Pathology 1979; 11:5.
26. Aure JC, Hoeg K, Kalstad P: Clinical and histologic studies of ovarian carcinoma: Long-term follow-up of 990 cases. Obstet Gynecol 1971; 37:1.
27. Tazelaar HD, Bostwick DG, Ballon SC, et al.: Conservative treatment of borderline ovarian tumors. Obstet Gynecol 1985; 66:417.
28. Lim-Tan SK, Cajigas HE, Scully RE: Ovarian cystectomy for serous borderline tumors: A follow-up study of 35 cases. Obstet Gynecol 1981; 72:775.
29. Gershenson DM, Silva EG: Serous ovarian tumors of low malignant potential with peritoneal implants. Cancer 1990; 65:578.
30. Young RC, Walton LA, Ellenberg SS, et al.: Adjuvant therapy in stage I and stage II epithelial ovarian cancer. Results of two prospective randomized trials. N Engl J Med 1990; 322:1021.
31. Munnell EW, Jacox HW, Taylor HC: Treatment and prognosis in cancer of the ovary. Am J Obstet Gynecol 1957; 74:1187.
32. Delclos L, Quinlan EJ: Malignant tumors of the ovary managed with postoperative megavoltage irradiation. Radiology 1969; 93:659.
33. Griffiths CT: Surgical resection of tumor bulk in the primary treatment of ovarian carcinoma: Seminar on ovarian cancer. NCI Monogr 1975; 42:101.
34. Griffiths CT, Parker LM, Fuller AF: Role of cytoreductive surgical treatment in the management of advanced ovarian cancer. Cancer Treat Rep 1979; 63:235.
35. Wharton JT, Herson J: Surgery for common epithelial tumors of the ovary. Cancer 1981; 48:582.
36. Hacker NF, Berek JS, Lagasse LD, et al.: Primary cytoreductive surgery for epithelial ovarian cancer. Obstet Gynecol 1983; 61:413.
37. Young RC, Chabner BA, Hubbard SP, et al.: Advanced ovarian adenocarcinoma: A prospective clinical trial of melphalan (L-PAM) versus combination chemotherapy. N Engl J Med 1978; 299:1261.
38. Greco FA, Julian CG, Richardson RL, et al.: Advanced ovarian cancer: Brief intensive combination chemotherapy and second-look operation. Obstet Gynecol 1981; 58:199.
39. Ehrlich CE, Einhorn L, Williams SD, et al.: Chemotherapy for stage III–IV epithelial ovarian cancer with cis-dichlorodiamineplatinum II, Adriamycin, and cyclophosphamide: A preliminary report. Cancer Treat Rep 1979; 63:281.
40. Skipper HE: Adjuvant chemotherapy. Cancer 1978; 41:936.
41. Skipper HE: Stepwise progress in the treatment of disseminated cancer. Cancer 1983; 5:1773.
42. Goldie JH, Coldman AJ: A mathematical model for relating the drug sensitivity of tumors to their spontaneous mutation rate. Cancer Treat Rep 1979; 63:1727.
43. Piver MS, Baker T: The potential for optimal (≤2 cm) cytoreductive surgery in advanced ovarian carcinoma at a tertiary medical center: A prospective study. Gynecol Oncol 1986; 24:1.
44. Chen SS, Bochner R: Assessment of morbidity and mortality in primary cytoreductive surgery for advanced ovarian carcinoma. Gynecol Oncol 1985; 20:190.
45. Blythe JG, Wahl TP: Debulking surgery: Does it increase the quality of survival? Gynecol Oncol 1982; 14:396.
46. Heintz APM, Hacker NF, Berek JS, et al.: Cytoreductive surgery in ovarian carcinoma: Feasibility and morbidity. Obstet Gynecol 1986; 67:783.
47. Berek JS, Hacker NF, Lagasse LD: Rectosigmoid colectomy and reanastomosis to facilitate resection of primary and recurrent gynecologic cancer. Obstet Gynecol 1984; 64:715.
48. Soper JT, Couchman G, Berchuck A, Clarke-Pearson D: The role of partial sigmoid colectomy for debulking epithelial ovarian carcinoma. Gynecol Oncol 1991; 41:239.
49. Berek JS, Hacker NF, Lagasse LD, Leuchter RS: Lower urinary tract resection as part of cytoreductive surgery for ovarian cancer. Gynecol Oncol 1982; 13:87.
50. Scarabelli C, Campagnutta E, Perin A, et al.: La splenectomia nel trattameno chirurgico radicale del carcinoma ovarico. Minerva Ginecol 1985; 37:37.
51. Joyeux H, Szawlowski A, Saint-Aubert B, et al.: Aggressive regional surgery for advanced ovarian carcinoma. Cancer 1986; 57:142.
52. Sonnendecker EW, Guidozzi F, Margolius KA: Splenectomy during primary maximal cytoreductive surgery for epithelial ovarian cancer. Gynecol Oncol 1989; 35:301.
53. Deppe G, Zbella EA, Skogerson K, Dumitru I: The rare indication for splenectomy as part of cytoreductive surgery in ovarian cancer. Gynecol Oncol 1983; 16:282.
54. Malfetano JH: Splenectomy for optimal cytoreduction in ovarian cancer. Gynecol Oncol 1986; 24:392.
55. Morris M, Gershenson DM, Burke TW, et al.: Splenectomy

in gynecologic oncology: Indications, complications, and technique. Gynecol Oncol 1991; 43:118.
56. Deppe G, Malviya V, Boike G, Hampson A: Surgical approach to diaphragmatic metastases from ovarian cancer. Gynecol Oncol 1986; 24:258.
57. Montz FJ, Schlaerth JB, Berek JS: Resection of diaphragmatic peritoneum and muscle: Role in cytoreductive surgery for ovarian cancer. Gynecol Oncol 1989; 35:338.
58. Fiorica JV, Hoffman MS, LaPolla JP, et al.: The management of diaphragmatic lesions in ovarian carcinoma. Obstet Gynecol 1989; 74:927.
59. Kapnick SJ, Griffiths CG, Finkler NJ: Occult pleural involvement in stage III ovarian carcinoma: Role of diaphragm resection. Gynecol Oncol 1990; 39:135.
60. Brand E, Pearlman N: Electrosurgical debulking of ovarian cancer: A new technique using the argon beam coagulator. Gynecol Oncol 1990; 39:115.
61. Adelson MD, Baggish MS, Seifer DB, et al.: Cytoreduction of ovarian cancer with the Cavitron Ultrasonic Surgical Aspirator. Obstet Gynecol 1988; 72:140.
62. Deppe G, Malviya VK, Malone JM: Debulking surgery for ovarian cancer with the Cavitron Ultrasonic Surgical Aspirator (CUSA): A preliminary report. Gynecol Oncol 1988; 31:223.
63. Deppe G, Malviya VK, Boike G, Malone JM: Use of Cavitron surgical aspirator for debulking of diaphragmatic metastases in patients with advanced carcinoma of the ovaries. Surg Gynecol Obstet 1989; 168:455.
64. Adelson MD: Cytoreduction of diaphragmatic metastases using the Cavitron Ultrasonic Surgical Aspirator. Gynecol Oncol 1991; 41:220.
65. Deppe G, Malviya VK, Malone JM, Christensen CW: Debulking of pelvic and para-aortic lymph node metastases in ovarian cancer with the Cavitron Ultrasonic Surgical Aspirator. Obstet Gynecol 1990; 76:1140.
66. Brand E, Wade ME, Lagasse LD: Resection of fixed pelvic tumors using the Nd:YAG laser. J Surg Oncol 1988; 37:246.
67. Wangensteen OH, Lewis FJ, Tongen LA: The "second-look" in cancer surgery. Lancet 1951; 71:303.
68. Schwartz P, Smith J: Second-look operations in ovarian cancer. Am J Obstet Gynecol 1980; 138:1124.
69. Webb M, Snyder J, Williams T, Decker D: Second-look laparotomy in ovarian cancer. Gynecol Oncol 1982; 14:285.
70. Roberts W, Hodel K, Rich W, DiSaia P: Second-look laparotomy in the management of gynecologic malignancy. Gynecol Oncol 1982; 13:345.
71. Luesley D, Chan K, Fielding J, et al.: Second-look laparotomy in the management of epithelial ovarian carcinoma: An evaluation of fifty cases. Obstet Gynecol 1984; 64:421.
72. Smirz L, Stehman F, Ulbright T, et al.: Second-look laparotomy after chemotherapy in the management of ovarian malignancy. Am J Obstet Gynecol 1985; 152:661.
73. Podczaski E, Stevens C, Manetta A, et al.: Use of second-look laparotomy in the management of patients with ovarian epithelial malignancies. Gynecol Oncol 1987; 28:205.
74. Barnhill D, Hoskins W, Heller P, Park R: The second-look surgical reassessment for epithelial ovarian carcinoma. Gynecol Oncol 1984; 19:148.
75. Berek J, Hacker N, Lagasse L, et al.: Second-look laparotomy in stage III epithelial ovarian cancer: Clinical variables associated with disease status. Obstet Gynecol 1984; 64:207.
76. Podratz K, Malkasian G, Hilton J, et al.: Second-look laparotomy in ovarian cancer: Evaluation of pathologic variables. Am J Obstet Gynecol 1985; 152:230.
77. Miller D, Ballon S, Teng N, et al.: A critical reassessment of second-look laparotomy in epithelial ovarian carcinoma. Cancer 1986; 57:530.
78. Chambers S, Chambers J, Kohorn E, et al.: Evaluation of the role of second-look surgery in ovarian cancer. Obstet Gynecol 1988; 72:404.
79. Lund B, Williamson P: Prognostic factors for outcome of and survival after second-look laparotomy in patients with advanced ovarian carcinoma. Obstet Gynecol 1990; 76:617.
80. Copeland L, Gershenson D, Wharton JT, et al.: Microscopic disease at second-look laparotomy in advanced ovarian cancer. Cancer 1985; 55:472.
81. Gershenson D, Copeland L, Wharton JT, et al.: Prognosis of surgically determined complete responders in advanced ovarian cancer. Cancer 1985; 55:1129.
82. Copeland L, Silva E, Gershenson D, et al.: The significance of muellerian inclusions found at second-look laparotomy in patients with epithelial ovarian neoplasms. Obstet Gynecol 1988; 71:763.
83. Copeland L, Gershenson DM: Ovarian cancer recurrences in patients with no macroscopic tumor at second-look laparotomy. Obstet Gynecol 1986; 68:873.
84. Podratz K, Malkasian G, Wieand H, et al.: Recurrent disease after negative second-look laparotomy in stages III and IV ovarian carcinoma. Gynecol Oncol 1988; 29:274.
85. Rubin S, Hoskins W, Hakes T, et al.: Recurrence after negative second-look laparotomy for ovarian cancer: Analysis of risk factors. Am J Obstet Gynecol 1988; 159:1094.
86. Luesley D, Chan K, Lawton F, et al.: Survival after negative second-look laparotomy. Eur J Surg Oncol 1989; 15:205.
87. Rubin S, Hoskins W, Saigo P, et al.: Prognostic factors for recurrence following negative second-look laparotomy in ovarian cancer patients treated with platinum-based chemotherapy. Gynecol Oncol 1991; 42:137.
88. Gershenson DM, Copeland L, DelJunco G, et al.: Second-look laparotomy in the management of malignant germ cell tumors of the ovary. Obstet Gynecol 1986; 67:789.
89. Smith W, Day T, Smith J: The use of laparoscopy to determine the results of chemotherapy for ovarian cancer. J Reprod Med 1977; 18:257.
90. Ozols R, Fisher R, Anderson T, et al.: Peritoneoscopy in the management of ovarian cancer. Am J Obstet Gynecol 1981; 140:611.
91. Berek S, Griffiths CT, Leventhal J: Laparoscopy for second-look evaluation in ovarian cancer. Obstet Gynecol 1981; 58:192.
92. Lele S, Piver MS: Interval laparoscopy as predictor of response to chemotherapy in ovarian carcinoma. Obstet Gynecol 1986; 68:345.
93. Stern J, Buscema J, Rosenshein N, Siegelman S: Can computed tomography substitute for second-look operation in ovarian carcinoma? Gynecol Oncol 1981; 11:82.
94. Goldhirsch A, Triller J, Greiner R, et al.: Computed tomography prior to second-look operation in advanced ovarian cancer. Obstet Gynecol 1983; 62:630.
95. Brenner D, Shaff M, Jones H, et al.: Abdominopelvic computed tomography: Evaluation in patients undergoing second-look laparotomy for ovarian carcinoma. Obstet Gynecol 1985; 65:715.
96. Clarke-Pearson D, Bandy L, Dudzinski M, et al.: Computed tomography in evaluation of patients with ovarian carcinoma in complete clinical remission. Correlation with surgical-pathologic findings. JAMA 1986; 255:627.
97. Stehman F, Calkins A, Wass J, et al.: A comparison of findings at second-look laparotomy with preoperative computed tomography in patients with ovarian cancer. Gynecol Oncol 1988; 29:37.
98. Reuter K, Griffin T, Hunter R: Comparison of abdominopelvic computed tomography results and findings at second-look laparotomy in ovarian carcinoma patients. Cancer 1989; 63:1123.
99. Lund B, Jaconsen K, Rasch L, et al.: Correlation of abdominal ultrasound and computed tomography scans with second- or third-look laparotomy in patients with ovarian carcinoma. Gynecol Oncol 1990; 37:279.
100. Niloff JM, Bast RC, Schaetzl EM, et al.: Predictive value of CA-125 antigen levels at second-look procedures in ovarian cancer. Am J Obstet Gynecol 1985; 148:1057.
101. Berek J, Knapp R, Malkasian G, et al.: CA-125 serum levels correlated with second-look operations among ovarian cancer patients. Obstet Gynecol 1986; 67:685.
102. Patsner B, Orr J, Mann W, et al.: Does serum CA-125 level prior to second-look laparotomy for invasive ovarian abenocarcinoma predict size of residual disease? Gynecol Oncol 1990; 37:319.
103. Ho AG, Beller U, Speyer J, et al.: A reassessment of the role of second-look laparotomy in advanced ovarian cancer. J Clin Oncol 1987; 5:1316.

104. Young RC: A second look at second-look laparotomy (editorial). J Clin Oncol 1987; 5:1311.
105. Sonnendecker EW: Is routine second-look laparotomy for ovarian cancer justified? Gynecol Oncol 1988; 31:249.
106. Friedman J, Weiss N: Second thoughts about second-look laparotomy in advanced ovarian cancer. N Engl J Med 1990; 322:1079.
107. Morris M, Gershenson DM, Wharton JT: Secondary cytoreductive surgery in epithelial ovarian cancer: Nonresponders to first-line therapy. Gynecol Oncol 1989; 33:1.
108. Morris M, Gershenson DM, Wharton JT, et al.: Secondary cytoreductive surgery for recurrent epithelial ovarian cancer. Gynecol Oncol 1989; 34:334.
109. Jacob JH, Gershenson DM, Morris M, et al.: Neoadjuvant chemotherapy and interval debulking for advanced epithelial ovarian cancer. Gynecol Oncol 1991; 42:146.
110. Griffiths CT, Parker LM, Fuller AF: Role of cytoreductive surgical treatment in the management of advanced ovarian cancer. Cancer Treat Rep 1979; 63:235.
111. Wils J, Blijham G, Naus A, et al.: Primary or delayed debulking surgery and chemotherapy consisting of cisplatin, doxorubicin, and cyclophosphamide in stage III–IV epithelial ovarian carcinoma. J Clin Oncol 1986; 4:1068.
112. Neijt JP, ten Bokkel, Huinink WW, van der Burg ME, et al.: Randomized trial comparing two combination chemotherapy regimens (CHAP-5 v CP) in advanced ovarian carcinoma. J Clin Oncol 1987; 5:1157.
113. Lawton FG, Redman CW, Leusley DM, et al.: Neoadjuvant (cytoreductive) chemotherapy combined with intervention debulking surgery in advanced, unresected epithelial ovarian cancer. Obstet Gynecol 1989; 73:61.
114. Varma R, Redman CW, Blackledge G, et al.: Early second surgery in bulky epithelial ovarian cancer (EOC) does not improve survival: Results of a randomized study (abstract). Second meeting of the International Gynecologic Cancer Society, Toronto, October 1989, p. 29.
115. Raju KS, McKinna JA, Barker GH, et al.: Second-look operations in the planned management of advanced ovarian carcinoma. Am J Obstet Gynecol 1982; 144:650.
116. Wiltshaw E, Raju KS, Dawson I: The role of cytoreductive surgery in advanced carcinoma of the ovary: An analysis of primary and second surgery. Br J Obstet Gynecol 1985; 92:522.
117. Stuart GC, Jeffries M, Stuart JL, Anderson RJ: The changing role of "second-look" laparotomy in the management of epithelial carcinoma of the ovary. Am J Obstet Gynecol 1982; 142:612.
118. Podratz KC, Schwarz MF, Wieand HS, et al.: Evaluation of treatment and survival after positive second-look laparotomy. Gynecol Oncol 1988; 31:9.
119. Dauplat J, Ferriere JP, Monique G, et al.: Second-look laparotomy in managing epithelial ovarian carcinoma. Cancer 1986; 57:1627.
120. Berek JS, Hacker NF, Lagasse LD, et al.: Survival of patients following secondary cytoreductive surgery in ovarian cancer. Obstet Gynecol 1983; 61:189.
121. Hoskins WJ, Rubin SC, Dulaney E, et al.: Influence of secondary cytoreduction at the time of second-look laparotomy on the survival of patients with epithelial ovarian carcinoma. Gynecol Oncol 1989; 34:365.
122. Castaldo TW, Petrilli ES, Ballon SC, Lagasse LD: Intestinal operations in patients with ovarian carcinoma. Am J Obstet Gynecol 1981; 139:80.
123. Krebs HB, Goplerud DR: Surgical management of bowel obstruction in advanced ovarian carcinoma. Obstet Gynecol 1983; 61:327.
124. Clarke-Pearson DL, Chin N, DeLong ER, et al.: Surgical management of intestinal obstruction in ovarian cancer. Gynecol Oncol 1987; 26:11.
125. Clarke-Pearson DL, DeLong ER, Chin N, et al.: Surgical management of intestinal obstruction in ovarian cancer. II. Analysis of factors associated with complications and survival. Arch Surg 1988; 123:42.
126. Larson JE, Podczaski ES, Manetta A, et al.: Bowel obstruction in patients with ovarian carcinoma: Analysis of prognostic factors. Gynecol Oncol 1989; 35:61.
127. Rubin SC, Hoskins WJ, Benjamin I, Lewis JL: Palliative surgery for intestinal obstruction in advanced ovarian cancer. Gynecol Oncol 1989; 34:16.
128. Krebs HB, Goplerud DR: The role of intestinal intubation in obstruction of the small intestine due to carcinoma of the ovary. Surg Gynecol Obstet 1984; 158:467.
129. Malone JM, Koonce T, Larson DM, et al.: Palliation of small bowel obstruction by percutaneous gastrostomy in patients with progressive ovarian carcinoma. Obstet Gynecol 1986; 68:431.
130. Piccart MJ, Speyer JL, Markman M, et al.: Intraperitoneal chemotherapy: Technical experience at five institutions. Semin Oncol 1985; 3:90.
131. Rubin SC, Hoskins WJ, Markman M, et al.: Long-term access to the peritoneal cavity in ovarian cancer patients. Gynecol Oncol 1989; 33:46.

Assisted Reproductive Technology (ART): Surgical Aspects

29

Lawrence Grunfeld
Janis H. Fox

HISTORY

In vitro fertilization (IVF) resulted in the birth of Louise Brown following Steptoe and Edwards' successful transfer of a human embryo in 1978.[1] This procedure represented a milestone as the first treatment for women with surgically uncorrectable fallopian tubes. Steptoe and Edwards were able to retrieve an oocyte and fertilize it in vitro by closely monitoring the patient's spontaneous luteinizing hormone (LH) surge. Trounson and colleagues increased the efficiency of the procedure by utilizing clomiphene to induce the development of several mature eggs.[2] The Norfolk group popularized menotropins to improve the oocyte yield.[3] The use of drugs to induce a controlled ovarian hyperstimulation (COH) is now routine in IVF therapy.

Although IVF was originally devised as a therapy for fallopian tube disease, it is currently used for a wide range of disorders, including immunologic, male factor, and unexplained infertility. The extension of indications to include women with patent fallopian tubes has resulted in the development of several newer procedures. An improved success was demonstrated by Asch and associates when gametes (sperm and oocytes) were transferred into the ampullary fallopian tube (gamete intrafallopian transfer [GIFT]).[4] Oocytes that are fertilized in the fallopian tubes are provided with an environment that is favorable for early embryo development. Furthermore, embryos residing in the fallopian tube enter the endometrial cavity at a more advanced developmental stage than when embryo transfer (ET) is performed following IVF. More recently, the transfer of zygotes into the fallopian tube (zygote intrafallopian transfer [ZIFT]) has been shown to produce higher implantation rates.[5]

The procedures that involve insemination, in vitro fertilization, and the transfer of gametes and zygotes are encompassed under the term assisted reproductive technology (ART) and are summarized in Figure 29–1. This chapter outlines the indications and techniques involved in ART.

INSEMINATION (Fig. 29–2)

Insemination was first successfully performed in 1770 by John Hunter in a couple in whom the husband could not ejaculate into the vagina because of hypospadias.[6] Although this classic indication still exists, it is the minority of patients who suffer from ejacu-

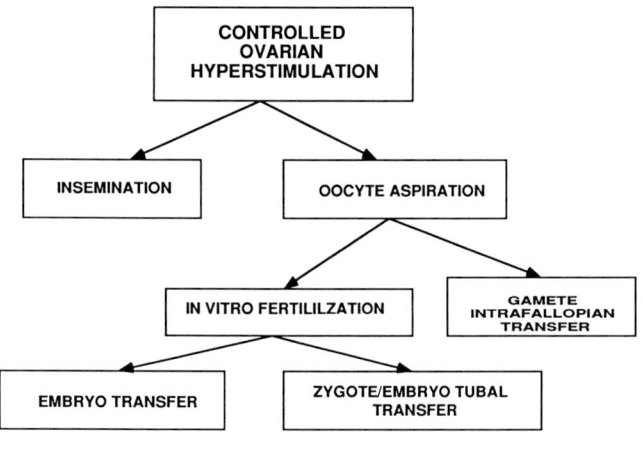

Figure 29–1
The steps in assisted reproductive technology (ART).

latory disturbances. Current indications for insemination include donor insemination, cervical mucus–sperm interaction abnormalities, oligoasthenospermia, antisperm antibodies, and unexplained infertility.

Cervical Insemination

The simplest form of insemination involves the placement of unprocessed semen into the cervical canal. Cervical insemination is most commonly utilized for the transfer of donor or cryopreserved semen. Also, when ejaculatory or sexual dysfunction precludes proper placement of semen into the vagina during coitus, cervical insemination is indicated.

Technique

Unprocessed semen is injected into the cervical canal following liquefaction at room temperature. Various devices are available to retain the semen in close proximity to the external os. An inert sponge, which is removed by the patient after several hours, can be inserted into the vagina following insemination. Alternatively, the cervical insemination cup (Milex Products, Inc., Chicago, IL) can be utilized (Fig. 29–2A). The cup allows the semen to be injected directly into the cervix through a stem that also serves as a handle that the patient withdraws after several hours.

Intrauterine Insemination

Patient Selection

The combination of COH with intrauterine insemination (IUI) has been shown by some authors to be an effective therapy for unexplained infertility, en-

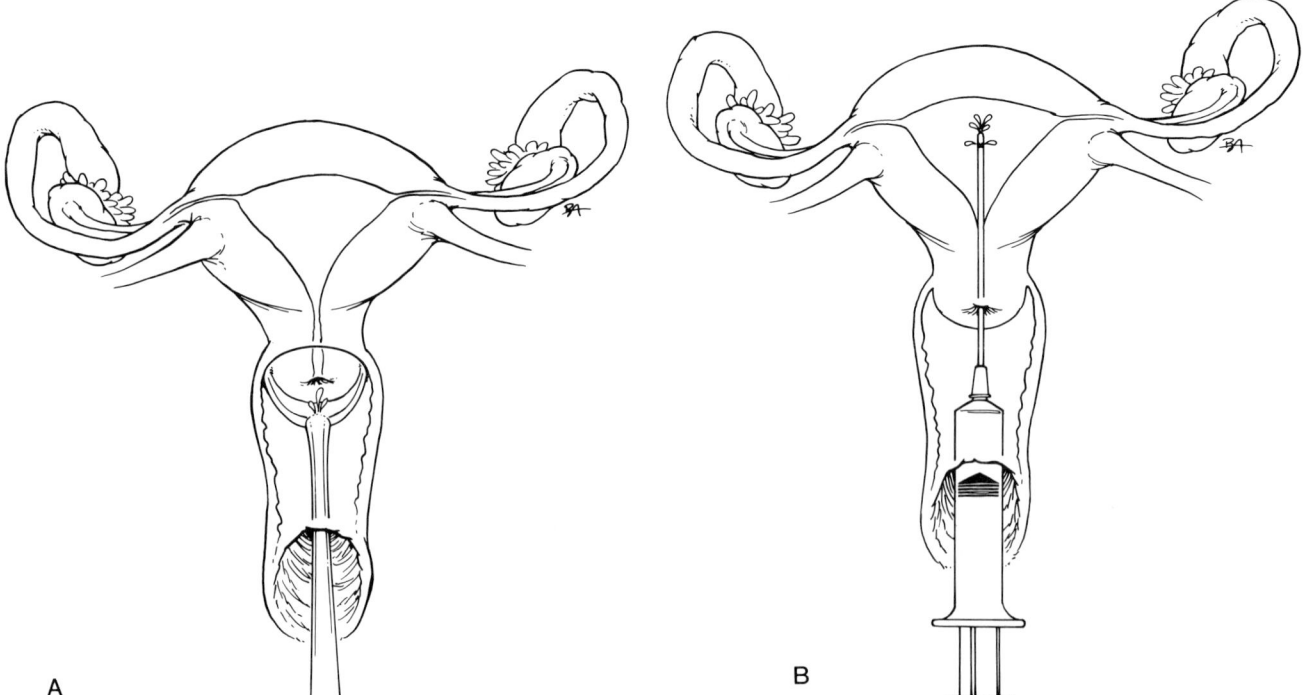

Figure 29–2
Forms of insemination. A, Cervical cup. A cervical cup is used to introduce semen into the cervix. The stem can be used to introduce sperm and also serves as a handle for withdrawal. B, Intrauterine insemination. Washed sperm are introduced into the uterine cavity.

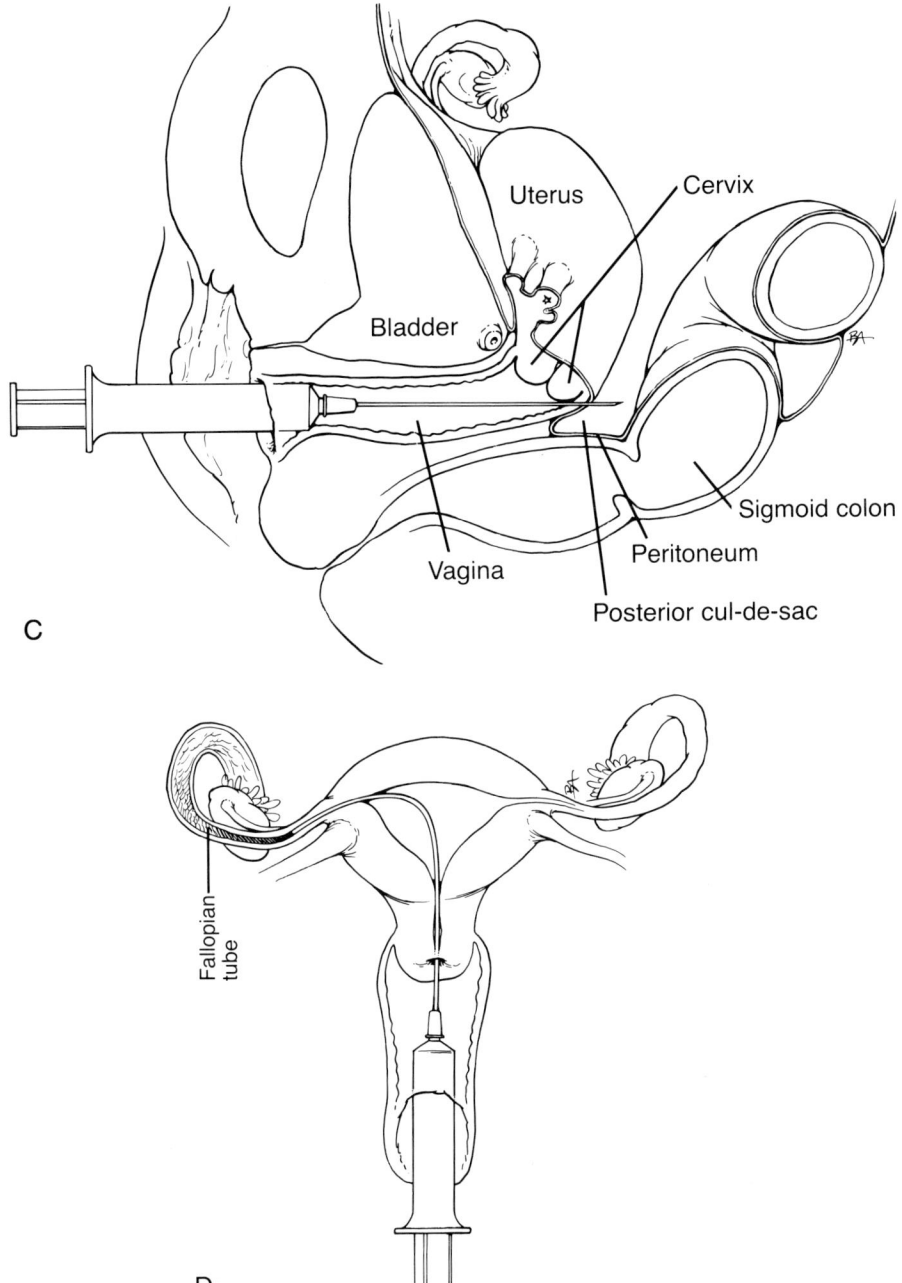

Figure 29–2 *Continued*
C, Intraperitoneal insemination. Washed sperm are introduced into the cul-de-sac. *D*, Intratubal insemination. A small volume of washed sperm are introduced into the ampullary fallopian tube, transcervically.

dometriosis, and possibly male factor infertility.[7-9] The term controlled ovarian hyperstimulation distinguishes the therapeutic production of several mature oocytes from ovarian hyperstimulation syndrome, a complication of menotropin therapy. Although the effectiveness of IUI for male factor infertility has been questioned,[10] most authors conclude that the procedure is indicated when there is poor penetration of the sperm through the cervical mucus.

Concern about human immunodeficiency virus (HIV) contamination of donated semen has mandated the cryopreservation of semen with a 6-month quarantine.[11] Compromised pregnancy rates have been reported following cervical insemination with cryopreserved semen. For this reason, some authors have suggested that all cryopreserved semen be inseminated into the uterus.[12]

Technique

Unprocessed semen can safely be deposited into the cervical canal, but the introduction of semen into the uterus is associated with intense cramping, hypotension, and infection. Therefore, only processed semen, in which the seminal plasma has been removed and the spermatozoa have been resuspended in tissue culture media, can safely be used for IUI. Sperm washing removes not only seminal plasma but also bacteria from the spermatozoa. In cases of oligo-asthenospermia, techniques to extract a concentrated, motile fraction of sperm may be employed ("swim-up"). A detailed description of the sperm washing technique is available in the IVF literature.[13] Unfortunately, sperm washing is ineffective for the removal of antibodies bound to sperm as a result of the avid binding of antisperm antibodies.

Insemination catheters allow the transfer of spermatozoa directly into the uterine cavity. One catheter, designed by Makler, has a round tip and side ports for injection (see Fig. 29–2B). The rigidity of the catheter allows for easy passage of the catheter into the uterus without cervical manipulation. It is important not to cleanse the cervix with spermicidal materials such as povidone-iodine (Betadine), or lubricants.[14] Catheters produced by Rocket of London consist of a 4 Fr catheter and a rigid cervical introducer (Fig. 29–3A). Another catheter commonly utilized for this purpose is the Tom Cat catheter (Sherwood Medical, St. Louis, MO) (Fig. 29–3B). This catheter is a simple device consisting of a flexible 3.5 Fr polyethylene tubing. The catheter is rigid and maintains a memory that allows a gentle curve to be placed into the tip. Alternatively, cervical traction with a tenaculum will straighten the cervical canal and allow introduction of the catheter.

With the patient in the lithotomy position, the insemination catheter is introduced beyond the cervix into the endometrial cavity. Attention to the depth of insertion confirms that the catheter has traversed the cervical canal and resides in the endometrial cavity before the sperm are expelled. If the internal os cannot be traversed, a catheter employing a cervical introducer may be utilized (Fig. 29–4). When injecting the sperm, it is important to remember that volumes in excess of 0.5 ml will usually be expelled through the cervix.

Intraperitoneal Insemination

Intraperitoneal insemination (IPI) may be indicated when IUI fails[15] (see Fig. 29–2C). In this technique, washed semen is injected through the posterior fornix into the pouch of Douglas. If intraperitoneal

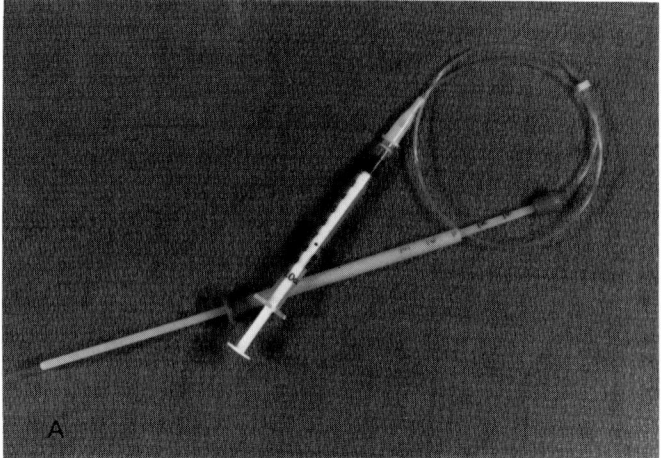
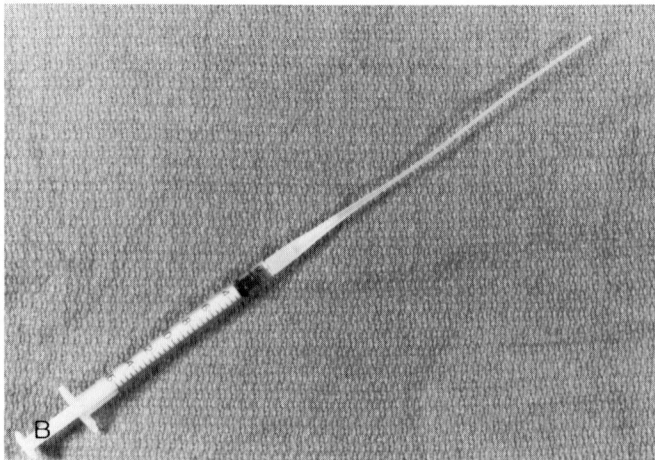

Figure 29–3
Insemination catheters. A, The catheter provided by Rocket consists of a rigid cervical introducer and a flexible polyethylene tubing. B, The Tom Cat catheter consists of a 3.5 Fr polyethylene tubing.

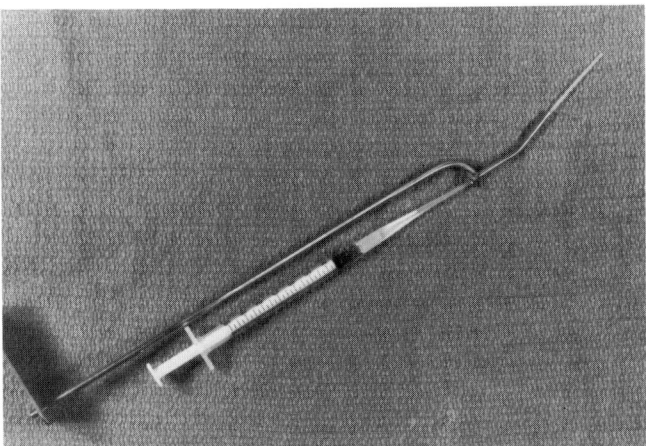

Figure 29–4
Tom Cat catheter with cervical introducer. When the catheter does not pass readily through the internal os an introducer may be employed to guide the catheter through the cervix.

sperm gain entry into the fallopian tube, fertilization may occur. Success rates of 15–40% are reported, but IPI is a newer addition to ART and there are no controlled studies demonstrating its effectiveness.[16] Its major advantage is the lower level of technology necessary when compared with intratubal insemination.

Intratubal Insemination

Patient Selection

Fertilization normally occurs in the ampullary fallopian tube, and deposition of spermatozoa into the ampulla is the ultimate goal of all insemination techniques. Jansen and colleagues described a transcervical technique that directly placed sperm into the fallopian tube under ultrasound guidance.[17] This procedure introduces a catheter into the interstitial portion of the tube, transcervically (see Fig. 29–2D). The catheter can be advanced into the ampullary fallopian tube, where sperm can be expelled.

The indications for fallopian tube insemination are identical to those for intrauterine insemination. A prerequisite for this procedure is normalcy of the fallopian tube. Because the technique is relatively new, success rates are impossible to calculate. As the success rate becomes apparent, intratubal insemination may become a viable alternative to more invasive fallopian tube transfer techniques such as GIFT.

Technique

A major limitation of transcervical ultrasound-guided tubal catheterization is the poor echogenicity of the fallopian tube. The junction of the endometrial cavity and interstitial tube, however, is apparent by transvaginal sonography. Following the endometrial cavity to the fundus of the uterus places the catheter in the tubal ostia. Current catheters are being modified with enhanced echogenicity to aid visibility when the catheter has passed beyond the uterus and is in the fallopian tube. A characteristic loss of resistance is described by both the patient and the physician as the interstitial tube is traversed. Most catheters consist of a coaxial system in which a rigid introducer is placed into the endometrial cavity up to the fundus. A flexible catheter measuring 1–3 Fr is passed through the introducer and into the tube. The fallopian tube can only accommodate a small volume of sperm, and volumes in excess of 80 µl will be expelled into the peritoneal cavity.

IN VITRO FERTILIZATION

Patient Selection

IVF was originally developed for patients with absent or irreparably damaged fallopian tubes. As IVF evolved, its indications widened. Currently, IVF is performed to treat disorders such as unexplained infertility, immunologic infertility, male factor infertility, and endometriosis. The minimal requirements for successful IVF is a normal uterine cavity, a source of oocytes, and enough sperm to achieve fertilization. A brief list of indications is included in this chapter (Table 29–1 and Fig. 29–5).

Tubal Disease

Tubal damage secondary to infection accounts for 20–30% of female infertility.[18] Microsurgical techniques have resulted in favorable outcomes for many types of tubal disease, but surgery for severely damaged fallopian tubes does not commonly result in pregnancy. Factors associated with poor results following surgical repair include dense adnexal adhesions, fixation of the ovary and tube, absence of fimbriae, bipolar disease, and massive dilatation of the fallopian tube.[19] Repeated attempts at corrective surgery are also associated with poor outcomes,[20] and better success can be achieved through IVF.

In some cases, better success can be achieved through surgery than by IVF. For example, sterilization procedures that retain more than 6 cm of the fallopian tube and preserve the fimbriae are best treated with a microsurgical anastomosis. A midsegment anastomosis offers pregnancy rates of over 60%, whereas a tubocornual anastomosis results in pregnancy in 45–50% of patients.[21] In distal tubal disease, when the fimbriae are preserved and the tube is not dilated, lysis of adhesions may be fol-

Table 29–1
Diagnostic Categories and Indications for Assisted Reproductive Technology (ART)

Etiology of Infertility	COH + IUI	IVF	GIFT	Ovum Donation
Tubal disease	Not helpful	Indicated	Mild disease	For inaccessible ovaries
Unexplained	Indicated	Indicated	Indicated	For oocyte abnormalities
Male factor	Mild disease	Indicated	Mild disease	—
Endometriosis	Mild disease	Indicated	Mild disease	—
Immunologic	Indicated	Indicated	?	—
DES	Indicated	Indicated	Indicated	—
Cervical factor	Indicated	Indicated	Indicated	—
Ovarian failure	Not helpful	Not helpful	Not helpful	Indicated
Resistant anovulation	—	Indicated	Probably indicated	Possibly indicated

COH, controlled ovarian hyperstimulation; IUI, intrauterine insemination; IVF, in vitro fertilization; GIFT, gamete intrafallopian transfer; DES, diethylstilbestrol. Modified from Navot D, Laufer N: Assisted reproductive technology. J Repro Med 1989; 34:3.

lowed by pregnancy in over 50% of individuals.[22] Because even several cycles of IVF cannot match these success rates, microsurgical anastomosis is a better choice under these circumstances.

Endometriosis

Endometriosis is present in 20–40% of women with infertility.[23] The mechanism of infertility in severe disease is due to mechanical impedance of oocyte pickup. In mild disease, the etiology of infertility is less clear. Theories that have been presented include luteal phase dysfunction, abnormal intraperitoneal macrophage function, and possibly premature luteinization of follicles.[24] Surgical correction of severe disease results in pregnancy rates of 30–40%,[23] rates that compete favorably with IVF. Mild endometriosis has been shown by Seibel and associates to have similar success when managed expectantly as when managed with danazol.[25]

Following surgical or medical failure, patients with endometriosis may be treated with ART. Those

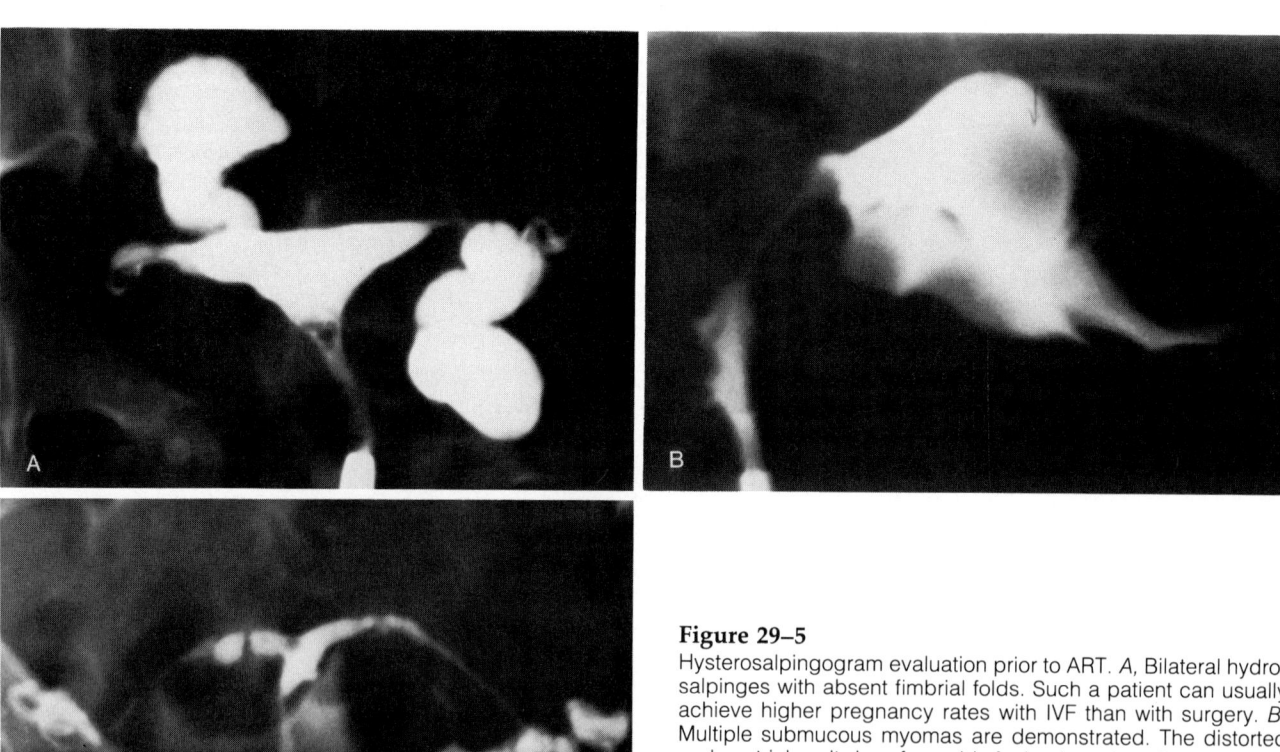

Figure 29–5
Hysterosalpingogram evaluation prior to ART. A, Bilateral hydrosalpinges with absent fimbrial folds. Such a patient can usually achieve higher pregnancy rates with IVF than with surgery. B, Multiple submucous myomas are demonstrated. The distorted endometrial cavity is unfavorable for implantation. C, A T-shaped uterus characteristic of diethylstilbestrol (DES) exposure. This uterus carries an unfavorable prognosis for sustained pregnancy.

patients who have undergone IVF are able to achieve normal fertilization and pregnancy rates, regardless of the extent of their disease.[26]

Unexplained Infertility

Fifteen per cent of infertile couples will not have a cause of their infertility identified, despite exhaustive investigation. Over 50% of these couples will become pregnant without therapy after 4 years.[27] In such couples, superovulation with intrauterine insemination is able to achieve a fecundity of 7–19% per cycle.[7, 8] When medical therapy fails, ART is usually attempted. Furthermore, when no explanation is apparent for infertility, IVF is important diagnostically as well as therapeutically. Fertilization failure is demonstrated in 14% of couples with unexplained infertility.[28]

Male Factor Infertility

IVF allows close approximation of sperm and oocytes, so that fewer sperm are necessary to achieve fertilization. Unfortunately, some sperm will be unable to fertilize oocytes even under ideal conditions. When fewer than 1 million motile sperm per ejaculate are available for insemination following semen processing, fertilization rates will usually be compromised.[29] Fortunately, once fertilization has been achieved, implantation rates are normal.[30]

Many women seeking ART for male factor infertility will have normal fallopian tubes. As a result, this group composes a large proportion of patients undergoing fallopian tube transfer.

Immunologic

Women whose serum contains antibodies directed against spermatozoa will have fewer oocytes fertilized than individuals whose serum does not contain antibodies.[31] Substituting serum with either bovine albumin or serum that does not contain antibodies will restore fertilization to normal. Antisperm antibodies do not seem to affect implantation, because normal pregnancy rates are usually achieved when embryos are transferred into the uterus.[32]

Ovarian Failure

Pregnancies have been reported to occur spontaneously and on estrogen replacement[33] in women with ovarian failure, but the fecundity is low. A more productive maneuver to achieve pregnancy is to provide oocytes to the patient from a fertile donor. Because the recipient's endometrium is stimulated under controlled conditions and the oocytes are retrieved from younger individuals, these patients are able to achieve pregnancy rates comparable with the most favorable group undergoing IVF-ET.[34]

Techniques

Follicular Recruitment and Timing of Oocyte Retrieval

The first human pregnancy conceived in vitro was achieved through the retrieval of an oocyte that matured in a natural cycle. This method is inefficient because of difficulties in synchronizing oocyte retrieval with the spontaneous LH surge. Furthermore, efficiency is improved when more than one embryo is transferred into the endometrial cavity. Although the natural cycle is still utilized for certain disorders,[35] human chorionic gonadotropin (hCG) is usually used along with controlled ovarian hyperstimulation to mature several oocytes and to time oocyte retrieval (Fig. 29–6). This allows for oocyte maturation without premature LH surges. Ovarian stimulation is continued until the follicles measure at least 15 mm on ultrasound examination. Follicles smaller than 11 mm rarely contain mature oocytes.[36] Oocyte retrieval is timed to an injection of hCG, which is administered 34–36 hours prior to oocyte retrieval.

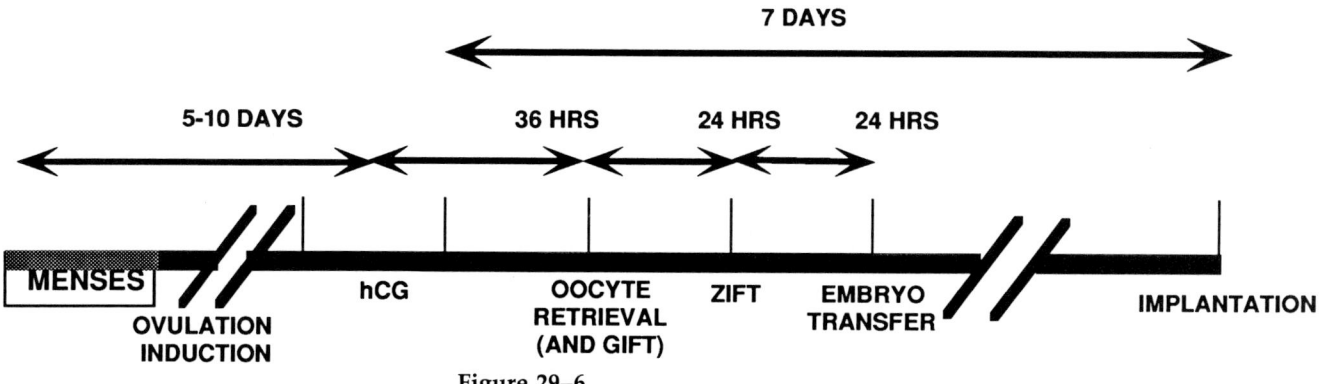

Figure 29–6
Timing of assisted reproductive technology.

Laparoscopic Oocyte Aspiration

The oocyte that ultimately resulted in a live birth in 1978 was retrieved through a laparoscopic procedure. A major limitation of this technique is that the ovary is inaccessible when there are dense peritoneal adhesions. Furthermore, general anesthesia is required for laparoscopic oocyte retrieval. The laparoscopic technique is able to recover oocytes from 60–90% of follicles.[37]

When laparoscopy is utilized to retrieve oocytes, the lithotomy position is not routinely used (Fig. 29–7). Uterine manipulation is avoided during assisted reproductive cycles so that the endometrium will not be disrupted. At least two punctures are employed, with the second puncture placed in the midline above the pubic symphysis. A self-retaining grasping forceps is used to grasp the utero-ovarian ligament, allowing ovarian manipulation and providing access to the entire surface of the ovary. Care is exercised when manipulating the ovary so that follicles do not rupture. When the ovary is densely adherent to adjacent structures, it is more prudent to switch to a transvaginal ultrasound-guided oocyte retrieval than to lyse adhesions and risk follicular rupture.

The oocyte aspiration needle is usually placed in the midline midway between the pubic bone and the umbilicus. The ovaries are turned so that the maximum diameter of the follicle is presented to the aspiration needle. Suction with a controlled suction device is begun prior to entry into the follicle. The follicular fluid is usually straw colored when aspiration begins, but rapidly becomes bloody as the follicle empties. A gentle curettage of the follicle wall is performed with the aspiration needle to remove oocytes that may be adherent. The ovary should be mapped by the operator, because follicles rapidly fill with blood and may appear to be unpunctured. Follicles that yield only blood have usually already been emptied.

Some bleeding is invariably observed from the site of follicle puncture. This rarely requires more than observation to ensure that hemostasis is achieved. Aspiration of the cul-de-sac will help identify persistent bleeders.

Ultrasound-Guided Oocyte Aspiration

Transabdominal Ultrasound. The first attempt at recovering oocytes under ultrasound guidance was reported by Lenz and Lauritsen, who described a technique that traversed the full bladder and entered the ovary at the posterior vesical wall.[38] This procedure was a major advance because of the diminished anesthesia requirement and because ovaries that could not be reached by other techniques were now accessible. Transvesical puncture is, however, associated with cystitis and hematuria. Furthermore, the procedure has limitations when the ovary is adherent behind the uterus and is inaccessible. Since the advent of transvaginal ultrasound-guided oocyte retrieval, this procedure is rarely utilized.

Transabdominal oocyte retrieval can be performed under either a conductive anesthesia or sedation. The bladder is emptied and is then filled with ap-

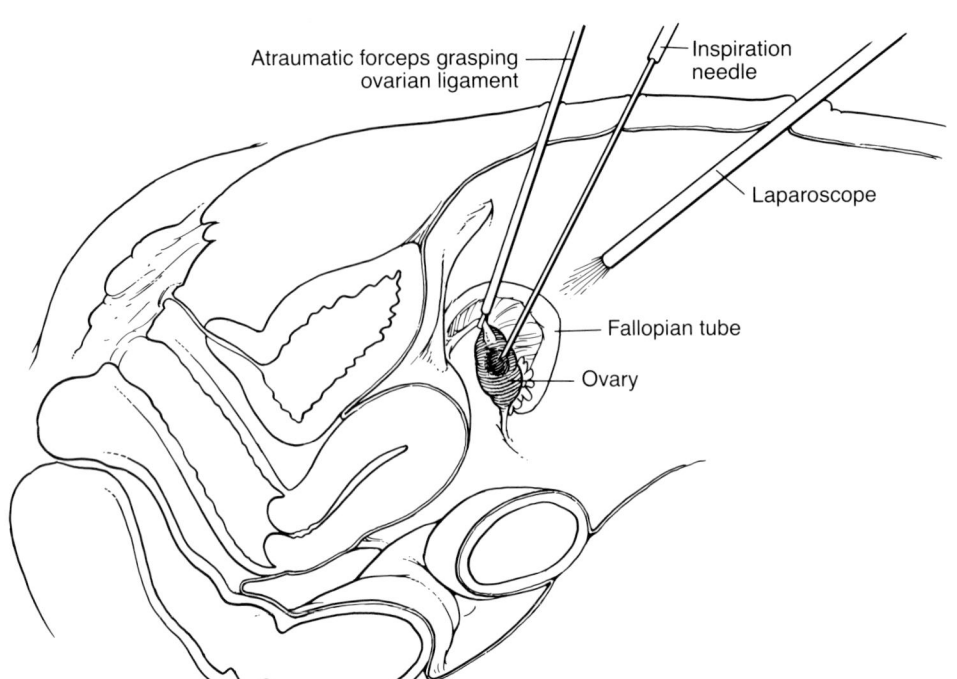

Figure 29–7
Laparoscopic follicle aspiration. The laparoscope is placed through the umbilicus. A grasping forceps is placed suprapubically. The aspiration needle is placed midway between the other two instruments.

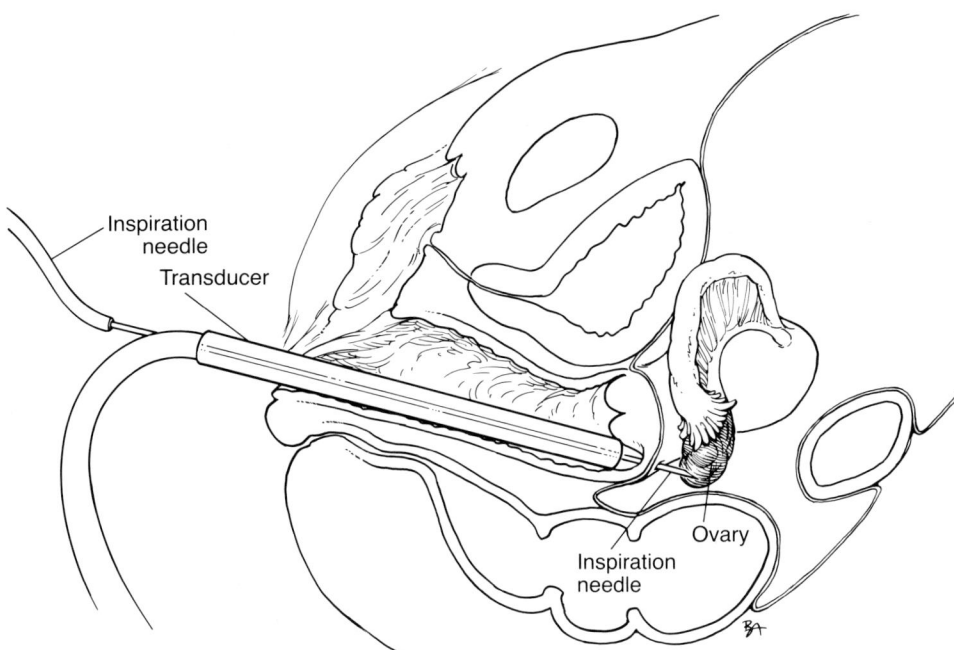

Figure 29–8
Transvaginal ultrasound-guided follicle aspiration. The ovary is entered through the posterior fornix. The ovary usually is located in the cul-de-sac, even when there are dense peritoneal adhesions.

proximately 500 ml of physiologic saline. An abdominal transducer (3.5 MHz) with a fixed needle guide is used. A stab wound is made through the abdominal wall to facilitate needle entry. The needle traverses the anterior and posterior bladder walls and enters the ovary. The bladder is emptied following completion of the procedure, and a Foley catheter is left in place for several hours, until clear urine is obtained.

Transvaginal Ultrasound. A major improvement in oocyte recovery occurred with the advent of endovaginal ultrasound[39] (Fig. 29–8). The proximity of the transducer to the pelvic organs allowed the use of higher-frequency transducers with a resultant increase in resolution. Furthermore, the absence of bowel gas in the cul-de-sac allows for direct visualization of the ovaries without the need for bladder filling to act as a sonic window. Oocyte recovery rates with this technique compare favorably with direct visualization of the ovary under laparoscopy.[37] In fact, under certain conditions, such as when the ovary is severely hyperstimulated, follicles present within the substance of the ovary can be visualized better under ultrasound guidance.

Dense pelvic adhesions are no longer a barrier to oocyte recovery, because the ovary is usually fixed to the cul-de-sac immediately adjacent to the vaginal fornix. Under certain circumstances, the ovary may be adherent to the fundus of the uterus and may be difficult to reach transvaginally. Alternatives such as laparoscopic, transvesical, or transurethral retrievals may be utilized as a backup, but the authors prefer to use a vaginal approach in all cases. Ovaries that are adherent to the fundus of the uterus can be reached through a transmyometrial approach.

Patients undergoing transvaginal ultrasound-guided oocyte aspiration are placed in the lithotomy position following adequate sedation. General anesthesia is unnecessary, and a combination of midazolam (1–4 mg) and fentanyl (50–200 µg) is utilized. If an anesthesiologist is present, supplementation with barbiturates provides ideal sedation in difficult cases.

A 5–7.5 MHz transvaginal transducer with a fixed needle guide is utilized. The needle that the authors prefer for this procedure is a 17-gauge, 11-inch long needle. Scoring the tip enhances echogenicity and allows visualization under ultrasound. The authors have found that scoring the needle with a file achieves superior visualization to commercially scored echo tip needles.

A vinyl glove filled with Aquasonics sterile jelly as a coupling material is used as a probe cover. Vaginal cleansing is necessary to limit infectious complications from the procedure.[40] The authors have found that cleansing the vagina with povidone-iodine (Betadine), followed by copious saline irrigation, does not affect oocyte health. The needle traverses the vaginal fornix and enters each follicle individually. As with laparoscopic retrievals, the follicular fluid is first straw colored and later becomes bloody. There is little confusion between follicles already emptied, because blood-filled follicles appear echogenic under ultrasound. Each follicle is aspirated separately until all follicles are emptied. The needle is left in each follicle and is rotated to ensure that complete emptying is achieved. A single vaginal

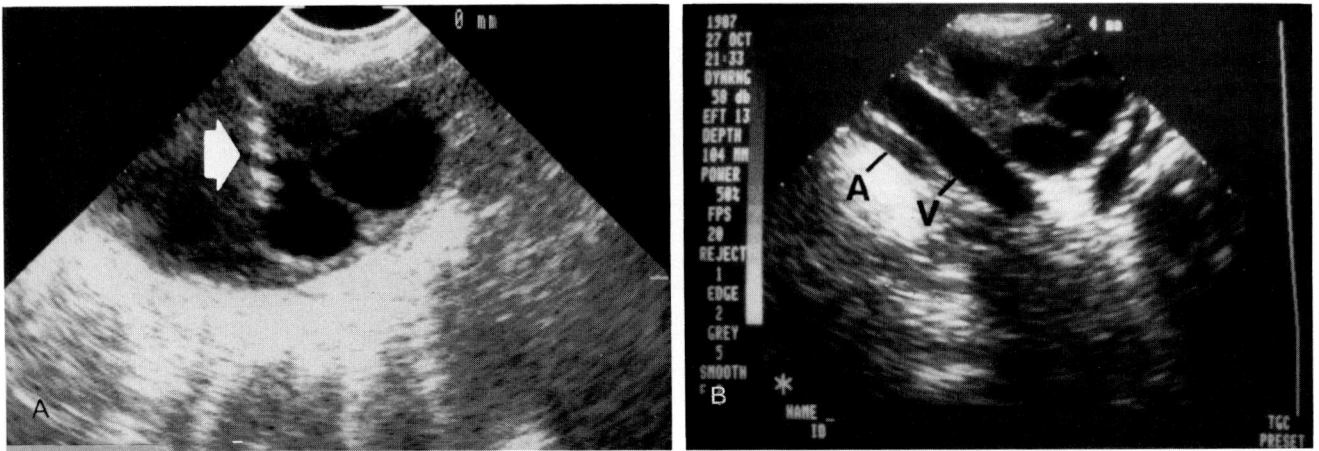

Figure 29-9
A, The ovary is demonstrated on transvaginal sonography. The needle is easily visualized in the ovary (arrow). B, The ovary is usually located near the hypogastric vessels (A, artery; V, vein). Care is exercised in transvaginal oocyte retrieval to avoid these structures.

puncture is usually adequate for each ovary, but multiple passes within the ovary may be necessary. Manipulation of the transducer allows visualization of the entire ovary without the need for a separate puncture.

Occasionally, ultrasonic monitoring detects the needle inside the follicle but fluid is not aspirated. One cause for this is clogging of the aspiration needle with blood clots. More often, however, this is an artifact of superimposition of the needle next to a follicle with the follicular contents. It is important to maximally demonstrate the follicle prior to its puncture so that the needle approaches the center of the follicle.

The hypogastric vessels are a reliable landmark usually found lateral to the ovary (Fig. 29-9). It is best to traverse the ovary parallel to the hypogastric vessels to avoid injury. When a perpendicular ap-

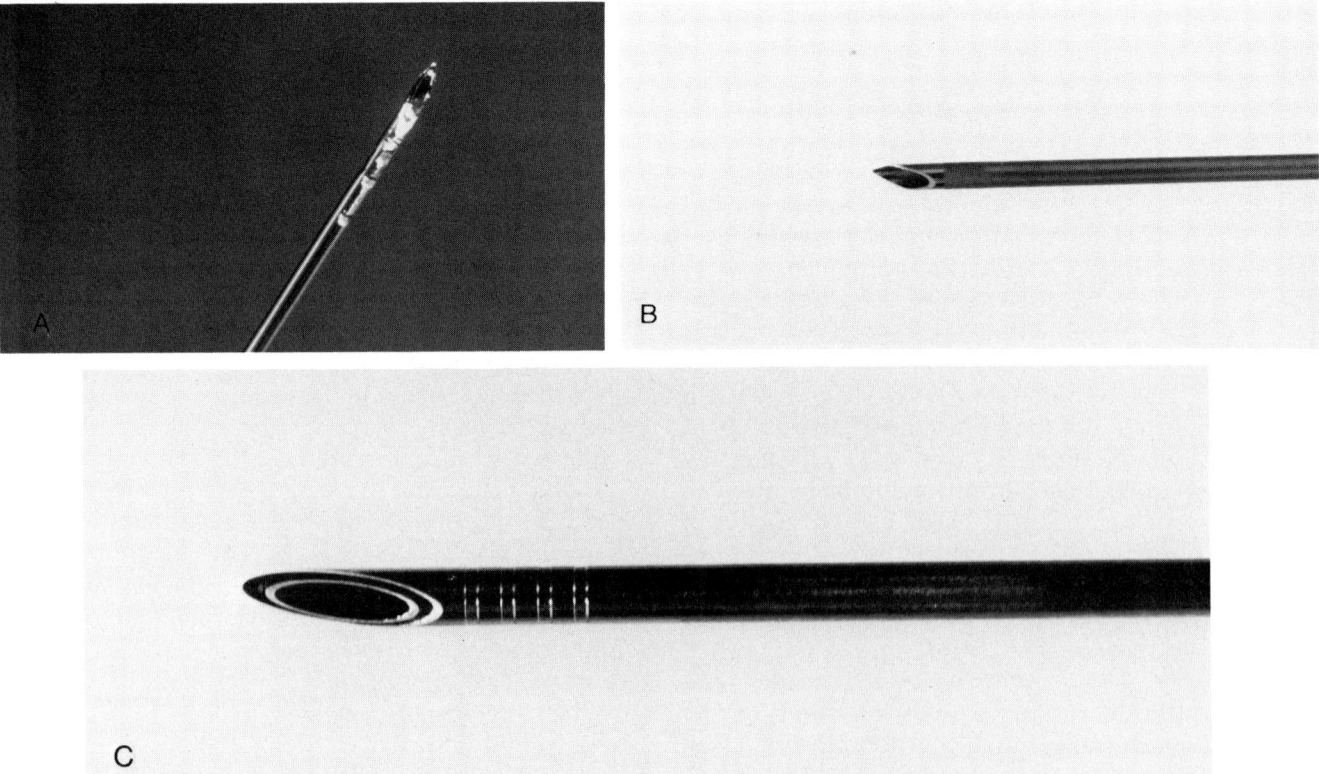

Figure 29-10
Oocyte aspiration needles. A, Single-lumen needle. The markings are mechanically scored and provide excellent echogenicity under ultrasound. B, Single-lumen needle. Commercial scoring. C, Double-lumen needle. The outer channel is used for flushing the follicles.

proach is necessary, care should be exercised not to traverse the vessels. Because the needle tip is visible at all times, avoidance of vascular structures is possible.

Aspiration Needles

Needles used for oocyte recovery are designed to maximize oocyte yield (Fig. 29–10). Too small a needle will traumatize the oocyte, whereas too large a diameter risks trauma to the ovary. Jones and colleagues found that a 2.16-mm (14-gauge) needle yielded more oocytes than when a 1.2-mm needle was used for laparoscopic oocyte retrieval.[41] The texture of the needle is also important, because fine needles with 1.4-mm inner diameters were found to be more efficient than coarse needles with diameters of 2.2 mm.[42] Double-lumen needles allow flushing of the follicles under continuous flow while aspiration is being performed. Under routine conditions, the complexity of this set-up is not rewarded with increased oocyte yields.[43] When single follicles are punctured, such as in the natural cycle, double-lumen needles are utilized.

The authors' program performs laparoscopic oocyte retrievals only when they are combined with other laparoscopic procedures such as GIFT and the ovary is inaccessible vaginally. A 14-gauge needle is utilized for laparoscopic oocyte retrieval. This set-up consists of the needle connected to sterile extension tubing. Fluid is collected in a DeLee suction trap. An oocyte recovery rate of 83% has been demonstrated with this apparatus[38] (Fig. 29–11). Various other commercially manufactured needles and suction traps are available. Suction is attached to the collection trap to maintain a controlled suction of approximately 100 mm Hg. Pressures higher than 200 mm Hg are associated with damaged oocytes.[44]

Anesthesia

Laparoscopic procedures are usually performed under general anesthesia, whereas ultrasound-guided follicle aspiration requires less analgesia. Transvesical puncture of the ovary was originally performed with local anesthesia and sedation, although some authors recommend regional anesthesia.[45] Transvaginal procedures are usually performed under sedation.[46] When only a single follicle is punctured, the procedure can be performed comfortably with no anesthesia except for local infiltration of the vaginal fornix.[47] Although 90% of patients found sedatives to be effective analgesia, some patients do require heavier analgesia. Hammarberg and colleagues found that 70% of patients achieved acceptable pain relief with premedication, 20% required additional sedatives, and 10% required heavier sedation.[48] For this reason, the authors prefer to perform all ultrasound-guided follicle aspiration in an operating room where analgesia is monitored by an anesthesiologist.

The oocytes seem to perform equally well when general anesthesia is administered as they do with regional techniques. Fertilization rates, embryo cleavage rates, and pregnancy rates are comparable in all studies whether embryo retrieval is performed laparoscopically under general anesthesia or vaginally under sedation, or under regional anesthesia.[13]

Complications

Dellenbach and associates have reported no major complications in over 800 transvaginal procedures,[49] although pelvic infections occurred in approximately 1–3% of procedures performed by Howe and colleagues.[50] In order to minimize the risk of infection, some authors have recommended prophylactic antibiotics.[51] Additionally, every attempt should be made to avoid entry into hydrosalpinges or endometriomas. Vaginal preparation followed by vigorous saline flush is also recommended. Initial concerns about oocyte toxicity in transvaginal punctures were allayed once pregnancy rates comparable with those of laparoscopic oocyte retrieval were achieved.

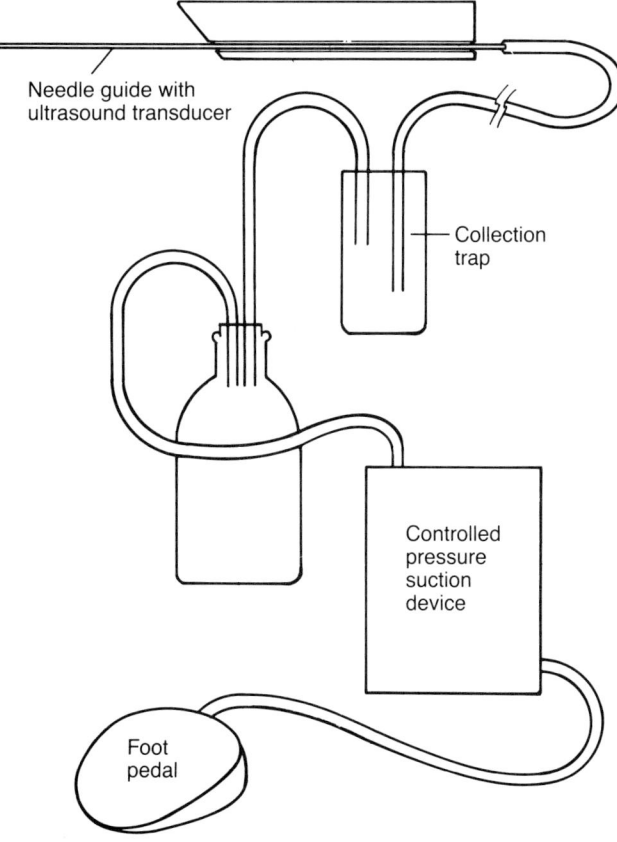

Figure 29–11
Instruments required for ultrasound-guided follicle aspiration. The needle is attached to a needle guide that is fixed to the ultrasound transducer. Fluid is collected in a specimen trap under controlled suction pressure.

Major hemorrhage occurs infrequently, and when hemoperitoneum does occur, bleeding tends to originate in the ovarian cortex. In a series of 181 retrievals, Evers and associates reported bleeding from the vaginal puncture site in 24% of cases, but only in 2 cases (0.5%) did the bleeding require intervention.[52] The hypogastric vessels are clearly visualized and avoided with transvaginal ultrasound scanning, but one case of traumatic injury to the ureter has been reported.[53] The hypogastric vessels serve as a reliable landmark for localizing the ovary, which usually is found medial to these structures.

Transvesical oocyte retrieval poses the additional complication of bladder puncture. Although this procedure has been replaced by transvaginal ultrasound, it may still be considered in cases in which the ovary is difficult to reach because it is adherent to the fundus of the uterus. When transvesical oocyte retrieval is employed, there is a 5% incidence of hematuria and urinary tract infection added to the risks previously described for transvaginal ultrasound-guided techniques.[54]

Ovarian hyperstimulation syndrome occurs more commonly when ovaries are aggressively stimulated, such as in the newer stimulation protocols. This complication is felt to be reduced when oocyte aspiration is performed because of the aspiration of granulosa cells. Nevertheless, cases of severe hyperstimulation syndrome requiring hospitalization have been reported.[55, 56] Safety limits for ovarian hyperstimulation and oocyte retrieval are not yet available.

EMBRYO TRANSFER (ET)

Oocyte retrieval is relatively efficient, with recovery rates of 60–90%.[13] When sperm are normal, 70% of oocytes will be fertilized in vitro and will be available for ET. The transfer step is less effective, with pregnancy rates of 20% or less per ET procedure. The reasons for this are poorly understood and may be due to deficiencies in embryo quality or endometrial receptivity.

Implantation failure following ET may be an expression of the fundamental inefficiency of human reproduction. Twenty five per cent of fertile couples will become pregnant following a single cycle of unprotected coitus.[57] Thus, IVF-ET technology results in success rates comparable with those achieved in nature.

Timing of Transfer

In natural conceptions, the embryo reaches the uterus at the 8–16 cell stage, approximately 96 hours from the peak LH surge.[58, 59] ET following in vitro fertilization occurs at the 2–6 cell stage, which is 84 hours from hCG injection. Mitotic arrest frequently occurs by day 3 in culture,[57] and any advantage achieved in culturing embryos for an additional day is offset by the loss of embryos, owing to inadequate culture conditions. Transfer of embryos at a less advanced stage does not appear to adversely affect implantation. Similar pregnancy rates are achieved when transfers are performed at 24 and 48 hours following oocyte retrieval (60–84 hours post-hCG).[60] The authors perform embryo transfers 48 hours after oocyte retrieval to allow morphologic assessment of embryo quality.

In addition to the stage of embryo development, endometrial receptivity is important in the timing of ET. Based on data derived from the replacement of donor embryos, the window of uterine receptivity for 2–12 cell embryos appears to be days 16–19 (48–120 hours) from LH peak.[61]

Instruments

ET is performed utilizing a transcervical approach to the endometrial cavity. Many devices are available to deliver the embryos through the cervical os and into the uterus. The authors' program utilizes the Tom Cat catheter, which was first introduced for use in humans by Kerin and coworkers in 1981[62] (see Fig. 29–4). The catheter is 11.5 cm in length with a 1-mm external diameter at the tip. This widens to 3 mm at the 8 cm mark. The base opening is 6 mm in diameter and easily fits into a 1-ml plastic disposable syringe. It is made of polyethylene and demonstrates no toxic effects on embryos.

Another commonly used catheter was developed by Jones and coworkers, who reported considerable success utilizing a side-loaded 20-gauge Teflon catheter that is inserted through a steel inducer.[63] This catheter is larger (1.47 mm external diameter) and more rigid than the Tom Cat and is often successful when there is an acute angle to the endocervical canal that cannot be negotiated by the Tom Cat. In general, larger volumes (i.e., 50–90 µl of media) are required to load the Jones catheter, and this may be associated with increased risk of ectopic pregnancy.[64]

Although there are reports of transfundal, ultrasonically guided transfer of human embryos (which required either general anesthesia or intravenous sedation)[65] and of transcervical replacement of embryos utilizing general anesthesia in order to relax the uterus and/or patient during the procedure,[66] success rates are no higher than with nonsurgical, transcervical ET under no sedation.

Patient Position

Initially, the most common practice was to place the patient in a position that resulted in dependency of the uterine fundus.[57] Subsequently, it was found that there was no difference in pregnancy rates between the two patient positions.[67] Because most patients are far more comfortable supine, the authors routinely perform all of their transfers with the patient in the lithotomy position.

Most programs recommend some period of rest following the ET; however, there is no consensus regarding the proper duration. The authors' patients remain in bed for 4 hours following transfer. There is tremendous variation among programs, and studies are unavailable demonstrating proper activity level following ET.

Technique

The authors recommend beginning with a "dry run," during which time an empty catheter is introduced into the fundus. The patient is placed in the lithotomy position with 15–20 degrees of Trendelenburg. A sterile bivalve speculum is placed in the vagina, and the cervix is washed with sterile culture media.

The Tom Cat catheter has a slight curve, which can be easily adjusted to a more acute angle, if necessary, to negotiate the cervical canal. In general, the Tom Cat easily and gently passes into the uterine cavity and the operator can feel when the internal os is negotiated. When difficulty is encountered passing through the internal os, placement of a tenaculum on the cervix and providing gentle traction to straighten the cervical canal may help pass the catheter into the uterus. If this maneuver fails, a metal introducer can be used to help guide the catheter past the internal os (see Fig. 29–4).

Once the "dry run" has been successful and the operator is certain he or she can easily guide the Tom Cat into the proper position, a new Tom Cat is loaded. Embryos are suspended in 50% serum supplemented medium to enhance stickiness (Fig. 29–12). The column with the embryos (20–30 µl) is placed between two smaller columns of medium (5–10 µl) and air (5–10 µl). Some investigators suggest that by completely filling the syringe and the catheter with medium, there is a greater control of the volume injected (i.e., the air column is not compressed behind the embryos) and the incidence of retained embryos is decreased.[68] In the authors' experience, most cases of retained embryos are associated with release of pressure on the plunger of the syringe prior to withdrawal, or with contact by the tip of the Tom Cat with the uterine fundus and subsequent "plugging" of the catheter tip prior to depositing the embryos.

Low embryo transfers result in pregnancies as commonly as high embryo transfers,[69] but high insertion of the transfer catheter (on or quite near the uterine fundus) is associated with a higher ectopic pregnancy rate.[70] When depositing the embryos, the operator must be careful to hold the plunger of the syringe tightly against the base of the catheter so that a vacuum is not created whereby the embryos can be aspirated back into the catheter.

After the transfer has been completed, the catheter and syringe are examined under the microscope to detect retained embryos. If embryos are discovered, the catheter is reloaded and the transfer repeated. Examination of the transfer catheter as well as the cervical mucus in women immediately following ET revealed embryos in 17% of transfers, with 40% of these retained in the cervical mucus.[71] Apparently, embryo loss is caused by their adherence to mucus on the sides of the catheter, allowing them to get "dragged" out upon withdrawal of the catheter.

Number of Embryos

Numerous statistical analyses and mathematical models have been proposed in order to determine the optimal number of embryos to transfer.[72, 73] Improved pregnancy rates achieved with the transfer of many embryos are offset by the increased risk for multifetal gestation. It appears from these analyses that only 10% of embryos have the potential to produce pregnancy.

Multiple ET improves pregnancy rates,[57] but this benefit must be weighed against the risk for multiple gestation. In general, it appears that the transfer of four embryos will provide a 25% pregnancy rate with a twinning rate of 15% and a triplet rate of 2–5%. The risk of multiple gestation is very real in the age of new reproductive technology, and the management of such an outcome is addressed in the section Multifetal Pregnancy Reduction.

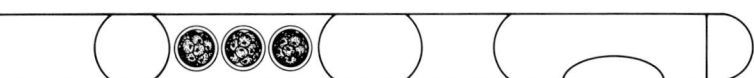

Figure 29–12
Embryo transfer catheter. The embryos are loaded in the transfer catheter in between two small bubbles of air. This allows easy visualization of the transferred medium to ensure that the embryos are expelled. (From Haselten F, Laufer N: *In vitro* fertilization. In DeCherney AH, Polan ML (eds.): Reproductive Surgery. Chicago, Year Book Medical Publishers, 1987, p. 314.)

GAMETE INTRAFALLOPIAN TRANSFER (GIFT)

Patient Selection

Asch and colleagues demonstrated that in patients with at least one normal fallopian tube, transferring gametes in the ampullary portion of the tube (gamete intrafallopian transfer [GIFT]) achieved higher pregnancy rates than those for IVF.[74] The likely mechanism for the improved pregnancy rate is the physiologic synchronization of ET to the stage of endometrium development. In IVF, embryos are usually transferred to the endometrial cavity on day 17.5 of the cycle at the 2–8 cell stage (3.5 days following hCG administration). Normally, embryos enter the endometrial cavity as late morulas or early blastocysts on day 19–20.[58] The longer residence of embryos fertilized in the ampullary fallopian tube may allow for healthier embryos.

GIFT enhances pregnancy rates only when the tubes are normal. Attempts to transfer embryos to patent fallopian tubes following corrective surgery results in poor success.[75] Immunologic problems are also not ideally treated with this technology, because the sperm will be exposed to antibodies in the female reproductive tract. Male factor infertility has been demonstrated to have a 33% pregnancy rate with GIFT and unexplained infertility a 19% rate.[76] A major disadvantage of this procedure, however, is the loss of diagnostic information about fertilization. Although excess oocytes can be utilized to test sperm-oocyte interaction, the rate of fertilization in vitro does not correlate well with the outcome of the GIFT procedure.[77]

GIFT Combined with Diagnostic Laparoscopy

One novel approach toward the work-up of unexplained infertility is to combine the diagnostic laparoscopy with GIFT. When the screening laparoscopy is combined with a GIFT procedure, Barad and co-workers found normal anatomy in 50% of cases and a clinical pregnancy rate of 40% was obtained when gamete transfer could be performed.[78] When unsuspected fallopian tube disease is encountered, IVF and reparative surgery can be performed. Patients in whom endometriosis or pelvic adhesions were encountered may anticipate success rates similar to those with normal anatomy, even when operative endoscopy was performed.[79] Although reparative surgery has been performed at the time of egg retrieval with favorable outcomes,[80] the hyperstimulated ovary results in conditions that are not ideal for pelvic reconstruction.

Techniques

Laparoscopy

The standard technique for fallopian tube catheterization for gamete transfer is through laparoscopy (Fig. 29–13). In the authors' program, oocyte retrieval is performed under ultrasound guidance and the laparoscopy is not performed until the number of oocytes is known. When fertilization of oocytes must be observed, such as with male factor or unexplained infertility, IVF is a better treatment for the patient when there are limited numbers of oocytes.

The semen must be prepared prior to the laparoscopy by one of the standard sperm separation techniques. Gametes are loaded into the GIFT catheter, which is threaded into the ampullary fallopian tube. Catheterization of the fallopian tube is best accomplished under laparoscopic guidance. The laparoscopy is performed in a fashion similar to that described for laparoscopic oocyte retrieval. The patient may be supine or in lithotomy, but cervical manipulation is not utilized. An atraumatic grasping forceps is placed suprapubically to support the fimbriae (Fig. 29–14). The best approach is to grasp the fimbriae across their full thickness from mucosa to serosa.

Placement of the transfer catheter is important for expeditious transfer of gametes. The authors utilize a high entry by placing an introducer near the umbilicus lateral to the rectus muscle. The high introduction of the catheter allows the fallopian tube to be stretched so that the path of gamete passage is in a straight line. When the fallopian tube is unusually lengthy, a higher entry of the catheter introducer may allow for a more expeditious catheterization of the fallopian tube.

Fimbrial narrowing is commonly encountered during GIFT. Catheterization of the tube is challenging when false passages of fimbrial folds simulate the tubal ostia. If this is unrecognized, the gametes will be expelled into the peritoneal cavity and pregnancy will not occur. It is important to confirm that the fallopian tube has been catheterized before expelling the gametes. One way of testing this is to place the introducer catheter into the fallopian tube. CO_2 should not escape when the catheter has adequately passed into the fallopian tube. More reliably, the tube should be inspected at the level of the ampulla to reveal the bulge of the transfer catheter.

Once the introducer is placed into the fallopian tube, the gametes are loaded in a Teflon catheter. Limiting the volume to approximately 100 µl of solution ensures that fluid does not reflux out the tubal ostia. The sperm are loaded first so that they will be expelled last into the fallopian tube. The gametes are transferred through the introducer and

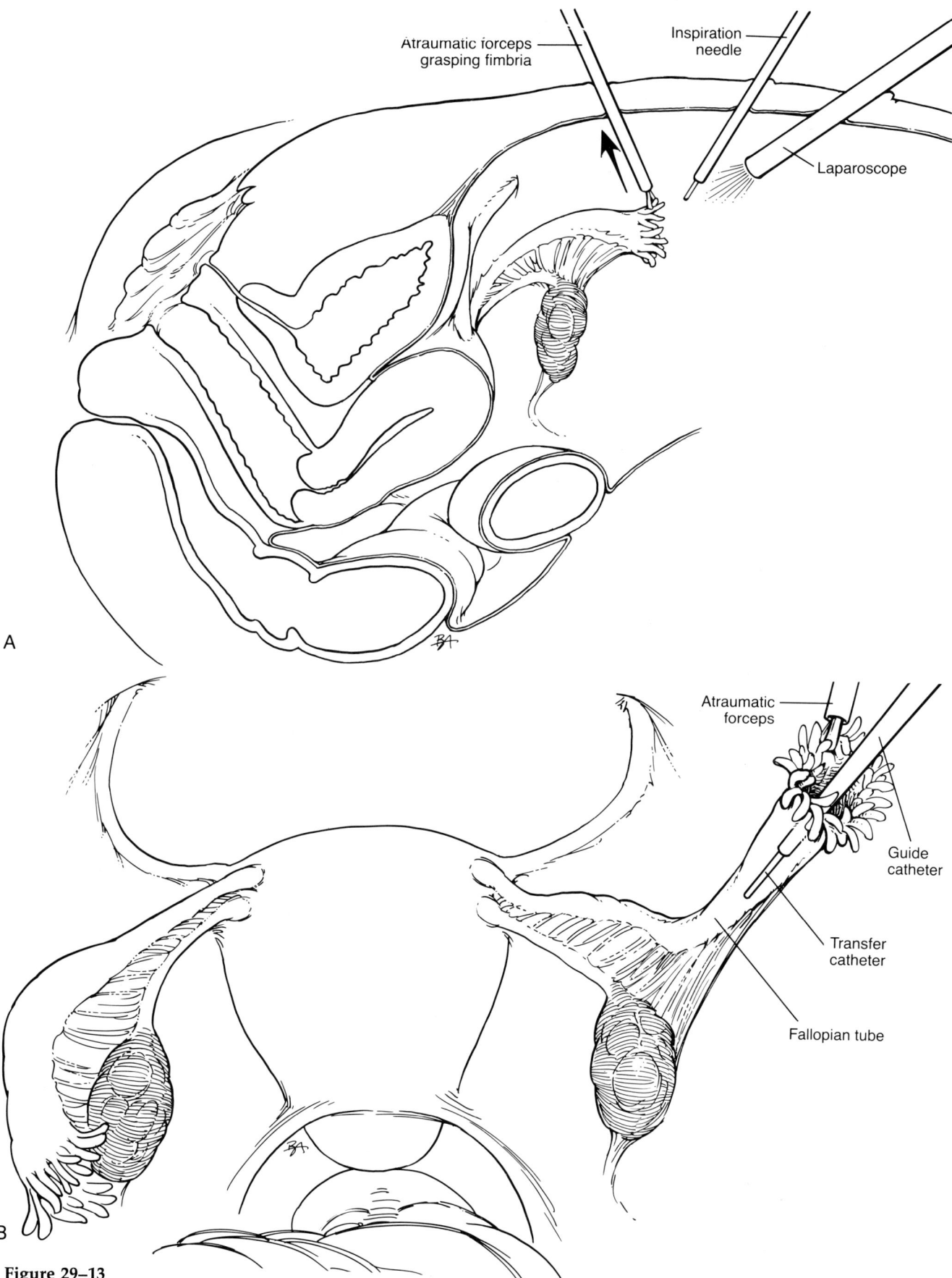

Figure 29–13
Fallopian tube catheterization for GIFT or ZIFT (laparoscopic approach). *A,* The fallopian tube is grasped with an atraumatic grasping forceps. The catheter introducer is best placed high in the abdominal wall, near the umbilicus. *B,* Stretching the fallopian tube creates a straight passage for the transfer of gametes and facilitates tubal cannulation.

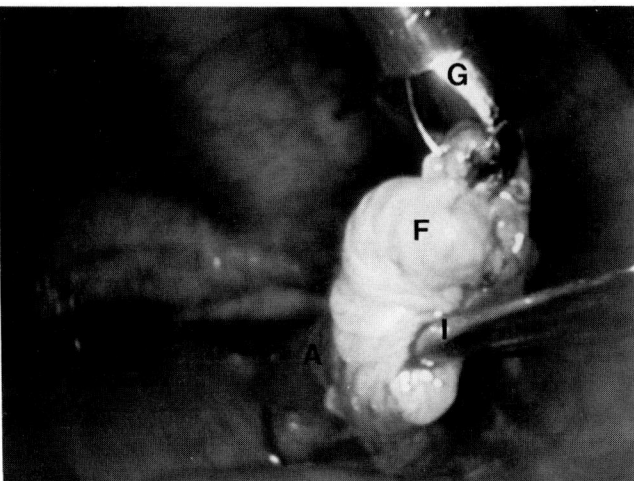

Figure 29–14
GIFT-ZIFT fallopian tube catheterization. The fimbriae (F) are grasped with atraumatic grasping forceps (G). The catheter introducer (I) is first passed into the proximal ampulla. The catheter is threaded through the catheter introducer into the isthmic-ampullary junction (A).

passed into the ampullary fallopian tube. When the isthmic-ampullary junction is encountered, resistance will be met. It is wise to withdraw the introducer slightly to ensure that the gametes are not expelled into the introducer.

Transcervical GIFT

A nonsurgical approach to gamete transfer has been reported by Jansen and coworkers.[17] The technique is identical to that already described for fallopian tube insemination (Fig. 29–15). In one review, Bustillo and Schulman summarized the world's experience with this technique.[81] Although fallopian tube catheterization was successful 92% of the time, the pregnancy rate in the first series was 13%, which is considerably lower than that achieved with laparoscopic GIFT. It is early in the evolution of this technique to determine whether it will ultimately replace laparoscopic GIFT.

Complications

Because GIFT requires COH and oocyte retrieval, complications previously described for IVF apply. In addition, a laparoscopy and fallopian tube catheterization are performed. Pelvic adhesions following oocyte aspiration have been reported.[82] Because of the greater efficiency of implantation in GIFT, there is an additional concern of multiple pregnancy with this procedure.[83] Prevention of this complication is best accomplished by limiting the number of eggs transferred and fertilizing all extra oocytes in vitro. Ectopic pregnancy seems to occur less commonly following GIFT (approximately 1%) than following IVF (approximately 5%), probably because patients are selected for normalcy of their fallopian tubes.[84]

ZYGOTE INTRAFALLOPIAN TRANSFER–TUBAL EMBRYO TRANSFER

Patient Selection

ZIFT differs from IVF only in the mechanism of embryo transfer. IVF embryo transfers are performed without anesthesia, through the cervix and into the endometrial cavity. In ZIFT, the zygotes are transferred into the fallopian tube. When transfer is delayed until syngamy (48 hours post-retrieval), the procedure is called tubal embryo transfer (TET).

Any patient who requires IVF and has normal fallopian tubes may undergo tubal zygote or embryo transfer. The primary indication for this is when GIFT should not be performed because of concern over sperm-oocyte interaction. This is true when there are antisperm antibodies, when there is a male factor infertility, or when there is unexplained infer-

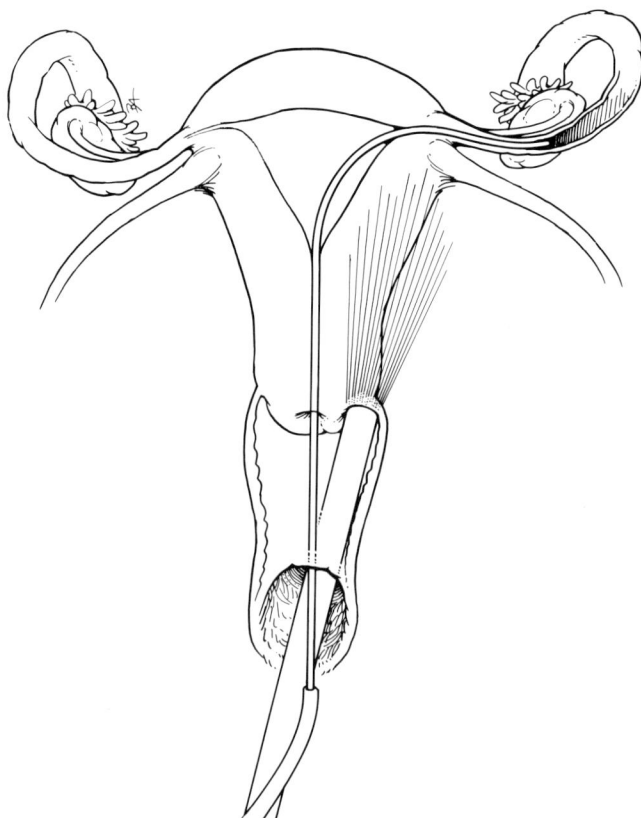

Figure 29–15
Fallopian tube catheterization for GIFT or ZIFT (transcervical approach). Under ultrasound guidance, the proximal portion of the fallopian tube is catheterized. The catheter is advanced into the ampullary fallopian tube, where the gametes are expelled.

tility. The justification for the more involved ET is the higher implantation rates reported for tubal ETs.[85]

Techniques

The technique for transferring zygotes or embryos is identical to that described for GIFT. Both laparoscopic- and ultrasound-guided transcervical techniques have been reported.[86, 87] Fertilization occurs in the laboratory, and fertilized zygotes or embryos are transferred instead of gametes.

MULTIFETAL PREGNANCY REDUCTION

With the introduction of COH, the incidence of multifetal pregnancies has increased tremendously. The Australian in vitro collaborative group reported a 21% incidence of multiple births, including a 35% incidence of triplets and one set of quadruplets in 902 pregnancies.[88]

As previously noted, the transfer of multiple embryos improves pregnancy rates, but also increases the chances for multiple gestations. Craft and colleagues report that during GIFT procedures, patients who received four or fewer oocytes conceived only singletons or twins, while those receiving more than five oocytes had a 5.7% incidence of three or more fetuses.[89]

The most important complication of multifetal pregnancy is prematurity, and this risk is directly proportional to the number of fetuses within the uterus. Reduction in the number of fetuses has been proposed as a way to improve perinatal outcome in this setting.

Technique

Multifetal pregnancy reduction was first utilized in the second trimester in twins where one had a congenital anomaly. Aberg and colleagues utilized cardiac puncture with exsanguination by aspiration.[90] Rodeck embolized air into the fetal circulation under fetoscopic visualization.[91] More recently, most second-trimester terminations are performed by percutaneous fetal cardiac or umbilical vein puncture and injection of a cardiotoxic substance such as potassium chloride.[92]

In 1986, Dumez and Oury reported a first-trimester multifetal pregnancy reduction.[93] This was performed by selective transcervical aspiration of one or more sacs under ultrasound guidance. Konkhai and associates utilized an ultrasonic-guided thoracic puncture in a quintuplet pregnancy.[94] At Mount Sinai, intrathoracic injection of potassium chloride under ultrasound guidance via a transabdominal approach has been utilized. In 85 reduction procedures, 8 of 53 pregnancies (15%) were lost.[95]

Fetuses were "selected" merely on the basis of their proximity to the maternal abdominal wall. The sac immediately adjacent to the uterine os was never selected for fear that devitalizing the membranes in that sac could result in their rupture and thus set the stage for an ascending uterine infection. Fetuses with obvious abnormalities or a significantly smaller crown-rump length than their siblings are preferentially selected for termination. Monochorionic twins should either both be terminated or both left intact.

Transvaginal cardiac injections, in the first trimester, have been reported more recently.[96, 97] The advantage of earlier reduction procedures is debatable, since there is a spontaneous loss rate even after cardiac activity has been detected. Most investigators agree that there is no advantage in delaying the procedure beyond 12 gestational weeks, because spontaneous losses after this time are unlikely.

Patients participating in ART need to be aware of the risk of multifetal pregnancy and of the availability of multifetal pregnancy reduction as an option for management. The decision to perform multifetal pregnancy reduction should be based upon an evaluation of the risk of maintaining the pregnancy as compared with the risk of its termination. Multifetal

Table 29–2

Results of In Vitro Fertilization–Embryo Transfer (IVF-ET) and Gamete Intrafallopian Transfer (GIFT)

	IVF Pregnancy/ET (%)		GIFT Pregnancy/Procedure (%)	
Etiology	Clinical Pregnancies	Deliveries	Clinical Pregnancies	Deliveries
Tubal disease	16	12	14	12
Female unexplained	14	10	24	24
Female immune	13	9	33	27
Endometriosis	15	11	27	21
Male unexplained	9	7	26	23
Male immune	25	19	23	19
Male sperm abnormalities	16	11	24	20

Data from reference 98.

Table 29-3

IVF and GIFT Pregnancy Rate (%) by Age

	IVF				GIFT			
Age	Clinical Pregnancies	Abortions	Ectopic Pregnancies	Deliveries	Clinical Pregnancies	Abortions	Ectopic Pregnancies	Deliveries
<25	40	0	9	40				
25–29	19	32	6	13				
30–34	17	22	4	13	29	14	6	25
35–39	15	24	4	11	23	29	4	17
40+	10	60	5	4	14	38	0	9
Totals	16	25	4	12	27	20	4	22

Data from reference 98.

pregnancy reduction is currently available for couples who in the past were forced to accept the risk of extreme prematurity, or terminate the entire pregnancy.

RESULTS

IVF results are usually calculated as clinical pregnancy per oocyte retrieval or per embryo transfer. Reduced success would be obtained if only live-born pregnancies are counted, whereas exaggerated statistics would be obtained if all positive pregnancy tests are measured. In an effort to standardize statistical analysis, the Society for Assisted Reproductive Technology (SART) has created a registry for the collection of IVF data, which are presented in Tables 29–2 and 29–3.[98]

References

1. Steptoe PC, Edwards RG: Birth after re-implantation of a human embryo. Lancet 1978; 2:366.
2. Trounson AO, Leeton JF, Wood C, et al.: Pregnancies in human by fertilization in vitro and embryo transfer in the controlled ovulatory cycle. Science 1981; 212:681.
3. Jones HW, Jones GS, Andrews MC, et al.: The program for in vitro fertilization at Norfolk. Fertil Steril 1982; 38:14.
4. Asch RH, Ellsworth LR, Balmaceda JP, Wong PC: Pregnancy after translaparoscopic gamete intrafallopian transfer. Lancet 1984; 2:1034.
5. Devroey P, Braeckmans P, Smitz J, et al.: Pregnancy after laparoscopic zygote intrafallopian transfer in a patient with sperm antibodies. Lancet 1986; 1:1329.
6. Loy RA, Seibel MM: Therapeutic insemination. In Seibel MM (ed.): Infertility: A comprehensive text. Norwalk, CT, Appleton & Lange, 1990, p. 100.
7. Dodson WC, Whitesides DB, Hughes CL, et al.: Superovulation with intrauterine insemination in the treatment of infertility: A possible alternative to gamete intrafallopian transfer and in vitro fertilization. Fertil Steril 1987; 48:441.
8. Welner S, DeCherney AH, Polan ML: Human menopausal gonadotropins: A justifiable therapy in ovulatory women with long-standing idiopathic infertility. Am J Obstet Gynecol 1988; 158:111.
9. Serhal PF, Katz M, Little V, Woronowski H: Unexplained infertility—the value of Pergonal superovulation combined with intrauterine insemination. Fertil Steril 1988; 49:602.
10. Ho PC, Poon IML, Chan SYW, Wang C: Intrauterine insemination is not useful in oligo-asthenospermia. Fertil Steril 1989; 51:682.
11. Moghissi KS: Reflections on the new guidelines for the use of semen donor insemination. Fertil Steril 1989; 53:399.
12. Byrd W, Bradshaw K, Carr B, et al.: A prospective randomized study of pregnancy rates following intrauterine and intracervical insemination using frozen sperm. Fertil Steril 1990; 53:521.
13. Laufer N, Grunfeld L, Garrissi GJ: In vitro fertilization. In Seibel MM (ed.) Infertility: A Comprehensive Text. Norwalk, CT, Appleton & Lange, 1990, p. 481.
14. Boyers SP, Corrales MD, Huszar G, DeCherney AH: The effects of Lubrin on sperm motility in vitro. Fertil Steril 1987; 47:882.
15. Studd J, Lim-Howe D, Dooley M, Savvas M: Direct intraperitoneal insemination. Lancet 1987; 1:326.
16. Forrier A, Dellenbach P, Nisand I, et al.: Direct intraperitoneal insemination in unexplained and cervical infertility. Lancet 1986; 1:916.
17. Jansen RPS, Anderson JC, Radonic I, et al.: Pregnancies after ultrasound-guided fallopian tube insemination with cryostored donor semen. Fertil Steril 1988; 49:920.
18. Soules MR: Infertility surgery. In DeCherney AH (ed.): Reproductive Failure. New York, Churchill Livingstone, 1986, p. 117.
19. Trimbos-Kemper TCM, Trimbos JB, Van Hall EV: Conscientious evaluation of tubal surgery results. In DeCherney AH, Polan ML (eds.): Reproductive Surgery. Chicago, Year Book Medical Publishers, 1987, p. 74.
20. Thie JL, Williams TJ, Coulam CB: Repeat tuboplasty compared with primary microsurgery for post inflammatory tubal disease. Fertil Steril 1986; 45:784.
21. Soules MR: Infertility surgery. In DeCherney AH (ed.): Reproductive Failure. New York, Churchill Livingstone, 1986, p. 117.
22. Bateman BG, Nunley WC, Kitchen JK: Surgical management of distal tubal obstruction—are we making progress? Fertil Steril 1987; 48:523.
23. Webster BW, Wentz AC, Maxson WS: Endometriosis. In DeCherney AH, Polan ML (eds.): Reproductive Surgery. Chicago, Year Book Medical Publishers, 1987, p. 221.
24. Olive DL, Haney AF: Endometriosis. In DeCherney AH (ed.): Reproductive Failure. New York, Churchill Livingstone, 1986, p. 153.
25. Seibel MM, Berber MJ, Weinstein FB, et al.: The effectiveness of danazol on subsequent fertility in minimal endometriosis. Fertil Steril 1982; 38:534.
26. Matson PL, Yovich JL: The treatment of infertility associated with endometriosis by in vitro fertilization. Fertil Steril 1986; 46:432.
27. Rosseau S, Lord J, Lepage Y, Campenhout JV: The expectancy of pregnancy for "normal" infertile couples. Fertil Steril 1983; 40:768.
28. Mahadevan MM, Trounson AO, Leeton JF: The relationship of tubal blockage, infertility of unknown cause, suspected

male infertility, and endometriosis to success of in vitro fertilization and embryo transfer. Fertil Steril 1983; 40:755.
29. Battin D, Vargyas JM, Sato F, et al.: The correlation between in vitro fertilization of human oocytes and semen profile. Fertil Steril 1985; 44:835.
30. Englert Y, Vekemans M, Lejeune B, et al.: Higher pregnancy rates after in vitro fertilization and embryo transfer in cases with sperm defects. Fertil Steril 1987; 48:254.
31. Mandelbaum SL, Diamond MP, DeCherney AH: Relationship of antisperm antibodies to oocyte fertilization in in vitro fertilization–embryo transfer. Fertil Steril 1987; 47:644.
32. Aybaliotis B, Bronson R, Rosenfeld D, Cooper G: Conception rates in couples where autoimmunity to sperm is detected. Fertil Steril 1985; 43:739.
33. Shangold MM, Turkson RN, Bashford RA, Hammond B: Pregnancy following the "insensitive ovary syndrome." Fertil Steril 1981; 28:1179.
34. Rosenwaks Z, Navot D, Veeck L, et al.: Oocyte donation. The Norfolk Program. Ann NY Acad Sci 1988; 541:728.
35. Garcia J: Return to the natural cycle for in vitro fertilization. J In Vitro Fertil Embryo Transf 1989; 6:67.
36. Scott RT, Hofmann GE, Muasher SJ, et al.: Correlation of follicular diameter with oocyte recovery and maturity at the time of transvaginal follicular aspiration. J In Vitro Fertil Embryo Transf 1989; 6:73.
37. Lavy G, Restrepo-Candelo H, Diamond M, et al.: Laparoscopic and transvaginal ova recovery: The effect on ova quality. Fertil Steril 1988; 49:1002.
38. Lenz S, Lauritsen JG: Ultrasonically guided percutaneous aspiration of human follicles under anesthesia. A new method of collecting oocytes for in vitro fertilization. Fertil Steril 1982; 38:673.
39. Gleicher N, Friberg J, Fullan N, et al.: Egg retrieval for in vitro fertilisation by sonographically controlled vaginal culdocentesis. Lancet 1983; 1:508.
40. Meldrum DR: Antbiotics for vaginal oocyte aspiration. J In Vitro Fertil Embryo Transf 1989; 6:1.
41. Jones HW, Acosta AA, Garcia J: A technique for the aspiration of oocytes from human ovarian follicles. Fertil Steril 1982; 37:26.
42. Renou P, Trounson AO, Wood C, Leeton JF: The collection of human oocytes for in vitro fertilization. I. An instrument for maximizing oocyte recovery rate. Fertil Steril 1981; 35:409.
43. Scott RT, Hofmann GE, Muasher SJ, et al.: A prospective randomized comparison of single and double lumen needles for transvaginal follicular aspiration. J In Vitro Fertil Embryo Transf 1989; 6:98.
44. Lopata A, Johnston IWH, Leeton JF, et al.: Collection of human oocytes at laparoscopy and laparotomy. Fertil Steril 1974; 25:1030.
45. Kogosowski A, Lessing J, Amit A, et al.: Epidural block: A preferred method of anesthesia for ultrasonically guided oocyte retrieval. Fertil Steril 1987; 47:166.
46. Schulman J, Dorfmann A, Jones S, et al.: Outpatient in vitro fertilization using transvaginal oocyte retrieval and local anesthesia. N Engl J Med 1985; 312:1639.
47. Ramseawak SS, Kumar A, Welsby R, et al.: Is analgesia required for transvaginal single follicle aspiration in in vitro fertilization? A double blind study. J In Vitro Fertil Embryo Transf 1990; 7:103.
48. Hammarberg K, Enk L, Nilsson L, Wikland M: Oocyte retrieval under the guidance of a vaginal transducer: Evaluation of patient acceptance. Hum Reprod 1987; 2:487.
49. Dellenbach P, Nisand I, Moreau L, et al.: The transvaginal method for oocyte retrieval. An update on our experience (1984–87). Ann NY Acad Sci 1988; 541:111.
50. Howe RS, Wheeler C, Mastroianni L, et al.: Pelvic infection after transvaginal ultrasound guided ovum retrieval. Fertil Steril 1988; 49:726.
51. Meldrum DR: Antibiotics for vaginal oocyte aspiration. J In Vitro Fertil Embryo Transf 1989; 6:1.
52. Evers J, Larsen J, Gnany G, Sieck U: Complications and problems in transvaginal sector scan guided follicle aspiration. Fertil Steril 1988; 49:278.
53. Jones WR, Haines CJ, Matthews CD, Kirby CA: Traumatic ureteric obstruction secondary to oocyte recovery for in vitro fertilization: A case report. J In Vitro Fertil Embryo Transf 1989; 6:185.
54. Ashkenazi J, BenDavid M, Feldberg D, et al.: Abdominal complications following ultrasonically guided percutaneous transvesical collection of oocytes for in vitro fertilization. J In Vitro Fertil Embryo Transf 1987; 4:316.
55. Friedman CI, Schmidt GE, Chang FE, Kim MH: Severe ovarian hyperstimulation following follicular aspiration. Am J Obstet Gynecol 1984; 150:436.
56. van der Merwe JP, Michell WL, Kruger TF: Severe ovarian hyperstimulation after follicular aspiration. S Afr Med J 1988; 73:426.
57. Jones HW: Embryo transfer. Ann NY Acad Sci 1985; 442:375.
58. Croxatto HB, Ortiz ME, Diaz S, et al.: Studies on the duration of egg transport by the human oviduct. Am J Obstet Gynecol 1978; 132:629.
59. Bustillo M, Buster JE, Cohen SW, et al.: Nonsurgical ovum transfer as a treatment in infertile women. JAMA 1984; 251:1171.
60. Feichtinger W, Kemeler P. Organization and computerized analysis of in vitro fertilization and embryo transfer programs. J In Vitro Fertil Embryo Transf 1984; 1:34.
61. Navot D, Anderson TL, Droesch K, et al.: Hormonal manipulation of endometrial maturation. J Clin Endocrinol Metab 1989; 68:801.
62. Kerin JFP, Warnes GM, Jeffrey R, et al.: A simple technique for human embryo transfer into the uterus. Lancet 1981; 2:726.
63. Jones HW Jr, Acosta AA, Garcia JE, et al.: On the transfer of conceptuses from oocytes fertilized in vitro. Fertil Steril 1983; 39:241.
64. Yovich JL, Turner SR, Murphy AJ: Embryo transfer technique as a cause of ectopic pregnancy in in vitro fertilization. Fertil Steril 1985; 44:318.
65. Lenz S, Leeton J, Rogers P, Trounson A: Transfundal transfer of embryo using ultrasound. J In Vitro Fertil Embryo Transf 1987; 4:13.
66. Fishel S, Webster J, Faratian B, Jackson P: General anesthesia for intrauterine placement of human conceptuses after in vitro fertilization. J In Vitro Fertil Embryo Transf 1987; 4:260.
67. Englert Y, Puissant F, Camus M, et al.: Clinical study on embryo transfer after human in vitro fertilization. J In Vitro Fertil Embryo Transf 1986; 3:243.
68. Poindexter AN III, Thompson JD, Gibbons WE, et ai.: Residual embryos in failed embryo transfer. Fertil Steril 1986; 46:262.
69. Meldrum DR, Chetkowski R, Steingold KA, et al.: Evolution of a highly successful in vitro fertilization embryo transfer program. Fertil Steril 1987; 48:86.
70. Yovich JL, Turner SR, Murphy AJ: Embryo transfer technique as a cause of ectopic pregnancies in in vitro fertilization. Fertil Steril 1985; 44:318.
71. Poindexter AN, Thompson DJ, Gibbons WE, et al.: Residual embryos in failed embryo transfer. Fertil Steril 1986; 46:262.
72. Speirs A, Lopata A, Gronow MJ, et al.: Analysis of the benefits of multiple embryo transfer. Fertil Steril 1983; 39:468.
73. Walters DE, Edwards RG, Meistrich ML: A statistical evaluation of implantation when replacing one or more human embryos. Reprod Fertil 1985; 74:557.
74. Asch RH, Balmaceda JP, Ellsworth LR, Wong PC: Preliminary experiences with gamete intrafallopian transfer (GIFT). Fertil Steril 1986; 45:366.
75. Corson SL, Dickey RP, Gocial B, et al.: Outcome in 242 in vitro fertilization–embryo replacement or gamete intrafallopian transfer–induced pregnancies. Fertil Steril 1989; 51:644.
76. Leeton J, Rogers P, Caro C, et al.: A controlled study between the use of gamete intrafallopian transfer (GIFT) and in vitro fertilization and embryo transfer in the management of idiopathic and male infertility. Fertil Steril 1987; 48:605.
77. Guzick DS, Balmaceda JP, Ord T, Asch RH: The importance of egg and sperm factors in predicting the likelihood of pregnancy from gamete intrafallopian transfer. Fertil Steril 1989; 52:795.
78. Barad DH, Bartfai G, Barg P, et al.: Gamete intrafallopian transfer (GIFT): Making the laparoscopy more than "diagnostic." Fertil Steril 1988; 50:928.
79. Gindoff PR, Hall JL, Nelson LM, Stillman RJ: Efficacy of assisted reproductive technology during diagnostic and operative laparoscopy. Obstet Gynecol 1990; 75:299.

80. Tureck RW, Ben-Rafael Z, Blasco L, et al.: Follicular aspiration and in vitro fertilization associated with pelvic reconstructive surgery. Fertil Steril 1988; 50:447.
81. Bustillo M, Schulman JD: Transcervical ultrasound guided intrafallopian placement of gametes, zygotes, and embryos. J In Vitro Fertil Embryo Transf 1989; 6:321.
82. Ashkenazi J, Feldberg D, Ben David M, et al.: Ovum pickup for in vitro fertilization: A cause of mechanical infertility? J In Vitro Fertil Embryo Transf 1987; 4:242.
83. Batzer FR, Gocial B, Corson SL, et al.: Multiple pregnancies with gamete intrafallopian transfer (GIFT): Complications of a new technique. J In Vitro Fertil Embryo Transf 1988; 5:35.
84. Asch RH, Balmaceda JP, Ellsworth LR, Wong PC: Preliminary experiences with gamete intrafallopian transfer (GIFT). Fertil Steril 1986; 45:366.
85. Devroey P, Staessen C, Camus M, et al.: Zygote intrafallopian transfer as a successful treatment for unexplained infertility. Fertil Steril 1989; 52:246.
86. Devroey P, Braeckmans P, Smitz J, et al.: Pregnancy after laparoscopic zygote intrafallopian transfer in a patient with sperm antibodies. Lancet 1986; 1:1329.
87. Jansen RPS, Anderson JC, Sutherland PD: Nonoperative embryo transfer to the fallopian tube. N Engl J Med 1988; 319:288.
88. Australian in vitro fertilization collaborative group. In vitro fertilization pregnancies in Australia and New Zealand, 1979–1985. Med J Aust 1988; 148:429.
89. Craft I, Brinsden P, Simon I: How many oocytes/embryos should be transferred? Lancet 1987; 2:109.
90. Aberg A, Miterion F, Conty M, Geliler J: Cardiac puncture of fetus with Hurler's disease avoiding abortion of unaffected co-twin. Lancet 1978; 2:990.
91. Rodeck CH: Fetoscopy in the management of twin pregnancies discordant for a severe abnormality. Acta Genet Med Gemellol (Roma) 1984; 33:57.
92. Chitkara U, Berkowitz RL, Wilkins IA, et al.: Selective mid-trimester termination of the anomalous fetus in twin pregnancies. Obstet Gynecol 1989; 73:690.
93. Dumez Y, Oury JF: Method for first trimester selective abortion in multiple pregnancy. Contrib Gynecol Obstet 1986; 15:50.
94. Konkhai HHH, von Rijssel EJC, Meerman RJ, Bennebrack Gravenhorst J: Selective termination in quintuplet pregnancy during the first trimester. Lancet 1986; 1:1447.
95. Lynch L, Berkowitz RL, Chitkara U, Alvarez M: First trimester transabdominal multifetal pregnancy reduction: A report of 85 cases. Obstet Gynecol 1990; 75:735.
96. Itskovitz J, Bolds R, Thaler I, et al.: Transvaginal ultrasonography guided aspirations of gestational sacs for selective abortion in multiple pregnancy. Am J Obstet Gynecol 1989; 160:215.
97. Shalev J, Frenkel Y, Goldenberg M, et al.: Selective reduction in multiple gestations: Pregnancy outcome of the transvaginal and transabdominal needle guided procedures. Fertil Steril 1989; 52:416.
98. Medical Research International and Society for Assisted Reproductive Technology: In vitro fertilization–embryo transfer in the United States: 1988 results from the IVF-ET registry. Fertil Steril 1990; 53:13.

Surgery for Endometriosis

30

Randall A. Loy
Alan H. DeCherney

Endometriosis, one of the most prevalent of gynecologic disorders, has remained a perplexing clinical entity since its original description in the late nineteenth century. John A. Sampson, a private practitioner in Albany, New York, later coined the term "endometriosis" to denote the "presence of ectopic tissue which possesses the histologic structure and function of uterine mucosa. It also includes the abnormal conditions which may result not only from the invasion of organs and other structures by this tissue, but also from its reaction to menstruation."[1] Although "internal endometriosis" (adenomyosis) was originally thought to be the myometrial variant of endometriosis, it is now recognized to be a distinct disease, differing in etiology, affected population, and clinical course.[2] The last 100 years have been fraught with efforts to develop effective medical and surgical therapies; however, controversy regarding the management of endometriosis persists. An abundance of anecdotal data, poorly designed clinical trials, and practitioner bias all have contributed to the general uncertainty regarding endometriosis.[3] In this chapter, following a limited discussion of the pathogenesis of endometriosis, the salient clinical features and the various surgical treatments of the disease will be discussed. Individualized care is paramount in both the establishment of the diagnosis and the operative management of endometriosis—a puzzling disease that exists as a clinical continuum.

EPIDEMIOLOGY

The prevalence of endometriosis cannot be known with certainty owing to the fact that the diagnosis is established at the time of surgery. Asymptomatic and subclinical cases, therefore, remain undiagnosed, and the cases that are reported are subject to individual and institutional surgical selection bias. As the use of diagnostic laparoscopy has been liberalized over the past decade, however, there has undoubtedly been closer approximation to the true prevalence of disease: probably 2–5% of the general population.[4,5] Typically, symptomatic patients are in the third to fourth decades of life, with the two commonest complaints being infertility and pelvic pain. Histologically proven endometriosis has been demonstrated in 18.7% and 38% of laparotomies in two series involving a total of approximately 3000 patients.[6,7] The disease is also seen frequently among teenaged patients, especially in association with congenital uterine anomalies,[8] pelvic pain, or both. Goldstein and colleagues[9] have diagnosed endometriosis by laparoscopy and biopsy in 52% of adolescent women who presented with chronic pelvic pain. These young women were predominantly of lower socioeconomic status, with ages ranging from 10–19 years. Moreover, established endometriosis may persist into the climacteric and postmenopausal years, especially in patients prescribed estrogen hormone replacement therapy or with increased endogenous estrogen secondary to obesity.[10] Although apparently rare, malignancy arising in endometriosis associated with estrogen replacement (unopposed by progestin) has been reported.[11]

Endometriosis probably has a multifactorial or polygenic mode of inheritance. A familial clustering of endometriosis was first proposed in 1943,[12] and recent retrospective genetic studies of first-degree relatives of patients with known endometriosis have confirmed that this disease has a genetic transmission.[13, 14] These investigators found that 5.8% of the sisters and 8.1% of the mothers of these patients also had endometriosis. With respect to severe endometriosis, the familial group was more than twice as likely to be affected than the nonfamilial group (61% versus 24%).

Despite some early studies on the demographic aspects of ectopic endometrial tissue, there are no data to support an increased frequency of disease in individuals of certain races, socioeconomic strata, geographic locations, body habitus types, or with particular personality characteristics.

HISTOGENESIS

Von Recklinghausen[15] (1896) ascribed the origin of endometriosis to the adult remains of wolffian tubules, whereas Cullen[16] (1896) suggested a müllerian origin. Early in the century, other morphologists (Iwanoff, Pick, and Meyer) further developed the müllerian theory and proposed that the endometrium-like nodules in and on the pelvic organs were due to metaplasia of the original coelomic mesothelium, that is, the differentiation of one mature tissue type (peritoneum or ovarian germinal epithelium) into another (endosalpinx, endometrium, or endocervix).[17–22] This early theory could explain, on an embryologic basis, the findings of extrapelvic endometriosis; however, it has not been validated experimentally and therefore remains primarily of historical interest. Present tenable hypotheses on the histologic origin include lymphatic and hematogenous spread, iatrogenic dissemination, and implantation following retrograde menstruation.

Lymphatic and Hematogenous Metastases

Metastasis of endometrial tissue via the pelvic lymphatics may account for some presentations of endometriosis, but this mode probably cannot explain disease in all locations. In 1922 Sampson histologically demonstrated the invasion of pelvic lymph vessels by endometrial tissue that had penetrated the broad ligament from its peritoneal surface in one case, and the sigmoid colon in another, and he suggested the possibility of lymphatic spread.[15] Halban,[23] however, was actually the first to postulate lymphatic dissemination as a mechanism for all forms of endometriosis, based on five cases involving endometrial glands in regional lymph nodes. Other authors have subsequently confirmed the lymphatic vessels as routes for endometriosis propagation.[24]

In 1927 Sampson[25] observed the presence of endometrium in the venous sinuses. He believed that during menses extravasated venous capillary blood from the mucosa may return to the venous circulation, carrying minute bits of endometrium that become embolic to other points in the pelvis.[25] Venous embolization may best explain the rare endometriotic foci in the extremities, pleura, lungs, and brain.

Iatrogenic Dissemination

Endometriosis may occur by direct implantation of tissue in surgical incision sites following gynecologic procedures. Endometrial tissue may be implanted iatrogenically in the abdominal wall incision, amniocentesis track, episiotomy site (Fig. 30–1), vulvar incision, or cervix following conization or ablation operations. This type of endometriosis spread has been demonstrated in the subhuman primate model as well as in humans; these investigations give further credence to the viability and implantation potential of endometrial fragments.[26]

Retrograde Menstruation

In 1921 Sampson presented his first paper on "Perforating Haemorrhagic (Chocolate) Cysts of the Ovary"[27] and emphasized the endometrial character of these cysts and the associated peritoneal lesions. Much further work by Sampson resulted in his "implantation theory of endometriosis," that is, the retrograde passage of uterine or tubal fluid containing desquamated endometrium, with subsequent implantation and growth on the pelvic structures most

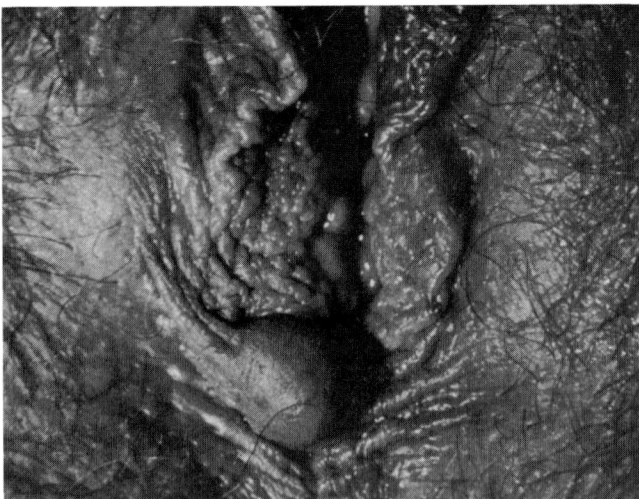

Figure 30–1
Endometriosis of the vulva after direct implantation in an episiotomy incision. (Courtesy of James L Breen, MD, Saint Barnabas Medical Center, Livingston, NJ.)

affected by such fluid.[28-37] In that menstrual detritus contains viable endometrial cells,[38] in that menstrual effluent commonly passes retrograde in normally cycling women,[39] and in that direct implantation of endometrial cells from menstrual fluid has been shown to yield endometriosis,[26] the retrograde menstruation theory best explains most cases of peritoneal and ovarian endometriosis. Whether all women have the same susceptibility for the development of endometriosis is under investigation. There may, in fact, be unique features in women who develop the disease, such as an altered immune response or an enhanced receptivity of the pelvic tissues to the transplanted endometrial fragments.[5]

PATHOLOGY

Microscopic Appearance

The histologic picture of endometriosis is highly variable, with only the occasional lesion demonstrating features of normal eutopic endometrium. Classically the microscopic diagnosis of endometriosis has required the presence of ectopic endometrial glands associated with endometrial stroma, with or without pseudoxanthoma cells (macrophages containing hemosiderin, lipid, and ceroid pigment) (Figs. 30–2 to 30–4). More typically, however, there is a differential response among endometriotic foci to the endocrine changes of the menstrual cycle, resulting in an inconstant epithelial cell and glandular morphology, frequent focal stromal hemorrhage, inflammatory infiltrate, and surrounding fibrous tissue[40] (Fig. 30–5). Metaplasia and hyperplasia of endometriotic glandular elements may occur, yielding tubal, clear cell, squamous, and mucinous types of epithelium.[41] Metaplasia is also common in the stroma, especially smooth muscle metaplasia in ovarian endometriotic cyst walls. The epithelial lining as well as the stroma of an endometrioma frequently reflects

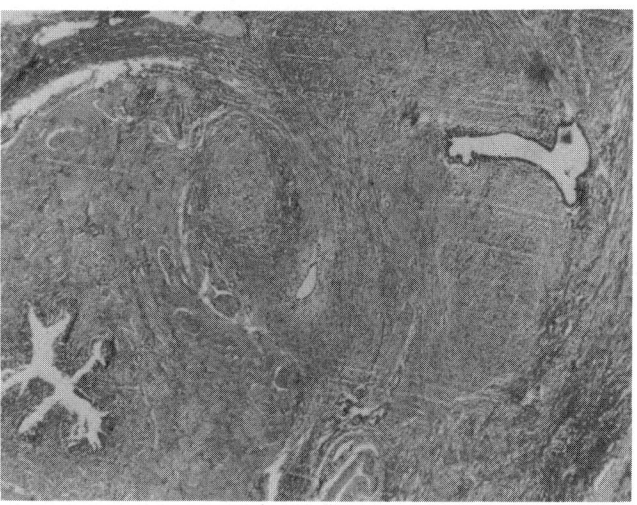

Figure 30–3
Endometriosis and associated fibrosis adjacent to the ureter. (Courtesy of James L Breen, MD, Saint Barnabas Medical Center, Livingston, NJ.)

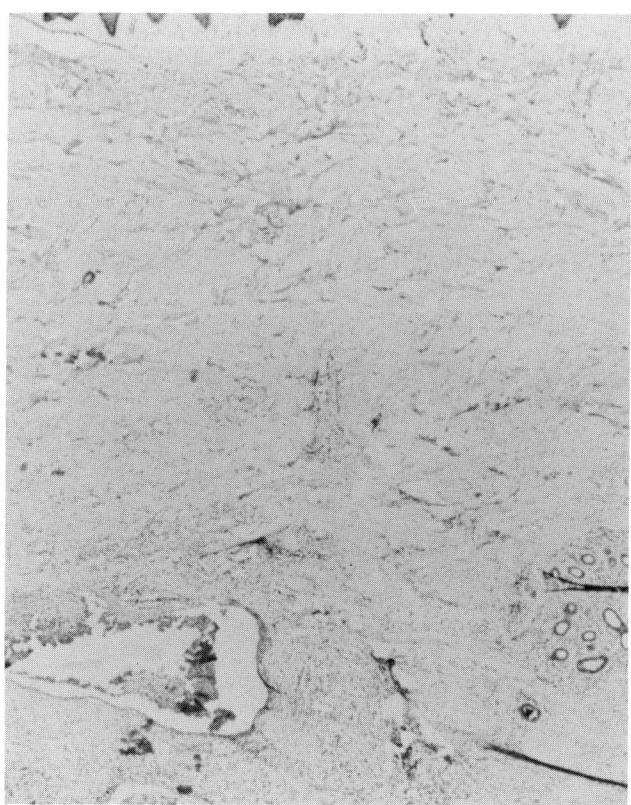

Figure 30–2
Microscopic features of endometriosis in an episiotomy scar. (Courtesy of James L Breen, MD, Saint Barnabas Medical Center, Livingston, NJ.)

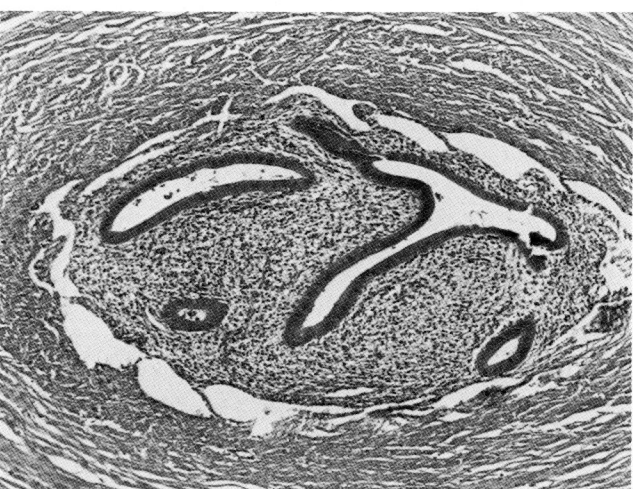

Figure 30–4
Fallopian tube endometriosis. (From Clement, PB: Endometriosis, lesions of the secondary müllerian system, and pelvic mesothelial proliferations. In Kurman RJ (ed.): Blaustein's Pathology of the Female Genital Tract. New York, Springer-Verlag, 1987.)

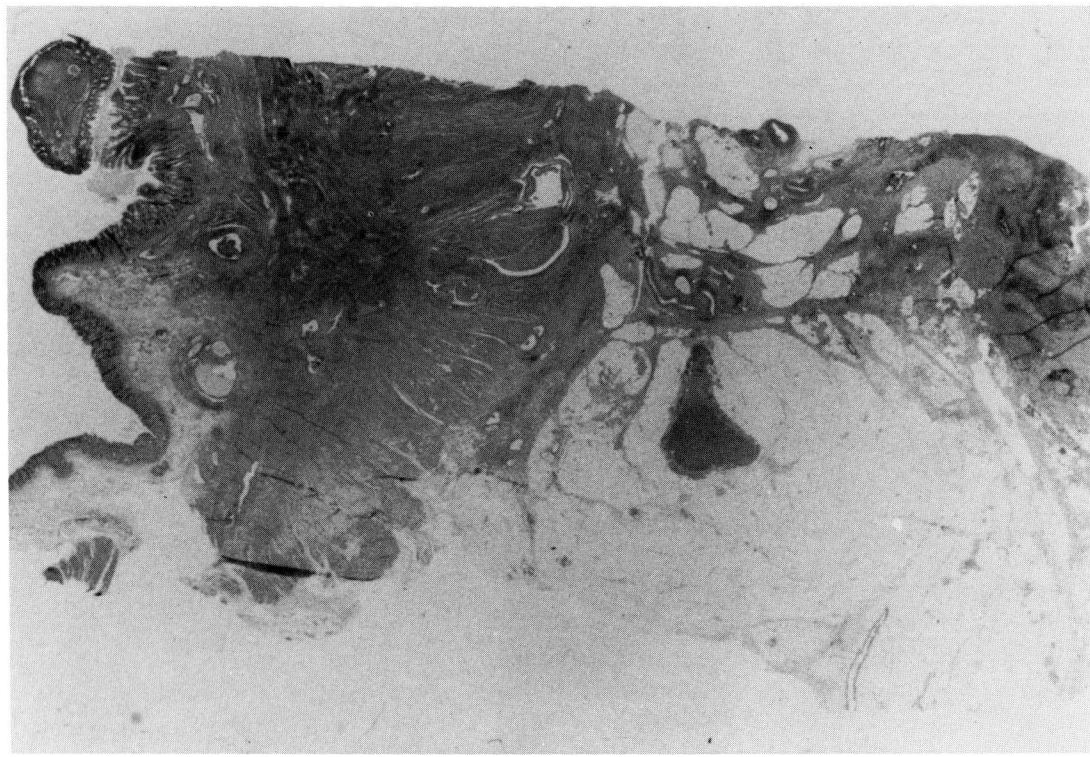

Figure 30–5
Endometriosis of the colon with thickening and fibrosis of the muscularis layer. (Courtesy of Robert Maier, MD, Medical College of Georgia.)

pressure-related flattening, such that the cyst lining is a single columnar or cuboidal cell layer, and may retain no specific features of endometriosis.[42]

Gross Appearance

The macroscopic appearance of the disease is dependent on the age of the lesion, its location, and any underlying pathophysiology. Perhaps the earliest morphologic change associated with retrograde menstruation is the brown-colored hemosiderin discoloration of affected peritoneal surfaces (hence the descriptive term "tobacco staining"). Once active glandular disease is established, the fresh lesions may appear as clusters of red, blue, or brown vesicles, as papules, or as hemorrhagic velvety to fibrous tufts covering serosal and germinal epithelia. Uncommonly, lesions are nonpigmented.[43] With progressive inflammatory response, the surrounding serosa be-

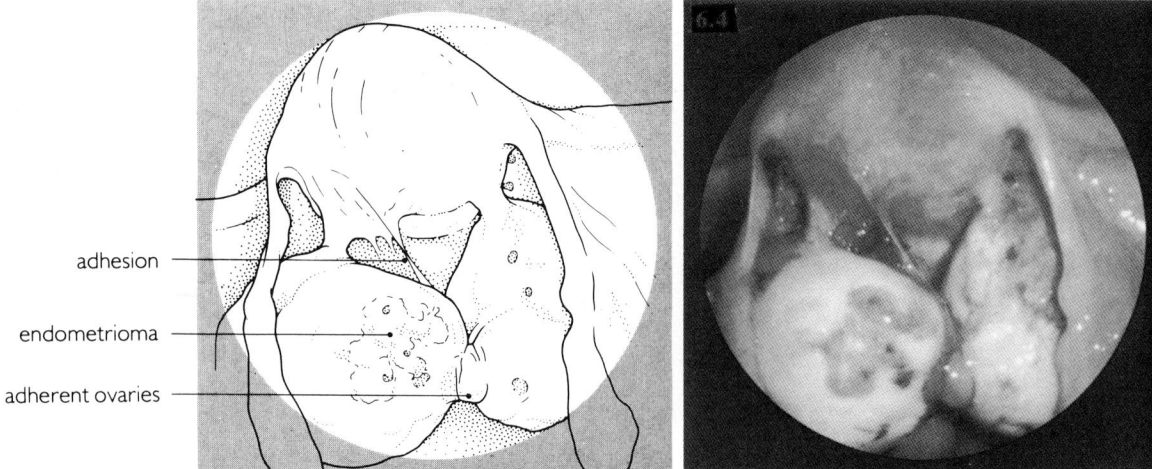

Figure 30–6
Bilateral endometriosis with adherent ovaries in the midline. (From Gordon AG, Lewis BV: Gynecologic Endoscopy. Philadelphia, JB Lippincott, 1988.)

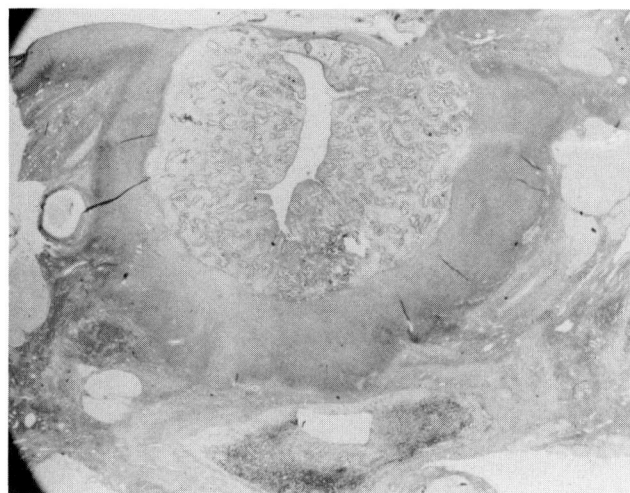

Figure 30–7
Endometriosis of the surface of the ovary. (Courtesy of James L Breen, MD, Saint Barnabas Medical Center, Livingston, NJ.)

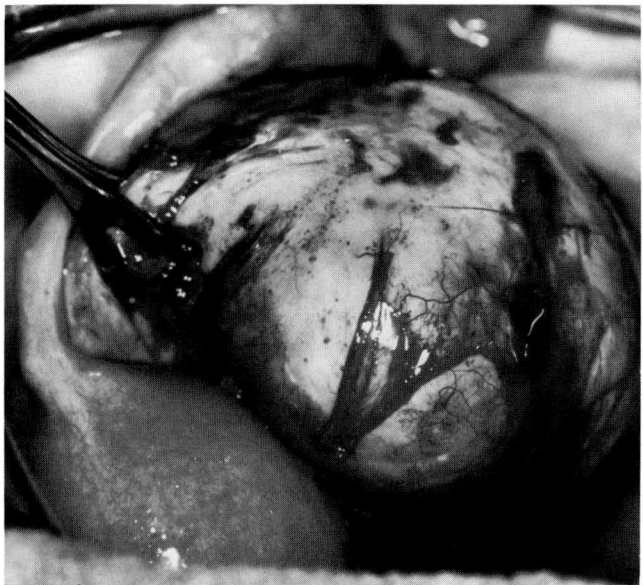

Figure 30–8
Endometriotic ovarian cyst at time of laparotomy. Note size of cyst relative to size of uterine corpus.

comes fibrotic, with peritoneal puckering or scarring. Older encapsulated papules often have a bluish-black appearance and have been labeled "powder burns," and these entrapped foci of endometriosis may enlarge to produce nodules or cysts. Dense fibrous adhesions are often associated with endometriotic implants (Fig. 30–6).

The ovary is the most commonly affected pelvic structure among infertile women. Thereafter, in approximate decreasing incidence of involvement, are the posterior broad ligament, the uterosacral ligaments and posterior cul-de-sac peritoneum, the anterior peritoneal surfaces, the fallopian tubes, and the bowel.[44] The coelomic epithelium of the ovary, however, appears to have a certain proclivity for, or susceptibility to, the development of endometriosis. Ovarian surface lesions may become embedded and cystic and may nearly completely replace normal ovarian anatomy (Fig. 30–7). Endometriotic cysts (endometriomas, "chocolate cysts") occur bilaterally in one-third to one-half of patients[5, 45] and may become relatively large (10–15 cm) (Figs. 30–8 and 30–9). These cysts usually have a well-defined fibrotic wall, with a smooth hemosiderin-stained lining, and the contents are typically a viscous, chocolate-colored fluid. Dense investing adhesions often accompany endometriomas, and the inflammatory response may be especially marked if there has been cyst rupture with peritoneal leakage.

CLINICAL CHARACTERISTICS

As stated by Goodall, "Endometriosis has a wide range of manifestations, and its expression must in certain degree conform, as do all diseases, to the milieu in which it operates."[12] Although there are no pathognomonic presentations of endometriosis, there is better correlation between symptoms and location of disease rather than its extent. The symptoms, believed to be secondary to the cyclic menstrual inflammation and progressive peritoneal fibrosis, are most commonly infertility, dysmenorrhea, pelvic pain, and abnormal uterine bleeding.[46, 47]

Infertility

Infertility occurs in 30–40% of patients with endometriosis and is the single most common presenting complaint.[48, 49] Considered conversely, as many as 25% of infertile women may have endometriosis, and

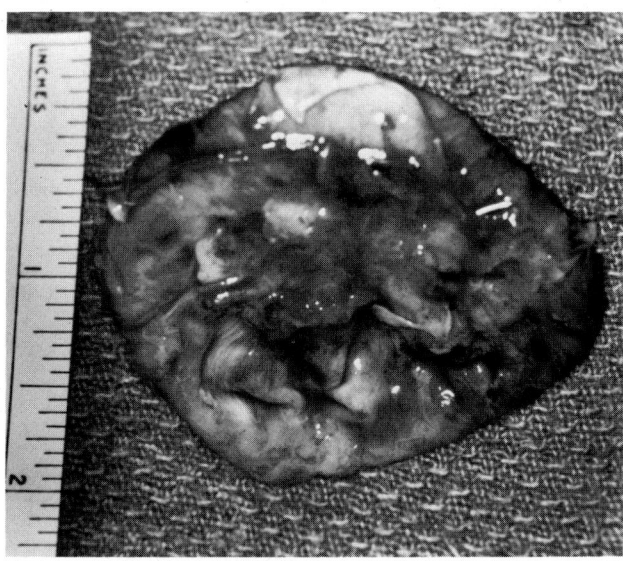

Figure 30–9
Capsule of excised endometrioma.

perhaps two-thirds of these have endometriosis as the only explanation for their inability to conceive.[50] In cases in which tubo-ovarian or peritoneal adhesions interfere with ovum pickup, or in which the ovarian architecture has been replaced by endometriotic cyst, the etiology of infertility may be explicable on an anatomic basis. Much less clearly understood, however, is the cause of subfertility in cases of "mild" endometriosis. Various putative factors have been proposed to account for the association of infertility in women who do not have adhesions or anatomic derangements, including ovulatory dysfunction,[51] luteinized unruptured follicle syndrome,[52] luteal phase insufficiency,[53–55] immunologic factors (increased peripheral and endometrial antibodies, increased complement factors, increased peritoneal cytokines, and defective peritoneal macrophage function),[56–60] and abnormal endometrial and peritoneal prostaglandin levels.[61–62] Endometriosis has also been associated with an increased risk of early spontaneous abortion, with a return to normal risk levels following medical or surgical treatment of disease.[63–65] This purported risk remains controversial, however, because of control group selection in these investigations.[66]

The current clinical significance of these proposed associations is in the diagnosis and therapy of the disease: in women with ovulatory dysfunction or spontaneous abortion the diagnosis of endometriosis should be borne in mind.[48]

Pelvic Pain

The clinical manifestations of pain vary widely, with pain present in most patients with endometriosis. The pain differs according to the site of disease and is frequently not well localized. It may be intermittent or constant, perceived as dull or as pressure, and may radiate to the lower back or upper thighs. Perimenstrually, in some patients, the discomfort may be exacerbated and manifested as dysmenorrhea, dyspareunia, or dyschezia. Moreover, there is little relationship between the extent of pelvic lesions and the amount and degree of pain; that is, women with minimal disease may have chronic debilitating pain, whereas others with severe disease may be asymptomatic. Menstrual enlargement of encapsulated peritoneal implants, fibrous fixation of adjacent structures (occasionally with functional derangement), and tension on pelvic adhesions are mechanisms thought to underlie endometriotic pain.

Atypical Presentations

Endometriosis may be diagnosed at the two extremes of the reproductive years. In the adolescent patient there is often a gastrointestinal, genitourinary, or reproductive tract anomaly,[67] and in the postmenopausal (or castrate) patient there is usually a history of previous endometriosis and estrogen replacement therapy. During the childbearing years, "postsalpingectomy endometriosis" may occur in the proximal stump of the interrupted fallopian tube, usually from one to several years following sterilization.[68] Extrapelvic endometriosis may produce unusual symptoms, often superimposed on the familiar background triad of pelvic pain, infertility, and a pelvic mass. Endometrial tissue may be directly implanted at the time of gynecologic surgery and may begin growth on the cervical or vaginal mucosa or in abdominal or vulvar scars. Cutaneous endometriosis is associated with pelvic endometriosis in one-fifth of cases. Areas of dermatologic involvement may present as painful hemorrhagic nodules, with possible catamenial enlargement or tenderness.[41]

Intestinal involvement occurs in an estimated 10–20% of patients with pelvic endometriosis, with the rectosigmoid colon most frequently involved, and appendiceal disease also common. The symptoms of bowel lesions are pain (frequently menstrual in onset); constipation, diarrhea, or both; obstipation; and, uncommonly, rectal bleeding.[69] Approximately 10% of patients with pelvic endometriosis have urinary tract disease. Endometriosis of the upper tract usually involves the lower one-third of the ureter, especially with peritoneal fibrosis, and may result in flank pain, hydroureter, hydronephrosis, hypertension, or renal failure. Lower tract disease typically involves the serosa of the bladder but may extend into the muscularis or mucosa, with attendant fibrosis, suprapubic pain, dysuria, and hematuria.[70] Pleural and pulmonic endometriosis are rare and usually present as menstrually related pneumothorax, hemothorax, or hemoptysis.[71] Rarer still are the reported cases of endometriosis in muscles of the extremities, inguinal and other lymph node groups, breast, bone, and brain, with organ-specific clinical manifestations.

DIAGNOSIS

The diagnosis of endometriosis can be made with surety by a careful gynecologic history, physical examination, and laparoscopic visualization of the pelvis. That is, endometriosis is a surgical diagnosis, and laparoscopy is the procedure of choice for making the diagnosis and monitoring the response to treatment.[72] The symptoms of endometriosis (considered previously) may or may not be corroborated by the classic signs of disease: a fixed retroflexed uterus, adnexal masses or tenderness, and uterosacral ligament tenderness and nodularity. The differential diagnosis of endometriosis is rather extensive and includes chronic pelvic inflammatory disease, peri-

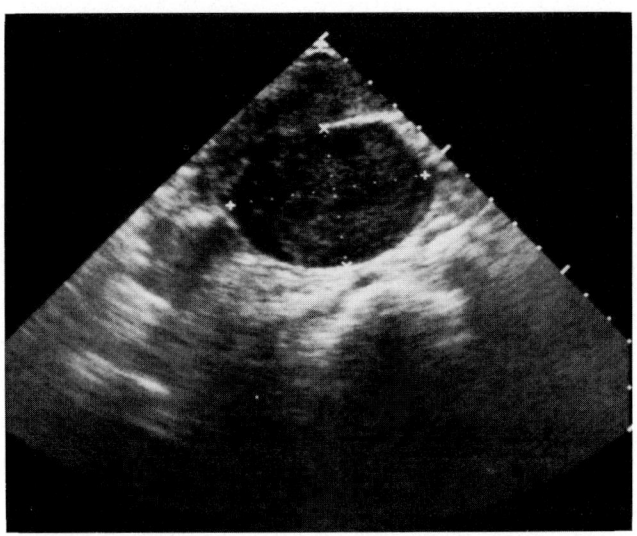

Figure 30–10
Transvaginal ultrasonography of ovarian endometriotic cyst (5-MHz transducer). Note homogeneous echogenic appearance of the cyst.

toneal adhesions, hemorrhagic ovarian cysts, neoplasia, and leiomyomas. If the symptoms and signs suggest the possibility of gastrointestinal or urinary tract involvement, appropriate imaging studies should be performed preoperatively.

Radiologic techniques (ultrasonography, computed tomography, and magnetic resonance imaging) are neither specific nor sensitive enough to make the diagnosis of endometriosis. These techniques, however, may be useful, in selected patients, in monitoring the response to medical therapy once the surgical diagnosis has been established[73] (Fig. 30–10).

CLASSIFICATION OF DISEASE

Analogous to cancer staging systems, various classification schema have been proposed and employed, based on fertility prognosis. A standardized characterization and categorization of endometriosis would provide for better communication, prognostication, treatment, and clinical research. Unfortunately, all systems that have been developed, to date, have been imperfect, several with heterogeneous parameters (active disease, residual or inactive disease, adhesions and endometriomas) considered in an integrated fashion.[3] In 1979 the American Fertility Society (AFS) developed a classification system that incorporated many of the anatomic changes of endometriosis, with points given for either endometriotic lesions or adhesions, and a range from mild to extensive disease. The AFS staging underwent some modifications in 1985, and currently the "Revised American Fertility Society Classification of Endometriosis" is the most commonly used system (Fig. 30–11). Both AFS staging systems, however, are arbitrary, clinically based point systems for anatomic changes only, with no real known correlation to fertility prognosis. Two patients with the same score may have very different disease patterns involving various lesion types, organs, and adhesions. Each stage of disease, then ("minimal, mild, moderate, and severe"), represents an entire spectrum of pathophysiology, with differing treatments and prognoses possible within a given stage. Therefore, a meticulous, detailed operative note and drawings or photographic documentation are essential for more accurate staging and add immeasurably to the simple AFS classification.

TREATMENT

Determinants that are relevant in the critical analysis of therapeutic series for endometriosis include patient selection, surgical methodology, and stage of disease; of these, the stage or degree of pelvic involvement is probably the single most important variable.[74] Furthermore, in the evaluation of therapeutic success, biologic end-points must be clearly defined. Generally, the patient who undergoes endometriosis therapy does so to obtain relief from pelvic pain, to become pregnant, or both; it is the statistical expression of achieving these goals that allows for accurate interpretations of the available literature. The monthly fecundity rate (the number of pregnancies divided by the number of months following therapy)[75] may be used for infertility cases and life table analysis may be employed with either infertility or pelvic pain cases. Life table analysis is a technique that gives an estimate of the proportions of a group of patients who will have a pregnancy (or pain relief) at different time intervals after initial observation as well as consideration of patients with incomplete follow-up.

Expectant Management

Endometriosis represents a relative, not an absolute, impediment to fertility. Therefore, as suggested by Olive and Haney,[3] in evaluating various surgical therapies for infertility for endometriosis, the standard against which success must be measured is the background pregnancy rate in couples "treated" with expectant management. In their review of six series (N = 183) of expectant management for mild disease, the overall pregnancy rate was an estimated 50.3%, using 12-month interval averages. Any successful treatment of mild endometriosis must, therefore, be compared with observational management. It has been recommended that infertility patients with mild

Revised American Fertility Society Classification of Endometriosis: 1985

The American Fertility Society*†

Birmingham, Alabama

Patient's Name ______ Date ______

Stage I (Minimal) - 1-5
Stage II (Mild) - 6-15
Stage III (Moderate) - 16-40
Stage IV (Severe) - >40
Total ______

Laparoscopy ______ Laparotomy ______ Photography ______
Recommended Treatment ______

Prognosis ______

PERITONEUM	ENDOMETRIOSIS	<1cm	1-3cm	>3cm
	Superficial	1	2	4
	Deep	2	4	6
OVARY	R Superficial	1	2	4
	Deep	4	16	20
	L Superficial	1	2	4
	Deep	4	16	20
	POSTERIOR CULDESAC OBLITERATION	Partial		Complete
		4		40
OVARY	ADHESIONS	<1/3 Enclosure	1/3-2/3 Enclosure	>2/3 Enclosure
	R Filmy	1	2	4
	Dense	4	8	16
	L Filmy	1	2	4
	Dense	4	8	16
TUBE	R Filmy	1	2	4
	Dense	4*	8*	16
	L Filmy	1	2	4
	Dense	4*	8*	16

*If the fimbriated end of the fallopian tube is completely enclosed, change the point assignment to 16.

Additional Endometriosis: ______ Associated Pathology: ______

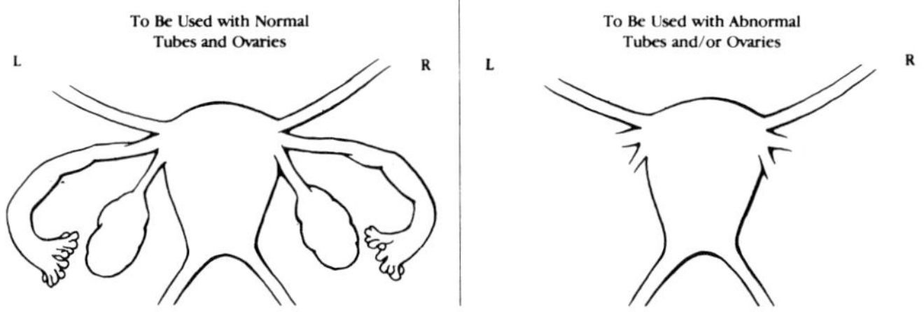

Figure 30–11
American Fertility Society Revised Classification of Endometriosis. (From Revised American Fertility Society Classification of Endometriosis. Fertil Steril 43:351, 1985. Reproduced with permission of the publisher, The American Fertility Society.)

endometriosis and no pelvic pain symptoms be managed on an expectant basis and that during the observation period other infertility factors be evaluated and treated. Patients who fail to conceive after 1 year, or older patients, may be better served with medical or surgical treatment.[76]

Medical Management

The pharmacologic basis of medical management is the hormonal suppression of ectopic endometrium. Multiple endocrine regimens have been prescribed, with variable success, including androgens, progestins, pseudopregnancy (high-dose estrogen-progestin combinations), and pseudomenopause (danazol and gonadotropin-releasing hormone analogues). Although an exhaustive discussion of medical management is beyond the scope of this chapter, it must be noted that there are no convincing data to suggest that any medical therapy for endometriosis enhances fertility more effectively than any other drug; that is, the question of efficacy cannot be adequately answered.[77] Current forms of hormonal treatment differ greatly with respect to side effects and costs, but none is definitive therapy for the infertility or pain associated with endometriosis. Suppression may be incomplete, fibrosis and adhesions are not affected, and recurrence is common after discontinuation of therapy.[78]

Operative Laparoscopy

The endoscopic era of pelvic surgery was boldly proclaimed in 1985, and over the ensuing years the burgeoning of operative laparoscopy has revolutionized gynecology.[79] Modern laparoscopy not only permits the accurate diagnosis and classification of disease but also allows for interventional procedures, including (1) adhesiolysis, (2) ablation of endometriotic implants, (3) ablation or excision of endometriomas, and (4) segmental ablation of the uterosacral ligaments.[80] Laparotomy may be delayed or avoided altogether. In each case of operative laparoscopy, however, informed consent should be obtained for laparotomy, thus allowing for appropriately aggressive surgery.[81] Optimally, laparoscopy should be performed during the proliferative phase of the menstrual cycle and should begin as a diagnostic procedure. A uterine manipulator-injector cannula should be placed via the cervix at the outset of the procedure. Then, the pelvis and abdomen are systematically explored with a two-puncture laparoscopic technique; the details of this observation, including AFS staging, are subsequently communicated in the operative note. Thereafter, extra puncture sites are located, as necessary, for the introduction of probes, grasping forceps, cautery, or laser. The surgeon should be trained with at least two- or three-puncture pelviscopic surgery and should be able to control unexpected bleeding with a variety of techniques (unipolar and bipolar coagulation, ligature placement, suturing, and surgical clip application).[81]

Electrocautery, now nearly supplanted by laser vaporization, was formerly a widely used laparoscopic treatment for endometriosis. Pregnancy rates from retrospective, noncontrolled studies with variable patient follow-up have ranged from 47.6%[83] to 57%[84] for mild endometriosis and from 34.5%[83] to 56%[84] for moderate disease. (The latter study included postoperative danazol use.) One controlled investigation of 90 infertility patients with moderate endometriosis revealed that 44% of patients who underwent electrocautery conceived, and 39% who were treated with danazol conceived during 7 months of follow-up ($P = 0.53$).[85] Because of the unpredictable depth of tissue penetration, electrocautery is a potentially dangerous technique, especially when used in close proximity to the bowel or ureters.

Four types of lasers have been applied laparoscopically for the treatment of endometriosis: carbon dioxide (CO_2); neodymium:yttrium-aluminum-garnet (Nd:YAG); argon; and potassium-titanyl-phosphate (KTP). The CO_2 laser is the most frequently used in laparoscopic surgery owing to its wide range of power output, relatively high efficacy, and nearly total absorption by cellular water (Fig. 30–12). Vaporization, the principal tissue effect of the CO_2 laser, is limited to 1 mm or less and may be precisely controlled, but there is only limited ability to stop active bleeding (Fig. 30–13). The three remaining laser types in gynecologic use can deliver their energies via flexible quartz fibers. The hemostatic effect of fiber lasers is greater than that of CO_2 lasers, and

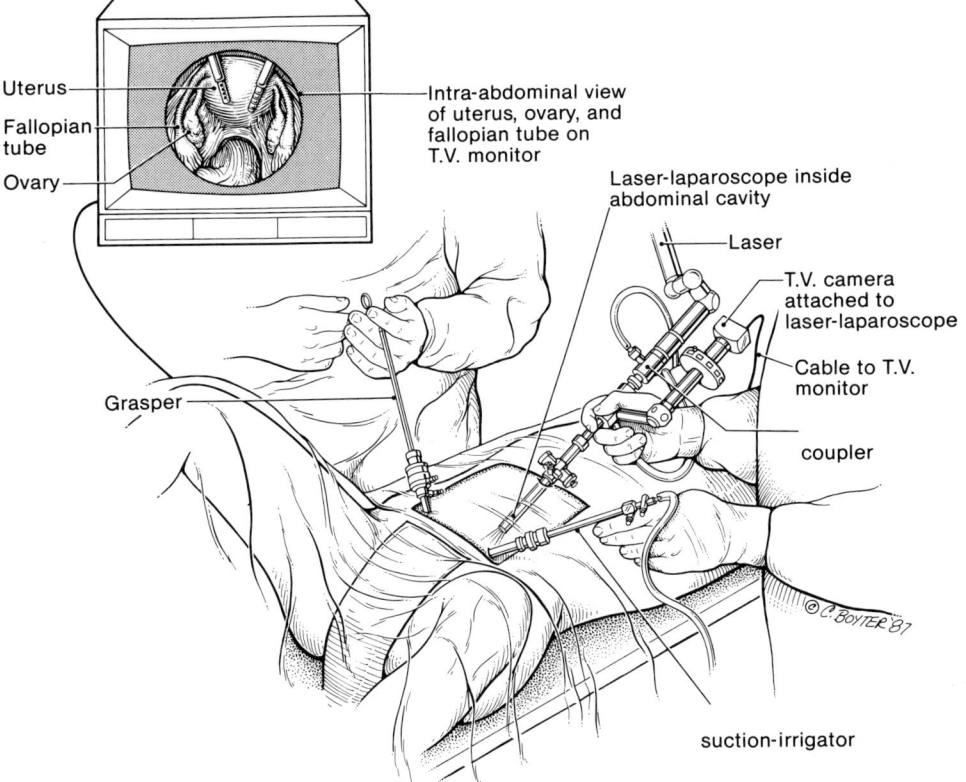

Figure 30–12
Operative set-up for laser laparoscopy using video display. (From Nezhat C, et al.: Endoscopic infertility surgery. J Reprod Med 1989; 34:127.)

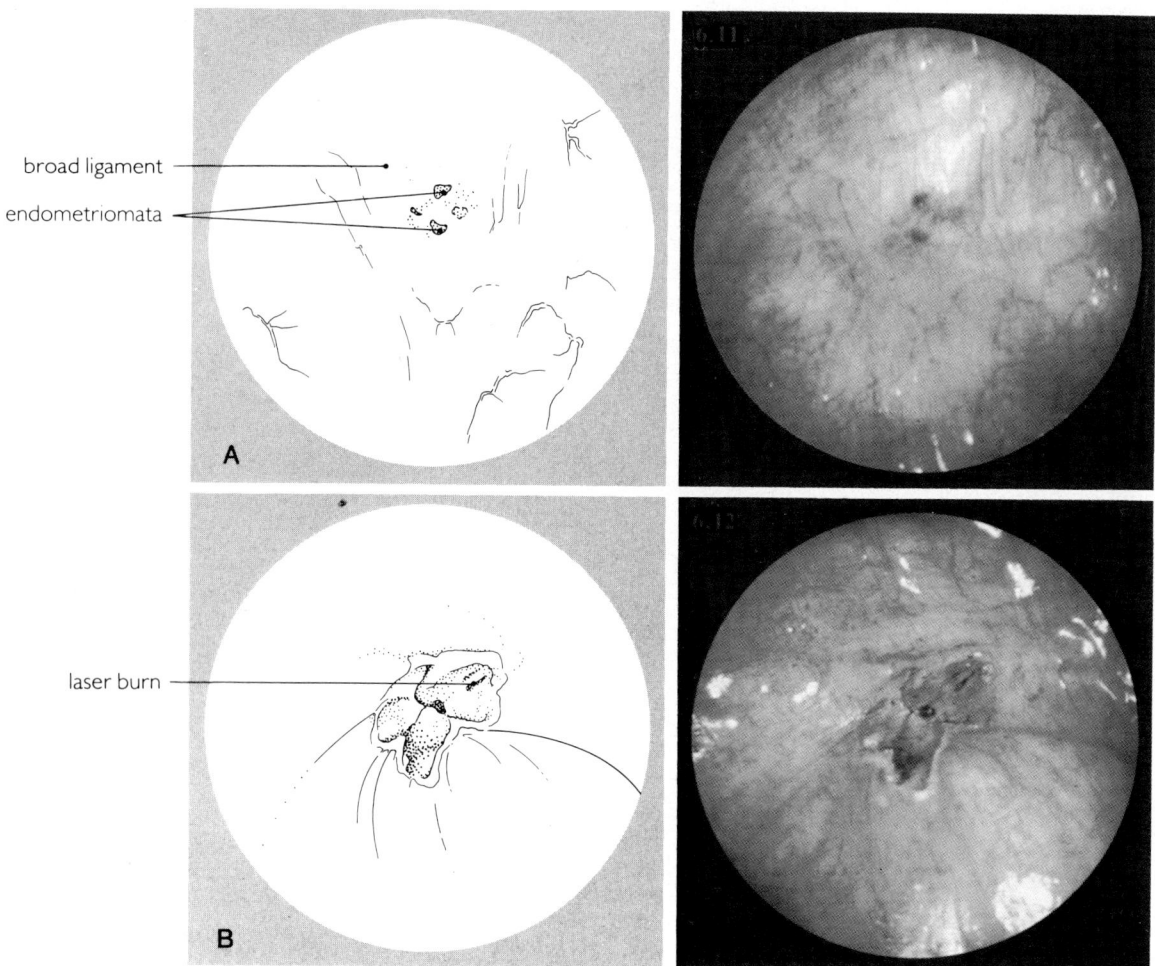

Figure 30–13
Laparoscopic view of peritoneal endometriosis prior to (*A*) and following (*B*) laser ablation. (From Gordon AG, Lewis BV: Gynecologic Endoscopy. Philadelphia, JB Lippincott, 1988.)

fiber lasers have a greater depth of penetration, are color-dependent, and have slight to moderate lateral beam scattering.

Lasers may be used endoscopically for incision or vaporization of pelvic adhesions, uterosacral ablation, vaporization of endometriotic implants, and incision of ovarian endometriomas (Fig. 30–14). These procedures, performed in the same surgical setting as that of the diagnostic laparoscopy, allow for restoration of the pelvic anatomy and often obviate the need for exploratory laparotomy and another anesthetic exposure.[82] In six series of laparoscopic laser vaporization of endometriosis (N = 437) (Table 30–1), the overall pregnancy rate was 59% (mild, 59.3%; moderate, 51.9%; severe, 61.5%). Unfortunately, there are no criteria by which to evaluate these data; that is, no controlled studies of staged endometriosis comparing laser vaporization with expectant management exist, making available "success" rates difficult to interpret.

Laparoscopic uterosacral neurolysis, performed for primary dysmenorrhea or dysmenorrhea associated with endometriosis, led to significant symptomatic improvement in 71% (30 of 42) of cases in one study.[85] Again, no controlled studies are available to compare "laser neurolysis" with observation, nonsteroidal anti-inflammatory agents, or presacral neurectomy.

Laparotomy

Prior to major abdominal surgery for infertility, the infertility evaluation should be complete, and all abnormalities in the husband and wife should be treated. "Conservative" surgery for endometriosis denotes excision or vaporization of all visible endometriosis and associated adhesions and the restoration of normal anatomic relationships, to maximize the potential for conception or pain relief. Laparotomy should be considered in cases in which there is distortion of reproductive anatomy or severe pelvic pain that is not amenable to medical or laparoscopic procedures. Conservative surgery, as a philosophy,

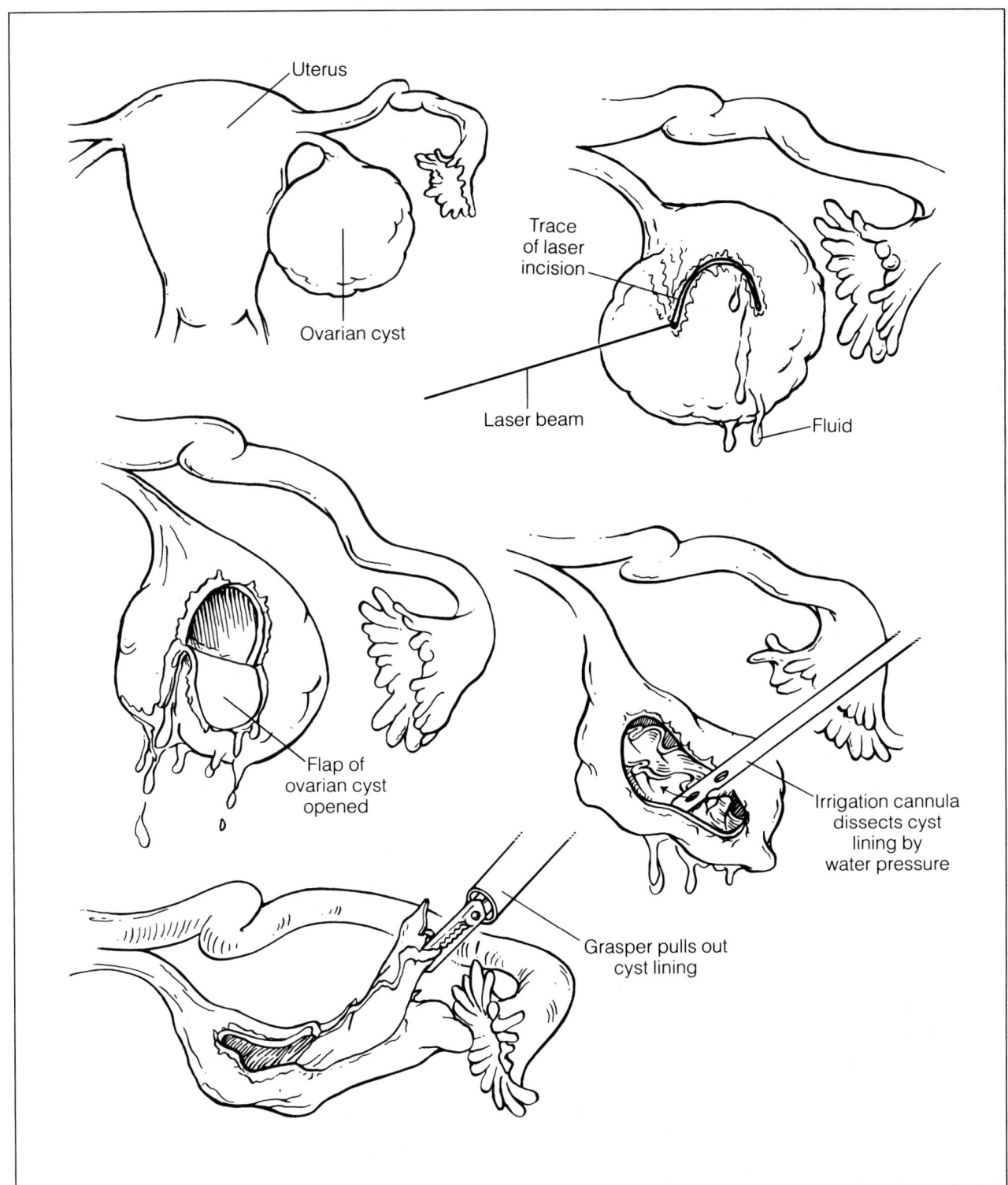

Figure 30–14
Technique for laparoscopic incision of endometriotic cyst and dissection of cyst wall from the ovarian stroma. The cyst lining is removed and extracted via the main laparoscopic sleeve. (From Baggish MS, et al.: Symposium: Performing safe laser laparoscopy. Contemp Obstet Gynecol, June 1990.)

Table 30-1

Pregnancies Following Laparoscopic Laser Vaporization of Endometriosis

		Pregnancies (%)				Total Monthly Fecundity Rate (%)
	N	Mild	Moderate	Severe	Total	
Kelly and Roberts[87] (1983)	10	3/3 (100)	3/7 (42.9)		6 (60.0)	
Feste[86] (1985)	58	24/47 (51.1)	4/6 (66.7)	2/5 (40.0)	30 (51.7)	
Martin and Olive[3] (1986)	80	18/45 (40.0)	7/22 (31.8)	8/13 (61.5)	33 (41.2)	3.5
Donnez[88] (1987)	70	26/42 (62.0)	11/21 (52.0)	3/7 (42.0)	40 (57.0)	
Nezhat et al.[89] (1989)	204	60/86 (69.8)	45/67 (67.2)	35/51 (68.6)	140 (68.6)	5.9
Shirk[90] (1989)	15	3/34 (100)	6/10 (60.0)	0/2 (0)	9 (60.0)	
TOTAL	437	134/226 (59.3)	66/133 (51.9)	48/78 (61.5)	258 (59.0)	

connotes microsurgical technique with gentle tissue handling, dedicated instruments, sharp dissection, tissue reconstruction, meticulous hemostasis, fine sutures, and the use of adjuvants to reduce the likelihood of postoperative adhesion formation (e.g., INTERCEED [TC7], oxidized regenerated cellulose adhesion barrier, or Gore-Tex) (Fig. 30-15).

For patients with a history of intractable, chronic pelvic pain, presacral neurectomy may be the procedure of choice. A retrospective analysis by Polan and DeCherney[91] demonstrated that 75% of patients with either pelvic inflammatory disease or endometriosis had significant relief of pain following presacral neurectomy, compared with only 26% of the control group who underwent laparotomy for infertility. Interruption of the presacral sensory nerves is often effective when medical therapy has failed and remains an alternative for women desiring maintenance of reproductive potential.[92] There is no evidence that this procedure independently enhances fertility, however.

Pregnancy rates following conservative surgery

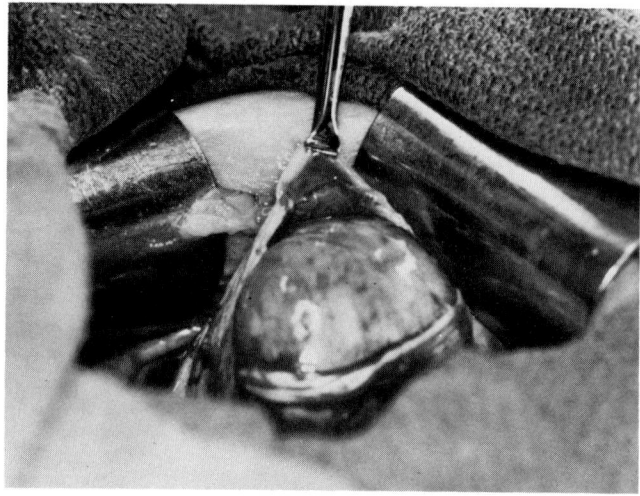

Figure 30-15
Dissection of ovarian endometriotic cyst at time of exploratory laparotomy. Following excision of the cyst, the ovary is repaired with fine, absorbable nonreactive suture, resulting in a functional, normal-appearing ovary.

are dependent largely on the extent and location of disease, the techniques used, the age of the patient, and the length of follow-up. In 2094 reported cases involving previously infertile women, an overall 52.7% pregnancy rate has been achieved.[3] For mild, moderate, and severe disease, the rates were 60.7%, 50.0%, and 39.2%, respectively. Few of these reviewed series were prospective, controlled, randomized trials; therefore, most are subject to various biases. One study of note, which employed life table analysis, compared results with danazol and conservative surgery in 224 women with AFS-staged mild and moderate disease. There were no significant differences between these treatments with respect to either cure rate or the monthly fecundity rate.[93]

The cumulative 3-year disease recurrence rate following conservative surgery has been reported to be 13.5%, with a 5-year recurrence rate of 40.3%, although severity of disease was not predictive of recurrence. Furthermore, the recurrent disease was not necessarily in the same location or of the same stage as the initial disease. This clinical report also documented a 47% pregnancy rate among infertile patients with recurrent endometriosis after a second conservative procedure.[94] If conception has not occurred by 12 to 18 months following conservative surgery for endometriosis, despite careful attention to other fertility factors, a second-look operative laparoscopy should be considered, because the majority of pregnancies occur within 18 months postoperatively.

The use of postoperative hormonal therapy (e.g., danazol or gonadotropin-releasing hormone [GnRH] analogues) remains controversial because of a lack of appropriate, controlled investigations. Buttram,[95] in a review following conservative surgery for endometriosis, found that of patients who conceived, 50% were pregnant within 6 months after surgery, and 86% were so after 15 months. These data indicate that suppressive treatment probably should be avoided during the early postoperative period, to allow for conception. On the other hand, Wheeler and Malinak[94] noted a 71% pregnancy rate at 18 months in women with severe endometriosis treated with conservative laparotomy followed by danazol therapy, compared with a 30% pregnancy rate in women who underwent surgery alone. In selected patients with AFS Stage III and IV disease, postoperative medical therapy is probably indicated for suppression of residual disease.

The Assisted Reproductive Technologies

In vitro fertilization (IVF), gamete intrafallopian transfer (GIFT), and zygote intrafallopian transfer (ZIFT) are surgical techniques indicated for endometriosis patients with infertility who have not conceived with more conservative treatments. Intuitively, it would seem that oocyte harvesting, fertilization and cleavage in vitro, and embryo replacement would overcome any detrimental effect of pelvic endometriosis; however, IVF treatment of women with severe disease has resulted in poorer pregnancy rates. Those patients with AFS Stage I and II disease have pregnancy rates per cycle comparable to tubal factor infertility patients,[96, 97] while reduced fertilization rates have been reported with IVF for severe endometriosis, especially in the presence of endometriomas. Patients with AFS Stage III and IV disease might benefit from medical or surgical treatment prior to commencing an IVF cycle.[98, 99] In women with low-grade endometriosis and normal-appearing fallopian tubes, GIFT or ZIFT is an alternative to IVF.

Definitive Surgery

Following uterine leiomyomas and genital prolapse, endometriosis is the third most common indication for hysterectomy in the United States, accounting for approximately 15% of all hysterectomies.[100] Available medical and conservative surgical modalities certainly do not represent curative therapy, and when endometriosis is symptomatic in women who have finished childbearing or in whom extensive disease is not remediable, total abdominal hysterectomy and bilateral salpingo-oophorectomy is the treatment of choice. Bowel and peritoneal lesions and adhesions should be removed at the time of extirpative surgery. Ovarian preservation is controversial in the definitive treatment of endometriosis but may be considered after well-informed consent in young women with little to no ovarian endometriotic involvement. In general, the risk of recurrent symptoms following hysterectomy and conservation of normal ovaries is approximately 3–6%.[7]

Hormone replacement therapy is not contraindicated in post-oophorectomy endometriosis patients. Physiologic estrogen-progestin doses only infrequently cause the persistence or recurrence of endometriosis. The effects of hormone replacement may be related to the bioactivity of exogenous estrogen, as well as endogenous circulating estrogen levels. Should symptoms recur while the patient is receiving estrogen therapy, a progestin-only regimen or relatively high-dose progestin with low-dose estrogen may be efficacious.

Treatment of Gastrointestinal Endometriosis

Endometriosis of the bowel has been estimated to occur in more than one-third of patients with pelvic endometriosis.[7] Most of these lesions involve the serosa of the sigmoid colon and rectum and are easily excised or vaporized by the gynecologic surgeon, but obstructive, full-thickness lesions often require bowel resection. Two recent series of endometriosis patients (N = 4646) revealed gastrointestinal involvement in 5.4%, with bowel resection necessary in approximately 1%.[69, 101] Excision of bowel was required owing to recurrent gastrointestinal symptoms (cyclic diarrhea, constipation, or rectal bleeding; dyschezia; and partial or complete bowel obstruction), the suspicion of malignancy, or both. Segmental resection of the colon for the treatment of deep bowel endometriosis is a safe procedure with acceptably low morbidity and good symptomatic relief.[102]

The absence of gastrointestinal symptoms appears to be predictive of the absence of clinically significant intestinal endometriosis.[69] Preoperative evaluation in the patient with bowel symptoms should include flexible sigmoidoscopy, barium enema, and consultation with a gastrointestinal surgeon. In addition, bowel preparation should be performed preoperatively on any patient with a clinical presentation suggestive of intestinal disease.

Treatment of Urinary Tract Endometriosis

Urinary tract involvement is usually confined to the visceral peritoneum of the bladder and is easily treatable with ablative surgery. Ureteral endometriosis is present only in approximately 1–2% of patients and is much more likely to consist of periureteral fibrosis and peritoneal scarring than of actual disease of the wall of the ureter.[103] Obstruction of a ureter may be slow and insidious, with clinically silent development of hydroureter, hydronephrosis, and renal destruction. The pelvic course of the ureters should be identified during any surgery for endometriosis and especially when there is dissection of

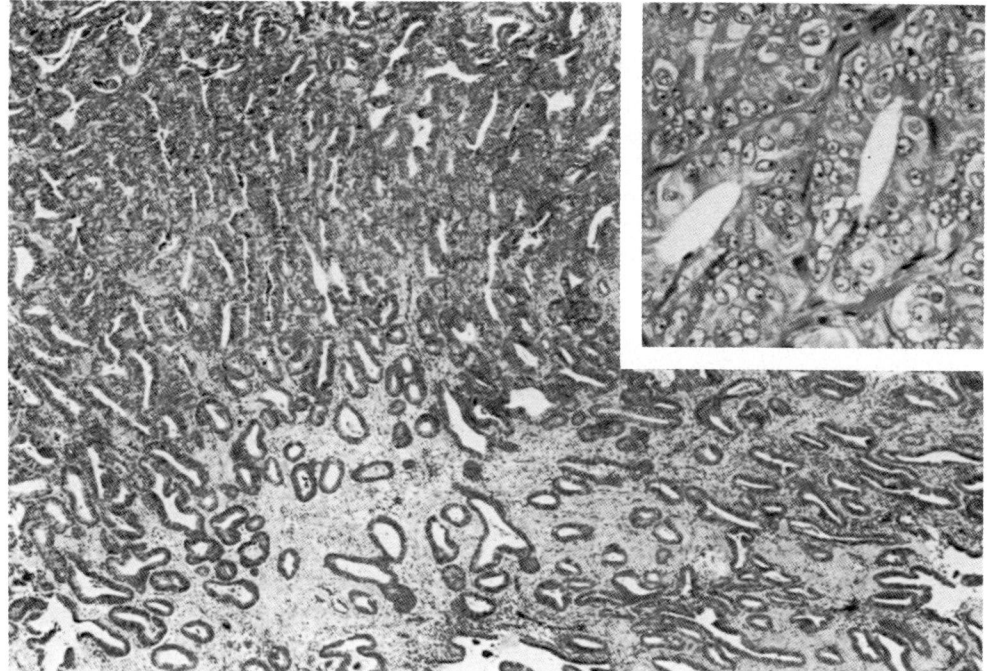

Figure 30–16
Endometrioid carcinoma arising in a focus of ovarian endometriosis. (From Clement PB: Endometriosis, lesions of the secondary müllerian system, and pelvic mesothelial proliferations. In Kurman RJ (ed.): Blaustein's Pathology of the Female Genital Tract. New York, Springer-Verlag, 1987.)

the lateral wall of the pelvis or broad ligament lesions. While ureteral obstruction is rarely diagnosed preoperatively in endometriosis patients, any woman presenting with upper urinary tract symptoms deserves intravenous pyelography and possible urologic consultation thereafter.

Malignancy

Malignancy arising from a nidus of endometriosis is a rare event, with approximately 75% of such tumors originating in the ovary.[104] Of the remaining 25% of reported cancers (fewer than 70 cases in the world literature), the most common sites are the rectovaginal septum, colon and rectum, vagina, and bladder. The actual incidence of malignancy arising from endometriosis is unknown, with the pathologic distinction difficult. Malignancy may also arise from a dormant focus of endometriosis after surgical castration or the climacteric, under the influence of unopposed estrogen replacement therapy.[11]

Endometrioid carcinoma is the most common tumor arising from endometriosis and microscopically has features of endometrial adenocarcinoma (Fig. 30–16). Other histologic types of malignancies arising within endometriosis include clear cell carcinoma, ovarian serous and mucinous tumors, and sarcomas (endometrial stromal sarcoma and mixed mesodermal tumor). These malignancies are clinically manifested most commonly as pelvic pain, a pelvic mass, or intra-abdominal bleeding. Because of their usual small size and low histologic grade, endometrioid carcinomas are common pathologic diagnoses in this setting and are thought to be less malignant than endometrioid carcinoma of the ovary seen in older women.

Review of Surgical Treatment

Surgical therapy for endometriosis must best serve the needs and desires of the individual patient. The patient's age, symptoms, signs, and childbearing plans are modifiers that must be taken into account when planning therapy. Women with AFS Stage I and II disease may be treated at the time of initial laparoscopy; expectant management and medical therapy are also options for minimal and mild disease. Stage III or IV endometriosis may be approached via laparoscopic surgery or conservative laparotomy in infertility patients. Close follow-up and scrupulous attention to other infertility factors are necessary owing to the unpredictable and often progressive course of endometriosis. Women with pain may be treated according to age, reproduction plans, and severity of symptoms. Ovarian preservation is often possible in young women with little to no endometriotic involvement of the ovaries.

Much regarding endometriosis remains unknown. Controlled, prospective, randomized clinical trials are needed for increased understanding of this most enigmatic disease.

References

1. Sampson JA: The development of the implantation theory for the origin of peritoneal endometriosis. Am J Obstet Gynecol 1940; 40:549.

2. Flowers CE Jr, Wilborn WH: New observations in the physiology of menstruation. Obstet Gynecol 1978; 51:16.
3. Olive DL, Haney AF: Endometriosis-associated infertility: A critical review of therapeutic approaches. Obstet Gynecol Surv 1986; 41:538.
4. Strathy JH, Molgaard CA, Coulam CG, Melton LH III: Endometriosis and infertility: A laparoscopic study of endometriosis among fertile and infertile women. Fertil Steril 1982; 38:667.
5. Haney AF: Pelvic endometriosis: Etiology and pathology. Semin Reprod Endocrinol 1988; 6:287.
6. Weed JC, Arquembourg PC: Endometriosis: Can it produce an autoimmune response resulting in infertility? Clin Obstet Gynecol 1980; 23:885.
7. Williams TJ, Pratt JH: Endometriosis in 1000 consecutive celiotomies: Incidence and management. Am J Obstet Gynecol 1977; 129:245.
8. Sanfilippo JS, Wakim NG, Schikler KN, Yussman MA: Endometriosis in association with a uterine anomaly. Am J Obstet Gynecol 1986; 154:39.
9. Goldstein DP, deCholnoky C, Emans SJ, Leventhal JM: Laparoscopy in the diagnosis and management of pelvic pain in adolescents. J Reprod Med 1980; 24:251.
10. Punnonen R, Klemi P, Nikkanen V: Postmenopausal endometriosis. Eur J Obstet Gynecol Reprod Biol 1980; 11:195.
11. Reimnitz C, Brand E, Nieberg RK, Hacker NF: Malignancy arising in endometriosis associated with unopposed estrogen replacement. Obstet Gynecol 1988; 71:444.
12. Goodall JR: A Study of Endometriosis, Endosalpingiosis, Endocervicosis and Peritoneo-ovarian Sclerosis: A Clinical and Pathological Study. Philadelphia, JB Lippincott, 1943, p. 119.
13. Simpson JL, Elias S, Malinak LR, Buttram VC, Jr: Heritable aspects of endometriosis. I. Genetic studies. Am J Obstet Gynecol 1980; 137:327.
14. Malinak LR, Buttram VC Jr, Elias S, Simpson JL: Heritable aspects of endometriosis. II. Clinical characteristics of familial endometriosis. Am J Obstet Gynecol 1980; 137:332.
15. Sutton LA: Endometriosis. In Davis CH (ed.): Gynecology and Obstetrics. Hagerstown, MD, WF Prior, 1946, p. 15.
16. Cullen TS: Adenomyoma of the round ligament. Bull Johns Hopkins Hosp 1896; 7:112.
17. Iwanoff NS: Druesiges cystenhaltiges Uterusfibromyom Kompliziert durch Sarcom und Carcinom. Monatsschr Geburtsh Gynaekol 1988; 7:295.
18. Pick L: Ueber Neubildungen am Genitale bei Zwittern, nebst Beitraegen zur Lehre von den Adenomen des Hodens und Eierstockes. Arch Gynaekol 1905; 76:192.
19. Meyer R: Zur genesis der Cystadeonome u Adenomyome des Uterus. Ztschr Geburtsh Gynaekol 1897; 43:130.
20. Meyer R: Ueber eine adenomatoese Wucherung der Serosa in einer Bauchnarbe. Ztschr Geburtsh Gynaekol 1903; 49:32.
21. Meyer R: Demonstration eines bis in die Wurzel des Mesocolon ausgedehnten heterotopen Darmepithels. Verh Dtsch Pathol Ges 1908; 12:48.
22. Meyer R: Ueber den Stand der Frage der Adenomyositis und Adenomyome im allgemeinen, und insbesonders ueber Adenomyositis seroepithelialis. Zentralbl Gynaekol 1919; 36:745.
23. Halban J: Hysteroadenosis metastatica (die Lymphogene Genese der sog Adenofibromatosis heterotopica). Wien Klin Wochenschr 1924; 37:1205.
24. Javert CT: Pathogenesis of endometriosis based on endometrial homeoplasia, direct extension, exfoliation and implantation, lymphatic and hematogenous metastasis. Cancer 1949; 2:399.
25. Sampson JA: Metastatic or embolic endometriosis: Due to menstrual dissemination of endometrial tissue into the circulation. Am J Pathol 1927; 3:93.
26. Ridley JH: The histogenesis of endometriosis. Obstet Gynecol Surg 1968; 23:1.
27. Sampson JA: Perforating haemorrhagic (chocolate) cysts of the ovary. Arch Surg 1921; 3:245.
28. Sampson JA: The life history of ovarian hematomas of endometrial type. Am J Obstet Gynecol 1922; 4:451.
29. Sampson JA: Intestinal adenomas of the endometrial type. Arch Surg 1922; 5:217.
30. Sampson JA: Benign and malignant endometrial implants in the peritoneal cavity and their relation to certain ovarian tumors. Surg Gynecol Obstet 1924; 38:287.
31. Sampson JA: Endometrial carcinoma of the ovary arising in endometrial tissue in that organ. Arch Surg 1925; 10:1.
32. Sampson JA: Inguinal endometriosis. Am J Obstet Gynecol 1925; 10:462.
33. Sampson JA: Heterotopic or misplaced endometrial tissue. Am J Obstet Gynecol 1925; 10:649.
34. Sampson JA: Peritoneal endometriosis due to the menstrual dissemination of endometrial tissue into the peritoneal cavity. Am J Obstet Gynecol 1927; 14:422.
35. Sampson JA: Endometriosis following salpingectomy. Am J Obstet Gynecol 1928; 16:461.
36. Sampson JA: Infected endometrial cysts of the ovary: A report of three cases. Am J Obstet Gynecol 1929; 18:1.
37. Sampson JA: Pelvic endometriosis and tubal fimbriae. Am J Obstet Gynecol 1932; 24:497.
38. Cron RS, Gey G: The viability of the cast-off menstrual endometrium. Am J Obstet Gynecol 1927; 43:645.
39. Halme J, Hammond MG, Hulka JF, et al.: Retrograde menstruation in healthy women and patients with endometriosis. Obstet Gynecol 1984; 64:151.
40. Bergquist A, Ljungberg O, Myhre E: Human endometrium and endometriotic tissue obtained simultaneously: A comparative histologic study. Int J Gynecol Pathol 1984; 3:135.
41. Clement PB: Endometriosis, lesions of the secondary müllerian system, and pelvic mesothelial proliferations. In Kurman RJ (ed.): Blaustein's Pathology of the Female Genital Tract. New York, Springer-Verlag, 1987, p. 523.
42. Fox H, Buckley CH: Current concepts of endometriosis. Clin Obstet Gynaecol 1984; 11:279.
43. Jansen RPS, Russell P: Nonpigmented endometriosis: Clinical, laparoscopic and pathologic definition. Am J Obstet Gynecol 1986; 155:1154.
44. Jenkins S, Olive DL, Haney AF: The location of endometriosis lesions in an infertile patient population. Obstet Gynecol 1986; 67:335.
45. Egger H, Weigmann P: Clinical and surgical aspects of ovarian endometriotic cysts. Arch Gynecol 1982; 233:37.
46. Holmes WR: Endometriosis. Am J Obstet Gynecol 1942; 43:255.
47. Stevenson CS, Campbell CG: The symptoms, physical findings, and clinical diagnosis of pelvic endometriosis. Clin Obstet Gynecol 1960; 3:441.
48. Muse K: Clinical manifestations and classification of endometriosis. Clin Obstet Gynecol 1988; 31:813.
49. Kistner RW: Endometriosis and infertility. Clin Obstet Gynecol 1979; 22:101.
50. Dmowski WP, Radwanska E: Endometriosis and infertility. Acta Obstet Gynecol Scand (Suppl) 1984; 123:73.
51. Soules M, Malinak L, Bury R, Poindexter A: Endometriosis and anovulation: A coexisting problem in the infertile female. Am J Obstet Gynecol 1976; 125:412.
52. Donnez J, Thomas K: Influence of the luteinized unruptured follicle syndrome in fertile women and in women with endometriosis. Eur J Obstet Gynecol Reprod Biol 1982; 14:187.
53. Pittaway D, Maxon W, Daniell J, et al.: Luteal phase defects in infertility patients with endometriosis. Fertil Steril 1983; 39:712.
54. Cheesman KL, Cheesman SD, Chatterton RT Jr, Cohen MR: Alterations in progesterone metabolism and luteal function in infertile women with endometriosis. Fertil Steril 1983; 40:590.
55. Ronnberg L, Kauppila A, Rajaniemi H: Luteinizing hormone receptor disorder in endometriosis. Fertil Steril 1984; 42:64.
56. Chihal H, Mathur S, Holtz G, Williamson H: An endometrial antibody assay in the diagnosis and management of endometriosis. Fertil Steril 1986; 46:408.
57. Badaway SZA, Cuenca V, Stitzel AB, et al.: Autoimmune phenomena in infertile patients with endometriosis. Obstet Gynecol 1984; 63:271.
58. Fakih H, Baggett B, Holtz G, et al.: Interleukin-1: A possible role in the infertility associated with endometriosis. Fertil Steril 1987; 47:213.
59. Eisermann J, Gast MJ, Pineda J, et al.: Tumor necrosis factor

in peritoneal fluid of women undergoing laparoscopic surgery. Fertil Steril 1988; 50:573.
60. Halme J, Becker S, Hammond MG, et al.: Increased activation of pelvic macrophages in infertile women with endometriosis. Am J Obstet Gynecol 1983; 145:333.
61. Dawood MA, Khan-Dawood FS, Wilson L Jr: Peritoneal fluid prostaglandins and prostanoids in women with endometriosis, chronic pelvic inflammatory disease, and pelvic pain. Am J Obstet Gynecol 1984; 148:391.
62. Vernon M, Beard J, Graves K, Wilson E: Classification of endometriotic implants by morphologic appearance and capacity to synthesize prostaglandin F. Fertil Steril 1986; 46:801.
63. Rock JA, Guzick DS, Sengos C, et al.: The conservative surgical treatment of endometriosis: Evaluation of pregnancy success with respect to extent of disease as categorized using contemporary classification systems. Fertil Steril 1981; 35:131.
64. Naples JD, Batt RE, Sadigh H: Spontaneous abortion rate in patients with endometriosis. Obstet Gynecol 1981; 57:509.
65. Wheeler JM, Johnston BM, Malinak LR: The relationship of endometriosis to spontaneous abortion. Fertil Steril 1983; 39:656.
66. Metzger DA, Olive DL, Stohs GF, Franklin RR: Association of endometriosis and spontaneous abortion: Effect of control group selection. Fertil Steril 1986; 45:18.
67. Muller P: Association of genital and urinary malformation in women. Gynaecologia 1968; 165:285.
68. Rock JA, Parmley TH, King TM, et al.: Endometriosis and the development of tuboperitoneal fistulas after tubal ligation. Fertil Steril 1981; 35:16.
69. Prystowsky JB, Stryker SJ, Ujiki GT, Poticha SM: Gastrointestinal endometriosis. Arch Surg 1988; 123:855.
70. Moore JG, Hibbard LT, Grodon WA, Schrifrin BS: Urinary tract endometriosis: Enigmas in diagnosis and management. Am J Obstet Gynecol 1979; 134:162.
71. Balasingham S, Arulkumaran S, Nadarajah K, Jayaratnam FJ: Catamenial pneumothorax. Aust NZ J Obstet Gynaecol 1986; 26:88.
72. Polan ML: Endometriosis. Semin Reprod Endocrinol 1984; 2:186.
73. Zawin M, McCarthy S, Scoutt L, Comite F: Endometriosis: Appearance and detection at MR imaging. Radiology 1989; 171:693.
74. Loy 5A, DeCherney AH: The impact of the assisted reproductive technologies on surgery of the fallopian tube. Semin Reprod Endocrinol 1990; 8:304.
75. Cramer DW, Walker AM, Schiff I: Statistical methods in evaluating the outcome of infertility therapy. Fertil Steril 1979; 32:80.
76. Schenken RS, Malinak LR: Conservative surgery versus expectant management for the infertile patient with endometriosis. Fertil Steril 1982; 37:183.
77. Miller MM, Rebar RW: An approach to patients with endometriosis. Clin Obstet Gynecol 1988; 31:883.
78. Kitchin JD III, Nunley WC Jr: Endometriosis. In Sciarra J (ed.): Gynecology and Obstetrics. Philadelphia, JB Lippincott, 1990, p. 14.
79. DeCherney AH: The leader of the band is tired... (editorial). Fertil Steril 1985; 44:299.
80. Gomel V: Operative laparoscopy: Time for acceptance. Fertil Steril 1989; 52:1.
81. Daniell J: Operative laparoscopy for endometriosis. Semin Reprod Endocrinol 1985; 3:353.
82. Wilson EA: Surgical therapy for endometriosis. Clin Obstet Gynecol 1988; 31:857.
83. Sulewski JM, Curcio FD, Bronitsky C, Stenger VG: The treatment of endometriosis at laparoscopy for infertility. Am J Obstet Gynecol 1980; 138:128.
84. Daniell JF, Christianson C: Combined laparoscopic surgery and danazol therapy for pelvic endometriosis. Fertil Steril 1981; 35:521.
85. Seiler JC, Gidwani G, Ballard L: Laparoscopic cauterization of endometriosis for fertility: A controlled study. Fertil Steril 1986; 46:1098.
86. Feste JR: Laser laparoscopy: A new modality. J Reprod Med 1985; 40:413.
87. Kelly RW, Roberts DK: CO_2 laser laparoscopy: A potential alternative to danazol in the treatment of Stage I and Stage II endometriosis. J Reprod Med 1983; 28:638.
88. Donnez J: CO_2 laser laparoscopy in infertile women with endometriosis and women with adnexal adhesions. Fertil Steril 1987; 48:390.
89. Nezhat C, Crowgey S, Nezhat F: Videolaparoscopy for the treatment of endometriosis associated with infertility. Fertil Steril 1989; 51:237.
90. Shirk GJ: Use of the Nd:YAG laser for the treatment of endometriosis. Am J Obstet Gynecol 1989; 160:1344.
91. Polan MK, DeCherney A: Presacral neurectomy for pelvic pain in infertility. Fertil Steril 1980; 34:557.
92. Lee RB, Stone K, Magelssen D, et al.: Presacral neurectomy for chronic pelvic pain. Obstet Gynecol 1986; 68:517.
93. Guzick DS, Rock JA: A comparison of danazol and conservative surgery for the treatment of infertility due to mild or moderate endometriosis. Fertil Steril 1983; 40:580.
94. Wheeler JM, Malinak LR: Recurrent endometriosis: Incidence, management, and prognosis. Am J Obstet Gynecol 1983; 146:247.
95. Buttram VC Jr: Conservative surgery for endometriosis in the infertile female: A study of 206 patients with implications for both medical and surgical therapy. Fertil Steril 1979; 31:117.
96. Chillik CF, Acosta AA, Garcia JE, et al.: The role of in vitro fertilization in infertile patients with endometriosis. Fertil Steril 1985; 44:56.
97. Matson PL, Yovich JL: The treatment of infertility associated with endometriosis by in vitro fertilization. Fertil Steril 1986; 46:432.
98. Wardle PG, McLaughlin EA, McDermott A, et al.: Endometriosis and ovulatory disorder: Reduced fertilization in vitro compared with tubal and unexplained infertility. Lancet 1985; 2:236.
99. Dlugi AM, Loy RA, Dieterle S, et al.: The effect of endometriomas on in vitro fertilization outcome. J In Vitro Fert Embryo Transf 1989; 6:338.
100. Pokras R, Hufnagel VG: Hysterectomy in the United States, 1965–84. Am J Public Health 1988; 78:852.
101. Weed JC, Ray JE: Endometriosis of the bowel. Obstet Gynecol 1987; 69:727.
102. Coronado C, Franklin RR, Lotze EC, et al.: Surgical treatment of symptomatic colorectal endometriosis. Fertil Steril 1990; 53:411.
103. Pratt JH, Williams TJ: Indications for complete pelvic operations and more radical procedures in the treatment of severe or extensive endometriosis. Clin Obstet Gynecol 1980; 23:937.
104. Brooks JJ, Wheeler JE: Malignancy arising in extragonadal endometriosis: A case report and summary of the world literature. Cancer 1977; 40:3065.

Operative Procedures for the Breast

31

Vicki Seltzer
Jeanne A. Petrek

During the past decade, it has become clear that the obstetrician-gynecologist has an expanding role in the field of breast disease. For many women, the obstetrician-gynecologist is the only physician whom they see and therefore is the person who is best able to have patients involved in programs for the early detection of breast cancer.

Breast cancer is the most common malignancy affecting American women. It is estimated that one of every nine women born in the United States today will develop breast cancer, and that there will be approximately 150,000 new cases in the United States each year. Breast cancer kills more women in the United States annually than all of the pelvic gynecologic malignancies combined.

During the past several decades, obstetrician-gynecologists have had their patients involved in programs for the early detection of invasive and preinvasive cervical neoplasia, and this has resulted in an enormous reduction in mortality. Whereas in the past it was more common for screening programs for breast disease to identify invasive than preinvasive lesions, programs for early diagnosis are extremely important and should ultimately contribute to a significant reduction in mortality from this disease.

The triad for most effective screening should include monthly breast self-examination, examination by a physician, and screening mammography. It is recommended that under typical circumstances a baseline mammogram should be obtained when the patient is 35 years of age, and that mammograms be performed every 1–2 years between the ages of 40 and 50, and then annually after the age of 50.

As Strax underscored in 1967, and as is still true today, both mammography and clinical evaluation are essential and are complementary.[1] Even with our current sophisticated technology, mammograms have a significant false-negative rate, and it is mandatory that when a breast abnormality is found, a normal mammogram must not impede further evaluation to determine the etiology of the mass.[2]

This chapter provides a detailed review of the surgical procedures performed for the diagnosis and treatment of breast disease.

CYST ASPIRATION

When a cystic breast mass is identified, in addition to focusing on evacuating the cyst, it is important to make certain that breast cancer is not present. A sonogram is often performed to confirm that the mass is cystic. In addition, unless the patient has had a current screening mammogram or unless she is under 30 years of age, a mammogram is usually performed.

For a cyst aspiration to be considered adequate treatment, the following criteria must be satisfied:

1. The cyst must fully collapse; there must be no residual mass following aspiration.
2. The cyst must not repeatedly reaccumulate.
3. The cyst fluid must be clear or cloudy (not red nor brown, which would be indicative of previous bleeding into the mass).

If the cyst does not fully collapse or if it reaccumulates, or if the cyst fluid is bloody, the patient should have a breast biopsy. Many physicians currently do not send the aspirated fluid for cytologic examination if it is not bloody, because the incidence of malignant cells being identified under these circumstances is so low when the cyst fully collapses and does not repeatedly reaccumulate. However, there is not completely uniform agreement that the fluid should be discarded. There is also not uniform agreement regarding whether a biopsy should be performed following a single reaccumulation of fluid or whether the same cyst can be aspirated more than once.

Procedure for Cyst Aspiration

1. The skin is prepared with povidone-iodine (Betadine).

2. The cyst is stabilized between the thumb and forefinger of the surgeon's nondominant hand.

3. A 20-gauge needle attached to a syringe is inserted into the cyst (Fig. 31–1).

4. The cyst is aspirated fully.

5. Pressure is applied to the area.

6. If the cyst fluid is bloody or brown, it should be sent for cytologic evaluation (if the fluid is clear or cloudy, this is optional).

7. The surgeon must make certain that the cyst has fully collapsed.

8. The patient is re-examined to make certain that the cyst has not recurred. If it has not, the patient is followed carefully.

9. If the cyst fluid is bloody or brown, if cytologic examination finds any abnormal cells, if the mass does not fully collapse, or if it reaccumulates following one or more aspirations, the patient must have an excision of the lesion.

ASPIRATION FOR CYTOLOGIC EVALUATION

Although needle aspiration of breast masses was a technique that was performed in the United States as early as the 1920s,[3] it has only been during the past two decades that it has been widely used in this country.

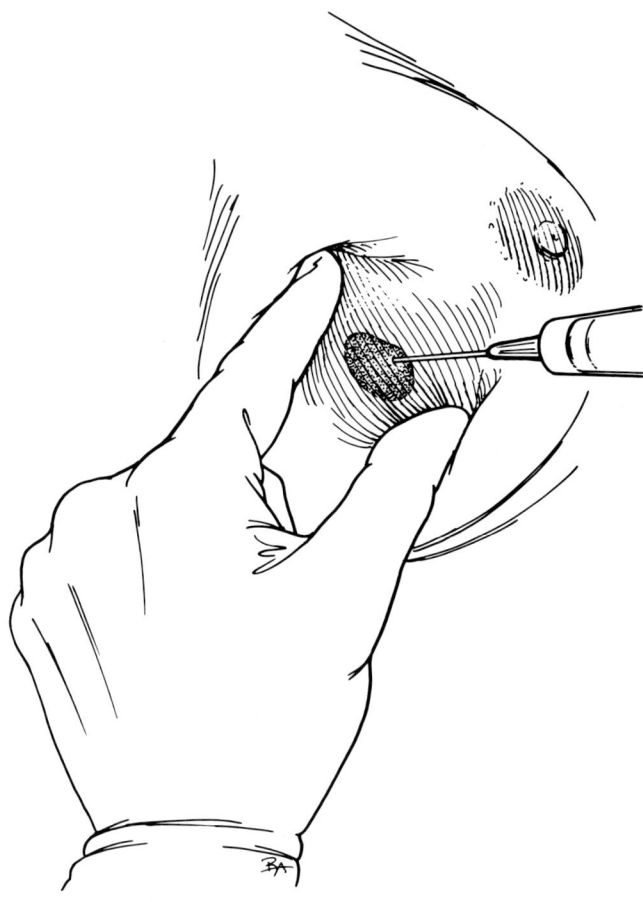

Figure 31–1

In 1975, Zajdela reported a series of 2772 breast masses in which aspiration cytology was performed, always with subsequent open biopsy.[4] There were 1745 histologically malignant tumors, 88% of which were diagnosed by aspiration cytology. There were 63 false-negative and 3 false-positives results. Zajdela's conclusion was that aspiration cytology is extremely reliable when the diagnosis is cancer. However, he warns that when no malignant cells are recovered, the aspiration cytology should be ignored, and an attempt to rule out malignancy must continue.

Several articles have also confirmed the value of needle aspiration in diagnosing malignant lesions of the breast.[5-7] Frable, in a series of 853 aspiration biopsies, found an 89% sensitivity for the diagnosis of breast cancer and a 97% specificity for the absence of breast cancer.[5] Palombini reported a sensitivity of 95.7% and a specificity of 89.6% in a series of 1956 fine-needle aspiration biopsies.[6] In addition to the excellent accuracy in identifying malignant lesions, Frable also noted that in his series there was at least an 85% correlation between histologic and cytologic identification of cancer type.[5] Lee concluded that this is a valuable diagnostic tool that can be safely employed by the practicing gynecologist.[7]

As has been repeatedly emphasized by other investigators, Frable underscores the fact that false-negative results do occur, and therefore all patients with solid breast masses but benign aspirates should have a surgical excision of the mass.[5]

Bottles performed fine-needle aspiration cytology in five pregnant women with dominant breast masses.[8] Three had benign adenomas, and two had ductal carcinoma. Unfortunately, there is occasionally a tendency by clinicians to underestimate the malignant potential of a breast mass found in pregnancy or during the puerperium, which creates the possibility of disastrous consequences. Bottles underscores the fact that more extensive use of fine-needle aspiration cytology when a breast mass is noted in this group of patients may decrease delays in the diagnosis of breast cancer.

Although the availability of fine-needle aspiration cytology has added immeasurably to our armamentarium of techniques to aid in the early diagnosis of breast cancer, the method has some limitations, and it is essential that these are recognized by both the physician and the patient. False-positive findings may occur, although they are uncommon, so that definitive histologic evaluation should be obtained prior to treatment. In addition, false-negative results occur, so that the presence of a negative result does not, with certainty, rule out a malignant lesion. On the other hand, aspiration is a simple technique that may help to hasten treatment planning decisions.

Procedure for Aspiration for Cytologic Evaluation

1. The skin is cleaned with Betadine.
2. The mass is stabilized between the thumb and forefinger of the nondominant hand.
3. A 22- or 25-gauge needle attached to a syringe is placed into the center of the mass.
4. Suction is applied.
5. While constant suction is maintained, the needle should be directed into several areas of the mass. This may be done in a clockwise fashion to make certain that the aspiration is systematically performed (Fig. 31–2). (It is important to be aware of the depth and location of the needle at all times, to avoid creating a pneumothorax.)
6. Before the needle is removed from the mass, the suction is discontinued so that the cells will not be drawn into the barrel.
7. The contents are expressed onto a glass slide (multiple slides will likely be used). A second slide is used to flatten the expressed material. The slides are fixed (Fig. 31–3).

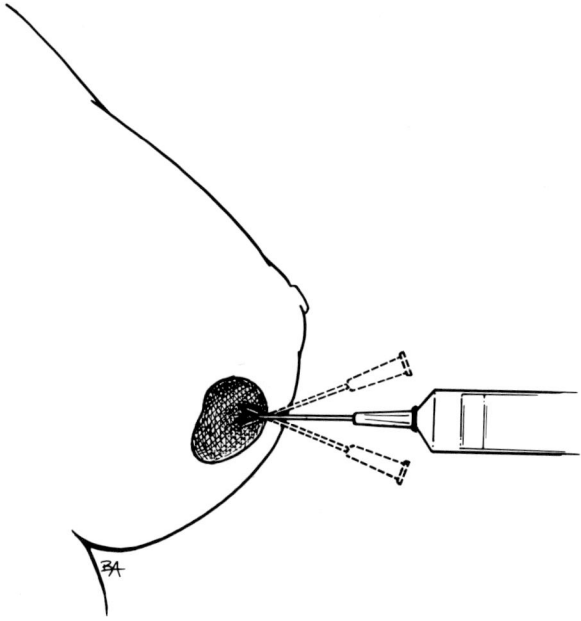

Figure 31–2

TRU-CUT NEEDLE BIOPSY

In the presence of a breast mass suspicious for malignancy, this instrument can be utilized to obtain a histologic diagnosis by a variant of incisional bi-

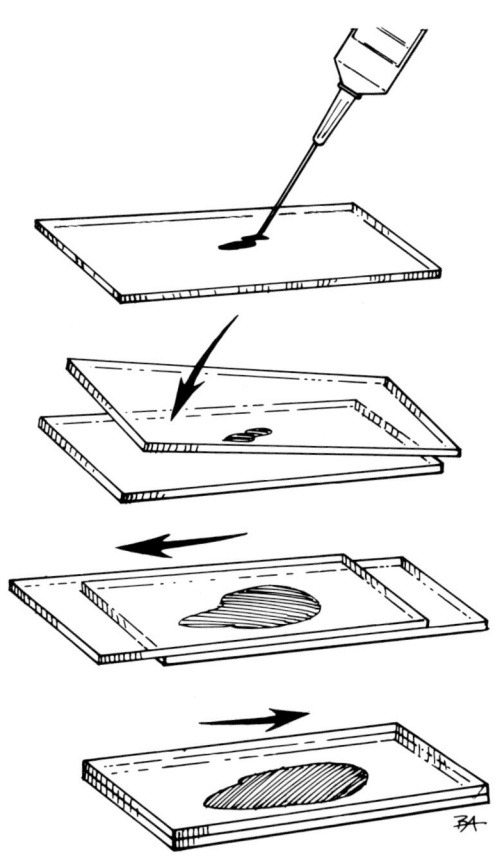

Figure 31–3

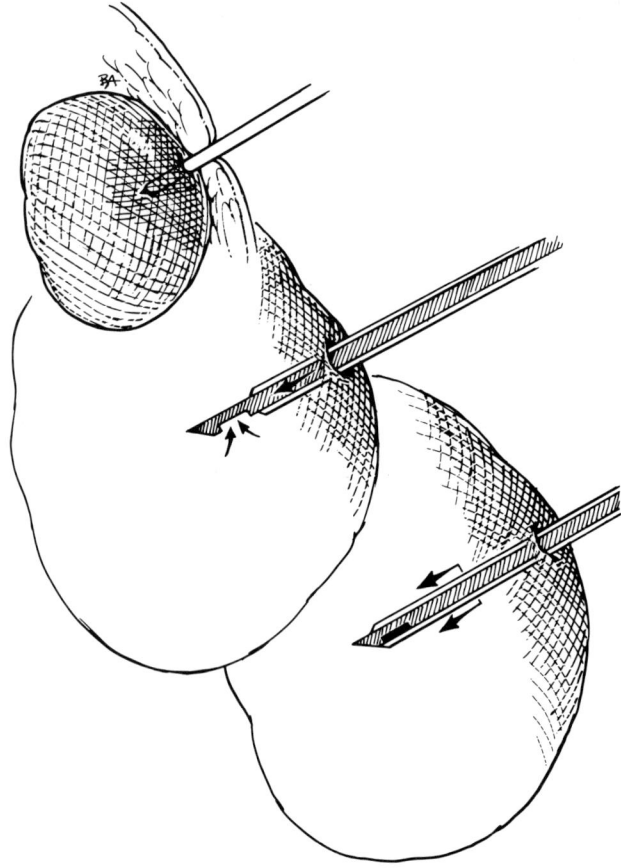

Figure 31–4

opsy. If the result is positive, treatment planning can be immediately discussed with the patient. If it is negative, an excisional biopsy must be performed to remove the lesion as well as to definitively rule out malignancy. The Tru-Cut needle is just one type of needle biopsy instrument. The following technique can be used for other instruments as well.

Procedure for Tru-Cut Needle Biopsy

1. The skin is prepared with Betadine.
2. Local anesthesia is employed.
3. The inner part of the Tru-Cut needle is inserted into the mass.
4. The needle point is advanced.
5. The outer sheath is then advanced. This has a sharp edge, which cuts the tissue as it advances (Fig. 31–4). The biopsied tissue remains in a small depression between the inner core and the outer sheath of the Tru-Cut needle.
6. The needle is now removed.
7. The biopsied tissue is put in formalin.

INCISIONAL BIOPSY

Tru-Cut needle biopsy is one type of incisional biopsy. Incisional biopsy may also be performed with a scalpel, utilizing local anesthesia. This might be utilized for a patient with a large malignancy, to make a diagnosis and obtain hormone receptor analysis prior to therapy.

Procedure for Incisional Biopsy

1. The area is prepared with Betadine, and local anesthesia is employed.
2. Langer's lines should be followed (Fig. 31–5).
3. A scalpel is used to make an incision into the area, making certain to obtain enough tissue to make a definitive diagnosis and to obtain hormone receptors (Fig. 31–6).
4. If it is possible that further surgery may eventually be performed the incision for the biopsy should be made within the area that would subsequently be removed.
5. Optimal hemostasis should be obtained, although this may be difficult if the patient has extensive necrotic tissue.
6. Depending upon the nature of the lesion and the friability of the tissue, subcuticular closure (which is cosmetically optimal under other circumstances) may be impossible.
7. If the incisional biopsy specimen does not confirm the clinical suspicion of malignancy, further surgery must be performed.

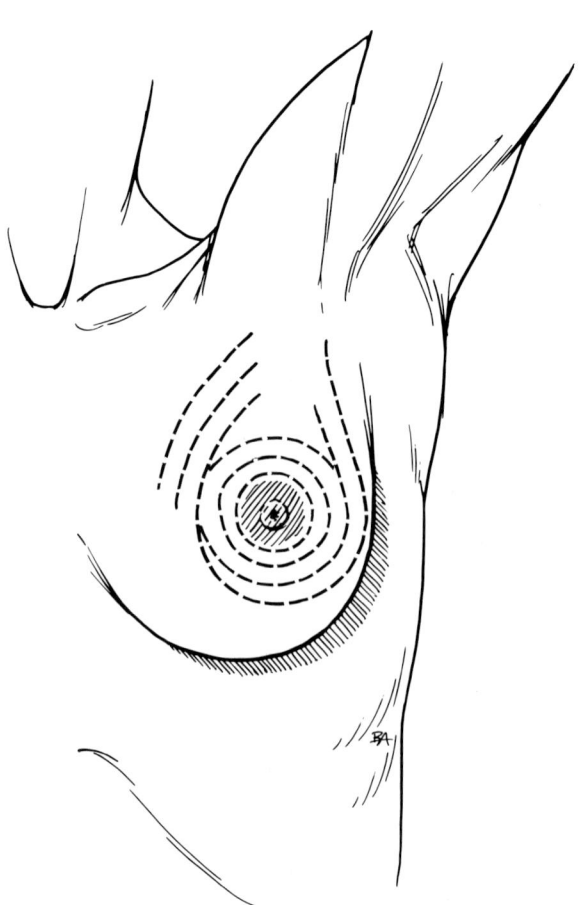

Figure 31–5

OPERATIVE PROCEDURES FOR THE BREAST

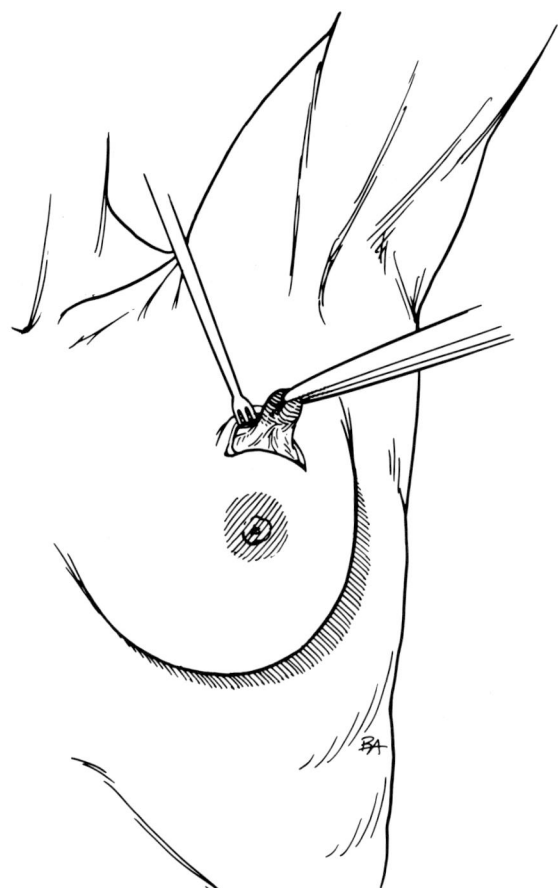

Figure 31–6

anesthesia is later infiltrated, a small mass may no longer be palpable.

2. The skin is prepared with Betadine, and local anesthesia is employed.

3. A circumareolar incision is optimal for a young woman if the physician believes that malignancy is unlikely. If malignancy is a significant probability, the incision should be made over the lesion, following Langer's lines. If the patient may be having further surgery, the incision should be made within the confines of the tissue that would be removed during a subsequent operation. For instance, if the patient would subsequently be having a mastectomy, the incision must be completely within the area that would be removed at mastectomy.

4. Dissection is carried out to the level of the mass, which is then entirely removed (Fig. 31–7).

5. Meticulous hemostasis is obtained.

6. A drain should not be employed unless the area is infected.

7. Subcuticular closure is employed.

EXCISIONAL BIOPSY

In the past decades, patients commonly had biopsies, immediately followed by mastectomies under the same general anesthetic, if the lesion was found to be malignant on frozen section. This is uncommon today in the United States because of the small likelihood of false-positive diagnosis, but, more importantly, because patients usually wish to know their diagnosis and then have the opportunity to weigh the treatment options that are available in their particular situations.

Therefore, breast biopsies are commonly performed in an ambulatory setting utilizing local anesthesia. General anesthesia may be employed for a patient who will require extensive dissection (for instance, a patient with a small lesion that is deep in the breast), when it is the patient's preference or need, or in the situation in which the patient requests an immediate mastectomy if malignancy is found.

NEEDLE LOCALIZATION

In 1982, approximately 15,000 American women had breast cancer diagnosed when the lesion was smaller

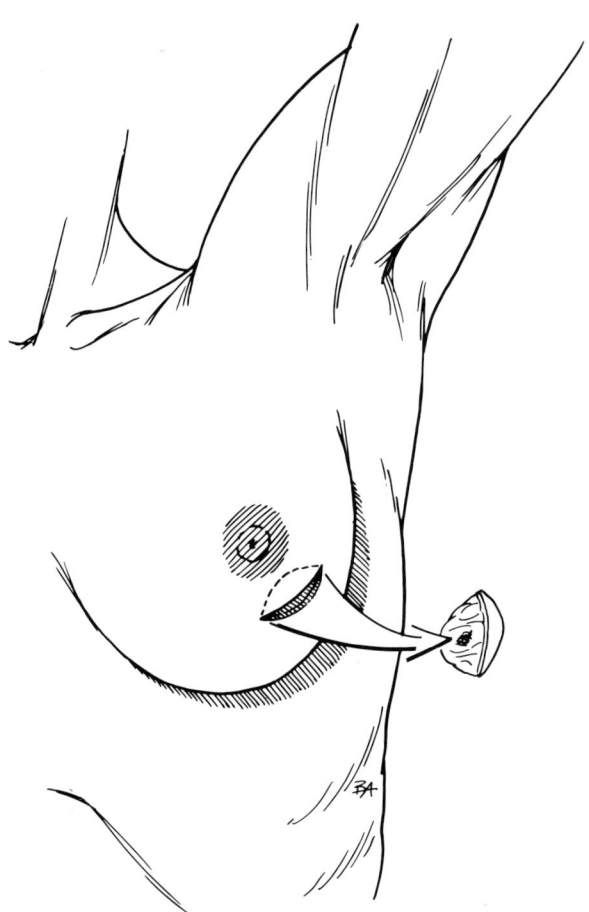

Figure 31–7

Procedure for Excisional Biopsy

1. The proposed incision is marked, as is the area directly over the mass. This is done because when local

than 2 cm. By 1986, there were 39,000 such cases diagnosed. Although the incidence of breast cancer has increased somewhat in the past decade, the main change has been the fact that a greater proportion of lesions are being diagnosed when they are smaller. Whereas some of this is attributable to increased clinical surveillance on the part of both the patient and the physician, a large number of the early breast cancers are diagnosed when they are nonpalpable, owing to the availability and utilization of the sophisticated screening mammography.

Smart and Beahrs reported on 280,000 volunteers who were screened for breast cancer as part of the Breast Cancer Detection Demonstration Project (BCDDP).[9] They found that physical examination and mammography were both suspicious in 47% of the cancers detected. However, at first screen, 44% of the cancers were detected only by mammography, and of those detected at second screen, 49% were suspicious only by mammography. In this study, with an aggressive screening program, 26% of the cancers diagnosed were noninfiltrative, and of the infiltrative cancers, 15% were less than 1 cm in diameter.

It is clear that screening mammography permits the identification of early breast abnormalities that can be detected radiographically but not clinically. The technology for percutaneous needle localization has been developed and refined so that after these lesions are identified with mammography they can be accurately localized, even though they are not palpable, and the radiographically abnormal area can be excised.

One of the earlier technologies that was developed to biopsy lesions that were suspicious on mammogram but not palpable was the injection of dye and/or contrast medium into the radiographically suspicious area.[10] The area was then excised. Because there is often diffusion of the injected material, a variety of other methods to identify the abnormal area at the time of surgery were sought.

In the mid 1970s, modifications and refinements of the earlier needle localization technique were described,[11-14] and some currently employed techniques are detailed below.

When needle localization is used to remove a nonpalpable lesion that was identified on mammogram as a result of suspicious calcifications, it is important to employ specimen radiography to ensure that the area that was found to be abnormal on mammography but is not palpable clinically has, in fact, been removed.[13, 15]

There has been interest in x-ray guided fine-needle aspiration for cytologic diagnosis of nonpalpable breast lesions.[16-18] Lofgren reported 215 such procedures, using a two-dimensional coordinate grid.[16] She reported a 92% sensitivity and a 95% specificity. She found that the predictive value of positive cytology was 88% and that the predictive value of negative cytology was 97%. Masood studied 20 females with nonpalpable breast lesions, using fine-needle aspiration biopsy under mammographic guidance followed by surgical excision.[18] Successful localization and aspiration was achieved in 90% of patients, and there was a 94% concordance between the histologic results of open biopsy specimens and the cytologic findings of aspirated specimens.[18] Further study with this technology is ongoing. Particularly because the lesions are nonpalpable, the potential for false-negative findings must constantly be borne in mind.

Procedure for Needle Localization Breast Biopsy

1. The skin is prepared with Betadine; the hooked needle is inserted into the mass, and its proper position is carefully confirmed radiographically in two planes (Fig. 31–8A).

2. If the dye technique is being utilized, dye is inserted at this point to stain the tissue in the area that is to be removed. Methylene blue (0.05 ml) and an equal amount

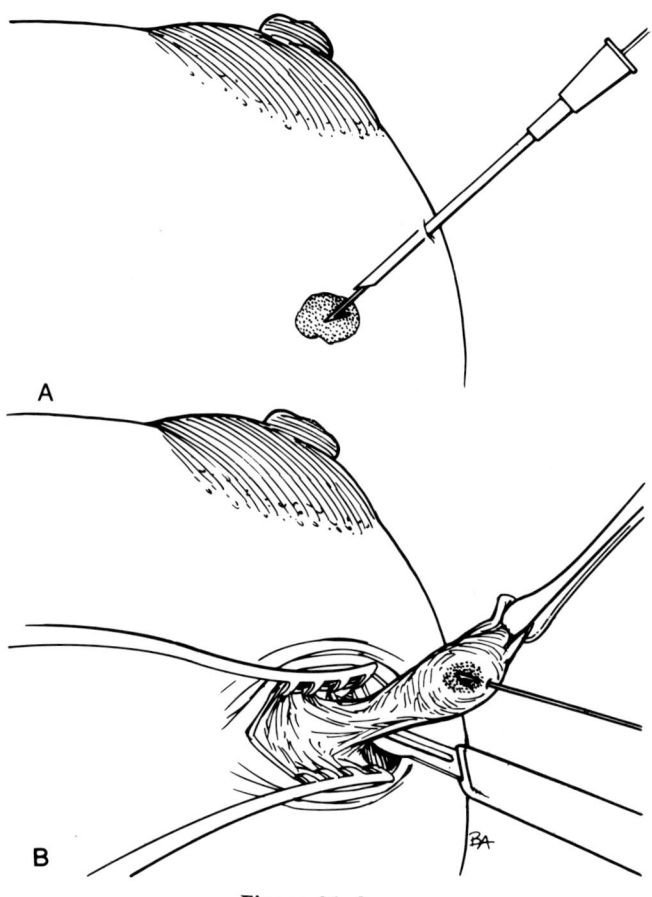

Figure 31–8

of radiopaque water-soluble contrast medium are inserted. A post-injection x-ray is taken to confirm the location.

3. The patient is brought to the operating room.
4. She is reprepped, and anesthesia is employed.
5. An incision is made next to the needle.
6. Dissection is carried down to the area just below the bottom of the needle (Fig. 31–8B).
7. The tissue surrounding the needle is removed.
8. An x-ray of the tissue is taken immediately to make certain that the area that was deemed suspicious on mammography has been removed. (If the abnormal area contained suspicious calcifications, these should be able to be identified in the tissue that has been excised.)
9. If the abnormalities that were identified on the mammogram are not found in the specimen, the abnormal tissue may not have been completely removed, and more tissue may need to be obtained.
10. Once it is clear to the surgeon that all appropriate tissue has been removed, hemostasis is obtained and the incision is closed.

MANAGEMENT OF NIPPLE DISCHARGE

Galactorrhea is the secretion of milk from the nipple unrelated to breast feeding. There are physiologic and pathologic causes of galactorrhea, and the etiology should always be evaluated. This section deals with nipple discharge other than galactorrhea.

Nipple discharge may occur in the presence of a benign or malignant breast lesion. There is no one type of discharge uniformly associated with malignancy. It may be watery, serous, serosanguineous, or bloody. All discharges should be investigated. Seltzer found that 12% of his patients with nipple discharge and no palpable mass had breast cancer, whereas 31% of his patients with nipple discharge and a palpable mass had breast cancer.[19] Obviously, nipple discharge must be fully investigated, even in the absence of a palpable mass.

Cytologic examination of the discharge should be obtained. A mammogram should be performed, but further evaluation is indicated even in the presence of a negative mammogram. When the breast tissue is compressed, the duct from which the discharge is emanating may be identified. It may be possible to remove the tissue surrounding a duct. More commonly, several ducts are removed.

Procedure for Duct Excision

1. The skin is prepared with Betadine, and anesthesia is employed.
2. A circumareolar incision is made (Fig. 31–9A).

3. A portion of the areola is retracted (Fig. 31–9B).
4. Dissection is then carried out to the base of the portion of the nipple that contains the dilated duct or ducts (Fig. 31–9C).
5. The tissue is then excised.
6. The flap of areola and nipple that was elevated and retracted is replaced.

MANAGEMENT OF AN ABSCESS

Mild postpartum mastitis is not an uncommon condition, and it can almost always be treated conservatively, without surgery. On the other hand, the presence of a defined breast abscess, either related to or remote from pregnancy, is a condition that is treated surgically. This will be described in detail below.

At this juncture, it is worthwhile to note a major pitfall that might result in the delayed diagnosis of breast cancer during pregnancy or the postpartum period. Inflammatory breast cancer may be mistaken for a postpartum mastitis, and it is essential that a careful history be obtained, a thorough physical performed, and that inflammatory breast cancer is considered in the differential diagnosis and its presence ruled out.

Procedure for Management of an Abscess

1. *It is often necessary to utilize general anesthesia, because finger dissection to make certain that all loculations have been entered and broken is important, and without general anesthesia this may be quite painful. On the other hand, for a small, superficial abscess, local anesthesia may be adequate.*
2. *The skin is prepared with Betadine.*
3. *If the abscess can be properly drained utilizing an incision in the lower portion of the breast, this is preferable, since scarring secondary to an abscess may be a problem (Fig. 31–10A).*
4. *An incision is made using Langer's lines, unless the abscess is pointing in such fashion that this is inappropriate (Fig. 31–10B).*
5. *Once the abscess has been entered, aerobic and anaerobic cultures should be obtained.*
6. *All loculations should be entered and broken manually (Fig. 31–10C).*
7. *The cavity should then be thoroughly irrigated and loosely packed with gauze.*
8. *The wound must be irrigated and the packing changed at least daily (more often if feasible) (Fig. 31–10D).*

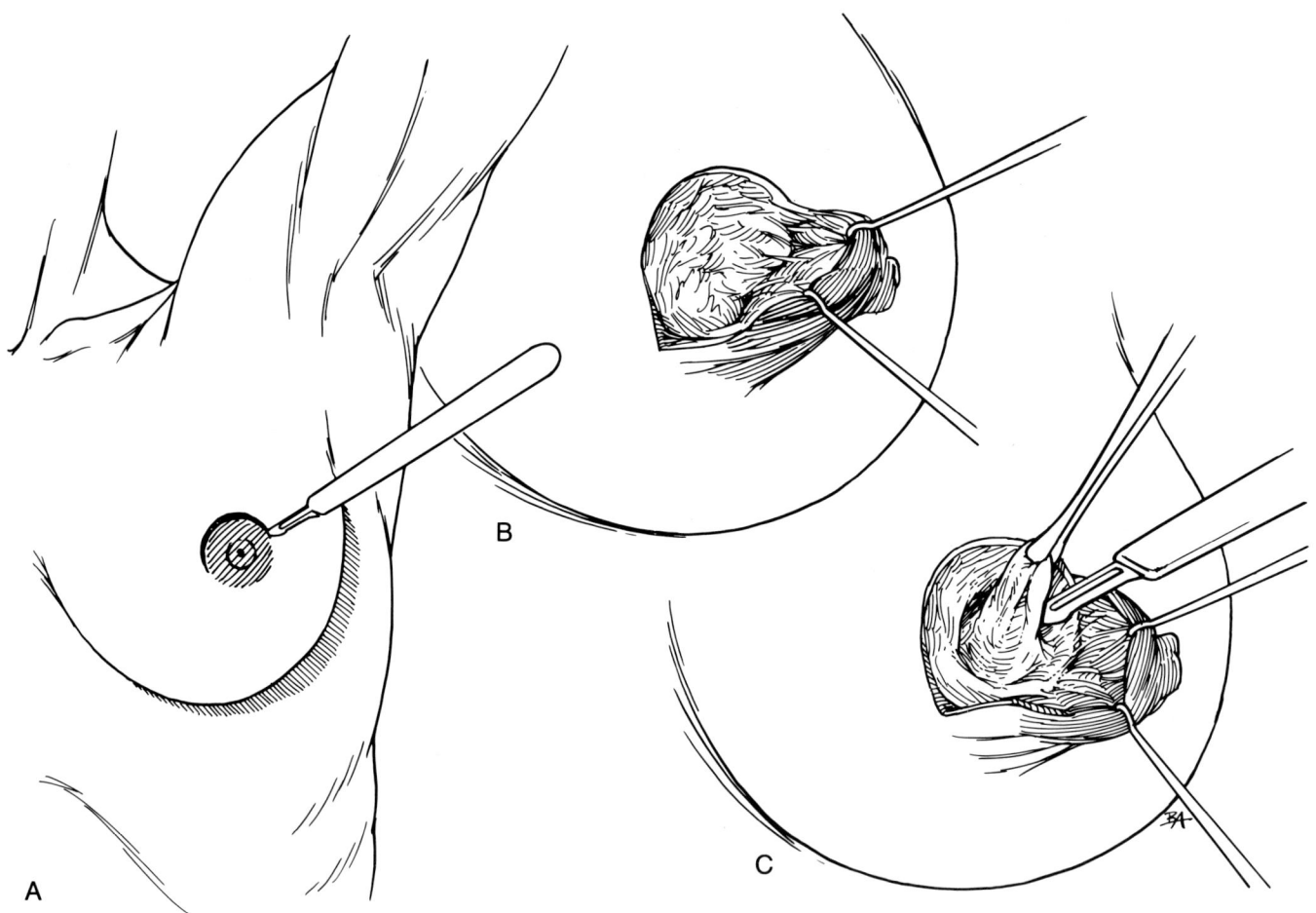

Figure 31–9

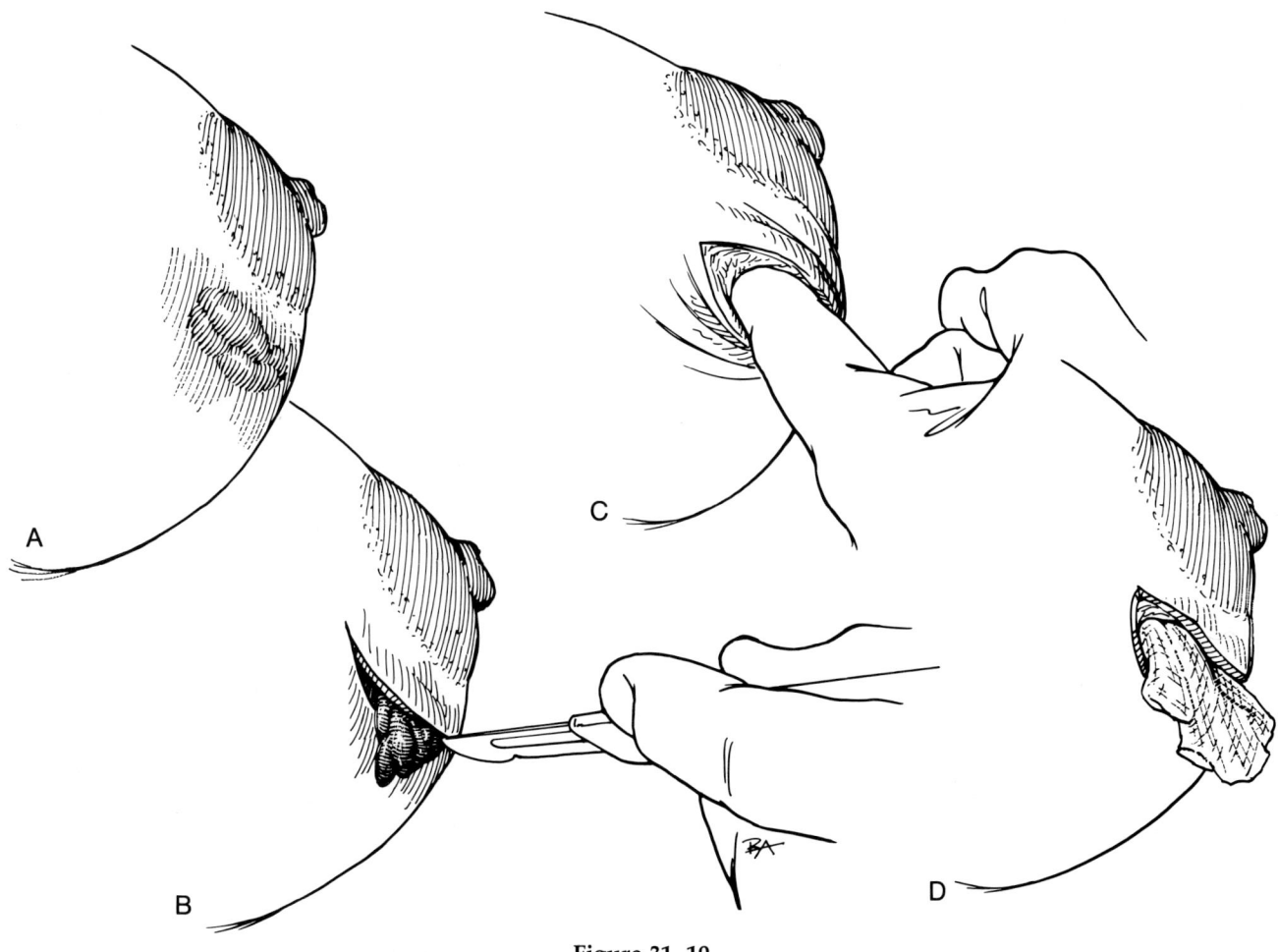

Figure 31–10

MANAGEMENT OF BREAST CANCER

Although there is historical reference to breast cancer dating back to 3000 B.C., it was not until 1882, when William Halsted, a Professor of Surgery at Johns Hopkins, developed and refined the technique of radical mastectomy, that a substantial number of women were cured of this disease. In his first 50 operations, Halsted reported a local-regional combined recurrence rate of only 24%. This enormous improvement when compared with previous results was responsible for the overwhelming acceptance of this procedure. Although removal of the pectoralis muscles caused significant cosmetic and functional difficulties for many women, this operation remained the cornerstone of breast cancer therapy for almost a century, because it enabled so many women to be cured of their disease.

However, once it became clear that a malignancy could be cured by radical therapy, the next step was to see whether similar cure rates could be achieved with less extensive therapy. Until 1970, approximately half of the American women who developed breast cancer were treated by radical mastectomy, and by 1976 only one-quarter of patients had radical surgery. By this time, it was coming to be accepted that mastectomy and axillary dissection and preservation of the pectoralis muscles could be equally curative but less debilitating for most women. Once it was determined that less radical treatment could result in equivalent cure rates for most patients, there was continued interest in pursuing treatment that could preserve the breast: lumpectomy, axillary dissection, and radiation.

The concept of treating breast cancer with radiation as primary therapy is not new. As early as the 1920s, Keynes treated breast cancer with radium needles, without mastectomy, and achieved good results. In Europe and Canada in the 1930s, there were series of patients treated with orthovoltage radiation. With this equipment, which is obviously far less sophisticated than that which is currently available, it was difficult to treat the cancers adequately without adverse effects on normal tissue, and therefore in some of the earlier studies the local recurrence rates were excessive.

At the Helsinki clinic, Rissanen reported patients under 50 years of age with T1, N0 lesions who were treated with orthovoltage between 1936 and 1956. Fifty-one patients had radical mastectomy, and forty had radiation. Although the 20-year survival rates were 78% in the radical mastectomy group and 73% in the radiation group, the group that had surgery had an 8% local recurrence rate and the radiation group had a 20% local recurrence rate.

Some other studies, even in these early years, reported excellent data with radiation. However, once megavoltage therapy became available, the results of studies using radiation as the primary treatment for breast cancer improved even further.

Two major studies that revolutionized the treatment of early primary breast cancer in the United States are those of Veronesi[20] and Fisher.[21] Veronesi's study involved 701 women with breast cancer at the National Cancer Institute in Milan who were treated in a randomized controlled study from 1973 to 1980. The women, who had breast cancers less than 2 cm in diameter and no palpable axillary lymph nodes, were randomized to have either a Halsted radical mastectomy or a quadrantectomy with axillary dissection and radiotherapy to the ipsilateral residual breast tissue. During the study period, there were four local recurrences, one in the quadrantectomy group and three in the Halsted group. Actuarial curves showed no difference in disease-free nor overall survival, whether the patient had Halsted radical mastectomy or quadrantectomy, axillary dissection, and radiation.[20]

In 1985, Fisher published the results of a collaborative study, initiated in 1976, in which 1843 women with stage I and II breast tumors, up to 4 cm in size, were enrolled in a prospective randomized study in which they would be treated either by total mastectomy, segmental mastectomy (removal of the tumor and only sufficient surrounding tissue to ensure margins free of tumor), or segmental mastectomy followed by breast irradiation. Every patient had an axillary dissection, and any patient with positive nodes received chemotherapy. Using life-table estimates, Fisher reported that patients who had segmental mastectomy, axillary dissection, and radiation had a better disease-free survival ($P = .04$) and overall survival ($P = .07$) than did patients with total mastectomy. He concluded that segmental mastectomy, axillary dissection, and breast radiation, with additional adjuvant chemotherapy in women with positive nodes, are appropriate therapy for stage I and II breast tumors up to 4 cm in size, as long as margins of resection are free of tumor.[21]

It has been accepted by most physicians that for most women with early breast cancer, lumpectomy, axillary dissection, and breast irradiation will result in cure rates equivalent to those of mastectomy, providing that there is no tumor at the resected margin. Decisions regarding optimal surgical therapy for any individual woman depend upon tumor characteristics, potential for multicentricity, potential for suboptimal cosmetic results, availability and accessibility of appropriate facilities, the patient's medical and psychologic status, and patient preference.

During the past decade, there has been increasing emphasis on the value of adjuvant chemotherapy and/or hormonal therapy for women with breast cancer.

In September 1985, the National Institutes of

Health held a Consensus Development Conference on Adjuvant Chemotherapy for Breast Cancer.[22] Because optimal therapy for any subset of patients still has not been defined, it is recommended that patients be encouraged to participate in clinical trials. For women not participating in clinical trials, the following recommendations were made regarding adjuvant therapy for women with breast cancer and positive nodes:

1. Premenopausal women should receive combination chemotherapy.
2. Postmenopausal women with positive hormone receptor levels should receive tamoxifen.
3. For postmenopausal women with negative hormone receptor levels, chemotherapy may be considered.

Despite the recommendations of the consensus conference, many physicians felt that postmenopausal women with positive nodes should receive combination chemotherapy and that those who are hormone receptor positive should have tamoxifen added to the regimen.

During the past few years, increasing attention has been given to the benefits of adjuvant therapy for patients with node-negative breast cancer. Although the majority of women with node-negative breast cancer were cured by their primary therapy, adjuvant therapy has been demonstrated to reduce the rate of recurrence.[23-27] The adverse effects of adjuvant therapy for these patients must be weighed against the potential for reduction in the rate of recurrence. Some physicians believe that almost all women with breast cancer should receive some form of adjuvant therapy. It is recommended that for all node-negative patients, the risks and benefits of adjuvant therapy should be explained. Patients should be informed of what is known about adjuvant therapy for node-negative breast cancer, as well as the fact that there are many questions that remain to be answered. It is important that patients who are willing to do so should be encouraged to participate in clinical trails so that appropriate therapy can be defined for all subsets of patients.

Lumpectomy

Lumpectomy is performed with axillary dissection and is followed by radiation therapy. Fisher has demonstrated that postoperative irradiation is important after the surgery, because it reduces the probability of local recurrence of tumor. Patients who were treated with radiation after lumpectomy and axillary dissection had a 90% likelihood of being free of tumor in the irradiated breast 8 years after surgery, as compared with a 61% likelihood of being free of cancer in the treated breast 8 years later if they did not receive postoperative irradiation.[28]

Procedure for Lumpectomy

1. The breast is prepared and draped in the normal fashion.
2. A curvilinear incision, usually running parallel to the areola, is made directly over the tumor, and, if a previous biopsy was performed, the previous biopsy site is excised with a thin margin of normal skin (Fig. 31–11A).
3. The incision is deepened through the subcutaneous tissue and breast fat, with careful manual attention, to a layer of normal tissue at least 1 cm, if not 2 cm, from the palpable edge of abnormality (Fig. 31–11B).
4. When this wide excision is accomplished, the fascia overlying the pectoralis muscle will be taken only if it is within the 1–2 cm distance (Fig. 31–11C).
5. After the specimen is removed, it is marked with stitches (usually a short stitch superiorly and a long stitch laterally) so that it will be able to be oriented in the pathologic laboratory for testing the margins of the specimen.
6. After careful hemostasis, usually only the skin is closed. This provides a much better cosmetic result than attempting to close the breast fat and subcutaneous tissue. Usually the skin is closed in a running subcuticular stitch, and a drain is avoided in almost all cases (Fig. 31–11D).
7. For optimal cosmetic results, the axillary dissection (section XII) is performed through a separate incision.

Axillary Dissection

Procedure

1. The arm on the affected side is draped sterile and free for the purposes of shoulder abduction during the procedure for increased visualization.
2. Many different incisions have been utilized to enter the axilla. With any of these incisions, the extent of skin flaps is as in the heavy dashed lines (Fig. 31–12A).
3. When the skin flaps are elevated, the lateral edge of the pectoralis major muscle is identified and dissected free in its extent to the lower edge of the axilla, which blends with the tail of the breast (Fig. 31–12B).
4. The free edge of the latissimus dorsi is identified, and at the superior extent the white tendon of the latissimus is found. The axillary vein is dissected free above this and cleared from the axillary fat, taking the tiny venous tributaries between steel clips or fine sutures. The axillary artery is not exposed (even though it is drawn in for purposes of orientation). Only the inferior portion of the axillary vein is seen as dissection proceeds towards the chest (Fig. 31–12C).

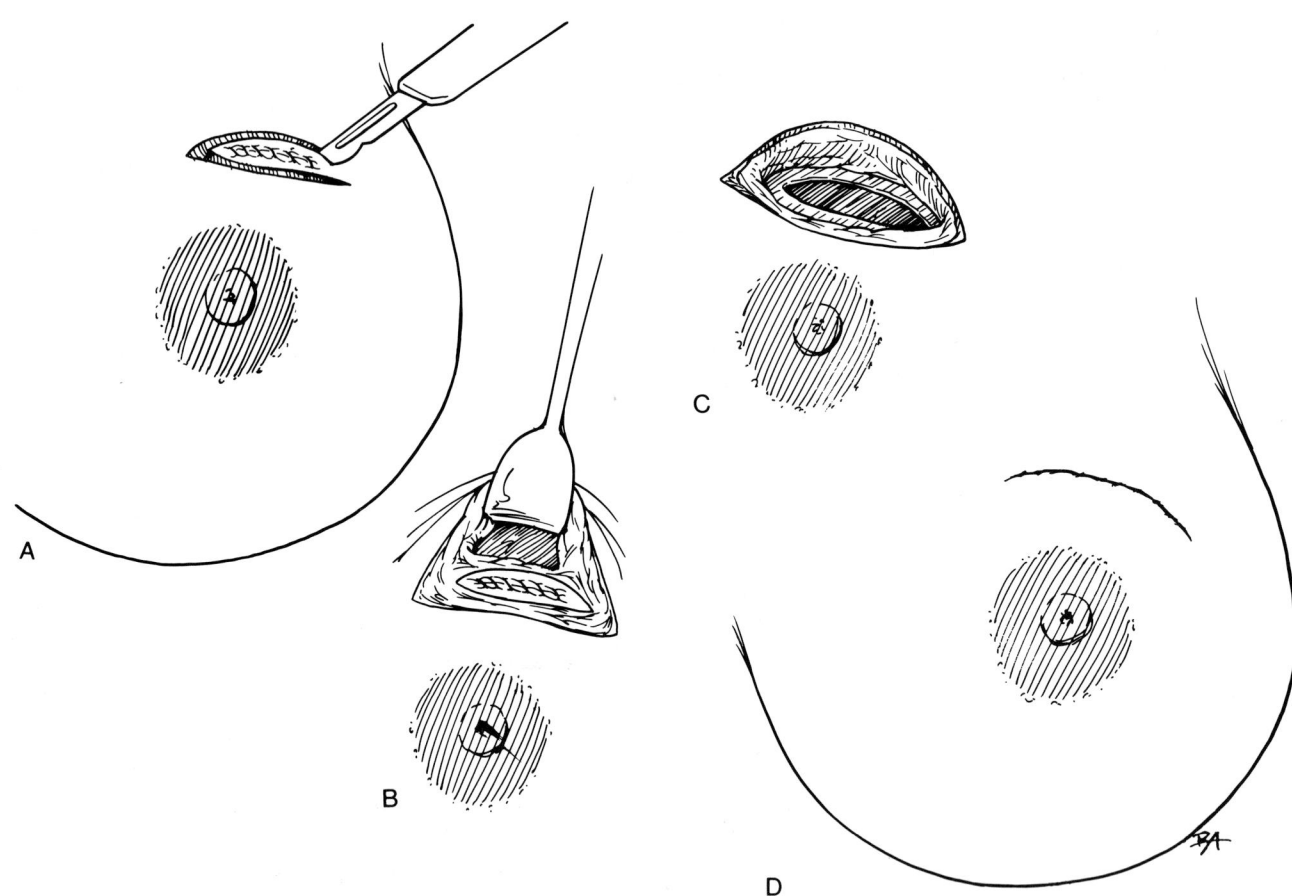

Figure 31–11

OPERATIVE PROCEDURES FOR THE BREAST 597

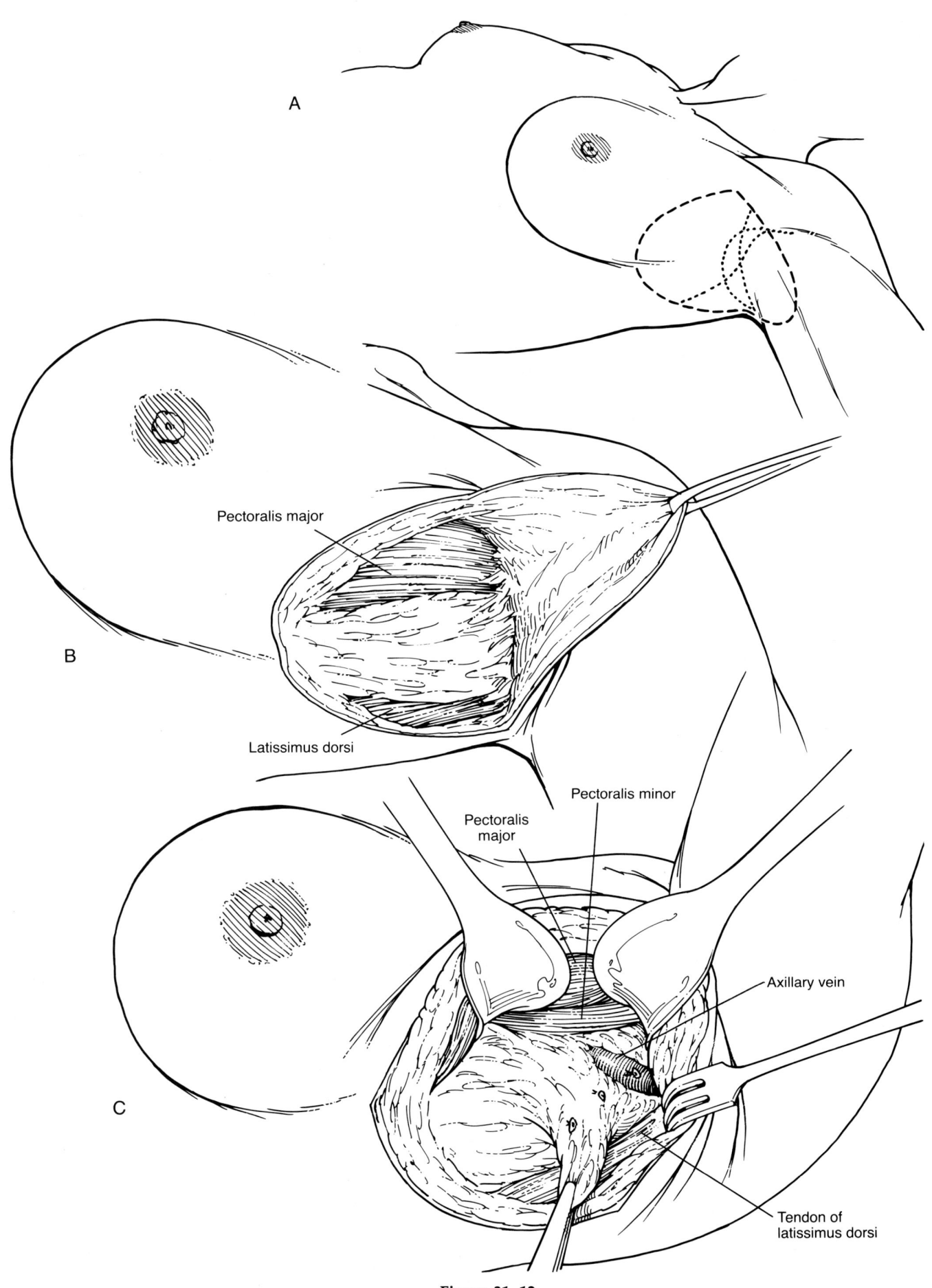

Figure 31–12

Illustration continued on following page

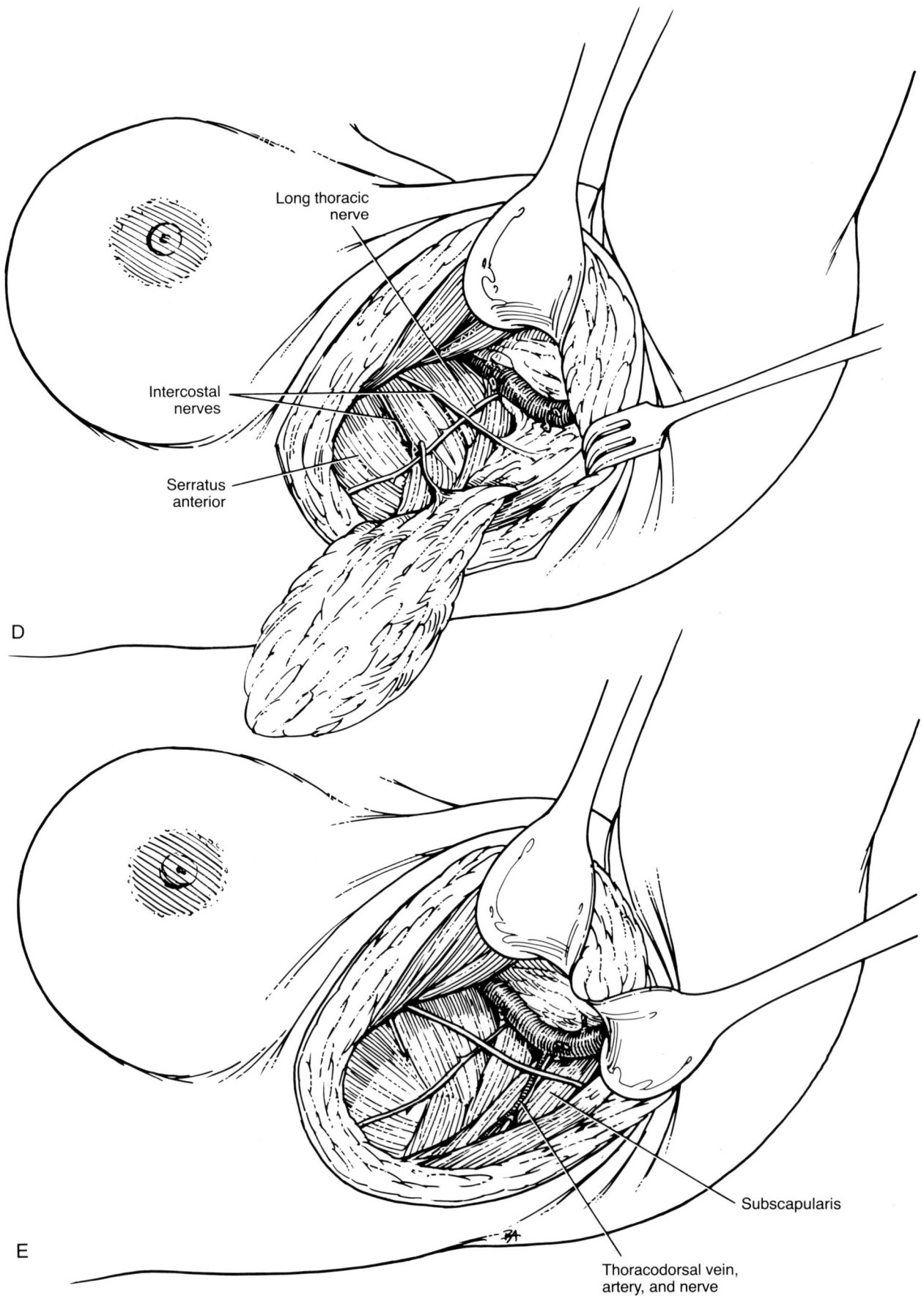

Figure 31–12 Continued

5. At the highest extent of the axillary vein where it goes under the costoclavicular ligament (joining the clavicle and the first rib), dissection stops at level III. Then the axillary contents are removed from the chest wall and the serratus anterior is seen in its extent.

6. After the intercostal brachial nerves are seen and either taken or preserved, dissection proceeds more slowly for the purposes of carefully identifying and preserving the long thoracic nerve (Fig. 31–12D).

7. Then dissection continues into the space between the latissimus dorsi muscle and the chest wall. For extensive nodal disease, the thoracodorsal nerve artery vein complex may be taken for a careful level I clean-out. Most surgeons prefer to save innervation to this muscle.

8. The specimen is carefully labeled with levels I and II. Usually it is not necessary to remove the highest lymph nodes of level III, and, when possible, it is best to save this area to avoid increased risk of lymphedema.

9. When the tissue has been sent to Pathology, the structures seen are as shown in Figure 31–12E.

10. A closed system suction drain is placed in the axilla with care being taken that it does not come into contact with the brachial plexus or the axillary artery or vein. It is brought out through a separate stab wound, usually placed inferiorly. The drain is sewn into place.

11. The skin flaps are usually closed with interrupted absorbable material, such as Dexon, to line up the incision, with running subcuticular Dexon or absorbable suture over that.

12. A dry sterile dressing is placed over the area.

Mastectomy

Procedure for Modified Radical Mastectomy

1. The arm on the affected side is draped sterile and free during the operation for the purposes of shoulder joint abduction for increased visualization of the axilla.

2. The incision is drawn and then made to include all of the previous biopsy incision (if any) and the nipple-areola complex. It is also drawn to include at least 4 cm from the periphery of the tumor.

3. Skin flaps are elevated superiorly above the second rib and slightly below the inferior edge of the clavicle, medially to the lateral border of the sternum, inferiorly to below the inframammary fold, and laterally to the free edge of the latissimus dorsi muscle (Fig. 31–13A).

4. The free edge of the latissimus dorsi is followed superiorly until its white tendon is visualized. The axillary vein is visualized immediately above the white tendon, and this marks the distal extent of the axillary dissection (Fig. 31–13B).

5. The specimen is dissected from the chest wall muscles with the pectoralis major fascia removed with the specimen. This dissection usually proceeds from superiorly to inferiorly and medially to laterally. The specimen is allowed to lie beside the patient's chest, still attached by the axillary contents (Fig. 31–13C).

6. The pectoralis major muscle is lifted by its lateral free edge with a retractor, and the pectoralis minor muscle is found and dissected free and visualized in its entirety.

7. The pectoralis minor muscle is incised, usually with cautery, high near the coracoid process, and then the muscle itself is usually removed from its attachments on the second, third, and fourth rib so as not to leave uninnervated and retracted muscle bulk.

8. The clavipectoral fascia is incised over the presumed site and course of the axillary vein to allow one into the axilla proper. The nerve going to the medial two-thirds of the pectoralis major muscle is seen on the underside of the pectoralis major muscle and is preserved (Fig. 31–13D).

9. The axillary vein is exposed, at least on the most inferior portion of its circumference, although the vein is shown completely dissected free for the purposes of illustration in Figure 31–13E.

10. If the highest level of axillary contents is to be dissected, the vein is cleared from axillary tissue inferiorly all the way up to the costoclavicular ligament (Halsted's ligament).

11. The axillary contents are dissected laterally; small venous tributaries are clamped, cut, and tied, or small steel clips are placed.

12. The long thoracic nerve is seen in its entirety, close to the chest wall, and carefully preserved. The intercostal brachial muscles exiting under the ribs (and providing sensation to the upper inner arm mainly) are usually sacrificed. The thoracodorsal nerve, artery, and vein (coursing to the latissimus) either are dissected free and preserved or are sacrificed, depending upon the extent of nodal disease (Fig. 31–13F).

13. Two Reliavac drains are usually placed in the depths of the incision and are usually let out through separate small incisions.

14. The mastectomy incision itself is closed with an interrupted suture to line up the incision.

15. A running subcuticular suture is used for closure.

Procedure for Radical Mastectomy

1. The arm of the affected side is draped sterile and free during the operation for the purposes of shoulder joint abduction for increased visualization of the axilla.

2. The incision is drawn and then made to include all of the previous biopsy incision (if any) and the nipple-areola complex. It is also drawn to be at least 4 cm from the site of any tumor.

3. Skin flaps are elevated superiorly to the inferior edge of the clavicle, medially to the lateral border of the sternum, inferiorly to below the inframammary fold, and laterally to the free edge of the latissimus dorsi muscle (Fig. 31–14A).

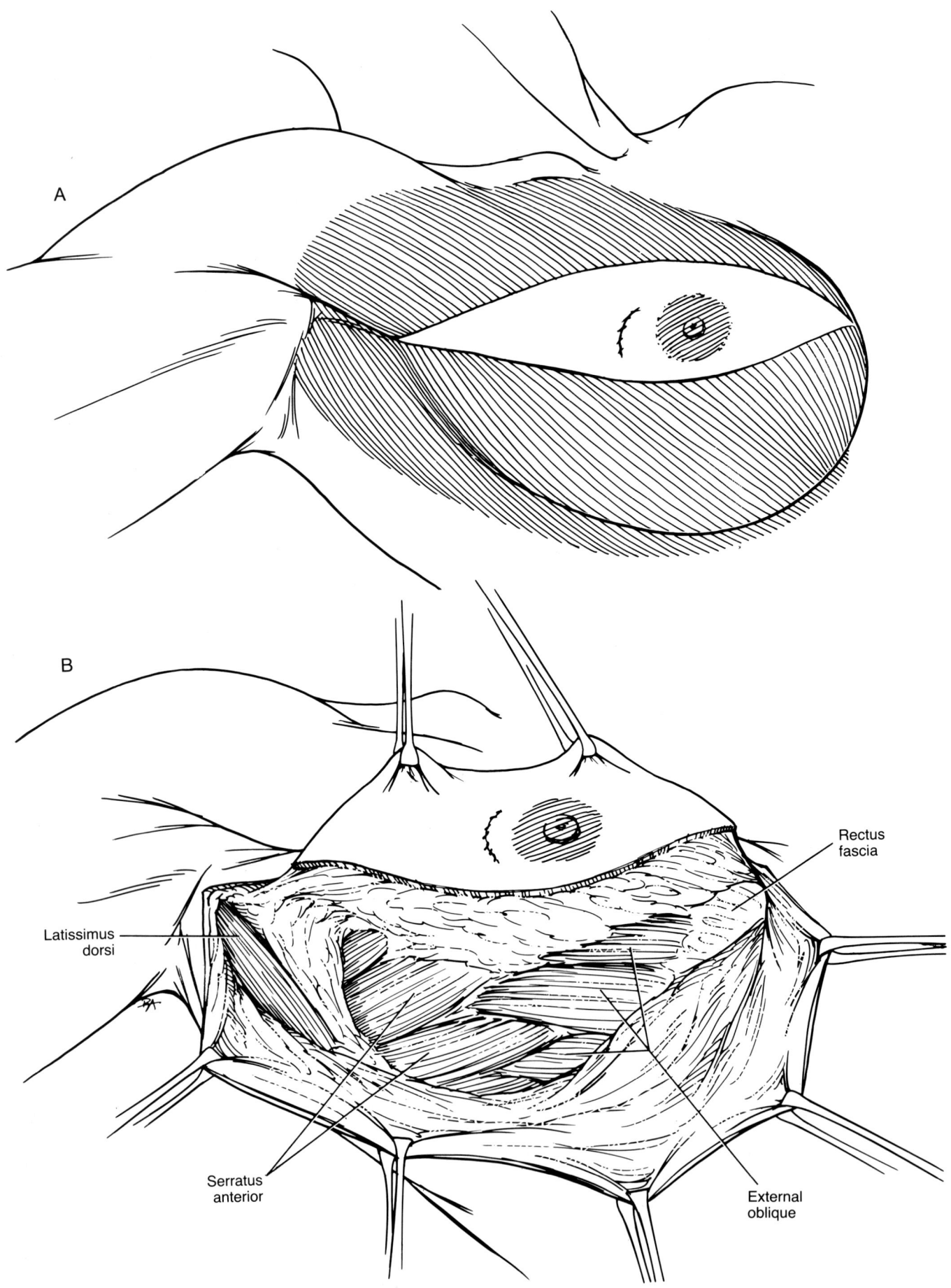

Figure 31–13

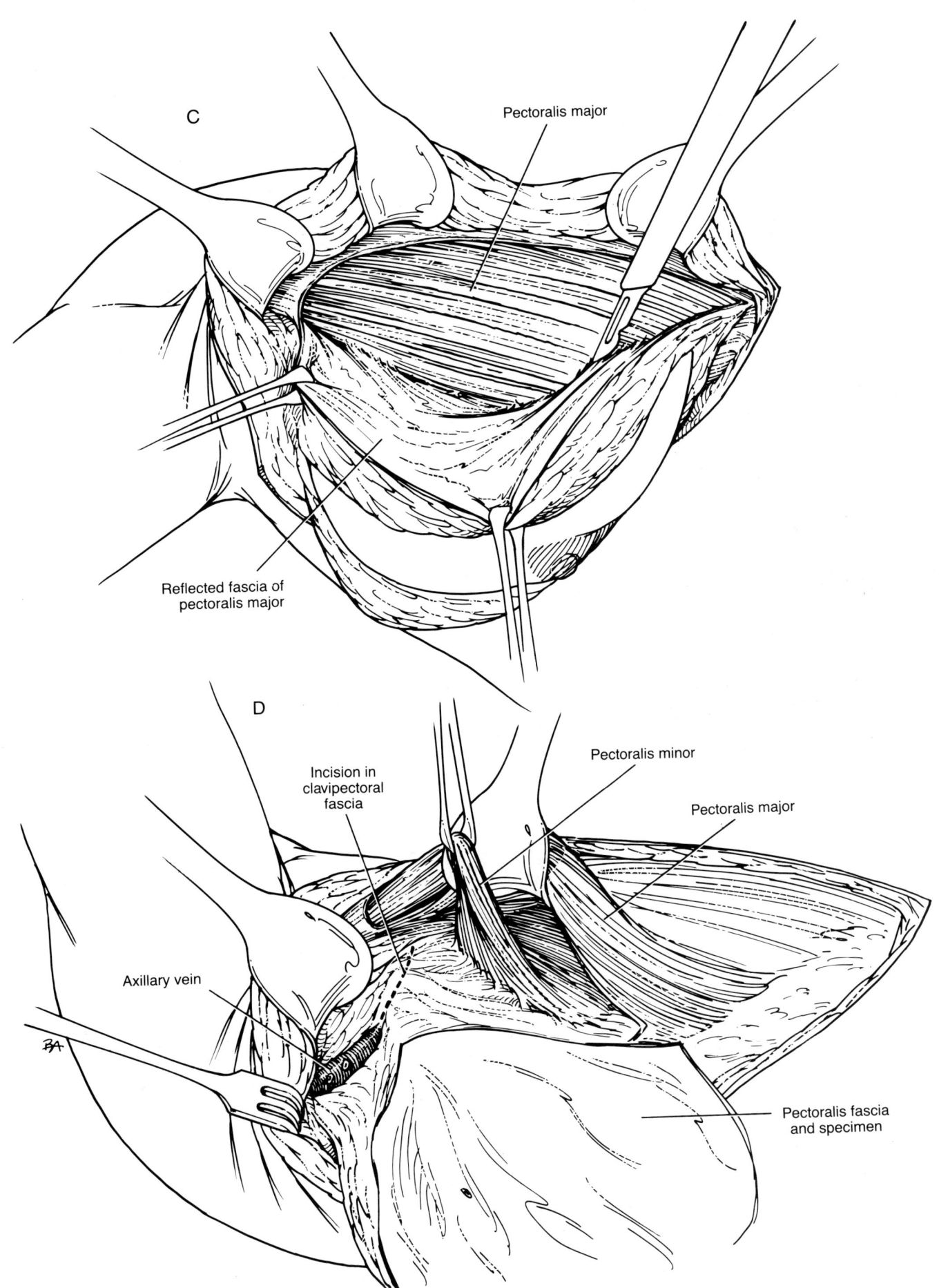

Figure 31–13 Continued

Illustration continued on following page

602 OPERATIVE PROCEDURES FOR THE BREAST

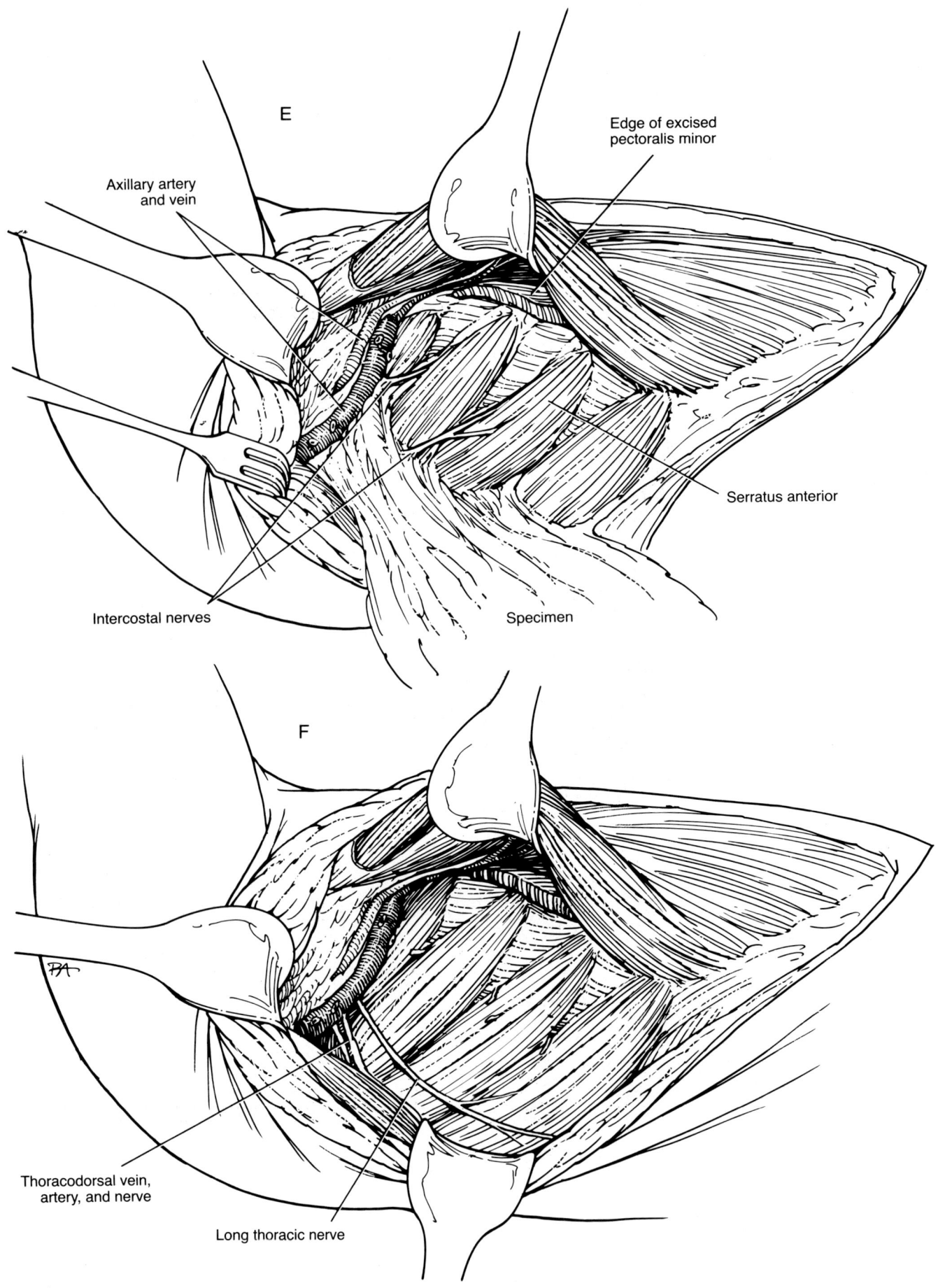

Figure 31–13 Continued

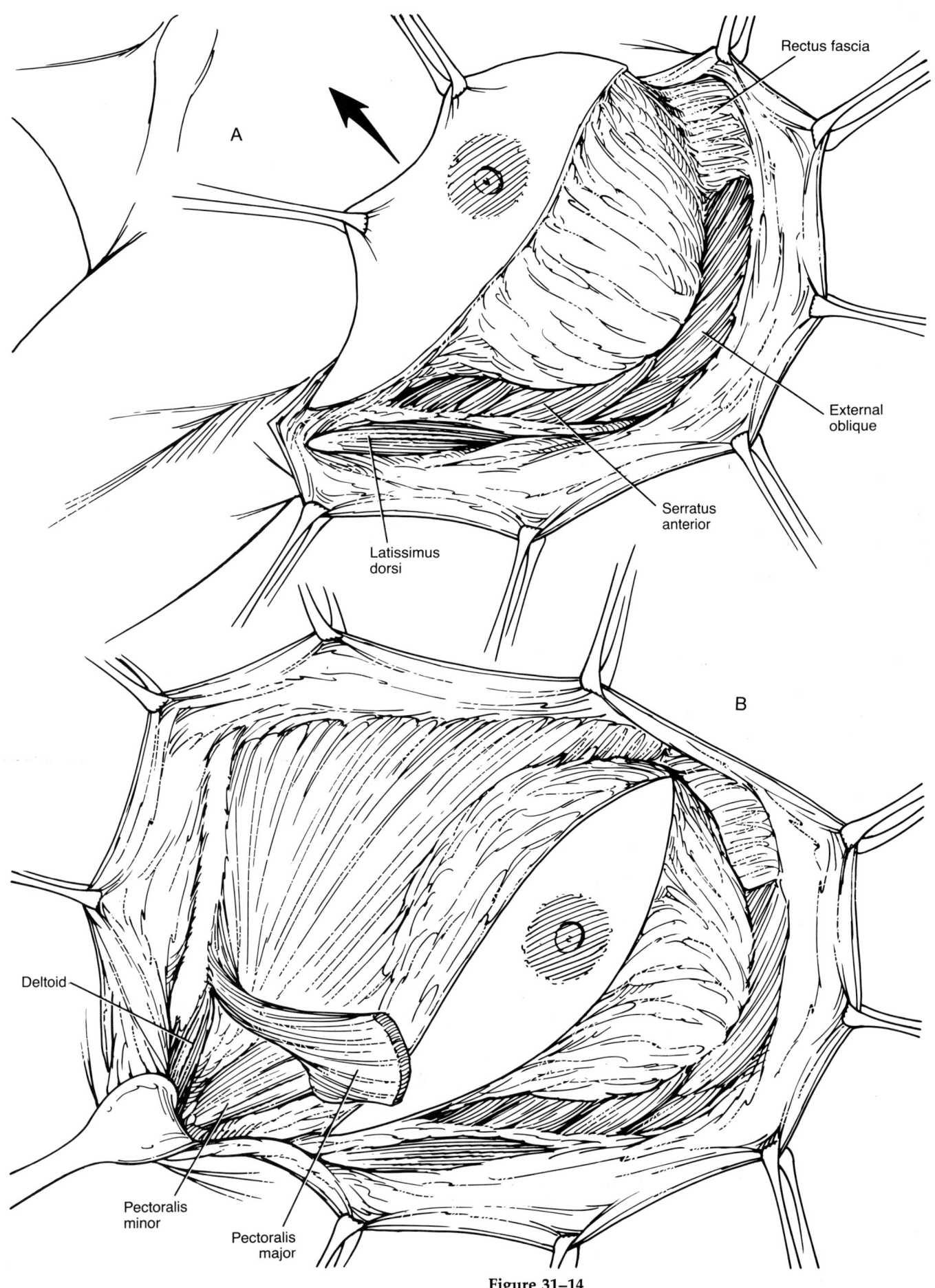

Figure 31–14

Illustration continued on following page

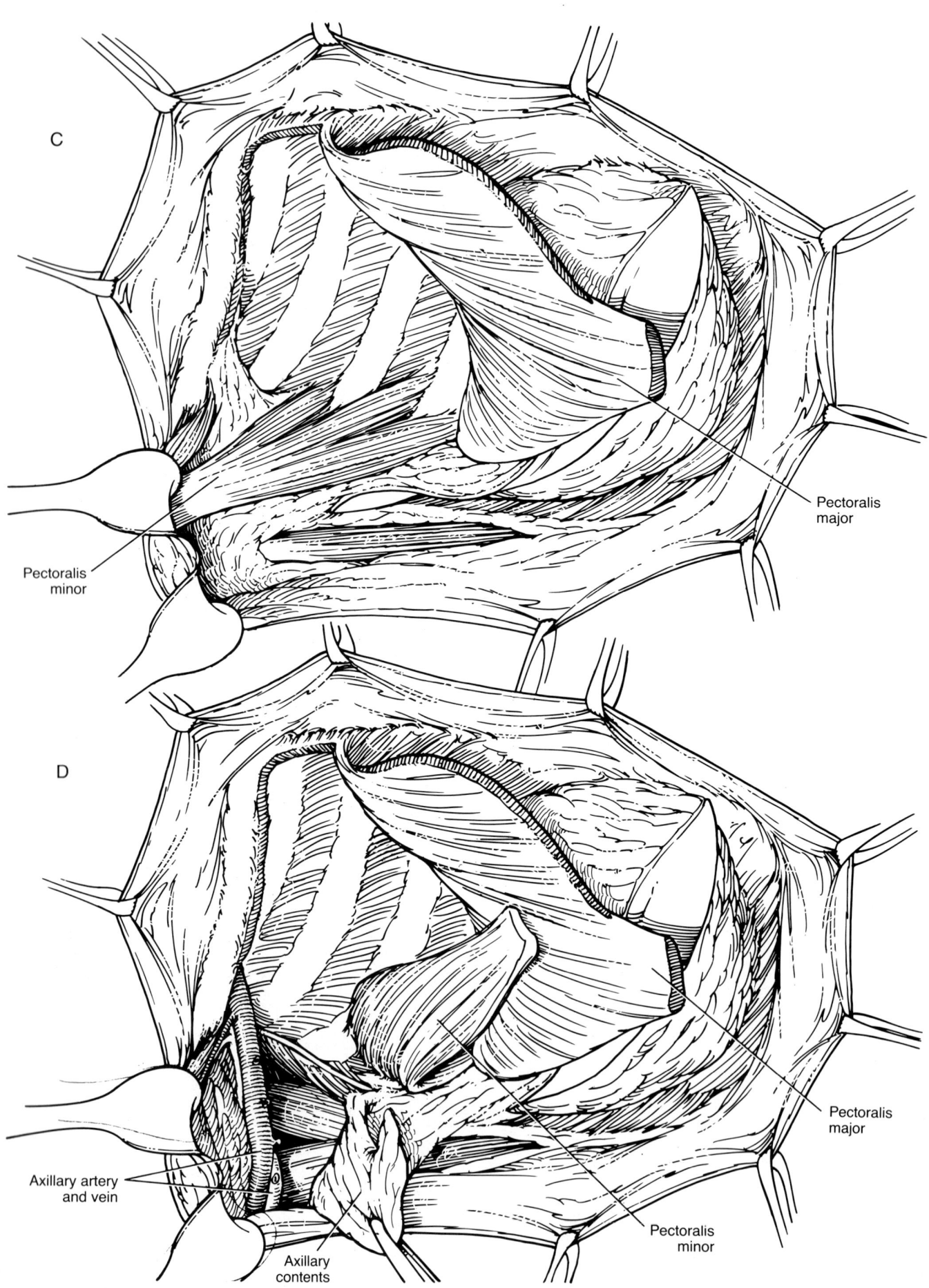

Figure 31–14 Continued

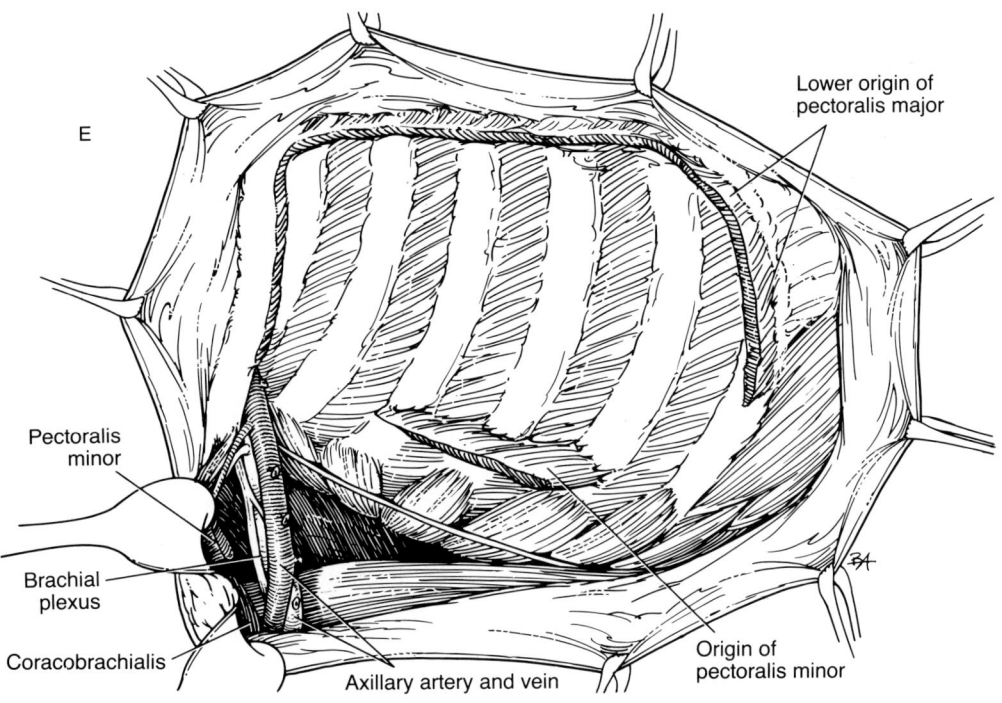

Figure 31–14 *Continued*

4. The free edge of the latissimus dorsi is followed superiorly until the area of the white tendon is visualized.

5. The latissimus free edge is exposed in its entirety, then the axillary vein is visualized immediately above the white tendon, and this marks the distal extent of the axillary dissection.

6. The pectoralis major muscle is separated and incised from the humerus at its tendinous insertion, and the upper muscle belly is folded caudally toward the clavicular origin. As necessary, the muscle from the clavicular origin is transsected between clamps and suture ligated (Fig. 31–14B).

7. The clavipectoral fascia overlying the pectoralis minor muscle is incised, and the muscle is transsected near the coracoid process. It is also folded caudally toward the pectoralis major muscle, and its blood and nerve supply are ligated and transsected (Fig. 31–14C).

8. At this point, the axillary contents may be dissected. The axillary vein is exposed by dividing the tissue above the axillary sheath, and all of the axillary fat and contents are removed from the highest level (level III) at the costoclavicular ligament (Halsted's ligament) and proceeding laterally. Small tributaries to the axillary vein are clamped, cut, and tied, or occluded with small steel clips (Fig. 31–14D).

9. Proceeding laterally, the intercostal brachial nerves are sacrificed, and then the long thoracic nerve in the subscapular fold is seen in its entirety and preserved.

10. Following along the inferior edge of the vein, the thoracodorsal vein is found, clamped, cut, and ligated, as well as the thoracodorsal artery and nerve.

11. The axillary contents are removed from the chest wall with the remaining Pectoralis major muscles towards the sternum and the rectus sheath. The perforators are clamped, cut, and tied at this point (Fig. 31–14E).

12. After irrigation and meticulous hemostasis, the incision is closed over internal suction drains brought out through separate incisions in the inferior flap.

References

1. Strax P, Venet L, Shapiro S, Gross S: Mammography and clinical examination in mass screening for cancer of the breast. Cancer 1967; 29:2184.
2. Burns PE: False-negative mammograms delay diagnosis of breast cancer. N Engl J Med 1978; 299:201.
3. Martin HE, Ellis EB: Biopsy by needle puncture and aspiration. Ann Surg 1930; 92:169.
4. Zajdela A, Ghossein NA, Pilleron JB, Ennuyer A: The value of aspiration cytology in the diagnosis of breast cancer: Experience at the Foundation Curie. Cancer 1975; 35:499–506.
5. Frable WJ: Needle aspiration of the breast. Cancer 1984; 53:671.
6. Palombini L, Fuleiniti F, Vetrani A, et al.: Fine needle aspiration biopsy of breast masses. Cancer 1988; 61:2273.
7. Lee GF: Fine needle aspiration of the breast: The outpatient management of breast lesions. Am J Obstet Gynecol 1987; 156:1532.
8. Bottles K, Taylor RN: Diagnosis of breast masses in pregnant and lactating women by aspiration cytology. Obstet Gynecol 1985; 66:76s.
9. Smart CR, Beahrs OH: Breast cancer screening results as viewed by the clinician. Cancer 1979; 43:851.
10. Simon N, Lesnick GJ, Lerer WN: Roentgenographic localization of small lesions of the breast by the spot method. Surg Gynecol Obstet 1972; 134:572.
11. Egan JF, Sayler CB, Goodman MJ: A technique for localizing occult breast lesions. CA 1976; 26:32.

12. Threatt B, Appelman H, Dow R, O'Rourke T: Percutaneous needle localization of clustered mammary microcalcifications prior to biopsy. Am J Roentgenol 1974; 121:839.
13. Libshitz HI, Feig SA, Fetouh S: Needle localization of nonpalpable breast lesions. Radiology 1976; 121:557.
14. Frank HA, Hall FM, Steer ML: Pre-operative localization of nonpalpable breast lesions demonstrated by mammography. New Engl J Med 1976; 295:259.
15. Snyder RE: Specimen radiography and pre-operative localization of nonpalpable breast cancer. Cancer 1980; 46:950.
16. Lofgren M, Andersson I, Bondeson L, Lindholm K: X-ray guided fine-needle aspiration for the cytologic diagnosis of nonpalpable breast lesions. Cancer 1988; 61:1032.
17. Dowlatshahi K, Gent HJ, Schmidt R, et al: Nonpalpable breast tumors: Diagnosis with stereotaxic localization and fine-needle aspiration. Radiology 1989; 170:427.
18. Masood S, Frykberg ER, Mitchum DG, et al.: The potential value of mammographically guided fine-needle aspiration biopsy of nonpalpable breast lesions. Am Surg 1989; 55:226.
19. Seltzer MH, Perloff LJ, Kelley RI, Fitts WT: The significance of age in patients with nipple discharge. Surg Gynecol Obstet 1970; 131:519.
20. Veronesi U, Saccozzi R, Del Vecchio M, et al.: Comparing radical mastectomy with quadratectomy, axillary dissection, and radiotherapy in patients with small cancers of the breast. N Engl J Med 1981; 305:6.
21. Fisher B, Bauer M, Margolese R, et al.: Five-year results of a randomized clinical trial comparing total mastectomy and segmental mastectomy with or without radiation in treatment of breast cancer. N Engl J Med 1985; 312:665.
22. Consensus Conference: Adjuvant chemotherapy for breast cancer. JAMA 1985; 254:3461.
23. Mansour EG, Gray R, Shatila AH, et al.: Efficacy of adjuvant chemotherapy in high-risk node-negative breast cancer. N Engl J Med 1989; 320:485.
24. Ludwig Breast Cancer Study Group: Prolonged disease-free survival after one course of perioperative adjuvant chemotherapy for node-negative breast cancer. N Engl J Med 1989; 320:491.
25. Fisher B, Costantino J, Redmond C, et al.: A randomized clinical trial evaluating tamoxifen in the treatment of patients with node-negative breast cancer who have estrogen-receptor-positive tumors. N Engl J Med 1989; 320:479.
26. Fisher B, Redmond C, Dimitrov NV, et al.: A randomized clinical trial evaluating sequential methotrexate and fluorouracil in the treatment of patients with node-negative breast cancer who have estrogen-receptor-negative tumors. N Engl J Med 1989; 320:473.
27. Merz B: Clinical alert gives breast cancer data, revises recommendations. JAMA 1988; 260:153.
28. Fisher B, Redmond C, Poisson R, et al.: Eight-year results of a randomized clinical trial comparing total mastectomy and lumpectomy with or without irradiation in the treatment of breast cancer. N Engl J Med 1989; 320:822.

Reconstructive Surgery in Gynecologic Oncology

32

Larry J. Copeland

As cancer treatments become more aggressive and more successful, increasing emphasis is directed toward improving patients' quality of life. Return to a normal lifestyle may depend on restoration of normal functional anatomy, and in recent years surgical reconstruction is commonly performed concurrently with radical cancer surgery. However, the management of tumor complications and treatment present the most challenging reconstructive problems. As in reconstructive surgery for benign diseases or congenital abnormalities, good surgical principles apply: the need to minimize trauma to tissue, close wounds without tension, secure hemostasis, and use drains prudently.

GENERAL PRINCIPLES

Relaxing Incisions or Band Releases

Distortions of the vaginal tube or introitus that cause dyspareunia can be corrected by cutting constricting bands transversely, undermining the local tissue, and closing longitudinally (Fig. 32–1).

Skin Flaps

Wound closures should be without significant tension on the sutures. Occasionally it is beneficial to mobilize adjacent skin and subcutaneous tissue, either to reduce tension with skin approximation or to close wound defects. Because the mobilized tissue should have good microvasculature, radiated tissue should be avoided if possible. Patients with diabetes or other microvascular diseases are at risk for tissue necrosis and poor wound healing. Also, the base of skin flaps should be at least one-half the length of the flap to ensure a satisfactory blood supply.

Depending on the characteristics of the defect, a variety of techniques can be used.

1. Z-plasty can be used to elongate contracted bands or scars (Fig. 32–2).[1]

2. Y-V plasty can be used to add width to an area of narrowing, either a flat surface or a luminal stricture (e.g., a ureteropelvic stricture) (Fig. 32–3).

3. Rhomboid or lateral transposition skin flaps are useful for closure of large defects if adjacent tissue offers good mobility. In the field of gynecologic oncology, the rhomboid flap has been used to close large vulvar defects, taking advantage of the supple, loose tissue of the medial thigh or buttocks (Fig. 32–4).

4. Axial translocation. This skin flap can be used to cover rectangular defects. Excision of two equilateral triangles allows for the mobilization of a broad-based flap without the formation of "dog-ears" (Fig. 32–5).

VAGINAL RECONSTRUCTION

A number of surgical techniques have been described for the various clinical situations in which vaginal

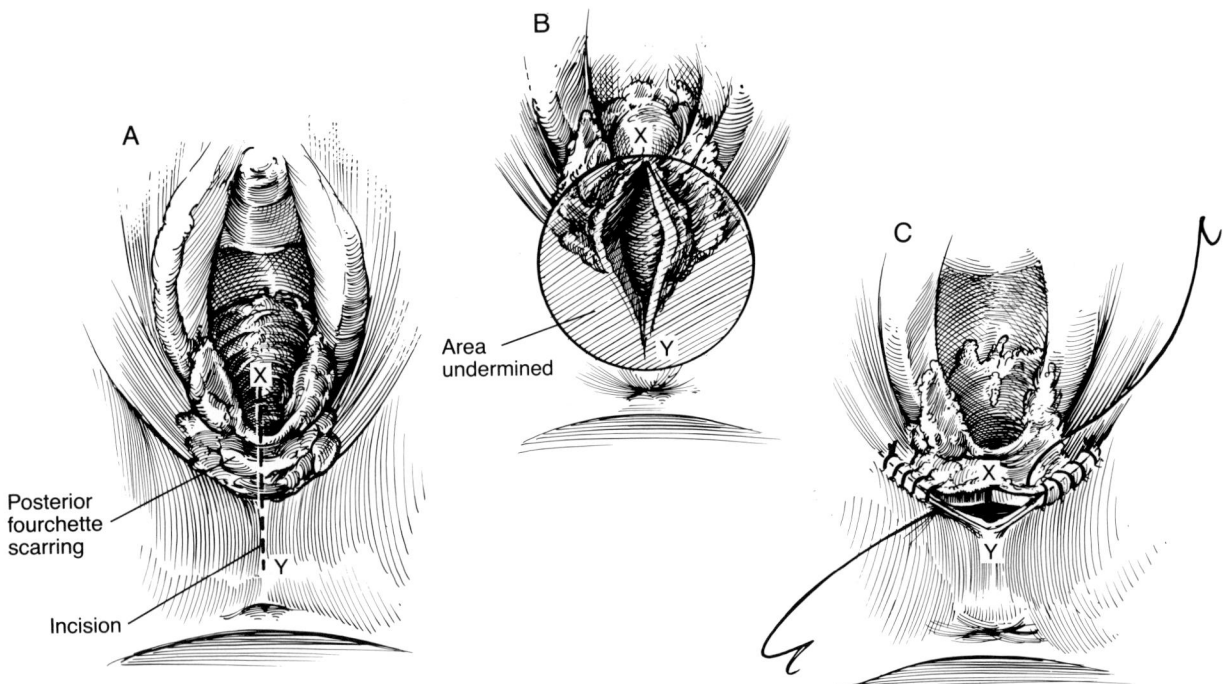

Figure 32–1
A to C, Scarring and retraction of the posterior fourchette is occasionally encountered after vulva surgery. This is best treated by transversely incising (X-Y) the band (A), undermining the adjacent local tissue (B), and closing the defect longitudinally (points X to Y) (C).

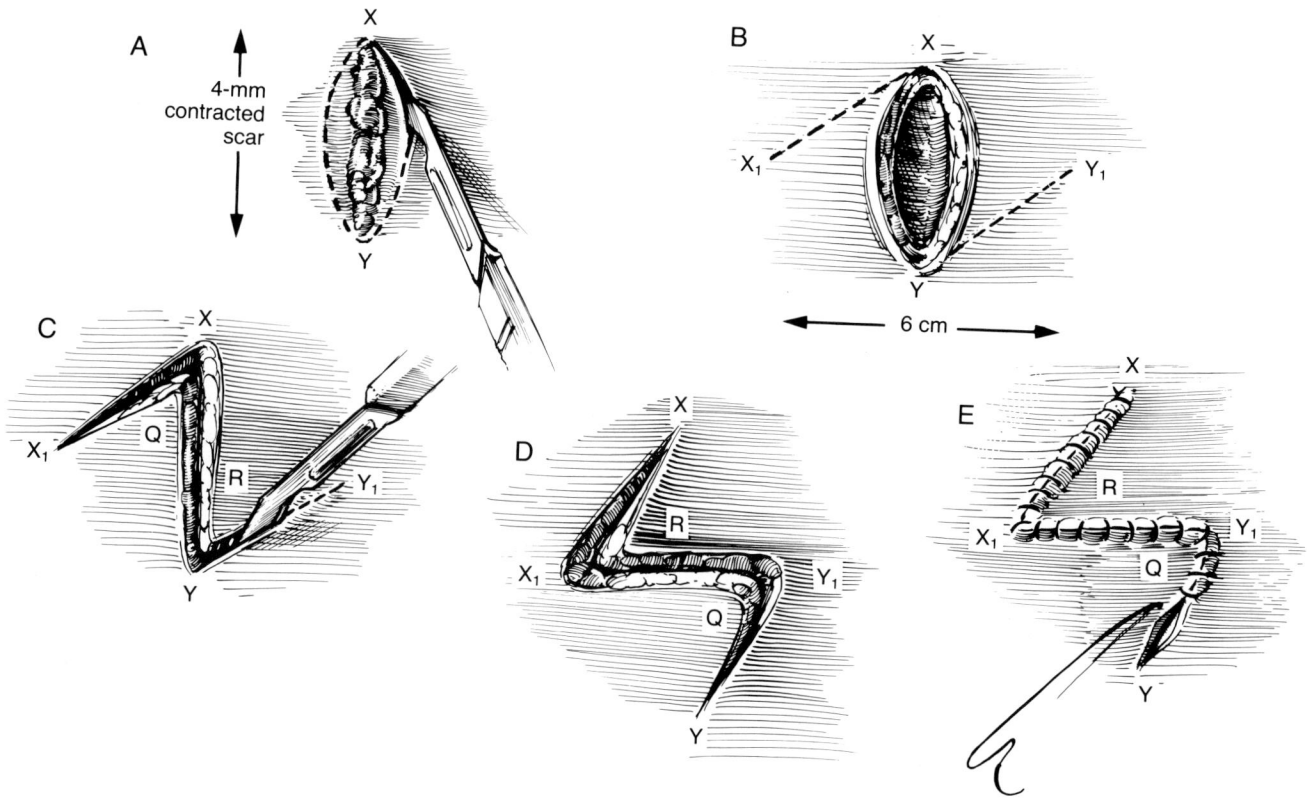

Figure 32–2
A to E, Z-plasty. The contracted scar (4 cm in length) is excised (XY); adjacent parallel incisions (X, X, and YY), with a horizontal width of about 6 cm, are made; and the underlying tissue is undermined to produce Q and R flaps, which are then exchanged for closure, thereby contributing more length between points X and Y.

RECONSTRUCTIVE SURGERY IN GYNECOLOGIC ONCOLOGY 609

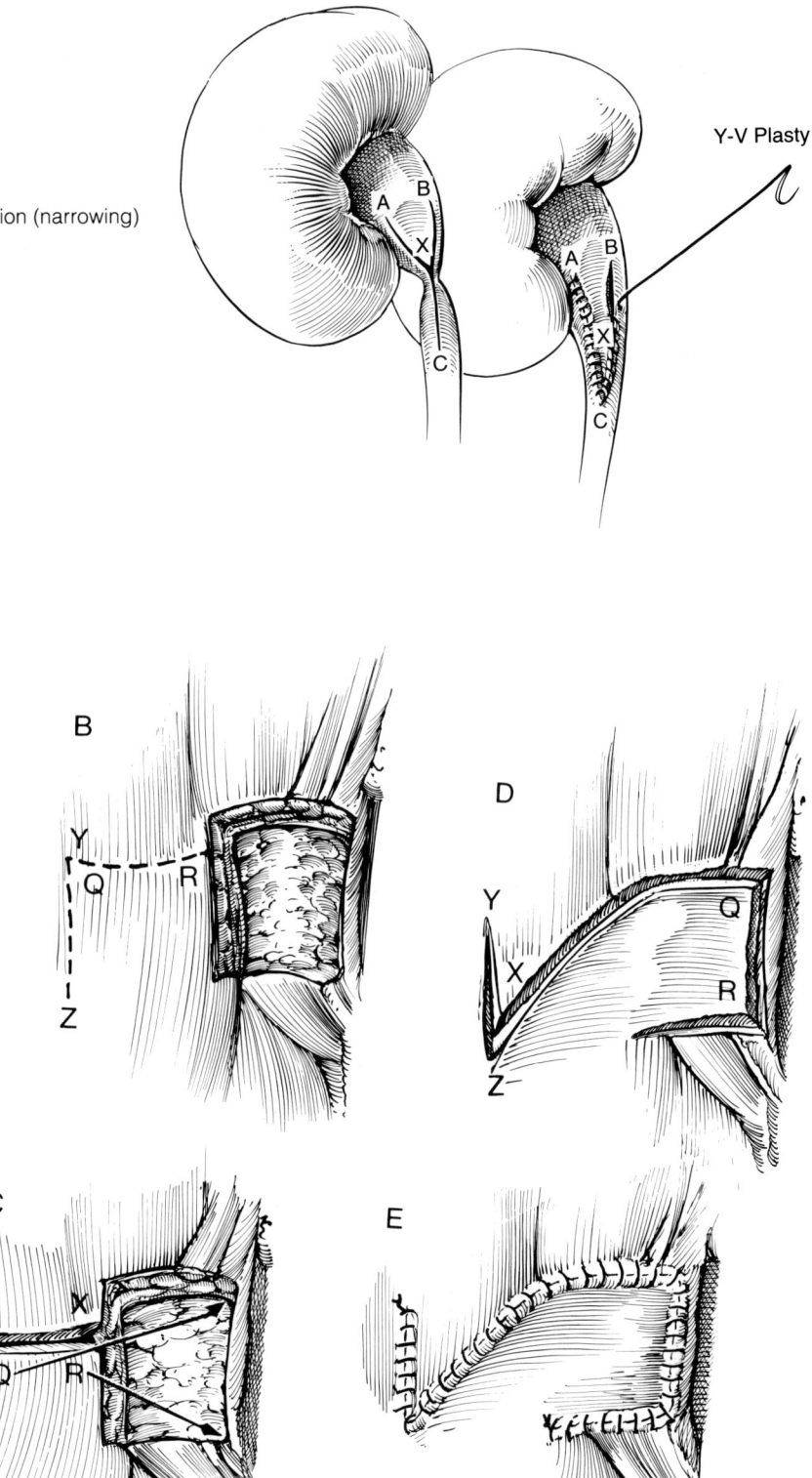

Figure 32–3
Y-V plasty procedure to manage an area of obstruction (narrowing) at the ureteropelvic junction.

Figure 32–4
A to *E*, A large defect to the right of the vagina is covered by an adjacent rhomboid flap (XYZ, where XY = XZ in length). This square or rhomboid is undermined and the flap (QR) is rotated 90 degrees, with point X closing in opposition to point Z.

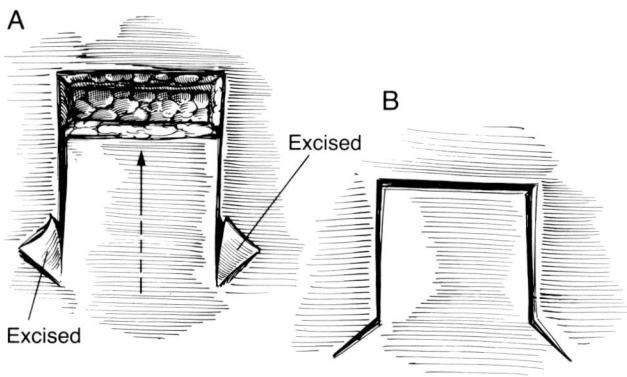

Figure 32–5
A and B, Axial translocation allows the direct sliding of an adjacent block of tissue into an uncovered defect. The resulting "dog-ears" of tissue are excised with equilateral triangles.

Table 32–1
Methods of Vaginal Reconstruction

Method	Clinical Situations	Advantages	Disadvantages
Frank nonoperative	Vaginal agenesis. Vaginectomy with residual soft perineal tissue.	Nonsurgical. Chronic stenting not always necessary. Steroid receptors physiologic.	Takes 4–6 mos. Requires highly motivated patient. May tend to stenosis if not dilated or used on a regular basis.
McIndoe	Vaginal agenesis and failed nonoperative procedure. Vaginectomy with perineal scar formation. Post-exenteration, especially if done in conjunction with an omental graft.	Can be functional within 4–6 wk.	Requires highly motivated patient to take care of prosthesis or stenting. Tends to stricture or contract. Donor site discomfort.
Williams	Vaginal agenesis. After exenteration with intact external genitalia.	Minor operative procedure. May be prelude to a successful Frank nonoperative neovagina.	Pouch in itself is not satisfactory as a functioning vagina because of vertical angle and hair within pouch.
Colon interposition	Procedure can be performed concurrently with pelvic exenteration.	Immediate restoration at time of exenteration. Shortening is not usually a problem. Does not require stenting.	Mucous discharge requires regular douching. Bleeding. Dyspareunia. Introital stenosis.
Bulbocavernosus myocutaneous	Partial exenteration (anterior or posterior)	Surgery limited and relatively easy with low rate of necrosis.	Requires stenting. Stenosis.
Gracilis myocutaneous	Concurrent with pelvic exenteration.	Does not extend operative time because abdominal reconstruction can be continued independent of vaginal reconstruction.	Usually requires bilateral flaps for complete neovagina.
Rectus abdominis myocutaneous	Procedure can be performed concurrently with pelvic exenteration.	Tissue is usually nonirradiated. Vascular supply and mobility are good. Only one flap need be developed.	Contributes to a longer operating time. Wound healing (tension) and stoma disruption are potential problems.
Free-flap procedure	Vaginal agenesis or after pelvic exenteration.	Tissue is nonirradiated. Self-dilatation not usually required.	Major surgical undertaking requiring 3 hr or more and therefore not appropriate to perform at same time as exenteration. Flap is denervated. Requires microvascular anastomosis training to perform.

reconstruction are needed (Table 32–1). Some techniques are applicable to a variety of clinical situations; others are better suited to specific circumstances.[2–4] Each technique is discussed below with regard to its clinical applications and limitations.

Frank Nonoperative Technique[5]

Although best suited to the patient with vaginal agenesis[6] and a perineal dimple, this technique may also be applied to those in whom a vaginectomy has been performed. The perineum should be soft, pliable, and nonirradiated to offer a reasonable opportunity for success. This technique is also effective in patients with transverse vaginal septa, post-hysterectomy cuff distortion, and contractures after a McIndoe procedure.

The technique involves the development of a perineal lumen over many weeks by blunt pressure. The initial pressure and dilatation is in a caudad direction with a blunt tube of small diameter, 1½ cm or less. After creation of a caudad pouch 2 to 3 cm in depth, the direction of the pressure is changed to cephalad (Fig. 32–6). When the depth is about 8 to 10 cm, the next step is to gradually increase the diameter of the dilators, usually up to a 3.5-cm diameter. A successful outcome may be made more likely by using this technique in conjunction with a bicycle seat, in which case the dilatation pressure is the weight of the body rather than digital.[7] Key to the success of this technique is strong patient motivation with physician supervision and encouragement. The technique usually requires 4 to 6 months or longer, and failure to progress may be the result of extensive fibrosis or scarring from previous sur-

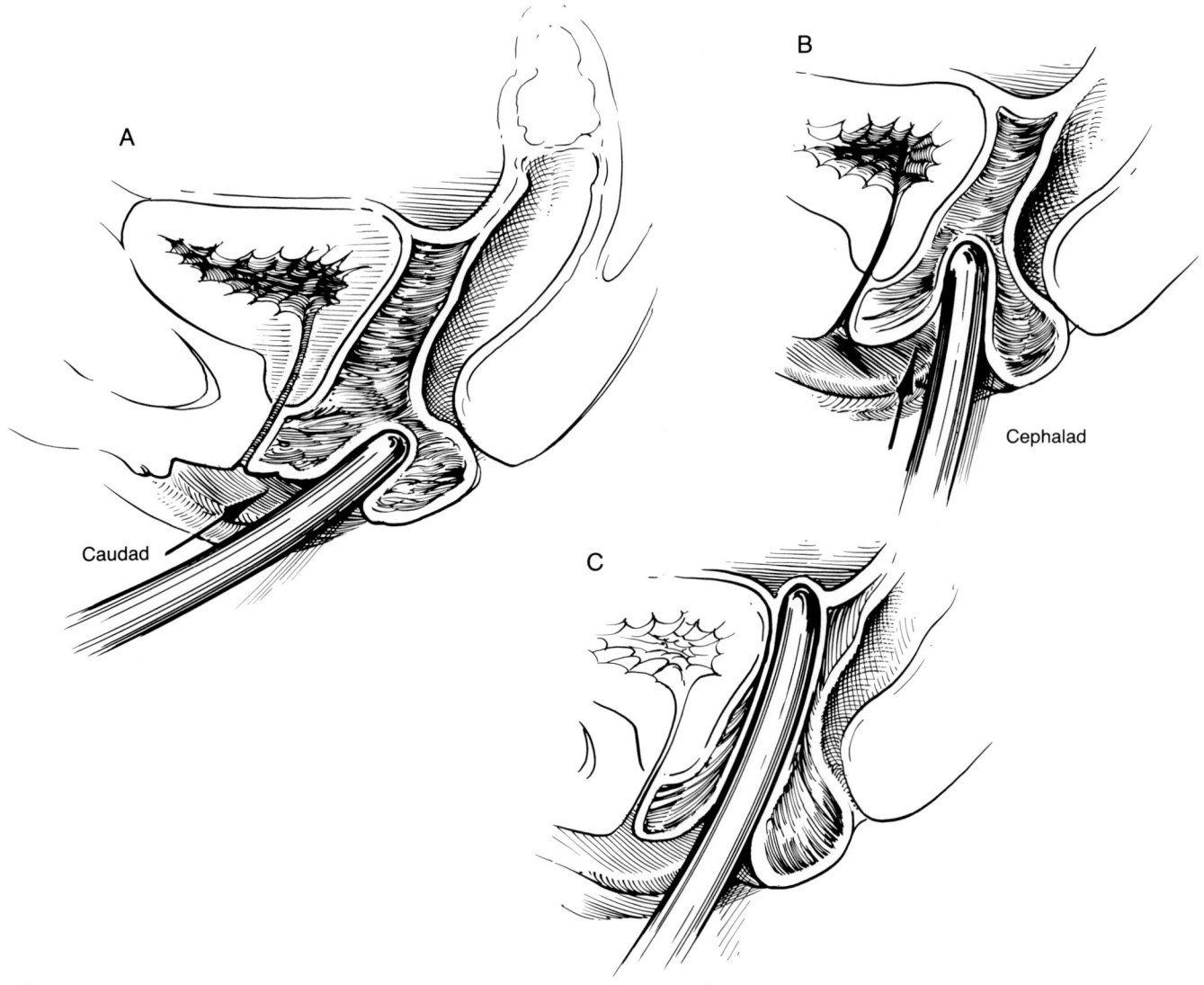

Figure 32–6
The Frank nonoperative vaginal reconstruction is developed by blunt dilatation directed initially in a caudad direction away from the urethra; after a 2- to 3-cm pouch has been created, the direction should be directed more cephalad.

gery or irradiation. There are rare reports of prolapse of a neovagina created by self-dilatation.[8]

McIndoe

Abbe in 1898 first described the technique of creating a vagina by cavitation and split-thickness skin grafts.[9] This technique was subsequently promoted and popularized by McIndoe[10, 11] and others.[12]

The McIndoe vaginal reconstruction consists of the formation of a vascular perineal pocket with the application of a split-thickness skin graft.[10, 11] This procedure is best suited to patients who have failed the Frank nonoperative method of reconstruction or to those who have had complete healing of the pelvis and perineum after pelvic cancer treatment. It has also been used as an interval procedure after pelvic exenteration.[13–15]

The perineal pouch is developed by sharp and blunt dissection, care being taken to avoid injury to the urethra, bladder, rectum, and bowel. The skin-graft donor site is chosen by the patient preoperatively. Most patients choose the posterior thigh-buttock area, which is cosmetically the most desirable. The only drawback is discomfort with sitting during the healing phase. Other sites for consideration are the anterior, posterior, or lateral thigh or the anterior abdomen. An electric dermatome is used to harvest a strip of split-thickness skin between 0.014 and 0.020 inch thick (Fig. 32–7A). The graft is then passed through a meshing device (Fig. 32–7B), which provides two advantages: the graft is more expansible, and therefore larger; and the fenestrations prevent serous drainage build-up behind the graft, so that there is a higher percentage of graft take. The graft is usually held in place by a soft inflatable stent (Fig. 32–7C and D), which is removed around the fourth or fifth postoperative day. The skin grafts, cornified epithelium, do not change to resemble normal vaginal mucosa, even with the use of local estrogen. The long-term vaginal lining tends to remain dry and nonmucosal, and desquamation can be problematic (Fig. 32–7E). Long-term stent management, usually in the form of a condom-covered balsa wood mold, is initiated before the patient's discharge from the hospital. The success of this procedure is very dependent on the patient's compliance with continuous stenting, except for brief intervals of removal for hygienic or functional purposes. Other types of materials, including lucite, Silastic, and polyurethane foam, have been used for dilators.[16] Also, substitutes for the split-thickness graft include peritoneum,[17] amnion,[18] and full-thickness skin.[19] There are rare reports of recurrent intraepithelial neoplasia developing in the grafted tissue.[20, 21]

When a normal upper genital tract coexists with vaginal agenesis, the establishment of an intact genital tract is possible and may permit future pregnancies.[22]

Omental McIndoe

In general the McIndoe technique was not particularly suited to post-exenteration patients because of the large pelvic cavity. The use of the omentum as a pelvic lid[23] or as a cylindrical pelvic graft,[24] has made this approach more successful. However, because the McIndoe procedure generally requires patients to be highly motivated and directly involved in stent management, this technique risks failure in post-exenteration patients because they are often too preoccupied and overwhelmed by the magnitude of the diagnosis and surgical procedure to give satisfactory attention to the vaginal restoration.

Williams

This vulvovaginoplasty technique, first described in 1964,[25] consists of developing a perineal pouch using labia majora (Fig. 32–8). The perineal pouch itself does not function as a satisfactory vagina because the pouch is at a vertical angle and sexual intercourse is not usually satisfactory. Patients also complain of discomfort from the hairy dry pouch and from excessive stimulation against the clitoris. The Williams vaginoplasty pouch also may tend to collect urine. Ideally, a shallow Williams pouch will encourage the patient to proceed with what in essence is a Frank nonoperative dilatation of a neovagina.[26, 27]

Three case reports described a satisfactory outcome of a variant of the Williams procedure, combined with cavitation and subsequent dilatation.[9]

Colon Interposition

The concept of constructing a neovagina from colon or ileum was first proposed in 1904,[28] advocated by Pratt in 1961,[29] and again more reported by Turner-Warwick and Kirby[30] (Fig. 32–9). Ileal and sigmoidal segments have been proposed, but the colocecal reconstruction appears to be the most reliable and functional.[30] This technique has not gained widespread acceptance because of problems with a continuous malodorous mucoid discharge that requires regular douching. Other patient complaints include dyspareunia, bleeding, and (in some) the development of introital stenosis that requires surgical intervention. Protrusion of the neovagina has also been reported.[30]

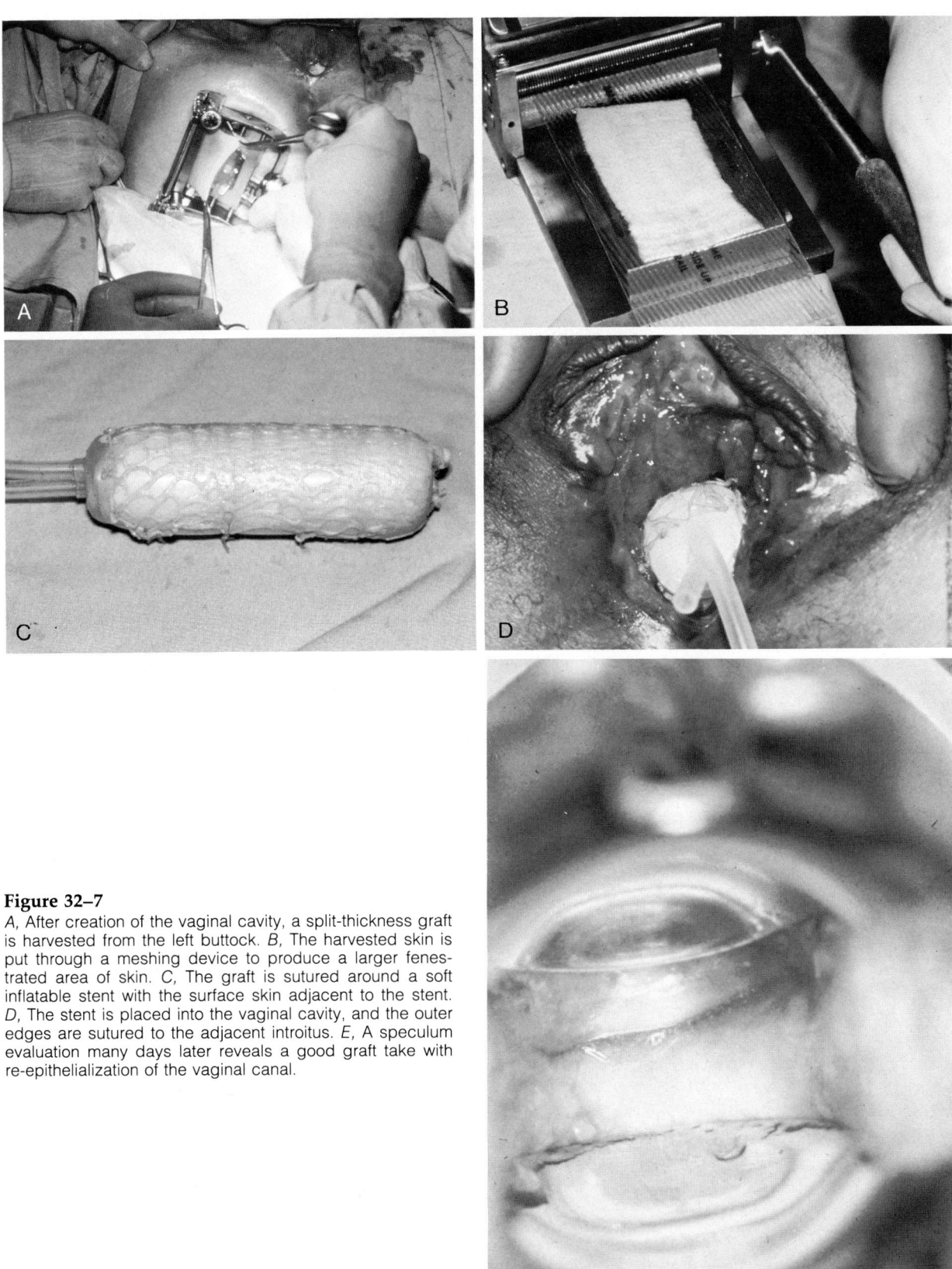

Figure 32–7
A, After creation of the vaginal cavity, a split-thickness graft is harvested from the left buttock. *B,* The harvested skin is put through a meshing device to produce a larger fenestrated area of skin. *C,* The graft is sutured around a soft inflatable stent with the surface skin adjacent to the stent. *D,* The stent is placed into the vaginal cavity, and the outer edges are sutured to the adjacent introitus. *E,* A speculum evaluation many days later reveals a good graft take with re-epithelialization of the vaginal canal.

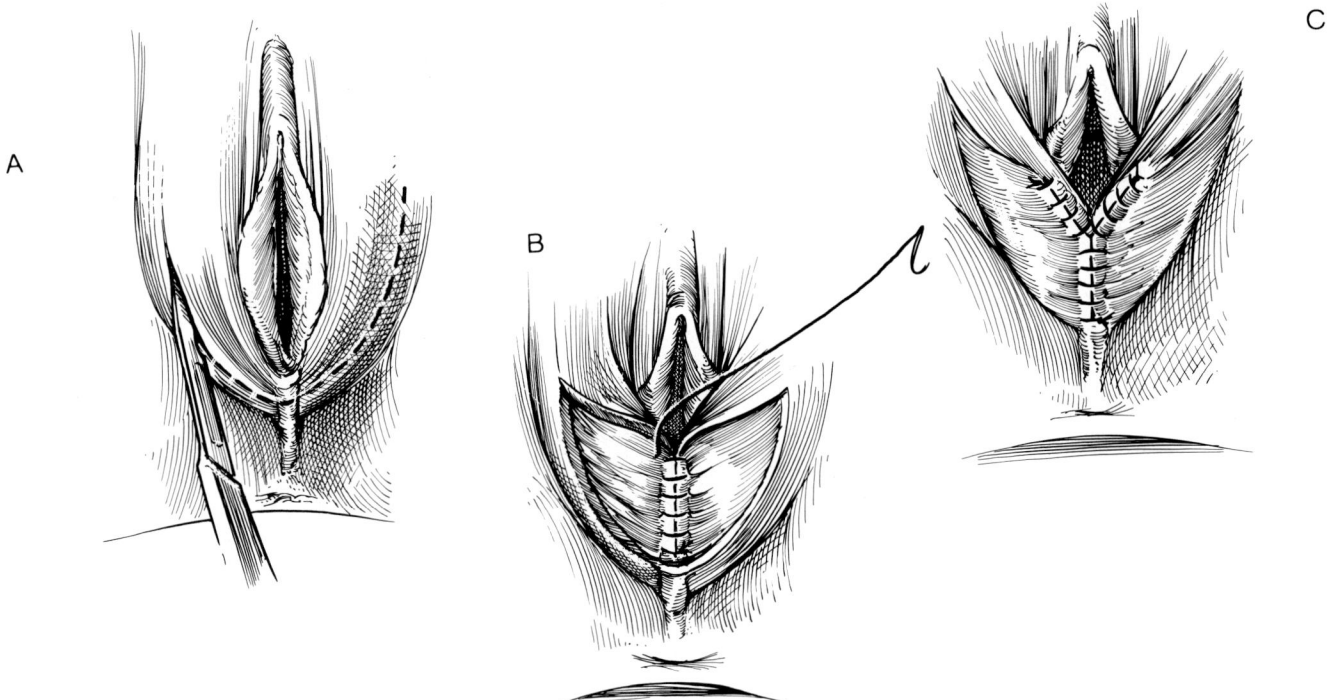

Figure 32–8
Williams vulvovaginoplasty. A posterior U-shaped incision of the labia majora and posterior fourchette (A), followed by approximation of the medial edges (B), followed by approximation of the lateral edges to form a shallow vulvar pouch at the vaginal introitus (C).

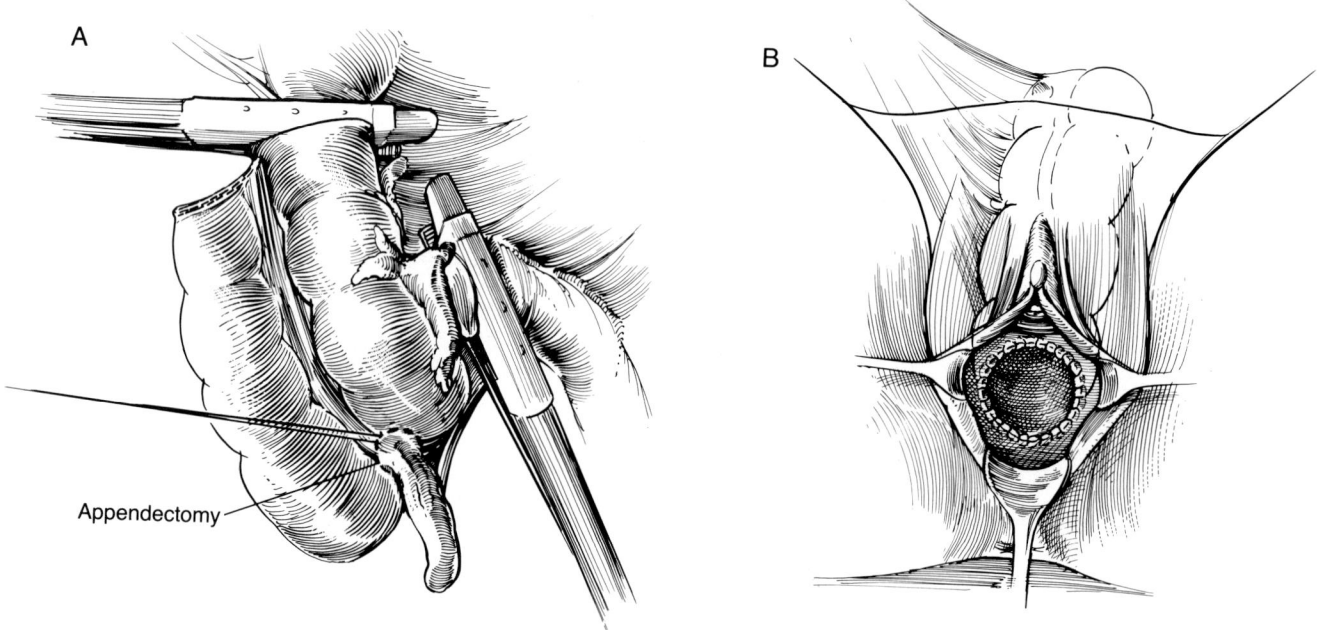

Figure 32–9
Colon interposition. The colocecum is isolated with its mesentery. An appendectomy is performed and the colonic segment is inverted and sutured to the vaginal introitus. An ileoascending enterocolostomy and closure of the mesenteric defect restores gastrointestinal continuity.

Bulbocavernosus (Martius)

The use of a posteriorly based pedicle of subcutaneous tissue, with or without bulbocavernous muscle from the labium majus as reported by Martius, is commonly used to provide well-vascularized tissue for the repair of fistulas involving the vagina, urethra, bladder, or rectum.[31] This technique is advantageous in the repair of irradiation injuries because the blood vascular supply (external pudendal) has usually received minimal irradiation.

The vulvobulbocavernosus myocutaneous neovaginal reconstruction reported by Hatch is reliable and easy to perform.[32] The use of this technique to construct a complete neovagina requires a significant amount of vulvar skin, and distortion of the vulva may occur. Also, the long pedicles are at risk for necrosis, especially at the end of the pedicle, in the area of the vaginal vault. Because of these limitations, this technique is best suited to patients in whom a portion of the normal vagina has been left intact. An example is when a posterior or anterior exenteration procedure allows for retention of the anterior or posterior vagina, respectively.

Gracilis Myocutaneous

McCraw and colleagues reported the gracilis myocutaneous vaginal reconstruction (Fig. 32–10) in 1976.[33] This technique offers the advantages of concurrent restoration, rapid healing, and less complicated management of the pelvic cavity in an exenteration patient. It has been shown that gracilis vaginal reconstruction concurrent with pelvic exenteration does not increase blood loss, operating time, or length of hospitalization.[34, 35] However, early experience with this technique presented problems of necrosis and prolapse.[34, 36] These complications and unsatisfactory results led to a number of modifications in the technique and subsequent improved outcomes.[34, 37] Alterations in technique include the use of smaller grafts (5–6 × 11–14 cm) and anchoring the grafts to the remaining levator fascia and retropubic fascia. Possibly the most important modification to the original technique is the division of the medial circumflex femoral artery, permitting higher mobilization of the grafts into the pelvis. The original[33] and subsequent reports[36, 38–40] emphasized the importance of this pedicle, later reports[34, 37] demonstrated that this restrictive vascular pedicle could be divided to provide better mobilization with no significant vascular compromise. The graft appears to receive sufficient anastomotic blood supply from the terminal branches of the obturator artery or possibly from retropubic vessels to the proximal gracilis insertion.[34, 37, 41]

The size of the grafts can be adjusted from the smaller paddles (5–6 × 11–14 cm) for replacement of the vagina only (Fig. 32–11) to larger paddles (7–10 × 15–18 cm) for replacement of the vagina and portions of the vulva (Fig. 32–12).

When a partial pelvic exenteration (anterior or posterior) or a supralevator exenteration is performed, it is usually necessary to use either smaller bilateral grafts or a unilateral graft in combination with a portion of remaining vaginal mucosa. A skin and fascia flap from the medial thigh has also been proposed for vaginal and vulvar reconstructions when a flap with less bulk than the gracilis flap is required.[42]

Rectus Abdominis Myocutaneous

Use of the rectus abdominis myocutaneous flap provides a reliable technique for vaginal reconstruction at the time of pelvic exenteration.[43–45] The rectus abdominis flap, initially described as a means of reconstructing abdominal wall defects,[46] is also used on occasion to reconstruct breasts[47] and perineal defects.[48] This flap is raised from the upper abdomen and is based on an inferior vascular pedicle, the inferior epigastric vessels, the artery arising from the external iliac artery, and the vein entering the external iliac vein (Fig. 32–13). Disruption to these vessels, e.g., during a pelvic lymphadenectomy, potentially poses a threat to flap viability.

Gluteal Thigh Flap

The gluteal thigh flap, either unilateral or bilateral, has been reported to offer results similar to those from the gracilis myocutaneous flaps in patients undergoing pelvic exenteration.[49]

Free-Flap Vaginoplasty

A successful free-flap vaginal reconstruction with a full-thickness graft from the scapular region and a microvascular anastomosis to vessels in the groin has been reported.[50]

VULVOPLASTY: VULVA AND GROINS

Femoral Vessel Coverage

Wound breakdown and necrosis after inguinofemoral lymphadenectomy rarely involves the femoral vessels. However, serious necrosis can lead to a femoral artery rupture (Fig. 32–14) and may result in the loss of a limb or exsanguination. Transposition of the sartorius muscle from the anterosuperior iliac spine

Text continued on page 620

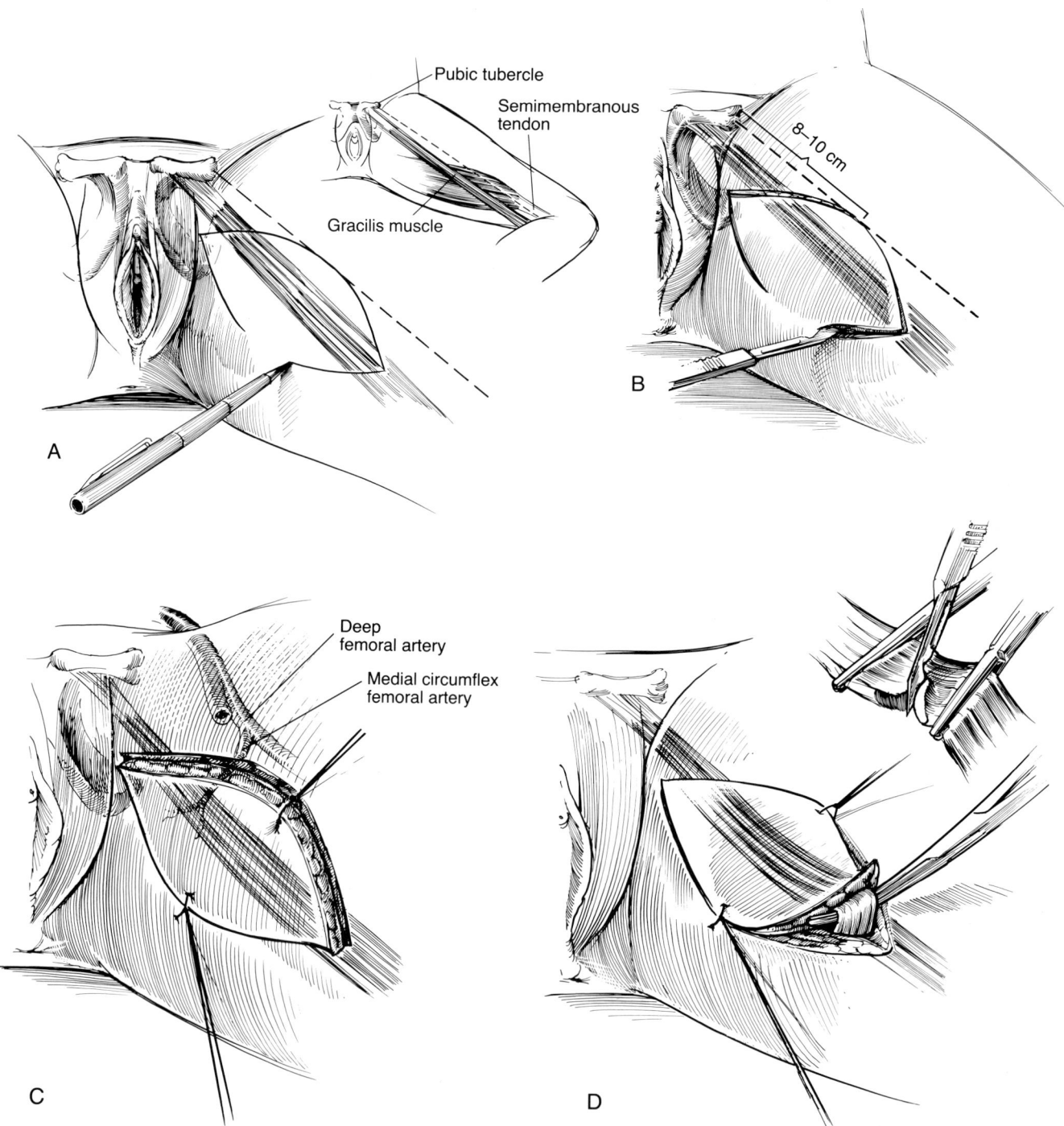

Figure 32–10

Gracilis myocutaneous vaginal reconstruction. *A,* The first step is to determine the topographical location of the gracilis muscle and the location of the skin paddle to be developed. The gracilis muscle is usually inferior to a line drawn between the pubic tubercle and the posterior insertion of the semimembranous muscle at the tibia (posterior medial popliteal fossa).
B, The skin, subcutaneous tissue, and fascia superior to the gluteal muscle are circumferentially incised and a neurovascular pedicle should be identified superiorly, about 8 to 10 cm from the pubic tubercle. The vessels are the medial circumflex femoral artery and vein, and very little additional mobility of the flap can be obtained by dissecting deeper. However, the adjacent nerve does mobilize out of the deeper tissue, and even if the vessels need to be sacrificed for mobility, the innovation of the flap can usually be maintained.
C, Since the skin and subcutaneous tissue are anchored only by small perforators from the fascia, it is advisable to place a few interrupted anchoring sutures between the deep fascia and the skin to prevent a shearing of the superficial tissue off the fascia.
D, The gracilis muscle distal to the myocutaneous graft is isolated, divided, and ligated. The muscle proximal to the graft (adjacent to the pubic tubercle) is not divided because it may contain a significant component of the graft's blood supply.

RECONSTRUCTIVE SURGERY IN GYNECOLOGIC ONCOLOGY 617

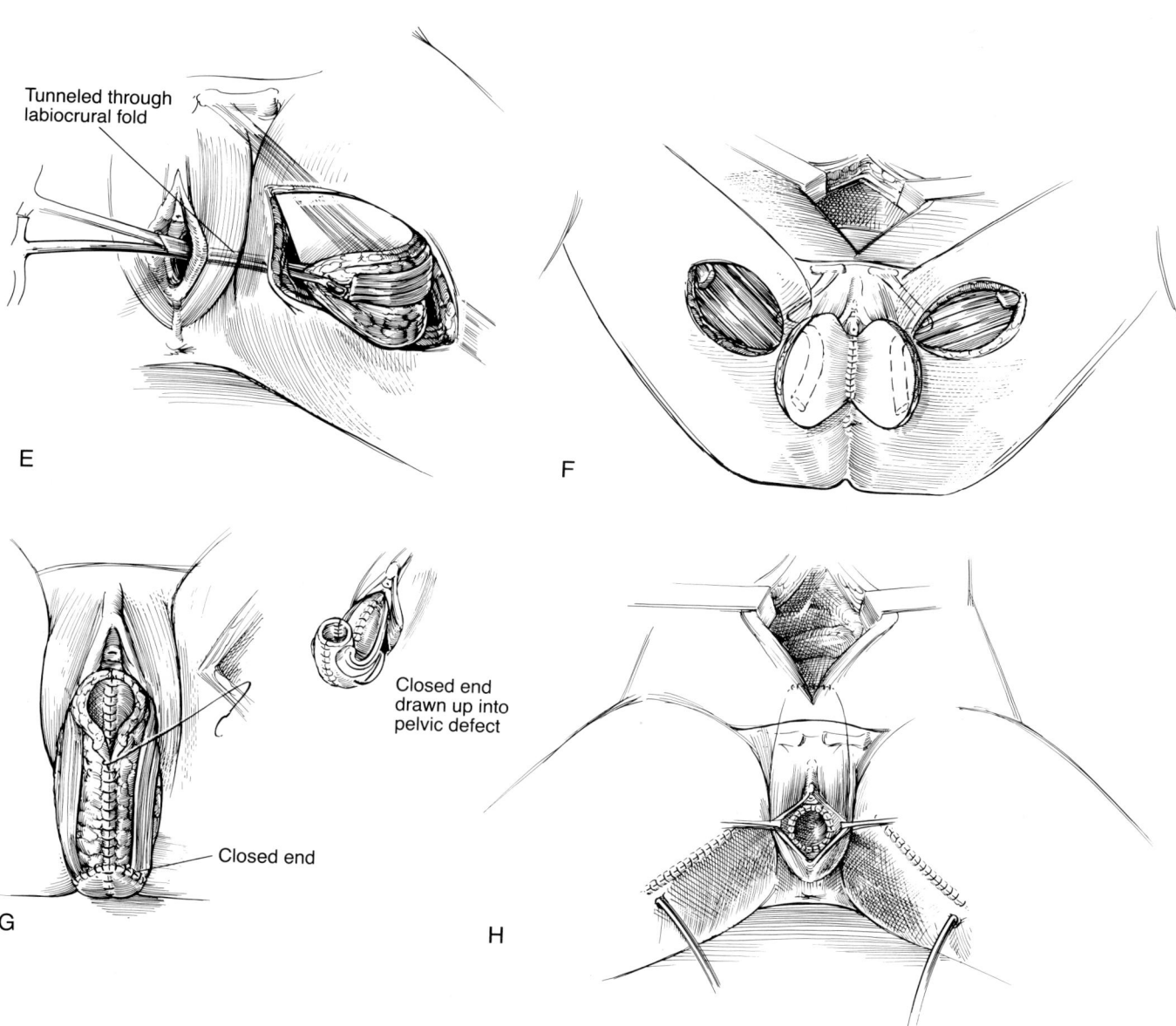

Figure 32–10 *Continued*
E, The distal end of the graft is then grasped with a Babcock instrument and guided through the subcutaneous labiocrural tunnel. The procedure is performed on both legs, producing bilateral grafts, which are then opposed and the skin edges sutured, except the proximal (upper) portions of the grafts as they lie in front of the perineum.
F, The two grafts are sutured into a tubal structure.
G, The inferior (closed) end is then drawn up into the pelvic defect.
H, The graft is then anchored laterally to the pelvic fascia and the retropubic fascia. The open end of the tube is circumferentially sutured to the skin surrounding the introitus. The thigh wounds are closed in layers over subfascial suction drains.

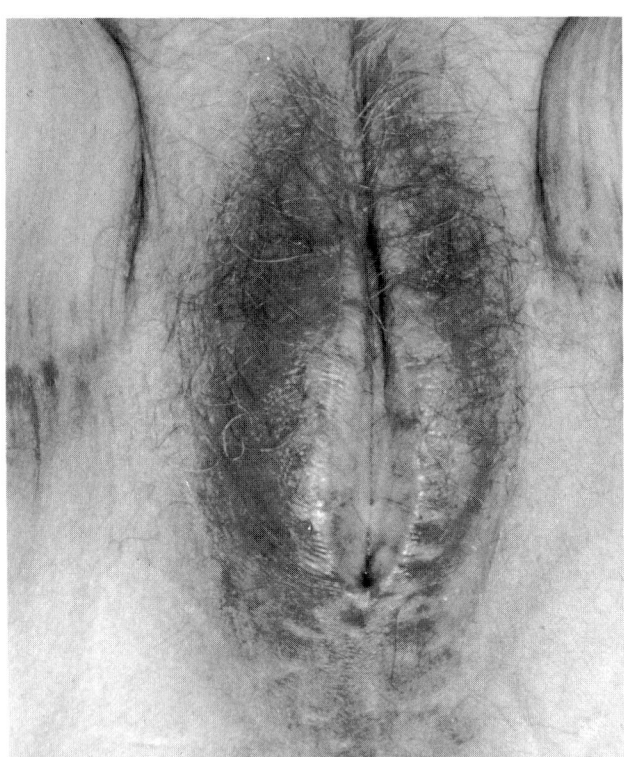

Figure 32–11
Postoperative appearance of the vulva after a bilateral gracilis myocutaneous vaginal reconstruction using small grafts.

Figure 32–12
Postoperative appearance of the vulva after a bilateral gracilis myocutaneous vaginovulva reconstruction using larger grafts.

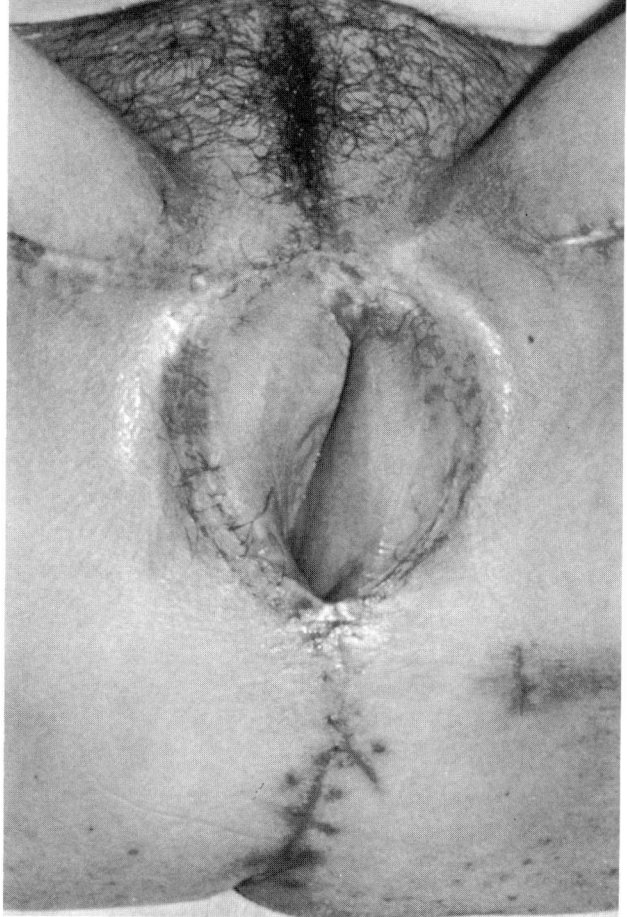

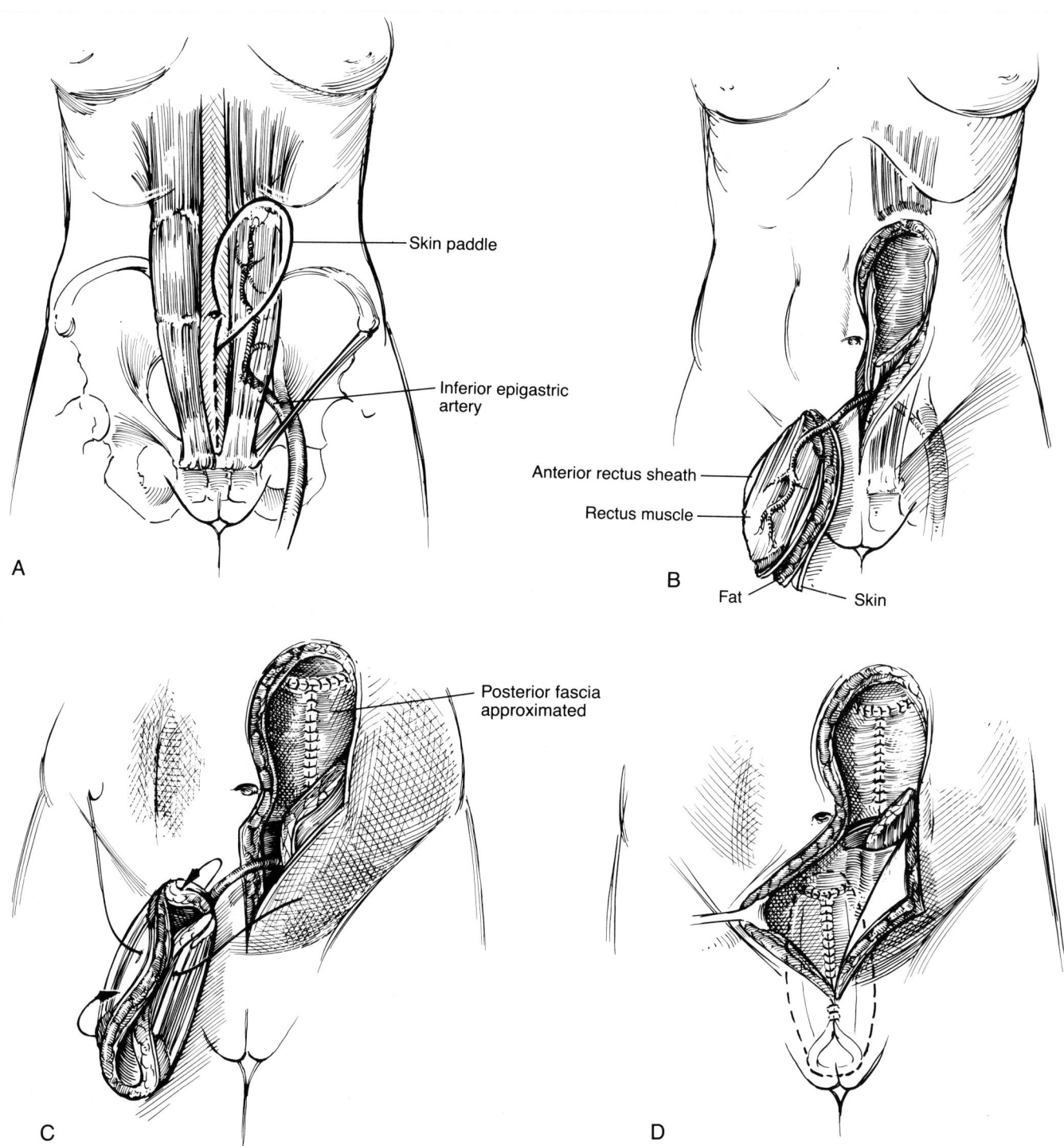

Figure 32–13
A, The rectus abdominis is based on an inferior pedicle with the vascular supply from the inferior epigastric vessels off the external iliacs. *B*, The paddle is usually 10 to 14 cm in horizontal width and 14 to 20 cm in vertical length, and the upper border is adjacent to the inferior costal margin. The rectus abdominis muscle is transected superiorly and dissected free from its fascial bed (although the anterior rectus fascia adjacent to the paddle is mobilized with the paddle). *C*, The vaginal tube is then developed by inverting the lateral and inner margins. *D*, The neovagina is sutured into place and the abdomen closed.

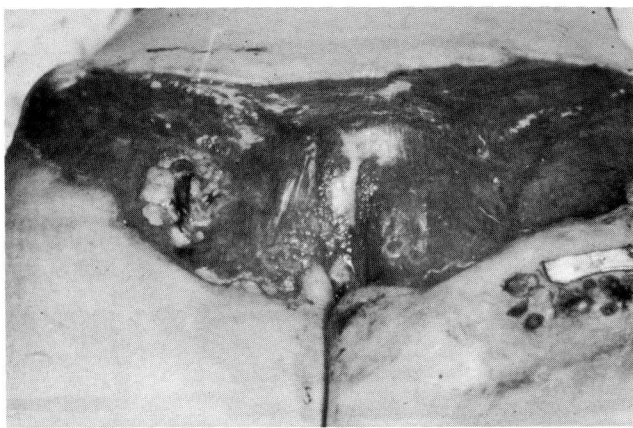

Figure 32–14
Extensive necrosis of groin wounds with resultant right femoral artery necrosis and rupture. An attempt has been made to repair with a venous patch and pinch skin grafts.

to the inguinal ligament, adjacent to the femoral vessels, provides a protective covering and padding for the femoral vessels (Fig. 32–15).[51] There are no clinical data supporting the use of this technique with every femoral lymphadenectomy. Ramasastry and colleagues described the use of a number of local flaps for the management of difficult wounds of the groin.[52]

Reports of the use of freeze-dried dura mater for femoral vessel coverage described a safe and effective alternative (Fig. 32–16) to the technically more difficult sartorius muscle transposition.[53, 54] In reports of Creutzfeldt-Jakob disease,[55] it appears to be most commonly associated with the use of the graft for intracranial repairs.[56] There have been no reported cases of hepatitis or human immunodeficiency virus transmission as a result of using the dura mater patch.

Rhomboid and Adjacent Pedicle Flaps

Split-thickness grafting to areas where only skin has been removed is satisfactory,[57] but it is necessary to use tissue that will provide subcutaneous padding when more radical excisions are performed. Rhomboid flaps have already been described (see Fig. 32–4) and are useful in providing coverage for moderate defects, especially in the vulvar area.[58]

Excellent results have been reported from a ped-

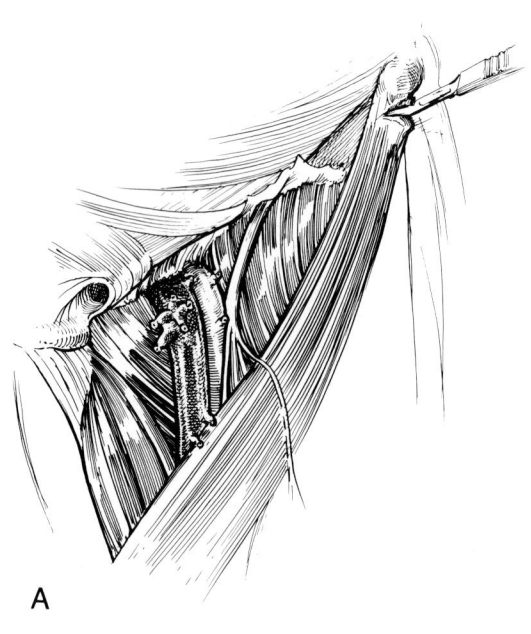
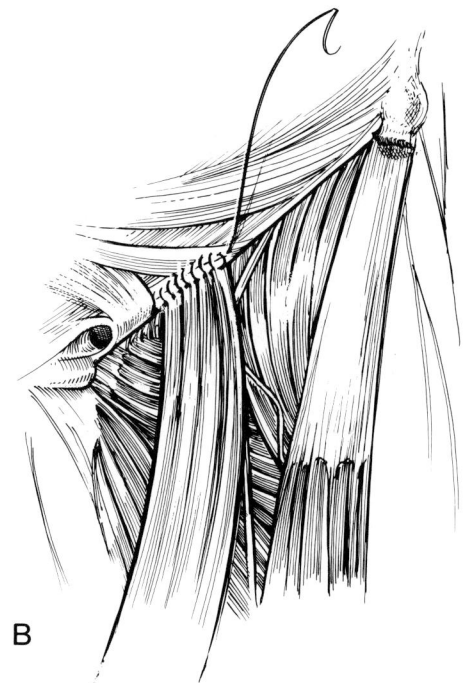

Figure 32–15
A, Sartorius muscle transposition. The anterosuperior iliac spine insertion of the sartorius muscle is divided and the loose lateral attachments are dissected free, permitting the sartorius to be mobilized medially. B, The sartorius muscle is sutured to the inguinal ligament, covering the femoral vessels in the process.

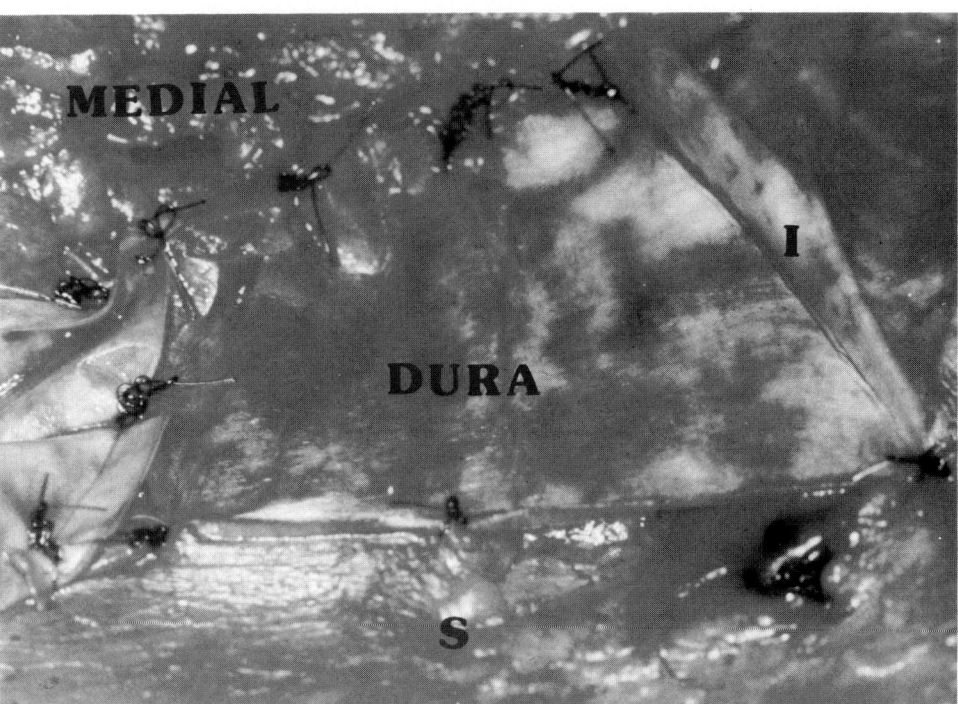

Figure 32–16
Dura mater, sutured to the inguinal ligament superiorly (I), the sartorius laterally (S), and the adductor longus medially, provides coverage of the entire femoral triangle. (From Fiorica JV, Roberts WS, LaPolla JP, et al.: Femoral vessel coverage with dura mater after inguinofemoral lymphadenectomy. Gynecol Oncol 1991; 42:217.)

icle flap based on the superficial external pudendal artery[59] (Fig. 32–17). Rectus abdominis flaps can also be developed to cover perineal defects.[48] Gluteal thigh flaps based on an inferior gluteal artery can cover perineal and buttock defects.[60]

Tensor Fasciae Latae Flaps

Large wounds or defects in the area of the thighs, vulva,[61] buttocks, and lower abdomen are possibly amenable to coverage with a tensor fasciae latae (TFL) flap.[62–64] This flap (Fig. 32–18) is developed from the lateral aspect of the leg, and the blood supply is based on the lateral circumflex femoral artery, a branch of the profundus femoral artery traversing laterally beneath the rectus femoris muscle and entering the tensor fasciae latae approximately 8 to 10 cm inferior to the anterosuperior iliac spine.

ABDOMINAL WALL

Gynecologic oncologic complications necessitating reconstructive procedures for the abdominal wall include large hernia defects, radiation ulcerations, and, rarely, large, abdominal wall defects secondary to tumor-reductive surgery.

Rectus Abdominis Myocutaneous

As previously described, a large myocutaneous graft can be developed from the upper abdomen and used for a vaginal reconstruction. Similarly, this graft can be used as a full-thickness graft to replace an excised area of lower abdomen (Fig. 32–19).

Tensor Fasciae Latae

Although less suited than the rectus abdominis flap for full-thickness abdominal wall defects, the TFL flap offers an alternative tissue source (Fig. 32–20). Depending on patient fat distribution variance, the graft may be too thin or too thick for repair of an abdominal defect.

Layered Reconstruction

Full-thickness abdominal defects may be covered by means of a combination of techniques to reconstruct the various abdominal wall layers.[65] Figure 32–21 illustrates one such situation. The abdominal fascia is replaced by a strong, synthetic, nonabsorbable material such as Mersilene, dura mater,[66] or Gore-Tex (Fig. 32–21A). Depending on the size of the defect, a rhomboid, lateral transposition or axial flap can be used to cover the synthetic material with the subcutaneous and skin layers. In other situations, the omentum, in the form of an omental pedicle graft, may be considered. Figure 32–21B demonstrates the use of a long omental pedicle brought through a suprapubic defect and layered over the synthetic fascial layer. The surface of this "neo-

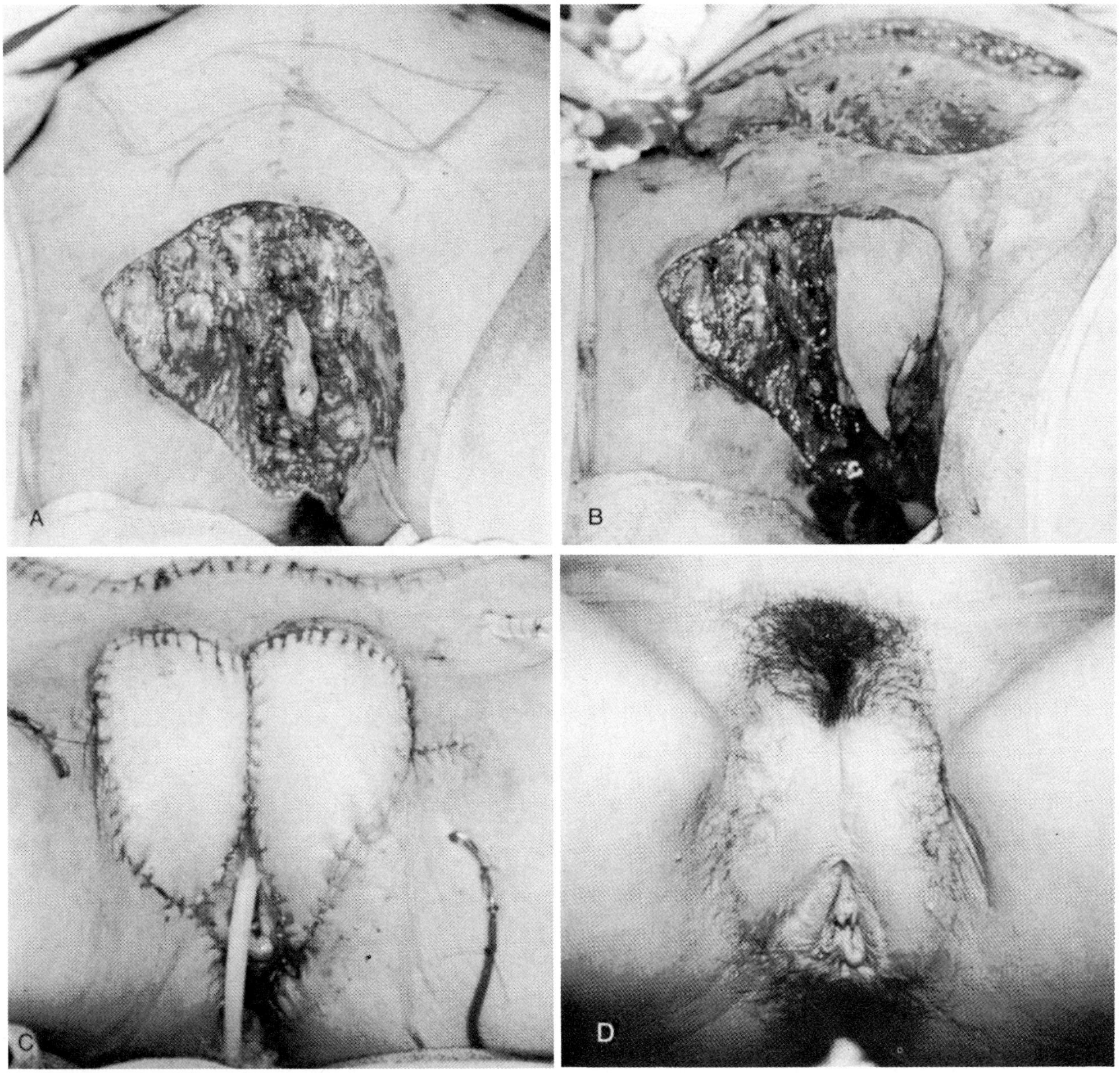

Figure 32–17
Vulvar reconstruction with a pedicle flap based on the superficial external pudendal artery. *A*, The outline of the flap and estimated course of the superficial external pudendal artery are indicated. *B*, After the flap is raised, it is rotated down to the perineum through a subcutaneous tunnel. *C*, The flaps are secured and suction drains placed. *D*, Long-term results are satisfactory. (Reprinted with permission from The American College of Obstetricians and Gynecologists [Obstetrics and Gynecology 1991; 78:964].)

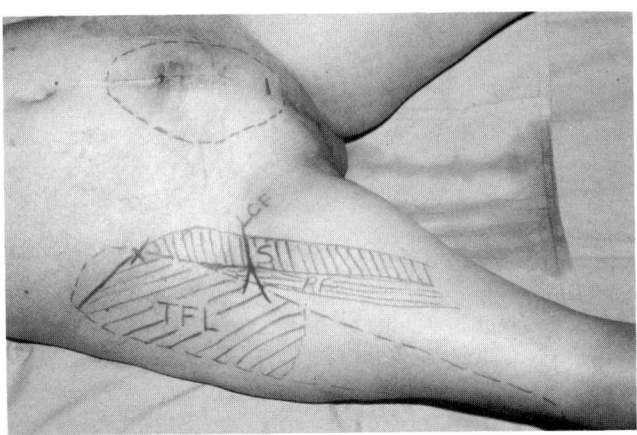

Figure 32–18
Preoperative topographical markings for a right tensor fasciae latae (TFL) flap anticipated to be necessary for closure of an abdominal wall defect.

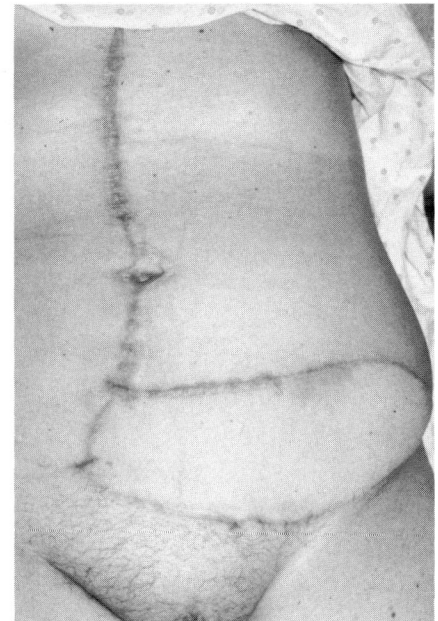

Figure 32–19
Rectus abdominis graft repair of a left lower abdominal wall defect after wide excision of a recurrent tumor.

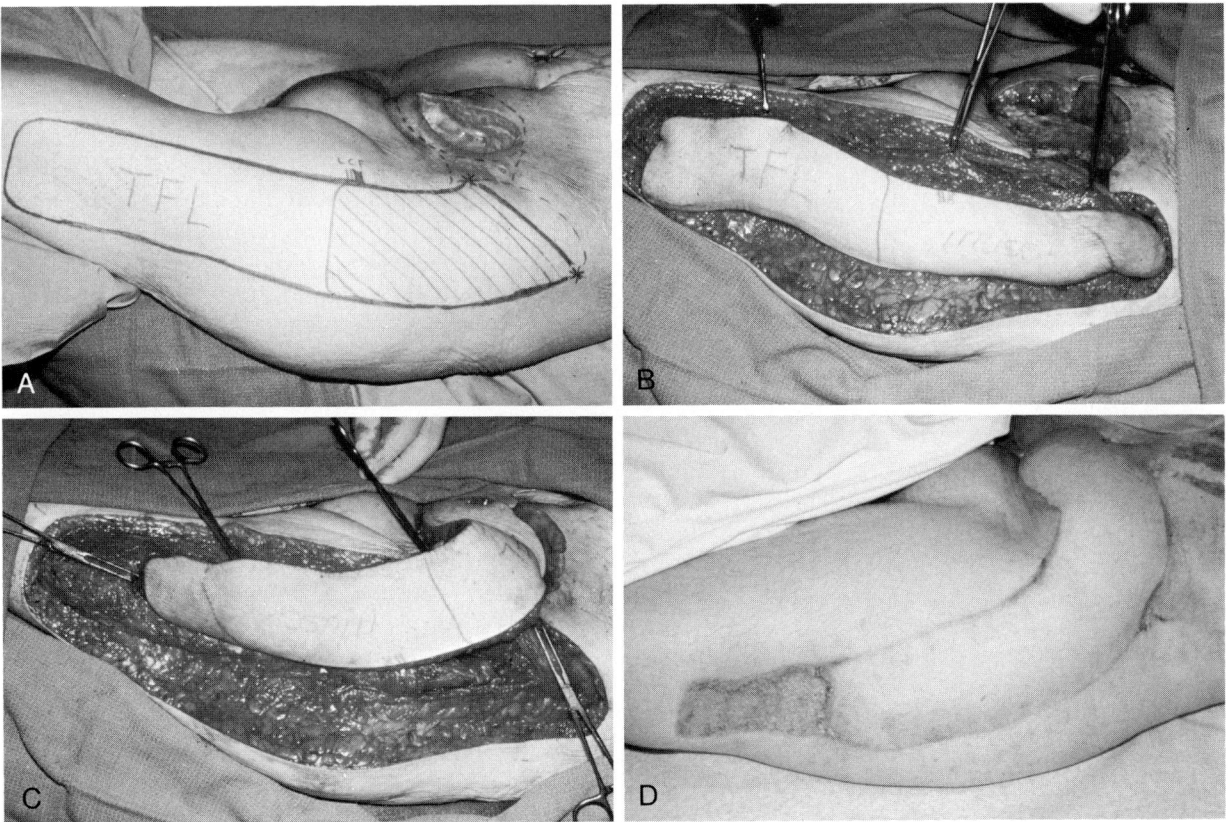

Figure 32–20
A TFL flap covers an abdominal wall defect. *A*, A left lower quadrant abdominal wall wound is within a cobalt radiation field and a TFL reconstruction is planned. *B*, The radiation ulcer is débrided and the TFL flap developed. *C*, The TFL flap is rotated 180 degrees on its lateral circumflex femoral vascular pedicle. *D*, The distal donor site is covered by a split-thickness graft and the abdominal defect by the TFL graft.

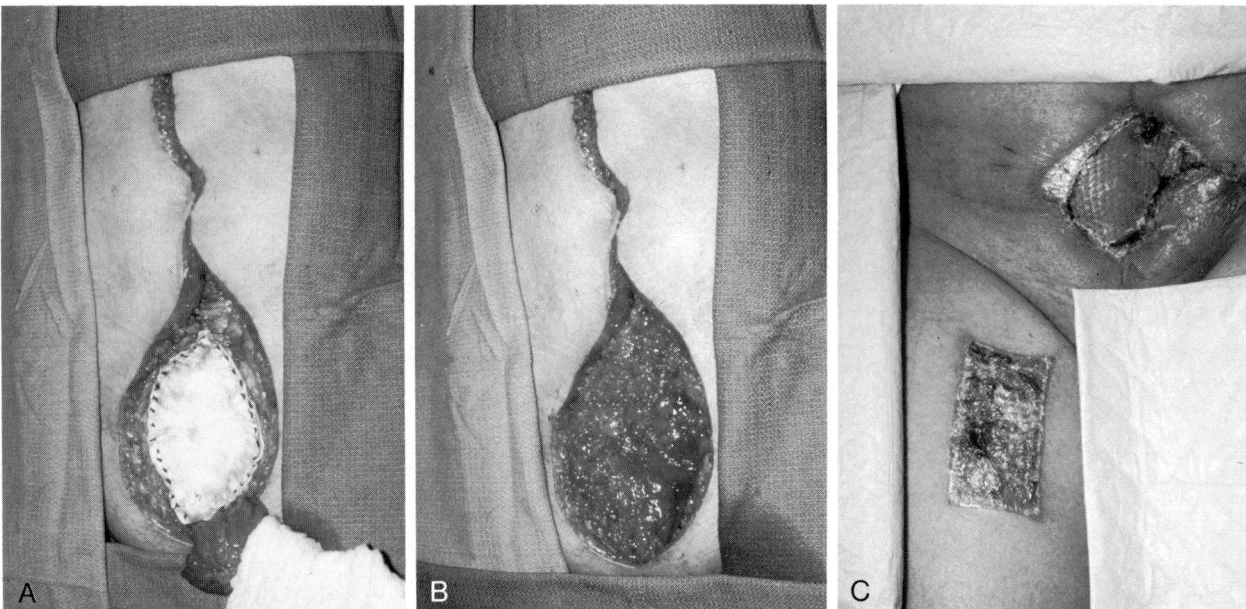

Figure 32–21
A layered abdominal wall reconstruction in a patient undergoing resection of the central lower abdomen. *A*, The fascial defect is closed with a large patch of Gore-Tex. *B*, The subcutaneous tissue is built up with the development of a long omental pedicle that was brought out through an opening adjacent to the pubic symphysis. *C*, The reconstruction is completed with a split-thickness skin graft.

subcutaneous" layer can then be covered by a split-thickness skin graft (Fig. 32–21C).

PELVIC FLOOR

One early and major postoperative problem encountered after total pelvic exenteration was prolapse of the abdominal contents through the pelvic floor, the perineal defect frequently resulting in bowel obstruction or fistula formation. Subsequently, techniques to provide pelvic floor support have been developed. One of the advantages of the gracilis myocutaneous vaginal reconstruction is that the perineal defect is obliterated and the bulky flaps also provide support to the superior abdominal contents. Techniques specifically designed to provide pelvic floor support include use of the omental pedicle or synthetic material.[53, 67–69]

SACRUM

Pressure sores (decubiti) are problematic for immobilized or chronically ill patients, but the most challenging gluteal or sacral defects are those that develop within radiation fields (Fig. 32–22). Radiation-related defects or ulcerations invariably require a new source of blood supply. Because of the problem of radiation-related endarteritis, free flaps are risky in view of the likelihood of damage to the local major vascular pedicles. Rotational myocutaneous grafts are therefore preferable. The previously described tensor fasciae latae and gracilis myocutaneous flaps have the potential to reach and cover sacral or gluteal defects. However, the most locally accessible tissue is the gluteus maximus, a myocutaneous source that can be developed through a rotational[70] method (Fig. 32–23) or an island pedicle[71, 72] (Fig. 32–24).

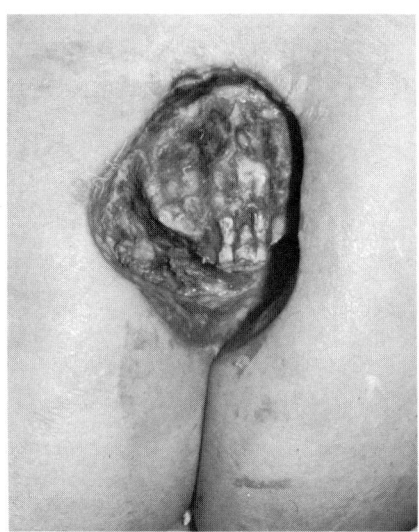

Figure 32–22
A large necrotic ulcerated radiation wound over the sacrum.

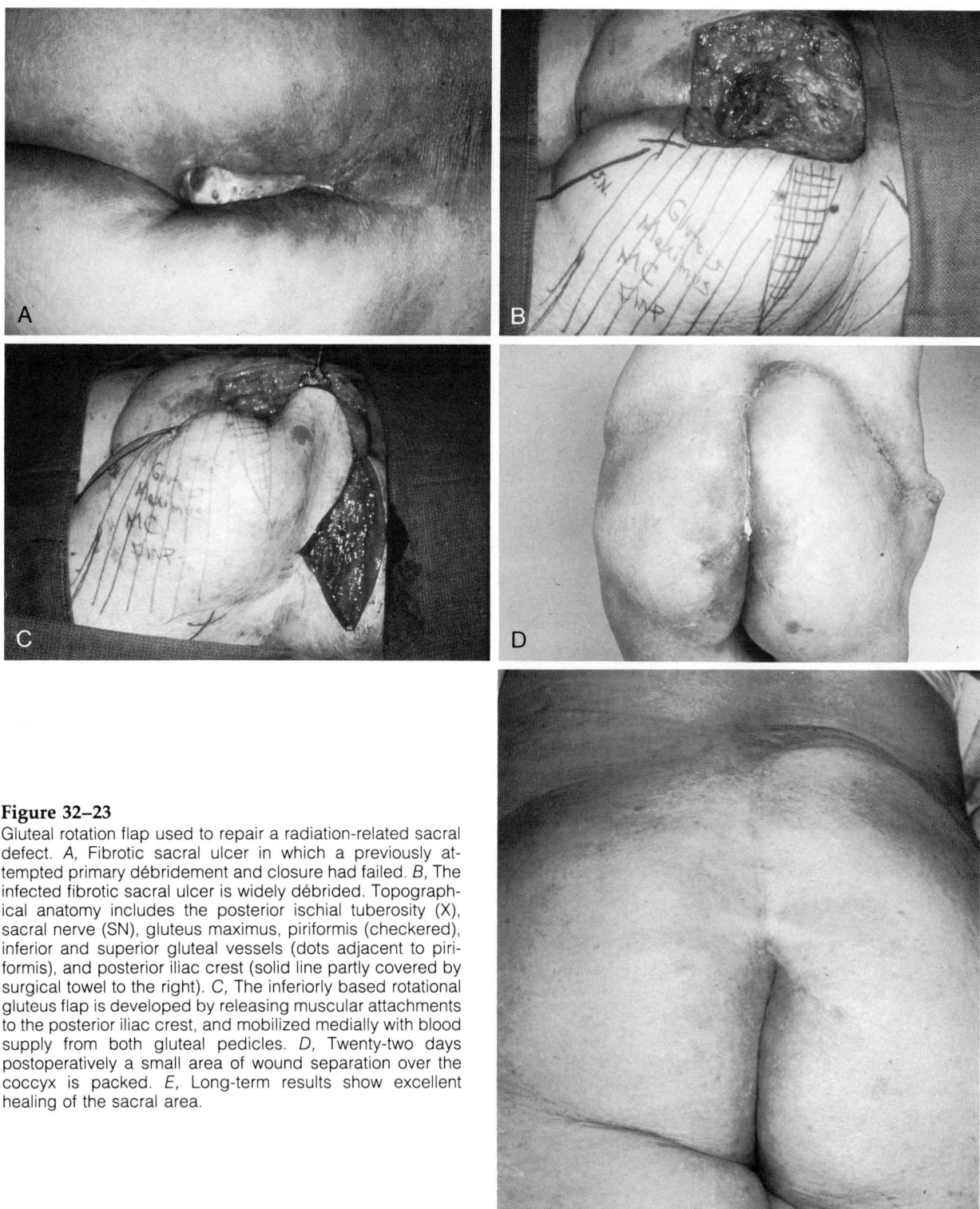

Figure 32–23
Gluteal rotation flap used to repair a radiation-related sacral defect. *A,* Fibrotic sacral ulcer in which a previously attempted primary débridement and closure had failed. *B,* The infected fibrotic sacral ulcer is widely débrided. Topographical anatomy includes the posterior ischial tuberosity (X), sacral nerve (SN), gluteus maximus, piriformis (checkered), inferior and superior gluteal vessels (dots adjacent to piriformis), and posterior iliac crest (solid line partly covered by surgical towel to the right). *C,* The inferiorly based rotational gluteus flap is developed by releasing muscular attachments to the posterior iliac crest, and mobilized medially with blood supply from both gluteal pedicles. *D,* Twenty-two days postoperatively a small area of wound separation over the coccyx is packed. *E,* Long-term results show excellent healing of the sacral area.

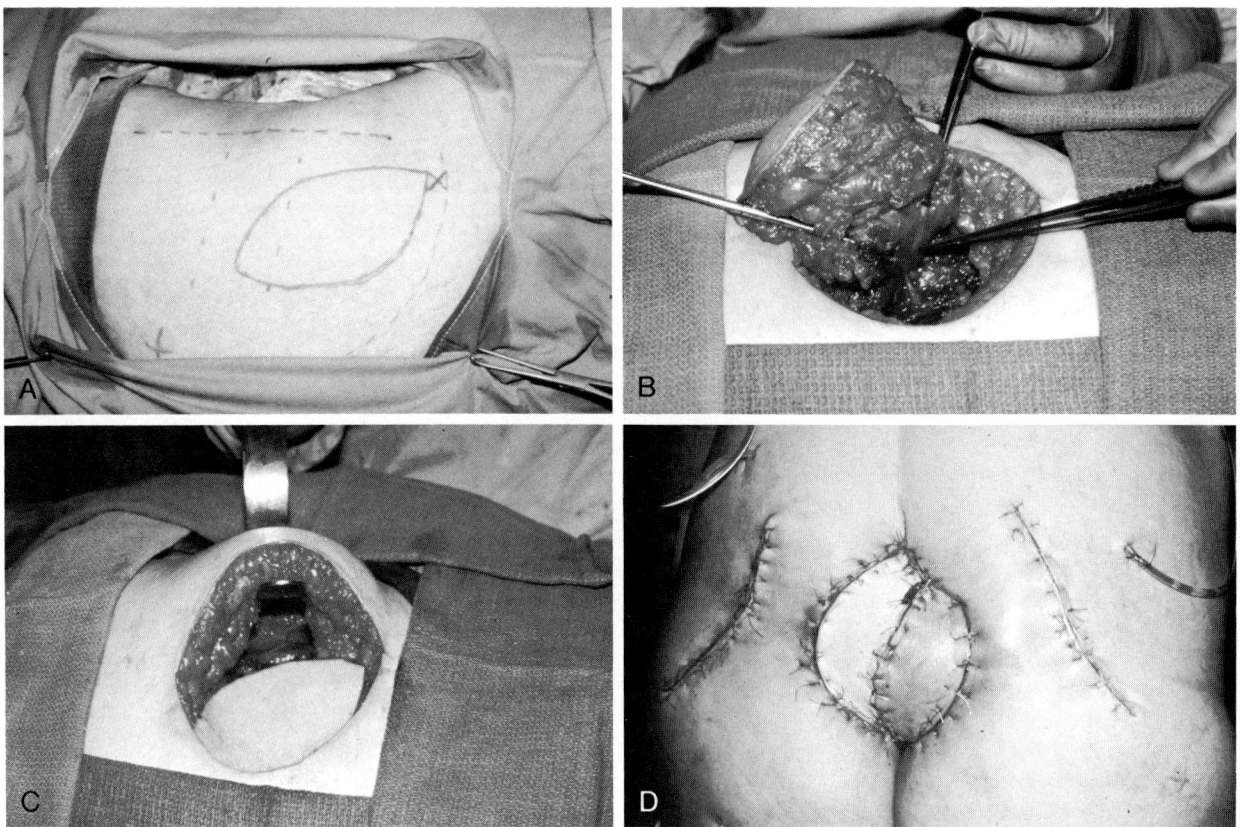

Figure 32–24
Large radiation-related ulcerative sacral defect. *A,* The superior gluteal island flap is outlined by the solid elliptical line. The posterior iliac spine and posterior iliac crest are outlined superiorly and the borders of the piriformis are also marked. *B,* The vascular forceps point to the vascular pedicle, the superior gluteal vessels, that will support this flap. *C,* The island flap is then transferred into the débrided ulcer defect through a subcutaneous tunnel. *D,* The procedure can be performed bilaterally for large defects. The donor sites are drained and closed primarily.

References

1. Wilkinson EJ: Introital stenosis and Z-plasty. Obstet Gynecol 1971; 38:638.
2. Capraro VJ, Gallego MB: Vaginal agenesis. Am J Obstet Gynecol 1976; 124:98.
3. Magrina JF, Masterson BJ: Vaginal reconstruction in gynecologic oncology: A review of techniques. Obstet Gynecol Surv 1981; 36:1.
4. Smith MR: Vaginal aplasia: Therapeutic options. Am J Obstet Gynecol 1983; 146:488.
5. Frank RT: The formation of an artificial vagina without operation. Am J Obstet Gynecol 1938; 35:1053.
6. Broadbent TR, Woolf RM: Congenital absence of vagina: Reconstruction without operation. Br J Plast Surg 1977; 30:118.
7. Ingram JM: The bicycle seat stool in the treatment of vaginal agenesis and stenosis: A preliminary report. Am J Obstet Gynecol 1981; 140:867.
8. Peters WA III, Uhlir JK: Prolapse of a neovagina created by self-dilatation. Obstet Gynecol 1990; 76:904.
9. O'Brien BM, Mellow CG, MacIsaac CG, MacIsaac IA, et al: Treatment of vaginal agenesis with a new vulvovaginoplasty. Plast Reconstr Surg 1990; 85:942.
10. McIndoe AH, Banister JB: An operation for the cure of congenital absence of the vagina. J Obstet Gynaecol Br Comm 1938; 45:490.
11. McIndoe AH: The treatment of congenital absence and obliterative conditions of the vagina. Br J Plast Surg 1950; 2:254.
12. Thompson JD, Wharton LR, Telinde RW: Congenital absence of the vagina. An analysis of thirty-two cases corrected by the McIndoe operation. Am J Obstet Gynecol 1957; 74:397.
13. Berek JS, Hacker NF, Lagasse LD, Smith ML: Delayed vaginal reconstruction in the fibrotic pelvis following radiation or previous reconstruction. Obstet Gynecol 1983; 61:743.
14. Morley GW, Lindernauer SM, Youngs D: Vaginal reconstruction following pelvic exenteration: Surgical and psychological considerations. Am J Obstet Gynecol 1973; 116:996.
15. Beemer W, Hopkins MP, Morley GW: Vaginal reconstruction in gynecologic oncology. Obstet Gynecol 1988; 72:911.
16. Rock JA, Jones HW Jr: Vaginal forms for dilatation or to maintain vaginal patency. Fertil Steril 1984; 42:187.
17. Tamaya T, Yamamoto T, Nakata Y, et al.: The use of pelvic peritoneum in the construction of a vagina: 10 cases. Asia Oceania J Obstet Gynaecol 1984; 10:439.
18. Dhall K: Amnion graft for the treatment of congenital absence of the vagina. Br J Obstet Gynaecol 1984; 91:279.
19. Liford RJ, Sharpe DT, Thomas DFM: Use of tissue expansion techniques to create skin flaps for vaginoplasty. Case report. Br J Obstet Gynaecol 1988; 95:402.
20. Lathrop JC, Ree HJ, McDuff HC: Intraepithelial neoplasia of the neovagina. Obstet Gynecol 1985; 65:91s.
21. Cox SM, Kaufman RH, Kaplan A: Recurrent carcinoma in situ of the vulva in a skin graft. Am J Obstet Gynecol 1986; 155:177.
22. Broadbent TR, Woolf RM, Hebertson R: Nonoperative construction of the vagina: Two unusual cases. Plast Reconstr Surg 1984; 73:117.
23. Berek JS, Hacker NF, Lagasse LD: Vaginal reconstruction performed simultaneously with pelvic exenteration. Obstet Gynecol 1984; 63:318.
24. Wheeless CR Jr: Neovagina constructed from an omental J flap and a split thickness skin graft. Gynecol Oncol 1989; 35:224.
25. Williams EA: Congenital absence of the vagina: A simple operation for its relief. J Obstet Gynaecol Br Comm 1964; 71:511.

26. Day TG, Stanhope CR: Vulvovaginoplasty in gynecologic oncology. Obstet Gynecol 1977; 50:361.
27. Schellhas HF, Fidler JP: Vaginal reconstruction after total pelvic exenteration using a modification of the Williams procedure. Gynecol Oncol 1975; 3:21.
28. Baldwin JF: The formation of an artificial vagina by intestinal transplantation. Ann Surg 1904; 40:398.
29. Pratt JH: Sigmoidovaginostomy: A new method of obtaining satisfactory vaginal depth. Am J Obstet Gynecol 1961; 81:535.
30. Turner-Warwick R, Kirby RS: The construction and reconstruction of the vagina with the colocecum. Surg Gynecol Obstet 1990; 170:132.
31. Martius H: Die operative wiederherstellung der vollkommen fehlenden Harnröhre und des Schiessmuskels derselben. Zentralbl Gynakol 1928; 52:480.
32. Hatch KD: Construction of a neovagina after exenteration using vulvobulbocavernosus myocutaneous graft. Obstet Gynecol 1984; 63:110.
33. McCraw JB, Massey FM, Shanklin KD, Horton CE: Vaginal reconstruction with gracilis myocutaneous flaps. Plast Reconstr Surg 1976; 58:176.
34. Copeland LJ, Hancock KC, Gershenson DM, et al.: Gracilis myocutaneous vaginal reconstruction concurrent with total pelvic exenteration. Am J Obstet Gynecol 1989; 160:1095.
35. Lacey CG, Stern JL, Feigenbaum S, et al.: Vaginal reconstruction after exenteration with use of gracilis myocutaneous flaps: The University of California, San Francisco experience. Am J Obstet Gynecol 1988; 158:1278.
36. Morrow CP, Lacey GC, Lucas WE: Reconstructive surgery in gynecologic oncology employing the gracilis myocutaneous pedicle graft. Gynecol Oncol 1979; 7:176.
37. Soper JT, Larson D, Hunter VJ, et al.: Short gracilis myocutaneous flaps for vulvovaginal reconstruction after radical pelvic surgery. Obstet Gynecol 1989; 74:823.
38. Becker DW Jr, Massey FM, McCraw JB: Musculocutaneous flaps in reconstructive pelvic surgery. Obstet Gynecol 1979; 54:178.
39. Ballon SC, Donaldson RC, Roberts JA, Lagasse LD: Reconstruction of the vulva using myocutaneous graft. Gynecol Oncol 1979; 7:123.
40. Wheeless CR Jr, McGibbon B, Dorsey JM, Maxwell GP: Gracilis myocutaneous flap in reconstruction of the vulva and female perineum. Obstet Gynecol 1979; 54:97.
41. Radke HM: Arterial circulation of the lower extremity. In Strandness DE Jr (ed.): Collateral Circulation in Clinical Surgery. Philadelphia, WB Saunders Co., 1969; pp. 308–334.
42. Wang T-N, Whetzel T, Mathes SJ, Vasconez LO: A fasciocutaneous flap for vaginal and perineal reconstruction. Plast Reconstr Surg 1987; 80:95.
43. Tobin GR, Day TG: Vaginal and pelvic reconstruction with distally based rectus abdominis myocutaneous flap. Plast Reconstr Surg 1988; 81:62.
44. Tobin GR, Pursell SH, Day JG Jr: Refinements in vaginal reconstruction using rectus abdominis flaps. Clin Plast Surg 1990; 17:705.
45. Lilford RJ, Johnson N, Batchelor A: A new operation for vaginal agenesis: Construction of a neovagina from a rectus abdominis musculocutaneous flap. Br J Obstet Gynaecol 1989; 96:1089.
46. Mathes SJ, Bostwock J: A rectus abdominal myocutaneous flap to reconstruct abdominal wall defects. Br J Plast Surg 1977; 30:2892.
47. Webster DJT, Hughes LE: The rectus abdominis myocutaneous island flap in breast cancer. Br J Surg 1983; 70:71.
48. Shukla HS, Hughes LE: The rectus abdominis flap for perineal wounds. Ann R Coll Surg Engl 1984; 66:337.
49. Achauer BM, Braly P, Berman ML, et al.: Immediate vaginal reconstruction following resection for malignancy using the gluteal thigh flap. Gynecol Oncol 1984; 19:79.
50. Johnson N, Lilford RJ, Batchelor A: The free-flap vaginoplasty: A new surgical procedure for the treatment of vaginal agenesis. Br J Obstet Gynecol 1991; 98:184.
51. Way S: Carcinoma of the vulva. Am J Obstet Gynecol 1968; 79:692.
52. Ramasastry SS, Liang MD, Hurwitz DJ: Surgical management of difficult wounds of the groin. Surg Gynecol Obstet 1989; 169:418.
53. Jarrell MA, Malinin TI, Averette HE, et al.: Human dura mater allografts in repair of pelvic floor and abdominal wall defects. Obstet Gynecol 1987; 70:280.
54. Fiorica JV, Roberts WS, LaPolla JP, et al.: Femoral vessel coverage with dura mater after inguinofemoral lymphadenectomy. Gynecol Oncol 1991; 42:217.
55. Prichard J, Thadani V, Kalb R, et al.: Rapidly progressive dementia in a patient who received a cadaveric dura mater graft. JAMA 1987; 257:1036.
56. Leads from the MMWR: Creutzfeldt-Jakob disease in a second patient who received a cadaveric dura mater graft. JAMA 1989; 261:1118.
57. Rutledge F, Sinclair M: Treatment of intraepithelial carcinoma of the vulva by excision and graft. Am J Obstet Gynecol 1968; 102:806.
58. Barnhill DR, Hoskins WJ, Metz P: Use of rhomboid flap after partial vulvectomy. Obstet Gynecol 1983; 62:444.
59. Mayer AR, Rodriguez RL: Vulvar reconstruction using a pedicle flap based on the superficial external pudendal artery. Obstet Gynecol 1991; 78:964.
60. Hurwitz DJ, Swartz WM, Mathes SJ: The gluteal thigh flap: A reliable sensate flap for the closure of buttock and perineal wounds. Plast Reconstr Surg 1981; 68:521.
61. Chafe W, Fowler WC, Walton LA, Currie JL: Radical vulvectomy with use of tensor fascia lata myocutaneous flap. Am J Obstet Gynecol 1983; 145:207.
62. Nahai F: The tensor fascia lata flap. Clinic Plast Surg 1980; 7:51.
63. Nahai F: Muscle and musculocutanous flaps in gynecologic surgery. Clin Obstet Gynecol 1981; 24:1277.
64. Nahai F, Hill HL, Hester TR: Experiences with the tensor fascia lata flap. Plast Reconstr Surg 1979; 63:788.
65. Franklin EW III, Bostwick J III, Burrell MO, Powell JL: Reconstructive techniques in radical pelvic surgery. Am J Obstet Gynecol 1977; 129:285.
66. Quilici PJ, Vieta JO, Privilera L: The use of dura mater allograft in the surgical repair of large defects of the abdominal wall. Surg Gynecol Obstet 1985; 161:47.
67. Symmonds RE, Pratt JH, Webb MJ: Exenterative operations: Experience with 198 patients. Am J Obstet Gynecol 1975; 121:907.
68. Delmore JE, Turner DA, Gershenson DM, Horbelt DV: Perineal hernia repair using human dura. Obstet Gynecol 1987; 70:507.
69. Donato D, Jarrell M, Averette H, et al.: Reconstructive techniques in gynecologic oncology: The use of human dura mater allographs. Eur J Gynecol Oncol 1988; 9:135.
70. Minami RT, Mills R, Pardoe R: Gluteus maximus myocutaneous flaps for repair of pressure sores. Plast Reconstr Surg 1977; 60:242.
71. Maruyama Y, Tajima S: Gluteus maximus muscle island flaps for repair of sacral radiation ulcers. Keio J Med 1978; 27:533.
72. Maruyama Y, Nakajima H, Wada M, et al: A gluteus maximus myocutaneous island flap for the repair of a sacral decubitus ulcer. Br J Plast Surg 1980; 33:150.

Operative Radiotherapeutic Procedures for Gynecologic Cancers

33

Luis Delclos
J. Taylor Wharton
David M. Gershenson

In 1948, Drs. Felix N. Rutledge and Gilbert H. Fletcher organized the gynecology and radiotherapy services at The University of Texas M. D. Anderson Cancer Center to provide comprehensive care for women with gynecologic cancer. From the beginning, they established excellent communication between the two services, a factor essential to the kind of treatment envisioned, and organized joint clinical conferences that are still conducted regularly today.

In many instances, the treatment plan for gynecologic cancers includes or consists entirely of radiotherapy. Specifically, radiotherapy is frequently the treatment of choice for malignant tumors of the uterine cervix, endometrium, and vagina and for pelvic wall recurrences of gynecologic and other cancers. In this chapter we describe the use of external-beam, intracavitary, and interstitial radiation to treat these cancers.

CANCER OF THE UTERINE CERVIX

Early-stage carcinoma confined to the cervix, of small volume, and in young patients is treated mainly by surgery so as to preserve the ovaries; with few exceptions, however, more advanced cervical cancer is treated by radiation. Well-planned radiotherapy offers only a small risk of complications, which can include urinary or rectal fistula, bladder dysfunction, shortening of the vagina, and risk of death from acute surgical complication. Adenocarcinoma of the cervix seems to have the same radiosensitivity as cervical squamous cell carcinoma when tumor volume, rather than International Federation of Gynecology and Obstetrics (FIGO) stage, is considered the defining factor and when tumor volume is small. In contrast, large tumors, some histologic varieties, and poorly differentiated tumors have a different biologic aggressiveness; their site of origin, pattern of growth, and rate of dissemination may also differ.[1] The volume of the primary tumor and the results of computed tomography (CT) or lymphangiography, neither of which is reflected in the FIGO classification system, are the most important prognostic factors.

When radiation is chosen as treatment for cervical cancer, it is administered by combining external with intracavitary irradiation. Intracavitary irradiation delivers the greatest dose to the primary site and surrounding tissues, which form the central component of the tumor, while sparing the most sensitive tissues such as the urinary bladder and the anterior

---

These investigations were supported in part by grant CA-06294 and CA-16672, awarded by the National Cancer Institute, United States Department of Health and Human Services.

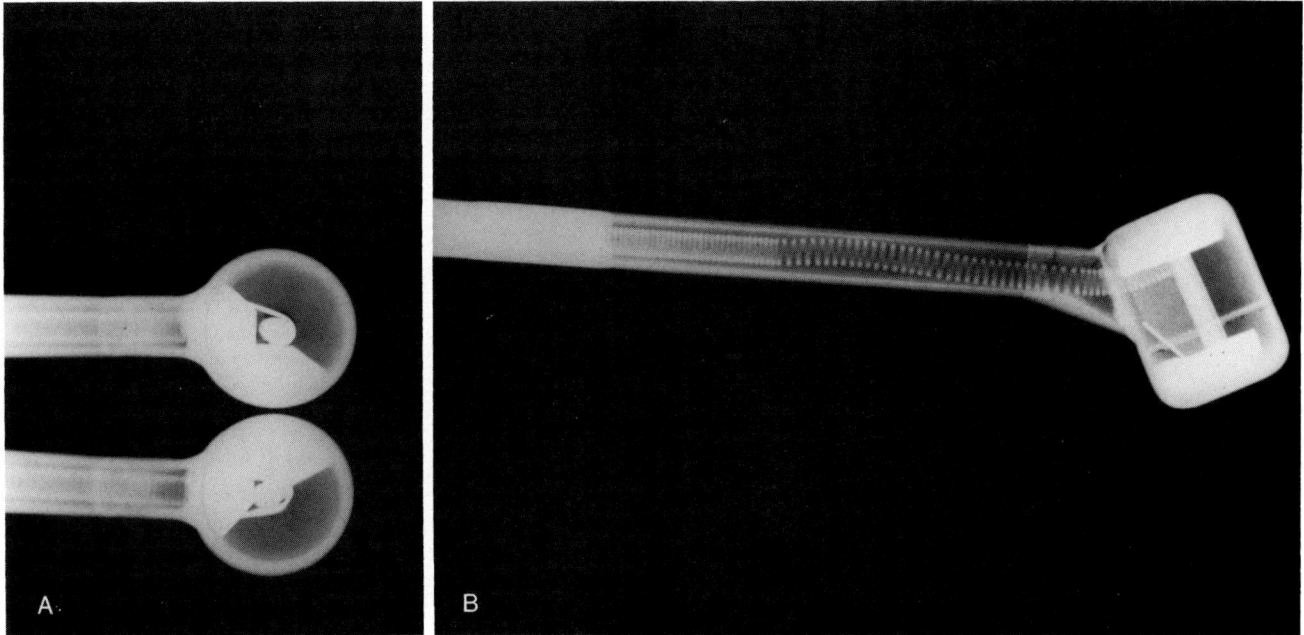

Figure 33–1
Roentgenogram of a round-handled colpostat for manual afterloading. Because of the shape of the colpostat, the position of the sources, and the shielding, the dose to the bladder and rectum is reduced. (From SH Levitt: Technological Basis of Radiation Therapy: Practical Clinical Applications. Philadelphia, Lea & Febiger, 1992. Used with permission.)

wall of the rectum. For this purpose, it is necessary that the applicators used be well designed (Fig. 33–1) and that the patient's anatomy be not distorted by such factors as congenital anomalies, age, previous surgery, and infections. External-beam irradiation is added in various sequences, both to sterilize tumor in the regional lymph nodes and to reduce the tumor volume in order to make intracavitary irradiation more effective. Variables to be considered in treatment planning are listed in Table 33–1.[2]

External-Beam Irradiation

External-beam irradiation generally precedes intracavitary treatment. Its purpose is both to decrease the tumor volume so that intracavitary radiation can be more effective and to treat possible tumor extension into the lymphatic vessels and pelvic structures around the uterus. Accordingly, the radiation field is set to encompass the primary tumor and the lymphatics of the pelvis.[3-9]

External-beam radiation can be delivered with cobalt-60 or 4- and 6-MeV units, but the authors recommend the use of higher energies, preferably 18- to 25-MeV photons; 10- and 15-MeV units can be used as a compromise. The advantages of high-energy beams are not only better tissue tolerance during the treatment but also better dose distribution throughout the pelvis; the dosage to some areas of the bladder and rectum is lower even when only two parallel-opposed fields are used. The choice of two parallel-opposed fields (anteroposterior and posteroanterior) or a four-field technique ("box" and modifications of the box) is a matter of personal preference at dose levels up to 40 Gy. Two parallel-opposed fields are easier to set and reproduce daily, but four fields are preferred when doses of 50 Gy or more are planned for the whole pelvis. Four fields are not indicated, however, when the patient has a wide pelvis or when disease extends along the vagina to the lower third; in these instances, parallel-opposed fields should be used.

Extended fields, above the level of the top of the interspace between L4 and L5, are necessary when the treatment field includes the whole common iliac node group; the portals are then extended to the top of L4 (L3–L4 interspace). When the para-aortic nodes are involved, the portals are extended to the top of T12. When the fields extend above the top of L5, the authors recommend a maximal dose to the extended fields of 45 Gy in 25 fractions over 5 weeks.[2]

Transvaginal irradiation is an important component of treatment that is very effective in reducing a large exophytic tumor of the portio vaginalis. Transvaginal irradiation is administered before or along with external-beam radiation, so that when the external-beam pelvic treatment is complete after 4 or 5 weeks, the exophytic tumor has disappeared or is smaller, allowing proper placement of intracavitary devices. Transvaginal irradiation is extremely well tolerated because the dose falls off very rapidly, both in depth and laterally. The authors use 125 or 250 kV, depending on the size of the exophytic compo-

Table 33–1
Factors Affecting Cervical Cancer Treatment Planning
Stage to be Ignored
Tumor histology
Invasiveness
Type: Squamous cell carcinoma or adenocarcinoma
Location of lesion on cervix
Exocervix, endocervix: Always irradiate whole pelvis first
Dilatation and curettage positive: Load tandem more heavily or perform hysterectomy
Tumor volume
Tumor effectively treatable with radium only
or
Tumor requires flattening before radium insertion: Perform additional hysterectomy in endocervix
Irrespective of volume, external-beam radiation may be necessary to irradiate cervix and paracervical area adequately
Bleeding intensity
Vault size and uterine cavity length
Determine need for external-beam irradiation to central pelvis
Invasion, degree of
Vaginal fornices minimal: Colpostats adequate
Vaginal walls: Individualized gamma-ray therapy required
Parametria
Pelvic wall(s) fixation
Ureter(s) blocked
Lymphatics
Lymphangiography, celiotomy to determine which node area(s) are involved
Involved nodes may need to be removed
Age and general condition

From Fletcher GH: Textbook of Radiotherapy, 3rd ed. Philadelphia; Lea & Febiger, 1980, p. 731.

nent of the tumor. This form of treatment is also effective in reducing vaginal hemorrhage that originates in the cervical tumor.[2]

Intracavitary Irradiation

Intracavitary Sources

Although radium sources are still in use, they are being replaced by cesium rods (slugs) or cesium spherical sources (Fig. 33–2) employing afterloading techniques, either manual[11–14] or remote.[10] These new radioactive sources are just as effective as the radium tubes while offering advantages in the manipulation of materials and in safety for the personnel attending the patient during the insertion.

Either source, inserted into a well-designed applicator (Figs. 33–3 and 33–4) and introduced into the intrauterine cavity and the vagina, is able to deliver a high dose of radiation to the primary tumor. This high dose falls off rapidly following the inverse-square law. The goal is to encompass all palpable tumor with a "volumetric isodose" of about 60 to 63 Gy in two intracavitary insertions (Fig. 33–5).[15] However, when the tumor is too large, this is not possible because a high dose would also be delivered to normal extrauterine tissues that cannot tolerate the doses tolerated by the uterus. The dose must therefore be a compromise, balancing the chances of tumor sterilization against the tolerance of such surrounding tissues as the urinary bladder, rectum, and small and large bowel. Although the upper vagina tolerates higher doses than the above-mentioned organs, the dose reaching this area should also be limited.

To optimize dose distribution, the applicators used must be placed with extreme care, both in the intrauterine canal (using a "tandem") and in the upper vagina (using a "colpostat"). The colpostats, which were originally designed by Fletcher, have since been modified by Suit and colleagues,[11] Green and colleagues,[12] and Delclos and colleagues[10, 13, 14] for afterloading. They are designed so that the dose to the anterior and posterior vaginal walls is lower than that to the lateral wall; the urinary bladder and rectum therefore receive a lesser dose than the paracervical tissues. In addition to the bladder and rectal "points of reference" recommended by other clinicians,[15] the authors have established some reference points at the lateral vaginal fornices.[16] None of these points has an absolute value, but all of them are considered to be guidelines of tolerance. By taking them all into account, it is possible to optimize treatment by giving an adequate dose to the tumor according to its volume and patterns of spread.

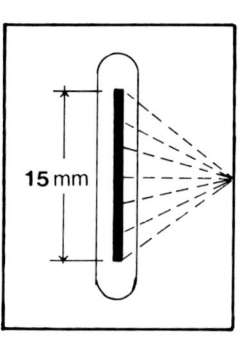
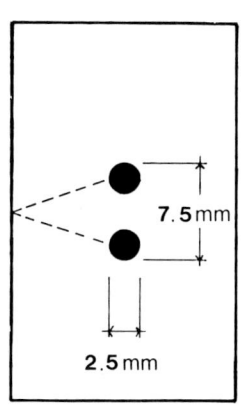

Figure 33–2
Comparison of a radium tube on a "small" hand, loaded Fletcher-Suit-Delclos (F-S-D) colpostat (a cesium rod would be shorter) loaded with cesium pellets with the Selectron remotely loaded F-S-D colpostats. MDAH, M. D. Anderson Cancer Center. (From Delclos L, Cundiff J: The Fletcher colpostat system as adapted to the Selectron LDR: A progress report. In Mould RF (ed.): Brachytherapy 2. Leersum, Nucletron International B.V., 1989, pp. 142–146.)

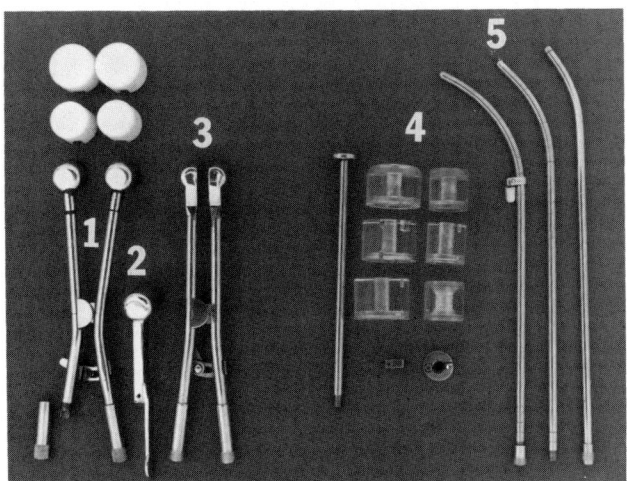

Figure 33–3
Left to right: (1) Fletcher-Suit-Delclos colpostats for manual afterloading. Teflon or nylon caps convert the small colpostats (10-mm radius) to medium (12.5-mm radius) and large (15-mm radius). (2) Single colpostats (same diameters as double colpostats). (3) Minicolpostats (8-mm radius, flat medially) to be used only when the vagina is too constricted to allow larger colpostats. Loading is reduced in the minicolpostats to maintain doses to the bladder and rectal points within tolerance. (4) Vaginal cylinders to extend irradiation along the vaginal axis; doses to the vagina are reduced as the length of the irradiated vagina is extended distally. (5) Intrauterine tandems (four curvatures are available; only three are illustrated). (From SH Levitt: Technological Basis of Radiation Therapy: Practical Clinical Applications. Philadelphia, Lea & Febiger 1984. Used with permission.)

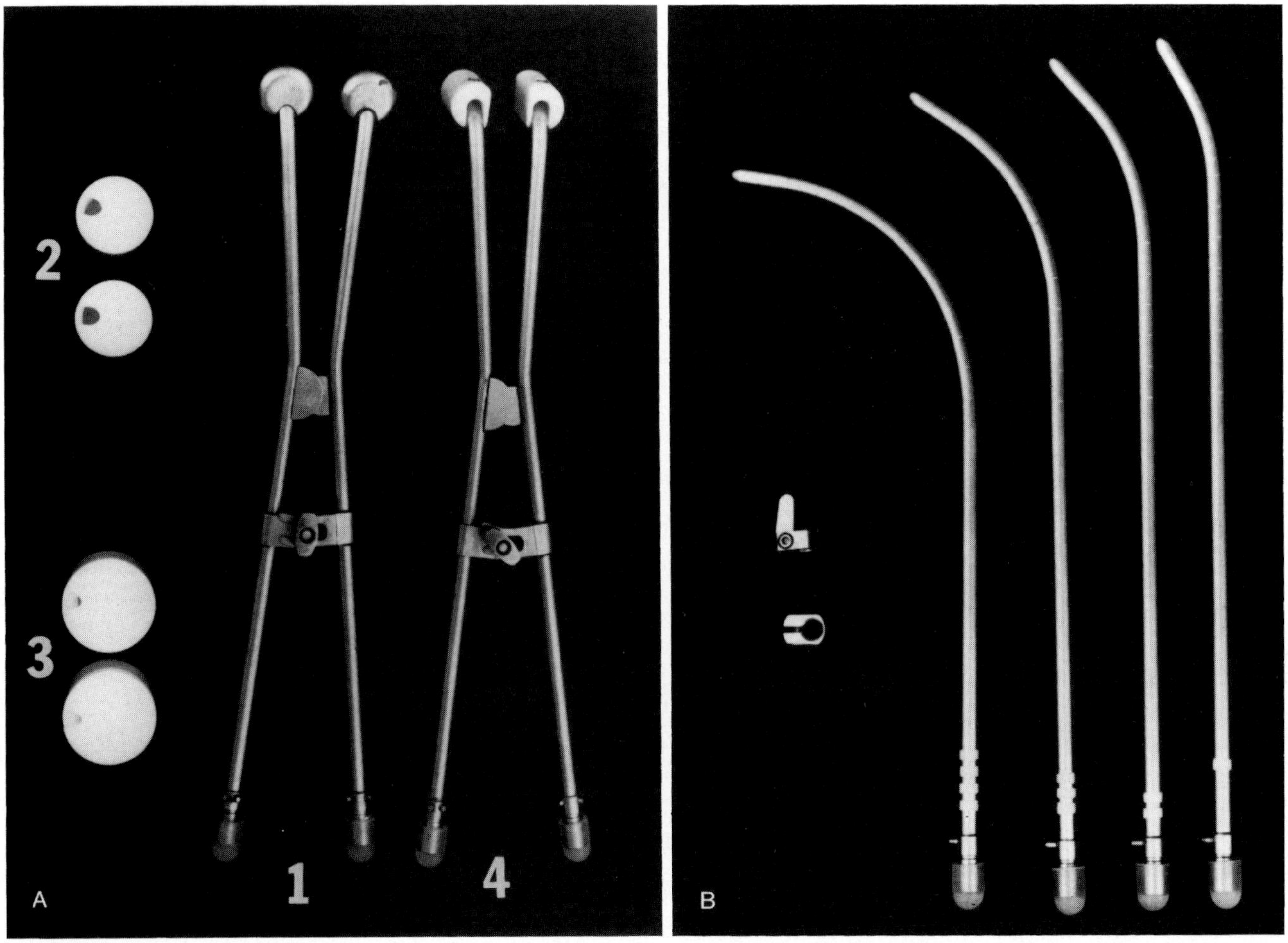

Figure 33–4
A, Fletcher colpostats adapted to a remote-controlled Selectron low-dose-rate unit. (1) Small colpostats (2-cm diameter) with incorporated tungsten shielding; (2) medium caps (2.5-cm diameter); (3) large caps (3.0-cm diameter); (4) minicolpostats (0.8-cm radius, flat medially, no shielding incorporated in this model). B, The intrauterine tandem is available in one curvature of four different lengths. (From Delclos L, Cundiff J: The Fletcher colpostat system as adapted to the low dose rate remotely controlled Selectron unit: A second progress report. In Martinez AA, Orton CG, Mould RF (eds.): Brachytherapy HDR and LDR. Leersum, Nucletron International B.V., 1990, pp. 83–92.)

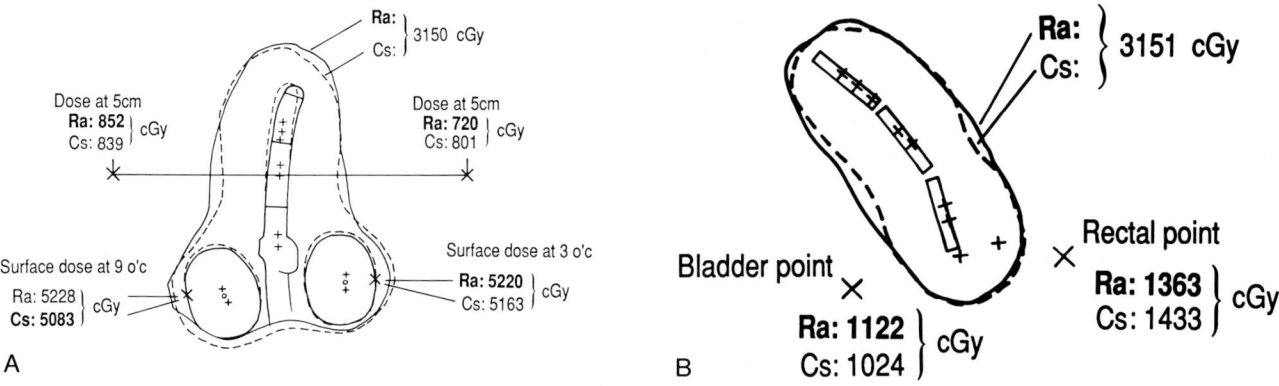

Figure 33-5
Selection of loading. Cesium sources are selected that produce isodoses resembling as closely as possible those obtained with radium tubes (A). For the cesium source (B), the authors determine the dose at selected vaginal points (3 o'clock on the left colpostat and 9 o'clock on the right colpostat) and recommend a total dose (intracavitary radiation alone or a combination with external-beam radiation) not less than 100 Gy and not more than 120 Gy. In addition, the dose is calculated to bladder and rectal points, as recommended in the ICRU Report 38, page 11, Fig. 3.2.[15] (From Delclos L, Cundiff J: The Fletcher colpostat system as adapted to the Selectron LDR: A progress report. In Mould RF (ed.): Brachytherapy 2. Leersum, Nucletron International B.V., 1989, pp. 142-146.)

Vaginal cylinders[17] have been designed to irradiate the vagina when the tumor extends to the middle and lower third.

Figures 33-6 and 33-7 show the instruments for inserting afterloading intrauterine tandems and colpostats.[14] The position of the applicators, types of applicators, and loading must be modified to fit the individual circumstance. Figure 33-8 shows a lateral-view radiograph of an intrauterine tandem and vaginal cylinders designed to irradiate tumor extension along the posterior vaginal wall.

Inserting the Intrauterine Tandem and Colpostats

Applicators are inserted in the operating room, with the patient in the lithotomy position and under general anesthesia. After rectovaginal and bimanual examination to confirm tumor volume and extension, the surgeon exposes the cervix, using vaginal retractors. While the cervix is held with one or two tenacula, the surgeon probes the uterine cavity with a hysterometer to determine its length and then dilates the endocervical canal to 6 mm (dilator No. 6).[18] Figure 33-9 illustrates the sequence of intrauterine tandem and colpostat placement.[16, 19]

The operating room must be equipped with a powerful x-ray unit to take orthogonal films of the pelvis (Fig. 33-10). These films are taken as many times as required to determine the correctness of the intracavitary insertion and to make adjustments as necessary. Selection of radioactive sources of the appropriate strength and distribution is made in the operating room so that the afterloadable applicators can be loaded as soon as the patient returns to her room. Loading the intrauterine tandem and colpostats with cesium rods (slugs) or spherical sources is prescribed in terms of radium-equivalency, and those cesium sources that produce isodoses resembling the ones obtained with radium tubes are selected. The duration of the insertion is the same as for radium, but when remotely controlled units are used the radioactive sources are removed from the carriers (applicators) 10% of the time to allow for nursing care and family visits.

The radioactive sources are initially selected on

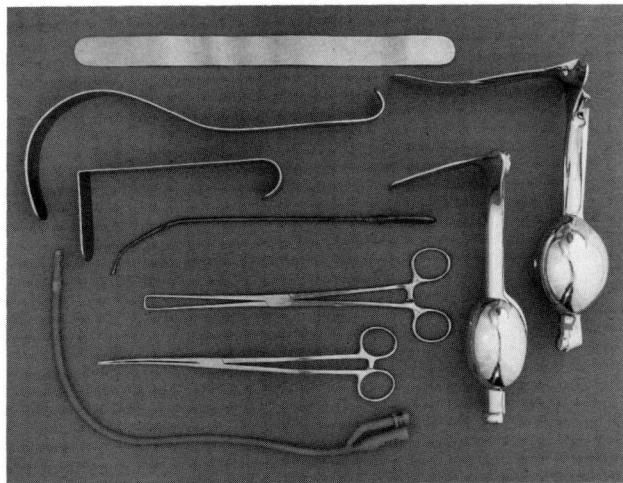

Figure 33-6
Instruments for inserting afterloadable intrauterine tandems and colpostats. *From top,* (1) Flexsteel ribbon retractor, which should be available in 1-, 1 1/2-, and 2-inch widths; (2) Deaver retractor, available in 1-, 1 1/2-, and 2-inch widths (two of each); (3) Heaney or Kristeller retractors, available in 1-, 1 1/2-, and 2-inch widths (two of each); (4) Auvard weighted retractors, 3, 4, and 5 inches long (one of each); (5) malleable hysterometer (one); (6) Braun or Duplay uterine tenaculum (two); (7) Boseman or DeLee uterine packing forceps (two); (8) No. 16-18 Foley catheter with a 5-ml balloon. (From SH Levitt: Technological Basis of Radiation Therapy: Practical Clinical Applications. Philadelphia, Lea & Febiger, 1984. Used with permission.)

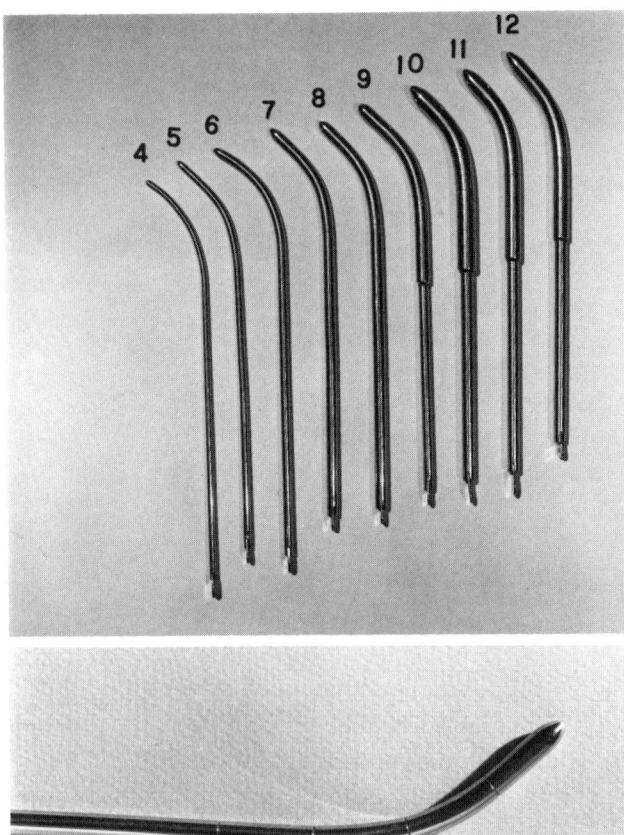

Figure 33–7
Uterine cervix dilators of intermediate curvature. Calibrated along their long axis in centimeters or inches, they are used to check the depth of the uterine cavity during dilatation, thereby minimizing the incidence of uterine perforation. The dilator number, as in the Hegar, represents its diameter. (From Delclos L: Uterine cervix dilator designed to be used before insertion of intrauterine tandems and/or capsules. Radiology 1969; 93:1201–1202.)

Figure 33–8
Radiograph of an intrauterine tandem with three vaginal cylinders along its vaginal component. Note the silver seeds in the anterior and posterior cervical lip and two in the posterior vaginal wall, marking the lower extent of the vaginal tumor extension. The position of the cylinders and dummy sources in relation to the tumor can be identified easily, allowing proper placement of the radioactive sources. The cylinders have lead incorporated anteriorly to reduce radiation to the bladder and urethra. (Reprinted from Delclos L, Fletcher GH, Moore EB, Sampiere VA: Minicolpostats, dome cylinders, and other additions and improvements of the Fletcher-Suit afterloadable system: Indications and limitations of their use. Int J Radiat Oncol Biol Phys 1980; 6:1203. With permission from Pergamon Press Ltd, Headington Hill Hall, Oxford OX3 0BW, UK.)

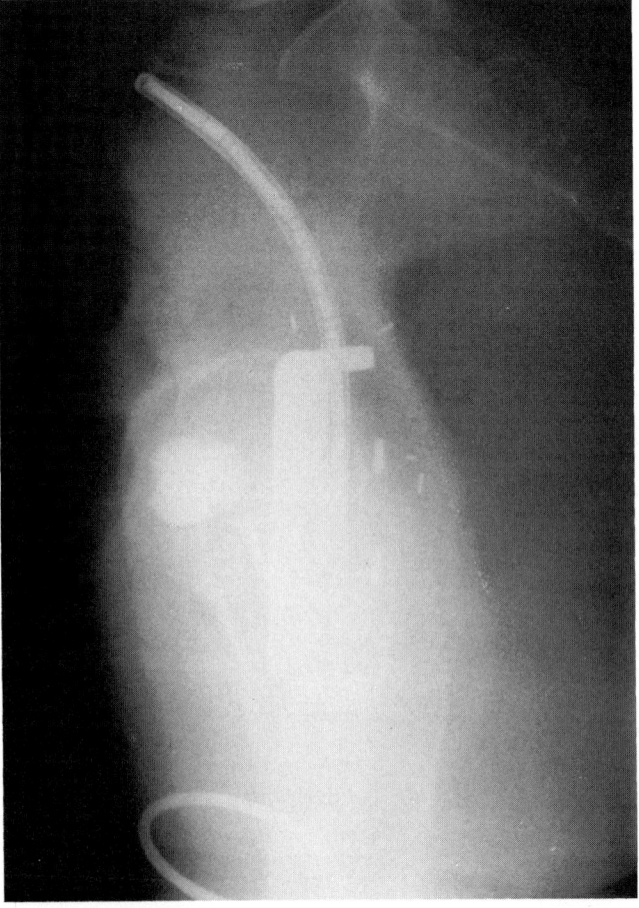

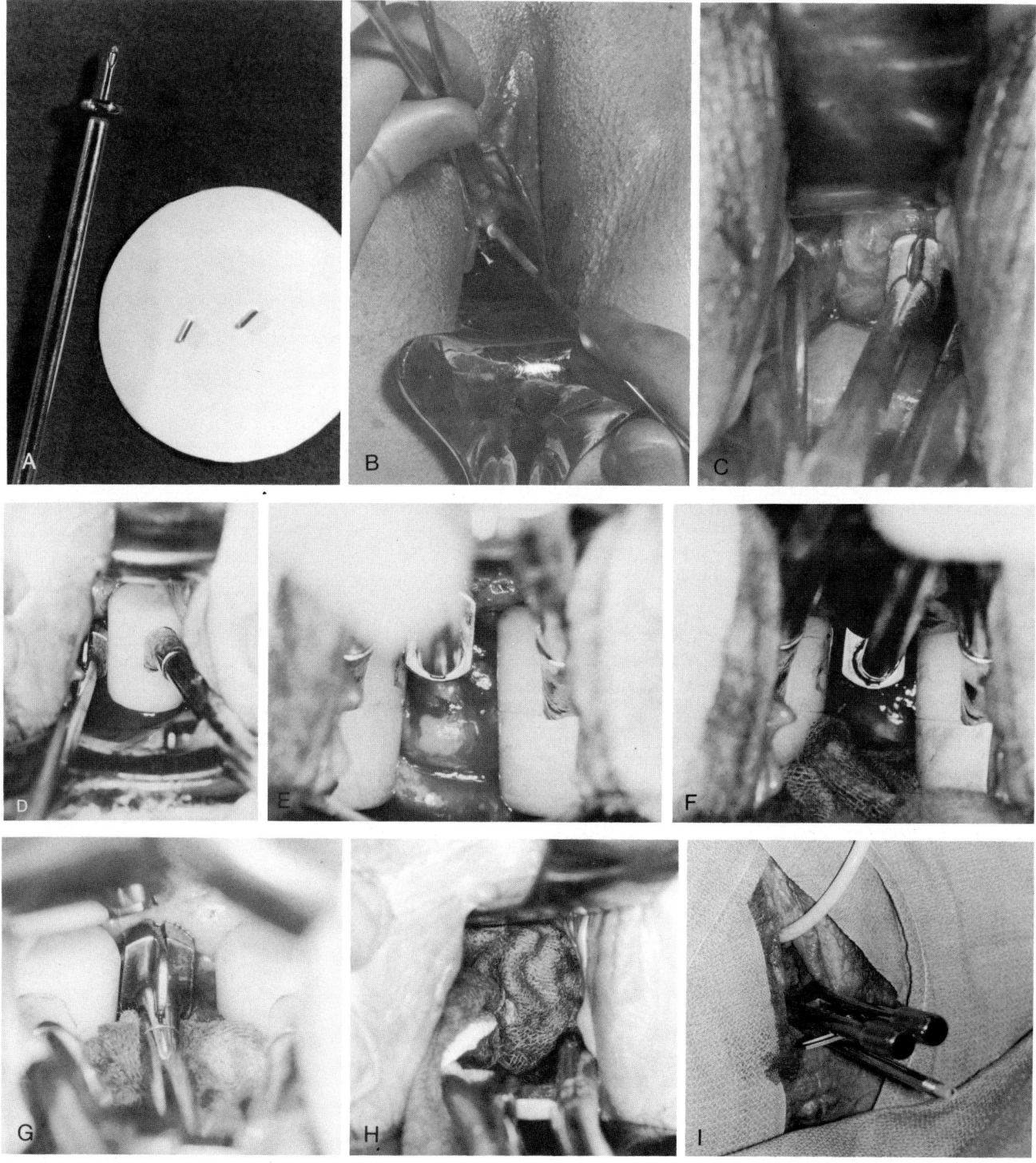

Figure 33–9
Sequence for inserting of afterloadable intrauterine tandem and colpostats. *A*, Seeds, silver or gold, are implanted *(B)* in the anterior and posterior cervical lip (or at the lower edge of the vaginal extent of the disease). *C*, The intrauterine tandem, with the keeled flange set at the selected tandem length, is introduced into the uterine canal. *D*, The left-handled ovoid is placed in the left lateral fornix. *E*, The right-handled ovoid is placed in the right fornix, and the handles are fastened together. *F* and *G*, The ovoids and tandem are maintained in the selected position by the packing, starting under the colpostats and tandem posteriorly and *(H)* filling between the ovoids. Packing also fills the spaces around the keeled flange to minimize tandem rotation. Finally, the whole vagina is filled with packing. *I*, Applicators in place (manual afterloading). The labia are sutured only if the fourchette does not support the packing; they are always sutured when vaginal or dome cylinders are used, and when the remote-controlled Selectron is used. A Foley catheter is inserted into the urinary bladder. The position of the applicators is checked with orthogonal radiographs taken in the operating room. (From SH Levitt: Technological Basis of Radiation Therapy: Practical Clinical Applications. Philadelphia: Lea & Febiger, 1984. Used with permission.)

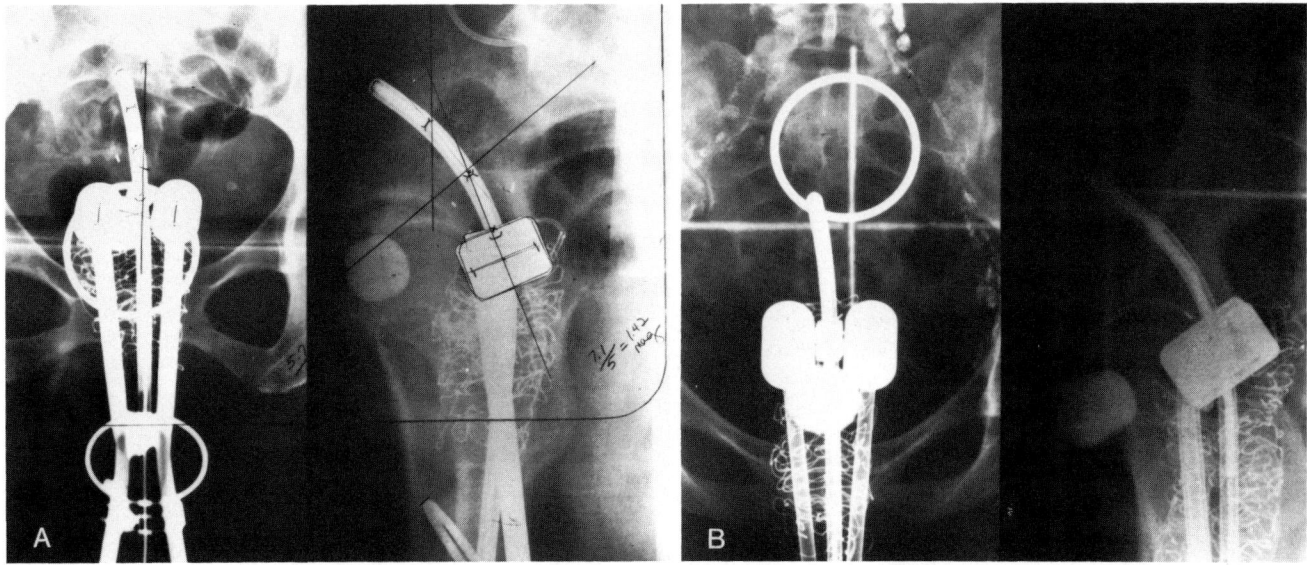

Figure 33–10
Orthogonal radiographs comparing two insertions of intrauterine tandems and colpostats. *A*, Regular Fletcher colpostat for manual afterloading (radium tubes or cesium rods). *B*, Remote-controlled Fletcher colpostats for a Selectron unit with cesium pellets. (From Delclos L, Cundiff J: The Fletcher colpostat system as adapted to the Selectron LDR: A progress report. In Mould RF (ed.): Brachytherapy 2. Leersum, Nucletron International B.V., 1989, pp. 142–146.)

Table 33–2

Summary of Combination of External and Intracavitary Irradiation in Carcinoma of the Cervix with Intact Uterus

Tumor Size	Whole Pelvis	Radium* hr	Radium* mg/hr	Parametrial	Comment
≤1 cm	None	72–2 wk–48	10,000	None	If anatomy is not good, radium is reduced and additional treatment is given with external irradiation
1–3 cm lesions of exocervix with little or no extension to parametria or fornices	None 2000 rad 4000 rad	72–2 wk–48 48–2 wk–72† 48–2 wk–48	≤9000 ≤7500 ≤5500	≤4000 rad§ ≤2000 rad§ None	Amount of whole pelvis and parametrial irradiation depends on (1) extent of disease, (2) patient anatomy, and (3) geometry and location in pelvis of radium system
Endocervical tumor or disease of moderate bulk >3 cm to ≤6 cm with or without extention to medial parametrium	4000 rad	48–2 wk–48	5500–6500‡	None	If regression is poor and there is no parametrial involvement, one single radium insertion (72 hr or 5000 mg/hr, whichever comes first) followed by extrafascial hysterectomy
Bulky central disease >6 cm "barrel-shaped" endocervical tumor	4000 rad	72	5000	None	Extrafascial hysterectomy performed 6 wk after irradiation
Bulky central disease >6 cm extending near or to pelvis wall(s) and/or lower vagina	4000 rad 5000 rad	48–2 wk–48 72 or 58–2 wk–24–48	5500–6600‡ 4000–5000‡	May add 1000 rad to side of major involvement	When major involvement is restricted to only one side, whole pelvis may be stopped at 4000 rad and involved side boosted through parametrial field
	6000 rad	72 or 48–2 wk–24	3000–4000‡		After 5000 rad, reduce fields to ≤12 cm × ≤12 cm
Massive disease or bladder or rectal involvement	Up to 7000 rad	None	None	None	After 5000 rad, reduce fields to ≤12 cm × ≤12 cm After 6000 rad, reduce fields to ≤10 cm × ≤10 cm

*Use whichever maximum comes first, either the time or mg/hr.
†May use longer time first if vault size may not permit colpostats at second application.
‡The larger figures for radium are used if lesions have not clinically disappeared at the time of the second radium; the lesser figures are used if there has been excellent regression of disease.
§Reduce parametrial irradiation by 500 rad for patients with previous pelvic surgery or pelvic inflammatory disease.

the basis of experience and can be adjusted once the isodose calculations become available, generally the following day. Further corrections can be made at the second insertion, which takes place 2 to 3 weeks later. Table 33-2 shows guidelines for combining external-beam and intracavitary irradiation.

"Subclinically" involved pelvic nodes require a dose of about 50 Gy to sterilize tumor to the 90% level, whereas lymph nodes large enough to be identified in the lymphangiogram require higher doses. Because the lymph nodes are in the pelvic wall, away from the applicators (colpostat and tandem), additional radiation (boost) is delivered with external beams. Unfortunately, the presence of small and large bowel in the area limits the dose level that can be delivered. When nodes are visualized in a lymphangiogram, the prognosis is worse and justifies trials that may include limited additional surgical procedures, extended-field irradiation, or chemotherapeutic agents.

Fine points in technique, applicator loading, and dosage are not discussed in this chapter. For further information the reader is referred to radiotherapy textbooks and papers on the subject.[2, 16]

Complications

Superficial vaginal vault necrosis or bladder and rectal ulcers are rare but can occur, most often in a patient with a distorted anatomy requiring the use of very small colpostats or cylinders. These complications are also more frequent when the tumor extends to the middle and lower thirds of the vagina, requiring extended vaginal irradiation. In addition to dosage and anatomic distortions, other significant contributing factors are old age, previous pelvic inflammatory disease, and previous surgical procedures that have created adhesions. Improved technology and the availability of computerized dosimetry make it possible to optimize dose distribution and minimize the occurrence of severe complications such as necrosis and fistulization. However, a certain risk has to be accepted in treating large tumors and tumor extensions that require radical therapy.[20]

Results

Table 33-3 emphasizes the importance of tumor volume rather than FIGO stage in determining treatment. Tables 33-4 and 33-5 analyze central and vaginal failures.

ADENOCARCINOMA OF THE ENDOMETRIUM

Intracavitary Preoperative Irradiation: History and Rationale

For patients with clinical Stages I and II (FIGO 1988) adenocarcinoma of the endometrium, M.D. Anderson Cancer Center in 1948 established a program

Table 33-3

Five-Year Survival Rates for Patients with Carcinoma of the Endocervix, 1955–1969 (n = 464) (Analysis 1976)*

Stage	Tumor Size	No. of Patients	% Survival	P Value
IB		239	87	
	<6 cm	201	91	.000
	>6 cm	38	63	
IIA		63	81	
	<6 cm	48	91	.005
	>6 cm	15	50	
IIB		192	70	
	<6 cm	103	72	.547
	>6 cm	89	69	

*Seven patients with severe hydroureter are included.
From Wilson W, et al.: Personal communication, 1978.

Table 33-4

Central Failures in Patients with Squamous Cell Carcinoma of the Cervix and an Intact Uterus Who Were Treated by Radiation (n = 916*) January 1964–December 1969 (Analysis August 1974)

	Failures			Reason	
Stage	%	No.	No Apparent	Less than Optimal Treatment	Massive Disease
IB + IIA	2	(11/494)	3	8	0
IIB	5	(10/204)	1	3	6
III	14	(31/218)	0	12	19
IIIA	12	(19/160)	0	12	7
IIIB	20.5	(12/58)	0	0	12

*Excluding seven analyzable patients with Stages IVA and IVB disease and eight with Stage IB disease treated surgically.
From Jampolis S, Andras EJ, Fletcher GH: Analysis of sites and causes of failures of irradiation in invasive squamous cell carcinoma of the intact uterine cervix. Radiology 1975; 115:681.

Table 33–5

Squamous Cell Carcinoma of the Cervix on Intact Uterus Treated by Irradiation (n = 916*), January 1964–December 1969 (Analysis August 1974)

Stage	Failures		Parametrial	Parametrial		Correlation of Dose at 5 cm	
	%	No.		Nodal	+Nodal		
IB + IIA	4.5	(23/494)	18	5	0	12	11
IIB	13	(27/204)	20	3	4	17	10
III	19	(41/218)	28	6	7	11	30
IIIA	17	(27/160)	16	6	5	10	17
IIIB	24	(14/58)	12	0	2	1	13

*Excluding seven analyzable patients with Stage IVA and IVB disease and eight Stage IB patients surgically.
From Jampolis S, Andras EJ, Fletcher GH: Analysis of sites and causes of failures of irradiation in invasive squamous cell carcinoma of the intact uterine cervix. Radiology 1975; 115:681.

combining preoperative irradiation followed by a simple extrafascial hysterectomy.[21] Previous reports indicated that the incidence of vaginal recurrences (5.4–17.7%) was sufficiently high to cause concern and justify preoperative irradiation.

The preoperative program established[22] was very elaborate. For patients with Stage I disease, it consisted mainly of intracavitary radium (two intracavitary insertions 3 weeks apart) followed by extrafascial hysterectomy 6 weeks later. Through the years, modifications were made, and an intrauterine tandem and Fletcher colpostats were added to the existing Heyman packing technique.[23] Vaginal irradiation was reduced to the upper fourth or third of the vagina when it became evident that vaginal recurrences in the lower third were rare after preoperative radium treatment. The dose to the uterus was increased in milligrams per hour. External-beam radiation preceded intracavitary radium treatment when the patient had an enlarged uterus, a Stage I undifferentiated (Grade 3) tumor, or a Stage II tumor (extension to the uterine cervix). All suitable patients underwent a simple extrafascial hysterectomy 4 to 6 weeks later.[24]

Published data from other centers, plus analysis of 43 patients treated at M. D. Anderson[25] with a single radium insertion followed by immediate simple hysterectomy, showed that the M. D. Anderson preoperative program was perhaps too elaborate and lengthy for patients who had well-differentiated tumors (Grade 1) and for those with a normal-size uterus; a randomized study was therefore conducted to determine the best technique for patients whose tumors were clinical Stage IA, Grades 2 and 3 and for all those with Stage IB disease. The authors concluded from the study that, for patients with clinical Stage IB well- (Grade 1) or moderately (Grade 2) differentiated tumors, one intracavitary insertion of radium or cesium for 72 hours, delivering a surface dose of 70 Gy to the upper vagina and 3250 mg/hr to the uterine cavity, followed by a simple extrafascial hysterectomy during the same hospital admission, was as effective as the earlier more elaborate treatment program. Patients with Grade 3 tumors had a significantly poorer prognosis, usually developing metastases intraperitoneally or at other sites. This finding agreed with those in other reports.

The current practice at M. D. Anderson Cancer Center[26] consists of (1) exploratory laparotomy, hysterectomy, and bilateral salpingo-ovariectomy for patients who have clinical Stage I, Grade 1 tumors; and (2) preoperative intracavitary irradiation for 72 hours as outlined earlier, followed by extrafascial hysterectomy during the same hospitalization, for patients with all other clinical Stage I tumors (Stage IA, Grades 2 and 3) and all tumors of clinical Stage IB. For those whose disease is clinical Stage II (tumor extension to the portio vaginalis cervicis), the authors still deliver preoperative pelvic radiation (18-MeV photon beam) to 40 Gy in 20 fractions over 4 weeks, and follow this with one intracavitary insertion for 72 hours and an extrafascial hysterectomy 4 to 6 weeks later. However, some patients with early Stage II disease (minimal endocervical involvement only) are treated in the same manner as those with Stage I.

Techniques of Preoperative Intracavitary Irradiation

Intrauterine Tandem and Colpostats in a Normal-Size Uterus

Insertion. The applicators are inserted in the operating room with the patient in the lithotomy position under general anesthesia. A rectovaginal and bimanual examination is performed first. When exposure by retractors is adequate, the cervix is held with one or occasionally two tenacula and the uterine cavity is probed with the hysterometer to determine its length. This is followed by cervical dilatation to 6 mm (dilator No. 6). The sequence of intrauterine

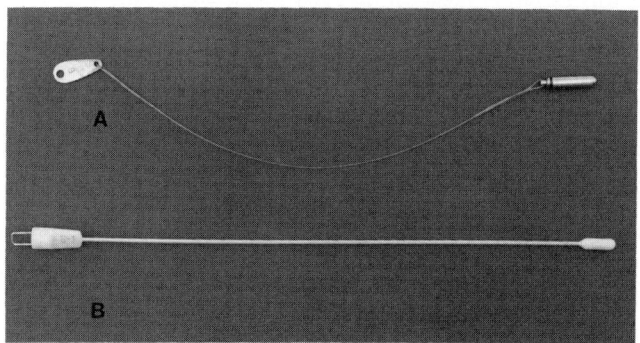

Figure 33–11
A, Heyman capsule. This No. 2 capsule is preloaded with radium tubes or a cesium rod. It is inserted in the operating room and followed by an afterloadable intrauterine tandem and colpostats. This capsule is preferred for very large uterine cavities because of its flexibility (it is attached to a flexible wire). B, Simon-Heyman capsule. This afterloadable capsule is also inserted empty in the operating room, followed by the afterloadable tandem and colpostats; these are not loaded until the patient returns to her room.

tandem and colpostat placement is the same as that described in the section on cervical cancer.

Selection of Loading. Loading the intrauterine tandem with cesium rods (manual afterloading) or with cesium spherical sources (remote afterloading) is different from the loading procedure used for carcinoma of the uterine cervix; to load a 3-inch tandem, we use 20-15-10 mg radium-equivalent cesium. The insertion remains in place for approximately the same length of time as does radium (72 hours). When the Selectron remote-controlled unit is used, the sources are withdrawn about 10% of the time to allow nursing care and visiting.

Simon-Heyman Capsules in an Enlarged Uterus

Modified Heyman packing with Simon capsules (Fig. 33–11) is used in large uterine cavities. The capsules are inserted into the uterus first, followed by an intrauterine tandem and the colpostats (Fig. 33–12).

Patients for Whom Hysterectomy Is Medically or Surgically Unsuitable

Hysterectomy is inappropriate when there is parametrial involvement. Treatment of such patients employs only radiation and is similar to treatment for carcinoma of the uterine cervix. Intrauterine irradiation is increased by loading the uterine tandem more heavily or by employing Simon-Heyman capsules.

Patients who are poor surgical risks, even though their disease be only Stage I or II, are also treated by radiotherapy alone.

Postoperative Radiation

Postoperative radiation is given only to patients who did not receive intracavitary irradiation preoperatively and who are found at surgery to have myometrial invasion. The vaginal vault is treated to a 60-Gy surface dose in 72 hours by means of a dome cylinder (Fig. 33–13) if myometrial invasion is limited to the inner half. However, when more than half the myometrium is involved, such patients receive external-beam irradiation as described for cancer of the cervix, complemented with vaginal irradiation to an additional 30-Gy surface dose in 49 to 50 hours.

Postoperative treatment for patients who have undergone preoperative intracavitary irradiation and hysterectomy and have tumor in more than 50% of the myometrium consists of pelvic radiation to 40 or 50 Gy in 20 to 25 fractions over 4 to 5 weeks; systemic chemotherapy is added if tumor is found in the fallopian tubes, ovaries, pelvic nodes, or abdomen. Whole-abdomen irradiation is a possible alternative.

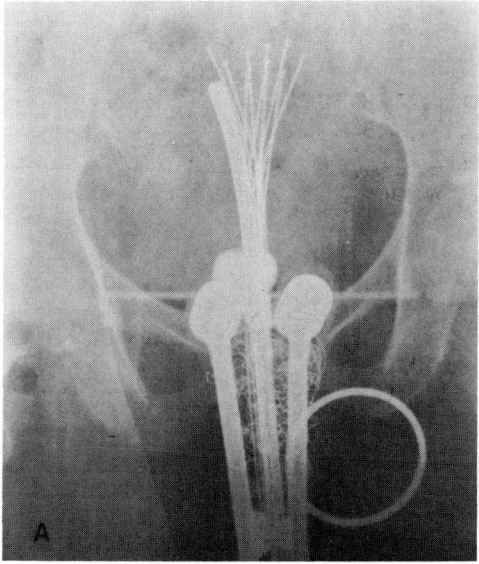
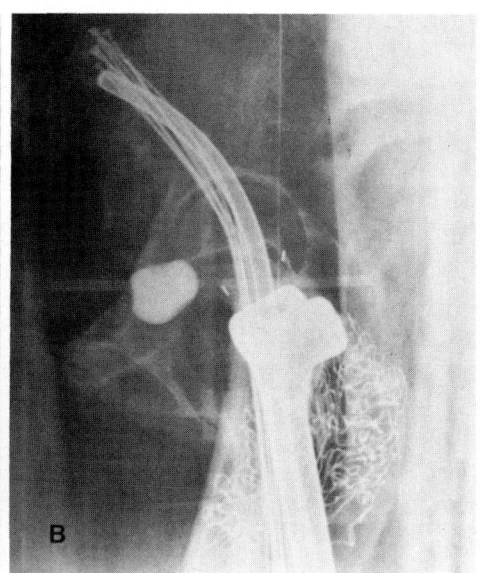

Figure 33–12
Orthogonal radiographs. A, Uterovaginal insertion with Simon-Heyman capsules. B, Intrauterine tandem with Fletcher colpostats. The whole "system" is afterloadable. Because of the limited flexibility of the capsule stem, these capsules do not spread as well as the preloadable classical Heyman capsules. (From GH Fletcher: Textbook of Radiotherapy, 3rd edition. Philadelphia, Lea & Febiger, 1980. Used with permission.)

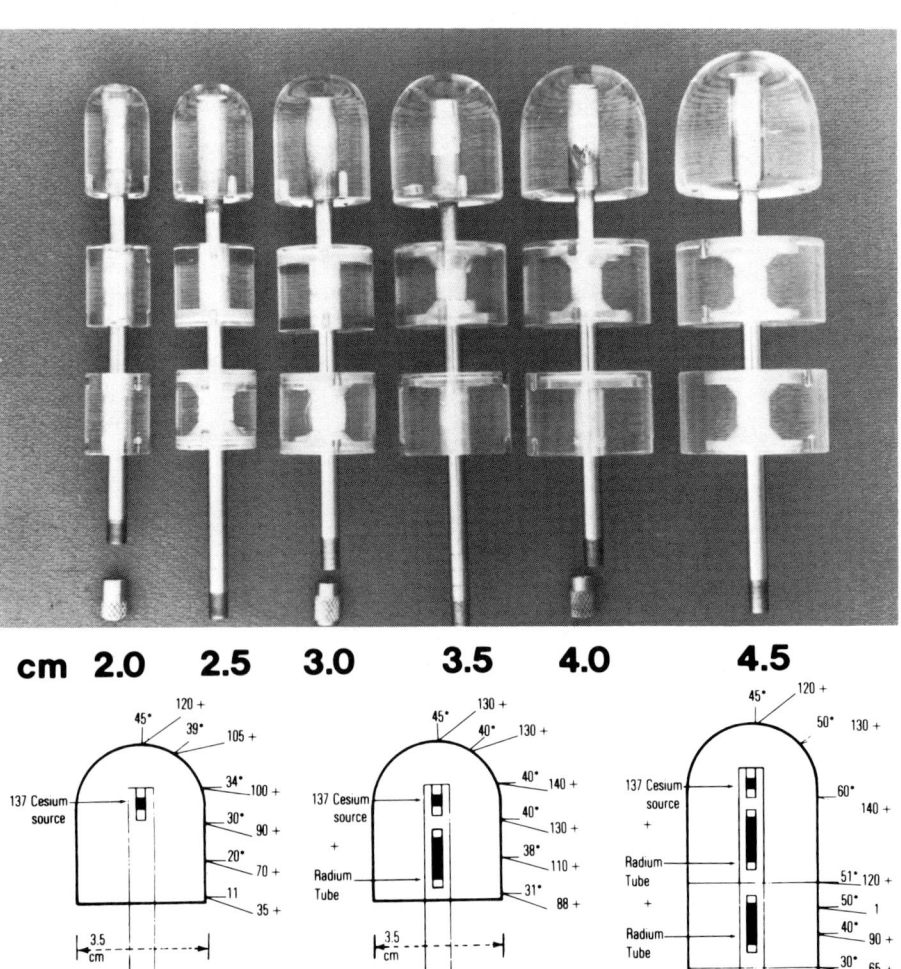

Figure 33–13
"Dome" cylinders, which are available for manual and remote loading. The top source is always a "point" source. The dome is shaped as a hemisphere to follow the isodose of the point source. This point source may be combined with radium tubes or cesium rods to treat a selected length of the vagina. (From Fletcher GH, Delclos L, Wharton JT, Rutledge FN: Tumors of the vagina and female urethra. In Fletcher GH (ed.): Textbook of Radiotherapy, 3rd ed. Philadelphia, Lea & Febiger, 1980, p. 814.)

For patients in whom positive cells are found only in the peritoneal cavity, the use of any postoperative treatment (chemotherapy or radiotherapy) is still being debated.

MALIGNANT TUMORS OF THE VAGINA

Malignant vaginal tumors are rare. Most are squamous cell carcinomas; adenocarcinomas occur, but are less frequent. Rare tumors include sarcomas and melanomas in adult women and clear cell carcinomas in young women. Some rare tumors such as sarcoma botryoides and endodermal sinus tumor can occur in children, but neither of these is treated by radiation. Metastatic vaginal tumors may also develop from a primary in the endometrium, the uterine cervix (squamous cell carcinoma or adenocarcinoma), or the gastrointestinal tract. Disease in any of these sites may also be the source of direct extension or recurrences in the vagina from tumor in the urinary bladder, urethra, or paraurethral glands, including Bartholin's glands. Another possibility is a vaginal metastasis from a primary tumor in the breast or lung.

Lymphatic Spread

The lymphatic drainage systems of the upper and lower vagina are different, although there is communication between them. Tumors involving the proximal half of the vagina spread like carcinoma of the cervix; tumors involving the distal half spread more like carcinoma of the vulva. This drainage difference is important in planning treatment. However, the radiation field need not encompass the common iliac lymphatics, even when the tumor is in the proximal vagina, because when radiation is limited to small fields that do not even include the lateral pelvic walls, the incidence of pelvic node failure is low.[28] When a tumor is in the distal half, it is important to include the midinguinal nodes, because tumors in the distal vagina can metastasize to this area.

Baseline studies should include a lower-extremity lymphangiogram. A positive lymphangiogram is particularly important because it identifies the location and volume of the positive nodes. Visibly positive nodes require a higher dose of radiation.

Treatment Planning

The FIGO staging[29] accepted by the American Joint Committee on Staging is not useful for therapy planning because it does not take into account the extent, volume, or location of the tumor. The importance of location, especially upper versus lower vagina, must be emphasized. It is also important to identify anterior, posterior, or lateral locations because of the proximity of the bladder and urethra to the anterior vaginal wall, and of the rectum and anus to the posterior wall. The presence or absence of the uterus is another important factor; when the uterus is present, tumors of the upper vagina can be treated like tumors of the uterine cervix, by inserting radioactive sources into the uterus and, if necessary, in the lateral fornices.

It is stressed that treatment of vaginal tumors must be highly individualized, and many factors must be considered in planning. Forty per cent of these tumors occur in patients treated earlier by surgery or radiation for cancer of the uterine cervix, which obviously affects subsequent treatment. Another important factor is the desire to conserve the bladder, urethra, rectum, and vagina. Because anatomic limitations do not allow sufficient surgical margins for conservative surgery, radiation is generally the treatment of choice.

Treatment Options

External-beam irradiation, used alone or combined with either (1) intracavitary or transvaginal irradiation for tumors of the upper half of the vagina or (2) interstitial irradiation, using stainless steel needle guides (Fig. 33–14) afterloaded with iridium wires

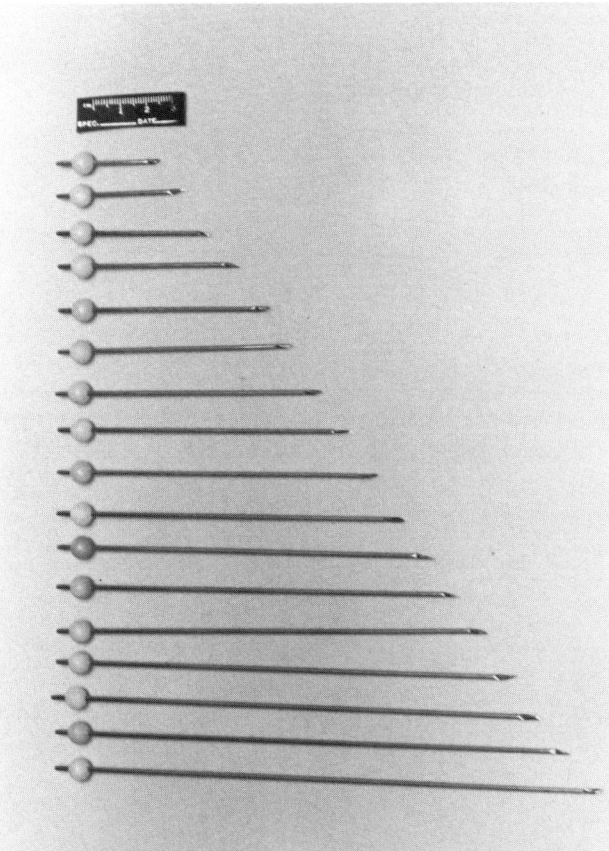

Figure 33–14
Needle guides with Teflon balls. Lengths range from 2 to 6 cm, increasing 0.5 cm at a time, or from 6 to 20 cm, increasing 1 cm at a time.

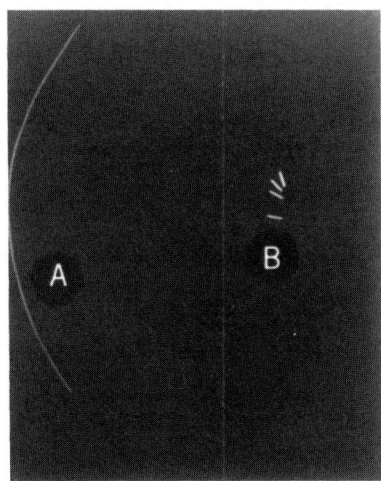
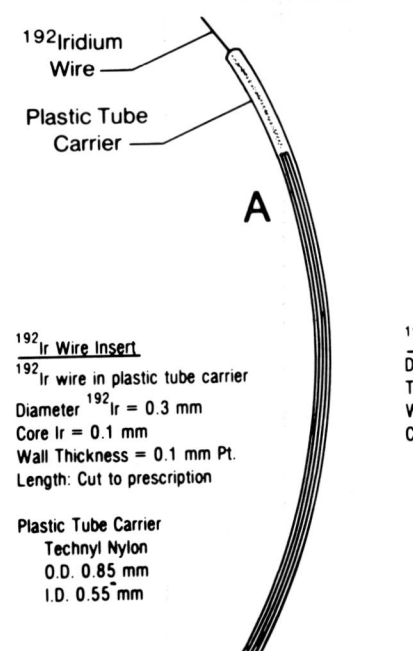

Figure 33–15
Isotopes used for interstitial irradiation at M. D. Anderson Cancer Center include ^{192}Ir wires (A) and ^{198}Au grains (B). The ^{192}Ir wire is thin and flexible and can be tailored to any length; its cross-section is excellent (750 barns), and its half-life is acceptable for treatment times of 2 to 8 days. For safe and easier manipulation, the iridium wire is mounted inside a nylon or Teflon tube carrier. (Iridium seed chains in Teflon may also be used, but the intensity per seed is higher.) The ^{198}Au seeds (gold grains) are small and therefore can be inserted in thin mucosa overlying bone and in narrow spaces. Although these are used for permanent implants, the short half-life of the gold allows it to deliver most of the dose in the first 5 to 10 days.

Table 33–6

Survival Data of Patients Treated for Primary Squamous Cell Carcinoma of the Vagina at M. D. Anderson Cancer Center, 1948–1972 (Analysis 1972)*

Stage	No. of Patients Treated	Patients Alive and Disease Free at 5 yr		Therapy Failures Within 5 yr		
		No.	%	Recurrences in Treated Area†	Distant Metastases	Unknown
I	25	16	64	4	2	1
II	39	23	59	6	1	1
III	28	10	36	6	—	—
IV	20	8	40	6	5	—
Total	112	57	50			2

*Includes patients treated with radiation, surgery, or both.
†With or without distant metastases.

(Fig. 33–15) or seed chains, has enhanced the outlook for patients with vaginal cancer. Table 33–6 details the survival data for a group of patients treated at M. D. Anderson Cancer Center over the last three decades.

External-beam irradiation for patients with a negative CT scan or lymphangiogram employs portals that extend from the midsacrum to the vaginal introitus, which has been marked previously with a silver seed that is visualized on the simulation films. The portals extend about 1.5 cm lateral to the pelvic brim, thus including the whole vagina and the lymphatics of the pelvis (paracolpal and parametrial, external iliac, hypogastric, and junctional nodes) but not the common iliac nodes. If the tumor is in the lower (distal) half of the vagina, the fields have to be extended downward to cover the introitus or part of the vulva and laterally to cover the midinguinal nodes. The location of the midinguinal nodes is determined by clinical and radiologic examination, including lymphangiography.

The authors prefer to use an 18-MeV photon beam unless the inguinal nodes are clinically involved, in which case an anterior 6-MeV photon beam and a posterior 18-MeV photon beam are used. Treatment portals are similar to the ones employed for postoperative treatment of carcinoma of the vulva (Fig. 33–16). A dose of 40 Gy is given in 20 fractions over 4 weeks to the midline of the pelvis.

For tumors of the upper half of the vagina (proximal), intracavitary radiation from intrauterine and vaginal sources is usually added (several colpostats are available), generally in two insertions of 48 hours each 2 weeks apart; if the tumor extends to the middle third of the vagina, it may require interstitial radiation also (Fig. 33–17). When the uterus is absent, the authors may continue with external-beam radiation and reduce the portals, delivering a total midline dose of 64 to 66 Gy at 2 Gy per fraction. To this may be added a "dome colpostat" (see Fig. 33–13) or ovoids to increase the dose to the upper vagina. In selected patients, interstitial irradiation is used, adding 40 Gy in 3 to 5 days from the implant to the 40 Gy from the external beam; interstitial irradiation requires a laparotomy to guide the needles.

For lesions of the lower half of the vagina (distal), interstitial irradiation is given with stainless steel needle guides loaded with iridium wires or seed chains, either alone or after external-beam treatment to 40 Gy in 20 fractions over 4 weeks. This area is vulnerable to radiation reactions, sequelae, and complications because the tissues of the vaginal introitus, vulva, and perineal area tolerate radiation poorly and are also exposed to constant irritation from perspiration, urine, and soiling. It is therefore vital to minimize radiation to the normal surrounding areas.

Iridium Implants

An example of an implant of the lateral wall is shown in Figure 33–18. An empty plastic cylinder is inserted, both to protect the uninvolved vagina and to maintain the needles in place.

To implant the anterior vaginal wall, the bladder

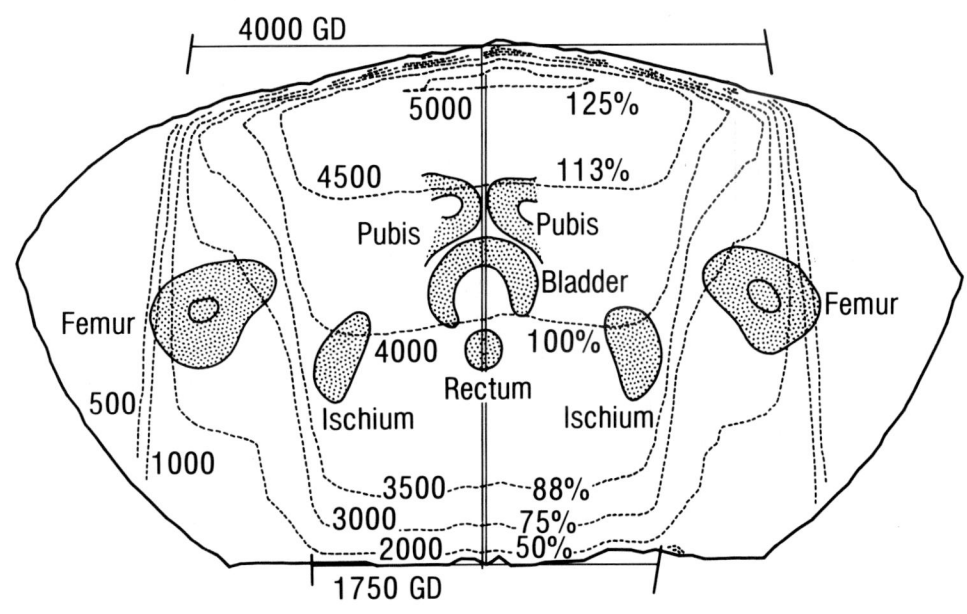

Figure 33–16
Combination of parallel fields as employed in treating tumors of the vulva and lower vagina. Note that different photon energies are used to increase the dose to the inguinal areas and spare the rectum, presacral area, and coxofemoral joints.

AP: 6 Mev Photons
PA: 18 Mev Photons

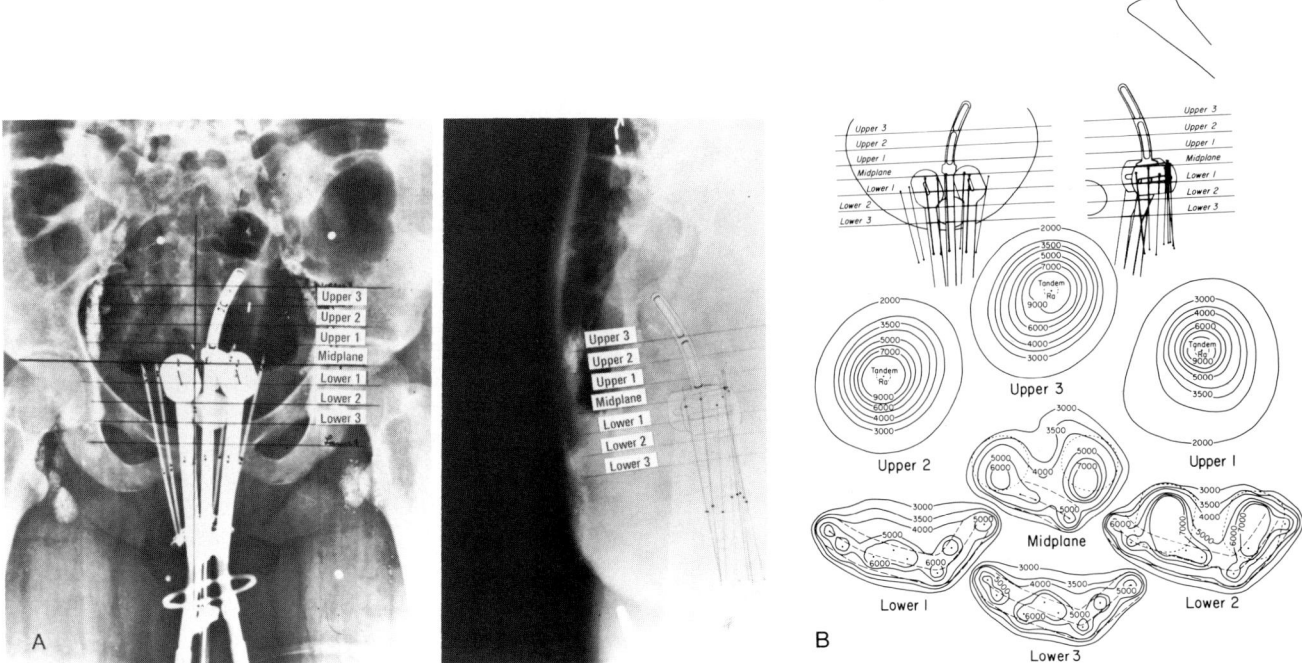

Figure 33–17
A 24-year old-white woman referred to the authors in March, 1975, after a clear cell carcinoma of the vagina in the anterior vaginal wall had been locally excised. A long scar extended from the anterior fornix, close to the anterior cervical lip, to 1 cm from the introitus. Our treatment began with 20 Gy administered in 10 fractions (2 weeks) to the anterior vaginal wall from a 24-MeV photon beam via a 12.5-cm parallel-opposed field. The posterior vaginal wall was partially shielded with a lead block on a Lucite rod. This was followed with a ^{192}Ir implant of the anterior vaginal wall (6 × 9 cm active-Length ^{192}Ir wires on afterloading stainless steel needles) delivering 30 to 40 Gy at about 5 mm outside the implant in 72 hours. In addition, a 7.5-cm intrauterine tandem (loaded with 15-10-10 mg of radium) and two small afterloading Fletcher-Suit ovoidal colpostats (loaded with 5-mg radium each) were left in for 72 hours (technique and dose illustrated in A and B). The patient was disease free in December 1977; she had a moderate amount of atrophy of the upper third of the vagina with some telangiectasis. This case illustrates the complexity and degree of individualization employed to minimize the risk of sequelae and complications.

is first filled with methylene blue diluted in water or saline. Since the needles are open at the end, the tinted fluid flows through the needle if the bladder or urethra is entered during the needle implant, in which case the needle is withdrawn and reimplanted. An example of an implant of the anterior vaginal wall is shown in Figure 33–19. Implants of the posterior wall (Fig. 33–20) require the needles to be guided by the index finger of the opposite hand inserted in the rectum. In some instances, a finger is needed in both vagina and rectum to guide the needles (Fig. 33–21).

Although most implants are single plane, it is occasionally necessary for large tumors to use more than one plane (Figs. 33–21 and 33–22).

Clear Cell Carcinoma in a Young Woman

Clear cell adenocarcinoma can occur in a young woman in either the vagina or the uterine cervix. Some of these have been associated with maternal use of diethylstilbestrol during early gestation, but identical cancers can occur in patients who have had no exposure.

Tumor volume, location, and extent are the primary factors in treatment planning. To preserve fertility in these young women, the authors treat small tumors (<3 cm in diameter) with interstitial or transvaginal radiation to spare the uterus and ovaries. Large lesions are treated in the same way as the carcinomas in older women, and the treatment techniques and doses are the same as those for squamous carcinomas.

Complications of Irradiation

Treatment complications are documented in Table 33–7. Some vaginal stenosis may occur; however, because large portions of the vagina are left untreated, the vagina retains considerable elasticity and compensates for the radiation-induced scarring. Delayed healing must be treated conservatively, resisting the temptation to subject the area to repeated biopsies, with resultant necrosis.

Lateral Pelvic Wall Recurrence: Treatment with Intraoperative Gold-Grain Implants

Gold-grain implants have been used since 1956 at M. D. Anderson Cancer Center to treat noncentral pelvic

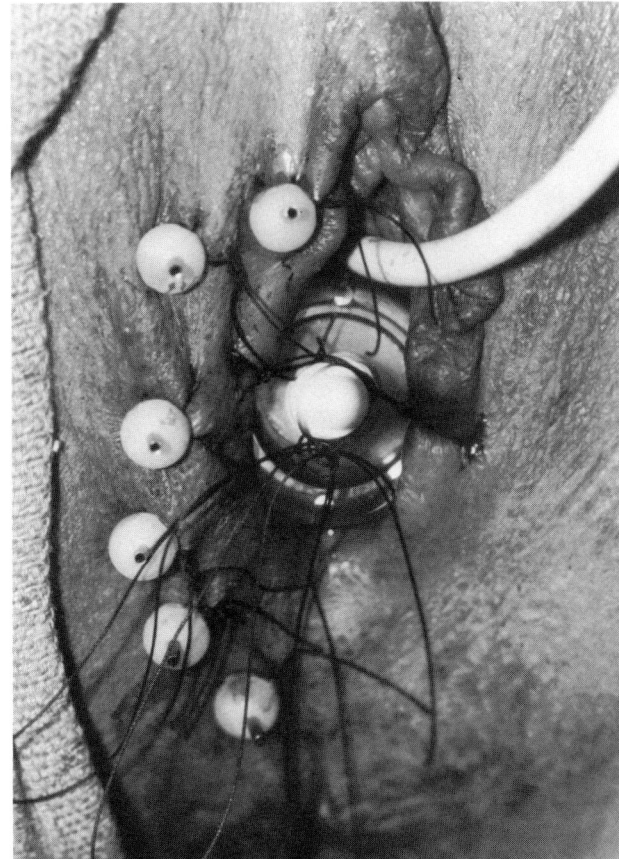

Figure 33–18
Single-plane implant of the right vaginal wall. The spacing of the stainless steel needles (to be loaded with ^{192}Ir wires) is closed to 2 cm in this patient, allowing a satisfactory uniform dose as prescribed at 1 cm from the needles. The empty vaginal cylinder maintains the needles in stable position and displaces the opposite vaginal wall away from the implant.

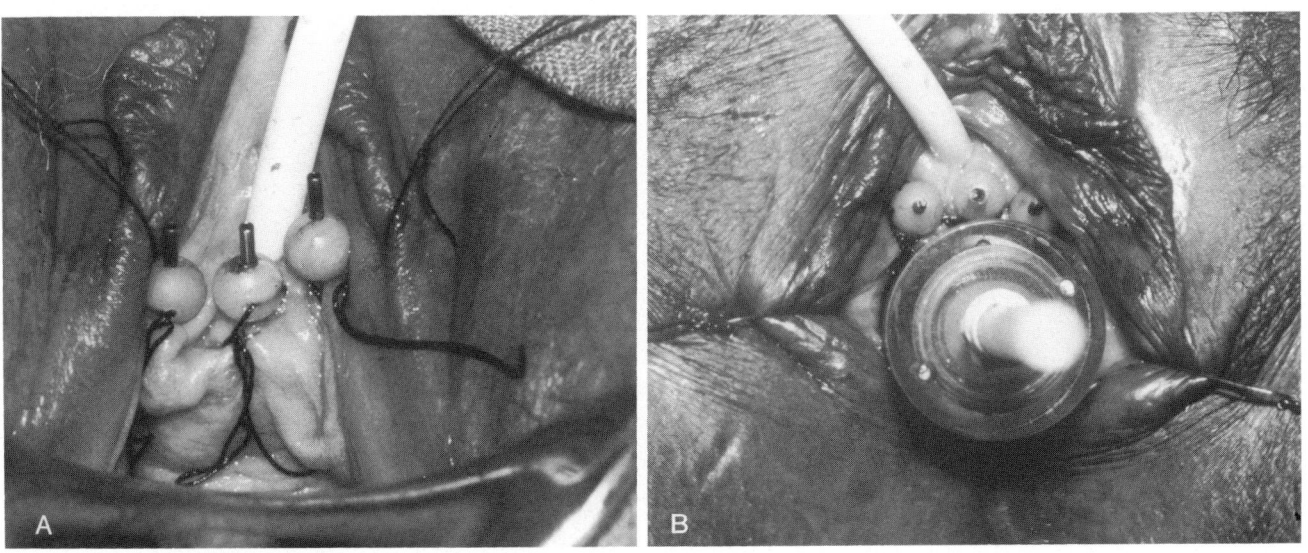

Figure 33–19
Implant of the anterior vaginal wall (suburethral area) without *(A)* and with *(B)* a vaginal cylinder.

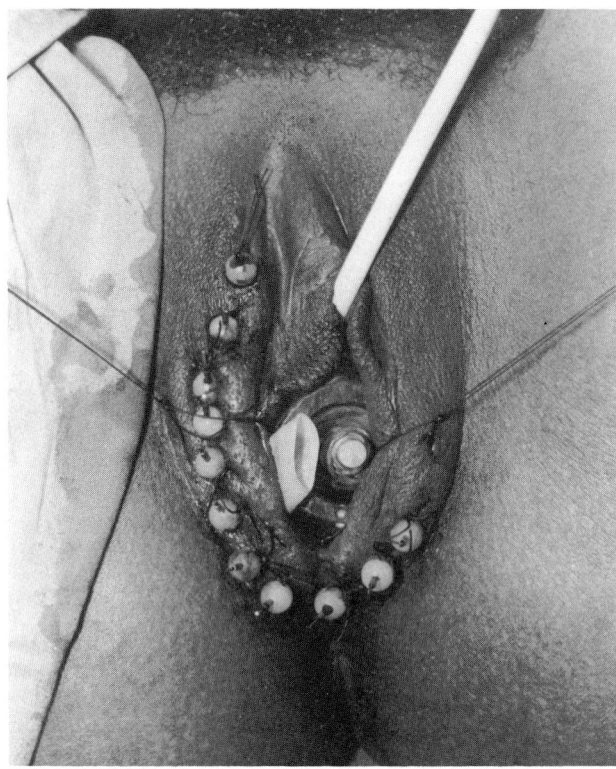

Figure 33–20
Large single-plane implant for a tumor that extended down from the 10 o'clock to the 6 o'clock position. The needles are 1.5 cm apart and the dose is prescribed to 0.75 cm from the needles' plane. The empty vaginal cylinder maintains the position of the needles and pushes away the anterior and left areas of the vaginal wall.

Figure 33–21
Volume (or three-plane) implant for a large tumor of the left side of the vagina and rectovaginal septum. The index finger is inserted into the vagina and the midfinger in the rectum to guide the needles during the implant and to verify that they are not entering the vagina or rectum.

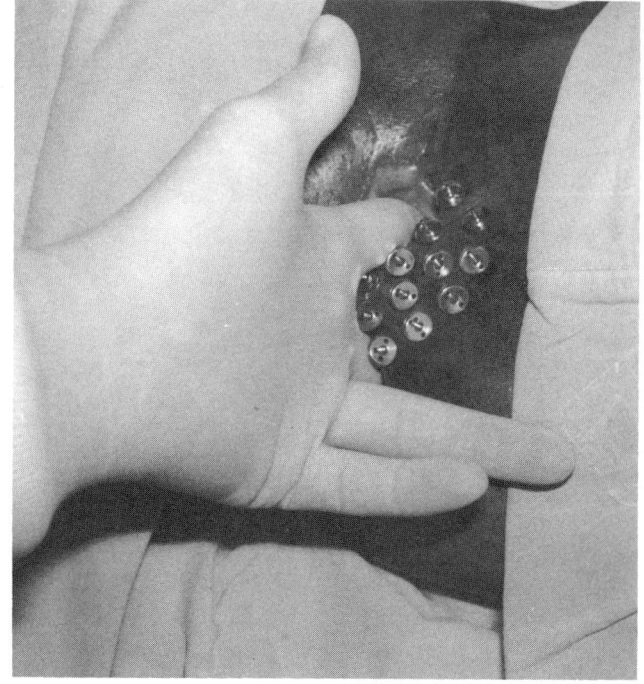

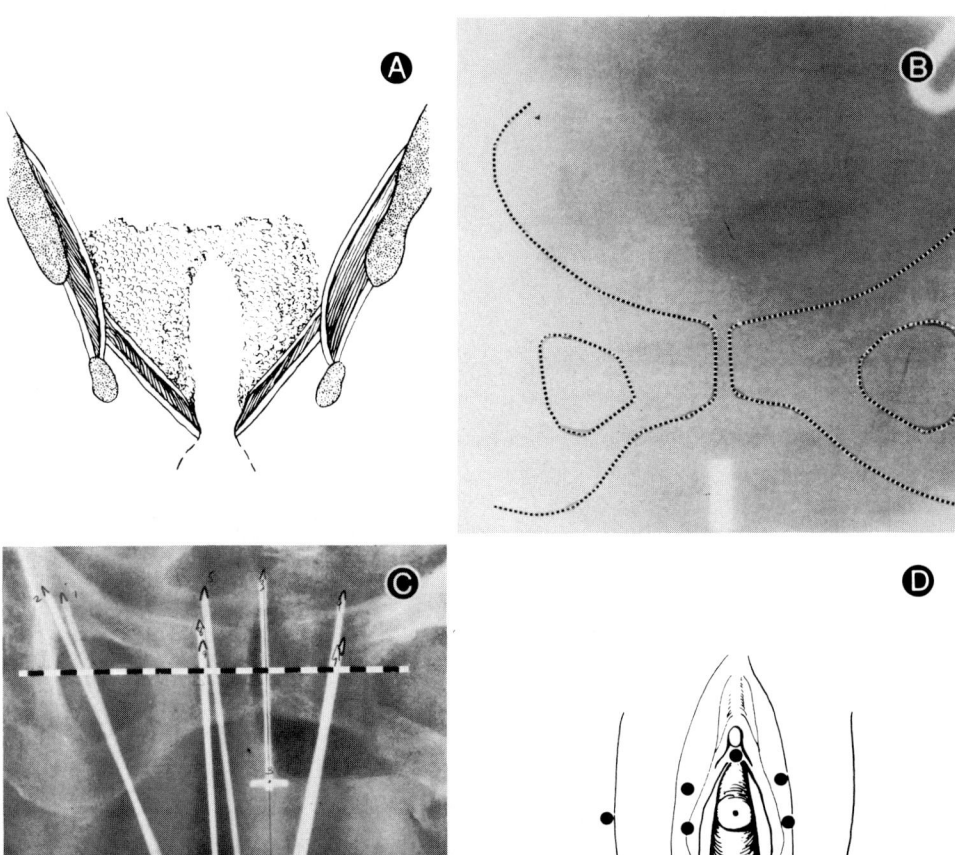

Figure 33–22
In 1961 a 71-year-old woman underwent a total abdominal hysterectomy and bilateral salpingo-oophorectomy for carcinoma in situ of the uterine cervix. She did well for 9 years. In May, 1970, she was found to have an extensive squamous cell carcinoma of the vagina. The lesion (A) involved the entire vagina and extended to both paracolpal areas, being fixed to the right pelvic wall. There was a crater at the apex of the vagina. The patient was treated by a combination of external-beam and interstitial radiation. From May 13, 1970 to June 9, 1970, she received 40 Gy in 20 fractions by means of a 22-MeV photon beam in parallel-opposed fields (B). On June 17, 1970, a ¹⁹²Ir implant was placed in an open bladder, shown in C, an anteroposterior x-ray film and diagram of the isodose distribution of the implant, and D, diagram of the implant placement. A dose of 40 Gy was administered in 73 hours (55 Gy/hr isodose). The patient was disease free in July, 1975. (From Fletcher GH, Delclos L, Wharton JT, Rutledge FN: Tumors of the vagina and female urethra. In Fletcher GH (ed): Textbook of Radiotherapy, 3rd ed. Philadelphia, Lea & Febiger, 1980, pp. 812–828.)

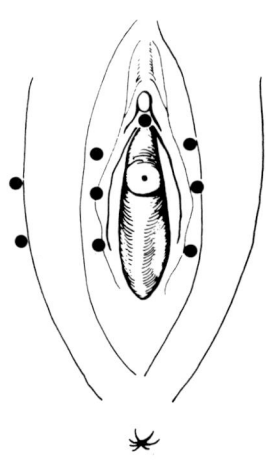

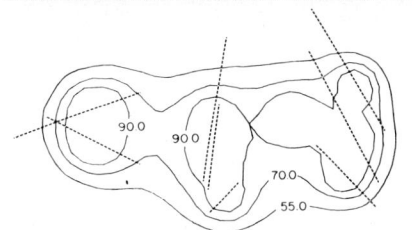

Table 33–7

Complications of Squamous Cell Carcinoma of the Vagina in Patients Without Recurrent Disease at M. D. Anderson Cancer Center, January 1955–December 1982 (n = 115)

Minimal and moderate reactions (treated conservatively)		
Cystitis	6	(4/6 developed vaginal fibrosis)*
Proctitis	6	
Vaginal necrosis	2	
Total	14/115 (12%)	
Sequelae		
Vaginal fibrosis*	11	(2/11 urethral stenosis)
Total	11/115 (10%)	
Severe complications		
Rectosigmoid stenosis	4	
Rectosigmoid hemorrhage	1	
Multiple fistulas	1	
Total	6/115 (5%)	

*Vaginal fibrosis developed in 15 of the 115 patients (13%).

recurrences that develop after irradiation. In 1966, Miller[30] reported 18 patients (16 with intact uteri and two with cervical stumps) in whom radioactive gold grains had been implanted as treatment for noncentral pelvic recurrence of squamous carcinoma of the uterine cervix. His analysis concluded that, for selected patients, gold-grain implantation to a dose of 70 to 110 Gy was a useful procedure that relieved some of the symptoms caused by an unremovable pelvic wall recurrence (a swollen, painful lower extremity on the same side as the pelvic mass was the most common presentation). Pain was substantially or completely relieved in 11 of the 18 patients for periods ranging from 2 to 23 months. Lower-limb edema was reduced in 10 of the 18 patients for 17 to 68 months. Ureteral obstruction was relieved, at least partially, in three of the eight patients who did not have a ureteral ligation. Three developed complications: one a ureterocutaneous fistula, one a pelvic abscess, and one wound dehiscence.[30]

One patient was alive with no evidence of disease at 5 years; 2 died at 2 years and 1 at 1 year. All the other patients (14) died in less than 1 year, 10 of them within 6 months. A dose of at least 70 Gy and up to 110 Gy increased the survival span (eight of 13 patients) over that of doses less than 70 Gy (one of five patients). This increase was the result of the combination of implants plus supplemental external-beam irradiation when required. Miller concluded with a recommendation to use gold grains of 0.38 to 0.67 radon-equivalencies to achieve a dosage of at least 70 Gy.

Since 1972, the authors have used gold grains of 0.4-mc radon-equivalent strength. An attempt is made to implant the seeds 1 cm apart, and the distribution follows the tumor mass (Fig. 33–23). If the dose within the tumor is too low, the dose is increased to 100 or 120 Gy with additional external-beam irradiation. Over the years, the authors have used implants for pelvic wall recurrences that developed after radiotherapy and after surgery. In addition to recurrences of squamous cell carcinomas, implants have been made for recurrences of adenocarcinomas of the uterus and of sarcomas.

To date, the authors have used the gold-grain implanter to treat 25 patients (Figs. 33–24 and 33–25).[31] Seven patients benefited definitively from the

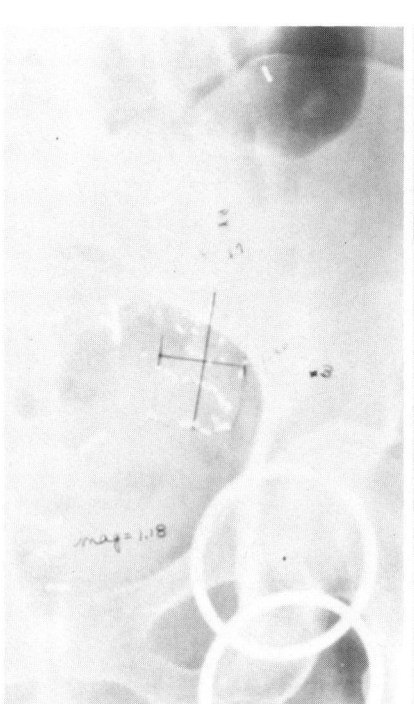
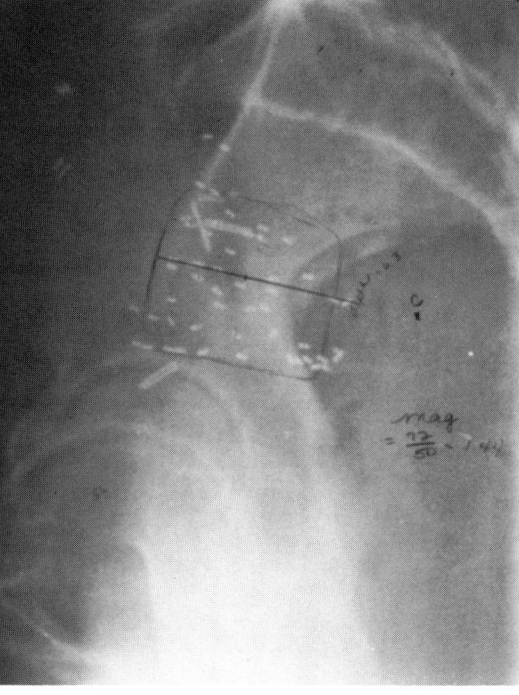

Figure 33–23
Radioactive gold-grain implant of a pelvic wall recurrence.

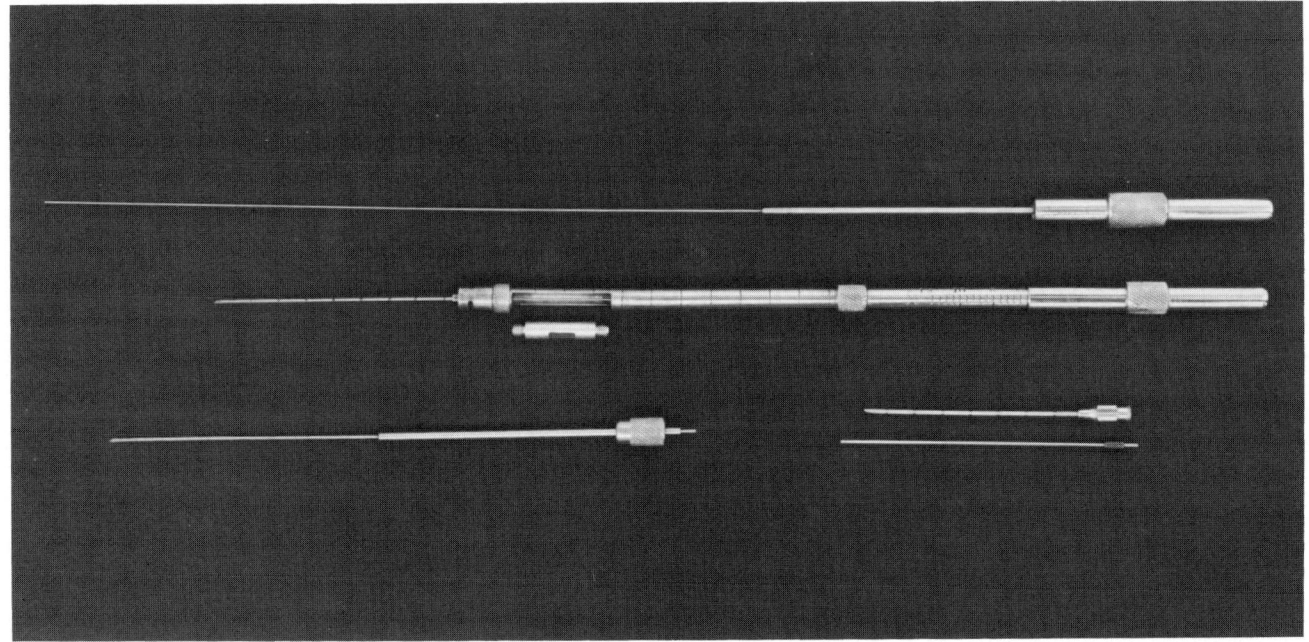

Figure 33–24
Gold-grain implanter. (From Delclos L, Moore EB: A slim 198 gold-grain implanter loaded with standard royal Marsden 14-grain magazines. Cancer 1979; 43:1021–1024.)

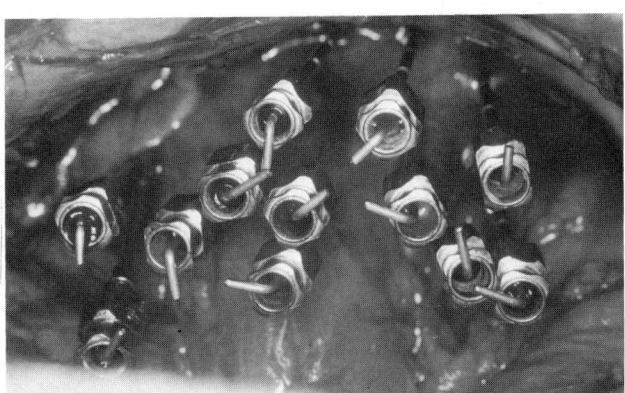

Figure 33–25
Needle guides for the gold-grain implanter. (From Delclos L, Moore EB: A slim 198 gold-grain implanter loaded with standard royal Marsden 14-grain magazines. Cancer 1979; 43:1021–1024.)

Table 33–8

Results of Gold-Grain Implants in the Lateral Pelvis Wall, January 1972–May 1986 (n = 25)

No. of Patients	Result	Survival Duration
4	Lost to follow-up	<1 yr
1	Pain relief; died from tumor	<1 yr
14	No palliation; died	<6 mo
1	Disease free	17 yr
1	Disease free	8 yr
1	Disease free	6 yr
1	Disease free	3 yr
2	Died from tumor	3 yr

treatment; six survived with symptoms relief for 3 (three patients), 6, 8, and 17 years, respectively (Table 33–8). One patient experienced pain relief but died of progressive disease at 1 year. Fourteen patients died in less than 6 months, and the degree of palliation was difficult to evaluate.[32]

To prevent complications, some essential details of this technique must be mastered: for example, correct placement of the omentum, which should be positioned on top of the implant to protect the bowel around it, and the occasional need to ligate a ureter.

References

1. Eifel PJ, Morris M, Oswald MJ, et al.: Adenocarcinoma of the uterine cervix: Prognosis and patterns of failure of 367 cases treated at the M. D. Anderson Cancer Center between 1965 and 1985. Cancer 1990; 65:2507.
2. Fletcher GH: Textbook of Radiotherapy, 3rd ed. Philadelphia, Lea & Febiger, 1980.
3. Rouviere H: Anatomie des Lymphatiques de l'Homme. Paris: Masson & Cie, 1932, p. 406.
4. Wall JA, Arnold H: Preliminary observations on retroperitoneal lymphadenectomies. Tex State J Med 1953; 49:93.
5. Wallace S, Jing B: Clinical Lymphangiography. Baltimore, Williams & Wilkins, 1977.
6. Durrance FY, Fletcher GH: Computer calculations of dose distribution to regional lymphatic from gynecological radium insertions. Radiology 1968; 91:140.
7. Fabian CE, Benninghoff DL: Lymphangiography as an adjunct to pelvic radium dosimetry. Am J Roentgenol 1966; 96:197.
8. Henriksen E: The lymphatic spread of carcinoma of the cervix and body of the uterus; study of 420 necropsies. Am J Obstet Gynecol 1949; 58:924.
9. Meigs JV: Radical hysterectomy with bilateral pelvic lymph node dissections: A report of 100 patients operated on five or more years ago. Am J Obstet Gynecol 1951; 62:854.
10. Delclos L, Cundiff J: The Fletcher colpostat system adapted to the low dose rate remotely controlled Selectron unit: A second progress report. In Martinez AA, Orton CG, Mould RF (eds.): Brachytherapy HDR and LDR. Leersum, Nucletron International B.V., 1990, pp. 83–92.
11. Suit HD, Moore EB, Fletcher GH, Worsnop R: Modification of Fletcher ovoid system for afterloading using standard sized radium tubes (milligram and microgram). Radiology 1963; 81:126.
12. Green AE, Broadwater JR, Hancock JA: Afterloading vaginal ovoids. Am J Roentgenol 1969; 105:609.
13. Delclos L, Fletcher GH, Sampiere V, Grant WH: Can the Fletcher gamma ray colpostat system be extrapolated to other systems? Cancer 1978; 41:970.
14. Delclos L, Fletcher GH, Moore EB, Sampiere VA: Minicolpostats, dome cylinders, and other additions and improvements of the Fletcher-Suit afterloadable system: Indications and limitations of their use. Int J Radiat Oncol Biol Phys 1980; 6:1195.
15. International Commission on Radiological Units and Measurement: Dose and volume specifications for reporting intracavitary therapy in gynecology. ICRU Report 38. Bethesda, MD, ICRU, 1985.
16. Delclos L, Fletcher GH: Gynecologic cancers: Pelvic examination and treatment planning. In Levitt SH (ed.): Technological Basis of Radiation Therapy: Practical Clinical Applications. Philadelphia, Lea & Febiger, 1992, pp. 263–289.
17. Delclos L, Fletcher GH, Suit HD, et al.: Technical notes: Afterloading vaginal irradiators. Radiology 1970; 96:666.
18. Delclos L: Uterine cervix dilator designed to be used before insertion of intrauterine tandems and/or capsules. Radiology 1969; 93:1201.
19. Delclos L: Uterine cervix marker. Radiology 1969; 93:695.
20. Fletcher GH, Shukovsky LJ: The interplay of radiocurability and tolerance in the irradiation of human cancers. J Radiol Electrol 1975; 56:383.
21. Rutledge FN, Tan SK, Fletcher GH: Vaginal metastasis from adenocarcinoma of the corpus uteri. Am J Obstet Gynecol 1958; 75:167.
22. Chau PM: Technic and evaluation of preoperative radium therapy in adenocarcinoma of the uterine corpus. In a collection of papers presented at the Fifth Annual Clinical Conference on Cancer, 1960, at The University of Texas MD Anderson Hospital and Tumor Institute. Carcinoma of the Uterine Cervix, Endometrium, and Ovary. Chicago, Year Book Medical Publishers, 1962, pp. 235–256.
23. Delclos L, Fletcher GH: Malignant tumors of the endometrium: Evaluation of some aspects of radiotherapy. In a collection of papers presented at the Eleventh Annual Clinical Conference on Cancer, 1966, at The University of Texas MD Anderson Hospital and Tumor Institute. Cancer of the Uterus and Ovary. Chicago, Year Book Medical Publishers, 1969, pp. 62–77.
24. Fletcher GH, Rutledge FN, Delclos L: Adenocarcinoma of the uterus. In Fletcher GH (ed.): Textbook of Radiotherapy, 3rd ed. Philadelphia, Lea & Febiger, 1980, pp. 789–808.
25. Delclos L, Fletcher GH, Landgren RC, et al.: The place of radiotherapy in adenocarcinoma of the endometrium. Rev Interam Radiol 1978; 3:199.
26. Delclos L, Wharton JT, Rutledge FN, et al.: Preoperative radiation in the treatment of adenocarcinoma of the endometrium, stage I: The U. T. M. D. Anderson Hospital experience. In Rutledge FN, Freedman RS, Gershenson DM (eds.): Gynecologic Cancer: Diagnosis and Treatment Strategies. Austin, University of Texas Press, 1987, pp. 317–326.
27. Fletcher GH, Delclos L, Wharton JT, Rutledge FN: Tumors of the vagina and female urethra. In Fletcher GH (ed.): Textbook of Radiotherapy, 3rd ed. Philadelphia, Lea & Febiger, 1980, pp. 812–828.
28. Dancuart F, Delclos L, Wharton JT, Silva EG: Primary squamous cell carcinoma of the vagina treated by radiotherapy: A failure analysis. The M. D. Anderson experience 1955–1982. Int J Radiat Oncol Biol Phys 1988; 14:745.
29. Petterson F (ed.): Annual report on the results of treatment in gynecological cancer. Radiumhemmet 1988; 18:13.
30. Miller LS: Palliation with radiogold grains for postradiation recurrences. In Cancer of the Uterus and Ovary. Chicago, Year Book Medical Publishers, 1969, pp. 323–330.
31. Delclos L, Moore EB: A slim 198 gold-grain implanter loaded with standard royal Marsden 14-grain magazines. Cancer 1979; 43:1021.
32. Delclos L, Edwards C: Intraoperative gold-grain implants for lateral pelvic wall recurrences (gyn. malignancies). A preliminary communication of the MDACC experience (1972–1988). Acta Radiol Portug 1990; 2:95.

Index

Note: Page numbers in *italics* indicate illustrations; page numbers followed by t indicate tables.

Abdominal pregnancy, 496
Abdominal sacral colpopexy, in vaginal prolapse, 331–332
Abdominal wall, anatomy of, 21, *22*, 23, *23*, 127–129, *128–130*
  blood supply to, 128–129, *129*, *130*
  closure of. See *Closure*.
  innervation of, *22*, 129, *130*
  opening of. See *Incisions*.
  reconstruction of, 621, *623*, 624, *624*
Abdominis muscles, *22*, 127–128, *128*
Ablation, endometrial, 367, 369, 510
Abortion, endometriosis and, 574
  incomplete, D & C in, 258
    suction curettage in, 263
  tubal, 491
Abscess, breast, 591, *593*
  intra-abdominal, 49
  parastomal, 416
  vulvar, 161–162
Acid-base balance, 35
  postoperative disorders of, 39–41, 41t
Acidosis, 40–41, 41t
Addison's disease, 60–61
Adenocarcinoma, endometrial. See *Endometrium, adenocarcinoma of*.
  vaginal, 201, 207–208
  vulvar, 195
Adenosquamous carcinoma, vulvar, 195
Adhesions, 147–158
  adnexal, 471, *472*, 474–475, *475*
    classification of, *483*
  anticoagulants and, 153
  anti-inflammatory agents and, 153
  barriers against, 154–155
  incidence of, 147–148, 148t, *149*
  laparoscopy and, 152–153

Adhesions *(Continued)*
  lasers and, 152
  microsurgery and, 152
  pathogenesis of, 148–151, *150*, *151*
  pregnancy and, 155–157
  reduction of, 151t, 151–152
  reproductive surgery and, 94–95, 147, 155–157, *156*
  small bowel obstruction and, 52
  sutures and, 110
  thrombolytic agents and, 154
Adnexa, adhesions of, 471, *472*, 474–475, *475*
  classification of, *483*
  hysterectomy and, 338, *339*, *340*, 345, *346*
  surgery on, 513–521. See also specific procedure.
Adult respiratory distress syndrome (ARDS), 75–76
Aesculapius, 2–3
Aetius of Amida, 5
Aldosterone, 35
Aldridge sling modification, 302, 304, *304*
Alexandrian school, 4
Alkalosis, 40, 40t, 41t
Allergy, preoperative evaluation of, 29
Analgesia, front-loading for, 42, 43t
  intraspinal, 43–44
  patient-controlled, 42–43
    problems with, 43t
  postoperative, 41–44
Anastomosis, intestinal, 399–402. See also *Anastomosis, large bowel*; *Anastomosis, small bowel*.
  disruption of, 405, 407, 412, 412t
  hand-sewn, 400, *400*

Anastomosis *(Continued)*
  in radiation injury, 421
  principles of, 399–400
  stapled, 400–401, *401*, *402*
  large bowel, 407, *407*, 409–411, *409–411*
    complications of, 412, 412t
    protective colostomy and, 411, 412t
  small bowel, 402, *402–405*, 405, 407
    care after, 405
    complications of, 405, 407
  tubal, for sterilization reversal, 460–461, 461t
    isthmic, *459*, 459–460, *460*, 494–495
    success rates of, 460t
    vs. IVF, 553–554
  ureteral, 434, *434*–435, *435*
    leakage from, 446
Anatomy, abdominal wall, 21, *22*, 23, *23*, 127–129, *128–130*
  gastrointestinal, 395–396, *396*
  isthmic tubal, 453–454, *454*
  landmarks in, *23*
  nerve injury and, 26–27
  of connective tissue spaces, 316, *317*
  of pelvic support structures, 314–316, *315*, *316*
  pelvic, 23–26, *24–26*
  peripheral nervous system, 26–27
  presacral, 25–26, *26*
  urinary tract, 427–430, *428*, *429*
  uterine, 354–355
  vaginal, 26, *26*, 314
  vulvar, 26, *26*, 173–176, *174*, *175*
Anemia, 68
Anesthesia, consent for, 31–32
  epidural, 43–44
  for D & C, 259

651

Anesthesia *(Continued)*
　history of, 10, *11*
　in oocyte recovery, 559
　intraspinal, 43–44
　liver disease and, 78, 79
Angiography, multigated, 63
Anion gap, 40
Anoproctectomy, 191
Anterior abdominal wall. See *Abdominal wall.*
Anterior colporrhaphy, 322–324, *322–324*
Antibiotics. See also specific drug or class.
　history of, 16–17
　in abscess, 49
　in COPD, 74
　prophylactic, 44–45, 51
　　before gastrointestinal surgery, 398
　　before hysterectomy, 274, 336
　　for bacterial endocarditis, 66t
Anticholinergic agents, in asthma, 72
Anticoagulants. See also *Heparin.*
　adhesions and, 153
Antidiuretic hormone, 35
　inappropriate secretion of, 38
　postoperative levels of, 39
Antihypertensive agents, 67t
Anti-inflammatory agents, adhesions and, 153
Antisepsis, history of, 14
Aortic stenosis, 65t, 65–66
Appendicitis, vs. ovarian torsion, 516
Arcuate line, 128
ARDS (adult respiratory distress syndrome), 75–76
Argon beam coagulator, 536
Argon laser, 121, 122
　properties of, 122t
Aristotle, 3, 353
Arrhythmias, 65
ART. See *Assisted reproductive technology (ART).*
Artificial insemination. See *Insemination.*
Ascherman's syndrome, 265
Ascites, 78
Aspiration cytology, in endometrial adenocarcinoma evaluation, 376
　of breast mass, 586–587, *587*
　　cystic, 585–586, *586*
　　nonpalpable, 590
Aspirator-irrigators, 114, *115*
Aspirators, 104, *104*, 536, *537*
Assisted reproductive technology (ART), 549–567
　embryo transfer in, 560–561, *561*
　GIFT in, 88t, 549, 562, *563*, 564, *564*
　　results of, 565t, 566t
　history of, 549
　in endometriosis, 554–555, 581
　in immunologic infertility, 555
　in male factor infertility, 555
　in ovarian failure, 555
　in tubal disease, 553–554
　in unexplained infertility, 555
　indications for, 554, 554t
　insemination in, 549–553
　　cervical, 550, *550*
　　intraperitoneal, 551, 552–553
　　intratubal, *551*, 553
　　intrauterine, 550, *550*, 552, *553*
　multiple gestation in, 561
　　reduction of, 565–566
　oocyte recovery in, 555–560
　　anesthesia for, 559
　　complications of, 559–560
　　laparoscopic, 556, *556*
　　needles for, 558, *559*

Assisted reproductive technology (ART) *(Continued)*
　　timing of, 555, *555*
　　ultrasound-guided, 556–559, *557–559*
　patient selection for, 553–555
　procedures in, 550t
　results of, 565t, 566, 566t
　ZIFT in, 564–565
Asthma, 71–72
Atelectasis, 74–75
　treatment of, 75t
Avicenna, 5
Axial translocation, 607, *610*
Axillary dissection, in breast cancer, 595, *597*, *598*, 599

Bacteria, in pulmonary infections, 47
　in salpingitis, 469
　in urinary tract infections, 47
　indigenous, 44t
Bacterial endocarditis, prophylaxis of, 66t
Bacteriology, 14
Bartholin's gland, 161, 174
　carcinoma of, 194, *194*
　cyst of, 161–163, *163*
　　vs. cyst of canal of Nuck, 163
　excision of, 163
　incision of, 161–162, *162*
　marsupialization of, 162–163, *163*
Basal cell carcinoma, vulvar, 195
Battery procedure, 14
Benign ovarian teratoma, 513–516
Berengarius of Bologna, 15
Beta-adrenergic agonists, in asthma, 72
Beta blockade, perioperative, 64
Bilateral groin incisions, 139, *140*
Biopsy. See also *Cone biopsy.*
　breast, excisional, 589, *589*
　　incisional, 588, *588*, 589
　　needle localization in, 589–591, *590*
　　Tru-Cut needle in, 587–588, *588*
　cervical. See *Cervix, biopsy of.*
　endometrial, 265, 374, *374*
　　in infertility, 90
　hysteroscopic, 509, *510*
　in ovarian cancer surgery, second-look, 537, *538*
　　staging, 527
　scalene fat pad, 288, *289*
　vulvar, 160
　wedge, ovarian, 520–521, *521*
Bladder. See also *Vesico-* entries.
　anatomy of, 429, 429–430
　injury to, 440–441, *441*
　　during hysterectomy, 339, 440
　　radiation, 449, 451
　mobilization of, in hysterectomy, 338–340, *340*
　ovarian cancer and, 534
　pelvic anatomy and, 23–24, *24*
　prolapse of, 317, *318*, 320–322
　　treatment of, 322–324, *322–324*
　repair of, 441, *441*
　resection of, 205, *207*
　suprapubic drainage of, 281
Bleeding, abnormal, D & C and, 257–259
　endometrial ablation and, 367, 369
　endometrial adenocarcinoma and, 259, 372, *372*
　leiomyomas and, 356
　postmenopausal, 259, 372
　after conization, 268–269
　after D & C, 265
　after hysterectomy, 348
　after oocyte recovery, 560

Bleeding *(Continued)*
　after surgical staging, 387
　stomal, 416
Bleeding time, 69
Blood circulation. See also *Blood supply.*
　endometriosis and, 570
　Harvey on, 7–8, *8*
Blood loss, 70
　fluid replacement and, 36
　from esophageal varices, 80
　heparin prophylaxis and, 55
　myomectomy and, 358
Blood supply, abdominal wall, 128–129, *129*, *130*
　bladder, 430
　gastrointestinal, 395–396, *396*, *397*
　pelvic, 25, *25*
　ureteral, *428*, 429
　uterine, 25, *25*, 354–355
　vulvovaginal, 26, 174, 314
Blood transfusions, 70
　anemia and, 68
　autologous, 336
　hepatitis and, 79
　in renal disease, 76
　platelets in, 69, 70
Boari flap, 435, 438, *438*
Body weight, 33
Bowel preparation, 51, 51t
　before fistula repair, 219
　before gastrointestinal surgery, 397–399, 398t
　before ovarian cancer surgery, 524–525
Bowenoid papillosis. See *Vulvar intraepithelial neoplasia (VIN).*
Brachytherapy. See *Radiotherapy.*
Breast, 585–606
　abscess of, 591, *593*
　aspiration of, 586–587, *587*
　biopsy of, excisional, 589, *589*
　　incisional, 588, *588*, 589
　　needle localization in, 589–591, *590*
　　Tru-Cut needle in, 587–588, *588*
　cancer of, 585, 594–605
　　adjuvant therapy for, 594–595
　　axillary dissection in, 595, *597*, *598*, 599
　　lumpectomy in, 594, 595, *596*
　　mastectomy in, history of, 594
　　　modified radical, 599, *600–602*
　　　radical, 599, *603–605*, 605
　　screening for, 585
　cyst of, 585–586, *586*
　discharge from, 591, *592*
Broders, A. C., 9
Bronchitis, chronic, 73
Bronchodilators, 72
Bulbocavernous flap technique, in fistula repair, 217, *217*, 226
　in vaginal reconstruction, 615
Bupivicaine, 44–45
Burch procedure, 300, *301*, 302
Bypass, intestinal, *420*, 420–421

CA-125, in endometriosis, 91
　in ovarian cancer, 539
Calcium, blood transfusions and, 70
　daily requirements of, 36t
Calf compression, postoperative, 56
Caloric requirements, preoperative, 32t
Canal of Nuck cyst, 163
Carbohydrates, daily requirements of, 36t
Carbon dioxide laser, 121–125, 505
　delivery system of, 123–124

INDEX 653

Carbon dioxide laser *(Continued)*
  in endometriosis, 577
  properties of, 122t
Carcinoma in situ (CIS). See also *Cervical intraepithelial neoplasia (CIN)*.
  defined, 232–233
  natural history of, 231–232
Carcinomatosis, intestinal obstruction and, 423
Cardiac output, 67–68
Cardinal ligaments, 314, 355
  in hysterectomy, 341, 343, *344*
Cardiovascular disease, 61–68
  hemodynamic monitoring in, 67–68
  preoperative evaluation in, 61, 62–63
Caruncle, urethral, 309, *309*
Catheter(s), embryo transfer, 560, 561, *561*
  insemination, 552, *552*, 553, *553*
  pulmonary artery, 67–68
  Swan-Ganz, 67
Catheterization, fallopian tube, for GIFT, 562, *563*, 564, *564*
  phlebitis and, 47–48
  pulmonary artery, 68
  urinary tract infections and, 47
Cavitron ultrasonic surgical aspirator, 104, *104*, 536, *537*
Cellulitis, vaginal cuff, 48
Central venous pressure, 67
Cephalosporins, prophylactic, 45
Cervical dilators, *260*, 260–261, *634*
  gauge conversion scale for, 261t
Cervical intraepithelial neoplasia (CIN), 231–244
  clinical management of, 234, *235*
  defined, 232
  epidemiology of, 233–234
  natural history of, 231–232
  risk factors for, 233–234
  treatment of, cone biopsy in, 241–242, *242, 243*, 244
    cryosurgery in, 235t, 235–236, *236*
    electrocautery in, 238, *239*, 239t
    interferon in, 240, 240t
    laser in, 236–238, *237*, 237t
    vs. cryosurgery, 238t
    LEEP in, 240–241, *241*, 241t
    cone biopsy with, 242, *243*, 244
Cervical pregnancy, 496
Cervicitis, chronic, 265–266
Cervix. See also *Cervical intraepithelial neoplasia (CIN)*.
  anatomy of, 354
  biopsy of, 234, *235*
    cone, 241–242, *242, 243*, 244, 265–269
      cold knife in, 241–242, *242*, 267, *267*–268
      complications of, 268–269
      in cancer, 271, *272*
      in pregnancy, 269
      indications for, 266, 266t
      interpretation of, 268
      laser in, 242, *243*, 268
      LEEP in, 242, *243*, 244
      transformation zone and, 266, *266*–267, *267*
    in CIN, 234, *235*
  cancer of, 271–296
    barrel-shaped, 282, *282*
    cone biopsy in, 271, *272*
    exenteration in, 288–290, *291*–*293*, 294
    hysterectomy in, 273, 274–275, *276*–*280*, 281–282
      extrafascial, 282–283, 283t, *284*–*285*
      para-aortic lymphadenectomy with, 283, 286, 286t, *287*, 288

Cervix *(Continued)*
  microinvasive, 271, *272*, 273, 273–274
    defined, 271
    lymph nodes and, 273, *273*, 273t, 274
  radiotherapy in, 629–637
    complications of, 637
    external-beam, 630–631
    guidelines for, 636t
    instruments for, *630*, 631, *632*–*636*
    intracavitary, 631, *631*, 633, 637
    planning for, 631t
    results of, 637t, 638t
    sources of, 631, *631*, 633
    scalene fat pad biopsy in, 288, *289*
    urinary tract and, 430
  circumcision of, 343, *343*
  support of, 314–315
  transition zone of, 267
Cesarean section, history of, 6–7
Cesium sources, 631, *631*, 633, *633*, 640
Chain, Ernst, 17
Chemotherapy, in breast cancer, 594–595
  in endometrial adenocarcinoma, 388t
  in ovarian cancer, cytoreduction with. See *Cytoreduction*.
    intraperitoneal, 544
  in vaginal sarcoma, 209
  in VAIN, 247, *247*
  in VIN, 251
  in vulvar carcinoma, 192
  in vulvar rhabdomyosarcoma, 196
Cherney's incision, *134*, 134–135, *135*
Chest films, preoperative, 71
  in infertility, 91
  in ovarian cancer, 524
Childbirth, after myomectomy, 360
  cystocele and, 321
  prolapse and, 319, 321, 324
  rectocele and, 324
  sterilization after, 518, *519*
Child's classification of liver dysfunction, 78t
Chlamydia trachomatis, in salpingitis, 469
Chromopertubation, 473, *473*
Chronic bronchitis, 73
Chronic obstructive pulmonary disease (COPD), 73–74
Cilia, tubal, 467, *467*, 468
CIN. See *Cervical intraepithelial neoplasia (CIN)*.
Circulation, blood. See also *Blood supply*.
  endometriosis and, 570
  Harvey on, 7–8, *8*
Circumflex artery, 129, *129*, 130
Cirrhosis, 78, 79
  postoperative care in, 80
CIS. See *Carcinoma in situ (CIS)*.
Clamps, 97, *98*, 101–102, *102*
  for reproductive surgery, 111, *111*
Clear cell carcinoma, vaginal, 201, 644, *644*
Clips, surgical, 104, *104*, 105
Clitoris, 173–174, *174*
  lesions of, 179
Cloquet's node, 175
Clostridium difficile, in postoperative diarrhea, 53
Closure, delayed primary, 48, 143–144
  instruments for, 105, *105*
  of large defects, in vulvar carcinoma, 186, *187*–*190*, 188
  of midline incision, *136*, 136–138, *137*, 137t
  of vaginal vault, 348

Closure *(Continued)*
  sutures for, 105, 131–132, 132t, 134, *136*, 136–138, 137t
Coagulation disorders, 68–69
  in liver disease, 77–78, 80
  in renal disease, 76
  postoperative, 70
Colectomy, care after, 411
  partial, with re-anastomosis, 407, *407*
    complications of, 412, 412t
  sigmoid, 408–411, *408*–*411*
Colles' fascia, 26
Colon, blood supply to, *397*
  endometriosis of, *572*, 581
    symptoms of, 574
  in vaginal reconstruction, 612, *614*
  obstruction of, ovarian cancer and, 543–544
    postoperative, 53
    radiation-induced, 418
  perforation of, 418
  preparation of, 51, 51t, 397–399, 398t
    before fistula repair, 219
    before ovarian cancer surgery, 524–525
  radiation injury to, 417–419, *418*
  surgery on, *406*–411, *407*–*412*. See also *Colostomy*.
    care after, 411, 412t
    complications of, 412, 412t
    in ovarian cancer debulking, 532–533, *533*
  urinary diversion to, 442–443, 444–445, *445*
Colostomy, 408, *408*
  counseling before, 397
  in postoperative rectovaginal fistula, 54, 229
  loop, 414–416, *415*, *416*
  ovarian cancer and, 533, 543–544
  protective, 411, 412t
  re-anastomosis and, 407, *407*, 408–411, *408*–*411*
  stoma formation in, 412–417, *413*–*416*
    complications of, 416–417
    in end colostomy, 412–413, *413*, *414*
    in loop colostomy, 414–416, *415*, *416*
    J-loop, 413–414
    mucous fistula with, 414
    site for, 412
    with EEA instrument, 413, *414*
Colpocleisis, partial, in fistula repair, 226
Colpopexy, abdominal sacral, in vaginal prolapse, 331–332
Colporrhaphy, anterior, 322–324, *322*–*324*
  posterior, 325–327, *325*–*327*
Colposcope, 234, *234*
Colposcopy, in CIN, 234, *235*, 266
Colpostats, *630*, 631, *632*, *639*
  insertion of, 633, *633*–*636*, 637
Computed tomography (CT), in endometrial adenocarcinoma evaluation, 375, 376
  in ovarian cancer, diagnostic, 524
  vs. second-look laparotomy, 539
  of urinary tract, 431
Conduits, urinary, 443–446
  colonic, 444–445, *445*
  complications of, 445–446
  ileal, 443–444, *444*
  preoperative preparation for, 443
Condylomata, vulvar, 160–161
Cone biopsy, 241–242, *242, 243*, 244, 265–269
  cold knife in, 241–242, *242*, 267, *267*–268

Cone biopsy *(Continued)*
  complications of, 268–269
  in cancer, 271, *272*
  in pregnancy, 269
  indications for, 266, 266t
  interpretation of, 268
  laser in, 242, *243*, 268
  LEEP in, 242, *243*, 244
  transformation zone and, 266, 266–267, *267*
Congestive heart failure, 64–65
  signs and symptoms of, 64t
Connective tissue spaces, 316, *317*
Consent, informed, 30–32
  for reproductive surgery, 87–88
Continent urinary diversion, 446–447, *447–449*, 449
COPD (chronic obstructive pulmonary disease), 73–74
Coronary artery disease, 61–64
Corticosteroids, 61
  in asthma, 72
  perioperative, 59, 61
Counseling, before exenteration, 290
  before hysterectomy, 350
  before intestinal resection, 397
  before ovarian cancer surgery, 524, 528
  before reproductive surgery, 89
  before sterilization, 517
Cromolyn sodium, 72
Cryosurgery, in CIN, 235t, 235–236, *236*
  vs. laser treatment, 238t
CT. See *Computed tomography (CT)*.
Culdocentesis, in ectopic pregnancy, 490
Cullen's sign, 489
Curettage, 262–263, *263*. See also *Dilatation and curettage (D & C)*.
Curettes, 262, *263*
  suction, 263
Cutaneous ureterostomy, 442
Cylinders, dome, 639, *640*
  vaginal, *632, 634, 645, 646*
Cyst(s), Bartholin's gland, 161–163, *162*
  vs. cyst of canal of Nuck, 163
  breast, aspiration of, 585–586, *586*
  canal of Nuck, 163
  embryology of, 21, *22*
  endometriotic, 514, *515*, 571–573, *573*
  Gartner's duct, 21, *22*
  ovarian, 513–516
    benign (teratoma), 513–516
      bilateral, 514
      surgery in, *514*, 514–516
    functional, 513
    laparoscopy for, 515–516
    malignant germ cell tumors with, 528–529
  parovarian, 21, *22*
  vulvar, 161–163, *162, 163*
Cystitis, hemorrhagic, radiation-induced, 449, 551
Cystocele, 317, *318*, 320–322
  repair of, 322–324, *322–324*
Cystoscopy, preoperative, 431
Cystourethrocele, 317, *318*
Cystourethropexy, Gittes, *307*, 307–308
Cytoreduction, in ovarian cancer, new techniques for, 536, *537*
  primary, 529–536
    diaphragmatic tumor resection in, *535*, 535–536
    efficacy of, 530
    exploration in, 530–531
    lymph node resection in, 536
    omentectomy in, 531, *531, 532*

Cytoreduction *(Continued)*
    pelvic tumor resection in, 531–532, *532*
    rectosigmoid resection in, 532–533, *533*
    splenectomy in, *534*, 534–535, *535*
  secondary, 540–542
    after suboptimal debulking, 541–542
    at second-look laparotomy, 542
    for chemotherapy nonresponders, 540–541
    for recurrent disease, 541
  in uterine cancer, 380, 386
  instruments for, 104, *104*, 536
Czerney, Vincenz, 15

D & C. See *Dilatation and curettage (D & C)*.
Debulking. See *Cytoreduction*.
Decompression, in intestinal obstruction, 423, 543
Deep venous thrombosis, postoperative, 54–58
  management of, 56–58
  prophylaxis of, 54–56
  risk factors for, 54
Dehiscence, 144–145
  incision type and, 134
  sutures and, 137, 137t
Dermatofibrosarcoma, vulvar, 197
Dermoid cyst, ovarian, 513–516
DES (diethylstilbestrol), clear cell carcinoma associated with, 201
  embryologic development and, 20–21, *21*
Dextran-70, 94, 154–155, 509
Diabetes, 58–59
Dialysis, 77
Diaphragm, ovarian cancer and, *535*, 535–536
  pelvic, 315–316
  urogenital, 316
Diarrhea, postoperative, 53
  radiation-induced, 418, 419
Diethylstilbestrol (DES), clear cell carcinoma associated with, 201
  embryologic development and, 20–21, *21*
Dilatation and curettage (D & C), anesthesia for, 259
  complications of, *264*, 264–265
  curettage in, 262–263, *263*
  dilatation in, 260–262, *260–262*
    passive, 261–262
  endometrial biopsy and, 265
  history of, 257
  indications for, 257–259, 490–491
  patient positioning for, 260
  ultrasound guidance with, *263*, 263–264
Dilators, cervical, *260*, 260–261
  gauge conversion scale for, 261t
Dipyridamole-thallium scale, 63
Distal fallopian tube. See *Fallopian tube(s), distal*.
Distention media, 94, 154–155, 509
Diversion, urinary. See *Urinary diversion*.
Diverticulum, urethral, 309, *310*, 311
Diverting colostomy, 411, 412t
Documentation, 502
Dome cylinders, 639, *640*
Drainage, 132–133, *133*
  in abdominal abscess, 49
  in Bartholin's duct abscess, 162

Drainage *(Continued)*
  in hysterectomy, 275, 281
  suprapubic bladder, 281
Drugs. See also specific drug or class.
  allergy to, 29
  liver disease and, 78
  platelets and, 69
  preoperative evaluation of, 29
  renal disease and, 76–77
Duct excision, breast, 591, *592*
Dura mater, for femoral vessel coverage, 620, *621*
Dysmenorrhea, D & C in, 259

Ectopic pregnancy, 487–499
  abdominal, 496
  cervical, 496
  clinical presentation in, 488–489
  D & C in, 258, 490–491
  diagnosis of, 489–491
  epidemiology of, 487
  fertility after, 497t, 497–498
  interstitial, 496
  isthmic tube, 456–459, *457–459*, 493, 494–495
    vs. ampullary ectopics, 457, *457*
  laparoscopy in, 491–492, 496
  medical therapy of, 458, 491
  ovarian, 496
  pathophysiology of, 457, 487–488
  persistent, 497
  recurrent, 488
  Rh factor and, 496–497
  SIN and, 455–456, 488
  sites of, 488
  surgery in, 457–459, *457–459*, 491–496, *492–495*
Edema, leg, after vulvar carcinoma surgery, 188
  pulmonary, 64–65
    cardiogenic, 75
    noncardiogenic, 75–76
Egyptian medicine, 2–3
Ehrlich, Paul, 16
Elastic stockings, 55–56
Electrocardiography, postoperative, 63–64
  preoperative, in infertility, 92–93
Electrocautery, 104. See also *Electrosurgery*.
Electrodes, 118, 120
Electrolyte balance, 35–37
  disease states and, 35
  maintenance of, 36, 36t
  postoperative management of, 38–39
  preexisting disorders of, 37–38
  urinary diversion and, 446
Electrolyte replacement, 36–38
Electrons, 120, *120*
Electrosurgery, 116–118, *117–120*, 120
  cytoreductive, 536
  in CIN, 238, *239*, 239t, 240–241, 241t
  cone biopsy with, 242, *243*, 244
  in endometriosis, 577
  instruments for, 113, *114*, 116, 118, 120, 505, *505*, 508
  lasers vs., 125
  principles of, 117–118, *117–120*
  unipolar vs. bipolar cautery in, 117–118, *119*
Embolism, pulmonary, postoperative, 54–58, 281–282
  management of, 57–58
  prophylaxis of, 54–56
  risk factors for, 54

INDEX 655

Embryo transfer, 560–561, *561*. See also *Gamete intrafallopian transfer (GIFT)*; *Zygote intrafallopian transfer (ZIFT)*.
Embryology, 19–21
  mesonephric remnants and, 21, *22*
  of endometriosis, 570
  of female genital tract, 20–21, *21*
  of ovary, 19–20
Emphysema, 73
Encephalopathy, hepatic, 80
Endocarditis, bacterial, prophylaxis of, 66t
Endodermal sinus tumors, vulvar, 197
Endometrioma, 514, *515*, 571–573, *573*
  laparotomy and, *580*
  laser incision of, 578, *579*
Endometriosis, 569–584
  ART in, 554–555, 581
  classification of, 575, *576*
  clinical characteristics of, 573–574
  diagnosis of, 574–575, *575*
  epidemiology of, 569–570
  fallopian tube, 456, *571*
  gastrointestinal tract, *572*, 574, 581
  histogenesis of, 570–571
    by lymphatic spread, 570
    by retrograde menstruation, 570–571
    iatrogenic, 570, *570*
  hysterectomy in, 581
  infertility and, 554–555, 573–574
  malignancy and, 582, *582*
  ovarian, 514, *515*, *572*, 573, *573*, 578, *579*, *580*
  pathology of, gross, *572*, 572–573, *573*
    microscopic, *571*, 571–572, *572*
  presacral neurectomy in, 580
  treatment of, 575–582
    definitive, 581
    expectant, 575–576
    laparoscopic, 576–578, *577–579*
      pregnancy after, 580t
    laparotomy in, 578, *580*, 580–581
    medical, 88–89, 576
  urinary tract, 574, 581–582
Endometrium, ablation of, 367, 369, 510
  adenocarcinoma of, 371–389
    abnormal bleeding and, 259, 372, *372*
    advanced, 378, 391
    chemotherapy for, 333t
    clinical presentation of, 372, 372–373, *373*
    diagnosis of, 374, *374*
    epidemiology of, 371
    estrogen and, 371–372
    hormonal therapy for, 388t
    preoperative evaluation and staging of, 374–376, *375*, 377t
    prognosis in, 376–379, *377*, 377t
    radiotherapy of, 376, 388t, 388–389, 637–640
      instruments for, *639*, *640*
      postoperative, 639–640, *640*
      preoperative, 638–639, *639*
    recurrence sites of, 389, 390–391
    spread of, *373*, 373–374
    surgery in, extended staging, 380–381, *381–385*, 386–388
      for primary tumor, *379*, 379–380, *380*
    surgical staging of, 377t, 377–381, *378*, *381–385*, 386–388
      advantages of, 387
      disadvantages of, 387–388
      risks of, 386–387
    urinary tract and, 430
  anatomy of, 354, *355*
  biopsy of, 265, 374, *374*

Endometrium *(Continued)*
  in infertility, 90
Enteral fistulas, 422
Enteral nutrition, 33, 405
Enterocele, 317–318, *318*
  prevention of, 346–347, *347*
  repair of, 328–329, *329*
Enterocutaneous fistula, 422
  postoperative, 53–54
Enterostomal therapist, 412, 443
Enterovaginal fistula, anatomy of, *214*
Epidural anesthesia, 43–44
Epigastric vessels, 22, 23, *23*, 128–129, *129*, *130*
Episiotomy, 164–165, *166*, 167
  endometriosis at site of, *570*, 571
  mediolateral, 165, 167
  midline, 164–165
Esmolol, 67t
Esophageal varices, 80
Estrogen, and endometrial adenocarcinoma, 371–372
Estrogen-progestin therapy, in functional ovarian cyst, 513
Evaluation, preoperative. See *Preoperative evaluation and care*.
Evisceration, 136, 144–145
  suturing and, 136–137
Exenteration, 288–290, *292–293*, 294
  anterior, 288–289
  complications of, 294
  contraindications to, 290
  counseling before, 290
  in uterine carcinoma, 380, 391
  in vaginal carcinoma, 207, *208*
  low rectal anastomosis and, 289
  reconstruction after. See *Reconstructive surgery*.
  survival after, 294t
  urinary conduits in. See *Urinary diversion*.
Exercise testing, preoperative, 62–63
External oblique muscle, 22, 127–128, *128*, *130*
External pneumatic leg compression, postoperative, 56
Extraperitoneal approaches, for incisions. See *Incisions, for extraperitoneal approaches*.

Fabiola, 4
Fallopian tube(s). See also *Ectopic pregnancy*.
  ampullary, 467
    surgery on, *492*, 492–494
  catheterization of, for GIFT, 562, *563*, 564, *564*
  distal, 465–485
    disease of, classification of, 469, *470*
    laparoscopy of, 479, *480*, 481
      instruments for, 479t
    surgery on, 469, 471t
      adhesiolysis in, 474–475, *475*
      care after, 481
      closure in, 479
      contraindications to, 471t
      definitions of, 471t
      evaluation before, 469, 471, *471*, 472, 472t, 473
      fertility after, 481, 482t, 484
      fimbrioplasty in, 476, *478*
      historical aspects of, 465, 465t, *466*, 467
      incision for, 474, *474*

Fallopian tube(s) *(Continued)*
      instruments for, 473, 473t
      laparotomy in, 473–476, *473–478*
      laser in, 479t
      salpingostomy in, 475–476, *476–478*, 477
  endometriosis of, 456, *571*
  endoscopy of, 461–462, 510–511
  function of, 453, 467
  isthmic, 453–463
    anatomy of, 453–454, *454*
    epithelium of, 454, *454*
    function of, 453
    surgery on, 454–461
      anastomosis in, *459*, 459–460, *460*, 460t, 494–495
      in ectopic pregnancy, 456–459, *457–459*, *493*, 494–495
      in endometriosis, 456
      in PID, 456
      in SIN, 455–456
  patency of, evaluation of, 92, *92*, *93*, 110–111, *111*, *112*
  pathology of, 455–456, *467*, 467–469, *468*
  PID and, 456, 457, 469
  probes for, 111, *112*
  salvage of, 520, 553–554
  sterilization and, 460–461, 517–518, *518*, *519*. See also *Sterilization*.
  surgical repair of, vs. IVF, 553–554
Fallopius, Gabriel, 6, 465
Falloposcopy, 510–511
  training in, 511–512
Fascia, 22, 26, 127–128, *128*
Fascia lata, in stress incontinence sling procedure, 304, *305*
Fasciitis, necrotizing, 49–51
  clinical data in, 50t
Fatio, J., 12
Femoral artery, *25*
Femoral nerve, surgical injury to, 27
Femoral vessels, necrosis of, 615, 620, *620*
  coverage in, 615, 620, *620*, *621*
Fertility. See *Infertility*.
Fever, post-hysterectomy, 348
  postoperative, 46
  fistula and, 53
Fiberoptics, 124, *124*
Fibrin, adhesions and, 150–151
Fibroid. See *Leiomyoma*.
FIGO staging, of endometrial adenocarcinoma, 375, 375t, 377t
  of ovarian cancer, 526t
  of vaginal cancer, 526t
  of vulvar carcinoma, 176, 176t
Fimbria, adhesions and, *149*
Fimbrial expression, in ectopic pregnancy, 493–494
Fimbriectomy, Kroener, 518, *518*
Fimbrioplasty, 476, *478*
  defined, 471t
Fine-needle aspiration cytology, in breast mass evaluation, 586–587, *587*
  nonpalpable, 590
  in endometrial adenocarcinoma evaluation, 376
Fistula, 213–229. See also specific type.
  anatomy of, *214*
  postoperative, 53–54, 281, 281t
  urinary diversion with, 217–218
Fleming, Alexander, 16
Florey, Howard, 17
Fluid balance, 35–37
  disease states and, 35
  maintenance of, 36, 36t

Fluid balance (Continued)
  postoperative management of, 38–39
  preexisting disorders of, 37
Fluid replacement, 36–37
Fluorouracil, in VAIN, 247, 247
  in VIN, 251
Forceps, 101
  hysteroscopic, 510
  laparoscopic, 113, 113, 503, 504
    for tissue removal, 507–508, 508
  tissue, 109, 109
Frank nonoperative technique, 610t, 611, 611–612
Free flap, 615
French scale, 261
Futh-Mayo technique, 216

Galactorrhea, 591
Galen, 4
Gamete intrafallopian transfer (GIFT), 88t, 549, 562, 563, 564, 564
  complications of, 564
  in endometriosis, 581
  indications for, 554t
  laparoscopic, 562, 563, 564
  patient selection for, 562
  results of, 565t, 566t
  transcervical, 564, 564
Gartner's duct cyst, 21, 22
Gastrointestinal fistula, 422
  postoperative, 53
    TPN and, 34, 53–54
Gastrointestinal fluid, composition of, 36, 37t
  replacement of, 36–37
Gastrointestinal tract, anatomy of, 395–396, 396, 397
  endometriosis of, 581
    symptoms in, 574
  fistulas in, 422
    postoperative, 53
      TPN and, 34, 53–54
  injury to, during hysterectomy, 349–350
    during surgical staging, 387
    radiation-induced, 417–421, 418–421
  obstruction of, 422–424
    ovarian cancer and, 542–544, 544
  surgery on, 402, 402–411, 405, 407–412. See also such procedures as Colostomy.
    anastomosis in, 399–402
      disruption of, 405, 407, 412, 412t
      hand-sewn, 400, 400
      in radiation injury, 421
      principles of, 399–400
      stapled, 400–401, 401, 402
      stricture of, 412
    bypass, 420, 420–421
    care after, 405, 411, 412t
    complications of, 405, 407, 412, 412t
    gastrostomy and, 417
    history of, 399
    in enteral fistula, 422
    ovarian cancer surgery and, 524–525, 532–534, 533
    preparation before, 51, 51t, 397–399, 398t
    sling, 421, 421
    urinary diversion. See Urinary diversion.
Gastrostomy, 417, 543, 544
Generators, 118
Genital hiatus, 315, 315
Genital prolapse. See Prolapse.

Genital tract, female. See also specific organ.
  embryology of, 20–21, 21
Genital warts, 160–161
Germ cell tumors, 528–529
  second-look laparotomy in, 539
GIFT. See Gamete intrafallopian transfer (GIFT).
Gittes cystourethropexy, 307, 307–308
Gluteus maximus myocutaneous graft, 186, 188, 190, 615
  for sacral defects, 624, 625, 626
GnRH (gonadotropin-releasing hormone), agonists to, before hysterectomy, 336
  before myomectomy, 359
  preoperative, 88–89
Goebell-Frangenheim-Stoeckel procedure, 302, 303
Gold-grain implanter, 649
  needle guides for, 649
Gold-grain implants, in recurrent vaginal cancer radiotherapy, 642, 644, 648, 648, 649, 650
  results of, 650t
GoLYTELY, 51, 51t, 398, 398t
Gonadotropin-releasing hormone (GnRH), agonists to, before hysterectomy, 336
  before myomectomy, 359
  preoperative, 88–89
Gore-Tex mesh, in stress incontinence sling procedures, 304, 305
Gracilis myocutaneous graft, 186, 187–188, 615, 616–618
Granulosa cell tumors, 529
Greek medicine, 3–4, 353
Groin, bilateral incisions of, 139, 140
  dissection of, in vulvar carcinoma, 179–182, 181, 182
    radical vulvectomy with, 183, 183, 184, 185
  reconstructive surgery on, 615, 620, 620–621

Halothane, liver disease and, 78, 79
Halsted, William, 14, 594
Harris uterine manipulator, 111, 111
Hartmann pouch, 408, 408
Harvey, William, 7–8, 8
hCG (human chorionic gonadotropin), in abnormal pregnancy, 258
  ectopic, 489
  in IVF, 555
  reference standards for, 490
Headlamps, 100, 101
Heart, output of, 67–68
Heart block, surgery and, 65
Heart failure, congestive, 64–65
  signs and symptoms of, 64t
Heart valve disorders, 65–66
  signs and symptoms of, 65t
Hematologic disorders, 68–70
  in renal disease, 76
Hematometra, 167
Hemodynamic monitoring, 67–68
  in ARDS, 76
Hemorrhage. See Bleeding.
Hemorrhagic cystitis, radiation-induced, 449, 551
Hemostasis, in conization, 267
  in hysterectomy, 342
  instruments for, 103–104, 104
Heparin, adhesions and, 153

Heparin (Continued)
  in postoperative thromboembolism, 57
  prophylactic, 54–56, 281–282
Hepatic encephalopathy, 80
Hepatitis, 78, 79
  halothane-induced, 79
  post-transfusion, 79
Hepatorenal syndrome, 79–80
Hernia. See also Prolapse.
  peristomal, 416
Herophilus of Chalcedon, 353
Heyman capsule, 639
Hippocrates, 3, 3–4, 353
History, patient medical. See Medical history.
  surgical, 1–18
    ancient, 2–4, 353
    early modern, 7–10
    genital prolapse treatment in, 313
    intestinal resection in, 399
    medieval, 5
    modern, 10–17
    Renaissance, 6–7
    tubal operations in, 465, 465t, 466, 467
    uterine operations in, 353–354
Holmes, Oliver Wendell, 14, 16
Hormonal therapy, in breast cancer, 594–595
  in endometrial adenocarcinoma, 388t
  in endometriosis, 576
    postoperative, 580–581
Hormones. See also specific hormones.
  ectopic pregnancy and, 488
  leiomyomas and, 355–356
  tubal contractility and, 453–454
Hospice, origin of, 2–3
Hospitals, origin of, 4
Human chorionic gonadotropin (hCG), in abnormal pregnancy, 258
  ectopic, 489
  in IVF, 555
  reference standards for, 490
Human papilloma virus (HPV), and CIN, 233–234
Humoral balance theory, 5
  decline of, 9
Hydatid of Morgagni, 21, 22
Hydatidiform mole, D & C in, 258
  evaluation of, 263
Hydrocortisone, perioperative, 59, 61
Hydrosalpinx, 90, 92, 467, 468, 468, 471
  infertility treatment and, 554
Hydrotubation, 94
Hymen, 174
  imperforate, 167, 168
Hyperbaric oxygen, in necrotizing fasciitis, 50
Hyperkalemia, 38
  in renal disease, 77
Hypernatremia, 38
Hypertension, 66
  agents against, 67t
  portal, 80
Hyperthyroidism, 59–60
Hypokalemia, 38
Hyponatremia, 37
Hypothyroidism, 60
Hyskon, 94, 154–155, 509
Hysterectomy, 335–351
  abdominal, 337–342, 338–342
    adnexal management in, 338, 339, 340
    bladder mobilization in, 338–340, 340
    cardinal and uterosacral ligaments in, 341
    exploration in, 337–338

INDEX 657

Hysterectomy *(Continued)*
  hemostasis and reperitonealization in, 342
  incision for, 337
  round ligament in, 338, *339*
  traction in, 338, *338*
  uterine vessel ligation in, 340–341, *341*
  vaginal cuff in, 341–342, *342*
  vs. vaginal hysterectomy, 335, 351
 antibiotics before, 44–45, 274, 336
 autologous blood transfusion in, 336
 bladder injury during, 349, 440
 complication(s) of, 281t, 281–282, 283t, 348–350
  fever as, 348
  gastrointestinal injury as, 349–350
  hemorrhage as, 348
  urinary tract injury as, 349, *349*, 431–432
 enterocele and, 328
 GnRH agonists before, 336
 history of, 14–16
 in cervical cancer, 273, 274–275, *276–280*, 281–282
  extrafascial, 282–283, 283t, *284–285*
  para-aortic lymphadenectomy with, 283, 286, 286t, *287*, 288
 in endometrial adenocarcinoma, 378–380, *379*, *380*
 in endometriosis, 581
 infection after, operative site and, 46t
 prolapse prevention in, 350
 prolapse repair with, 320
 prophylactic oophorectomy and, 336–337
 psychological response to, 350
 ureteral injury during, 349, *349*, 431–432
 vaginal, 342–348, *343–348*
  adnexal management in, 345, *346*
  anterior peritoneum in, 344, *345*
  cervical circumcision in, 343, *343*
  enterocele prevention in, 346–347, *347*
  intramyometrial coring in, 345, *346*
  positioning for, 342, *343*
  uterine vessels in, 344–345
  uterosacral and cardinal ligaments in, 343, *344*
  vault suspension and closure in, *347*, 347–348, *348*
  vs. abdominal hysterectomy, 335, 351
 vaginectomy with, *206*
 workup before, 335–336
Hysterosalpingography, in distal tubal disease, 471, *471*
 in infertility, before ART, *554*
  before reconstructive surgery, 90, 92, *92*, *93*
 salpingoscopy with, 461–462
Hysteroscope, 509, *510*
Hysteroscopy, instruments for, 115–116, *116*, 508–510, *510*
 metroplasty with, 366
  results of, 368t
 myomectomy with, 359–360
 procedures with, 511t
 salpingoscopy with, 461–462
 training in, 511–512

Ileal urinary conduit, 443–444, *444*
Ileocecal reservoir, 447, *448–450*, 449
Ileocolectomy, *406*, *407*, 533

Ileostomy, stoma formation in, 413–414, *415*
Ileum. See also *Gastrointestinal tract*.
 in ureteral repair, 438–439, *439*
 lesions of, *402*
Ileus, postoperative, 51–52, 405
 gastrostomy and, 417
Iliac artery, 25, *25*
Iliohypogastric nerve, 22, 129, *130*
Ilioinguinal nerve, 22, 129, *130*
Immunologic infertility, 555
Impedance plethysmography, in postoperative thromboembolism, 56–57
Imperforate hymen, 167, *168*
In vitro fertilization (IVF), 88, 88t, 553–556. See also *Assisted reproductive technology (ART)*.
 embryo transfer in, 560–561, *561*
 history of, 549
 in endometriosis, 554–555, 581
 in male factor infertility, 555
 in ovarian failure, 555
 in tubal disease, 553–554
 in unexplained infertility, 555
 indications for, 554t
 multiple gestation in, 561
  reduction of, 565–566
 oocyte recovery for, 555–560
  anesthesia in, 559
  complications of, 559–560
  laparoscopic, 556, *556*
  needles in, *558*, 559, *559*
  timing of, 555, *555*
  ultrasound-guided, 556–559, *557–559*
 ovarian cancer surgery and, 528
 patient selection for, 553–555
 results of, 565t, 566, 566t
Incisions, abdominal, for obese patient, 138, *139*
 transverse, 134, 134–136, *135*
 vertical, *136*, 136–138, *137*
 for Bartholin's duct drainage, 162, *162*
 for distal tube surgery, 474, *474*
 for extraperitoneal approaches, 138–142, *140–143*
  bilateral groin, 139, *140*
  extended (OIPE), 142, *142*
  J-shaped, 139–140, *140*
  midline, 140–142, *141*, *142*
  sunrise, 142, *143*
  upper abdominal, 142
 for hysterectomy, 337
 for transperitoneal approaches, 143, *144*
Incontinence. See *Stress incontinence; Urinary incontinence*.
Indiana pouch, 447, *448–450*
Infection, after D & C, 265
 catheter-related, 47–48
 diabetes and, 58
 nosocomial, 46
 postoperative, 45–51
 wound, 48
  obesity and, 138
  prevention of, 133–134
  wound classification and, 131, 131t
Infertility. See also *Assisted reproductive technology (ART); Pregnancy*.
 after adhesiolysis, 155–157, *156*
 after ectopic pregnancy, 497t, 497–498
 after salpingostomy, 481, 482t, 484
  linear laparoscopic, 457–458
 after sterilization reversal, 461t
 endometriosis and, 554–555, 573–574
 evaluation of, 89–94, 553–555
 immunologic, 555

Infertility *(Continued)*
 leiomyomas and, 356–358
 male factor, 89, 90–91, 555
 müllerian anomalies and, 363–364, 367, 368t
 ovarian failure and, 555
 reconstructive surgery in. See *Reproductive reconstructive surgery*.
 SIN and, 455
 tubal disease and, 553–554
 unexplained, 555
Inflammatory bowel disease, rectovaginal fistula and, 218
Informed consent, for reproductive surgery, 87–88
Inguinal-femoral lymph nodes, 174–176, *175*
Inguinal ligament, *128*
Innervation, abdominal wall, 22, 129, *130*
 isthmic tube, 453–454
 vulvar, 174
Insemination, 549–553
 cervical, 550, *550*
 intraperitoneal, *551*, 552–553
 intratubal, *551*, 553
 intrauterine, 550, *550*, 552, *553*
Instruments. See also *specific instrument*.
 ancient, 2
 early, 9, 98
 for closure, 105, *105*
 for cytoreduction, 104, *104*, 536
 for electrosurgery, 118, 120
 for embryo transfer, 560
 for endometrial biopsy, 265, 374, *374*
 for establishing tubal patency, 110–111, *111*, *112*
 for exploration, 100–101, *101*
 for exposure, 99, 99–100, *100*
 for hemostasis, 103–104, *104*
 for hysteroscopy, 115–116, *116*, 508–510, *510*
 for insemination, 552, *552*, *553*
 for laparoscopy. See *Laparoscopy, instruments for*.
 for laparotomy, 107–112, *108–112*
 for laser surgery, 121–124, 504–505
 for magnification, 107–109, *108*, 114–115
 for microsurgical salpingostomy, 473, 473t
 for oocyte recovery, *558*, 559, *559*
 for operative radiotherapy, in cervical cancer, 630, 631, *632–636*
  in endometrial adenocarcinoma, 639, *640*
  in vaginal cancer, 641, *642*, 645–649
 for resection, 101–102, *102*
 for stapling, 102–103, *103*, 400–401, *401*, *402*
 for tissue handling, 109, *109*
 patient positioning and, 98, *99*
 special, 105, *105*, *106*, *107*
Insufflation, 502–503
Insulin, perioperative management of, 58–59
INTERCEED (TC7), 155, 515
Interferon, in CIN, 240, 240t
Internal oblique muscle, 22, 127–128, *128*, *130*
Internal pudendal artery, 174
International Federation of Gynecology and Obstetrics (FIGO) staging. See *FIGO staging*.
Intestinal bypass, 420, 420–421
Intestinal resection. See *Gastrointestinal tract, surgery on*.
Intestinal sling procedure, 421, *421*

Intestine. See *Colon; Small bowel.*
Intra-abdominal abscess, 49
Intraepithelial neoplasia. See site-specific entries, e.g., *Cervical intraepithelial neoplasia (CIN).*
Intramyometrial coring, 345, *346*
Intraspinal anesthesia, 43–44
Intrauterine tandems, 631, *632, 634, 639*
  insertion of, 633, *633–636,* 637
Iodine, perioperative, 59
Iodine sensitivity, 29
Iridium sources, in vaginal cancer radiotherapy, *642,* 643–644, *644–647*
Irrigation, 133
  adhesions and, 154–155
  bladder, 449
  for laparoscopy, 114, *115,* 481, 503
  for laparotomy, 112, 474
Irving procedure, 518, *518*
Isthmic tube. See *Fallopian tube(s), isthmic*
IVF. See *In vitro fertilization (IVF).*

Jejunostomy, tube, after small bowel surgery, 405
J-loop stoma, 413–414
Jones metroplasty, 364, *364, 366*
J-shaped incision, 139–140, *140*

Kelly-Kennedy procedure, 298, *299*
Ketosis, 41
Kidney, disease of, 76–77
  liver dysfunction and, 79–80
  fluid and electrolyte balance and, 35
  leiomyomas and, 356
  scan of, preoperative, 431
  ureteral damage and, 433
Knots, in laparoscopic suturing, 505–506, *506, 507*
Kock pouch, 446–447, *447*
Kroener fimbriectomy, 518, *518*
KTP-532 laser, 121, 122
  properties of, 122t

Labetolol, 67t
  perioperative, 64
Labia, 173, *174*
  sarcoma of, 196
Laboratory studies, in infertility, 91
  in liver disease, 77–78
  in ovarian cancer, 523–524
  in postoperative fever, 46
  in postoperative thromboembolism, 56–57
  preoperative, 30
    before hysterectomy, 335–336
Laceration, perineal, 164–165, *166*
Lactic acidosis, 40–41
Laminaria, 261–262
Landmarks, retropubic, 23
Langenbeck, C. J. M., 15
Laparoscope, 501–502, *502*
Laparoscopy, 501–508
  adhesions and, 152–153
  care after, 94
  energy source for, 503
  GIFT by, 562, *563,* 564
  in distal tubal disease, 471, *472,* 479, *480,* 481
  in ectopic pregnancy, 491–492, 496
  in endometriosis, 576–578, *577–579*

Laparoscopy *(Continued)*
  diagnostic, 574
  pregnancy after, 580t
  instruments for, 112–115, *113–115,* 479t, 501–508
    ablative, 508
    basic, 501–503, *502*
    incising, 113, *113, 504,* 504–505, *505*
    manipulative, 113, *113,* 503, *504*
    suction-irrigation, 503
    tissue-approximating, 113–114, *114,* 505–507, *506, 507*
    tissue-removing, 507–508, *508*
  laser, 125
  lighting for, 502
  oocyte recovery by, 556, *556*
  ovarian cyst removal by, 515–516
  procedures with, 511t
  salpingostomy with, 457–459, 471, *472, 472,* 479, *480,* 481
    instruments for, 479t
  second-look, adhesions and, 94–95, 147–148, 148t, *149,* 156
    in ovarian cancer, 539
  sheaths for, 508
  training in, 511–512
  trocars for, 508
  video, 108–109, 114–115, 502
    camera for, 502
Laparotomy, care after, 94
  distal tube surgery with, 473–476, *473–478*
  fertility after, 481, 482t, 484
  in endometriosis, 578, *580,* 580–581
  instruments for, 107–112, *108–112,* 473, 473t
  second-look, defined, 536–537
    in ovarian cancer, 536–540
      alternatives to, 539
      assessment before, 537
      benefits of, 539–540
      biopsy with, 537, *538*
      complications of, 537
      cytoreduction with, 542
      results of, 537–539, 538t
Large bowel. See *Colon.*
Lasers, *120,* 120–125, *121, 123, 124,* 504–505, 508
  adhesions and, 152
  clinical considerations with, 124–125
  components of, 122–123
  delivery systems of, *123,* 123–124, *124*
  electrosurgery vs., 125
  endometrial ablation with, 367, 369, 510
  in CIN, 236–238, *237,* 237t
    cone biopsy with, 242, *243,* 268
    vs. cryosurgery, 238t
  in endometriosis, 577, 577–578, *578*
  in ovarian cancer surgery, 536
  in VAIN, 247, *247, 248*
  in VIN, 251, *252–253,* 253
  metroplasty with, 366
  myomectomy with, 360
  principles of, *120,* 120–122, *121,* 504–506
  types of, 122t, 122–122
Latzko's technique, 216, *216,* 226
LEEP (loop electrosurgical excision procedure), in CIN, 235, 240–241, *241,* 241t
  cone biopsy with, 242, *243,* 244
Leeuwenhoek, Anton van, 8
Leiomyoma, 355–356
  fertility and, 356–358
  medical treatment of, 88–89
  recurrent, 360
  surgical treatment of. See *Myomectomy.*

Leiomyoma *(Continued)*
  symptoms associated with, 356
  ultrasonography of, 356, *357*
Leiomyosarcoma, uterine, 390
  vaginal, 209
  vulvar, 196
Leonardo da Vinci, 6, 353
Levator plate, 315, *315*
Levator sling, 26
Lichen sclerosus, vulvar, 160
Ligaments, 314–315, 355. See also specific ligaments.
Ligatures, history of, 7
Light waves, 120–121, *121*
Lighting, 100, *101,* 502
Linea alba, 128
Linear salpingostomy, in ampullary ectopic pregnancy, *492,* 492–493
  in isthmic ectopic pregnancy, 457–459, *458*
Liver disease, 77–80
  classification of, 78t
  postoperative, 79
Loop electrosurgical excision procedure (LEEP), in CIN, 235, 240–241, *241,* 241t
  cone biopsy with, 242, *243,* 244
Loupes, 107–108, *108*
Lumpectomy, 594, *595, 596*
  axillary dissection with, 595, *597–598,* 599
Luzzi, Mondino dei, 353
Lymph nodes. See also specific lymph nodes.
  axillary, dissection of, 595, *597–598,* 599
  in cervical cancer, 273, *273,* 273, 273t, 274
    radiotherapy of, 637
    scalene fat pad biopsy in, 288, *289*
    staging of, 283, 286, 286t, *287,* 288
    ureteral obstruction by, 430
  in endometrial adenocarcinoma, 373
    metastasis to, 386
    preoperative evaluation of, 375–376
    surgical staging and, 377t, 377–379, *378,* 380–381, *383–385,* 386–388
  in ovarian cancer, 527, 528, 536
  vaginal cancer and, 202, 640–641
  vulvar cancer and, 177t, 177–178, 178t, 180–183, *182,* 185–186
Lymphadenectomy. See also *Lymph nodes.*
  complete pelvic, 381
  selective. See *Para-aortic lymph node sampling; Pelvic lymph node sampling.*
  urinary tract injury and, 432
Lymphatic system, 26, *26*
  endometriosis and, 570
  vaginal, 202
    cancer and, 640–641
  vulvar, 174–176, *175*
Lymphocysts, pelvic, 281t, 282
Lymphoma, vulvar, 197

Machaon, 3
Magnesium, daily requirements of, 36t
Magnetic resonance imaging (MRI), in cervical cancer staging, 274
  in infertility, 92
  in ovarian cancer diagnosis, 524
  in postoperative thromboembolism, 57
Magnification, 107–109, *108*
  for laparoscopy, 114–115
Male, fertility evaluation of, 89, 90–91
  IVF and, 555

Mammography, screening, 585
  needle localization and, 590
Marshall-Marchetti-Krantz procedure, 300, *301*
Martius' bulbocavernous flap technique, in fistula repair, 217, *217*, 226
  in vaginal reconstruction, 615
Mastectomy, radical, 599, *603–605*, 605
  history of, 594
  modified, 599, *600–602*
Mastitis, 591
Maylard incision, *135*, 135–136
McDowell, Ephraim, 12–13, *13*
McIndoe technique, 612, *613*
  omental, 612
MEAC (minimum effective analgesic concentration), 42
Mechanical ventilation, in ARDS, 76
Medical history, before hysterectomy, 335
  preoperative, 29–30
  in cardiovascular disease, 61
  in infertility, 90–91
Medications. See *Drugs*.
Medieval medicine, 5
Melanoma, vaginal, 208
  vulvar, *192*, 192–194
    prognosis in, 192–194
    staging of, 193, 193t
    treatment of, 193
Meltauer, John Peter, 12
Menopause, bleeding after, 259
Menstruation, abnormal, D & C in, 259
  leiomyomas and, 356
  retrograde, and endometriosis, 570–571
Merkel cell carcinoma, vulvar, 197
Mesonephric remnants, 21, *22*
Methotrexate, in ectopic pregnancy, 491
Methylxanthines, in asthma, 72
Metroplasty, 364, *364–366*, 366–367
  abdominal uterine unification, 364, *364–366*, 366
  evaluation before, 361, 363, *363*
  laser, 366
  transcervical hysteroscopic, 366–367
  results of, 368t
Microcolpostats, *632*
Microelectrodes, 118, *120*
Microscope, operating, 108, *108*
Midline incision, 136–138
  closure of, *136*, 136–138, *137*, 137t
  for extraperitoneal node sampling, 140–142, *141*, *142*
Minimum effective analgesic concentration (MEAC), 42
Mitral stenosis, 65t, 66
Modern surgical history, 7–17
Modinus of Bologna, 5
Molar pregnancy, D & C in, 258
  evaluation of, 263
Mons veneris, 173
Morcellators, 114, *115*, 507, *508*
Morton, Thomas Green, 10, *11*
MRI (magnetic resonance imaging), in cervical cancer staging, 274
  in infertility, 92
  in ovarian cancer diagnosis, 524
  in postoperative thromboembolism, 57
Mucous fistula, 414
Müller, Johannas Peter, 354
Müllerian anomalies, 360–369
  classification of, *362*
  fertility and, 363–364, 367, 368t
  surgery for, 360–361, 364, *364–366*, 366–367
    evaluation before, 361, 363, *363*
    results of, 368t

Müllerian anomalies *(Continued)*
  types of, 360–361, *361*
Müllerian ducts, embryology of, 20
Müllerian tumors, uterine, 390
Multigated angiography, 63
Muscle(s). See also specific muscles.
  abdominal wall, 127–128, *128*
  isthmic tube, 453, *454*
Muscle mass, 33
Musculophrenic artery, 129, *129*
Myocardial infarction, 61–64
  perioperative, diagnosis of, 63–64
  risk factors for, 62t, 62–63
Myocutaneous grafts. See *Skin flaps and grafts*.
Myomectomy, 355–360, *357*
  evaluation before, 358
  fertility after, 357–358
  indications for, 356
  laser, 360
  obstetrical management after, 360
  recurrence after, 360
  technique for, 358–360
  timing of, 356–357
  transcervical hysteroscopic, 359–360
  ultrasonography and, 356, *357*

Narcotics, postoperative, 44
Nasogastric tube, for intestinal decompression, 52, 543
  in ileus, 52
Nd:YAG (neodymium-yttrium-aluminum-garnet) laser, 121–122
  in ovarian cancer surgery, 536
  properties of, 122t
Necrosis, bladder, 451
  femoral vessel, 615, 620, *620*
    coverage in, 615, 620, *620*, *621*
  ovarian torsion and, 516
  sigmoid, radiation-induced, 418
  stomal, 416
Necrotizing fasciitis, 49–51
  clinical data in, 50t
Needle(s), for oocyte recovery, *558*, 559, *559*
  Tru-Cut, 587–588, *588*
Needle guides, in vaginal cancer radiotherapy, *641*, 645, *646*, 649
Needle holders, 110, *110*, 113
Needle suspension procedures, 304, *305–307*, 306–308
Neodymium-yttrium-aluminum-garnet (Nd:YAG) laser, 121–122
  in ovarian cancer surgery, 536
  properties of, 122t
Neoplasia, intraepithelial. See site-specific entries, e.g., *Vulvar intraepithelial neoplasia (VIN)*.
Neovagina. See *Vagina, reconstruction of*.
Nephrostomy, 441–442
Nephrotoxicity, 77
Nerves, surgical injury to, 26–27
Nifedipine, 67t
  postoperative, 64
Nipple discharge, 591, *592*
Nitrates, 67t
  perioperative, 64
Noble-Mengert-Fish procedure, 226, *228–229*
Nosocomial infection, 46
  pulmonary, 47
Nufer, Jacob, 6–7
Nutrition, CIN and, 233
  enteral, 33, 405

Nutrition *(Continued)*
  in patient with enteral fistula, 422
  parenteral, 33–35
  postoperative, 34–35
    after intestinal anastomosis, 405, 411
    after radiation injury repair, 421
    gastrostomy and, 417
  preoperative, 33–34, 398–399
    assessment of, 32t, 32–33

Obesity, incisions in, 138, *139*
  sutures in, 134
Oblique muscles, 22, 127–128, *128*, 130
Obstruction, colonic, postoperative, 53
  radiation-induced, 418
  ovarian cancer and, 424, 542–544, *544*
  small bowel, 422–424
    postoperative, 52–53
    TPN and, 34–35
  tubal, 92–93. See also *Fallopian tube(s)*.
  ureteral, 430, 432, 433
    after urinary diversion, 446
    radiation-induced, 451
Obturator nerve, surgical injury to, 27
OIPE approach (one-incision, pararectal, extraperitoneal approach), 142, *142*
Omentectomy, 531, *531*, 532
One-incision, pararectal, extraperitoneal approach (OIPE approach), 142, *142*
Oocyte recovery, 555–560
  anesthesia for, 559
  complications of, 559–560
  laparoscopic, 556, *556*
  needles for, *558*, 559, *559*
  timing of, 555, *555*
  ultrasound-guided, 556–559, *557–559*
Oophorectomy, 518, 520, *520*
  history of, 12–14
  indications for, 518
  prophylactic, 336–337, 518
Oophoropexy, 516, *517*
Operating microscope, 108, *108*
Osiander of Gottingen, 15
Osmolarity, 35, 37
  normal serum, 37
Ovarian arteries, 25, *25*, 354
Ovarian function, adhesions and, 156, *156*, 156–157
Ovarian pregnancy, 496
Ovarian remnant syndrome, 20
Ovary, adhesions and, 149
  cancer of, 523–547
    bilateral, 529
    borderline, 529
    endometriosis and, 582, *582*
    intestinal obstruction and, 424, 542–544, *544*
    intraperitoneal therapy for, 544
    malignant germ cell, 528–529, 539
    metastasis sites in, 527t
    primary surgery for, 523–536
      conservative, 528t, 528–529
      cytoreductive, 529–536
      evaluation before, 523–525, *524*
      exploration in, 530–531
      lymph node resection in, 536
      new techniques in, 536, *537*
      omentectomy in, 531, *531*, 532
      pelvic tumor resection in, 531–532, *532*
      rectosigmoid resection in, 532–533, *533*
      small intestine resection in, 533–534
      urinary tract resection in, 534

660 INDEX

Ovary (Continued)
   secondary surgery for, 536–542
      alternatives to, 539
      assessment before, 537
      benefits of, 539–540
      biopsy with, 537, 538
      complications of, 539
      cytoreductive, 540–542
      definition of, 536–537
      results of, 537–539, 538t
      technique for, 537
   serum markers for, 539
   sex cord-stromal, 529
   surgical staging of, 525–528, 526t
      incomplete, 525–526
      malignancy category and, 526t
      survival in, 526t, 529, 530t
      urinary tract and, 430
   cysts of, 513–516
      benign (teratoma), 513–516
         bilateral, 514
         surgery in, 514, 514–516
      functional, 513
      laparoscopy for, 515–516
      malignant germ cell tumors with, 528–529
   embryology of, 19–20
   endometriosis of, 514, 515, 572, 573, 573
      cyst dissection in, 578, 579, 580
      malignancy arising from, 582, 582
   hyperstimulation of, 560
   postmenopausal, 337
   removal of. See Oophorectomy.
   supernumerary, 19, 20
   torsion of, 516, 517
   wedge biopsy of, 520–521, 521
Ovulation, abnormal bleeding and, 258–259
   evaluation of, 90
Ovum donation, indications for, 554t
   ovarian failure and, 555
Oxygen, hyperbaric, in necrotizing fasciitis, 50

Pacemaker, surgery and, 65
Packing, 100
   for microsalpingostomy, 474, 474
Paget's disease, vulvar, 194–195
Pain, postoperative, 41–44
Papanicolaou, George, 9, 10
Papanicolaou smear, abnormal, D & C and, 259
   endometrial adenocarcinoma and, 372, 373
   cone biopsy and, 266
Para-aortic lymph node sampling, 283, 286, 286t, 287, 288
   extraperitoneal approach to, 138–142, 140–143
      complications of, 286t
      incisions in, bilateral groin, 139, 140
         extended (OIPE), 142, 142
         J-shaped, 139–140, 140
         midline, 140–142, 141, 142
         sunrise, 142, 143
         upper abdominal, 142
      in endometrial adenocarcinoma, 384, 384, 385, 386
   transperitoneal approaches to, 143, 144
Paramedian incision, 136
Pararectal spaces, 316, 317
Paraumbilical veins, 130
Paravaginal defect repair, in stress incontinence, 308

Paravesical spaces, 316, 317
Pare, Ambroise, 7, 7
Parovarian cyst, 21, 22
Pasteur, Louis, 14
Pathology, history of, 9
Patient-controlled analgesia, 42–43
   problems with, 43t
Patient positioning, 98, 99
   for embryo transfer, 560–561
   for hysterectomy, 342, 343
Paulus Aegina, 5
Pedicle flap, 620–621, 622
Pelvic abscess, 49
Pelvic connective tissue spaces, 316, 317
Pelvic diaphragm, 315–316
Pelvic dissection, in ovarian cancer, 531–532, 532
Pelvic examination, in infertility, 91
   rectovaginal, in enterocele, 328
   in rectocele, 325
Pelvic exenteration. See Exenteration.
Pelvic inflammatory disease (PID), 456, 467–468, 469
Pelvic lymph node sampling, in endometrial adenocarcinoma, 380–381, 381–384
Pelvic lymphocysts, 281t, 282
Pelvic relaxation. See Prolapse.
Pelvis, adhesions and, 149
   anatomy of, 23–26, 24–26
   bony, 316
Pereyra-Raz procedure, 304, 305, 306
Perianal intraepithelial neoplasia. See Vulvar intraepithelial neoplasia (VIN).
Perineal body, 316
   defects of, 327
Perineorrhaphy, 327
Perineum, 174
Peritoneum, healing of, 148–151, 150, 151
   in hysterectomy, 343, 344, 345
Pfannenstiel incision, 23, 134
Phlebitis, postoperative, 47–48
Physical examination, before hysterectomy, 335
   in cardiovascular disease, 61
   in infertility, 90–91
PID (pelvic inflammatory disease), 456, 467–468, 469
Plasminogen activator, 151, 154
Platelets, 68–69
   transfusions of, 69, 70
Plethysmography, in postoperative thromboembolism, 56–57
Pliny the Elder, 4
Pneumonia, 47
Pomeroy technique, 518, 519
Port-A-Cath, 544
Portal hypertension, 80
Positioning, 98, 99
   for embryo transfer, 560–561
   for hysterectomy, 342, 343
Postcoital test, 90
Posterior colporrhaphy, 325–327, 325–327
Postoperative care, acid-base disorders and, 39–41, 41t
   after anterior colporrhaphy, 324
   after distal tube surgery, 481
   after hysterectomy, 275
   after intestinal anastomosis, 405, 411
   after reproductive reconstructive surgery, 94–95
   after stress incontinence surgery, 298, 300
   fluid and electrolyte management in, 38–39
   hemodynamic monitoring in, 67–68

Postoperative care (Continued)
   in adrenal insufficiency, 61
   in arrhythmias, 65
   in coronary artery disease, 64
   in hematologic disorders, 68–70
   in hypertension, 66
   in hyperthyroidism, 60
   in hypothyroidism, 60
   in liver disease, 77–80
   in myocardial infarction, 63–64
   in pulmonary disease, 70–76
      predictors in, 71t
   in renal disease, 76–77
   in steroid suppression, 60–61
   in valvular heart disease, 65–66
   in vulvar carcinoma, 188
   nutritional, 34–35
   of complications, 51–58. See also specific complication.
   of infection, 45–51
   pain management in, 41–44
   thromboembolism management in, 56–58
   thromboembolism prevention in, 54–56
Potassium, daily requirements of, 36t
   preexisting disorders of, 38
Pregnancy, abnormal, D & C in, 257–258
   hCG and, 258, 489
   after adhesiolysis, 155–157
   after ectopic pregnancy, 497t, 497–498
   after endometriosis treatment, 575–578, 580t, 580–581
   after metroplasty, 367, 368t
   after myomectomy, 357–358
   after salpingostomy, 457–458, 481, 482t, 484
   after tubal sterilization reversal, 461t
   breast mass in, 587
   cone biopsy in, 269
   ectopic. See Ectopic pregnancy.
   molar, D & C in, 258
      evaluation of, 263
   müllerian anomalies and, 363–364
   multiple, with IVF, 561
      reduction of, 565–566
Preinvasive disease, 231–232, 253. See also site-specific entries.
Preoperative evaluation and care, antibiotic prophylaxis in, 44–45, 51
   before distal tubal surgery, 469, 471, 471, 472, 472t, 473
   before hysterectomy, 274, 335–337
   before müllerian anomaly repair, 361–362
   before myomectomy, 358, 359
   before ovarian cancer surgery, primary, 523–525, 524
      secondary, 537
   before sterilization, 517
   before urinary diversion, 443
   bowel preparation in, 51, 51t, 397–399, 398t
   fluid and electrolyte management in, 35–37
   hemodynamic monitoring in, 67–68
   in adrenal insufficiency, 61
   in arrhythmias, 65
   in cardiovascular disease, 61, 62, 63, 65–66, 66t
   in congestive heart failure, 64
   in diabetes, 58–59
   in endometrial adenocarcinoma, 374–376, 375t
   in hematologic disorders, 68–70
   in hypertension, 66
   in hyperthyroidism, 59–60

Preoperative evaluation and care (Continued)
  in hypothyroidism, 60
  in liver disease, 77–80
  in pulmonary disease, 70–76
  in renal disease, 76–77
  in steroid suppression, 60–61
  informed consent in, 30–32
  laboratory studies in, 30
  medical history in, 29–30
  nutritional, 32–34
  of urinary tract, 431
Presacral area, anatomy of, 25–26, 26
Presacral neurectomy, in endometriosis, 580
Prevesical space, 134, 134–135, 135, 316, 317
Probes, laparoscopic, 503
  tubal, 111, 112
Proctosigmoiditis, radiation-induced, 417–418
Progesterone, in abnormal pregnancy diagnosis, 489–490
Prognostic nutritional index, 33–34
Prolapse, 313–333
  anatomical considerations in, 314–316, 315, 317
  choice of operation in, 319–320
  classification of, 316–318, 318
  exenteration and, 624
  into rectovaginal space, 317, 328
    prevention of, 346
  of bladder, 317, 318, 320–322
    repair of, 322–324, 322–324
  of bladder and urethra, 317, 318
  of posterior cul-de-sac peritoneum, 317–318, 318, 328
    prevention of, 346–347, 347
    repair of, 328–329, 329
  of rectum, 317, 318, 324–325
    repair of, 325–327, 325–327
  of stoma, 416–417
  of urethra, 309, 309
  of uterus, 318, 318
  of vaginal vault, 318, 329
    hysterectomy and, 350
    repair of, 330–332
  pathophysiology of, 319
  perineal body defects and, 327
  signs and symptoms of, 318–319
Prophylaxis, antibiotic, before gastrointestinal surgery, 398
  before hysterectomy, 274, 336
  for bacterial endocarditis, 66t
  heparin, 54–56, 281–282
  oophorectomy in, 336–337, 518
  pulmonary, 73–74
Propranolol, perioperative, 59–60
Propylthiouracil, perioperative, 59
Protein reserve, 33
Prothrombin time, in liver disease, 77–78
Pruritus, vulvar, 160
Psoas hitch, 435, 437
Psychologic factors. See also Counseling.
  exenteration and, 290
  hysterectomy and, 350
Pubic symphysis, 22
Pudendal artery, internal, 174
Pudendal nerve, surgical injury to, 27
Puerperal fever, 14
Pulmonary artery catheter, 67–68
Pulmonary disease, 70–76. See also specific disease.
  postoperative, predictors of, 71t
Pulmonary edema, 64–65
  cardiogenic, 75
  noncardiogenic, 75–76

Pulmonary embolism, postoperative, 54–58, 281–282
  management of, 57–58
  prophylaxis of, 54–56
  risk factors for, 54
Pulmonary function testing, 73
Pulmonary infections, postoperative, 47
  preoperative, 74
Pyelography, preoperative, 431
Pyramidalis muscle, 128

Radiation therapy. See Radiotherapy.
Radical mastectomy, 599, 603–605, 605
  history of, 594
  modified, 599, 600–602
Radiography, in postoperative ileus, 52
  preoperative, 30
  chest films in, 71, 91
  in infertility, 91–92
  in ovarian cancer, 524, 524
Radiotherapy, extrafascial hysterectomy with, 282–283
  complications of, 282–283, 283t
  gastrointestinal injury from, 417–421
  in breast cancer, 594
    after lumpectomy, 595
  in cervical cancer, 629–637
    complications of, 637
    external-beam, 630–631
    guidelines for, 636t
    instruments for, 630, 631, 632–636
    intracavitary, 631, 631, 633, 637
    planning for, 631t
    results of, 637t, 638t
    sources of, 631, 631, 633, 633
  in clitoral lesions, 179
  in endometrial adenocarcinoma, 376, 388t, 388–389, 391, 637–640
    instruments for, 639, 640
    postoperative, 639–640, 640
    preoperative, 638–639, 639
    surgical staging and, 387
  in vaginal cancer, 202–203, 640–650
    complications of, 644, 648t
    gold-grain implants in, 642, 644, 648, 648, 649
    results of, 650t
    instruments for, 641, 642, 645–649
    iridium implants in, 642, 643–644, 644–647
    lymph nodes and, 640–641
    options in, 641, 643, 643, 644
    planning for, 641
  in VAIN, 244
  in VIN, 253
  in vulvar carcinoma, 180–181, 182
    advanced, 191
  of para-aortic lymph node metastases, 288t
  sacral injury from, 624, 624–626
  sigmoid injury from, 417–419, 418
  small bowel injury from, 419, 419–421, 420
    sling procedure for, 421, 421
  urologic complications of, 449, 451
Radium sources, 631, 631, 633, 633, 640
Re-anastomosis, colonic, 407, 407, 408–411, 408–411
  care after, 411, 412t
  complications of, 412, 412t
Reconstructive surgery, 607–627. See also Reproductive reconstructive surgery.
  abdominal wall, 621, 623, 624, 624
  pelvic floor, 624

Reconstructive surgery (Continued)
  sacral, 624, 624–626
  vaginal, 290, 607, 610, 611
    band release in, 607, 608
    cancer arising at site of, 209
    colon interposition for, 612, 614
    Frank technique for, 611, 611–612
    free flap in, 615
    gluteal thigh flap in, 615
    gracilis myocutaneous graft in, 615, 616–618
    Martius bulbocavernous technique for, 615
    McIndoe technique for, 612, 613
    rectus abdominis myocutaneous flap in, 615, 619
    skin flaps in, 607, 608–610, 611
    Williams technique for, 612, 614
  vulvar, 615, 618, 620–621
    femoral vessel coverage in, 615, 620, 620, 621
    pedicle flaps for, 620–621, 622
Rectocele, 317, 318, 324–325
  repair of, 325–327, 325–327
Rectoscopy, 510
  metroplasty with, 366
  myomectomy with, 359–360
Rectovaginal examination, in enterocele, 328
  in rectocele, 325
Rectovaginal fistula, 218–229
  anatomy of, 214
  classification of, 218
  diagnosis of, 218–219
  etiology of, 218
  postoperative, 54
  radiation-induced, 418–419
  treatment of, 219, 219t
    surgical, abdominal approach in, 226, 229
      anorectal approach in, 226
      bowel preparation before, 219
      colostomy and, 229
      vaginal approach in, 219–220, 220–225, 226, 227–229
Rectovaginal space, 316, 317
  prolapse into, 317, 328
    prevention of, 346
Rectum, prolapse of, 317, 318, 324–325
  repair of, 325–327, 325–327
  surgical injury to, 350
Rectus abdominis muscle, 22, 127–128, 128
  blood supply and, 130
  in reconstructive surgery, 615, 619, 621, 623
Relaxation, pelvic. See Prolapse.
Renaissance medicine, 6–7
Renal disorders, 76–77
  leiomyomas and, 356
  liver dysfunction and, 79–80
Renal scan, preoperative, 431
Reproductive reconstructive surgery, 87–96
  adhesions and, 94–95, 147
  alternatives to, 87, 88, 89. See also Assisted reproductive technology (ART).
  care after, 94–95
  conception after, 95
  counseling before, 89
  evaluation before, 89–94
  informed consent for, 87–88
  instruments for, 107–126
    electrosurgical, 116–118, 116–120, 120
    hysteroscopic, 115–116, 116
    laparoscopic, 112–115, 113–115

Reproductive reconstructive surgery (Continued)
  laparotomy, 107–112, *108–112*
  laser, *120*, 120–125, *121*, 122t, *123*, *124*
Resection, intestinal. See *Gastrointestinal tract, surgery on.*
Residual ovary syndrome, 337
Respiratory tract infections, postoperative, 47
Retraction, stomal, 416
Retractors, *99*, 99–100, *100*
  for reproductive surgery, 112, *112*
Retroperitoneal lymph nodes, in ovarian cancer, 527, 528, 536
Retrorectal space, 316, *317*
Rh factor, ectopic pregnancy and, 496–497
Rhabdomyosarcoma, vaginal, 208–209
  vulvar, 196
Rhomboid flap, 186, 607, *609*, 620
Right-angle clamp, 101–102, *102*
Roeder loop, 114, *114*
Roman medicine, 4, 353
Round ligaments, 24, *24*, *128*, 355
  hysterectomy and, 338, *339*
Rufus of Ephesus, 4, 353

Sacrospinous ligament suspension, in vaginal prolapse, 330–331
Sacrum, reconstructive surgery on, 624, *624–626*
Salerno school, 5
Salpingectomy, in ectopic pregnancy, 457, 494–495, *495*
Salpingitis, 468–469
Salpingitis isthmica nodosa (SIN), 455–456, 488
Salpingocentesis, 491
Salpingo-ovariolysis, defined, 471t
Salpingoscopy, 461–462
Salpingostomy, defined, 471t
  fertility after, 481, 482t, 484
  laparoscopic, 457–459, 471, *472*, 472t
    in distal tubal surgery, 479, *480*, 481
  laser, 479t
  linear, in ampullary ectopic pregnancy, *492*, 492–493
    in isthmic ectopic pregnancy, 457–459, *458*
  microscopic, 472t
    in distal tubal surgery, 473–476, *473–478*
      adhesiolysis with, 474–475, *475*
      closure in, 479
      fimbrioplasty with, 476, *478*
      incision for, 474, *474*
      instruments for, 473, 473t
Salpingotomy, 493
Sarcoma, urinary tract, 430
  uterine, 371, 389–390, *390*
  vaginal, 208–209
  vulvar, 196
Sartorius muscle transposition, 615, 620, *620*
Scalene fat pad biopsy, 288, *289*
Scalpels, 98
  for conization, *267*
  laparoscopic, 504
  wound infection and, 133–134
Schuchardt incision, 165, 167
Sciatic nerve, surgical injury to, 27
Scientific method, 7–8
Scissors, 101, *102*
  for reproductive surgery, *109*, 109–110, 113, *113*

Scissors (Continued)
  laparoscopic, 113, *113*, 504, *505*
Scrubbing, 133
Second-look procedures. See *Laparoscopy, second-look; Laparotomy, second look.*
Segmental resection, in isthmic ectopic pregnancy, 458, 459, *459*, 493, 494–495
Semen, analysis of, 89–90
  processed, 552
Semmelweis, Ignaz Philipp, 14, *15*
Sengstaken-Blakemore tube, 80
Sertoli-Leydig cell tumor, 529
Serum tumor markers, for ovarian cancer, 539
Sex cord-stromal tumor, 529
Sexual function, evaluation of, 90–91
  exenteration and, 289–290
  prolapse repair and, 320, 330
Shaving, preoperative, 133
Sheaths, 508
Shellfish allergy, 29
Sigmoid urinary conduit, 444–445, *445*
Simon-Heyman capsule, *639*
Sims, James Marion, 10, 12, *12*
Sims-Emmet technique, *215*, 215–216, *216*
SIN (salpingitis isthmica nodosa), 455–456, 488
Skin flaps and grafts, axial translocation, 607, *610*
  Boari, 435, 438, *438*
  free, 615
  gluteus maximus, 186, 188, *190*, 615
    for sacral defects, 624, *625*, *626*
  gracilis, 186, *187–188*, 615, *616–618*
  in exenteration, 290, 610t
  in fistula repair, 217, *217*, 226, *227–229*
  in reconstructive surgery, 607, *608–610*, 611
  pedicle, 620–621, *622*
  rhomboid, 186, 607, *609*, 620
  tensor fascia lata, 186, *189*, 621, *622*, *623*
  Warren, 226, *227*
  Y-V plasty, 607, *609*
  Z-plasty, 607, *608*
Skin grafts. See *Skin flaps and grafts.*
Skin preparation, preoperative, 133
Sling procedures, for stress incontinence, 302, *303–305*, 304
  fascia lata or artificial materials in, 304, *305*
  intestinal, 421, *421*
Small bowel, injury to, during hysterectomy, 349–350
  during surgical staging, 387
  radiation-induced, *419*, 419–421, *420*
  obstruction of, 422–424
    ovarian cancer and, 543–544
    postoperative, 52–53
    TPN and, 34–35
  surgery on, 402, *402–405*, 405, 407
    bypass, *420*, 420–421
    care after, 405
    complications of, 405, 407
    ovarian cancer surgery and, 533–534
    sling, 421, *421*
Small cell carcinoma, vaginal, 209
Smead-Jones closure, 137
Smoking, 73–74
Sodium, daily requirements of, 36t
  imbalance of, 37–38
Somatostatin, in management of postoperative gastrointestinal fistula, 34, 54
Soranus of Ephesus, 4, 353

Space of Retzius, *134*, 134–135, *135*, 316, *317*
Speculum, history of, 12, *12*
Spirometry, preoperative, 71
Spleen, ovarian cancer and, *534*, 534–535, *535*
Splenectomy, 534–535
  complications of, 535
Squamous cell carcinoma, cervical, radiotherapy results in, 637t, 638t
  vaginal, 201–202, 204–205, *205–208*, 207
    radiotherapy in, *647*
      complications of, 644, 648t
      survival in, 642t
  vulvar, 176–192
    advanced, 188, *191*, 191–192
    clinical features of, 177
    diagnosis of, 177
    early (T1, N0-1), 178–182, *179–182*
    large defect closure in, 186, *187–190*, 188
    N2, N3, 185–186
    postoperative complications in, 188
    postoperative management in, 188
    prognosis in, 192, 192t
    radical vulvectomy in, 183, *183*, *184*, 185
    recurrent, 191–192
    spread of, 177t, 177–178, 178t
    staging of, 176, 176t
    vulvar conservation in, 185
    vulvar dystrophy with, 179
Squamous cell hyperplasia, vulvar, 160
Staging, FIGO, of endometrial adenocarcinoma, 375, 375t, 377t
  of ovarian cancer, 526t
  of vaginal cancer, 202, 202t
  of vulvar carcinoma, 176, 176t
  of vaginal cancer, 202, 202t
  of vulvar carcinoma, 176, 176t
  of vulvar melanoma, 193, 193t
  surgical, of cervical cancer, 283, 286, 286t, *287*, 288, *289*
    of endometrial adenocarcinoma, 377t, 377–379, *378*, 380–381, *381–385*, 386–388
      advantages of, 387
      disadvantages of, 387–388
      risks of, 386–387
    of ovarian cancer, 525–528, 526t
      incomplete, 525–526
      malignancy category and, 526t
Stamey procedure, *306*, 306–307
Staplers, 400–401, *401*, *402*
Stapling, 102–103, *103*, 105, *105*, 399
  laparoscopic, 506–507
  of anastomosis, 400–401
  side-to-side, 405, *405*
Stenosis, aortic, 65t, 65–66
  mitral, 65t, 66
  stomal, 416, 446
Stenting, ureteral, 432–433, *434*, *435*
  in ileal conduit, 444
Sterilization, 460–461, 517–518, *518*, *519*
  evaluation before, 517
  reversal of, 460–461
    evaluation before, 90, 92
    success of, 461t
Steroids, 61
  in asthma, 72
  perioperative, 59, 61
Stirrups, 98, *99*
Stockings, elastic, 55–56
Stoma formation, 412–417, *413–416*
  complications of, 416–417, 446
  in end colostomy, 412–413, *413*, *414*

INDEX 663

Stoma formation *(Continued)*
  in loop colostomy, 414–416, *415, 416*
  J-loop, 413–414
  mucous fistula with, 414
  site for, 412
  with EEA instrument, 413, *414*
Stomach, blood supply to, *396*
Strassman metroplasty, 364, *364, 365, 366*
Stress incontinence, 297–309
  abdominal approach in, 300, *301,* 302
  cystocele and, 320, 321–322
  needle suspension procedures for, 304, *305–307,* 306–308
  paravaginal defect repair in, 308
  sling procedures for, 302, *303–305,* 304
    fascia lata or artificial materials in, 304, *305*
  surgical results in, 308
  vaginal procedures for, 298, *299*
Stress testing, preoperative, 62–63
Stricture, anastomotic, 412
Suction, 133
  curettage with, 263
  for laparoscopy, 114, *115,* 503
Sunrise incision, 142, *143*
Surgeon, endoscopic, 512
  fingers of, 101
Surgery. See also *Postoperative care; Preoperative evaluation and care.*
  caloric needs before, 32t
  gastrointestinal. See *Gastrointestinal tract, surgery on.*
  in patient with previous operations, 29–30
  reconstructive, 607–627. See also *Reconstructive surgery; Reproductive reconstructive surgery.*
  urinary diversion. See *Urinary diversion.*
  urinary tract injury due to, 431–434, 440–441. See also *Ureter(s), injury to.*
Surgical clips, 104, *104,* 105
Surgical history. See *History.*
Sutures, 103–104
  evisceration and, 136–137, 145
  for anastomosis, 400
  for closure, 105, 131–132, 132t, 134
    of midline incision, *136,* 136–138, 137t
  for episiotomy, 165
  for laparoscopy, 113–114, *114,* 505–506, *506, 507*
  for reproductive surgery, 110, 113–114, *114*
  wire, 131–132
  history of, 12
Swan-Ganz catheter, 67

Tampon Moir test, in fistula diagnosis, 214, 219
Tandems, intrauterine, 631, *632, 634, 639*
  insertion of, 633, *633–636,* 637
Taping, 105, *105*
Teflon rods, 111, *112*
Tenaculum, 260
Tensor fascia lata myocutaneous graft, 186, *189,* 621, *622, 623*
Teratomas, benign ovarian, 513–516
  embryology of, 20
Thoracic vessels, *130*
Thoracoabdominal nerves, 129
Thorwald, Jurgen, 10
Thrombocytopenia, 68–69
Thromboembolism, postoperative, 54–58
  management of, 56–58

Thromboembolism *(Continued)*
  prophylaxis of, 54–56
  risk factors for, 54
Thrombolytic agents, adhesions and, 154
Thyroid storm, postoperative, 60
Tissue forceps, 109, *109*
Torsion, ovarian, 516, *517*
Total parenteral nutrition (TPN), in patient with enteral fistula, 422
  postoperative, 34–35, 405, 411, 421
  preoperative, 33–34, 398–399
TPN. See *Total parenteral nutrition (TPN).*
Trachelorrhaphy, 266
Transureteroureterostomy, *439,* 439–440
Transverse incisions, *134,* 134–136, *135*
Transversus abdominis muscle, 22, 127–128, *128*
Trocars, 508
Tubes, Fallopian. See *Fallopian tube(s); Ectopic pregnancy.*

Ultrasonography, for cytoreduction, 104, *104,* 536, *537*
  in abnormal pregnancy, 258
    ectopic, 490, *490*
  in D & C, 263, 263–264
  in endometriosis, 575, *575*
  in leiomyoma evaluation, 356, *357*
  in müllerian anomalies, 361, *363*
  in oocyte retrieval, 556–559, *557–559*
  in ovarian cancer diagnosis, 524, *524*
  in ovarian torsion, 516
  in postoperative thromboembolism, 57
  of urinary tract, 431
Umbilical fold, *128*
Umbilical ligament, *128*
Upper abdominal incision, 142
Ureter(s), anatomy of, 427–429, *428, 429*
  endometriosis and, *571,* 574, 581–582
  injury to, 431–434
    detection of, 432–434
    during hysterectomy, 349, *349,* 431–432
    repair of, 434–435, *434–439,* 438–440
    stenting in, 432–433, *434, 435,* 440
  malignant involvement of, 430
  obstruction of, 430, 432, 433
    after urinary diversion, 446
    radiation-induced, 451
  ovarian cancer surgery and, 534
  pelvic anatomy and, 23–24, *25*
Ureteral fistula, 433
Ureteroileoneocystostomy, 438–439, *439*
Ureteroneocystostomy, 434–435, *436*
Ureterosigmoidostomy, 442, 442–443
Ureterostomy, cutaneous, 442
Ureteroureterostomy, 434, *434, 435*
Ureterovaginal fistula, 433–434
  after hysterectomy, 281, 281t
  anatomy of, *214*
Urethra, caruncle of, 309, *309*
  diverticulum of, 309, *310, 311*
  prolapse of, 309, *309*
Urethrovaginal fistula, anatomy of, *214*
Urinary bladder. See *Bladder; Vesico-* entries.
Urinary diversion, 289, 441–447, *442–445, 447–449,* 449
  conduits for, 443–446
    colonic, 444–445, *445*
    complications with, 445–446
    ileal, 443–444, *444*
    preoperative preparation for, 443
  continent, 446–447, *447–450,* 449

Urinary diversion *(Continued)*
  cutaneous ureterostomy for, 442
  in fistula management, 217–218
  nephrostomy for, 441–442
  ureterosigmoidoscopy for, *442,* 442–443
Urinary incontinence, 297. See also *Stress incontinence.*
  vesicovaginal fistula and, 214
Urinary tract. See also *Urinary diversion.*
  anatomy of, 427–430, *428, 429*
  benign conditions of, 430
  endometriosis of, 581–582
    symptoms in, 574
  gynecological cancers and, 430
  müllerian anomalies and, 360
  ovarian cancer surgery and, 534
  postoperative infection of, 46–47
    after urinary diversion, 446
  preoperative evaluation of, 431
    before urinary diversion, 443
  radiation injury to, 449, 551
  surgical injury to, 431–434, 440–441. See also *Ureter(s), injury to.*
Urinoma, 433, 440
Urodynamic testing, in cystocele, 321
Urogenital diaphragm, 316
Urogynecology, 309
Uterine adnexa. See *Adnexa.*
Uterine arteries, 25, *25,* 354
  ligation of, 340–341, *341,* 344–345
Uterine cervix. See *Cervix.*
Uterosacral ligaments, 314–315, 355
  in hysterectomy, 341, 343, *344*
Uterus. See also *Cervix; Endometrium.*
  abnormal bleeding from, D & C and, 258–259
  adenocarcinoma of, 371–389. See also *Endometrium, adenocarcinoma of.*
  anatomy of, *24,* 354–355
  bicornuate, *361, 363,* 363
    surgery for, 364, *364, 365, 366*
  blood supply to, 25, *25,* 354–355
  cancer of, 371–389, 372t, 389–390
    endometrium as site of, 371–389. See also *Endometrium, adenocarcinoma of.*
    mixed müllerian, 390
    recurrent, 390–391
  endometrium of. See *Endometrium.*
  endoscopy of. See *Hysteroscopy.*
  leiomyoma of, 355–356
    fertility and, 356–358
    medical treatment of, 88–89
    myomectomy for, 355–360
    recurrent, 360
    symptoms associated with, 356
    ultrasonography of, 356, *357*
  leiomyosarcoma of, 390
  müllerian anomalies of, 360–369
    classification of, *362*
    fertility and, 363–364
    surgery for, 360–361, 364, *364–366,* 366–367
      evaluation before, 361, *363*
      results of, 368t
    types of, 360–361, *361*
  perforation of, D & C and, *264,* 264–265
  prolapse of, 318, *318*
  resection of. See *Hysterectomy.*
  sarcoma of, 371, 389–390, *390*
  septate, 92, *93, 361, 363*
    surgery for, 364, *364, 366,* 366–367
  support system of, 355

Vagina, adenocarcinoma of, 201, 207–208
  benign tumors of, 209, 210t
  cancer of, 201–204, 205–208, 207–209
    diagnosis of, 202
    etiology of, 201–202
    metastatic, 209
    pathology of, 203–204, 204t
    prognosis in, 202, 203t
    radiotherapy of, 640–650
      complications of, 644, 648t
      gold-grain implants in, 642, 644, 648, 648, 649, 650, 650t
      instruments for, 641, 642, 645–649
      iridium implants in, 642, 643–644, 644–647
      lymph nodes and, 640–641
      options in, 641, 643, 643, 644
      planning for, 641
    staging of, 202, 202t
    survival in, 642t
    treatment of, 202–203, 203t, 204t
  clear cell carcinoma of, 201, 644, 644
  embryology of, 20
  eversion involving. See *Prolapse, into rectovaginal space; Prolapse, of vaginal vault.*
  melanoma of, 208
  pelvic anatomy and, 23–24, 26, 26, 314
  prolapse involving. See *Prolapse, into rectovaginal space; Prolapse, of vaginal vault.*
  reconstruction of, 290, 607, 610t, 611
    band release in, 607, 608
    cancer arising in, 209
    colon interposition for, 612, 614
    Frank technique for, 611, 611–612
    free flap in, 615
    gluteal thigh flap in, 615
    gracilis myocutaneous graft in, 615, 616–618
    Martius bulbocavernous technique for, 615
    McIndoe technique for, 612, 613
    rectus abdominis myocutaneous flap in, 615, 619
    skin flaps in, 607, 608–610, 611
    Williams technique for, 612, 614
  sarcoma of, 208–209
  septae of, 167, 168–170, 169, 171
    longitudinal, 169, 170, 171
    transverse, 167, 168, 169
  small cell carcinoma of, 209
  squamous cell carcinoma of, 201–202, 204–205, 205–208, 207
    radiotherapy in, 647
      complications of, 644, 648t
      survival in, 642t
  support system of, 314–316, 315
Vaginal cuff, cellulitis of, 48
  in hysterectomy, 341–342, 342
  stapling across, 103
Vaginal cylinders, 632, 634, 645, 646
Vaginal intraepithelial neoplasia (VAIN), 244–248
  clinical management of, 244
  epidemiology of, 244
  treatment of, 244, 245t
    chemotherapy in, 247, 247
    electrocautery in, 247
    laser in, 247, 247, 248
    radiation therapy in, 244
    surgery in, 246, 247
Vaginectomy, 204–205, 205–207, 246
  hysterectomy with, 206

VAIN. See *Vaginal intraepithelial neoplasia (VAIN).*
Valvular heart disorders, 65–66
  signs and symptoms of, 65t
Varices, esophageal, 80
Venous stasis, postoperative, 55–56
Ventilation, in ARDS, 76
Verapamil, 67t
Verrucous carcinoma, vulvar, 195–196, 196
Vesalius, Andreas, 6, 6, 353–354
Vesicocervicovaginal fistula, anatomy of, 214
Vesicoureterovaginal fistula, radiation-induced, 451
Vesicovaginal fistula, 213–218
  after hysterectomy, 281, 281t
  anatomy of, 214
  diagnosis of, 214
  etiology of, 213–214
  treatment of, 214–215, 215t
    surgical, 215–217, 215–218
      abdominal approach in, 217
      history of, 10, 12
      vaginal approach in, 215–217, 215–217
    urinary diversion with, 217–218
Vesicovaginal space, 316, 317
Vestibular glands, major (Bartholin's glands), 161, 174
  carcinoma of, 194, 194
  cyst of, 161–163, 162
    vs. cyst of canal of Nuck, 163
  excision of, 163
  incision of, 161–162, 162
  marsupialization of, 162–163, 163
  minor, 163
Video laparoscopy, 108–109, 114–115, 502
  camera for, 502
VIN. See *Vulvar intraepithelial neoplasia (VIN).*
Virchow, Rudolf, 9
Viruses, and CIN, 233–234
  and genital carcinoma, 176–177, 201
Vital capacity, postoperative, 74, 74
Vitamin K, in liver dysfunction, 77–78, 80
Vulva. See also *Vestibular glands, major (Bartholin's glands).*
  adenocarcinoma of, 195
  anatomy of, 26, 26, 173–176, 174, 175
  basal cell carcinoma of, 195
  biopsy of, 160
  blood supply to, 174
  cancer of, 173–200
    staging of, 176, 176t
    types of, 176t
  condylomata of, 160–161
  cysts of, 161–163, 162, 163
  dermatofibrosarcoma of, 197
  endodermal sinus tumor of, 197
  examination of, 159
  innervation of, 174
  lesions of, 159–160
  lichen sclerosus of, 160
  lymphatic system of, 174–175, 175
  lymphoma of, 197
  melanoma of, 192, 192–194
    prognosis in, 193–194
    staging of, 193, 193t
    treatment of, 193
  Merkel cell carcinoma of, 197
  Paget's disease of, 194–195
  reconstruction of, 615, 618, 620–621

Vulva (Continued)
  femoral vessel coverage in, 615, 620, 620, 621
  pedicle flaps for, 620–621, 622
  sarcoma of, 196
  squamous cell carcinoma of, 176–192
    advanced, 188, 191, 191–192
    clinical features of, 177
    diagnosis of, 177
    early (T1, N0–1), 178–182, 179–182
    large defect closure in, 186, 187–190, 188
    N2, N3, 185–186
    postoperative complications in, 188
    postoperative management in, 188
    prognosis in, 192, 192t
    radical vulvectomy in, 183, 183, 184, 185
    recurrent, 191–192
    spread of, 177t, 177–178, 178t
    staging of, 176, 176t
    vulvar conservation in, 185
    vulvar dystrophy with, 179
  squamous cell hyperplasia of, 160
  verrucous carcinoma of, 195–196, 196
  wide local excision of, 160, 251
Vulvar intraepithelial neoplasia (VIN), 248–253
  clinical analysis of, 248
  epidemiology of, 248
  treatment of, 249t
    chemotherapeutic, 251
    laser, 251, 252–253, 253
    radiation, 253
    surgical, 250, 251, 251
Vulvectomy, radical, 183–184
  anoproctectomy with, 191
  superficial skinning, 250
Vulvovaginectomy, 207
Vulvovaginoplasty, Williams, 612, 614

Warfarin, perioperative, 66
Warren flap, in fistula repair, 226, 227
Warts, genital, 160–161
Waveforms, 117, 117, 118
Way's incision, 183, 183
Wedge biopsy, ovarian, 520–521, 521
Weight, body, 33
White blood cell count, 69–70
Whole gut lavage, 51, 398
Wound closure. See *Closure.*
Wound dehiscence, 144–145
  incision type and, 134
  sutures and, 137, 137t
Wound healing, 131
  adhesions and, 148–151, 150, 151
  wound classification and, 131t
Wound infection, 48
  obesity and, 138
  prevention of, 133–134
  wound classification and, 131, 131t

Y-V plasty, 607, 609

Z-plasty, 607, 608
Zygote intrafallopian transfer (ZIFT), 564–565
  in endometriosis, 581